CLINICAL
PHARMACOLOGY

'Nature is not only odder than we think, but it is odder than we can think.'
  J B S Haldane 1893–1964

'Patients may recover in spite of drugs or because of them.'
  J H Gaddum 1959

'But know also, man has an inborn craving for medicine … the desire to take medicine is one feature which distinguishes man the animal, from his fellow creatures. It is really one of the most serious difficulties with which we have to contend … the doctor's visit is not thought to be complete without a prescription.'
  William Osler 1894

'Morals do not forbid making experiments on one's neighbour or on one's self … among the experiments that may be tried on man, those that can only harm are forbidden, those that are innocent are permissible, and those that may do good are obligatory.' 'Men who have excessive faith in their theories or ideas are not only ill prepared for making discoveries; they make very poor observations … they can see in [their] results only a confirmation of their theory … This is what made us say that we must never make experiments to confirm our ideas, but simply to control them.' 'Empiricism is not the negation of science, as certain physicians seem to think; it is only its first stage.'

'Medicine is destined to get away from empiricism little by little; like all other sciences, it will get away by the scientific method.'

'Considered in itself, the experimental method is nothing but reasoning by whose help we methodically submit our ideas to experience — the experience of facts.'
  Claude Bernard 1865

'I do not want two diseases — one nature-made, one doctor-made.'
  Napoleon Bonaparte 1820

'The ingenuity of man has ever been fond of exerting itself to varied forms and combinations of medicines.'
  William Withering 1785

'All things are poisons and there is nothing that is harmless, the dose alone decides that something is no poison.'
  Paracelsus 1493–1541

'First do no harm.'
'It is a good remedy sometimes to use nothing.'
  Hippocrates 460–355 B.C.

CLINICAL PHARMACOLOGY

P. N. Bennett MD FRCP
Reader in Clinical Pharmacology, University of Bath, and Consultant Physician, Royal United Hospital, Bath, UK

M. J. Brown MA MSc MD FRCP
Professor of Clinical Pharmacology, University of Cambridge; Consultant
Physician, Addenbrooke's Hospital, Cambridge and Director of Clinical Studies
Gonville and Caius College, Cambridge, UK

NINTH EDITION

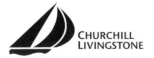
CHURCHILL
LIVINGSTONE

EDINBURGH LONDON NEW YORK OXFORD PHILADELPHIA ST LOUIS SYDNEY TORONTO 2003

CHURCHILL LIVINGSTONE
An imprint of Elsevier Science Limited

Commissioning Editor: Timothy Horne
Project Development Manager: Colin Arthur
Copy Editor: Leslie Smillie
Project Controller: Nancy Arnott
Designer: Erik Bigland

First edition 1960
Second edition 1962
Third edition 1966
Fourth edition 1973
Fifth edition 1980
Sixth edition 1987
Seventh edition 1992
Eighth edition 1997

Previous editions translated into
Italian, Chinese, Spanish,
Serbo-Croat, Russian

Standard edition ISBN 0443064806

International Student Edition ISBN 0443064814

British Library Cataloguing in Publication Data
A catalogue record for this book is available from the
British Library

Library of Congress Cataloging in Publication Data
A catalog record for this book is available from the
Library of Congress

The
publisher's
policy is to use
**paper manufactured
from sustainable forests**

Printed in Spain

Preface

For your own satisfaction and for mine, please read this preface![1]

Professor D. R. Laurence was either author or co-author of this textbook from its 1st edition in 1960 to its 8th in 1997. This is a long life for any textbook. Its achievement bears testimony to a style of presentation that strives to be clear and readable, and to retain the reader's interest whilst imparting information about a subject that can be at times both complex and confusing. As he withdraws from active involvement in the book it is opportune to pay tribute in this 9th edition to an achievement in authorship sustained over four decades, during which 'Laurence's pharmacology' became the aid, advisor and companion to generations of students and doctors seeking guidance in the vital field of medicinal therapeutics.

> This book is about the scientific basis and practice of drug therapy. It is particularly intended for medical students and doctors, and indeed for anyone concerned with evidence-based drug therapy and prescribing.

The scope and rate of drug innovation increases. Doctors are now faced with a professional lifetime handling drugs that are new to themselves — drugs that do new things as well as drugs that do old things better; drugs that become familiar during training will be superseded.

We do not write only for readers who, like us, have a special interest in pharmacology. We try to make pharmacology understandable for those whose primary interests lie elsewhere but who recognise that they need some knowledge of pharmacology if they are to meet their moral and legal 'duty of care' to their patients. We try to tell them what they need to know without burdening them with irrelevant information and we try to make the subject interesting. We are very serious, but seriousness does not always demand wearying solemnity. An author, poet and critic said that he judged fiction thus: 'Could I read it? If I could read it, did I believe it? If I believed it, did I care about it, what was the quality of my caring, and did it last?'[2] It would be presumptuous for us to aspire to satisfy the criteria for fiction but we have been mindful of them in producing this book.

All who prescribe drugs would be wise to keep in mind that the expectations of patients and of society in general are becoming ever more exacting and that doctors who prescribe casually or ignorantly now face not only increasing criticism but also civil (or even criminal) legal charges. The ability to handle new developments depends, now more than ever, on comprehension of the principles of pharmacology. These principles are not difficult to grasp and are not so many as to defeat even the busiest doctors who take on themselves the responsibility of introducing manufactured medicines into the bodies of their patients.

The principles of pharmacology and drug therapy will be found in chapters 1–8 and they are applied in the subsequent specialist chapters which are offered as a reasonably brief solution to the problem of combining practical clinical utility with some account of the principles on which clinical practice rests.

How much practical technical detail to include is difficult to decide. In general, where therapeutic practices that are complex, potentially dangerous and commonly up-dated, e.g. anaphylactic shock, we provide more detail together with web-sites that list the latest advice; less, or even no detail is given on therapy that is generally conducted only by specialists, e.g. anticancer drugs and i.v. oxytocin. But always, especially with modern drugs with which the prescriber may not be familiar, formularies, approved guidelines, or the manufacturer's current literature should be consulted.

---

[1] St Francis of Sales: Preface to *Introduction to the devout life* (1609)

[2] Philip Larkin: 1922–85

Use of the book. Students are, or should be, concerned to understand and to develop a rational, critical attitude to drug therapy and they should therefore chiefly concern themselves with how drugs act and interact in disease and with how evidence of therapeutic effect is obtained and evaluated. To this end they should read selectively and should not impede themselves by attempts to memorise lists of alternative drugs and doses and minor differences between them, which should never be required of them in examinations. Thus the text has not been encumbered with exhaustive lists of preparations which properly belong in a formulary, although it is hoped that enough have been mentioned to cover much routine prescribing, and many drugs have been included solely for identification.

The role and status of a textbook. If a book is to be a useful guide to drug use it must offer clear conclusions and advice. If it is to be of reasonable size, alternative acceptable courses of action will often have to be omitted. What is recommended should be based on sound evidence where this exists, and on an assessment of the opinions of the experienced where it does not.

Increasingly, the selection of drugs is influenced by guidelines produced by specialist societies and national bodies. We have provided or made reference to these as representing a consensus of best practice in particular situations. Similarly, it is assumed that the reader possesses a formulary, local or national, which will provide guidance on the availability, including doses, of a broad range of drugs. But the practice of therapeutics by properly educated and conscientious doctors working in settings complicated by intercurrent disease, metabolic differences or personality, involves challenges beyond the rigid adherence to published recommendations. The role of a textbook is to provide the satisfaction of understanding the basis for a recommended course of action so that an optimal result may be achieved by informed selection and use of drugs.

The guide to further reading at the end of each chapter generally comprises a few references to original papers, to referenced editorials and review articles from a small range of English language journals that are likely to be available in most hospital libraries in order to enable anyone, anywhere, to gain access to the original literature and to informed opinion, and also to provide interest and sometimes amusement. We urge readers to select a title that looks interesting and to read the article. We do not attempt to document all the statements we make, which would be impossible in a book of this size.

Bath, Cambridge   P.N.B.,
2003   M.J.B.

Farewell

This book originated in 1957 when I, then senior lecturer in the Department of Pharmacology and in the Department of Medicine at University College and Medical School London, told the Professor of Medicine that there was no book on Clinical Pharmacology that I could recommend to our medical students. He replied that if that was so then I should get down to it and write such a book. I doubted that I could accomplish the task. He marched me off to a nearby medical publisher and a contract was soon signed. Without this pressure and the long-sustained support of Max Rosenheim (later Lord Rosenheim of Camden and President of the Royal College of Physicians of London) this book would not have materialised in its first edition in 1960. Since that date, both in collaboration and alone, there have been eight editions. I am deeply grateful to my collaborators.

Now, after above 40 years with the book, and in my eightieth year, the time has come to stand aside.

I have seen too many elderly academics become unable, or unwilling, to recognise that they are no longer quite the people that they once were and that they have become an embarrassment to their younger colleagues, who are often too kind to enlighten them; though they may murmur behind their senior's back. I long ago decided that I must not join that group, and I hope I may just have escaped doing so.

Perhaps my greatest reward has been the kindness of people from all over the world who have taken the trouble to communicate to me that they have not only profited from, but have actually enjoyed, reading *Clinical Pharmacology.*

The world of clinical pharmacology has greatly changed since 1957 when I took up my pen, and I wish my successors well.

D R Laurence, Professor Emeritus of Pharmacology and Therapeutics, University College London

Contributors

It is not possible for two individuals to cover the whole field of drug therapy from their own knowledge and experience. For the first time in this 9th edition, we invited selected experts to review chapters in their specialty. They were given free rein to add, delete or amend existing text as they deemed appropriate. As a result, some chapters exhibit substantial changes from the 8th edition, and all have benefited greatly from the knowledge and experience of these individuals. We are deeply indebted for their contributions. They are:

Nigel S Baber BSc, FRCP, FRCPEd, FFPM, Dip Clin Pharmacol
Head of Renewals, Reclassification and Patient Safety, Medicines Control Agency, London, UK and Visiting Professor, Queen Mary and Westfield College, University of London, London, UK

Chapter 3.   *Discovery and development of drugs*
Chapter 4.   *Evaluation of drugs in man*
Chapter 5.   *Official regulation of medicines*
Chapter 6.   *Classification and naming of drugs*

Mark Farrington MA, MB, BChir, FRCPath
Consultant Microbiologist, Addenbrooke's Hospital, Cambridge, UK

Chapter 11.   *Chemotherapy of infections*
Chapter 12.   *Antibacterial drugs*
Chapter 13.   *Chemotherapy of bacterial infections*
Chapter 14.   *Viral, fungal, protozoal and helminthic infections*

Nicola J Minaur BSc, MB ChB, PhD
Specialist Registrar in Rheumatology, Royal National Hospital for Rheumatic Diseases, Bath, UK

Neil John McHugh MB, ChB, FRACP, MD, FRCP
Consultant Rheumatologist, Royal National Hospital for Rheumatic Diseases, Bath, UK

Chapter 15.   *Inflammation, arthritis and nonsteroidal anti-inflammatory drugs*

Christopher R Lovell MD FRCP
Consultant Dermatologist, Royal United Hospital, Bath, UK

Chapter 16.   *Drugs and the skin*

G R Park MD, DMedSci
Director of Intensive Care Research, Addenbrooke's Hospital, Cambridge, UK

J Grewal MBBS
SHO, The John Farman Intensive Care Unit, Addenbrooke's Hospital, Cambridge, UK

Chapter 17.   *Pain and analgesics*

Jerry Nolan FRCA
Consultant in Anaesthesia and Intensive Care, Royal United Hospital, Bath, UK

Chapter 18.   *Anaesthesia and neuromuscular block*

Simon J C Davies MA (Oxon), MBBS (Lond), MRCPsych
Clinical Research Fellow, University of Bristol, Bristol, UK

Sue Wilson PhD
Research Fellow, University of Bristol, Bristol, UK

David J Nutt MB BChir, MA, DM, FRCP, FRC Psych, FMedSci
Professor of Psychopharmacology, Head of the Department of Clinical Medicine, Dean of Clinical Medicine and Dentistry, University of Bristol, Bristol, UK

Chapter 19.   *Psychotropic drugs*

D Bateman MD FRCP
Consultant Neurologist, Royal United Hospital NHS Trust, Bath, UK

Chapter 20.   *Epilepsy, parkinsonism and allied conditions*

Kevin M O'Shaughnessy MA, BM, BCh, DPhil, FRCP
University Lecturer in Clinical Pharmacology and Honorary Consultant Physician, Addenbrooke's Hospital, Cambridge, UK

Andrew Grace PhD, FRCP, FACC
Consultant Cardiologist, Papworth Hospital, Cambridge, UK

Charles R J Singer BSc, MB, ChB, FRCP, FRCPath
Consultant Haematologist, Royal United Hospital, Bath, UK

Pippa G Corrie PhD, FRCP
Consultant and Associate Lecturer in Medical Oncology, Addenbrooke's Hospital and University of Cambridge, Cambridge, UK

Charles R J Singer BSc, MB, ChB, FRCP, FRCPath
Consultant Haematologist, Royal United Hospital, Bath, UK

Michael Davis MD FRCP, Consultant Gastroenterologist, Royal United Hospital, Bath, UK

D C Brown MD, MSc, FRCP
Consultant Endocrinologist, Cromwell Hospital, London, UK

Acknowledgements

Aditionally, we express our gratitude to others who have, with such good grace, given us their time and energy to supply valuable facts and opinions for this and previous editions; they principally include: Dr E S K Assem, Dr Stella Barnass, Dr N B Bennett, Dr Noeleen Foley, Dr Sheila Gore, Professor J Guillebaud, Professor D H Jenkinson, Dr H Ludlam, Professor P J Maddison, Dr P T Macgee, the late Professor Sir William Paton, Professor B N C Prichard, Dr J P D Reckless, Dr Catriona Reid, Dr Andrew Souter, Professor P L Weissberg.

Other acknowledgements are made in the appropriate places.

Much of any merit this book may have is due to the generosity of those named above as well as others too numerous to mention who have put their knowledge and practical experience of the use of drugs at our disposal. We hope that this collective acknowledgement will be acceptable. Errors are our own.

In addition, permission to quote directly from the writings of some authorities has been generously granted and we thank the authors and their publishers who have given it. If we have omitted any acknowledgement that ought to have been made we will make such amends as we can as soon as we can.

P.N.B.
M.J.B.

Note from the authors and publisher

Medical knowledge is constantly changing. Standard safety precautions must be followed, but as new research and clinical experience broaden our knowledge, changes in treatment and drug therapy may become necessary or appropriate. Readers are advised to check the most current product information provided by the manufacturer of each drug to be administered to verify the recommended dose, the method and duration of administration, and contraindications. It is the responsibility of the practitioner, relying on experience and knowledge of the patient, to determine dosages and the best treatment for each individual patient. Neither the Publisher nor the authors assumes any liability for any injury and/or damage to persons or property arising from this publication.

Contents

CONTENTS

SECTION 1

GENERAL

1

Topics in drug therapy

The therapeutic situation

> Poisons in small doses are the best medicines; and useful medicines in too large doses are poisonous (William Withering, 'discoverer' of digitalis, 1789).

The use of drugs[1] to increase human happiness by elimination or suppression of diseases and symptoms and to improve the quality of life in other ways is a serious matter and involves not only technical, but also psychosocial considerations.

Overall, the major benefits of modern drugs are on **quality** of life (measured with difficulty), and exceed those on **quantity** of life (measured with ease).[2]

We therefore begin this book with a series of essays on what we think are important topics.

---

[1] A World Health Organization Scientific Group has defined a drug as 'any substance or product that is used or intended to be used to modify or explore physiological systems or pathological states for the benefit of the recipient'. WHO 1966 Technical Report Series no. 341: 7. A less restrictive definition is 'a substance that changes 'a biological system by interacting with it'.

A *drug* is a single chemical substance that forms the active ingredient of a *medicine* (a substance or mixture of substances used in restoring or preserving health). A medicine may contain many other substances to deliver the drug in a stable form, acceptable and convenient to the patient. The terms will be used more or less interchangeably in this book. To use the word 'drug' intending only a harmful, dangerous or addictive substance is to abuse a respectable and useful word.

Medicines are part of our way of life from birth, when we enter the world with the aid of drugs, to death where drugs assist (most of) us to depart with minimal distress and perhaps even with a remnant of dignity. In between these events we regulate our fertility, often, with drugs. We tend to take such usages for granted.

But during the intervals remaining, an average family experiences illness on one day in four and between the ages of 20 and 45 years a lower-middle-class man experiences approximately one life-endangering illness, 20 disabling (temporarily) illnesses, 200 non-disabling illnesses and 1000 symptomatic episodes: the average person in the USA can expect to have about 12 years of bad health in an average lifespan.[3] And medicines play a major role in these. 'At any time, 40–50% of adults [UK] are taking a prescribed medicine.'[4]

Before treating any patient with drugs, doctors should have made up their minds on eight points:

1. Whether they should interfere with the patient at all and if so —
2. What alteration in the patient's condition they hope to achieve.
3. That the drug they intend to use is best capable of bringing this about.
4. How they will know when it has been brought about.
5. That they can administer the drug in such a way that the right concentration will be attained in the right place at the right time and for the right duration.
6. What other effects the drug may have and whether these may be harmful.
7. How they will decide to stop the drug.

8. Whether the likelihood of benefit, and its importance, outweighs the likelihood of damage, and its importance, i.e. to consider benefit versus risk, or efficacy in relation to safety.

> **Drug therapy** involves a great deal more than matching the name of the drug to the name of a disease; it requires knowledge, judgement, skill and wisdom, but above all a sense of responsibility.

A book can provide knowledge and can contribute to the formation of judgement, but it can do little to impart skill and wisdom, which are the products of example of teachers and colleagues, of experience and of innate and acquired capacities.

'It is evident that patients are not treated in a vacuum and that they respond to a variety of subtle forces around them in addition to the specific therapeutic agent.'[5] *When a patient is given a drug the responses are the resultant of numerous factors:*

- The pharmacodynamic effect of the drug and interactions with any other drugs the patient may be taking
- The pharmacokinetics of the drug and its modification in the individual due to genetic influences, disease, other drugs
- The physiological state of the end-organ — whether, for instance, it is over- or underactive
- The act of medication, including the route of administration and the presence or absence of the doctor
- The doctor's mood, personality, attitudes and beliefs
- The patient's mood, personality, attitudes and beliefs
- What the doctor has told the patient
- The patient's past experience of doctors
- The patient's estimate of what has been received and of what ought to happen as a result
- The social environment, e.g. whether supportive or dispiriting.

The relative importance of these factors varies according to circumstances. An unconscious patient

---

[2] Consider, for example, the worldwide total of suffering relieved and prevented *each day* by anaesthetics (local and general) and by analgesics, not forgetting dentistry which, because of these drugs, no longer strikes terror into even the most stoical as it has done for centuries.

[3] Quoted in: Anderson J A D (ed) 1979 Self medication. MTP Press, Lancaster; USA Public Health Service 1995.

[4] George C F 1994 Prescribers' Journal 34: 7. A moment's reflection will bring home to us that this is an astounding statistic which goes a long way to account for the aggressive promotional activities of the highly competitive international pharmaceutical industry; the markets for medicines are colossal.

[5] Sherman L J 1959 American Journal of Psychiatry 116: 208.

with meningococcal meningitis does not have a personal relationship with the doctor, but patients sleepless with anxiety because they cannot cope with their family responsibilities may be affected as much by the interaction of their own personalities with that of the doctor as by the anxiolytics prescribed by the latter; and the same applies to appetite suppressants in food addicts.

The physician may consciously use all of the factors listed above in therapeutic practice. But it is still not enough that patients get better, it is essential to know **why** they do so. This is because potent drugs should only be given if their pharmacodynamic effects are needed; many adverse reactions have been shown to be due to drugs that are not needed, including some severe enough to cause hospital admission.

Drugs can do good

Medically this good may sometimes seem trivial, as in the avoidance of a sleepless night in a noisy hotel or of social embarrassment from a profusely running nose due to seasonal pollen allergy (hay-fever). Such benefits are not necessarily trivial to recipients, concerned to be at their best in important matters, whether of business, of pleasure or of passion, i.e. with quality of life.

Or the good may be literally life-saving, as in serious acute infections (pneumonia, septicaemia) or in the prevention of life-devastating disability from severe asthma, from epilepsy or from blindness due to glaucoma.

Drugs can do harm

This harm may be relatively trivial, as in hangover from an hypnotic or transient headache from glyceryl trinitrate used for angina.

The harm may be life-destroying, as in the rare sudden death following an injection of penicillin, rightly regarded as one of the safest of antibiotics, or the destruction of the quality of life that occasionally attends the use of drugs that are effective in rheumatoid arthritis (adrenocortical steroids, penicillamine), and Parkinson's disease (levodopa).

There are risks in taking medicines just as there are risks in food and transport. There are also risks in not taking medicines when they are needed, just as there are risks in not taking food or in not using transport when they are needed.

Efficacy and safety do not lie solely in the molecular structure of the drug. Doctors must choose which drugs to use and must apply them correctly in relation not only to their properties, but also to those of the patients and their disease. Then patients must use the prescribed medicine correctly (see Compliance/concordance).

Uses of drugs/medicines

Drugs are used in three principal ways:

- to cure disease: primary and auxiliary
- to suppress disease
- to prevent disease: (prophylaxis): primary and secondary.

Cure implies primary therapy (e.g. in bacterial and parasitic infections) when the disease is eliminated and the drug is withdrawn; or auxiliary therapy (as with anaesthetics and with ergometrine and oxytocin in obstetrics).

Suppression of diseases of symptoms is used continuously or intermittently to maintain health without attaining cure (as in hypertension, diabetes mellitus, epilepsy, asthma) or to control symptoms (such as pain and cough) whilst awaiting recovery from the causative disease.

Prevention (prophylaxis). In *primary prevention,* the person does not have the condition and is to be prevented from getting it. In malaria, vaccinations and contraception the decision to treat healthy people is generally easy.

In *secondary prevention* the patient has the disease and the objective is to reduce risk factors and to retard progression (e.g. aspirin and lipid-lowering drugs in atherosclerosis and post-myocardial infarction). In breast cancer, the use of tamoxifen, which can itself rarely cause endometrial cancer (which is detectable and treatable), raises complex scientific and socioeconomic issues.

PHYSICIAN-INDUCED (IATROGENIC) DISEASE

The most shameful act in therapeutics, apart from actually killing a patient, is to injure a patient who is but little disabled or who is suffering from a self-limiting disorder. Such iatrogenic disease,[6] induced by misguided treatment, is far from rare.

Doctors who are temperamentally extremist will do less harm by therapeutic nihilism than by optimistically overwhelming patients with well-intentioned polypharmacy. If in doubt whether or not to give a drug to a person who will soon get better without it, don't.

In 1917 the famous pharmacologist, Sollmann, felt able to write:

> Pharmacology comprises some broad conceptions and generalisations, and some detailed conclusions, of such great and practical importance that every student and practitioner should be absolutely familiar with them. It comprises also a large mass of minute details, which would constitute too great a tax on human memory, but which cannot safely be neglected.[7]

The doctor's aim must be not merely to give the patient what will do good, but to give only what will do good, or at least more good than harm.

BENEFITS AND RISKS

Benefits of drugs are manifest to doctor and patient and also, it might be thought, obvious to even the most unimaginative healthy people who find themselves dismayed by some aspects of modern technology.

Modern technological medicine has been criticised, justly, for following the tradition of centuries by waiting for disease to occur and then trying to cure it rather than seeking to prevent it from occurring in the first place.

Although many diseases are partly or wholly preventable by economic, social and behavioural

means, these are too seldom adopted and also are slow to take effect. In the meantime people continue to fall sick and to need and to deserve treatment.

In any case we all have eventually to die of something and, even after excessive practising of all the advice on how to live a healthy life, the likelihood that the mode of death for most of us will be free from pain, anxiety, cough, diarrhoea, paralysis (the list is endless) seems so small that it can be disregarded. Drugs already provide immeasurable solace in these situations, but better drugs are needed and their development should be encouraged.

Doctors know the sick are thankful for drugs just as even the most dedicated pedestrians and environmentalists struck down by a passing car are thankful for a motor ambulance to take them to hospital.

Benefits of drugs in individual diseases are discussed throughout this book and will not be further expanded here. But a general discussion of risk of adverse events is appropriate.

Unavoidable risks

A risk-free drug would be one for which:

- The physician knew exactly what action was required and used the drug correctly
- The drug did that and nothing else, either by true biological selectivity or by selective targeted delivery
- Exactly the right amount of action—not too little, not too much—was easily achieved.

These criteria may be **completely** fulfilled, e.g. in a streptococcal infection sensitive to penicillin in patients whose genetic constitution does not render them liable to an allergic reaction to penicillin.

These criteria are **partially** fulfilled in insulin-deficient diabetes. But the natural modulation of insulin secretion in response to need (food, exercise) does not operate with injected insulin and even sophisticated technology cannot yet exactly mimic the normal physiological responses. The criteria are still further from realisation in, for example, some cancers and schizophrenia.

The reasons why criteria for a risk-free drug are not met are as follows:

- *Drugs may be insufficiently selective.* As the concentration rises, a drug that is highly

---

[6] Iatrogenic means 'physician-caused', i.e. disease consequent on following medical advice or intervention (from the Greek *iatros*, physician).

[7] Sollman T A 1917 Manual of pharmacology. Saunders, Philadelphia.

The information explosion of recent decades is now being brought under better control such that prescribers can, from their desktop computer terminals, enter the facts about their patient (e.g. age, sex, weight, principal and secondary diagnoses) and receive suggestions for which drugs should be considered, with proposed doses and precautions.

selective at low concentrations will begin to affect other target sites (receptors, enzymes); a disease process (cancer) is so close to normal cellular mechanisms that perfectly selective cell kill is impossible.

- *Drugs may be highly selective*, but the mechanism affected has widespread functions and interference with it cannot be limited to one site only, e.g. atenolol, aspirin.
- *Prolonged modification of cellular mechanisms* can lead to permanent change in structure and function, e.g. carcinogenicity.
- *Insufficient knowledge of disease processes* (some cardiac arrhythmias) and of drug action can lead to interventions that, though undertaken with the best intentions, are harmful.
- *Patients are genetically heterogeneous* to an enormous degree and may have unpredicted responses to drugs.
- *Dosage adjustment* according to need is often unavoidably imprecise, e.g. in depression.
- *Ignorant and casual* prescribing.

Reduction of drug risk

This can be achieved by:

- *Better knowledge of disease* (research); as much as 40% of useful medical advances derive from basic research that was not funded with a practical outcome in view.
- *Site-specific effect:* by molecular manipulation.
- *Site-specific delivery:* drug targeting
  — by topical (local) application
  — by target-selective carriers.
- *Informed*, careful and responsible prescribing.

Two broad categories of risk

First are those that we accept by deliberate choice, even if we do not exactly know their magnitude, or we know but wish they were smaller, or, especially where the likelihood of harm is sufficiently remote though the consequences may be grave, we do not even think about the matter. Such risks include transport and sports, both of which are inescapably subject to potent physical laws such as gravity and momentum, and surgery to rectify disorders that could either be tolerated or treated in other ways, e.g. hernia, much cosmetic surgery.

Second are those risks that are imposed on us in the sense that they cannot be significantly altered by individual action. Risks such as those of food additives (e.g. preservatives, colouring), air pollution and some environmental radioactivity are imposed by man. But there are also risks imposed by nature, such as skin cancer due to excess ultraviolet radiation in sunny climes, as well as some radioactivity.

It seems an obvious truth that unnecessary risks should be avoided, but there is disagreement on what risks are truly unnecessary and, on looking closely at the matter, it is plain that many people habitually take risks in their daily and recreational life that it would be a misuse of words to describe as necessary.

It is also the case that some risks, though known to exist, are, in practice, ignored other than by conforming to ordinary prudent conduct. These risks are negligible in the sense that they do not influence behaviour, i.e. they are neglected.[8]

Risk has two elements

- The likelihood or probability of an adverse event
- Its severity

In general it has been suggested that, in medical cases, concern ceases when risks fall below about 1 in 100 000 so that the procedure then becomes regarded as 'safe'. In such cases, when disaster occurs, it can be difficult indeed for individuals to accept that they 'deliberately' accepted a risk; they feel 'it should not have happened to me' and in their distress they may seek to lay blame on others where there is no fault or negligence, only misfortune (see Warnings).

The benefits of chemicals used to colour food verge on or even attain negligibility, although some are known to cause allergy in man. Yet our society permits their use.

There is general agreement that drugs prescribed for disease are themselves the cause of a significant amount of disease (adverse reactions), of death, of permanent disability, of recoverable illness and of

---

[8] Sometimes the term *minimal risk* is used to mean risk about equal to going about our ordinary daily lives; it includes travel on public transport, but not motor bicycling on a motorway.

minor inconvenience, e.g. in one study (USA) 3% of hospital emergency room visits were attributable to adverse drug reactions.

Three major grades of risk

These are: *unacceptable, acceptable* and *negligible*. In the presence of life-threatening disease and with sufficient information on both the disease and the drug, then decisions, though they may be painful, present relatively obvious problems. But where the disease risk is remote, e.g. mild hypertension, or where drugs are to be used to increase comfort or to suppress symptoms that are, in fact, bearable, or for convenience rather than for need, then the issues of risk acceptance are less obvious.

Risks should not be considered without reference to benefits any more than benefits should be considered without reference to risks.

> Risks are among the facts of life. In whatever we do and in whatever we refrain from doing, we are accepting risk. Some risks are obvious, some are unsuspected and some we conceal from ourselves. But risks are universally accepted, whether willingly or unwillingly, whether consciously or not.[9]

Whenever a drug is given a risk is taken

The risk is made up of the properties of the drug, of the prescriber, of the patient and of the environment; it is often so small that second thoughts are hardly necessary, but sometimes it is substantial. The doctor must weigh the likelihood of gain for the patient against the likelihood of loss. There are often insufficient data for a rational decision to be reached, but a decision must yet be made, and this is one of the greatest difficulties of clinical practice. Its effect on the attitudes of doctors is often not appreciated by those who have never been in this situation. The patients' protection lies in the doctors' knowledge of the drug and of the disease, and experience of both, together with knowledge of the patient.

Drugs that are capable of killing or disabling patients at doses within the therapeutic range

continue to be used where the overall balance of benefit and risk is judged favourable. This can be very difficult for the patient who has suffered a rare severe adverse reaction to understand and to accept (see below).

In some chronic diseases in which suppressive drugs will ultimately be needed they may not benefit the patient in the early stages. For example, victims of early parkinsonism or hypertension may be little inconvenienced or hazarded by the disease, as yet, and the premature use of drugs can exact such a price in side-effects that patients prefer the untreated state; what patients will tolerate depends on their personality, their attitude to disease, their occupation, mode of life and relationship with their doctor (see Compliance).

PUBLIC VIEW OF DRUGS AND PRESCRIBERS

The current public view of modern medicines, ably fuelled by the mass media, is a compound of vague expectation of 'miracle' cures with outrage when anything goes wrong. It is also unreasonable to expect the public to trust the medical profession (in collaboration with the pharmaceutical industry) to the extent of leaving to them all drug matters.

The public wants benefits without risks and without having to alter its unhealthy ways of living; a deeply irrational position. But it is easy to understand that a person who has taken into his body a chemical with intent to relieve suffering, whether or not it is self-induced, can feel profound anger when harm ensues.

Expectations have been raised and now, at the beginning of the 21st century, with the manifest achievement of technology all around us, the naive expectation that happiness can be a part of the technological package is increasingly seen to be unrealisable.

Patients are aware that there is justifiable criticism of the standards of medical prescribing, indeed doctors are in the forefront of this; as well as justifiable criticism of promotional practices of the profitably rich, aggressive, international pharmaceutical industry.

There are obvious areas where some remedial action is possible:

[9] Pochin E E 1975 British Medical Bulletin 31: 184.

- *Improvement of prescribing* by doctors, including better communication with patients, i.e. doctors must learn to feel that introduction of foreign chemicals into their patients' bodies is a serious matter, which the majority do not seem to feel at present.[10]
- Introduction of *no-fault compensation schemes* for serious drug injury (some countries already have these; see p. 10).
- *Informed* public discussion of the issues between the medical profession, industrial drug developers, politicians and other 'opinion-formers' in society, and patients (the public).
- *Restraint* in promotion *by the pharmaceutical industry* including self-control by both industry and doctors in their necessarily close relationship, which the public is inclined to regard as a conspiracy, especially when the gifts and payments made to doctors get into the news.

If restraint by both parties is not forthcoming, and it may not be, then both doctor and industry can expect more control to be exercised over them by politicians responding to public demand. If doctors do not want their prescribing to be restricted, they should prescribe better.

Medication errors

It is a salutary thought that each year medical errors kill an estimated 44 000–98 000 Americans (more than die in motor vehicle accidents) and injure 1 000 000.[11] Evidence from both the USA and Australia shows that among inpatients about half of the injuries caused by medical mismanagement result from surgery but that therapeutic mishaps

and diagnostic errors are the next most common. In one survey of adverse drug events, 1% were fatal, 12% life threatening, 30% serious and 57% significant.[12] About half of the life threatening and serious events were preventable. Errors of prescribing account for one half and of administering drugs for one quarter of these. Inevitably, a proportion of lapses result in litigation and in the UK, 20–25% of complaints received by the medical defence organisations about general practitioners follow medication errors.

CRITICISMS OF MODERN DRUGS

Extremist critics have attracted public attention for their view that modern drug therapy, indeed modern medicine in general, does more harm than good; others, whilst admitting some benefits from drugs, insist that this is medically marginal. These opinions rest on the undisputed fact that favourable trends in many diseases preceded the introduction of modern drugs and were due to economic and environmental changes, sanitation, nutrition and housing. They also rest on the claim that drugs have not changed *expectation of life* or *mortality* (as measured by national mortality statistics) and that drugs can cause illness (adverse reactions).

If something is to be measured then the correct criteria must be chosen. Overall mortality figures are an extremely crude and often an irrelevant measure of the effects of drugs whose major benefits are so often on quality of life rather than on its quantity.

Two examples of inappropriate measurements will suffice:
1. In the case of many infections it is not disputed that environmental changes have had a greater beneficial effect on health than the subsequently introduced antimicrobials. But this does not mean that environmental improvements alone are sufficient in the fight against infections. When comparisons of illnesses in the pre- and post-antimicrobial eras are made, like is not compared with like. Environmental changes achieved their results when mortality from

---

[10] Doctors who seek to exculpate themselves from serious, even fatal, prescribing errors by appealing to undoubted difficulties presented by the information explosion of modern times, allied to pressures of work, are unlikely to get sympathy, and increasingly are more likely to be told, 'If you can't stand the heat, get out of the kitchen' (a dictum attributed to Harry S Truman, US President 1948–52, though he assigns it to US Army General Harry Vaughn). Pharmacists and nurses stand ready and willing to relieve doctors of the burden of prescribing.

[11] Kohn L, Corrigan J, Donaldson M (eds) for the Committee on Quality of Health Care in America, Institute of Medicine 2000 To err is human: building a safer health system. Washington: National Academy Press.

[12] Bates DW et al. 1995 incidence of adverse drug events and potential adverse drug events. Journal of the American Medical Association 274: 29–34.

infections was high and antimicrobials were not available; antimicrobials were introduced later against a background of low mortality as well as of environmental change; decades separate the two parts of the comparison, and observers, diagnostic criteria and data recording changed during this long period. It is evident that determining the value of antimicrobials is not simply a matter of looking at mortality rates.

2. About 1% of the UK population has diabetes mellitus and about 1% of death certificates mention diabetes. This is no surprise because all must die and insulin is no cure[13] for this lifelong disease. A standard medical textbook of 1907 stated that juvenile-onset 'diabetes is in all cases a grave disease, and the subjects are regarded by all assurance companies as uninsurable lives: life seems to hang by a thread, a thread often cut by a very trifling accident'. Most, if not all, life insurance companies now accept young people with diabetes with no or only modest financial penalty, the premium of a person 5–10 years older. Before insulin replacement therapy was available few survived beyond 3 years[14] after diagnosis; they died for lack of insulin. It is unjustified to assert that a treatment is worthless just because its mention on death certificates (whether as a prime or as a contributory cause) has not declined. The relevant criteria for juvenile onset diabetes are change in the age at which the subjects die and the quality of life between diagnosis and death, and both of these have changed enormously.

DRUG-INDUCED INJURY[15] (see also Ch. 8)

Responsibility for drug-induced injury raises important issues affecting medical practice and development of needed new drugs, as well as of law and of social justice.

---

[13] A cure eliminates a disease and may be withdrawn when this is achieved.

[14] Even if given the best treatment. 'Opium alone stands the test of experience as a remedy capable of limiting the progress of the disease', wrote the great Sir William Osler, successively Professor of Medicine in Pennsylvania, McGill, Johns Hopkins and Oxford Universities, in 1918, only three years before the discovery of insulin.

They used to have a more equitable contract in Egypt: for the first three days the doctor took on the patient at the patient's risk and peril: when the three days were up, the risks and perils were the doctor's.

But doctors are lucky: the sun shines on their successes and the earth hides their failures.[16]

Negligence and strict and no-fault liability

All civilised legal systems provide for compensation to be paid to a person injured as a result of using a product of any kind that is defective due to negligence (fault: failure to exercise reasonable care).[17] But there is a growing opinion that special compensation for serious personal injury, beyond the modest sums that general social security systems provide, should be automatic and not dependent on fault and proof of fault of the producer, i.e. there should be 'liability irrespective of fault', 'no-fault liability' or 'strict liability'.[18] After all, victims need assistance (compensation) regardless of the cause of injury and whether or not the producer and, in the case of drugs, the prescriber deserves censure. The question why a person who has suffered injury due to the biological accident of disease should have to depend on social security payments whilst and identical injury due to a drug (in the absence of fault) should attract special added compensation receives no persuasive answer except that this is what society seems to want.

Many countries are now revising their laws on liability for personal injury due to manufactured

---

[15] This discussion is about drugs that have been properly manufactured and meet proper standards, e.g. of purity, stability, as laid down by regulatory bodies or pharmacopoeias. A manufacturing defect would be dealt with in a way no different from manufacturing errors in other products.

[16] Michael de Montaigne 1533–92. French essayist.

[17] A plaintiff (person who believes he/she has been injured) seeking to obtain compensation from a defendant (via the law of negligence) must prove three things; 1, that the defendant owed a duty of care to the plaintiff; 2, that the defendant failed to exercise reasonable care; and 3, that the plaintiff has suffered actual injury as a result.

[18] The following distinction is made in some discussions of product liability. *Strict liability*: compensation is provided by the producer/manufacturer. *No-fault liability* or scheme: compensation is provided by a central fund.

products and are legislating Consumer Protection Acts (Statutes) which include medicines, for 'drugs represent the class of product in respect of which there has been the greatest pressure for surer compensation in cases of injury'.[19]

Issues that are central to the debate include:

- *Capacity to cause harm* is inherent in drugs in a way that sets them apart from other manufactured products; and harm often occurs in the absence of fault.
- *Safety,* i.e. the degree of safety that a person is entitled to expect, and adverse effects that should be accepted without complaint, must often be a matter of opinion and will vary with the disease being treated, e.g. cancer or insomnia.
- *Causation,* i.e. proof that the drug in fact caused the injury, is often impossible, particularly where it increases the incidence of a disease that occurs naturally.
- *Contributory negligence.* Should compensation be reduced in smokers and drinkers where there is evidence that these pleasure-drugs increase liability to adverse reactions to therapeutic drugs?
- *The concept of defect,* i.e. whether the drug or the prescriber or indeed the patient can be said to be 'defective' so as to attract liability, is a highly complex matter and indeed is a curious concept as applied to medicine.

Nowhere has a scheme that meets all the major difficulties yet been implemented. This is not because there has been too little thought, it is because the subject is so difficult.

COMPLEMENTARY AND TRADITIONAL MEDICINE

Because practitioners of complementary[21] and traditional medicine are severely critical of modern

---

Principles of a workable compensation scheme for injury due to drugs

- *New unlicenced drugs undergoing clinical trial in small numbers of subjects* (healthy or patient volunteers): the developer should be strictly liable for all adverse effects.
- *New unlicenced drugs undergoing extensive extensive trials* in patients who may reasonably expect benefit: the producer should be strictly liable for any serious effect.
- *New drugs after licencing by an official body:* liability for serious injury should be shared with the community, which is expected to benefit from new drugs.
- *Standard drugs in day-to-day therapeutics:*
  1. there should be a no-fault scheme, operated by or with the assent of government, that has authority, through tribunals to decide cases quickly and to make awards. This body would have authority to reimburse itself from others — manufacturer, supplier, prescriber — wherever that was appropriate. (The basic funding of the scheme would be via a levy on all manufacturers of medicinal products.) An award must not have to wait on the determinination of prolonged, vexatious, adversarial, expensive court proceedings.
  2. Patients would be compensated where:
     — causation was proven on 'balance of probability'[20]
     — the injury was serious
     — the event was rare and remote and not reasonably taken into account in making the decision to treat.

---

drugs, and because they use drugs according to their own special beliefs, it is appropriate to discuss drug use in complementary medical systems here.

---

[19] Royal Commission on Civil Liability and Compensation for Personal Injury 1978 HMSO, London: Cmnd. 7054. Although the Commission considered compensation for death and personal injury suffered by any person through manufacture, supply or use of products, i.e. all goods whether natural or manufactured, and included drugs and even human blood and organs, it made no mention of tobacco and alcohol.

[20] This is the criterion for (UK) civil law, rather than 'beyond reasonable doubt', which is the criterion of criminal law.
[21] The term *complementary* seems to make a less ambitious claim than *alternative* medicine, and is preferred. The definition adopted by the Cochrane Collaboration is: 'Complementary and alternative medicine (CAM) is a broad domain of healing resources that accompanies all health systems, modalities, and practices and their accompanying theories and beliefs, other than those intrinsic to the politically dominant health system of a particular society or culture in a given historical period. CAM includes all such practices and ideas self-defined by their users as preventing or treating illness or promoting health and well-being. Boundaries within CAM and between the CAM domain and that of the dominant system are not always sharp or fixed.'

Public disappointment that scientific medicine can neither guarantee happiness nor wholly eliminate the disabilities of degenerative diseases in long-lived populations, as well as the fact that drugs used in modern medicine can cause serious harm, naturally lead to a revival of interest in alternatives that alluringly promise efficacy with complete safety. These range from revival of traditional medicine to adoption of the more modern cults.[22]

A proposition belongs to science if we can say what kind of event we would accept as refutation (and this is easy in therapeutics). A proposition (or theory) that cannot clash with any possible or even conceivable event (evidence) is outside science, and this in general applies to cults: everything is interpreted in terms of the theory of the cult; the possibility that the basis of the cult is false is not entertained. This appears to be the case with medical cults, which join Freudianism, and indeed religions, as outside science (after Karl Popper). Willingness to follow where the evidence leads is a distinctive feature of conventional scientific medicine.

> A scientific approach does not mean a patient must be treated as a mere biochemical machine. It does not mean the exclusion of spiritual, psychological and social dimensions of human beings. But it does mean treating these in a rational manner.

Traditional or indigenous medicinal therapeutics has developed since before history in all societies. It comprises a mass of practices varying from the worthless to highly effective remedies, e.g. digitalis (England), quinine (South America), reserpine (India), atropine (various countries). It is the task of science to find the gems and to discard the dross,[23] and at the same time to leave intact socially valuable supportive aspects of traditional medicine.

Features common to *complementary medicine cults* are absence of scientific thinking, naive acceptance of hypotheses, uncritical acceptance of causation, e.g. reliance on anecdote, assumption that if recovery follows treatment it is due to the treatment, and close attention to the patient's personal feelings. Lack of understanding of how therapeutic effects may be measured is also a prominent feature. It is useful to list some common *false beliefs* of its practitioners:

- That synthetic modern drugs are toxic, but products obtained in nature are not.[24]
- That traditional (prescientific) medicines have special virtue.
- That scientific medicine will accept evidence that remedies are effective only where the mechanism is also understood.
- That scientific medicine recognises no form of evaluation other than the strict randomised controlled trial.
- That collection and formal analysis of data on

---

[22] A cult is a practice that follows a dogma, tenet or principle based on theories or beliefs of its promulgator to the exclusion of demonstrable scientific experience (definition of the American Medical Association). Scientific medicine changes in accord with evidence obtained by scientific enquiry applied with such intellectual rigour as is humanly possible. But this is not the case with cults, the claims for which are characterised by absence of rigorous intellectual evaluation and unchangeability of beliefs. The profusion of medical cults prompts the question why, if each cult has the efficacy claimed by its exponents, conventional medicine and indeed the other cults are not swept away. Some practitioners use conventional medicine and, where it fails, turn to cult practices. Where such complementary practices give comfort they are not to be despised, but their role and validity should be clearly defined. No community can afford to take these cults at their own valuation; they must be tested, and tested with at least the rigour required to justify a therapeutic claim for a new drug. It is sometimes urged in extenuation that traditional and cult practices do no harm to patients, unlike synthetic drugs. But even if that were true (which it is not), investment of scarce resources in delivering what may be ineffective, though sometimes pleasing, experiences, e.g. dance therapy, exaltation of flowers, and the admittedly inexpensive urine therapy, means that resources are not available for other desirable social objectives, e.g. housing, art subsidies, medicine. We do not apologise for this diversion to consider medical cults and practices, for the world cannot afford unreason, and the antidote to unreason is reason and the rigorous pursuit of knowledge, i.e. evidence-based medicine.

---

[23] Traditional medicine is being fostered particularly in countries where scientific medicine is not accessible to large populations for economic reasons, and destruction of traditional medicine would leave unhappy and sick people with nothing. For this reason governments are supporting traditional medicine and at the same time initiating scientific clinical evaluations of the numerous plants and other items employed, many of which contain biologically active substances. The World Health Organization is supportive to these programmes.

therapeutic outcomes, failures as well as successes, is inessential.

- That scientific medicine rests on acceptance of rigid and unalterable dogmas.
- That, if a patient gets better when treated in accordance with certain beliefs, this provides evidence for the truth of these beliefs (the *post hoc ergo propter hoc*[25] fallacy).

Exponents often state that comparative controlled trials of their medicines versus conventional medicines are impracticable because the classic double-blind randomised controlled designs are inappropriate and in particular do not allow for the individual approach characteristic of complementary medicine. But modern therapeutic trial designs can cope with this. There remain extremists who contend that they understand scientific method, and reject it as invalid for what they do and believe, i.e. their beliefs are not, in principle, refutable. This is the position taken up by magic and religion where subordination of reason to faith is considered a virtue.

Complementary medicine particularly charges that conventional medicine seriously neglects patients as whole integrated human beings (body, mind, spirit) and treats them too much as machines. Conventional practitioners may well feel uneasily that there has been and still is truth in this, that with the development of specialisation some doctors have been seduced by the enormous successes of medical science and technology and have become liable to look too narrowly at their patients where a much broader (holistic) approach is required. It is evident that such an approach is likely to give particular satisfaction in psychological and psychosomatic conditions for which conventional doctors in a hurry have been all too ready to think that a prescription meets all the patients' needs.

Complementary medicine does not compete with the successful mainstream of scientific medicine. Users of complementary medicine commonly have chronic conditions and have tried conventional medicine but found that it has not offered a satisfactory solution, or has caused adverse effects. A survey estimated that about 20% of the UK population had consulted a complementary practitioner in the previous year (in Germany the figure exceeds 60%).[26] Usage rises sharply among those with chronic, relapsing conditions such as cancer, multiple sclerosis, HIV infection, psoriasis and rheumatological diseases. The following will suffice to give the flavour of homoeopathy, the principal complementary medicine cult involving medicines, and the kind of criticism with which it has to contend.

Homoeopathy

Homoeopathy[27] is a system of medicine founded by Samuel Hahnemann (German physician: 1755–1843) and expounded by him in the Organon of the rational art of healing.[28] Hahnemann described his position:

> After I had discovered the weakness and errors of my teachers and books I sank into a state of sorrowful indignation, which had nearly disgusted me with the study of medicine. I was on the point of concluding that the whole art was vain and incapable of improvement. I gave myself up to solitary reflection, and resolved not to terminate

---

[24] Herbal teas containing pyrrolidizine alkaloids *(Senecio, Crotalaria, Heliotropium)* cause serious hepatic veno-occlusive disease. Comfrey *(Symphitum)* is similar but also causes hepatocellular tumours and haemangiomas. Sassafras (carminative, antirheumatic) is hepatotoxic. Mistletoe *(Viscum)* contains cytotoxic alkaloids. Ginseng contains oestrogenic substances which have caused gynaecomastia: long-term users may show 'ginseng abuse syndrome' comprising CNS excitation; arterial hypotension can occur. Liquorice *(Glycyrrhiza)* has mineralocorticoid action. An amateur 'health food enthusiast' made himself a tea from 'an unfamiliar [to him] plant' in his garden: unfortunately this was the familiar foxglove *(Digitalis purpurea)*: he became very ill but happily he recovered. Other toxic natural remedies include lily of the valley *(Convallaria)* and horse chestnut *(Aesculus)*. 'The medical herbalist is at fault for clinging to outworn historical authority and for not assessing his drugs in terms of today's knowledge, and the orthodox physician is at fault for a cynical scepticism with regard to any healing discipline other than his own' (Penn R G 1983 Adverse Drug Reaction Bulletin: no 102).

[25] Latin: after this, therefore on account of this.

[26] Ernst E 2000 The role of complementary and alternative medicine. British Medical Journal 32: 1133–1135.

[27] Greek: *homos:* same; *patheia:* suffering.

[28] 1810: trans. Wheeler C E 1913: Dent, London.

my train of thought until I had arrived at a definite conclusion on the subject.[29]

By understandable revulsion at the medicine of his time, by experimentation on himself (a large dose of quinine made him feel as though he had a malarial attack) and by search of records he 'discovered' a 'law' that is central to homoeopathy (and from which the name is derived):[30]

Similar symptoms in the remedy remove similar symptoms in the disease. The eternal, universal law of Nature, that every disease is destroyed and cured through the similar artificial disease which the appropriate remedy has the tendency to excite, rests on the following proposition: that only one disease can exist in the body at any one time.

In addition to the above, he 'discovered' that the effect of drugs but not of trace impurities is potentiated by dilution (provided the dilution is shaken correctly, i.e. by 'succussion', even to the extent that an effective dose may not contain a single molecule of the drug. It has been pointed out[29] that the 'thirtieth potency' (1 in 10^{60}), recommended by Hahnemann, provided a solution in which there would be one molecule of drug in a volume of a sphere of literally astronomical circumference. That a dose in which no drug is present (including sodium chloride prepared in this way) can be therapeutically effective is explained by the belief that there is a spiritual energy diffused throughout the medicine by the particular way in which the dilutions are shaken (succussion) during preparation, or that the active molecules leave behind some sort of 'imprint' on solvent or excipient.[31] The absence of potentiation of the inevitable contaminating impurities is attributed to the fact that they are not incorporated by serial dilution. It also seems that solid formulations may be inactivated during dispensing, by machine or hand counting carried out incorrectly.

Thus, writes a critic:

We are asked to put aside the whole edifice of evidence concerning the physical nature of materials and the normal concentration–response relationships of biologically active substances in order to accommodate homoeopathic potency.[32]

But no hard evidence that tests the hypothesis is supplied to justify this, and we are invited, for instance, to accept that sodium chloride merely diluted is no remedy, but that 'it raises itself to the most wonderful power through a well-prepared dynamisation process' and stimulates the defensive powers of the body against the disease.

Thus pharmacologists have felt that in the absence of conclusive evidence from empirical studies that homoeopathic medicines can reproducibly be shown to differ from placebo, there is no point in discussing its hypotheses. But empirical studies can be made without accepting any particular theory of causation; nor should the results of good studies be disregarded just because the proposed theory of action seems incredible or is unknown. A meta-analysis of 186 double-blind and/or randomised placebo-controlled trials of homoeopathic remedies found 89 had adequate data for analysis. The authors concluded that their results 'were not compatible with the hypothesis that the clinical effects are completely due to placebo' but also found 'insufficient evidence from these studies that homoeopathy is clearly efficacious for any single clinical condition'.[33]

Conclusion. There is a single fundamental issue between conventional scientific medicine and traditional and complementary medicine (though it is often obscured by detailed debates on individual practices); the issue is: *what constitutes acceptable evidence*, i.e. what is the nature, quality and interpretation of evidence that can justify general adoption of modes of treatment and acceptance of hypotheses? In the meantime, we depend on the accumulation of evidence from empirical studies to justify the allocation of resources for future research.

[29] Hahnemann S 1805 Aesculapius in the balance. Leipsic.
[30] Clark AJ 1937 General Pharmacology Hefter's Handbuch. Springer, Berlin.
[31] Homoeopathic practitioners repeatedly express their irritation that critics give so much attention to dilution. They should not be surprised considering the enormous implications of their claim.

[32] Cuthbert A W 1982 Pharmaceutical Journal 15 May: 547.
[33] Linde K et al, 1997 Are the clinical effects of homoeopathy placebo effects? A meta-analysis of placebo-controlled trials. Lancet 350: 834–843.

Prescribing, consumption and economics

The reasons for taking a drug history from patients are:

- Drugs are a cause of disease. Withdrawal of drugs, if abrupt, can cause disease, e.g. benzodiazepines, antiepilepsy drugs.
- Drugs can conceal disease, e.g. adrenal steroid.
- Drugs can interact causing positive adverse effect, or negative adverse effect, i.e. therapeutic failure.
- Drugs can give diagnostic clues, e.g. ampicillin and amoxicillin causing rash in infectious mononucleosis — a diagnostic adverse effect, not a diagnostic test.
- Drugs can cause false results in clinical chemistry tests, e.g. plasma cortisol, urinary catecholamine, urinary glucose.
- Drug history can assist choice of drugs in the future.
- Drugs can leave residual effects after administration has ceased, e.g. chloroquine, amiodarone.
- Drugs available for independent patient self-medication are increasing in range and importance.

(See also Appendix 2, The prescription.)
Prescribing should be **appropriate.**[34]

> Appropriate [prescribing is that] which bases the choice of a drug on its effectiveness, safety and convenience relative to other drugs or treatments (e.g. surgery or psychotherapy), and takes cost into account only when those criteria for choice have been satisfied. In some circumstances appropriateness will require the use of more costly drugs. Only by giving appropriateness high

priority will [health payers] be able to achieve their aim of ensuring that patients' clinical needs will be met (Report).

Prescribing that is **inappropriate** is the result of several factors:

- Giving in to patient pressure to write unnecessary prescriptions. The extra time spent in careful explanation will, in the long run, be rewarded.
- Continuing patients, especially the elderly, on courses of medicinal treatment over many months without proper review of their medication.
- Doctors 'frequently prescribe brand-name drugs rather than cheaper generic equivalents, even where there is no conceivable therapeutic advantage in so doing. The fact that the brand-name products often have shorter and more memorable names than their generic counterparts' contributes to this. (Report) (see also Ch. 6).
- 'Insufficient training in clinical pharmacology. Many of the drugs on the market may not have been available when a general practitioner was at medical school.[35] The sheer quantity of new products may lead to a practitioner becoming over-reliant on drugs companies' promotional material, or sticking to "tried and tested" products out of caution based on ignorance' (Report).
- Failure of doctors to keep up-to-date (see Doctor compliance).

Computerising prescribing addresses some of these issues, e.g. by prompting regular review of a patient's medication, by instantly providing generic names from brand names, by giving ready access to formularies and prescribing guidelines.

Cost-containment

Cost-containment in prescription drug therapy attracts increasing attention. It may involve two particularly contentious activities:

---

[34] The text on appropriate prescribing and some quotations (designated *Report*) are based on a UK Parliamentary Report (The National Health Service Drugs Budget 1994 HMSO London). Twelve Members of Parliament took evidence from up to 100 organisations and individuals orally and/or in writing. It is both a surprise and a pleasure to be able to continue to quote with approval from such a source. PNB, MJB.

[35] This statement illustrates a common and serious misunderstanding of the role of medical schools. Their role is to teach the scientific basis of clinical pharmacology and safe drug therapy so that doctors can handle existing and future drugs intelligently, using current data sheets, formularies, etc. It is not to attempt to teach enormous numbers of impossible-to-remember facts, the deadening effect of which on a thinking approach would be disastrous.

1. *Generic substitution,* where a generic formulation (p. 85) is substituted (by a pharmacist) for the proprietary formulation prescribed by the doctor.
2. *Therapeutic substitution,* where a drug of different chemical structure is substituted for the drug prescribed by the doctor. The substitute is of the same chemical class and is deemed to have similar pharmacological properties and to give similar therapeutic benefit. Therapeutic substitution is a particularly controversial matter where it is done without consulting the prescriber, and legal issues may be raised in the event of adverse therapeutic outcome.

The following facts and opinions are worth thinking about:

- The UK National Health Service (NHS) spending on drugs has been 9–11% per year (of the total cost) over nearly 50 years.
- 80% of the total cost of drugs is spent by general practitioners, i.e. in primary care.
- People over the age of 65 years receive on average 13 prescriptions per year — twice as many as the population in general.
- 'The average cost per head of medicines supplied to people aged over 75 is nearly five times that of medicines supplied to those below pensionable age (currently in UK women 60 years; men 65)' (Report).
- 'Underprescribing can be just as harmful to the health of patients as overprescribing.'

It is crucially important that incentives and sanctions address quality of prescribing as well as quantity: 'it would be wrong if too great a preoccupation with the cost issue in isolation were to encourage underprescribing or have an adverse effect on patient care' (Report).

Reasons for underprescribing include: lack of information or lack of the will to use available information (in economically privileged countries there is, if anything, a surplus of information); fear of being blamed for adverse reactions (affecting doctors who lack the confidence that a knowledge of pharmacological principles confers); fear of sanctions against over-costly prescribing. Prescrip-

tion frequency and cost per prescription are lower for older than for younger doctors. There is no reason to think that the patients of older doctors are worse off as a result.

Repeat prescriptions

About two-thirds of general (family) practice prescriptions are for repeat medication (half issued by the doctor at a consultation and half via the receptionist without patient contact with the doctor): 95% of patients' requests are acceded to without further discussion; 25% of patients who receive repeat prescriptions have had 40 or more repeats; 55% of patients aged over 75 years are on repeat medication (with periodic review).

Many patients taking the same drug for years are doing so for the best reason, i.e. firm diagnosis for which effective therapy is available, such as epilepsy, diabetes, hypertension, but some are not.

WARNINGS AND CONSENT

Doctors have a professional duty to inform and to warn, so that patients, who are increasingly informed and educated, may make meaningful personal choices, which it is their right to do (unless they opt to leave the choice to the doctor, which it is also their right to do).

> **Warnings to patients are of two kinds:**
> - Warnings that will affect the patient's choice to accept or reject the treatment
> - Warnings that will affect the safety of the treatment once it has begun, e.g. risk of stopping treatment, occurrence of drug toxicity.

Just as engineers say that the only safe aeroplane is the one that stays on the ground in still air on a disused airfield or in a locked hangar, so the only safe drug is one that stays in its original package. If drugs are not safe then plainly patients are entitled to be warned of their hazards, which should be **explained** to them, i.e. probability, nature and severity.

There is no formal legal or ethical obligation on doctors to warn all patients of all possible adverse consequences of treatment. It is their duty to adapt the information they give (not too little, and not so much as to cause confusion) so that the best interest of each patient is served. If there is a 'real' (say 1–2%) risk inherent in a procedure of some misfortune occurring, then doctors should warn patients of the possibility that the injury may occur, however well the treatment is performed. Doctors should take into account the personality of the patient, the likelihood of any misfortune arising and what warning was necessary for each particular patient's welfare.[36]

Doctors should consider what their particular individual patients would wish to know (i.e. would be likely to attach significance to) and not only what they think (paternalistically) that the patients ought to know. It is part of the professionalism of doctors to tell what is appropriate to the individual patient's interest. If things go wrong doctors must be prepared to defend what they did or, more important in the case of warnings, what they did not do, as being in their patient's best interest. Courts of law will look critically at doctors who seek to justify under-information by saying that they feared to confuse or frighten the patient (or that they left it to the patient to ask, as one doctor did). The increasing availability of patient information leaflets (PILs) prepared by the manufacturer indicates the increasing trend to give more information. Doctors should know what their patients have read (or not read, as is so often the case) when patients express dissatisfaction.

Evidence that extensive information on risks causes 'unnecessary' anxiety or frightens patients suggests that this is only a marginal issue and it does not justify a general policy of withholding of information.

Legal hazards for prescribers

Doctors would be less than human if, as well as trying to help their patients, they were not also concerned to protect themselves from allegations of malpractice (negligence) (see Regret avoidance). The legal position regarding a doctor's duty has been pungently put by a lawyer specialising in the field:

> The provision of information to patients is treated by (English) law as but one part of the way a

doctor discharges the obligation he owes to a patient to take reasonable care in all aspects of his treatment of that patient. The provision of information is a corollary of the patient's right to self-determination which is a right recognised by law. Failure to provide appropriate information will usually be a breach of duty and if that breach leads to the patient suffering injury then the basis for a claim for compensation exists.[37]

The keeping of appropriate medical records, written at the time of consultation (and which is so frequently neglected) is not only good medical practice, it is the best way of ensuring that there is an answer to unjustified allegations, made later, when memory has faded;[38] for example, allegations by patients that they would have declined a treatment that has done harm if the doctor had given a proper warning.

FORMULARIES, GUIDELINES AND 'ESSENTIAL' DRUGS

Increasingly, doctors recognise that they need guidance through the bountiful menu (thousands of medicines) so seductively served to them by the pharmaceutical industry. Principal sources of guidance

---

[37] Ian Dodds-Smith.

[38] A professor of clinical pharmacology who has made special studies of prescribing and patient information writes: 'What should a prescriber record in the notes?'

Given the existing format of general practitioner notes and the limited time available for each consultation, it seems unlikely that detailed information will be recorded in the notes. A compromise is therefore inevitable. My suggestion is that doctors should make a point of recording the fact that they have warned patients about treatments which are potentially hazardous. Specific examples include the description of dietary precautions to be taken if a monoamine oxidase inhibitor has been prescribed and the issue of steroid treatment cards to patients given prednisolone. Similarly, it would be wise to record that a young woman given a retinoid for acne is taking adequate contraceptive precautions, or that a patient taking carbimazole for thyrotoxicosis had been warned to report to the surgery in the event of a severe sore throat.

'Despite all of these uncertainties, the good news is that patients who receive leaflets are more satisfied than those who do not. Satisfied patients are less likely to complain, and are therefore presumably less likely to take legal action against prescribers' (George C F 1994 Prescribers' Journal 34: 7–11).

---

[36] Legal correspondent 1980 British Medical Journal 280: 575.

are the pharmaceutical industry ('prescribe my drug') and governments ('spend less'); also the developing (profit-making) managed care/insurance bodies ('spend less'); and the proliferating drug bulletins offering independent, and supposedly unbiased advice ('prescribe appropriately').

Even the pharmaceutical industry, in its more sober moments, recognises that their ideal world in which doctors, advised and informed by industry alone, were free to prescribe whatever they pleased,[39] to whomsoever they pleased, for as long as they pleased with someone other than the patient paying, is an unrealisable dream of a 'never-never land'.

The industry knows that it has to learn to live with restrictions of some kinds and one of the means of restriction is the **formulary,** a list of formulations of medicines with varying amounts of added information. A formulary may list all nationally licensed medicines prescribable by health professionals, or list only preferred drugs.

It may be restricted to what a third party payer will reimburse, or to the range of formulations stocked in a hospital (and chosen by a local drugs and therapeutics committee, which all hospitals or groups of hospitals should have), or the range agreed by a partnership of general practitioners or primary care health centre.

All restricted formularies are heavily motivated to keep costs down without impairing appropriate prescribing (p. 15). They should make provision for prescribing outside their range in cases of special need with an 'escape clause'.

Thus restricted formularies are in effect guidelines for prescribing. There is a profusion of these from national sources, hospitals, group practices and specialty organisations (epilepsy, diabetes mellitus).

'Essential' drugs. Economically disadvantaged countries may need help to construct formularies. Technical help has been forthcoming since 1977 from the World Health Organization (WHO) with its *Model List of Essential Drugs,* i.e. drugs (or representatives of classes of drugs) 'that satisfy the health care needs of the majority of the population; they should therefore be available at all times in adequate amounts and in the appropriate dosage forms'. Countries needing such advice can use the list as a basis for their own choices (WHO also publishes model prescribing information).[40] The list is updated every few years and contains about 300 items. The current list is provided as Appendix 1 to this chapter.

The pharmaceutical industry dislikes the concept that some drugs may be classed as essential and therefore others, by implication, are deemed inessential. But the WHO programme has attracted much interest and approval (see WHO Technical Report Series: The use of essential drugs: current edition).

Compliance

Successful therapy, especially if it is long-term, comprises a great deal more than choosing a standard medicine. It involves patient and doctor compliance.[41] The latter is liable to be overlooked (by doctors), for doctors prefer to dwell on the deficiencies of their patients rather than of themselves.

PATIENT COMPLIANCE

Patient compliance is the extent to which the actual behaviour of the patient coincides with medical advice and instructions: it may be complete, partial,

---

[39] It is difficult for us now to appreciate the naive fervour and trust in doctors that allowed them almost unlimited rights to prescribe (in the early years of the UK National Health Service: founded in 1948). Beer was a prescription item in hospitals until, decades later, an audit revealed that only 1 in 10 bottles reached a patient. More recently (1992): 'There could be fewer Christmas puddings consumed this year. The puddings were recently struck off a bizarre list of items that doctors were able to prescribe for their patients. They were removed by Health Department officials without complaint from the medics, on the grounds they had "no therapeutic or clinical value".' (Lancet 1992 340: 1531).

[40] There is an agency for WHO publications in all UN countries.

[41] The term **compliance** has been objected to as having overtones of obsolete, authoritarian attitudes, implying 'obedience' to doctors' 'orders'. The world **concordance** has been suggested as an alternative which expresses the duality of drug prescribing (by the doctor) and taking (by the patient). We retain **compliance,** pointing out that it applies equally to those doctors who neither keep up-to-date, nor follow prescribing instructions, and to patients who fail, for whatever reason, to keep to a drug regimen.

erratic, nil, or there may be overcompliance. To make a diagnosis and to prescribe evidence-based effective treatment is a satisfying experience for doctors, but too many assume that patients will gratefully or accurately do what they are told, i.e. obtain the medicine and consume it as instructed. This assumption is wrong.

The rate of **nonpresentation** (or redemption) of prescriptions[42] (UK) is around 5% but up to 20% or even more in the elderly (who pay no prescription charge). Where lack of money to pay for the medicine is not the cause, this is due to lack of motivation.

Having obtained the medicine, some 25–50% (sometimes even more) of patients either fail to follow the instruction to a significant extent (taking 50–90% of the prescribed dose), or they do not take it at all.

Patient noncompliance is identified as a major factor in therapeutic failure in both routine practice and in scientific therapeutic trials; but, sad to say, doctors, are too often noncompliant about remedying this. All patients are potential noncompliers;[43] good compliance cannot be reliably predicted on clinical criteria, but noncompliance often can be.

In addition to therapeutic failure, undetected noncompliance may lead to the best drug being deemed ineffective when it is not, leading to substitution by second-rank drugs.

Noncompliance may occur because:

- the patient has not understood the instructions, so cannot comply,[44] or
- understands the instructions, but fails to carry them out.

Prime factors for poor patient compliance are:

- *Frequency and complexity of drug regimen.* Many studies attest to compliance being inhibited by *polypharmacy*, i.e. more than three *drugs* to be taken concurrently or more than three *drug-taking occasions* in the day (the ideal of one occasion only is often unattainable).
- *Unintentional noncompliance,* or forgetfulness,[45] may be addressed by associating drug-taking with cues in daily life (breakfast, bedtime), by special packaging (e.g. calendar packs) and by enlisting the aid of others (e.g. carers, teachers).
- *'Intelligent' or wilful noncompliance.*[46] Patients

---

[44] **Cautionary tales**:

— A 62-year-old man requiring a metered-dose inhaler (for the first time) was told to 'spray the medicine to the throat'. He was found to have been conscientiously aiming and firing the aerosol to his anterior neck around the thyroid cartilage, four times a day for two weeks (Chiang A A, Lee J C 1994 New England Journal of Medicine 330: 1690).

— A patient thought that 'sublingual' meant able to speak two languages; another that tablets cleared obstructed blood vessels by exploding inside them (E A Kay) — reference, no doubt, to colloquial use of the term 'clot-busting drugs' (for thrombolytics).

— These are extreme examples, most are more subtle and less detectable. Doctors may smile at the ignorant naivety of patients, but the smile should be replaced by a blush of shame at their own deficiencies as communicators.

[45] Where noncompliance, whether intentional or unintentional, is medically serious it becomes necessary to bypass self-administration (unsupervised) and to resort to directly observed (i.e. supervised) oral administration or to injection (e.g. in schizophrenia).

[46] Of the many causes of failure of patient compliance the following case must be unique:

On a transatlantic flight the father of an asthmatic boy was seated in the row behind two doctors. He overheard one of the doctors expressing doubt about the long-term safety in children of inhaled corticosteroids. He interrupted the conversation, explaining that his son took this treatment; he had a lengthy conversation with one of the doctors, who gave his name. As a consequence, on arrival, he faxed his wife at home to stop the treatment of their son immediately. She did so, and two days later the well-controlled patient had a brisk relapse that responded to urgent treatment by the family doctor (who had been conscientiously following guidelines recently published in an authoritative journal). The family doctor later ascertained that the doctor in the plane was a member of the editorial team of the journal that had so recently published the guidelines that were favourable to inhaled corticosteroid (Cox S 1994 Is eavesdropping bad for your health? British Medical Journal 309: 718).

---

[42] Many factors are associated with prescription nonredemption. Perhaps the cameo of a person least likely to redeem a prescription is a middle-aged woman, not exempt from prescription charges (in UK National Health Service) who has a symptomatic condition requiring an 'acute' prescription that is issued by a trainee general practitioner on a Sunday (Beardon P H G et al 1994 British Medical Journal 307: 846).

[43] Even where the grave consequences of noncompliance are understood (glaucoma: blindness) (renal transplant: organ rejection), significant noncompliance has been reported in as many as 20% of patients; psychologists will be able to suggest explanations for this.

decide they do not need the drug or they do not like the drug, or take 2–3-day drug holidays.

- *Lack of information.* Oral instructions alone are not enough; one-third of patients have been found unable to recount instructions immediately on leaving the consulting room. Lucid and legible labelling of containers is essential, as well as patient-friendly information leaflets, which are increasingly available via doctors and pharmacists and as package inserts. (In hospitals, pharmacists have been known to throw away patient package inserts because they present problems for their administrative routine.)

- *Poor patient–doctor relationship and lack of motivation* to take medicines as instructed offer a major challenge to the prescriber whose diagnosis and prescription may be perfect, but yet loses efficacy by patient noncompliance. Unpleasant disease symptoms, particularly where these are recurrent and known by previous experience to be quickly relieved, provide the highest motivation, i.e. self-motivation, to comply. But particularly where the patient does not feel ill, adverse effects are immediate, and benefits are perceived to be remote, e.g. in hypertension, where they may be many years away in the future, then doctors must consciously address themselves to motivating compliance. The best way to motivate patients compliance is to cultivate the patient–doctor relationship. Doctors cannot be expected actually to like all their patients, but it is a great help (where liking does not come naturally) if they make a positive effort to understand how individual patients must be feeling about their illnesses and their treatments, i.e. to empathise with their patients. This is not always easy, but its achievement is the action of the true professional, and indeed is part of their professional duty of care.

Suggestions to doctors to enhance patient compliance are:

- Form a nonjudgemental alliance or partnership with the patient, giving the patient an opportunity to ask questions
- Plan a regimen with the minimum number of drugs and drug-taking occasions, adjusted to fit the patient's lifestyle. Use fixed-dose combinations or sustained-release (or injectable depot), as appropriate; arrange direct observation of each dose in exceptional cases
- Provide oral and written information adapted to the patient's understanding and medical and cultural needs
- Use patient-friendly packaging, e.g. calendar packs, where appropriate; or monitored-dose systems, e.g. boxes compartmented and labelled
- See the patient regularly and not so infrequently that the patient feels the doctor has lost interest
- Use computer-generated reminders for repeat prescriptions.

Directly observed therapy (DOT) (where a reliable person supervises each dose). In addition to the areas where it is obviously in the interest of patients that they be supervised, e.g. children, DOT is employed (even imposed) where free-living uncooperative patients may be a menace to the community, e.g. multiple-drug-resistant tuberculosis.

What every patient needs to know :

- An account of the disease and the reason for prescribing
- The name of the medicine
- The objective
  — to treat the disease and/or
  — to relieve symptoms, i.e. how important the medicine is, whether the patient can judge its efficacy and when benefit can be expected to occur
- How and when to take the medicine
- Whether it matters if a dose is missed and what, if anything, to do about it (see p. 23)
- How long the medicine is likely to be needed
- How to recognise adverse effects and any action that should be taken, including effects on car driving
- Any interaction with alcohol or other medicines.

A remarkable instance of noncompliance, with hoarding, was that of a 71-year-old man who attempted suicide and was found to have in his home 46 bottles containing 10 685 tablets. Analysis of his prescriptions showed that over a period of 17 months he had been expected to take 27 tablets of several different kinds daily.[48]

From time to time there are campaigns to collect all unwanted drugs from homes in an area. Usually the public are asked to deliver the drugs to their local pharmacies. In one UK city (600 000 population) 500 000 'solid dose units' (tablets, capsules, etc.) were handed in (see Opportunity cost); such quantities have even caused local problems for safe waste disposal.

Factors that are *insignificant* for compliance are: age[49] (except at extremes), gender, intelligence (except at extreme deficiency) and education level (probably).

Overcompliance. Patients (up to 20%) may take more drug than is prescribed, even increasing the dose by 50%. In diseases where precise compliance with frequent or complex regimens is important, e.g. in glaucoma where sight is at risk, there have been instances of obsessional patients responding to their doctors' overemphatic instructions by clock-watching in a state of anxiety to avoid the slightest deviance from timed administration of the correct dose, to the extent that their daily (and nightly) life becomes dominated by this single purpose.

Evaluation of patient compliance. Merely asking patients whether they have taken the drug as directed is not likely to provide reliable evidence;[50] and it can be assumed that anything that can happen to impair compliance, will happen sometimes. Estimations of compliance are based on studies using a variety of measures.

Requiring patients to produce containers when they attend the doctor, who counts the tablets, seems to do little more than show the patient that the doctor cares about the matter (which is useful); and a tablet absent from a container has not necessarily entered the patient's body. On the other hand, although patients are known to practise deliberate deception, to maintain effective deception successfully over long periods requires more effort than most patients are likely to make. The same applies to the use of monitored-dosage systems (e.g. compartmented boxes) as memory aids and to electronic containers that record times of opening.

Some pharmacodynamic effects, e.g. heart rate with beta-adrenoceptor blocker, provide a physiological marker as an indication of the presence of drug in the body.

Compliance in new drug development

Noncompliance, discovered or undiscovered, can invalidate therapeutic trials (in which it should always be monitored). In new drug development trials the diluting effect of undetected noncompliance (prescribed doses are increased) can result in unduly high doses being initially recommended (licensed) (with toxicity in good compliers after marketing), so that the standard dose has soon to be urgently reduced (this has probably occurred with some new nonsteroidal anti-inflammatory drugs).

DOCTOR COMPLIANCE

Doctor compliance is the extent to which the behaviour of doctors fulfils their professional duty:

- not to be ignorant
- to adopt new advances when they are sufficiently proved (which doctors are often slow to do)
- to prescribe accurately[51]
- to tell patients what they need to know

---

[47] After Drug and Therapeutics Bulletin 1981 19: 73.

Patient information leaflets. In economically privileged countries original or patient-pack dispensing is becoming the norm, i.e. patients receive an unopened pack just as it left the manufacturer. The pack contains a Patient Information Leaflet (PIL) (which is therefore supplied with each repeat prescription). Its content is increasingly determined by regulatory authority. The requirements to be comprehensive and, in this litigious age, to protect both manufacturer and regulatory authority, to some extent impair the patient-friendliness of PILs. But studies have shown that patients who receive leaflets are more satisfied than those who do not. Doctors need to have copies of these leaflets so that they can discuss with their patients what they are (or are not) reading.

[48] Smith S E et al 1974 Lancet 1: 937.

[49] But the elderly are commonly taking several drugs — a major factor in noncompliance — and monitoring compliance in this age group becomes particularly important. The over-60s (UK) are, on average, each receiving two or three medications.

---

[50] Hippocrates (5th cent. BC) noted that patients are liars regarding compliance. The way the patient is questioned may be all-important, e.g. 'Were you able to take the tablets?' may get a truthful reply where, 'Did you take the tablets?' may not, because the latter question may be understood by the patient as implying personal criticism (Pearson R M 1982 British Medical Journal 285: 757).

- to warn, i.e. to recognise the importance of the act of prescribing.

In one study in a university hospital, where standards might be expected to be high, there was an error of drug use (dose, frequency, route) in 3% of prescriptions and an error of prescription writing (in relation to standard hospital instructions) in 30%. Many errors were trivial, but many could have resulted in overdose, serious interaction or under-treatment.

In other hospital studies error rates in drug administration of 15–25% have been found, rates rising rapidly where four or more drugs are being given concurrently, as is often the case; studies on hospital inpatients show that each receives about six drugs, and up to 20 during a stay is not rare. Merely providing information (on antimicrobials) did not influence prescribing, but gently asking physicians to justify their prescriptions caused a marked fall in inappropriate prescribing.

On a harsher note, of recent years, doctors who have given drugs, of the use of which they have later admitted ignorance (e.g. route of administration and/or dose), have been charged with manslaughter[52] and have been convicted. Shocked by this, fellow doctors have written to the medical press offering under-standing sympathy to these, sometimes junior, colleagues; 'There, but for the grace of God, go I'.[53] But the public response is not sympathetic. Doctors put themselves forward as trained professionals who offer a service of responsible, competent provision of drugs which they have the legal right to prescribe. The public is increasingly inclined to hold them to that claim, and, where they seriously fail, to exact retribution.[54]

If you don't know about a drug, find out before you act, or take the personal consequences, which, increasingly, may be very serious indeed.

---

[51] Accuracy includes legibility: a doctor wrote Intal (sodium cromoglycate) for an asthmatic patient: the pharmacist read it as Inderal (propranolol): the patient died. See also, Names of drugs.
[52] Unlawful killing in circumstances that do not amount to murder (which requires an intention to kill), e.g. causing death by negligence that is much more serious than mere carelessness; reckless, breach of the legal duty of care.
[53] Attributed to John Bradford, an English preacher and martyr (16th cent), on seeing a convicted criminal pass by.

Underdosing

Use of suboptimal doses of drugs in serious disease, sacrificing efficacy for avoidance of serious adverse effects, has been documented. It particularly affects drugs of low therapeutic index (see Index), i.e. where the effective and toxic dose ranges are close, or even overlap, e.g. heparin, anticancer drugs, aminoglycoside antimicrobials. In these cases dose adjustment to obtain maximum benefit with minimum risk requires both knowledge and attentiveness.

The clinical importance of missed dose(s)

Even the most conscientious of patients will miss a dose or doses occasionally. Patients should therefore be told whether this matters and what they should do about it, if anything.

> **Missed dose(s) may lead to:**
> - loss of efficacy (acute disease)
> - resurgence (chronic disease)
> - rebound or withdrawal syndrome.

Loss of efficacy relates to the **pharmacokinetic properties** of the drugs. With some short $t_{\frac{1}{2}}$ drugs there is a simple issue of a transient drop in plasma concentration below a defined therapeutic level. But with others there may be complex issues such as recovery of negative feedback homoeostatic mechanisms, e.g. adrenocortical steroids. Therapeutic effect may not decline in parallel with plasma concentration. With some drugs a single missed dose may be important, e.g. oral contraceptives, with others (long $t_{\frac{1}{2}}$) several doses may be omitted before there is any serious decline in efficacy, e.g. thyroxine (levothyroxine).

---

[54] A doctor wrote a prescription for isosorbide ninitrate 20 mg 6-hourly but because of the illegibility of the handwriting the pharmacist dispensed felodipine in the same dose (maximum daily dose 10 mg). The patient died and a court ordered the doctor and pharmacist to pay compensation of $450 000 to the family. Charatan F 1999 British Medical Journal 319: 1456.

These pharmacokinetic considerations are complex and important, and are, or should be, taken into account by drug manufacturers in devising dosage schedules and informative Data Sheets. Manufacturers should aim at one or two doses per day (not more), and this is generally best achieved with drugs having relatively long biological effect $t\frac{1}{2}$, or where the biological effect $t\frac{1}{2}$ is short, by using sustained-release formulations.

Discontinuation syndrome (recurrence of disease, rebound, or withdrawal syndrome) may occur due to a variety of mechanisms (see Index).

Placebo medicines

> A **placebo**[55] is any component of therapy that is without specific biological activity for the condition being treated.

Placebo medicines are used for two purposes:

- As a control in scientific evaluation of drugs (see Therapeutic trials) (see p. 60)
- To benefit or please a patient, not by any pharmacological actions, but by psychological means.

All treatments have a psychological component, whether to please (placebo effect) or, occasionally, to vex (negative placebo or nocebo[56] effect).

A placebo medicine is a vehicle for 'cure' by suggestion, and is surprisingly often successful, if only temporarily.[57] All treatments carry placebo effect: physiotherapy, psychotherapy, surgery, entering a patient into a therapeutic trial, even the personality and style of the doctor; but the effect is most easily investigated with drugs, for the active and the inert can often be made to appear identical so that comparisons can be made.

The deliberate use of drugs as placebos is a confession of failure by the doctor. Failures however are sometimes inevitable and an absolute condemnation of the use of placebos on all occasions would be unrealistic.

> A **placebo-reactor** is an individual who reports changes of physical or mental state after taking a pharmacologically inert substance.

Placebo-reactors are suggestible people and likely to respond favourably to any treatment. They have misled doctors into making false therapeutic claims.

Negative reactors, who develop adverse effects when given a placebo, exist but, fortunately, are fewer.

Some 35% of the physically ill and 40% or more of the mentally ill respond to placebos. Placebo reaction is an inconstant attribute; a person may respond at one time in one situation and not at another time under different conditions. There is some consistency in the type of person who tends to react to any therapeutic intervention. In one study on medical students, psychological tests revealed that those who reacted to a placebo tended to be extraverted, sociable, less dominant, less self-confident, more appreciative of their teaching, more aware of their autonomic functions and more neurotic than their colleagues who did not react to a placebo under the particular conditions of the experiment.

It is of great importance that all who administer drugs should be aware that their attitudes to the treatment may greatly influence the result. Undue scepticism may prevent a drug from achieving its effect and enthusiasm or confidence may potentiate the actions of drugs.

---

[55] Latin: *placebo,* I shall be pleasing or acceptable.
[56] Latin: *nocebo,* I shall injure; the term is little used.

---

[57] As the following account by a mountain rescue guide illustrates: 'The incident involved a 15-year-old boy who sustained head injuries and a very badly broken leg. Helicopter assistance was unavailable and therefore we had to carry him by stretcher to the nearest landrover (several miles away) and then on to a waiting ambulance.

During this long evacuation the boy was in considerable distress and we administered Entonox (a mixture of nitrous oxide and oxygen, 50% each) sparingly as we only had one small cylinder. He repeatedly remarked how much better he felt after each intake of Entonox (approximately every 20 minutes) and after 7 hours or so we eventually got him safely into the ambulance and on his way to hospital.

On going to replace the Extonox we discovered the cylinder was still full of gas due to the equipment being faulty. There was no doubt that the boy felt considerable pain relief as a result of thinking he was receiving Entonox.'

Tonics are placebos. They may be defined as substances with which it is hoped to strengthen and increase the appetite of those so weakened by disease, misery, overindulgence in play or work, or by physical or mental inadequacy, that they cannot face the stresses of life. The essential feature of this weakness is the absence of any definite recognisable defect for which there is a known remedy. Since tonics are placebos, they must be harmless.[58]

Pharmacoeconomics

Even the richest societies cannot satisfy the appetite of their citizens for health care based on their real needs, on their wants and on their (often unrealistic) expectations.

Health care resources are rationed[59] in one way or another, whether according to national social policies or to individual wealth. The debate on supply is not about whether there should be rationing, but about what form rationing should take; whether it should be explicit or concealed (from the public).

Doctors prescribe, patients consume and, increasingly throughout the world, third (purchasing) parties (government, insurance companies) pay the bill with money they have obtained from increasingly reluctant healthy members of the public.

The purchasers of health care are now engaged in serious exercises to contain drug costs in the short term without, it is hoped, impairing the quality of medical care, or damaging the development of useful new drugs (which is an enormously expensive and long-term process). This can be achieved successfully only if reliable data are available on costs and benefits, both absolute and relative. The difficulties of generating such data, not only during development, but later under actual-use conditions, are enormous and are addressed by a special breed of professionals: the health economists.

> **Economics** is the science of the distribution of wealth and resources. Prescribing doctors, who have a duty to the community as well as to individual patients, cannot escape involvement with economics.

The economists' objective

The objective is to enable needs to be defined so that available resources may be deployed according to priorities set by society, which has an interest in fairness between its members. The question is whether resources are to be distributed in accordance with and unregulated power struggle between professionals and associations of patients and public pressure groups — all, no doubt, warm-hearted towards deserving cases of one kind or another, but none able to view the whole scene; or whether there is to be a planned evaluation that allows division of the resources on the basis of some visible attempt at fairness.

A health economist[60] writes:

> The economist's approach to evaluating drug therapies is to look at a group of patients with a particular disorder and the various drugs that could be used to treat them. The costs of the various treatments and some costs associated with their use (together with the costs of giving no treatment) are then considered in terms of impact on health status (survival and quality of life) and impact on other health care costs (e.g. admissions to hospital, need for other drugs, use of other procedures).
>
> Economists are often portrayed as people who want to focus on cost, whereas in reality they see everything in terms of a balance between costs and benefits.

Four economic concepts have particular importance to the thinking of every doctor who takes up a pen to prescribe, i.e. to distribute resources.

● *Opportunity cost* means that which has to be sacrificed in order to carry out a certain course of action, i.e. costs are benefits foregone elsewhere. If money is spent on prescribing, that money is not available for another purpose; wasteful prescribing can be seen as an affront to those

---

[58] Tonics (licensed) available in the UK include: Gentian Mixture, acid (or alkaline) (gentian, a natural plant bitter substance, and dilute HCl or sodium bicarbonate): Labiton (thiamine, caffeine, alcohol, all in low dose).

[59] The term rationing is used here to embrace the allocation of priorities as well as the actual withholding of resources (in this case, drugs).

[60] Prof Michael Drummond.

who are in serious need, e.g. institutionalised mentally handicapped citizens who everywhere would benefit from increased resources.

- *Cost-effectiveness analysis* is concerned with how to attain a given objective at minimum financial cost, e.g. prevention of postsurgical venous thromboembolism by heparins, warfarin, aspirin, external pneumatic compression. Analysis includes cost of: materials, adverse effects, any tests, nursing and doctor time, duration of stay in hospital (which may greatly exceed the cost of the drug).
- *Cost-benefit analysis* is concerned with issues of whether (and to what extent) to pursue objectives and policies; it is thus a broader activity than cost-effectiveness analysis and puts monetary values on the quality as well as on the quantity (duration) of life.
- *Cost-utility analysis* is concerned with comparisons between programmes, e.g. an antenatal drug treatment which saves a young life or a hip replacement operation which improves mobility in a man of 60 years. Such differing outcomes can be placed on the same basis for comparison by computing quality-adjusted life years (see below).

An allied measure is the *cost-minimisation analysis* which finds the least costly programme among those shown or assumed to be of equal benefit. Economic analysis requires that both quantity and quality of life be measured. The former is easy, the latter is hard.

Quality of life

Everyone is familiar with the measurement of the benefit of treatment in saving or extending life, i.e. life expectancy: the measure is the quantity of life (in years). But it is evident that life may be extended and yet have a low quality, even to the point that it is not worth having at all. It is therefore useful to have a unit of health measurement that combines the quality of life with its quality to allow individual and social decisions to be made on a sounder basis than mere intuition. To meet this need economists have developed the *quality-adjusted–life-year* (QALY); estimations of years of life expectancy are modified according to estimations of quality of life.

Quality of life has four principal dimensions:[61]
1. physical mobility
2. freedom from pain and distress
3. capacity for self-care
4. ability to engage in normal work and social interactions.

The approach to measure quality of life has been developed by questionnaire to measure what the subject perceives as personal health. The assessments are being refined to provide improved assessment of the benefits and risks of medicines to the individual and to society. The challenge is to ensure that these are sufficiently robust to make resource allocation decisions between, for example: the rich and the poor, the educated and the uneducated, the old and the young, as well as between groups of patients having very different diseases. Plainly, quality of life is a major aspect of what is called *outcomes research*.

Self-medication

To feel unwell is common, though the frequency varies with social and cultural circumstances. People commonly experience symptoms or complaints and commonly want to take remedial action. In one study of adults randomly selected from a large population, 9 out of 10 had one or more complaints in the 2 weeks before interview; in another of premenopausal women a symptom occurred as often as 1 day in 3; in both studies a medicine was taken for more than half these occurrences.

Self-medication and consumer rights

Increasingly, educated and confident consumers are aware of five consumer rights (United Nations charter):
- *access* (to a wide range of products)
- *choice* (self-determination)
- *information* (on which to base choice)
- *redress* (when things go wrong)
- *safety* (appropriate to the use of the product).

---

[61] Williams A 1983. In: Smith G T (ed) Measuring the social benefits of medicine. Office of Health Economics, London.

Modern consumers (patients) wish to take a greater role in the maintenance of their own health and are often competent to manage (uncomplicated) chronic and recurrent illnesses (not merely short-term symptoms) after proper medical diagnosis and with only occasional professional advice, e.g. use of histamine H_2-receptor blocker, topical corticosteroid and antifungal, and oral contraceptive. They are understandably unwilling to submit to the inconvenience of visiting a doctor for what they rightly feel they can manage for themselves, given adequate information.

Increased consumer autonomy leads to satisfied:

- consumers (above)
- governments (lower drug bill)
- industry (profits)
- doctors (reduced work load).

The pharmaceutical industry enthusiastically estimates that extending the use of self-medication to all potentially self-treatable illnesses could save 100–150 million general practitioner consultations per year (in the UK: population 57 million). But there will also be added costs as pharmacists extend their responsibilities for supply and information.

Regulatory authorities are increasingly receptive to switching hitherto prescription-only medicines (POM) for self-medication (over-the-counter, OTC, sale) via pharmacies (P) or via any retail outlet (general sale). The operation is known as POM-OTC or POM-P 'switch'. It requires particularly exacting standards of safety.

> **Self-medication is appropriate for:**
>
> - short-term relief of symptoms where accurate diagnosis is unnecessary
> - uncomplicated cases of some chronic and recurrent disease (a medical diagnosis having been made and advice given).

Safety in self-medication (an overriding requirement) depends on four items:

- *The drug* — its inherent properties, dose and duration of use, including its power to induce dependence
- *The formulation* — devised with unsupervised use in mind, e.g. low dose

- *Information* — available with all purchases (printed) and rigorously reviewed (by panels of potential users) for user-friendliness and adequacy for a wide range of education and intellectual capacity
- *Patient compliance.*

> Doctors must recognise the increasing importance of questioning about self-medication when taking a drug history.

GUIDE TO FURTHER READING

Barach P, Small S D 2000 Reporting and preventing medical mishaps: lessons from non-medical near miss reporting systems. British Medical Journal 320: 759–763.

de Craen A et al 1996 Effect of colour of drugs: systematic review of perceived effect of drugs and their effectiveness. British Medical Journal 313: 1624–1626

Editorial 1988 When to believe the unbelievable. Nature 333: 787 A report of an investigation into experiments with antibodies in solutions that contained no antibody molecules (as in some homoeopathic medicines). The editor of Nature took a three-person team (one of whom was a professional magician, included to detect any trickery) on a week-long visit to the laboratory that claimed positive results. Despite the scientific seriousness of the operation it developed comical aspects (codes of the contents of test tubes were taped to the laboratory ceiling); the Nature team, having reached an unfavourable view of the experiments 'sped past the [laboratory] common-room filled with champagne bottles destined now not to be opened'. Full reports in this issue of Nature (28 July 1988), including an acrimonious response by the original scientist, are highly recommended reading, both for scientific logic and for entertainment. See also Nature 1994 370: 322

Ernst E, Thompson J 2001 Heavy metals in traditional Chinese medicines: a systematic review. Clinical Pharmacology and Therapeutics 70: 497–504

Ferner R E 2000 Medication errors that have led to manslaughter charges. British Medical Journal 321: 1212–1216

Kleijnen J et al 1994 Placebo effect in double-blind clinical trials. Lancet 344: 1347–1349

Mead T (ed) 1998 Science-based complementary medicine. Royal College of Physicians of London; London

Meltzer M I 2001 Introduction to health economics for physicians. Lancet 358: 993–998 (and subsequent papers in this quintet).

Moynihan R et al 2000 Coverage by the news media of the benefits and risks of medications. New England Journal of Medicine 342: 1645–1650

Reason J 2000 Human error: models and management. British Medical Journal 320: 768–770

Thomas K B 1994 The placebo in general practice. Lancet 344: 1066

Urquhart J 2000 Erratic patient compliance with prescribed drug regimens: target for drug delivery systems. Clinical Pharmacology and Therapeutics 67: 331–334

Vickers A 2000 Complementary medicine. British Medical Journal 321: 683–686

Vickers A, Zollman C 1999 Homeoepathy. British Medical Journal 319: 1115–1118

Volmink J, Matchaba P, Garner P 2000 Directly observed therapy and treatment adherence. Lancet 355: 1345–1350

Weingart S N et al 2000 Epidemiology of medical error. British Medical Journal 320: 774–777

Zollman C, Vickers A 1999 What is complementary medicine? British Medical Journal 319: 693–696 (and other articles in this series).

Appendix 1: The World Health Organization model list of essential drugs[1]

We reprint the current list (by permission). Whilst the WHO programme (revised 1999) was instituted particularly to help less developed countries, the list has interest and lessons for all societies facing, as they now are, the problems of delivering economically affordable health care to all. We commend a study of the list to our readers (see also p. 18).

The list of essential drugs may be considered against the background of the available marketed medicines worldwide. Any national or local group of health workers wishing to produce a formulary to provide for the needs of their own community would be well advised to study the current version in addition to other sources.

A major standard reference work (Martindale 1996 The extra pharmacopoeia. 31st edn., Pharmaceutical Press, London), describes 62 500 preparations or groups of preparations from 17 different countries.

---

[1] WHO Drug Information Vol 13, No 4, 1999

Explanatory notes

We print the list in full.

Drugs marked* represent an example of a therapeutic group, i.e. various other drugs could serve as an alternative say, on cost grounds.

Complementary drugs are for use where, for any reason, drugs in the main list are unavailable, or there are exceptional medical circumstances, e.g. bacterial resistance, rare disorders.

Spelling of drug names. The World Health Organization devises recommended International Non-proprietary Names (rINN). These are becoming universal; most do not give rise to any confusion, but occasionally we insert an alternative name or spelling.

Not every entry in the list is discussed in this book. Conversely, the book may give drug treatments for specific conditions that differ from those listed here.

---

1. **Anaesthetics**

1.1 **General anaesthetics and oxygen**
ether, anaesthetic
halothane
ketamine
nitrous oxide
oxygen
* thiopental

1.2 **Local anaesthetics**
* bupivacaine
* lidocaine (lignocaine)
COMPLEMENTARY DRUG
ephedrine (in spinal anaesthesia during delivery to prevent hypotension)

1.3 **Preoperative medication and sedation for short-term procedures**
atropine

chloral hydrate
* diazepam
* morphine
* promethazine

2. **Analgesics, antipyretics, nonsteroidal anti-inflammatory drugs (NSAIDs), drugs used to treat gout and disease-modifying agents used in rheumatic disorders (DMARDs)**

2.1 **Non-opioids and NSAIDs**
acetylsalicylic acid (aspirin)
* ibuprofen
paracetamol

2.2 **Opioid analgesics**
* codeine
* morphine

COMPLEMENTARY DRUG
* pethidine

2.3 **Drugs used to treat gout**
allopurinol
colchicine

2.4 **Disease-modifying agents used in rheumatic disorders**
azathioprine
chloroquine
cyclophosphamide
methotrexate
penicillamine
sulfasalazine

3. **Antiallergics and drugs used in anaphylaxis**
* chlorphenamine
* dexamethasone
epinephrine (adrenaline)
hydrocortisone
prednisolone

4. Antidotes and other substances used in poisonings

4.1 Nonspecific
* charcoal, activated
ipecacuanha

4.2 Specific
acetylcysteine
atropine
calcium gluconate
deferoxamine
(desferrioxamine)
dimercaprol
* DL-methionine.
methylthioninium chloride
(methylene blue)
naloxone
penicillamine
potassium ferric
hexacyanoferrate(II). $2H_2O$
(Prussian blue)
sodium calcium edetate
sodium nitrite
sodium thiosulfate

5. Anticonvulsants/ antiepileptics
carbamazepine
* diazepam
ethosuximide
magnesium sulfate
phenobarbital (phenobarbitone)
phenytoin
valproic acid
COMPLEMENTARY DRUG
* clonazepam

6. Anti-infective drugs

6.1 Anthelminthics
6.1.1 *Intestinal anthelminthics*
albendazole
levamisole
* mebendazole
niclosamide
praziquantel
pyrantel

6.1.2 Antifilarials
diethylcarbamazine
ivermectin
COMPLEMENTARY DRUG
suramin sodium

6.1.3 *Antischistosomals and other antitrematode drugs*
praziquantel
triclabendazone

COMPLEMENTARY DRUG
oxamniquine

6.2 Antibacterials
6.2.1 *Beta-lactam drugs*
* amoxicillin
ampicillin
benzathine benzylpenicillin
benzylpenicillin
* cloxacillin
phenoxymethylpenicillin
procaine benzylpenicillin
RESTRICTED INDICATIONS
* amoxycillin + *clavulanic acid
ceftazidime
* ceftriaxone
imipenem + cilastatin

6.2.2 *Other antibacterials*
* chloramphenicol
* ciprofloxacin
* doxycycline
* erythromycin
* gentamicin
* metronidazole
nalidixic acid
nitrofurantoin
spectinomycin
* sulfadiazine
* sulfamethoxazole +
trimethoprim
trimethoprim
COMPLEMENTARY DRUGS
chloramphenicol
clindamycin
RESTRICTED INDICATIONS
vancomycin

6.2.3 *Antileprosy drugs*
clofazimine
dapsone
rifampicin

6.2.4 *Antituberculosis drugs*
ethambutol
isoniazid
pyrazinamide
rifampicin
streptomycin
COMPLEMENTARY DRUG
thioacetazone

6.3 Antifungal drugs
amphotericin B
* fluconazole
griseofulvin
nystatin
COMPLEMENTARY DRUGS
flucytosine
potassium iodide

6.4 Antiviral drugs
6.4.1 *Antiherpes drug*
aciclovir

6.4.2 *Antiretroviral drugs*
nevirapine
zidovudine

6.5 Antiprotozoal drugs
6.5.1 *Antiamoebic and antigiardiasis drugs*
* diloxanide
* metronidazole

6.5.2 *Antileishmaniasis drugs*
* meglumine antimoniate
pentamidine
COMPLEMENTARY DRUG
amphotericin B

6.5.3 *Antimalarial drugs*
(a) For curative treatment
* chloroquine primaquine
* quinine
COMPLEMENTARY DRUGS
* doxycycline (for use only in combination with quinine)
mefloquine
* sulfadoxine + pyrimethamine
RESTRICTED INDICATIONS
artemether
artesunate
(b) For prophylaxis
chloroquine
doxycycline
mefloquine
proguanil (for use only in combination with chloroquine)

6.5.4 *Antipneumocystosis and antitoxoplasmosis drugs*
pentamidine
pyrimethamine
sulfamethoxazole +
trimethoprim

6.5.5 *Antitrypanosomal drugs*
(a) African trypanosomiasis
melarsoprol
pentamidine
suramin sodium
COMPLEMENTARY DRUG
eflornithine
(b) American trypanosomiasis
benznidazole
nifurtimox

6.5 Insect repellent
diethyltoluamide

7. Antimigraine drugs

7.1 For treatment of acute attack
acetylsalicylic acid (aspirin)
ergotamine
paracetamol

7.2 For prophylaxis
* propranolol

8. Antineoplastic and immunosuppressant drugs and drugs used in palliative care

8.1 Immunosuppressant drugs
* azathioprine
* ciclosporin (for organ transplantation)

8.2 Cytotoxic drugs
asparaginase
bleomycin
calcium folinate
chlorambucil
chlormethine
cisplatin
cyclophosphamide
cytarabine
dacarbazine
daunorubicin
dactinomycin
* doxorubicin
etoposide
fluorouracil
levamisole
mercaptopurine
methotrexate
procarbazine
vinblastine
vincristine

8.3 Hormones and antihormones
* prednisolone
tamoxifen

8.4 Drugs used in palliative care
The drugs are included in the relevant sections of the model list, according to their therapeutic use, e.g. analgesics

9. Antiparkinsonism drugs
* biperiden
levodopa + *carbidopa

10. Drugs affecting the blood

10.1 Antianaemia drugs
ferrous salt
ferrous salt + folic acid (nutritional supplement for use during pregnancy)
folic acid
hydroxocobalamin
COMPLEMENTARY DRUG
* iron dextran

10.2 Drugs affecting coagulation
desmopressin
heparin sodium
phytomenadione
protamine sulfate
* warfarin

11. Blood products and plasma substitutes

11.1 Plasma substitutes
* dextran 70
* polygeline

11.2 Plasma fractions for specific uses
albumin, human
COMPLEMENTARY DRUGS
* factor VIII concentrate,
* factor IX complex (coagulation factors II, VII, IX, X) concentrate

12. Cardiovascular drugs

12.1 Antianginal drugs
* atenolol
glyceryl trinitrate
* isosorbide dinitrate
* verapamil

12.2 Antiarrhythmic drugs
* atenolol
digoxin
lidocaine
verapamil
COMPLEMENTARY DRUGS
epinephrine (adrenaline)
isoprenaline
* procainamide
* quinidine

12.3 Antihypertensive drugs
* atenolol
* captopril
* hydralazine
* hydrochlorothiazide
methyldopa
* nifedipine

* reserpine
COMPLEMENTARY DRUGS
prazosin
* sodium nitroprusside

12.4 Drugs used in heart failure
* captopil
digoxin
dopamine
* hydrochlorothiazide

12.5 Antithrombotic drugs
acetylsalicylic acid (aspirin)
COMPLEMENTARY DRUG
streptokinase

12.6 Lipid-lowering agents
HMG Co-A reductase inhibitors (statins) have been shown to reduce the incidence of fatal and non-fatal myocardial infarction, stroke and mortality (all causes), as well as the need for coronary artery bypass surgery. Since no single drug has been shown to be significantly more effective or less expensive than others in the group, none is included in the model list; the choice of drug for use in patients at highest risk should be decided at national level.

13. Dermatological drugs (topical)

13.1 Antifungal drugs
benzoic acid + salicylic acid
* miconazole
sodium thiosulphate
COMPLEMENTARY DRUG
selenium sulfide

13.2 Anti-infective drugs
* methylrosanilinium chloride (gentian violet)
* neomycin + *bacitracin
potassium permanganate
silver sulfadiazine

13.3 Anti-inflammatory and antipruritic drugs
* betamethasone
* calamine lotion
* hydrocortisone

13.4 Astringent drugs
aluminium diacetate

13.5 **Drugs affecting skin differentiation and proliferation**
benzoyl peroxide
coal tar
dithranol
fluorouracil
* podophyllum resin
salicylic acid
urea

13.6 **Scabicides and pediculicides**
* benzyl benzoate
permethrin

13.7 **Ultraviolet-blocking agents**
COMPLEMENTARY DRUGS
topical sun protection agent with activity against UVA and UVB cream, lotion or gel

14. **Diagnostic agents**

14.1 **Ophthalmic drugs**
fluorescein
* tropicamide

14.2 **Radiocontrast media**
* amidotrizoate
barium sulfate
* iohexol
* iopanoic acid
* propyliodone (for administration only into the bronchial tree)
COMPLEMENTARY DRUG
* meglumine iotroxate

15. **Disinfectants and antiseptics**

15.1 **Antiseptics**
* chlorhexidine
* ethanol
* polyvidone iodine

15.2 **Disinfectants**
* chlorine base compound
chloroxyenol
glutaral

16. **Diuretics**
* amiloride
* furosemide (frusemide)
* hydrochlorothiazide
spironolactone
COMPLEMENTARY DRUG
* mannitol

17. **Gastrointestinal drugs**

17.1 **Antacids and other antiulcer drugs**
aluminium hydroxide
* cimetidine
magnesium hydroxide

17.2 **Antiemetic drugs**
metoclopramide
* promethazine

17.3 **Antihaemorrhoidal drugs**
* local anaesthetic, astringent and anti-inflammatory drug

17.4 **Anti-inflammatory drugs**
hydrocortisone
* sulfasalazine

17.5 **Antispasmodic drugs**
* atropine

17.6 **Laxatives**
* senna

17.7 **Drugs used in diarrhoea**

17.7.1 Oral rehydration
oral rehydration salts (for glucose-electrolyte solution)

17.7.2 Antidiarrhoeal (symptomatic) drugs
* codeine

18. **Hormones, other endocrine drugs and contraceptives**

18.1 **Adrenal hormones and synthetic substitutes**
* dexamethasone
hydrocortisone
* prednisolone
COMPLEMENTARY DRUG
fludrocortisone

18.2 **Androgens**
COMPLEMENTARY DRUG
testosterone

18.3 **Contraceptives**

18.3.1 Hormonal contraceptives
* ethinylestradiol +
* levonorgestrel
* ethinylestradiol +
* norethisterone
levonorgestrel
COMPLEMENTARY DRUGS
* levonorgestrel
medroxyprogesterone acetate
norethisterone enantate

18.3.2 Intrauterine devices
copper-containing device

18.3.3 Barrier methods
condoms with or without spermicide (nonoxinol)
diaphragms with spermicide (nonoxinol)

18.4 **Estrogens**
* ethinylestradiol

18.5 **Insulins and other antidiabetic agents**
* glibenclamide
insulin injection (soluble)
intermediate-acting insulin
metformin

18.6 **Ovulation inducers**
* clomifene

18.7 **Progestogens**
norethisterone
COMPLEMENTARY DRUG
medroxyprogesterone acetate

18.8 **Thyroid hormones and antithyroid drugs**
levothyroxine
potassium iodide
* propylthiouracil

19. **Immunologicals**

19.1 **Diagnostic agents**
tuberculin, purified protein derivative (PPD)

19.2 **Sera and immunoglobulins**
anti-D immunoglobulin (human)
* antitetanus immunoglobulin (human)
antivenom serum
diphtheria antitoxin
immunoglobulin, human normal
* rabies immunoglobulin

19.3 **Vaccines**

19.3.1 For universal immunisation
BCG
diphtheria
pertussis
tetanus
hepatitis B
measles
poliomyelitis

19.3.2 For specific groups of individuals
influenza
meningitis
mumps
rabies
rubella

typhoid
yellow fever

20. Muscle relaxants (peripherally acting) and cholinesterase inhibitors
* alcuronium chloride
* neostigmine
  pyridostigmine bromide
  suxamethonium chloride
  COMPLEMENTARY DRUG
  vecuronium bromide

21. Ophthalmological preparations

21.1 Anti-infective agents
* gentamicin
* idoxuridine
  silver nitrate
* tetracycline

21.2 Anti-inflammatory agents
* prednisolone

21.3 Local anaesthetics
* tetracaine (amethocaine)

21.4 Miotics and antiglaucoma drugs
  acetazolamide
* pilocarpine
* timolol

21.5 Mydriatics
  atropine
  COMPLEMENTARY DRUG
  epinephrine (adrenaline)

22. Oxytocics and antioxytocics

22.1 Oxytocics
* ergometrine
  oxytocin

22.2 Antioxytocics
* salbutamol

23. Peritoneal dialysis solution
  intraperitoneal dialysis solution (of appropriate composition)

24. Psychotherapeutic drugs

24.1 Drugs used in psychotic disorders
* chlorpromazine
* fluphenazine
* haloperidol

24.2 Drugs used in mood disorders

24.2.1 Drugs used in depressive disorders
* amitryptiline

24.2.2 Drugs used in bipolar disorders
  carbamazepine
  lithium carbonate
  valproic acid

24.3 Drugs used in generalised anxiety and sleep disorders
* diazepam

24.4 Drugs used in obsessive-compulsive disorders and panic attacks
  clomipramine

25. Drugs acting on the respiratory tract

25.1 Antiasthmatic drugs
* aminophylline
* beclometasone
  epinephrine (adrenaline)
  ipratropium bromide
* salbutamol

theophylline
COMPLEMENTARY DRUG
* cromoglicic acid (sodium cromoglycate)

25.2 Antitussives
* dextromethorphan

26. Solutions correcting water, electrolyte and acid-base disturbances

26.1 Oral rehydration
  oral rehydration salts (glucose-electrolyte solution)
  potassium chloride

26.2 Parenteral
  glucose
  glucose with sodium chloride
  potassium chloride
  sodium chloride
  sodium hydrogen carbonate
* compound solution of sodium lactate

26.3 Miscellaneous
  water for injection

27. Vitamins and minerals
  ascorbic acid
* ergocalciferol
  iodine
* nicotinamide
  pyridoxine
* retinol
  riboflavin
* sodium fluoride
  thiamine
  COMPLEMENTARY DRUG
  calcium gluconate

Appendix 2: The prescription

The prescription is the means by which medicines that are not considered safe for sale directly to the public are delivered to patients. Its format is officially regulated to ensure precision in the interests of safety and efficacy and to prevent fraudulent misuse; full details will be found in national formularies and prescribers have a responsibility to comply with these.

Prescriptions of pure drugs or of formulations from the British National Formulary (BNF)[1] are satisfactory for almost all purposes. The composition of many of the preparations in the BNF is laid down in official pharmacopoeias, e.g. British Pharmacopoeia (BP). There are also many national and international pharmacopoeias.

Traditional extemporaneous prescription-writing art, defining drug, base, adjuvant, corrective, flavouring and vehicle is obsolete, as is the use of the Latin language. Certain convenient Latin abbreviations do survive for lack of convenient English substitutes (chiefly in hospitals where instructions are given to nurses and not to patients). They are listed below, without approval or disapproval.

> The elementary requirements of a prescription are that it should state what is to be given to whom and by whom prescribed, and give instructions on how much should be taken how often, by what route and for how long or total quantity to be supplied, as below.

---

1. **Date.**

2. **Address of doctor.**

3. **Name and address of patient:** *age* is also desirable for safety reasons; in the UK it is a legal requirement for children under age 12 years.

4. **℞**
   This is a traditional esoteric symbol[2] for the word 'Recipe' — 'take thou', which is addressed to the pharmacist. It is pointless; but since many doctors gain a harmless pleasure from writing it with a flourish before the name of a proprietary preparation of whose exact nature they are ignorant, it is likely to survive as a sentimental link with the past.

5. **The name and dose of the medicine.**
   Abbreviations. Only abbreviate where there is an official abbreviation. Never use unofficial abbreviations or invent your own; **it is not safe to do so.**
   Quantities (after BNF)
   — 1 gram or more: write 1 g etc.
   — Less than 1 g: write as milligrams: 500 mg, not 0.5 g.
   — Less than 1 mg: write as micrograms, e.g. 100 micrograms, not 0.1 mg.
   — For decimals a zero should precede the decimal point where there is no other figure, e.g. 0.5 mL, not .5 mL, or for a range, 0.5 to 1 g.
   — Do not abbreviate microgram, nanogram or unit.
   — Use millilitre, ml or mL, not cubic centimetre, cc.
   — Home/domestic measures, see below.

   State dose and dose frequency; for 'as required', specify minimum dose interval or maximum dose per day.

6. **Directions to the pharmacist,** if any: 'mix', 'make a solution'. Write the total quantity to be dispensed (if this is not stated in 5 above); or duration of supply.

7. **Instruction for the patient,** to be written on container by the pharmacist. Here brevity, clarity and accuracy are especially important. It is dangerous to rely on the patient remembering oral instructions. The BNF provides a list of recommended 'cautionary and advisory labels for dispensed medicines' representing a balance between 'the unintelligibly short and the inconveniently long', e.g. 'Do not stop taking this medicine except on your doctor's advice'.
   Pharmacists nowadays use their own initiative in giving advice to patients.

8. **Signature of doctor.**

Example of a prescription for a patient with an annoying unproductive cough.
   1,2,3, as above
   4. ℞
   5. Codeine Linctus, BNF, 5 ml
   6. Send 60 ml
   7. Label: Codeine Linctus [or NP]. Take 5 ml twice a day and on retiring.
   8. Signature of doctor.

---

[1] Supplied free to all doctors practising in the UK National Health Service.
[2] Derived from the eye of Horus, ancient Egyptian sun god.

Computer-issued prescriptions must conform to recommendations of professional bodies. If altered by hand (undesirable), the alteration must be signed.

Medicine containers. Reclosable child-resistant containers and blister packs are increasingly used, as is dispensing in manufacturers' original sealed packs containing a patient information leaflet. These add to immediate cost but may save money in the end (increased efficiency of use, and safety).

Unwanted medicines. Patients should be encouraged to return these to the original supplier for disposal.

Drugs liable to cause dependence or be the subject of misuse. Doctors have a particular responsibility to ensure that (1) they do not create dependence, (2) the patient does not increase the dose and create dependence, (3) they are not used as an unwitting source of supply to addicts. To many such drugs special prescribing regulations apply (see BNF).

Abbreviations (see also Weights and measures, below)

a.c.: ante cibum	before food
b.d.: bis in die	twice a day (bid is also used)
BNF	British National Formulary
BP	British Pharmacopoeia
BPC	British Pharmaceutical Codex
i.m.: intramuscular	by intramuscular injection
IU	International Unit
i.v.: intravenous	by intravenous injection
NP: nomen proprium	proper name
o.d.: omni die	every day
o.m.: omni mane	every morning
o.n.: omni nocte	every night
p.c.: post cibum	after food
p.o.: per os	by mouth
p.r.: per rectum	by the anal/rectal route
p.r.n.: pro re nata	as required. It is best to add the maximum frequency of repetition, e.g. Aspirin and Codeine Tablets, 1 or 2 prn, 4-hourly
p.v.: per vaginam	by the vaginal route
q.d.s.: quater die sumendus	4 times a day (qid is also used)
q. or q.q.: quaque	every, e.g. qq6 h = every 6 h
q.q.h.: quarta quaque hora	every 4 hours
q.s.: quantum sufficiat	a sufficiency, enough
rep: repetatur	let it be repeated, as in rep. mist(ura), repeat the mixture
s.c.: subcutaneous	by subcutaneous injection
s.o.s.: si opus sit	if necessary. It is useful to confine sos to prescriptions to be repeated once only and to use prn where many repetitions are intended
stat: statim	immediately
t.d.s.: ter (in) die sumendus	3 times a day (tid is also used).

Weights and measures

In this book doses are given in the metric system, or in international units (IU) when metric doses are impracticable.

Equivalents:
1 litre (l or L) = 1.76 pints
1 kilogram (kg) = 2.2 pounds (lb)

Abbreviations:
1 gram (g)
1 milligram (mg) (1×10^{-3} g)
1 microgram[3] (1×10^{-6} g)
1 nanogram[3] (1×10^{-9} g)
1 decilitre (dL) (1×10^{-1} l)
1 millilitre (mL) (1×10^{-3} l)

Home/domestic measures. A standard 5 ml spoon and a graduated oral syringe are available. Otherwise the following approximations will serve:
1 tablespoonful = 14 ml (or mL)
1 dessertspoonful = 7 ml (or mL)
1 teaspoonful = 5 ml (or mL)

---

[3] Spell out in full in prescribing.

Percentages, proportions, weight in volume

Some solutions of drugs (e.g. local anaesthetics, epinephrine/adrenaline) for parenteral use are labelled in a variety of ways: percentage, proportion, or weight in volume (e.g. 0.1%, 1:1000, 1 mg per mL). Also, dilutions may have to be made by doctors at the time of use. Such drugs are commonly dangerous in overdose and great precision is required, especially as any errors are liable to be by a factor of 10 and can be fatal. Doctors who do not feel confident with such calculations (because they do not do them frequently) should feel no embarrassment,[4] but should recognise that they have a responsibility to check their results with a competent colleague or pharmacist before proceeding.

---

[4] Called to an emergency tension pneumothorax on an intercontinental flight, two surgeons, who chanced to be passengers, were provided with lignocaine 100 mg in 10 ml (in the aircraft medical kit). They were accustomed to thinking in percentages for this drug and 'in the heat of the moment' neither was able to make the conversion. Chest surgery was conducted successfully with an adapted wire coat-hanger as a trocar ('sterilised' in brandy), using a urinary catheter. The patient survived the flight and recovered in hospital. Wallace W A 1995 Managing in-flight emergencies: A personal account. British Medical Journal 311: 374.

2

Clinical pharmacology

SYNOPSIS

Clinical pharmacology comprises all aspects of the scientific study of drugs in man. Its objective is to optimise drug therapy and it is justified in so far as it is of practical use.

Over recent years pharmacology has undergone great expansion resulting from technology that allows the understanding of molecular action and the capacity to exploit this. The potential consequences for therapeutics are enormous. All cellular mechanisms (normal and pathological), in their immense complexity are, in principle, identifiable. What seems almost an infinity of substances, transmitters, local hormones, cell growth factors, can be made, modified and tested to provide agonists, partial agonists, inverse agonists and antagonists. And interference with genetic disease processes is now possible. Increasingly large numbers of substances will deserve to be investigated in therapeutics and used for altering physiology to the perceived advantage (real or imagined) of humans.

But, with all these developments and their potential for good, comes capacity for harm, whether inherent in the substances or as a result of human misapplication.

Successful use of the power conferred (by biotechnology in particular) requires understanding of the enormous complexity of the *consequences of interference*. Willingness to learn the principles of pharmacology and how to apply them in individual circumstances of infinite variety is vital to success without harm: to maximise benefit and minimise risk. All these issues are the concern of clinical pharmacologists and are the subject of this book.

The drug and information 'explosion' of the past six decades combined with medical need has called into being the discipline, clinical pharmacology. The discipline is now recognised as both a health care and an academic specialty; indeed, no medical school can now be considered complete without a department or subdepartment of Clinical Pharmacology.

The clinical pharmacologist's role is to provide facts and opinions that are *useful* for optimising the treatment of patients. Therapeutic success with drugs is becoming more and more dependent on the user having at least an outline understanding of both pharmacodynamics and pharmacokinetics. And this outline is quite simple and easy to acquire. However humane and caring doctors may be, they cannot dispense with scientific skill.

Clinical pharmacology provides the scientific basis for:

- the general aspects of rational, safe and effective drug therapy
- drug therapy of individual diseases
- introduction of new medicines.

Pharmacology is commonly practised in concert with other clinical specialties. More detailed aspects comprise:

1. Pharmacology
   - *Pharmacodynamics*: how drugs, alone and in combination, affect the body (young, old, well, sick)
   - *Pharmacokinetics*: absorption, distribution, metabolism, excretion or, how the body, well or sick, affects drugs
2. Therapeutic evaluation
   - Whether a drug is of value
   - How it may best be used
   - Formal therapeutic trials
   - Surveillance studies for both efficacy and safety (adverse effects): pharmacoepidemiology and pharmacovigilance
3. Control
   - Rational prescribing and formularies
   - Official regulation of medicines
   - Social aspects of the use and misuse of medicines
   - Pharmacoeconomics.

If it is desired to single out a pioneer clinical pharmacologist it would surely be Harry Gold[1] (1899–1972) of Cornell University, USA, whose influential studies in the 1930s showed us how to be clinical pharmacologists. In 1952 he wrote in a seminal article:

a special kind of investigator is required, one whose training has equipped him not only with the principles and technics of laboratory pharmacology but also with knowledge of clinical medicine …

Clinical scientists of all kinds do not differ fundamentally from other biologists; they are set apart only to the extent that there are special difficulties and limitations, ethical and practical, in seeking knowledge from man.[2]

Pharmacology is the same science whether animal or man is investigated. The need for it grows rapidly as not only scientists, but now the whole community, can see its promise of release from distress and premature death over yet wider fields. The concomitant dangers of drugs (fetal deformities, adverse reactions, dependence) only add to the need for the systematic and ethical application of science to drug development, evaluation, and use, i.e. clinical pharmacology.

GUIDE TO FURTHER READING

Brater D C, Daly W J 2000 Clinical pharmacology in the middle ages: principles that presage the 21st century. Clinical Pharmacology and Therapeutics 67: 447–450

Breckenridge A 1995 Science, medicine and clinical pharmacology. British Journal of Clinical Pharmacology 40: 1–9

Breckenridge A 1999 Clinical pharmacology and drug regulation. British Journal of Clinical Pharmacology 47: 11–12

Dollery C T 1996 Clinical pharmocology: future prospects for the discipline. British Journal of Clinical Pharmacology 42: 137–141

---

[1] Gold H 1952 'The proper study of mankind is man', American Journal of Medicine 12: 619. The title is taken from An Essay on Man by Alexander Pope (English poet, 1688–1744); the whole passage is relevant to modern clinical pharmacology and drug therapy; it is best read aloud whether the reader be alone or in company.
Know then thyself, presume no God to scan,
The proper study of mankind is man,
Placed on this isthmus of a middle state,
A being darkly wise, and rudely great:
With too much knowledge for the sceptic side,
With too much weakness for the stoic's pride,
He hangs between; in doubt to act or rest;
In doubt to deem himself a god or beast;
In doubt his mind or body to prefer;
Born but to die, and reas'ning but to err;
Alike in ignorance, his reason such,
Whether he thinks too little or too much;
Chaos of thought and passion, all confused;
Still by himself abused, or disabused;
Created half to rise, and half to fall;
Great lord of all things, yet a prey to all;
Sole judge of truth, in endless error hurled;
The Glory, jest and riddle of the world!

[2] Self-experimentation has always been a feature of clinical pharmacology. A survey of 250 members of the Dutch Society of Clinical Pharmacology evoked 102 responders of whom 55 had done experiments on themselves (largely for convenience) (van Everdingen et al 1990 Lancet 336: 1448). A spectacular example occurred at the 1983 meeting of the American Urological Association at Las Vegas, during a lecture on pharmacologically-induced penile erection, when the lecturer stepped out from behind the lectern to demonstrate personally the efficacy of the technique (Zorgniotti A W 1990 Lancet 336: 1200).

Grahame-Smith D G 1991 Clinical Pharmacology. Roles and responsibilities in academic research. British Journal of Clinical Pharmacology 32: 151

Laurence D R 1989 Ethics and law in clinical pharmacology. British Journal of Clinical Pharmacology 27: 715–722

Reidenberg M M 1999 Clinical pharmacology: the scientific basis of therapeutics. Clinical Pharmacology and Therapeutics 66: 2–8

Walley T 1995 Drugs, money and society. British Journal of Clinical Pharmacology 39: 343–345

3

Discovery and development of drugs

SYNOPSIS

- Preclinical drug development. Discovery of new drugs in the laboratory is an exercise in prediction
- Techniques of discovery. Sophisticated molecular modelling allows precise design of potential new therapeutic substances and new technologies have increased the rate of development of potential medicines.
- Studies in animals and in humans
- Prediction. Failures of prediction occur and a drug may be abandoned at any stage, including after marketing. New drug development is a colossally expensive and commercially driven activity.
- Orphan drugs and diseases.

Preclinical drug development

Pharmacology and medicinal chemistry have transformed medicine from an intellectual exercise in diagnosis into a powerful force for the relief of human disease (C T Dollery 1994)[1]

The development of new medicines (drugs) is an exercise in **prediction** from laboratory studies in vitro and in vivo (animals), which forecast what the agent will do to man. Medicinal therapeutics rests on the **two great supporting pillars of pharmacology:**

- **Selectivity:** the desired effect alone is obtained; 'We must learn to aim, learn to aim with chemical substances' (Paul Ehrlich).[2]
- **Dose:** '…The dose alone decides that something is no poison' (Paracelsus).[3]

For decades the rational discovery of new medicines has depended on modifications of the molecular structures of increasing numbers of known natural chemical mediators. Often the exact molecular basis of drug action is unknown, and this book contains frequent examples of old drugs whose

---

[1] In this chapter we are grateful for permission from Professor Sir Colin Dollery to quote directly and indirectly from his Harveian Oration, 'Medicine and the pharmacological revolution' (1994) Journal of the Royal College of Physicians of London 28: 59–69.

[2] Paul Ehrlich (1845–1915), German scientist who pioneered the scientific approach to drug discovery. The 606th organic arsenical that he tested against spirochaetes (in animals) became a successful medicine (Salvarsan 1910); it and a minor variant were used against syphillis until superseded by penicillin in 1945.

[3] Paracelsus (1493–1541) was a controversial figure who has been portrayed as both ignorant and superstitious. He had no medical degree; he burned the classical medical works (Galen, Avicenna) before his lectures in Basel (Switzerland) and had to leave the city following a dispute about fees with a prominent churchman. He died in Salzburg (Austria) either as a result of a drunken debauch or because he was thrown down a steep incline by 'hitmen' employed by jealous local physicans. *But he was right about the dose.*

mechanism of action remains mysterious. The evolution of *molecular medicine* (including recombinant DNA technology) in the past 20 years has led to a new pathway of drug discovery: *pharmacogenomics*.[4] This broad term encompasses all genes in the genome that may determine drug response, desired and undesired. Completion of the Human Genome Project in 2001 has yielded a minimum of 30 000 potential drug targets, although the function of many of these genes remains unknown. In the future, drugs may be designed according to individual genotypes, thereby to enhance safey as well as efficacy.

The chances of discovering a truly novel medicine, i.e. one that does something valuable that had previously not been possible (or that does safely what could only previously have been achieved with substantial risk), are increased when the development programme is founded on precise knowledge, at molecular level, of the biological processes it is desired to change. The commercial rewards of a successful product are potentially enormous and provide a massive incentive to developers to invest and risk huge sums of money.

> Studies of signal transduction, the fundamental process by which cells talk to one another as intracellular proteins transmit signals from the surface of the cell to the nucleus inside, have opened an entirely new approach to the development of therapeutic agents that can target discrete steps in the body's elaborate pathways of chemical reactions. The opportunities are endless.[5]

The molecular approach to drug discovery should enable a 'molecular dissection' of any disease process. There are two immediate consequences:

- More potential drugs and therapeutic targets will be produced than can be experimentally validated in animals and man. A further risk is that this 'production line' approach could lead to a loss of integration of the established specialities

(chemistry, biochemistry, pharmacology), and an overall lack of understanding of how physiological and pathophysiological processes contribute to the interaction of drug and disease.

- New drugs could be targeted at selected groups of patients based on their genetic make-up.

This concept of 'the right medicine for the right patient' is the basis of *pharmacogenetics* (see p. 122), the genetically determined variability in drug response. Pharmacogenetics has gained momentum from recent advances in molecular genetics and genome sequencing, due to:

- Rapid screening for specific gene polymorphisms (see p. 122).
- Knowledge of the genetic sequences of target genes such as those coding for enzymes, ion channels, and other receptor types involved in drug response.

The expectations of pharmacogenetics and its progeny, *pharmacoproteomics* (understanding of and drug effects on protein variants), are high. They include:

- Identification of subgroups of patients with a disease or syndrome based on their genotype.
- Targeting specific drugs for patients with specific gene variants.

Consequences of these expectations include: smaller clinical trial programmes, better understanding of the pharmacokinetics and dynamics according to genetic variation, simplified monitoring of adverse events after marketing. A great challenge will be to determine the function of each polymorphic gene (or gene product) and whether it has pharmacological or toxicological importance. Some of the expectations for both pharmacogenomics and pharmacogenetics have been exaggerated: at the least, the timescale over which the expectations may be realised is longer than first thought.

Nevertheless, exploitation of the new technologies will create more potential medicines, and more doctors will become involved in clinical testing; it is expedient that they should have some acquaintance with the events and processes that precede their involvement.

---

[4]An example of the opportunity created by pharmacogenomics comes in the announcement by a major pharmaceutical company of plans to search the entire human genome for genetic evidence of intolerance to one of its drugs. If achieved, adverse reactions to the drug would be virtually eliminated.

[5]Culliton B J 1994 Nature Medicine 1:1

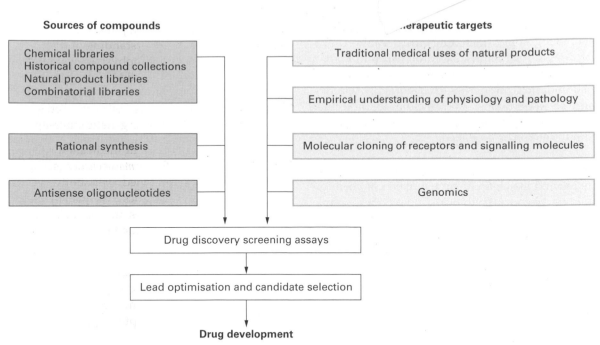

Fig. 3.1 Drug discovery sources in context. Different types of chemical compounds (top left) are tested against bioassays that are relevant to therapeutic targets, which are derived from several possible sources of information (right). The initial lead compounds discovered by the screening process are optimised by analogue synthesis and tested for appropriate pharmacokinetic properties. The candidate compounds then enter the development process involving regulatory toxicology studies and clinical trials.

New drug development proceeds thus:
- Idea or hypothesis
- Design and synthesis of substances
- Studies on tissues and whole animal (preclinical studies)
- Studies in man (clinical studies) (see Chapter 4)
- Grant of an official licence to make therapeutic claims and to sell (see Chapter 5)
- Postlicensing (marketing) studies of safety and comparisons with other medicines.

It will be obvious from the account that follows that drug development is an extremely arduous, highly technical and enormously expensive operation. Successful developments (1% of compounds that proceed to full test eventually become licensed medicines) must carry the cost of the failures (99%).[6] It is also obvious that such programmes are likely to be carried to completion only when the organisations and the individuals within them are motivated overall by the challenge to succeed and to serve society, as well as to make money.

TECHNIQUES OF DISCOVERY
(see Figure 3.1)

The newer technologies, the impact of which have yet to be fully felt include:

---

[6] The cost of development of a new chemical entity (NCE) (a novel molecule not previously tested in humans) from synthesis to market (general clinical use) is estimated at US$ 500 million; the process may take as much as 15 years (including up to 10 years of clinical studies), which is relevant to duration of patent life and so to ultimate profitability; if the developer does not see profit at the end of the process, the investment will not be made. The drug may fail at any stage, including the ultimate, i.e. at the official regulatory body after all the development costs have been incurred. It may also fail (due to adverse effects) within the first year after marketing, which constitutes a catastrophe (in reputation and finance) for the developer as well as for some of the patients.

Pirated copies of full regulatory dossiers have substantial black market value to competitor companies who have used them to leap-frog the original developer to obtain a licence for their unresearched copied molecule. Dossiers may be enormous, even one million pages or the electronic equivalent, the latter being very convenient as it allows instant searching.

Molecular modelling aided by three-dimensional computer graphics (including virtual reality) allows the design of structures based on new and known molecules to enhance their desired, and to eliminate their undesired, properties to create highly selective targeted compounds. In principle all molecular structures capable of binding to a single high-affinity site can be modelled.

Combinatorial chemistry involves the random mixing and matching of large numbers of chemical building blocks (amino acids, nucleotides, simple chemicals) to produce 'libraries' of all possible combinations. This technology can generate billions of new compounds that are initially evaluated using automated robotic high-throughput screening devices that can handle thousands of compounds a day.[7] These screens utilise radio-labelled ligand displacement on single human receptor subtypes or enzymes on nucleated (eukaryotic) cells. If the screen records a positive response the compound is further investigated using traditional laboratory methods, and the molecule is manipulated to enhance selectivity and/or potency (above).

Proteins as medicines: biotechnology. The targets of most drugs are proteins (cell receptors, enzymes) and it is only lack of technology that has hitherto prevented the exploitation of proteins (and peptides) as medicines. This technology is now available. But there are great practical problems in getting the proteins to the target site in the body (they are digested when swallowed and cross cell membranes with difficulty).

Biotechnology involves the use of recombinant DNA technology/genetic engineering to clone and express human genes, for example, in microbial, *Escherichia coli* or yeast, cells so that they manufacture proteins that medicinal chemists have not been able to synthesise; they also produce hormones and autacoids in commercial amounts (such as insulin and growth hormone, erythropoietins, cell growth factors and plasminogen activators, interferons, vaccines and immune antibodies). *Transgenic animals* (that breed true for the gene) are also being developed as models for human disease as well as for production of medicines.

The *polymerase chain reaction* (PCR) is an alternative to bacterial cloning. This is a method of gene amplification that does not require living cells; it takes place in vitro and can produce (in a cost-effective way) commercial quantities of pure potential medicines.

Genetic medicines. Synthetic oligonucleotides are being developed to target sites on DNA sequences or genes (double strand DNA: triplex approach) or messenger RNA (the antisense approach) so that the production of disease-related proteins is blocked. These oligonucleotides offer prospects of treatment for cancers and viruses without harming healthy tissues.[8]

Gene therapy of human genetic disorders is 'a strategy in which nucleic acid, usually in the form of DNA, is administered to modify the genetic repertoire for therapeutic purposes', e.g. cystic fibrosis. 'The era of "the gene as drug" is clearly upon us' (R G Crystal). Significant problems remain; in particular the methods of delivery. Three methods are available: an injection of 'naked' DNA; using a virus as carrier with DNA incorporated into its genome; or DNA encapsulated within a liposome.

Immunopharmacology. Understanding of the molecular basis of immune responses has allowed the definition of mechanisms by which cellular function is altered by a legion of local hormones or autacoids in, for example, infections, cancer, autoimmune diseases, organ transplant rejection. These processes present targets for therapeutic intervention. Hence the rise of immunopharmacology.

---

[7] 'It is too early to say what success these programmes may have but automation of assays, possibly coupled to similar automation of syntheses, promises to speed up the search for new leads which is the rate-limiting step in the introduction of really novel therapeutic agents. Their value in medicine will depend upon the significance of the control mechanism concerned in the pathogenesis of a disease process. Critics fear that the result may well be large numbers of drugs in search of a disease to treat' (CT Dollery, ibidem). The demand for competent clinical trialists, already great, will increase to meet the demand; the financial rewards to competent (and honest) clinical trialists are great, in the competitive world of drug introduction (see also McNamee D 1995 Lancet 345: 1167).

[8] Cohen J S, Hogan M E 1994 The new genetic medicines. Scientific American (Dec): 50–55.

Positron emission tomography (PET) allows non-invasive pharmacokinetic and pharmacodynamic measurements in previously inaccessible sites, e.g. the brain in intact humans and animals.

Older approaches to discovery of new medicines that continue in use include:

- *Animal models of human disease* or an aspect of it of varying relevance to man.
- *Natural products,* the basis for many of today's medicines for pain, inflammation, cancer, cardiovascular problems. Modern technology for screening has revived interest and intensified the search by multinational pharmaceutical companies which scour the world for leads from microorganisms (in soil or sewage or even from insects entombed in amber 40 million years ago), from fungi, plants and animals. Developing countries in the tropics (with their luxuriant natural resources) are prominent targets in this search and have justly complained of exploitation ('gene robbery'). Many now require formal profit-sharing agreements to allow such searches
- *Traditional medicine,* which is being studied for possible leads to usefully active compounds
- *Modifications of the structures of known drugs*; these are obviously likely to produce more agents having similar basic properties, but may deliver worthwhile improvements. It is in this area that the much-complained-of, *me-too* and *me-again* drugs are developed (sometimes purely for commercial reasons).
- *Random screening* of synthesised and natural products.
- New *uses for drugs already in general use* as a result of intelligent observation and serendipity,[9] or advancing knowledge of molecular mechanisms, e.g. aspirin for antithrombosis effect.

DRUG QUALITY

It is easy for an investigator or prescriber, interested in pharmacology, toxicology and therapeutics, to forget the fundamental importance of chemical and pharmaceutical aspects. An impure, unstable drug or formulation is useless. Pure drugs that remain pure drugs after 5 years of storage in hot, damp climates are vital to therapeutics. The record of manufacturers in providing this is impressive.

Preclinical studies in animals[10]

In general, the following tests are undertaken:

Pharmacodynamics: to explore actions relevant to the proposed therapeutic use, and other effects at a range of doses

Pharmacokinetics: to discover how the drug is distributed in and disposed of by, the body.

Toxicology: to see whether and how the drug causes injury (in vitro tests and intact animals) in:
— single-dose studies (acute toxicity)
— repeated-dose studies (subacute, intermediate, and chronic or long-term toxicology)

General toxicology studies are performed in two species, usually a rodent and dog. Regulatory requirements differ around the world but significant alignment has been made. Single and repeat dose study requirements are given in Tables 3.1 and 3.2. The dosing regimens are selected to produce a range of plasma concentrations, the highest of which will be several times greater than that achieved in man.

Special toxicology involves areas in which a particularly horrible drug accident might occur on a substantial scale; all involve interaction with genetic material or its expression in cell division.

Mutagenicity (genotoxicity) tests are designed to identify compounds that may induce genetic damage. A standard battery of tests is conducted and include:

- A test for gene mutation in bacteria, e.g. Ames test

---

[9] Serendipity is the faculty of making fortunate discoveries by general sagacity or by accident: the word derives from a fairy tale about three princes of Serendip (Sri Lanka) who had this happy faculty.

---

[10] Mouse, rat, hamster, guinea pig, rabbit, cat, dog, monkey *(not all used for any one drug).*

TABLE 3.1 Single and repeated dose toxicity requirements to support studies in healthy normal volunteers (Phase I) and in patients (Phase 2) in the European Union (EU), and Phases 1, 2 & 3 the USA and Japan[1]

Duration of clinical trial	Minimum duration of repeated dose toxicity studies	
	Rodents	Non-rodents
Single dose	2 weeks[2]	2 weeks
Up to 2 weeks	2 weeks	2 weeks
Up to 1 month	1 month	1 month
Up to 3 months	3 months	3 months
Up to 6 months	6 months	6 months
>6 months	6 months	chronic[3]

[1]In Japan, if there are no Phase 2 clinical trials of equivalent duration to the planned Phase 3 trials, conduct of longer duration toxicity studies is recommended as given in Table 3.2.
[2]In the USA, specially designed single dose studies with extended examinations can support single dose clinical studies.
[3]Regulatory authorities may request a 12-month study or accept a 6-month study, determined on a case-by-case basis.
See p. 56 for a description of a clinical trial.

TABLE 3.2 Repeated dose toxicity requirements to support Phase 3 studies in the EU, and marketing in all regions[1]

Duration of clinical trial	Minimum duration of repeated dose toxicity studies	
	Rodents	Non-rodents
Up to 2 weeks	1 month	1 month
Up to 1 month	3 months	3 months
Up to 3 months	6 months	3 months
>3 months	6 months	Chronic[2]

[1]When a chronic non-rodent study is recommended if clinical use >1 month.
[2]Regulatory authorities may request a 12-month study or accept a 6-month study, determined on a case-by-case basis.

- An in-vitro test with cytogenetic evaluation of chromosomal damage with mammalian cells or an in-vitro mouse lymphoma thymidine kinase (tK) assay
- An in-vivo test for chromosomal damage using rodent haematopoietic cells.

Usually the first two tests are performed before human exposure, but all must be complete prior to Phase II studies. Additional tests may be required.

Definitive **carcinogenicity** (oncogenicity) tests are often not required prior to the early studies in man unless there is serious reason to be suspicious of the drug, e.g. if the mutagenicity test is unsatisfactory; the molecular structure, including likely metabolites in man, gives rise to suspicion; or the histopathology in repeated-dose animal studies raises suspicions.

Full scale (most of the animal's life) carcinogenicity tests will generally be required only if the drug is to be given to man for above one year, or it resembles a known human carcinogen, or it is mutagenic (in circumstances relevant to human use) or it has major organ-specific hormonal agonist action.

It may be asked why any novel compound should be given to man before full-scale formal carcinogenicity studies are completed. The answers are that animal tests are uncertain predictors,[11] that such a requirement would make socially desirable drug development expensive to a seriously detrimental degree, or might even cause potentially valuable novel ventures to cease. For example, tests would have to be done on numerous compounds that are eventually abandoned for other reasons. This may seem right or wrong, but it is how things are at present.

Toxicology testing of biotechnology-derived pharmaceuticals. The standard regimen of toxicology studies is not appropriate for biotechnology-derived pharmaceuticals. The choice of species used will depend on the expression of the relevant receptor. If no suitable species exists, homologous proteins or transgenic animals expressing the human receptor may be studied. Additional immunological studies are also required, and the genotoxicity and carcinogenicity studies are modified.

Reproduction studies have to be extensive because of the diversity of physiological processes that may be affected, and because the consequences of error in this field are potentially horrific. Tests include

---

[11] A sardonic comment on the relevance for man or carcinogenicity tests in animals was made by investigators who induced cancer in animals using American 'dimes' (10 cent coin) and the plastic of credit cards. They advised the US Government to consider banning money as unsafe for humans (Moore GE et al 1977 Journal of the American Medical Association 238: 397)

effects on fertility, reproductive performance, fetal organogenesis, and peri- and postnatal development. Studies are in mammals, usually the rat. Embryo-fetal development studies are conducted in a non-rodent, usually the rabbit. Later development studies include growth, behaviour and intellectual function of progeny, and their fertility (second generation effects).

Local tolerability studies. In most acute and repeat dose studies, the test drug is administered by the oral route. Additional studies are required when the clinical route of administration is parenteral. There are two objectives. First, to determine if the drug is absorbed in sufficient quantities, e.g. by inhalation, and second to test for local tolerability, e.g. by the percutaneous or intravenous routes.

It is plain that all the above tests constitute a major laboratory exercise requiring great and diverse scientific skills and significant financial resource.

ETHICS[12]

No one will read the above scheme with satisfaction and some people will read it with disgust. Experienced toxicologists point out that:

> The majority of toxicity tests (which particularly are subject to ethical criticism) are firmly based on studies in whole animals, because only in them is it possible to approach the complexity of organisation of body systems in humans, to explore any consequences of variable absorption, metabolism and excretion, and to reveal not only direct toxic effects but also those of a secondary or indirect nature due to induced abnormalities in integrative mechanisms, or distant effects of a toxic metabolite produced in one organ that acts on another.[13]

The use of animals would be totally unjustified if results useful to man could not be obtained. In many known respects animals are similar to man, but in many respects they are not. Increasingly, the low-prediction tests are being defined and eliminated. It will be a long time before in-vitro tests become sufficiently robust to eliminate the need for tests in whole animals, but we welcome the progress that is being made towards this end. The incentive to eliminate whole animal tests is not only ethical, it is economic, for whole animals are very expensive to breed and house and keep in health. The European Union instructs researchers to choose non-(whole) animal methods if they are 'scientifically satisfactory [and] reasonably and practically available'.

Prediction

It is frequently pointed out that regulatory guidelines are not rigid requirements to be universally applied. But whatever the intention, they do tend to be treated as minimum requirements if only because research directors fear to risk holding up their expensive coordinated programmes with disagreements that result in their having to go back to the laboratory, with consequent delay and financial loss.

Knowledge of the *mode of action* of a potential new drug obviously greatly enhances prediction from animal studies of what will happen in man. Whenever practicable such knowledge should be obtained; sometimes this is quite easy, but sometimes it is impossible. Many drugs have been introduced safely without such knowledge, the later acquisition of which has not always made an important difference to their use, e.g. antimicrobials. Pharmacological studies are integrated with those of the toxicologist to build up a picture of the undesired as well as the desired drug effects.

In *pharmacological testing* the investigators know what they are looking for and choose the experiments to gain their objectives.

In *toxicological testing* the investigators have less clear ideas of what they are looking for; they are screening for risk, unexpected as well as predicted, and certain major routines must be done. Toxicity testing is therefore liable to become mindless routine to meet regulatory requirements to a greater extent than are the pharmacological studies. The

[12] An admirable discussion of the issues will be found in Paton W 1984 Man and mouse. Oxford, London and in Zbinden G 1990 Alternatives to animal experimentation. Trends in Pharmacological Sciences 11: 104
[13] Brimblecome R W, Dayan A D 1993 In: Burley D M, Clarke J M, Lasagna L (eds) Pharmaceutical Medicine. Arnold, London

predictive value of special toxicology (above) is particularly controversial.

All drugs are poisons if enough is given and the task of the toxicologist is to find out whether, where and how a compound acts as a poison to animals, and to give an opinion on the significance of the data in relation to risks likely to be run by human beings. This will remain a nearly impossible task until molecular explanations of all effects can be provided. Toxicologists are in an unenviable position. When a useful drug is safely introduced they are considered to have done no more than their duty. When an accident occurs they are invited to explain how this failure of prediction came about. When they predict that a chemical is unsafe in a major way for man, this prediction is never tested.

CONCLUSION ON PRECLINICAL TESTING

As drugs are developed and promoted for long-term use in more and relatively trivial conditions, e.g. minor anxiety, and affluent societies become less and less willing to tolerate small physical or mental discomforts, the demand for and the supply of new safer medicines will continue to increase. Only profound knowledge of molecular mechanisms will reduce risk in the introduction of new drugs. Occasional failures of prediction are inevitable, with consequent public outcry.

Limited resources of scientific manpower and money will not be used to the best advantage if the public shock over thalidomide (p. 81) and subsequent events is allowed to express itself in governmental regulations requiring a plethora of expensive tests (and toxicity testing is very expensive), many of them of dubious meaning for anything other than the animal concerned. Such a policy would prevent industrial laboratories from devoting resources to investigation of molecular mechanisms of drug action, in the knowledge of which alone lies health with safety.

When the preclinical testing has been completed to the satisfaction of the developer and of the national or international regulatory agency, it is time to administer the drug to man and so to launch the experimental programme that will decide whether the drug is only a drug or whether it is also a medicine. This is the subject of the next chapter.

Orphan drugs and diseases

A free market economy is liable to leave untreated, rare diseases, e.g. some cancers (in all countries) and some common diseases, e.g. parasitic infections (in poor countries).

Where a drug is not developed into a usable medicine because the developer will not recover the costs then it is known as an orphan drug, and the disease is an orphan disease; the sufferer is a health orphan.[14] Drugs for rare diseases inevitably must often be licensed on less than ideal amounts of clinical evidence.

The remedy for these situations lies in government itself undertaking drug development (which is likely to be inefficient) or in government-offered incentives, e.g. tax relief, subsidies, exclusive marketing rights, to pharmaceutical companies and, in the case of poor countries, international aid programmes; such programmes are being implemented.[15]

GUIDE TO FURTHER READING

Banks R E et al 2000 Proteomics: new perspectives, new biomedical opportunities. Lancet 356: 1749–1756

Beeley N, Berger A 2000 A revolution in drug discovery: combinatorial chemistry still needs logic to drive science forward. British Medical Journal 321: 581–582

Black J W 1986 Pharmacology: analysis and exploration. British Medical Journal 293: 252

Crystal R G 1995 The gene as a drug. Nature Medicine 1: 15

Di Masi J A 1995 Success rates for new drugs entering clinical testing in the United States. Clinical Pharmacology and Therapeutics 58: 1

---

[14] The cost of treating a patient having the rare genetic Gaucher's liposome storage disease with genetically engineered enzyme is US$ 145 000 to 400 000 per annum according to severity. Who can and will pay? More such situations will occur.

[15] Official recognition of *orphan drug status* is accorded in the USA (pop 240 million) where the relevant disease affects fewer than 200,000 people; in Japan (pop 121 million) for fewer than 50,000 people.

Dollery C T 1999 Drug discovery and development in the molecular era. British Journal of Clinical Pharmacology 47: 5–6

Fears R, Robert D, Poste G 2000 Rational or rationed medicine? The promise of genetics for improved clinical practice. British Medical Journal 320: 933

Gale E A M 2001 Lessons from the glitazones: a story of drug development. Lancet 357: 1870–1875

Graeme-Smith D G 1999 How will knowledge of the human genome affect drug therapy? British Journal of Clinical Pharmacology 47: 7–10

Lachmann P 1992 The use of animals in research. British Medical Journal 305: 1

Lasagna L 1982 Will all new drugs become orphans? Clinical Pharmacology and Therapeutics 31: 285

Meyer B R 1992 Biotechnology and therapeutics: Experimental treatments and limited resources. Clinical Pharmacology and Therapeutics 51: 359

Roses A D 2000 Pharmacogenetics and future drug development and delivery. The Lancet 355: 1358–1361

Smith A E 1999 Gene therapy — where are we? Lancet 354 (suppl 1): st1–4

Sykes R 1998 Being a modern pharmaceutical company. British Medical Journal 317: 1172

Wolf R C, Smith G, Smith R L 2000 Pharmacogenetics. British Medical Journal 320: 987–990

4

Evaluation of drugs in man

> We must be daring and search after Truth; even if we do not succeed in finding her, we shall at least come closer than we are at present (Galen AD 130–200)

SYNOPSIS

This chapter is about evidence-based drug therapy.

New drugs are gradually introduced by clinical pharmacological studies in rising numbers of healthy and/or patient volunteers until enough information has been gained to justify formal therapeutic studies. Each of these is usually a randomised controlled trial where a precisely framed question is posed and answered by treating equivalent groups of patients in different ways.

The key to the ethics of such studies is informed consent from patients, efficient scientific design and review by an independent research ethics committee. The key interpretative factors in the analysis of trial results are calculations of confidence intervals and statistical significance. The potential clinical significance needs to be considered within the confines of controlled clinical trials. This is best expressed by stating not only the percentage differences, but also the absolute difference or its reciprocal, the number of patients who have to be treated to obtain one desired outcome. The outcome might include both efficacy and safety.

SYNOPSIS (CONTINUED)

Surveillance studies and the reporting of spontaneous adverse reactions respectively determine the clinical profile of the drug and detect rare adverse events. Further trials to compare new medicines with existing medicines are also required. These form the basis of cost-effectiveness comparisons.

Topics include:
- Experimental therapeutics
- Ethics of research
- Rational introduction of a new drug
- Need for statistics
- Types of trial: design, size
- Meta-analysis
- Pharmacoepidemiology

Experimental therapeutics

As the number of potential medicines produced increases, the problem of whom to test them on grows. There are two main groups: healthy volunteers and volunteer patients (plus, rarely, nonvolunteer patients). Studies in healthy normal volunteers can help to determine the safety, tolerability, pharmacokinetics and for some drugs, e.g. anticoagulants and anaesthetic agents, their dynamic effect. For most drugs the dynamic effect and hence therapeutic potential can be investigated only in patients, e.g. drugs for parkinsonism and anti-microbials. These two groups of subjects for drug testing are complementary, not mutually exclusive in drug development. Introduction of novel agents into both groups poses ethical and scientific problems (see below).

There are four main reasons why doctors should have a grounding in the knowledge and application of the principles of experimental therapeutics:

1. The optimal selection of a specific dose of a drug for a specific patient should be based on good clinical research. To some extent, every new administration to a patient is an exercise in experimental therapeutics.
2. Increasingly, doctors are personally involved.
3. Good therapeutic research alters clinical practice.
4. Such study provides an exercise in ethical and logical thinking.

Plainly, doctors cannot read in detail and evaluate for themselves all the published studies (often hundreds) that *might* influence their practice. They therefore turn to specialist research articles and abstracts[1] including meta-analyses (p. 66) for guidance, but readers must approach these critically.

Modern medicine is sometimes accused of callous application of science to human problems and of subordinating the interest of the individual to those of the group (society).[2] Official regulatory bodies rightly require scientific evaluation of drugs. Drug developers need to satisfy the official regulators and they also seek to persuade an increasingly sophisticated medical profession to prescribe their products. Patients are also far more aware of the comparative advantages and limitations of their medicines than they used to be. For these reasons scientific drug evaluation as described here is likely to increase in volume and the doctors involved will be held responsible for the ethics of what they do even if they played no personal part in the study design.

Therefore we provide a brief discussion of some relevant ethical aspects (and particularly of the randomised controlled trial).

RESEARCH[3] INVOLVING HUMAN SUBJECTS

A distinction may be made between:

- **Therapeutic**: that which may actually have a therapeutic effect or provide information that can be used to help the participating subjects and
- **Nontherapeutic**: that which provides information that cannot be of direct use to them, e.g. healthy volunteers always and patients sometimes.

This is a somewhat artificial separation, because some trials that are 'therapeutic', i.e. involve use of new potential medicines, may by their design and intent have no therapeutic benefit for the participants. For example, a dose ranging study of an antihypertensive drug may employ four doses, one of which is expected to be too low and another too high, in order to describe the shape and position of

---

[1] Many review articles (and there are whole journals devoted to reviews) are of poor quality, merely reporting uncritically the opinions of the original authors. But high-quality critical reviews are to be treasured. A journal titled Evidence-Based Medicine was launched in 1995.

[2] Guidance to researchers in this matter is clear. *The World Medical Association* declaration of Helsinki (Edinburgh revision 2000) states that '…considerations related to the well-being of the human subject should take precedence over the interests of science and society.' *The General Assembly of the United Nations* adopted in 1966 the International Covenant on Civil and Political Rights, of which Article 7 states, 'In particular, no one shall be subjected without his free consent to medical or scientific experimentation.' This means that subjects are entitled to know that they are being entered into research even though the research be thought to be 'harmless'. But there are people who cannot give (informed) consent, e.g. the demented. The need for special procedures for such is now recognised, for there is a consensus that without research, they and the diseases from which they suffer will become therapeutic 'orphans'.

[3] 'The definition of research continues to present difficulties. The distinction between medical research and innovative medical practice derives from the *intent*. In medical *practice* the sole intention is to benefit the *individual patient* consulting the clinician, not to gain knowledge of general benefit, though such knowledge may incidentally emerge from the clinical experience gained. In medical *research* the primary intention is to advance knowledge so that *patients in general* may benefit; the individual patient may or may not benefit directly.' (Royal College of Physicians of London 1996 Guidelines on the practice of ethics committees in medical research involving human subjects).

the dose–response curve. Furthermore, many such trials are frequently too short to bring lasting benefit to participants even if the right dose is selected.

Research may also be *experimental* (involving psychologically intrusive or physically invasive intervention) or solely *observational* (sometimes called noninterventional) (including epidemiology).

Ethics of research in humans[4]

> People have the right to choose for themselves whether or not they will participate in research, i.e. they have the right to self-determination (the ethical principle of *autonomy*). They should be given whatever information is necessary for making an informed choice (consent) and the right to withdraw at any stage.

The issue of (informed) *consent*[5] looms large in discussions of the ethics of research involving human subjects and is a principal concern of the Research Ethics Committees that are now the norm in medical research.

Some dislike the word 'experiment' in relation to man, thinking that its mere use implies a degree of impropriety in what is done. It is better, however, that all should recognise the true meaning of the word, 'to ascertain or establish by trial',[6] that the benefits of modern medicine derive almost wholly from experimentation and that some risk is inseparable from much medical advance. The moral obligation of all doctors lies in ensuring that in their desire to help patients (the ethical principal of *beneficence*) they should never allow themselves to put the individual who has sought their aid at any disadvantage (the ethical principal of *non-maleficence*)

for 'the scientist or physician has no right to choose martyrs for society'.[7]

It is, of course, only proper to perform a therapeutic trial when the doctors genuinely do not know which treatment is best, and when they are prepared to withdraw individual patients or to stop the whole trial when at any time they become convinced that it is in the patients' interest to do so.

If it is truly not known whether one treatment is better than another, i.e. there is *equipoise*,[8] then nothing is lost, at least in theory, by allotting patients at random to those treatments under test, and it is in everybody's interest that good treatments should be adopted and bad treatments abandoned as soon as possible. It is, of course, more difficult to justify a new treatment when existing treatments are good than when they are bad, and this difficulty is likely to grow. It involves weighing the needs of future patients who may benefit from the results of a study against those of the patients who are actually taking part, some of whom will receive new (and possibly less effective) treatment, i.e. the ethical principle of *justice*.[9]

The ethics of the randomised and placebo controlled trial

History, including recent history, is replete with examples of even the best-intentioned doctors being wrong about the efficacy and safety of (new)

---

[4] For extensive practical detail, see *International ethical guidelines for biomedical research involving human subjects*; prepared by the Council for International Organisations of Medical Sciences (CIOMS) in collaboration with the World Health Organisation (WHO): Geneva, (1993, and revisions). (WHO publications are available in all UN member countries), also the *Guideline for Good Clinical Practice. International Conference on Harmonisation Tripartite Guideline.* EU Committee on Proprietary Medicinal Products (CPMP/ICH/135/95). Also: Smith T 1999 *Ethics in Medical Research. A Handbook of Good Practice.* Cambridge University Press, Cambridge.
[5] Consent procedures, e.g. information, especially on risks, loom larger in research, particularly where it is non-therapeutic, than they do in medical practice.

[6] Oxford English Dictionary.
[7] Kety S. Quoted by Beecher H K 1959 Journal of the American Medical Association 169:461.
[8] In this situation it has been urged that it need to be no concern of patients that they are entered into a research study. Even if it should be the case that there is true equipoise, this (convenient) belief does not allow the requirement for (informed) consent to be bypassed; and doctors often have opinions that would be of interest to patients if they were told of them, which they may not be.
[9] In a disabling disease having no proved treatment, the advent of a potentially effective medicine, unavoidably in *limited supply,* heightens the emotions of all concerned. This was the situation for the first study of interferon beta in multiple sclerosis. The manufacturer, seeking to be fair, arranged a lottery for patients (having a certified diagnosis) to enter a randomised placebo-controlled trial. Some patients, when they understood that they might be allocated placebo, became angry (and said so on television). (British Medical Journal 1993 307: 958; Lancet 1993 343: 169). It is not obvious how this situation could have been made fairer.

treatments and that this situation can and should be remedied by the ethical employment of science. This was well summarised in a Report.[10]

An analysis of the ethical problems of therapeutic trials might begin with a question long familiar to moral philosophy: what is the nature and degree of certitude required for an ethical decision? More precisely, is there any ethically relevant difference between the use of statistical methods and the use of other ways of knowing, such as experience, common sense, guessing, etc.? When decisions are to be made in uncertainty, is it more or less ethical to choose and abide by statistical methods of defining 'certitude' than to be guided by one's hunch or striking experience? These questions are raised by the assertion that it is ethically imperative to conclude a clinical trial when a 'trend' appears... the choice of statistical methods can constitute in many circumstances an acceptable ethical approach to the problem of decision in uncertainty.

The use of a placebo (or dummy) raises both ethical and scientific issues. There are clear-cut cases when its use would be ethically unacceptable and scientifically unnecessary e.g. drug trials in epilepsy and tuberculosis, when the control groups comprise patients receiving the best available therapy. But the use of a placebo does not necessarily require that patients be deprived of effective therapy (where it exists). New drug and placebo may be added against a background of established therapy e.g. in heart failure. This is the so-called 'add on' design.

The pharmacologically inert (placebo) treatment arm of a trial is useful:

- To distinguish the *pharmacodynamic effects* of a drug from the psychological effects of the act of medication and the circumstances surrounding it, e.g. increased interest by the doctor, more frequent visits, for these latter may have their placebo effect. These are common in trials of antidepressants, antiobesity drugs and antihypertensives.
- To distinguish *drug effects* from fluctuations in disease that occur with time and other external factors, provided active treatment, if any, can be ethically withheld. This is also called the 'assay sensitivity' of the trial.

- To avoid *false conclusions*. The use of placebos is valuable in Phase I healthy volunteer studies of novel drugs to help determine whether minor but frequently reported adverse events are drug-related or not. Placebos are also helpful to distinguish between real and imaginary responses in short-term trials with new analgesic agents.

While the use of a placebo treatment can pose ethical problems, it is often preferable to the continued use of treatments of unproven efficacy or safety. The ethical dilemma of subjects suffering as a result of receiving a placebo (or ineffective drug) can be overcome by designing clinical trials that provide mechanisms to allow them to be withdrawn ('escape') when defined criteria are reached, e.g. blood pressure above levels that represent treatment failure.

Investigators who propose to use a placebo or otherwise withhold effective treatment should specifically justify their intention. The variables to consider are:

- The severity of the disease
- The effectiveness of standard therapy
- Whether the novel drug under test aims to give symptomatic relief only, or has the potential to prevent or slow up an irreversible event, e.g. stroke or myocardial infarction
- The length of treatment
- The objective of the trial (equivalence, superiority or noninferiority, see p. 61)

Thus it may be quite ethical to compare a novel analgesic against placebo for 2 weeks in the treatment of osteoarthritis of the hip (with escape analgesics available). It would not be ethical to use a placebo alone as comparator in a 6-month trial of a novel drug in active rheumatoid arthritis, even with escape analgesia.

The precise use of the placebo will depend on the study design, e.g. whether *crossover*, when all patients receive placebo at some point in the trial, or *parallel group*, when only one cohort receives placebo. Generally, patients easily understand the concept of distinguishing between the imagined effects of treatment and those due to a direct action on the body. Provided research subjects are properly informed and freely give consent, they are not the subject of deception in any ethical sense; but a patient

---

[10] European Journal of Clinical Pharmacology 1980 18: 129.

given a placebo in the absence of consent is deceived and research ethics committees will, rightly, decline to agree to this. (But see Lewis et al. 2002, p. 71)

Injury to research subjects

The question of compensation for accidental (physical) injury due to participation in research is a vexed one. Plainly there are substantial differences between the position of healthy volunteers (whether or not they are paid) and that of patients who may benefit and, in some cases, who may be prepared to accept even serious risk for the chance of gain. There is no simple answer. But the topic must always be addressed in any research carrying risk, including the risk of withholding known effective treatment.

The CIOMS/WHO guidelines[4] state:

> Research subjects who suffer physical injury as a result of their participation are entitled to such financial or other assistance as would compensate them equitably for any temporary or permanent impairment or disability. In the case of death, their dependents are entitled to material compensation. The right to compensation may not be waived.
>
> Therefore, when giving their informed consent to participate, research subjects should be told whether there is provision for compensation in case of physical injury, and the circumstances in which they or their dependants would receive it.

Payment of subjects in clinical trials

Healthy volunteers are usually paid to take part in a clinical trial. The rationale is that they will not benefit from treatment received and should be compensated for discomfort and inconvenience. There is a fine dividing line between this and a financial inducement, but it is unlikely that more than a small minority of healthy volunteer studies would now take place without a 'fee for service' provision. It is all the more important that the sums involved are commensurate with the invasiveness of the investigations and the length of the studies. The monies should be declared and agreed by the ethics committee.

Patients are not paid to take part in clinical trials, though 'out of pocket' expenses are frequently met.

There is an intuitive abreaction by physicians to pay patients (compared with healthy volunteers), because they feel the accusation of inducement or persuasion could be levelled at them, and because they assuage any feeling of taking advantage of the doctor–patient relationship by the hope that the medicines under test may be of benefit to the individual. This is not an entirely comfortable position.

Rational introduction of a new drug to man

When studies in animals predict that a new molecule may be a useful medicine, i.e. effective and safe in relation to its benefits, then the time has come to put it to the test in man.

We devote substantial space to clinical evaluation of drugs because doctors need to be able to scan reports of therapeutic studies to decide whether they are likely to be reliable and deserve to influence their prescribing.

Moreover, most doctors will be involved in clinical trials at some stage of their career and need to understand the principles of drug development.

When a new chemical entity offers a possibility of doing something that has not been done before or of doing something familiar in a different or better way, it can be seen to be worth testing. But where it is a new member of a familiar class of drug, potential advantage may be harder to detect.

Yet these 'me-too' drugs are often worth testing. Prediction from animal studies of modest but useful clinical advantage is particularly uncertain and therefore if the new drug seems reasonably effective and safe in animals it is also reasonable to test it in man: 'It is possible to waste too much time in animal studies before testing a drug in man'.[11]

From the commercial standpoint, the investment in the development of a new drug can be in the order of £200 million but will be substantially less for a 'me-too' drug entering an already developed and profitable market.

---

[11] Brodie B B 1962 Clinical Pharmacology and Therapeutics 3: 374.

4 **EVALUATION OF DRUGS IN MAN**

PHASES OF CLINICAL DEVELOPMENT

Human experiments progress in a commonsense manner that is conventionally divided into four phases. These phases are divisions of convenience in what is a continuous expanding process. It begins with a small number of subjects (healthy subjects and volunteer patients) closely observed in laboratory settings and proceeds through hundreds of patients, to thousands before the drug is agreed to be a medicine by a national or international regulatory authority. It then is licenced for general prescribing (though this is by no means the end of the evaluation). The process may be abandoned at any stage for a variety of reasons including poor tolerability or safety, inadequate efficacy and commercial pressures.

- *Phase 1. Human pharmacology* (20–50 subjects)
  — Healthy volunteers or volunteer patients, according to the class of drug and its safety.
  — Pharmacokinetics (absorption, distribution, metabolism, excretion).
  — Pharmacodynamics (biological effects) where practicable, tolerability, safety, efficacy.
- *Phase 2. Therapeutic exploration* (50–300)
  — Patients.
  — Pharmacokinetics and pharmacodynamic dose-ranging, in carefully controlled studies for efficacy and safety,[12] which may involve comparison with placebo.
- *Phase 3. Therapeutic confirmation* (randomised controlled trials; 250–1000+)
  — Patients
  — Efficacy on a substantial scale; safety; comparison with existing drugs.
- *Phase 4. Therapeutic use* (post-licensing studies) (2000–10 000+)
  — Surveillance for safety and efficacy: further formal therapeutic trials, especially comparisons with other drugs, marketing studies and pharmacoeconomic studies.

OFFICIAL REGULATORY GUIDELINES AND REQUIREMENTS[13]

For studies in man (see also Chapter 5) these ordinarily include:

- Studies of *pharmacokinetics* and (when other manufacturers have similar products) of *bioequivalence* (equal bioavailability) with alternative products.
- *Therapeutic trials* (reported in detail) that substantiate the safety and efficacy of the drug under likely conditions of use, e.g. a drug for long-term use in a common condition will require a total of at least 1000 patients (preferably more), depending on the therapeutic class, of which at least 100 have been treated continuously for about one year.
- *Special groups.* If the drug will be used in, e.g. the elderly, then elderly people should be studied if there are reasons for thinking they may react to or handle the drug differently. The same applies to children and to pregnant women (who present a special problem) and who, if they are not studied, may be excluded from licenced uses and so become health 'orphans'. Studies in patients having disease that affects drug metabolism and elimination may be needed, such as patients with impaired liver or kidney function.
- *Fixed-dose combination* products will require explicit justification for each component.
- *Interaction studies* with other drugs likely to be taken simultaneously. Plainly, all possible combinations cannot be evaluated; an intelligent choice, based on knowledge of pharmacodynamics and pharmacokinetics, is made.

---

[13] Guidelines for the conduct and analysis of a range of clinical trials in different therapeutic categories are released from time to time by the Committee on Proprietary Medicinal Products (CPMP) of the European Commission. These guidelines apply to drug development in the European Union. Other regulatory authorities issue guidance, e.g. the Food and Drug Administration for the USA, the MHW for Japan. There has been considerable success in aligning different guidelines across the world through the International Conferences on Harmonisation (ICH). The CPMP Guidelines source is *info@mca.gsi.gov.uk* or EuroDirect Publications Officer, Medicines Control Agency, Room 10-238, Market Towers, 1 Nine Elms Lane, Vauxhall, London SW8 5NQ.

---

[12] Moderate to severe adverse events have occurred in about 0.5% of healthy subjects (Orme M et al 1989 British Journal of Clinical Pharmacology 27: 125; Sibille M et al 1992 European Journal of Clinical Pharmacology 42: 393).

- The application for a licence for general use (marketing application) should include a draft Summary of Product Characteristics[14] for prescribers. A Patient Information Leaflet must be submitted. These should include information on the form of the product (e.g. tablet, capsule, sustained-release, liquid), its uses, dosage (adults, children, elderly where appropriate), contraindications (strong recommendation), warnings and precautions (less strong), side-effects/adverse reactions, overdose and how to treat it.

The emerging discipline of *pharmacogenomics* seeks to identify patients who will respond beneficially or adversely to a new drug by defining certain genotypic profiles. Individualised dosing regimens may be evolved as a result. This tailoring of drugs to individuals is consuming huge resources from drug developers.

THERAPEUTIC INVESTIGATIONS

> **There are three key questions to be answered during drug development:**
>
> - Does the drug work?
> - Is it safe?
> - What is the dose?

With few exceptions, none of these is easy to answer definitively within the confines of a preregistration clinical trials programme. Effectiveness and safety have to be balanced against each other. What may be regarded as 'safe' for a new oncology drug in advanced lung cancer would not be so regarded in the treatment of childhood eczema. The use of the term 'dose', without explanation, is irrational as it implies a single dose for all patients. Pharmaceutical companies cannot be expected to produce a large array of different doses for each medicine, but the maxim to use the smallest effective dose that results in the desired effect holds true. Some drugs require titration, others have a wide safety margin so that one 'high' dose may achieve optimal effectiveness with acceptable safety.

There are two classes of endpoint or outcome of a therapeutic investigation.

- the therapeutic effect itself e.g. sleep, eradication of infection
- a surrogate effect, a short-term effect that can be reliably correlated with long-term therapeutic benefit e.g. blood lipids or glucose or blood pressure.

A surrogate endpoint might also be a pharmacokinetic parameter, if it is indicative of the therapeutic effect, e.g. plasma concentration of an anti-epilepsy drug.

Use of surrogate effects presupposes that the disease process is fully understood. They are employed (when they can be justified) in diseases for which the true therapeutic effect can be measured only by studying large numbers of patients over years. Such long-term outcome studies are indeed always preferable but may be impracticable on organisational, financial and sometimes ethical grounds prior to releasing new drugs for general prescription. It is in areas such as these that the techniques of large-scale surveillance for efficacy, as well as for safety, under conditions of ordinary use (below), would be needed to supplement the necessarily smaller and shorter formal therapeutic trials employing surrogate effects.

Surrogate endpoints are of particular value in early drug development to select candidate drugs from a range of agents. Over-zealous fixation on the use of surrogate endpoints can, however, lead to serious errors in decision-making.

Therapeutic evaluation

The aims of therapeutic evaluation are three-fold.

- To assess the efficacy, safety and quality of new drugs to meet unmet clinical needs.
- To expand the indications for the use of current drugs (or generic drugs[15]) in clinical and marketing terms.
- To protect public health over the lifetime of a given drug.

---

[14] Medicines need instruction manuals just as do domestic appliances.

[15] A drug for which the original patent has expired, so that anyone may market it in competition with the inventor. The term 'generic' has, however, come to be synonymous with the nonproprietary or approved name (see Chapter 6).

4 EVALUATION OF DRUGS IN MAN

TABLE 4.1 Process of therapeutic evaluation

	Preregistration		Postregistration	
	Pharmaceutical company	Regulatory authority	Pharmaceutical company	Regulatory authority
Purpose of therapeutic evaluation	To select best candidate for development and registration	To satisfy the regulatory authority on efficacy, safety and quality	To promote drug to expand the market	To add to indications (by variation to licence) and to add evolving safety information

The process of therapeutic evaluation may be divided into pre- and postregistration phases (Table 4.1), the purposes of which are set out below.

When a new drug is being developed, the first therapeutic trials are devised to find out the best that the drug can do (and how it looks) under conditions ideal for showing efficacy, e.g. uncomplicated disease of mild-to-moderate severity in patients taking no other drugs, with carefully supervised administration by specialist doctors. Interest lies particularly in patients who complete a full course of treatment. If the drug is ineffective in these circumstances there is no point in proceeding with an expensive development programme. Such studies are sometimes called *explanatory trials* as they attempt to 'explain' why a drug works (or fails to work) in ideal conditions.

If the drug is found useful in these trials, then it becomes desirable next to find out how closely the ideal may be approached in the rough and tumble of routine medical practice: in patients of all ages, at all stages of disease, with complications, taking other drugs and relatively unsupervised. Interest continues in all patients from the moment they are entered into the trial and it is maintained if they fail to complete, or even to start, the treatment; what is wanted is to know the outcome in all patients deemed suitable for therapy, not only in those who successfully complete therapy.[16] The reason some drop out may be related to aspects of the treatment and it is usual to analyse these according to the clinicians' *initial* intention (*intention-to-treat analysis*), i.e. investigators are not allowed to risk introducing bias by exercising their own judgement as to who should or should not be excluded from the analysis.

In these real life, or 'naturalistic', conditions the drug may not perform so well, e.g. minor adverse effects may now cause patient noncompliance, which had been avoided by supervision and enthusiasm in the early trials. These naturalistic studies are sometimes called *'pragmatic'* trials.

The *methods* used to test the therapeutic value depend on the stage of development, who is conducting the study (a pharmaceutical company, or an academic body or health service at the behest of a regulatory authority), and the *primary endpoint* or *outcome* of the trial. The methods include:

- Formal therapeutic trials
- Equivalence and noninferiority trials
- Safety surveillance methods

Formal therapeutic trials are conducted during Phase 2 and Phase 3 of preregistration development, and in the postregistration phase to test the drug in new indications. *Equivalence* trials aim to show the therapeutic equivalence of two treatments, usually the new drug under development and an existing drug used as a standard active comparator. Equivalence trials may be conducted before or after registration for the first therapeutic indication of the new drug (see p. 61 for further discussion). *Safety surveillance methods* use the principles of pharmacoepidemiology (see p. 68) and are mainly concerned with evaluating adverse events and especially rare events, which formal therapeutic trials are unlikely to detect.

Need for statistics

In order truly to know whether patients treated in one way are benefited more than those treated in another, is essential to use numbers. Statistics may be defined as 'a body of methods for making wise

---

[16] Information on both categories (*use effectiveness* and *method effectiveness*) is valuable. Sheiner L B et al 1995 Intention-to-treat analysis and the goals of clinical trials. Clinical Pharmacology and Therapeutics 57: 1.

decisions in the face of uncertainty'.[17] Used properly, they are tools of great value for promoting efficient therapy.

Over 100 years ago Francis Galton saw this clearly.

In our general impressions far too great weight is attached to what is marvellous … Experience warns us against it, and the scientific man takes care to base his conclusions upon actual numbers. The human mind is … a most imperfect apparatus for the elaboration of general ideas … General impressions are never to be trusted. Unfortunately when they are of long standing they become fixed rules of life, and assume a prescriptive right not to be questioned. Consequently, those who are not accustomed to original enquiry entertain a hatred and a horror of statistics. They cannot endure the idea of submitting their sacred impressions to cold-blooded verification. But it is the triumph of scientific men to rise superior to such superstitions, to devise tests by which the value of beliefs may be ascertained, and to feel sufficiently masters of themselves to discard contemptuously whatever may be found untrue … the frequent incorrectness of notions derived from general impressions may be assumed…[18]

CONCEPTS AND TERMS

Hypothesis of no difference

When it is suspected that treatment A may be superior to treatment B and the truth is sought, it is convenient to start with the proposition that the treatments are equally effective — the 'no difference' hypothesis (*null hypothesis*). After two groups of patients have been treated and it has been found that improvement has occurred more often with one treatment than with the other, it is necessary to decide how likely it is that this difference is due to a real superiority of one treatment over the other. To make this decision we need to understand two major concepts, *statistical significance* and *confidence intervals*.

A **statistical significance test**[19] (e.g. the Student's 't' test, the Chi-Square test) will tell how often an observed difference would occur due to chance (random influences) if there is, in reality, no difference between the treatments. Where the statistical significance test shows that an observed difference would only occur five times if the experiment were repeated 100 times, this is often taken as sufficient evidence that the null hypothesis is *unlikely* to be true. Therefore the conclusion is that there is (probably) a real difference between the treatments. This level of probability is generally expressed in therapeutic trials as: 'the difference was statistically significant', or 'significant at the 5% level' or, $P = 0.05$ (P = probability based on chance alone). Statistical significance simply means that the result is unlikely to have occurred if there is *no* genuine treatment difference, i.e. there probably *is* a difference.

If the analysis reveals that the observed difference, or greater, would occur only once if the experiment were repeated 100 times, the results are generally said to be 'statistically highly significant', or 'significant at the 1% level' or '$P = 0.01$'.

Confidence intervals. The problem with the P value is that it conveys no information on the *amount* of the differences observed or on the *range* of possible differences between treatments. A result that a drug produces a uniform 2% reduction in heart rate may well be statistically significant but it is clinically meaningless. What doctors are interested to know is the *size* of the difference, and what degree of assurance, or confidence, they may have in the *precision* (reproducibility) of this estimate. To obtain this it is necessary to calculate a confidence interval (see Figs 4.1 and 4.2).[20]

A confidence interval expresses a range of values, which contains the true value with 95% (or other chosen %) certainty. The range may be broad, indicating uncertainty, or narrow, indicating (relative) certainty. A wide confidence interval occurs when numbers are small or differences observed are variable and points to a lack of information, whether the difference is statistically significant or not; it is a

[17] Wallis W A et al 1957 Statistics, a new approach. Methuen, London.
[18] Galton F 1879 Generic images. Proceedings of the Royal Institution.

[19] Altman D et al 1983 British Medical Journal 286: 1489.
[20] Gardner M J, Altman D G 1986 British Medical Journal 292: 746.

warning against placing much weight on, or confidence in, the results of small or variable studies. Confidence intervals are extremely helpful in interpretation, particularly of small studies, as they show the degree of uncertainty related to a result. Their use in conjunction with nonsignificant results may be especially enlightening.[21] A finding of 'not statistically significant' can be interpreted as meaning there is no clinically useful difference only if the confidence intervals for the results are also stated in the report and are narrow. If the confidence intervals are wide, a real difference may be missed in a trial with a small number of subjects, i.e. absence of evidence that there is a difference is not the same as showing that there is no difference. Small numbers of patients inevitably give low precision and low power to detect differences.

Types of error

The above discussion provides us with information on the likelihood of falling into one of the two principal kinds of error in therapeutic experiments, for the hypothesis that there is no difference between treatments may either be accepted incorrectly or rejected incorrectly.

Type I error (α) is the finding of a difference between treatments when in reality they do not differ, i.e. *rejecting* the null hypothesis incorrectly. Investigators decide the degree of this error which they are prepared to tolerate on a scale in which 0 indicates complete rejection of the null hypothesis and 1 indicates its complete acceptance; clearly the level for α must be set near to 0. This is the same as the significance level of the statistical test used to detect a difference between treatments. Thus α (or $P = 0.05$) indicates that the investigators will accept a 5% chance that an observed difference is not a real difference.

Type II error (β) is the finding of no difference between treatments when in reality they do differ, i.e. *accepting* the null hypothesis incorrectly. The probability of detecting this error is often given

wider limits, e.g. $\beta = 0.1$–0.2, which indicates that the investigators are willing to accept a 10–20% chance of missing a real effect. Conversely, the *power* of the study $(1 - \beta)$ is the probability of avoiding this error and detecting a real difference, in this case 80–90%.

It is up to the investigators to decide the target difference[22] and what probability level (for either type of error) they will accept if they are to use the result as a guide to action.

Plainly, trials should be devised to have adequate *precision* and *power,* both of which are consequences of the size of study. It is also necessary to make an estimate of the likely size of the difference between treatments, i.e. the target difference. Adequate power is often defined as giving an 80–90% chance of detecting (at 1–5% statistical significance, $P = 0.01$–0.05) the defined useful target difference (say 15%). It is rarely worth starting a trial that has less than a 50% chance of achieving the set objective, because the power of the trial is too low; such small trials, published without any statement of power or confidence intervals attached to estimates reveal only their inadequacy.

Types of therapeutic trial

A therapeutic trial is:

a carefully, and ethically, designed experiment with the aim of answering some precisely framed question. In its most rigorous form it demands equivalent groups of patients concurrently treated in different ways or in randomised sequential order in crossover designs. These groups are constructed by the random allocation of patients to one or other treatment … In principle the method has application with any disease and any treatment. It may also be applied on any scale; it does not necessarily demand large numbers of patients.[23]

---

[21]Altman D G et al 1983 British Medical Journal 286: 1489.

[22]*The Target Difference.* Differences in trial outcomes fall into three grades (1) that the doctor will ignore, (2) that will make the doctor wonder what to do (more research needed), and (3) that will make the doctor act, i.e. change prescribing practice.

This is the classic randomised controlled trial (RCT), the most secure method for drawing a causal inference about the effects of treatments. Randomisation attempts to control biases of various kinds when assessing the effects of treatments. RCTs are employed at all phases of drug development and in the various types and designs of trials discussed below.

Fundamental to any trial are:

- An hypothesis
- Definition of the primary endpoint
- The method of analysis
- A protocol.

Other factors to consider when designing or critically appraising a trial are the:

- Characteristics of the patients
- General applicability of the results
- Size of the trial
- Method of monitoring
- Use of interim analyses[24]
- Interpretation of subgroup comparisons.

The aims of a therapeutic trial, not all of which can be attempted at any one occasion, are to decide:

- Whether a treatment is of value
- The magnitude of that value (compared with other remedies)
- The types of patients in whom it is of value
- The best method of applying the treatment (how often, and in what dosage if it is a drug)
- The disadvantages and dangers of the treatment.

Dose–response trials. Response in relation to the dose of a new investigational drug may be explored in all phases of drug development. Dose–response trials serve a number of objectives, of which the following are of particular importance.

- Confirmation of efficacy (hence a therapeutic trial)

[23]Bradford Hill A 1977 Principles of medical statistics. Hodder and Stoughton, London. If there is a 'father' of the modern scientific therapeutic trial, it is he.
[24]Particularly in large-scale outcome trials, a *monitoring committee* is given access to the results as these are accumulated; the committee is empowered to discontinue a trial if the results show significant advantage or disadvantage to one or other treatment.

- Investigation of the shape and location of the dose–response curve
- The estimation of an appropriate starting dose
- The identification of optimal strategies for individual dose adjustments
- The determination of a maximal dose beyond which additional benefit is unlikely to occur.

Superiority, equivalence and noninferiority in clinical trials. The therapeutic efficacy of a novel drug is most convincingly established by demonstrating superiority to placebo, or to an active control treatment, or by demonstrating a dose–response relationship (as above).

In some cases, however, the purpose of a comparison is to show not necessarily superiority, but either equivalence or noninferiority. The objectives of such trials are to avoid the use of a placebo, to explore possible advantages of safety, dosing convenience and cost, and to present an alternative or 'second-line' therapy.

Examples of possible outcome in a 'head to head' comparison of two active treatments appear in Figure 4.1.

There are in general, two types of equivalence trials in clinical development, *bio-* and *clinical* equivalence. In the former, certain pharmacokinetic variables of a new formulation have to fall within specified (and regulated) margins of the standard formulation of the same active entity. The advantage of this type of trial is that, if bioequivalence is 'proven' then proof of clinical equivalence is not required. Proof of clinical equivalence of a generic product to the marketed product can be much more difficult to demonstrate.

DESIGN OF TRIALS

Techniques to avoid bias

The two most important techniques are:

- Randomisation
- Blinding

Randomisation introduces a deliberate element of chance into the assignment of treatments to the subjects in a clinical trial. It provides a sound statistical basis for the evaluation of the evidence

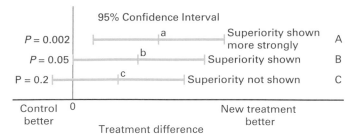

Fig. 4.1 Relationship between significance tests and confidence intervals for the comparisons between a new treatment and control. The treatment differences a, b, c are all in favour of 'New treatment', but superiority is shown only in A and B. In C, superiority has not been shown. This may be because the effect is small and not detected. The result, nevertheless, is compatible with equivalence or noninferiority. Adequate precision and power are assumed for all the trials.

relating to treatment effects, and tends to produce treatment groups that have a balanced distribution of prognostic factors, both known and unknown. Together with blinding, it helps to avoid possible bias in the selection and allocation of subjects.

Randomisation may be accomplished in simple or more complex ways such as:

- Sequential assignments of treatments (or sequences in crossover trials).
- Randomising subjects in blocks. This helps to increase comparability of the treatment groups when subject characteristics change over time or there is a change in recruitment policy. It also gives a better guarantee that the treatment groups will be of nearly equal size.
- By dynamic allocation, in which treatment allocation is influenced by the current balance of allocated treatments

Blinding. The fact that both doctors and patients are subject to bias due to their beliefs and feelings has led to the invention of the double-blind technique, which is a

control device to prevent bias from influencing results. On the one hand it rules out the effects of hopes and anxieties of the patient by giving both the drug under investigation and a placebo (dummy) of identical appearance in such a way that the subject (the first 'blind' man) does not know which he is receiving. On the other hand, it also rules out the influence of preconceived hopes of, and unconscious communication by, the investigator or observer by keeping him (the second 'blind' man) ignorant of whether he is

prescribing a placebo or an active drug. At the same time, the technique provides another control, a means of comparison with the magnitude of placebo effects. The device is both philosophically and practically sound.[25]

A nonblind trial is called an *open trial.*

The double-blind technique should be used wherever possible and especially for occasions when it might at first sight seem that criteria of clinical improvement are objective when in fact they are not. For example, the range of voluntary joint movement in rheumatoid arthritis has been shown to be greatly influenced by psychological factors, and a moment's thought shows why, for the amount of pain patients will put up with is influenced by their mental state.

Blinding should go beyond the observer and the observed. None of the investigators should be aware of treatment allocation, including those who evaluate endpoints, assess compliance with the protocol and monitor adverse events. Breaking the blind (for a single subject) should be considered only when the subject's physician deems knowledge of the treatment assignment essential in the subject's best interests.

Sometimes the double-blind technique is not possible, because, for example, side-effects of an active drug reveal which patients are taking it or tablets look or taste different; but it never carries a disadvantage ('only protection against biased data'). It is not, of course, used with new chemical entities

[25]Modell W 1958 Journal of the American Medical Association 167: 2190.

fresh from the animal laboratory, whose dose and effects in man are unknown, although the subject may legitimately be kept in ignorance (single-blind) of the time of administration. Single-blind techniques have a place in therapeutics research but only when the double-blind procedure is impracticable or unethical.

Ophthalmologists are understandably disinclined to refer to the double-blind technique; they call it double-masked.

SOME COMMON DESIGN CONFIGURATIONS

Parallel group design

This is the most common clinical trial design for confirmatory therapeutic (Phase 3) trials. Subjects are randomised, to one of two or more treatment 'arms'. These treatments will include the investigational drug at one or more doses, and one or more control treatments such as placebo and/or an active comparator. Parallel group designs are particularly useful in conditions that fluctuate over a short-term basis, e.g. migraine or irritable bowel syndrome, but are also used in chronic stable diseases such as Parkinson's disease and forms of cancer. The particular advantages of the parallel group design are simplicity, the ability to approximate more closely the likely conditions of use, and the avoidance of 'carry-over effects' (see below).

Crossover design

In this design, each subject is randomised to a sequence of two or more treatments, and hence acts as his/her own control for treatment comparisons. The advantage of this design is that subject-to-subject variation is eliminated from treatment comparison so that number of subjects is reduced.

In the basic crossover design each subject receives each of the two treatments in a randomised order. There are variations to this in which each subject receives a subset of treatments or ones in which treatments are repeated within the same subject (to explore the reproducibility of effects).

The main disadvantage of the crossover design is carry-over, i.e. the residual influence of treatments on subsequent treatment periods. This can be avoided to

some extent by separating treatments with a 'wash-out' period and, more importantly, by selecting treatment lengths based on a knowledge of the disease and the new medication. The crossover design is best suited for chronic stable diseases e.g. hypertension, chronic stable angina pectoris, where the baseline conditions are attained at the start of each treatment arm. The pharmacokinetic characteristics of the new medication are also important, the principle being that the plasma concentration at the start of the next dosing period is zero and no dynamic effect can be detected.

Factorial designs

In the factorial design, two or more treatments are evaluated simultaneously through the use of varying combinations of the treatments. The simplest example is the 2×2 factorial design in which subjects are randomly allocated to one of four possible combinations of two treatments A and B. These are: A alone, B alone, A + B, neither A nor B (placebo). The main uses of the factorial design are to:

- make efficient use of clinical trial subjects by evaluating two treatments with the same number of individuals
- examine the interaction of A with B
- establish dose–response characteristics of the combination of A and B when the efficacy of each has been previously established.

Multicentre trials

Multicentre trials are carried out for two main reasons. First, they are an efficient way of evaluating a new medication, by accruing sufficient subjects in a reasonable time to satisfy trial objectives. Second, multicentre trials may be designed to provide a better basis for the subsequent generalisation of their findings. Thus they provide the possibility of recruiting subjects from a wide population and of administering the medication in a broad range of clinical settings. Multicentre trials can be used at any phase in clinical development, but are especially valuable when used to confirm therapeutic value in Phase 3.

The main potential problem with a multicentre clinical trial is that heterogeneity of treatment effects between centres may create difficulty in arriving at a single interpretation. This is not as big a problem as it sometimes painted, however, and large-scale multi-centre trials using minimised data collection techniques and simple endpoints have been of immense value in establishing modest but real treatment effects that apply to a large number of patients e.g. drugs that improve survival after myocardial infarction.

Historical controls

Naturally there is a temptation simply to give a new treatment to all patients and to compare the results with the past, i.e. historical controls. Unfortunately this is almost always unacceptable, even with a disease such as leukaemia, for standards of diagnosis and treatment change with time, and the severity of some diseases (infections) fluctuates. The general provision stands that controls must be concurrent and concomitant. An exception to this rule is case-control studies (see p. 68)

SIZE OF TRIALS

Before the start of any controlled trial it is necessary to decide number of patients that will be needed to deliver an answer, for ethical, as well as practical reasons. This is determined by four factors:

1. The *magnitude* of the difference sought or expected on the primary efficacy endpoint (the target difference). For between-group studies, the focus of interest is the mean difference that constitutes a clinically significant effect.
2. The *variability* of the measurement of the primary endpoint as reflected by the standard deviation of this primary outcome measure. The magnitude of the expected difference (above) divided by the standard deviation of the difference, gives the *standardised difference* (see Fig. 4.2)
3. The defined *significance* level, i.e. the level of chance for accepting a Type I (α) error. Levels of 0.05 (5%) and 0.01 (1%) are common targets.
4. The *power* or desired probability of detecting the required mean treatment difference, i.e. the level of chance for accepting a Type II (β) error. For most controlled trials, a power of 80–90% (0.8–0.9) is frequently chosen as adequate, though higher power is chosen for some studies.

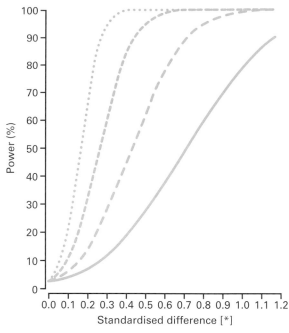

| Number of subjects per group | —— 16 | – – 40 |
| | ---- 100 | ···· 250 |

*Difference between treatments/standard deviation (based on a two-sided test at the 0.05 level)

Fig. 4.2 Power curves — an illustrative method of defining the number of subjects required in a given study. In practice the actual number would be calculated from standard equations. In this example the curves are constructed for 16, 40, 100 and 250 subjects per group in a two-limb comparative trial. The graphs can provide three pieces of information: (1) The number of subjects that need to be studied, given the power of the trial and the difference expected between the two treatments. (2) The power of a trial, given the number of subjects included and the difference expected. (3) The difference that can be detected between two groups of subjects of given number, with varying degrees of power. (With permission from: Baber N, Smith RN, Griffin JP, O'Grady J, D'Arcy (eds) 1998 Textbook of pharmaceutical medicine, 3rd edn. Belfast: Queen's University of Belfast Press.)

It will be intuitively obvious that a *small* difference in the effect that can be detected between two treatment groups, or a *large* variability in the measurement of the primary endpoint, or a *high* significance level (low *P* value) or a *large* power requirement, all act to increase the required sample size. Figure 4.2 gives a graphical representation of how the power of a clinical trial relates to values of clinically relevant standardised difference for varying numbers of trial subjects (shown by the individual curves). It is clear that the larger the number of subjects in a trial, the smaller is the difference that can be detected for any given power value.

The aim of any clinical trial is to have small Type I and II errors and consequently sufficient power to detect a difference between treatments, if it exists. Of the four factors that determine sample size, the power and significance level are chosen to suit the level of risk felt to be appropriate; the magnitude of the effect can be estimated from previous experience with drugs of the same or similar action; the variability of the measurements is often known from published experiments on the primary endpoint, with or without drug. These data will, however, not be available for novel substances in a new class and frequently the sample size in the early phase of development is chosen on a more arbitrary basis. As an example, a trial that would detect, at the 5% level of statistical significance, a treatment that raised a cure rate from 75% to 85% would require 500 patients for 80% power.

Fixed-sample size and sequential designs

Defining when a clinical trial should end is not as simple as it first appears. In the standard clinical trial the end is defined by the passage of all of the recruited subjects through the complete design. But, it is results and decisions based on the results that matter, not the number of subjects. The result of the trial may be that one treatment is superior to another or that there is no difference. These trials are of *fixed-sample size.* In fact, patients are recruited sequentially, but the results are analysed at a fixed time-point. The results of this type of trial may be disappointing if they miss the agreed and accepted level of significance.

It is not legitimate, having just failed to reach the agreed level (say, $P = 0.05$) to take in a few more patients in the hope that they will bring P value down to 0.05 or less, for this is deliberately not allowing chance and the treatment to be the sole factors involved in the outcome, as they should be.

An alternative (or addition) to repeating the fixed-sample size trial is to use a *sequential design* in which the trial is run until a useful result is reached.[26] These adaptive designs, in which decisions are taken on the basis of results to date, can assess results on a continuous basis as data for each subject that becomes available or, more commonly, on groups of subjects

(group sequential design). The essential feature of these designs is that the trial is terminated when a *predetermined* result is attained and not when the investigator looking at the results thinks it appropriate. Reviewing results in a continuous or interim basis requires *formal interim analysis* and there are specific statistical methods for handling the data, which need to be agreed in advance. Group sequential designs are especially successful in large long-term trials of mortality or major non-fatal endpoints when safety must be monitored closely.

Interim analyses can reduce the power of statistical significance tests to a serious degree if they are scheduled to occur more than, say, about four times in a trial. Such sequential designs recognise the reality of medical practice and provide a reasonable balance between statistical, medical and ethical needs. It is a necessity to have expert statistical advice when undertaking such trials; poorly designed and executed studies cannot be salvaged after the event.

SENSITIVITY OF TRIALS

Definitive therapeutic trials are expensive and tedious and may be so prolonged that aspects of treatment have been superseded by the time a result is obtained. A single trial, however well-designed, executed and analysed, can only answer the question addressed. The Regulatory Authorities give guidance as to the number and design of trials that, if successful, would lead to a therapeutic claim. But changing clinical practice in the longer term depends on many other factors, of which confirmatory trials in other centres by different investigators under different conditions are an important part.

Meta-analysis

The two main outcomes for therapeutic trials are to influence clinical practice and, where appropriate, to make a successful claim for a drug with the regulatory authorities. Investigators are eternally optimistic and frequently plan their trials to look for large effects. Reality is different. The results of a planned (or unplanned) series of clinical trials may

[26]Whitehead J 1992 The Design Analysis of Sequential Clinical Trials, 2nd Edition. Ellis Horwood, Chester.

vary considerably for several reasons but most significantly because the studies are too small to detect a treatment effect. In common but serious diseases such as cancer or heart disease, however, even small treatment effects can be important in terms of their total impact on public health. It may be unreasonable to expect dramatic advances in these diseases; we should be looking for small effects. Drug developers too should be interested not only in whether a treatment works, but also how well and for whom.

The collecting together of a number of trials with the same objective in a *systematic review*[27] and analysing the accumulated results using appropriate statistical methods is termed *meta-analysis*. The principles of a meta-analysis are that

- It should be comprehensive, i.e. include data from all trials, published and unpublished,
- Only randomised controlled trials should be analysed, with patients entered on the basis of 'intention to treat',[28]
- The results should be determined using clearly defined, disease-specific endpoints (this may involve a re-analysis of original trials).

There are strong advocates and critics of the concept, its execution and interpretation. Arguments that have been advanced against meta-analysis are:

- An effect of reasonable size ought to be demonstrable in a single trial,
- Different study designs cannot be pooled,
- Lack of accessibility of all relevant studies,
- Publication bias ('positive' trials are more likely to be published).

In practice, the analysis involves calculating an 'odds ratio' for each trial included in the meta-analysis. This is the ratio of the number of patients experiencing a particular endpoint, e.g. death, and the number who do not, compared with the equivalent figures for the control group. The number of deaths *observed* in the treatment group is then compared with the number to be *expected* if it is assumed that the treatment is ineffective, to give the 'observed minus expected' statistic. The treatment effects for all trials in the analysis are then obtained by summing all the 'observed minus expected' values of the individual trials to obtain the overall odds ratio. An odds ratio of 1.0 indicates that the treatment has no effect, an odds ratio of 0.5 indicates a halving and an odds ratio of 2.0 indicates a doubling of the risk that patients will experience the chosen endpoint.

From the position of drug development, the general requirement that scientific results have to be repeatable has been interpreted in the past by the Food and Drug Administration (the regulatory agency in the USA) to mean that two well-controlled studies are required to support a claim. But this requirement is itself controversial and its relation to a meta-analysis in the context of drug development is unclear.

In clinical practice, and in the era of cost-effectiveness, the use of meta-analysis as a tool to aid medical decision making and underpinning 'evidence-based medicine' is here to stay.

Figure 4.3 shows detailed results from 11 trials in which antiplatelet therapy after myocardial infarction was compared with a control group. The number of vascular events per treatment group is shown in the figures in the second and third columns and the odds ratios, with the point estimates (the value most likely to have resulted from the study) represented by black squares and their 95% confidence intervals (CI), in the fourth column.

The size of the square is proportional to the number of events. The diamond gives the point estimate and CI for overall effect.

Results: implementation

The way in which data from therapeutic trials is presented can influence doctors' perceptions of the advisability of adopting a treatment in their routine practice.

[27] A review that strives comprehensively to identify and synthesise all the literature on a given subject (sometimes called an overview). The unit of analysis is the primary study and the same scientific principles and rigour apply as for any study. If a review does not state clearly whether and how all relevant studies were identified and synthesised it is not a systematic review (The Cochrane Library, 1998).

[28] Reports of therapeutic trials should contain an analysis of all patients entered, regardless of whether they dropped out or failed to complete, or even started the treatment for any reason. Omission of these subjects can lead to serious bias (Laurence D R, Carpenter J 1998 A dictionary of pharmacological and allied topics. Elsevier, Amsterdam).

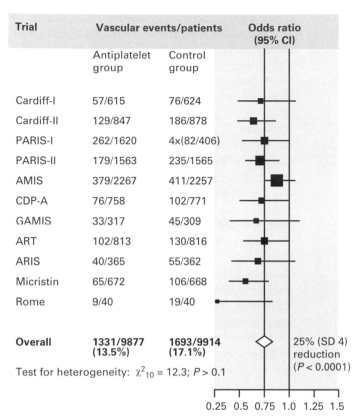

Fig. 4.3 A clear demonstration of benefits from meta-analysis of available trial data, when individual trials failed to provide convincing evidence. Reproduced with permission of Collins R 2001 Lancet 357: 373–380.

Trial	Vascular events/patients		Odds ratio (95% CI)
	Antiplatelet group	Control group	
Cardiff-I	57/615	76/624	
Cardiff-II	129/847	186/878	
PARIS-I	262/1620	4x(82/406)	
PARIS-II	179/1563	235/1565	
AMIS	379/2267	411/2257	
CDP-A	76/758	102/771	
GAMIS	33/317	45/309	
ART	102/813	130/816	
ARIS	40/365	55/362	
Micristin	65/672	106/668	
Rome	9/40	19/40	
Overall	**1331/9877 (13.5%)**	**1693/9914 (17.1%)**	25% (SD 4) reduction (P < 0.0001)

Test for heterogeneity: $\chi^2_{10} = 12.3$; $P > 0.1$

0.25 0.5 0.75 1.0 1.25 1.5

Relative and absolute risk

The results of therapeutic trials are commonly expressed as % reduction of an unfavourable (or % increase in a favourable) outcome, i.e. as *relative* risk, and this can be very impressive indeed until the figures are presented as the number of individuals actually affected per 100 people treated, i.e. as risk.

Where a baseline risk is *low,* a statement of relative risk alone is particularly misleading as it implies big benefit where actual benefit is small. Thus a reduction of risk from 2% to 1% is 50% relative risk reduction, but it saves only one patient for every 100 patients treated. But where the baseline is high, say 40%, a 50% reduction in relative risk saves 20 patients for every 100 treated.

Relative risk reductions can remain high (and thus make treatments seem attractive) even when susceptibility to the events being prevented is low (and the corresponding numbers needed to be treated are large). As a result, restricting the reporting of efficacy to just relative risk reductions can lead to great — and at times excessive — zeal in decisions about treatment for patients with low susceptibilities.[30]

A real-life example follows:

Antiplatelet drugs reduce the risk of future non-fatal myocardial infarction by 30% [relative risk] in trials of both primary and secondary prevention. But when the results are presented as the number of patients who need to be treated for one nonfatal

To make clinical decisions, readers of therapeutic studies need to know: how many patients must be treated[29] (and for how long) to obtain one desired result (*number needed to treat*). This is the inverse (or reciprocal) of absolute risk reduction.

[29] See Cooke R J, Sackett D L 1995 The number needed to treat: a clinically useful treatment effect. British Medical Journal 310: 452.
[30] Sackett D L, Cooke R J 1994 Understanding clinical trials: What measures of efficacy should journal articles provide busy clinicians? British Medical Journal 309: 755.

myocardial infarction to be avoided [absolute risk] they look very different.

In secondary prevention of myocardial infarction, 50 patients need to be treated for 2 years, while in primary prevention 200 patients need to be treated for 5 years, for one nonfatal myocardial infarction to be prevented. In other words, it takes 100 patient-years of treatment in primary prevention to produce the same beneficial outcome of one fewer nonfatal myocardial infarction.[31]

In the context of absolute risk, the question whether a low incidence of adverse drug effects is acceptable becomes a serious one.[31]

Nonspecialist, primary care doctors particularly, need and deserve clear and informative presentation of therapeutic trial results that measure the overall impact of a treatment on the patient's life, i.e. on clinically important outcomes such as morbidity, mortality, quality of life, working capacity, fewer days in hospital, etc. Without it, they cannot adequately advise patients.

Important aspects of therapeutic trial reports

Statistical significance and its clinical importance
Confidence intervals
Number needed to treat, or absolute risk

Pharmacoepidemiology

Pharmacoepidemiology is the study of the use and effects of drugs in large numbers of people. Some of the principles of pharmacoepidemiology are used to gain further insight into the efficacy, and especially the safety, of new drugs once they have passed from the limited exposure in controlled therapeutic pre-registration trials to the looser conditions of their use in the community. These (Phase 4) trials are not experimental (as is the randomised trial where entry and allocation of treatment are strictly controlled). They are *observational* in that the groups to be compared have been assembled from subjects who are, or who are not (the controls), taking the treatment in the ordinary way of medical care. Observational studies come into their own when sufficiently large randomised trials are logistically and financially impracticable. The following approaches are used.

Observational cohort[32] studies. Patients receiving the drug are followed up to determine the outcomes (therapeutic or adverse). This is usually forward-looking (prospective) research. *Prescription event monitoring* (below) is an example, and there is an increasing tendency to recognise that most new drugs should be monitored in this way when prescribing becomes general. Major differences include selection of an appropriate control group, the need for large numbers of subjects and for prolonged surveillance. This sort of study is scientifically inferior to the experimental cohort study (randomised controlled trial) and is cumbersome for research on drugs. Happily, clever epidemiologists have devised a partial alternative, the case-control study.

Case-control studies. This reverses the direction of scientific logic from forward-looking, 'what happens next' (*prospective*) to a backward-looking, 'what has happened in the past' (*retrospective*)[33] investigation. The investigator assembles a group of patients who have the condition it is desired to investigate, e.g. women who have had an episode of thromboembolism. A control group of women who have not had an episode of thromboembolism is then assembled, e.g. similar age, parity and smoking habits, from hospital admissions for other reasons, or primary care records. A complete drug history is taken from each group, i.e. the two groups are 'followed up' backwards to determine the proportion

---

[31] For example, drug therapy for high blood pressure carries risks, but the risks of the disease vary enormously according to severity of disease: 'Depending on the initial absolute risk, the benefits of lowering blood pressure range from preventing one cardiovascular event a year for about every 20 people treated to preventing one event for about every 20 people treated. The level of risk at which treatment should be started is debatable' (Jackson R et al 1993 Management of raised blood pressure in New Zealand: a discussion document. British Medical Journal 307: 107).

[32] Used here for a group of people having a common attribute, e.g. they have all taken the same drug.
[33] For this reason Feinstein has named these *trohoc* (cohort spelled backwards) studies.

in each group that has taken the suspect agent, in this case the oral contraceptive pill.

To investigate the question of thromboembolism and the combined oestrogen-progestogen contraceptive pill by means of an observational cohort study required enormous numbers of subjects[34] (the adverse effect is, happily, uncommon) followed over years. An investigation into cancer and the contraceptive pill by an observational cohort would require follow-up for 10–15 years. But a case-control study can be done quickly; it has the advantage that it begins with a much smaller number of cases (hundreds) of disease; though it has the disadvantage that it follows up subjects backwards and there is always suspicion of the intrusion of unknown and so unavoidable biases in selection of both patients and controls. Here again, independent repetition of the studies, if the results are the same, greatly enhances confidence in the outcome.

A major disadvantage of the case-control study is that it requires a definite hypothesis or suspicion of causality. A cohort study on the other hand does not; subjects can be followed 'to see what happens' (event recording). Case-control studies do not prove causation.[35] They reveal associations and it is up to investigators and critical readers to decide what is the most plausible explanation.

SURVEILLANCE SYSTEMS: PHARMACOVIGILANCE

When a drug reaches the market, a good deal is known about its therapeutic activity but rather less about its safety when used in large numbers of patients with a variety of diseases, for which they are taking other drugs. The term *pharmacovigilance* refers to the process of identifying and responding to issues of drug safety through the detection in the community of drug effects, usually adverse. Over a number of years increasingly sophisticated systems have been developed to provide surveillance of drugs in the postmarketing phase. For understandable reasons, they are strongly supported by governments. The position has been put thus:

> Four kinds of logic can be applied to drug safety monitoring:
> - to attempt to follow a complete cohort of (new) drug users for as long as it is deemed necessary to have adequate information.
> - to perform special studies in areas which may be predicted to give useful information
> - to try to gain experience from regular reporting of suspected adverse drug reactions from health professionals during the regular clinical use of the drug
> - to examine disease trends for drug-related causality.[36]

Drug safety surveillance relies heavily on the techniques of pharmacoepidemiology which include:

Voluntary reporting. Doctors, nurses and pharmacists are supplied with cards on which to record suspected adverse reaction to drugs. In the UK, this is called the 'Yellow Card' system and the Committee on Safety of Medicines collates the results and advises the government's Medicines Control Agency. It is recommended that for:

- newer drugs: all suspected reactions should be reported, i.e. any adverse or any unexpected event, however minor, which could conceivably be attributed to the drug
- established drugs: all serious suspected reactions should be reported, even if the effect is well recognised.

Inevitably the system depends on the intuitions and willingness of those called on to respond. Surveys suggest that not more than 10% of serious reactions are reported. Voluntary reporting is effective for identifying reactions that develop shortly after starting therapy, i.e. at providing early warnings of drug toxicity. Thus it is the first line in post-

---

[34] The Royal College of General Practitioners (UK) recruited 23 000 women takers of the pill and 23 000 controls in 1968 and issued a report in 1973. It found an approximate doubled incidence of venous thrombosis in combined-pill takers (the dose of oestrogen has been reduced since this study).

[35] Experimental cohort studies (randomised controlled trials) are on firmer ground with regard to causation. In the experimental cohort study there should be only *one* systematic difference between the groups (i.e. the treatment being studied). In case-control studies the groups may differ systematically in several ways.

[36] Edwards I R 1998 A prespective on drug safety. In: Edwards IR (ed) Drug Safety. Adis International, Auckland, p xii.

marketing surveillance. Reporting is particularly low, however, for reactions with long latency, such as tardive dyskinesia from chronic neuroleptic use. As the system has no limit of quantitative sensitivity it may detect the rarest events, e.g. those with an incidence of 1:5000–1:10 000. Voluntary systems are, however, unreliable for estimating the *incidence* of adverse reactions as this requires both a high rate of reporting (the numerator) and a knowledge of the rate of drug usage (the denominator).

Prescription event monitoring. This is a form of observational cohort study. Prescriptions for a drug (say, 20 000) are collected (in the UK this is made practicable by the existence of a National Health Service in which prescriptions are sent to a single central authority for pricing and payment of the pharmacist). The prescriber is sent a questionnaire and asked to report all events that have occurred (not only suspected adverse reactions) without a judgement about causality. Thus 'a broken leg is an event. If more fractures were associated with this drug they could have been due to hypotension, CNS effects or metabolic disease'.[37] By linking general practice and hospital records and death certificates, both prospective and retrospective studies can be done and unsuspected effects can be detected. Prescription event monitoring can be used routinely on newly licenced drugs, especially those likely to be widely prescribed in general practice, and it can also be implemented quickly in response to a suspicion raised, e.g. by spontaneous reports.

Medical record linkage allows computer correlation in a population of life and health events (birth, marriage, death, hospital admission) with history of drug use. It is being developed as far as resources permit. It includes prescription event monitoring (above). The largest UK medical record linkage is the General Practitioner Research Data Base at the Medicines Control Agency.

Population statistics, e.g. birth defect registers and cancer registers. These are insensitive unless a drug-induced event is highly remarkable or very frequent.

If suspicions are aroused then case-control and observational cohort studies will be initiated.

STRENGTH OF EVIDENCE

A number of types of clinical investigation are described in this chapter, and elsewhere in the book. When making clinical decisions about a course of therapeutic action, it is obviously relevant to judge the strength of evidence generated by different types of study. This has been summarised as follows, in rank order.[38]

1. Systematic reviews and meta-analysis
2. Randomised controlled trials with definitive results (confidence intervals that do not overlap the threshold of the clinically significant effect)
3. Randomised controlled trials with nondefinitive results (a difference that suggests a clinically significant effect but with confidence intervals overlapping the threshold of this effect)
4. Cohort studies
5. Case-control studies
6. Cross-sectional surveys
7. Case reports.

IN CONCLUSION[39]

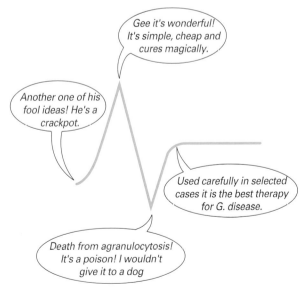

Fig. 4.4 Oscillations in the development of a drug.[40]

[37] Inman W H W et al 1986 Prescription-event monitoring. In: Inman WHW (ed) Monitoring for drug safety, 2nd edn. MTP, Lancaster, p 217.

[38] Guyatt G H et al 1995 Journal of the American Medical Association 274: 1800.

GUIDE TO FURTHER READING

Biomarkers Definitions Working Group 2001 Biomarkers and surrogate endpoints: preferred definitions and conceptual framework. Clinical Pharmacology and Therapeutics 69: 89–95

Bland J M, Altman D G 2000 Statistical notes. The odds ratio. British Medical Journal 320: 1468

Chalmers I 1995 What do I want from health research and researchers when I am a patient? British Medical Journal 310: 1315–1318

Chatellier G et al 1996 The numbers needed to treat: a clinically useful nomogram in its proper context. British Medical Journal 312: 426–429

Doll R 1998 Controlled trials: the 1948 watershed. British Medical Journal 317: 1217 (and following articles).

Egger M et al 1997 Meta-analysis. Principles and practice. British Medical Journal 315: 1533–1537 (See also other articles in the series entitled 'Meta-analysis'.)

Emanuel E J, Miller F G 2001 The ethics of placebo-controlled trials — a middle ground. New England Journal of Medicine 345: 915–919

Greenhalgh T 1997 Papers that report drug trials. British Medical Journal 315: 480–483 (See also other articles in the series entitled 'How to read a paper'.)

Hróbjartsson A, Gøtzsche P C 2001 Is the placebo powerless? An analysis of clinical trials comparing placebo with no treatment. New England Journal of Medicine 344: 1594–1602

Kaptchuk T J 1998 Powerful placebo: the dark side of the randomised controlled trial. Lancet 351: 1722–1725

Levy G 1992 Publication bias: Its implications for clinical pharmacology. Clinical Pharmacology and Therapeutics 52: 115–119

Lewis J et al 2002 Placebo-control led trials and the Declaration of Helsinki. Lancet 359: 1337–1340

Pogue J, Yusuf S 1998 Overcoming the limitations of current meta-analysis of randomized controlled trials. Lancet 351: 47–52

Silverman W A, Altman D G 1996 Patients' preferences and randomized trials. Lancet 347: 171–174

Sibbald B, Roland M 1998 Why are randomised controlled trials important? British Medical Journal 316: 201 (See also subsequent articles in this series entitled 'Understanding controlled trials'.)

Urquhart J 2001 Demonstrating effectiveness in a post-placebo era. Clinical Pharmacology and Therapeutics 70: 115–120

Waller P C, Jackson P R, Tucker G T, Ramsay L E 1994 Clinical pharmacology with confidence [intervals]. British Journal of Clinical Pharmacology 37: 309

---

[39] 'Quick, let us prescribe this new drug while it remains effective'. Richard Asher.

[40] By courtesy of Dr Robert H Williams and the Editor of The Journal of the American Medical Association.

5

Official regulation of medicines

SYNOPSIS

This chapter describes the background to why it became necessary to regulate the use and supply of drugs, and the ways in which these processes are managed.

- Basis for regulation: safety, efficacy, quality, supply
- Present medicines regulatory system
- Present day requirements
- Counterfeit drugs
- Appendix: the thalidomide disaster

Basis for regulation

Neither patients nor doctors are in a position to decide for themselves across the range of medicines that they use, which ones are *pure* and *stable*, and *effective* and *safe*.

They need assurance that the medicines they are offered fulfil these requirements and are supported by information that permits optimal use. The information about and the usage of medicines gets out of date, and there is an obligation on licence holders continually to review their licence with particular regard to safety. Marketing Authorisation Holders (MAH), i.e. pharmaceutical companies, can also change the efficacy claims to their licence, e.g. new indications, extension of age groups, or change the safety information e.g. add new warnings, or contraindications. The quality aspects may also need to be revised as manufacturing practices change. MAH's have strong profit motives for making claims about their drugs. Only governments can provide the assurance about all those aspects in the life of a medicine, (in so far as it can be provided).

The principles of official (statutory) medicines regulation are that

- No medicines shall be marketed without prior licensing by the government.
- A licence shall be granted on the basis of scientific evaluation[1] of:
  — **safety,** in relation to its use: evaluation at the point of marketing is provisional in the sense that it is followed in the community by a pharmacovigilance programme
  — **efficacy** (now often including quality of life)
  — **quality,** i.e. purity, stability (shelf-life)

---

[1] Except in the case of traditional herbal medicines (which can be ineffective and/or hazardous), as well as other substances used in the 'legitimate practice' of complementary medicine, for which this requirement cannot be met. Official regulators, finding themselves between 'the rock' of maintaining scientific principles and 'the hard place' of banning complementary medicines that are popular with the public (a political impossibility), have reacted in accordance with the highest traditions of their calling as civil servants. They have produced a compromise mix of reinterpreted regulations with circumspect labelling that will allow these products to continue to be sold without, it is hoped, misleading the public.

— **supply**: i.e. whether the drug is suitable to be unrestrictedly available to the public or whether it should be confined to sales through pharmacies or on doctors' prescriptions; and what printed information should accompany its sale (labelling, leaflets).

- A licence shall specify the clinical indications that may be promoted and shall be for a limited period (5 years), which is renewable on application.
- A regulatory authority may order a drug to be taken off the market at any time for good cause
- A licence may be varied by an application from the MAH to update efficacy, safety and quality sections.

Plainly manufacturers and developers are entitled to be told what substances are regulated and what are not[2] and what kinds and amounts of data are likely to persuade a regulatory authority to grant a marketing application (licence) and for what medical purpose. In summary, medicines regulation aims to provide an objective, rigorous and transparent assessment of efficacy, safety and quality in order to protect and promote public health but not to impede the pharmaceutical industry. It may be appreciated that an interesting tension exists between regulator and regulated.[3]

HISTORICAL BACKGROUND

The beginning of substantial government intervention in the field of medicines paralleled the prolifer-

ation of synthetic drugs in the early 20th century when the traditional and familiar pharmacopoeia[4] expanded slowly and then, in mid-century, with enormous rapidity.

The first comprehensive regulatory law that required premarketing testing was passed in the USA in 1938, following the death of about 107 people due to the use of diethylene glycol (a constituent of anti-freezes) as a solvent for a stable liquid formulation of sulphanilamide for treating common infections[5]. It was convenient for children to take; the toxicity (CNS, renal, hepatic) of ethylene glycol was already known. The only premarketing 'tests' were for appearance, fragrance and flavour. The procedure was compatible with the then-existing law in the USA. The head of the company said he was sorry for the deaths but he felt no responsibility.

Other countries did not take on board the lesson provided by the USA and it took the thalidomide disaster of 1961 (Chapter 5, Appendix) to make governments all over the world initiate comprehensive control over all aspects of drug introduction, therapeutic claims and supply. Those governments that already had some control system strengthened it.

In the UK two direct consequences were the development of a spontaneous adverse drug reaction reporting scheme (the Yellow Card system) and legislation to provide regulatory control on the safety, quality and efficacy of medicines through the systems of standards, authorisation, pharmcovigilance (see p. 69) and inspection (Medicines Act 1968). A further landmark was the establishment of the Committee on Safety of Medicines in 1971 to advise the Licensing Authority in the UK. Despite these protective systems, other drug disasters occurred. In 1974 the β-blocking agent practolol was withdrawn because of a rare but severe syndrome affecting the eyes and other mucocutaneous regions in the body (not

---

[2] It is obviously impossible to list substances that will be regulated if anybody should choose one day to synthesise them. Therefore regulation is based on the supply of 'medicinal products', i.e. substances are regulated according to their proposed use; and they must be defined in a way that will resist legal challenge (hence the stilted regulatory language). The following terms have gained informal acceptance for 'borderline substances' (which may or may not be regulated): *nutriceutical*: a food or part of a food that provides medicinal benefits *cosmeceutical*: a cosmetic that also has medicinal use.

[3] However much doctors may mock the bureaucratic 'regulatory mind', regulation provides an important service and it is expedient that doctors should have some insight into its working and some of the very real problems faced by public servants who are trying to do good without risking losing their jobs.

[4] Pharmacopoeia: a book (often official) listing drugs, their uses, standards of purity, etc.

[5] Report of the Secretary of Agriculture submitted in response to resolutions in the House of Representatives and Senate (USA). 1937 Journal of the American Medical Association 111: 583, 919. Recommended reading. A similar episode occurred as recently as 1990–1992: See Hanif M et al 1995 Fatal renal failure caused by diethylene glycol in paracetamol elixir: the Banglandesh epidemic. British Medical Journal 311: 88. Note: diethylene glycol is cheap.

detected by animal tests), and in 1982 benoxaprofen, a nonsteroidal anti-inflammatory drug, was found to cause serious adverse effects including onycholysis and photosensitivity in elderly patients. In 1995, the new European regulatory system was introduced (below).

CURRENT MEDICINES REGULATORY SYSTEMS

All countries where medicines are licenced for use have a regulatory system. From the point of view of a potential MAH (pharmaceutical company) seeking worldwide marketing rights, the regulatory bodies its programmes *must* satisfy include the Food and Drug Administration (FDA) of the USA, the European Medicines Evaluation Agency (EMEA) of the European Union (EU), and the Japanese Pharmaceutical Affairs Bureau. The national regulatory bodies of the individual EU members remain in place and work with the EMEA (see below). National licences can still be granted through individual member states, and they maintain particular responsibility for the public health issues in their own country. Some appreciation of the system in Europe is important. Up until 1995, applications for licences had to be made to these separate national authorities. This was enormously wasteful in time and manpower, as drug developers had to adapt their research and clinical development programmes to meet diverse national (often bureaucratic) requirements. In addition to the introduction of the European system, significant harmonisation of practices and procedures at a global level (especially Europe, Japan and the USA), have also been achieved through the International Conferences on Harmonisation (see p. 53, footnote 4).

In the European Union, drugs may be licensed in three ways:

- The centralised procedure allows applications to be made directly to the EMEA, which are then allocated for assessment to one member state (the rapporteur) assisted by a second member state (co-rapporteur). This approach is mandatory for biotechnology products and optional for new medicinal products.
- The mutual recognition (or decentralised) procedure allows applicants to nominate one member state (known as a reference member state), which assesses the application and seeks opinion from the other (concerned) member states. Granting the licence will ensure simultaneous mutual recognition in these other states, provided agreement is reached among them. There is an arbitration procedure to resolve disputes.
- A product to be marketed in a single country can have its licence applied for through the national route.

The European systems are conducted according to strict timelines and written procedures and there are regulations in place to handle disagreements between member states and rights of appeal for applications against refusals to licence.

Once a medicine is licenced for sale by one of the above procedures, its future regulatory life remains within that procedure. Licences have to be reviewed every 6 months for the first 2 years, then annually until 5 years, then renewed subsequently at 5-year intervals. The renewal of a licence is primarily the responsibility of the MAH but requires approval from the regulatory authority. This is the opportunity for MAHs to review, especially, the safety aspects to keep the licence in line with current clinical practice. Any major changes to licences must be made by variation of the original licence (safety, efficacy or quality, see below) and supported by data, which for a major indication, can be substantial.

Requirements

AUTHORISATION FOR CLINICAL TRIALS IN THE UK

The 1968 Medicines Act laid down the terms under which investigations of a new potential medicine could be undertaken in man. The Licensing Authority[6] does not have rigid requirements concerning all the data that must be provided before authorisation can be given for a clinical trial

---

[6] The Licensing Authority consists of the responsible Minister(s) and the Medicines Control Agency (MCA) — the executive arm in the Department of Health.

of a new drug. This is left to the judgement of the applicant but in any event will include a detailed clinical trial protocol and supporting experimental animal pharmacology and toxicology.

The MCA is advised by independent senior experts, sitting on the Committee on Safety of Medicines (CSM) and its subcommittees, on the suitability of the application. If the opinion is favourable, a Clinical Trial Certificate (CTC) is issued (valid for 2 years, and renewable) and the trial may start. Where clinical trial data on a drug already exist the process can be accelerated by submitting summarised preclinical and human volunteer data on pharmacokinetics and tolerability (the Clinical Trials Exemption or CTX procedure). If the MCA does not object within 35 days, the study may start. One further important aspect of regulation (or rather nonregulation) in the UK is that authorisation to start trials with a potential new medicine in healthy volunteers is not required, although local ethics review committee approval is required. This has provided incentive for novel drug investigation in humans but a European Union Directive, when in force, will remove this freedom and require that all clinical trials, i.e. including Phase 1, receive prior regulatory approval.

REGULATORY REVIEW OF A NEW DRUG APPLICATION

A drug regulatory authority requires the following:

- **Preclinical tests**
  - Tests carried out in animals to allow some prediction of potential efficacy and safety in man (see Chapter 4)
  - Chemical and pharmaceutical quality checks, e.g. purity, stability, formulation.
- **Clinical (human) tests (Phases 1, 2, 3)**
- The full process of regulatory review of a truly novel drug (new chemical entity) may take months.
- **Knowledge of the environmental impact of pharmaceuticals** Regulatory authorities expect manufacturers to address this concern in their application to market new chemical entities. Aspects include manufacture (chemical pollution), packaging (waste disposal), pollution in immediate use, e.g. antimicrobials and, more remotely, drugs

or metabolites entering the food chain or water where use may be massive, e.g. hormones. ˙

Regulatory review

Using one of the regulatory systems described above, an authority normally conducts a review in two stages:

1. Examination of preclinical data to determine whether the drug is safe enough to be tested for (predicted) human therapeutic efficacy.
2. Examination of the clinical studies to determine whether the drug has been shown to be therapeutically effective with safety appropriate to its use.[7]

If the decision is favourable, the drug is granted a marketing authorisation (for 5 years: renewable), which allows it to be marketed for *specified therapeutic uses.* The authority must satisfy itself of the adequacy of the information to be provided to prescribers in a Summary of Product Characteristics (SPC) and also a Patient Information Leaflet (PIL).

The PIL must also be approved by the licensing authority, be deemed fairly to represent the SPC, and be comprehensive and understandable to patients and carers. Where a drug has special advantage, but also has special risk, restrictions on its promotion and use can be imposed, e.g. isotretinoin and clozapine.

Central to the decision to grant a marketing authorisation is the assessment procedure under-taken by professional medical, scientific, statistical and pharmaceutical staff at one of the national agencies. In the UK these are employed as civil servants within the MCA and are advised by various independent expert committees (see above).

When a novel drug is granted a marketing autho-risation it is recognised as a medicine by independent critics and there is rejoicing amongst those who have spent many years developing it. But the testing is not over; the most stringent test of all is about to begin. It will be used in all sorts of people of all ages and sizes and having all sorts of other conditions. Its use can no longer be so closely supervised as hitherto. Doctors will prescribe it and patients will use it correctly and incorrectly. It will have effects that

---

[7] Common sense dictates that what, in regulatory terms is 'safe' for leukaemia would not be 'safe' for anxiety.

have not been anticipated. It will be taken in overdose. It has to find its place in therapeutics, through extended comparisons with other drugs available for the same diseases. Drugs used to prevent a long-term morbidity (e.g. stroke in hypertensive patients) can be proven effective only in outcome trials that are usually considered too expensive even to start until marketing of the drug is guaranteed. The effect of a drug at preventing rare occurrences requires many thousands of patients, more than are usually studied during development. Similarly rare adverse events cannot be detected prior to marketing, and it would be unethical to expose large numbers of trial patients to a novel drug for purely safety reasons.[8]

Postlicensing responsibilities

The pharmaceutical company is predominantly interested in gaining as widespread usage as fast as possible, based on the efficacy of the drug demonstrated in preregistration trials. The regulatory authorities are more concerned with the safety profile of the drug, and protection of public health. The most important source of safety data once the drug is in clinical use is spontaneous reporting of adverse events, which will generate 'signals' and raise suspicion of infrequent but potentially serious adverse events caused by the drug.[9] Proving the causal link from sporadic signals can be extremely difficult, and is entirely dependent on the number and quality of these spontaneous reports. In the UK, these reports are captured through the Yellow Card system (see p. 69), which may be completed by doctors, nurses or pharmacists. Other countries have their own systems. The importance of encouraging accurate spontaneous reporting of adverse events cannot be overemphasised.

Postmarketing (Phase 4) studies are not generally regulated by legislation, although in the EU, in exceptional circumstances, they may be a condition of the marketing authorisation. Voluntary guidelines are in use for postmarketing studies agreed between industry and the regulatory authorities. All company-sponsored trials that are relevant to the safety of a marketed medicine are included; they clearly state that such studies should not be conducted for the purposes of promotion. Other studies investigating the safety of a medicine that are not directly sponsored by the manufacturer may be identified from various organisations, e.g. The Drug Safety Research Unit (Southampton, UK) using Prescription-Event Monitoring (PEM), the Medicines Monitoring Unit (MEMO) (Tayside, UK), and the use of computerised record linkage schemes (in place in the USA for many years) such as the UK General Practice Research Database at the MCA. All these systems have the important capacity to obtain information on very large numbers of patients, 10 000–20 000, in *observational cohort* studies and *case-control* studies which complement the spontaneous reporting system (see Chapter 4).

In the UK, many new drugs are highlighted as being under special consideration by the regulatory authorities, by marking the drug with a symbol, the inverted black triangle ▼, in formularies. The regulatory authority communicates emerging data on safety of drugs to doctors through letters or papers in journals, through specialist journals e.g. *Current Problems in Pharmacovigilance* in the UK, and for very significant issues by direct ('Dear Doctor') letters, and fax messages.

Two other important regulatory activities that affect marketed drugs are:

- Variations to licences
- Reclassifications.

Variations are substantial changes instigated usually by pharmaceutical companies, but sometimes by the regulatory authority, to the efficacy, safety or quality aspects of the medicine. Most significant variations involve additions to indications or dosing regimens, or to the warnings and contraindication sections of the SPC. They need to be supported by evidence and undergo formal assessment.

Reclassification means change in the legal status of a medicine and is the process by which a prescription-only medicine can be converted to one

---

[8] Patients entering trials do not receive a novel drug because it may be the best drug for their condition: indeed, half (usually) are randomly assigned placebo or an alternate agent. After marketing, doctors should use a new drug only when they believe it an improvement (in efficacy, safety, convenience or cost) on the older alternatives.

[9] Waller P C, Wood S M 1998 Regulatory Aspects of Adverse Drug Reactions. In: Davies D M, Ferner R E, de Glanville H (eds) Davies's Textbook of Adverse Drug Reactions 5th edn, Chapman & Hall Medical, ch 3, pp 20–28.

that is available directly to the public through pharmacies and shops. It follows a rigorous assessment process with a particular stress on safety aspects of the medicine and involves advice from the Committee on Safety of Medicines, and requires a change in secondary legislation. The purpose of reclassification is to allow easier access of the general public to effective and safe medicines.

Discussion

It may be wondered why postlicensing/marketing surveillance and pharmacovigilance should be necessary. Common sense would seem to dictate that safety and efficacy of a drug should be fully defined before it is granted marketing authorisation. Prelicensing trials with very close supervision are commonly limited to hundreds of patients and this is unavoidable, chiefly because this close supervision is impracticable on a large scale for a very long time.

Postlicensing studies are increasingly regarded as essential to complete the definitive evaluation of drugs under conditions of ordinary use on a large scale, these programmes being preferable to attempts to enlarge and prolong formal therapeutic trials.

It would also seem sensible to require developers to prove that a new drug is not only effective but is actually *needed* in medicine before it is licensed. But a novel drug finds its place only after several, sometimes many, years, and to delay licensing is simply impracticable on financial grounds. This ought not to be so, but it is so. A 'need clause' in licensing is not generally practicable if drug developers are to stay in that business. This is why *comparative* therapeutic studies of a new drug with existing drugs are not required for licensing in countries having a research-based pharmaceutical industry. A 'need clause' is, however, appropriate for economically deprived countries (see World Health Organization Essential Drugs Programme); indeed such countries have no alternative.

The licensing authority in the UK is not concerned with the pricing of drugs or their cost effectiveness. The cost of medicines does however concern all governments, as part of the rising costs of national health services. A serious attempt to control costs on drug usage by the introduction of national guidelines on disease management (including the use of individual drugs) and the appraisal of new and established medicines for cost effectiveness now operate through a government funded body called NICE (National Institute for Clinical Excellence). The impact of its recommendations on health care, on costs and the pharmaceutical companies response to it are awaited.

Licensed medicines for unlicensed indications

Doctors may generally prescribe any medicine for any legitimate medical purpose.[10]

But if doctors use a drug for an indication that is not formally included in the Product Licence ('off-label' use) they would be wise to think carefully and to keep particularly good records for, if a patient is dissatisfied, prescribers may find themselves having to justify the use in a court of law. (Written records made at the time of a decision carry substantial weight, but records made later, when trouble is already brewing, lose much of their power to convince, and records that have been altered later are quite fatal to any defence.)

Manufacturers are not always willing to go to the trouble and expense of the rigorous clinical studies required to extend their licence unless a new use is likely to generate significant profits. They are prohibited by law from promoting an unlicenced use.

Unlicensed medicines and accelerated licensing

Regulatory systems make provision for supply of an unlicenced medicine, e.g. one that has not yet completed its full programme of clinical trials, for patients who, on the judgement of their doctors, have no alternative amongst licensed drugs. The doctor must apply to the manufacturer who may supply the drug for that particular patient and at the doctor's own responsibility. Various terms are used, e.g. supply on a 'named-patient' basis (UK); 'compassionate' drug use (USA). It is illegal to exploit this sensible loophole in supply laws to conduct research. Precise record-keeping of such use is essential.

---

[10] In many countries this excludes supply of drugs such as heroin or cocaine for controlled/supervised maintenance of drug addicts. In the UK such supply is permitted to doctors.

But there can be desperate needs involving large numbers of patients, e.g. AIDS, and regulatory authorities may respond by licensing a drug before completion of the usual range of studies (making it clear that patients must understand the risks they are taking). Unfortunately such well-intentioned practice discourages patients from entering formal trials and may, in the long run, actually delay the definition of lifesaving therapies.

Decision taking

> It must be remembered always that, though there are risks in taking drugs, there are also risks in not taking drugs, and there are risks in not developing new drugs.

The responsibility to protect public health on the one hand yet to allow timely access to novel medicines on the other, is one shared by drug regulators and developers. It is complicated by an ever increasing awareness of the risks and benefits (real, or perceived) of medicines by the general public.

Some new medicines are registered with the high expectation of effectiveness and with very little safety information; rare and unpredictable adverse events may take years to appear with sufficient conviction that causality is accepted.

In taking decisions about drug regulation, it has been pointed out that there is uncertainty in three areas.[11]

- Facts
- Public reaction to the facts
- Future consequences of decisions.

Regulators are influenced not only to avoid risk but to avoid regret later (*regret avoidance*) and this consideration has a profound effect whether or not the decision taker is conscious of it; it promotes defensive regulation.

It is self-evident that it is much harder to detect and quantitate a good that is not done, than it is to detect and quantitate a harm that is done. Therefore, although it is part of the decision-taker's job to facilitate the doing of good, the avoidance of harm looms larger. Attempts to blame regulators for failing to do good due to regulatory procrastination, the 'drug lag'[12] do not induce the same feelings of horror in regulators and their advisory committees that are induced by the prospect of finding they have approved a drug that has, or may have, caused serious injury and that the victims are about to appear on television.[13] The bitterness of people injured by drugs, whether or not there is fault could be much reduced by the institution of simple non-adversarial arrangements for compensation (see p. 10).

This is not to ridicule the regulators and their advisers. They are doing their best, and commonly make good and sensible decisions that receive no congratulations.

Counterfeit drugs

Fraudulent medicines make up as much as 6% of pharmaceutical sales worldwide. They present a serious health (and economic) problem in countries with weak regulatory authorities and lacking money to police drug quality. In these countries counterfeit medicines may comprise 20–50% of available products. The trade may involve false labelling of legally manufactured products, in order to play one national market against another; also low-quality manufacture of correct ingredients; wrong ingredients, including added ingredients (such as corticosteroids added to herbal medicine for arthritis); no active ingredient; false packaging.

The trail from raw material to appearance on a pharmacy shelf may involve as many as four countries, with the final stages (importer, wholesaler) quite innocent, so well has the process been obscured.

Developed countries have inspection and enforcement procedures to detect and take appropriate action on illegal activities.

---

[11] Lord Ashby 1976 Proceedings of the Royal Society of Medicine 69: 721.

[12] Nevertheless, regulatory authorities have responded by providing a facility for 'fast-tracking' drugs for which clinical need may be urgent, e.g. AIDS (see above).
[13] The very last thing a drug regulator wishes to be able to say is, 'I awoke one morning and found myself famous': Lord Byron (1788–1824) on the publication of his poem, Childe Harold's Pilgrimage.

GUIDE TO FURTHER READING

Baber N 1994 International conference on harmonization of technical requirements for registration of pharmaceuticals. British Journal of Clinical Pharmacology 37: 401–404

Brass E P 2001 Changing the status of drugs from prescription to over-the-counter availability. New England Journal of Medicine 345: 810–816

Collier J 1999 Paediatric prescribing: using unlicenced drugs and medicines outside their licensed indications. British Journal of Clinical Pharmacology 48: 5–8

Conroy S et al 2000 Survey of unlicenced and off label drug use in paediatric wards in European countries. British Medical Journal 320: 79–82

DiMasi J A, Seibring M A, Lasagna L 1994 New drug development in the United States from 1963 to 1992. Clinical Pharmacology and Therapeutics 55: 609–622

Gale E A M, Clark A 2000 A drug on the market? Lancet 355: 61–63

Medicines Control Agency 1994 Guidelines for company-sponsored Safety Assessment of Marketed Medicines (SAMM Guidelines). British Journal of Clinical Pharmacology 38: 95

Reichert J M 2000 New biopharmaceuticals in the USA: trends in development and marketing approvals 1995–1999. Trends in Biotechnology 18: 364–369

Richard B W et al 1987 Drug regulation in the United States and the United Kingdom: the Depo-Provera story. Annals of Internal Medicine 106: 886–891; (An analysis of how drug regulators in the USA and the UK came to opposite conclusions on the same data.)

ON THALIDOMIDE

Chamberlain G 1989 The obstetric problems of the [now adult] thalidomide children. British Medical Journal 298: 6

Dally A 1998 Thalidomide: was the tragedy preventable? Lancet 351: 1197–1199

Editorial 1981 Thalidomide: 20 years on. Lancet 2: 510

Mellin G W et al 1962 The saga of thalidomide. New England Journal of Medicine 267: 1184–1192, 1238–1244

Appendix: A tale to remember — the thalidomide disaster

Thalidomide has provided a terrible lesson to the world in regard to drug development, testing, naming, prescribing and consumption. It deserves to be remembered.

In 1960–61 in [West] Germany an outbreak of phocomelia occurred. Phocomelia means 'seal extremities'; it is a congenital deformity in which the long bones of the limbs are defective and substantially normal or rudimentary hands and feet arise on, or nearly on, the trunk, like the flippers of a seal; other abnormalities may occur. Phocomelia is ordinarily exceedingly rare.

Most [West] German clinics had no cases during the 10 years up to 1959. In 1959, in 10 clinics, 17 were seen in 1959, 126 in 1960, 477 in 1961. The European outbreak seemed confined to [West] Germany (though a similar but smaller occurrence was simultaneously noted in Australia), and this, with the steady increase, made a virus infection, such as rubella, seem an unlikely cause. Radioactive fall-out was considered and so were x-ray exposure of the mother, hormones, foods, food preservatives and contraceptives. One doctor, investigating his patients retrospectively with a questionnaire, found that 20% reported taking a proprietary medicine, Contergan, in early pregnancy. He questioned the patients again and 50% then admitted taking it; many said they had thought the drug too obviously innocent to be worth mentioning initially.[14]

In November 1961, the suggestion that a drug, unnamed, was the cause of the outbreak was publicly made by the same doctor at a paediatric meeting, following a report on 34 cases of phocomelia. That night a physician came up to him and said, 'Will you tell me confidentially, is the drug Contergan? I ask because we have such a child and my wife took Contergan'. Several letters followed, asking the same question, and it soon became widely known that the sedative drug thalidomide (Contergan, Distaval, Kevadon, Talimol, Softenon) was probably the cause.

It was withdrawn from the [West] German market in November and from the British market in December 1961. By that time reports had also come from other countries. A case-control study showed that of 46 cases of phocomelia 41 mothers had taken thalidomide and of 300 mothers with normal babies none had taken thalidomide between the fourth and ninth week of pregnancy.

Prospective observational cohort studies were quickly made in antenatal clinics where women had yet to give birth; though few, they provided evidence incriminating thalidomide. The worst had happened, a trivial new drug was the cause of the most grisly disaster in the short history of modern scientific drug therapy. Many thalidomide babies died, but many live on with deformed limbs, eyes, ears, heart and alimentary and urinary tracts.[15]

The [West] German Health Ministry estimated that thalidomide caused about 10 000 birth deformities in babies, 5000 of whom survived and 1600 of whom would eventually need artificial limbs. In Britain there were probably at least 600 live births of malformed children of whom about 400 survived. The world total of survivors was probably about 10 000.

Thalidomide had been marketed in [West] Germany in 1956, in Britain in 1958, and in other countries as a sedative and hypnotic and was recommended for use in pregnant women. It had not been tested on pregnant animals. When it was eventually tested it was at first difficult to induce fetal deformity (until it was used on New Zealand White Rabbits).

Thalidomide, skilfully promoted and credulously prescribed and taken by the public — it was also sold without prescription — achieved huge popularity; it 'became [West] Germany's baby-sitter'. It was a routine hypnotic in hospitals, was even recommended to help children adapt themselves to a convalescent home atmosphere and was sold mixed with other drugs for symptomatic relief of pain,

---

[14] Illustrating the problem of retrospective research, e.g. case-control studies; enquiries of patients are unreliable.

[15] For pictures of thalidomide deformities, see British Medical Journal 1962; 2: 646–647 and Journal of the American Medical Association 1962; 180: 1106–1114.

cough and fever. In 1960–61 it had become evident that prolonged use of thalidomide could cause hypothyroidism and peripheral neuritis. The latter effect was the principal reason why approval for marketing in the USA, as Kevadon, had been delayed by the US Food and Drug Administration. Approval had still not been given when the fetal effects were discovered and so general distribution was avoided. Nonetheless some 'thalidomide babies' were born in the USA following indiscriminate pre-marketing clinical trials.

Thalidomide has anti-inflammatory and immuno-suppressant actions and retains a limited specialist use in, for example, lepromatous leprosy,[16] and oral ulceration in AIDS (some cases).

The thalidomide disaster provided the impetus for the introduction of national drug regulatory authorities worldwide.

---

[16] Further cases of congenital malformations were reported in 1994 due to lax control of thalidomide use (Lancet 343: 433 and 344: 196). Thalidomide is available in the UK on a 'named-patient' basis only, with a detailed patient information leaflet and with signed patient consent.

6

Classification and naming of drugs

SYNOPSIS

In any science there are two basic
requirements — classification and
nomenclature (names):

- Classification: drugs cannot be classified and
  named according to a single rational system
  because the requirements of chemists,
  pharmacologists, and doctors differ.
- Nomenclature: nor is it practicable always to
  present each drug under a single name
  because the formulations in which they are
  presented as prescribable medicines may
  vary widely and commercial considerations
  are too often paramount.

Generic (nonproprietary) names should be
used as far as possible when prescribing except
where pharmaceutical bioavailability differences
have overriding importance.

Classification

It is evident from the way this book is organised
that there is no homogeneous system for classifying
drugs that suits the purpose of every user. Drugs
are commonly categorised according to the convenience of who is discussing them: clinicians,
pharmacologists or medicinal chemists.

Drugs may be classified by:

- *Body system*, e.g. alimentary, cardiovascular
- *Therapeutic use*, e.g. receptor blockers, enzyme
  inhibitors, carrier molecules, ion channels
- *Mode* or *site of action*
  - *molecular interaction*, e.g. glucoside, alkaloid,
    steroid.
  - *cellular site*, e.g. loop diuretic, catecholamine
    uptake inhibitor (imipramine)
- *Molecular structure*, e.g. glycoside, alkaloid,
  steroid.[1]

Nomenclature (names)

Any drug may have names in all three of the
following classes:

1. The *full chemical name*
2. A *nonproprietary (official, approved, generic) name*
   used in pharmacopoeias and chosen by official
   bodies; the World Health Organization (WHO)
   chooses recommended International
   Nonproprietary Names (rINN). The
   harmonisation of names began 50 years ago, and

---

[1] The ATC Classification System developed by the Nordic
countries and widely used in Europe meets most
classification requirements. Drugs are classified according to
their Anatomical, Therapeutic and Chemical characteristics
into five levels of specificity, the fifth being that for the single
chemical substance.

most countries have used rINNs for many years. The USA is an exception, but even here most USA National Names are the same as their rINN counterparts. In the UK, the British Approved Name (BAN) system is being progressively modified such that the rINN name is adopted; in many cases this involves only a trivial change. In a few cases, there is cause for concern that change of name could lead to confusion and constitute a public health risk, e.g. adrenaline is the BAN, epinephrine is the rINN name. In such instances, both rINN and BAN must currently appear in the manufacturer's literature. In general we use rINNs in this book and aim to minimise some unavoidable differences with, where appropriate, alternative names in the text and index.

3. A *proprietary (brand)* name that is the commercial property of a pharmaceutical company or companies.

Example on drug three names

1. 3-(10, 11-dihydro-5H-dibenz [b.*f*]-azepin-5-yl) propyldimethylamine
2. imipramine
3. Tofranil (UK), Prodepress, Surplix, Deprinol, etc (various countries)

In this book proprietary names are distinguished by an initial capital letter.

The full chemical name describes the compound for chemists. It is obviously unsuitable for prescribing.

A nonproprietary (generic,[2] approved) **name** is given by an official (pharmacopoeia) agency, e.g. WHO.

Three principles remain supreme and unchallenged in importance: the need for distinction in sound and spelling, especially when the name is handwritten; the need for freedom

from confusion with existing names, both nonproprietary and proprietary, and the desirability of indicating relationships between similar substances.[3]

The generic names **diazepam, nitrazepam, flurazepam** are all of benzodiazepines. Their proprietary names are Valium, Mogadon and Dalmane respectively. Names ending in *-olol* are adrenoceptor blockers; in *-pril* are ACE-inhibitors; in *-floxacin* are quinolone antimicrobials.

Any pharmaceutical company may manufacture a drug that has a well-established use and is no longer under patent restriction, in accordance with official pharmacopoeial quality criteria, and may apply to the regulatory authority for a licence to market. The task of authority is to ensure that these *generic* or *multisource pharmaceuticals* are interchangeable, i.e. they are pharmaceutically and biologically equivalent, so that a formulation from one source will be absorbed and give the same blood concentrations and have the same therapeutic efficacy as that from another. (Further formal therapeutic trials are not demanded for these well-established drugs.) A prescription for a generic drug formulation may be filled for any officially licensed product that the dispensing pharmacy has chosen to purchase (on economic criteria, see 'generic substitution' below).[4]

The proprietary name is a trade mark applied to particular formulation(s) of a particular substance by a particular manufacturer. Manufacture is confined to the owner of the trade mark or to others licensed by the owner. It is designed to maximise the difference between the names of similar drugs marketed by rivals for obvious commercial reasons. To add confusion, some companies give their proprietary products the same names as their generic products in an attempt to capture the prescription market, both proprietary and generic, and some market lower-priced generics of their own proprietaries. When a prescription is written for a proprietary product, pharmacists under UK law must dispense that product only. But by agreement

---

[2] The generic name is now widely accepted as being synonymous with the nonproprietary name. Strictly 'generic' (L. *genus*, race, a class of objects) should refer to a group or class of drug, e.g. benzodiazepines, but by common usage the word is now taken to mean the nonproprietary name of individual members of a group, e.g, diazepam.

[3] R B Trigg 1998 Chemical Nomenclature. Kluwer Academic, Dorerechat, pp 208–234.
[4] EU Medicines Evaluation Agency and USA Food and Drug Agency guidelines are available that give pharmacokinetic limits that must be met.

with the prescribing doctor, they may substitute an approved generic product (*generic* substitution). What is not permitted is the substitution of a different molecular structure deemed to be pharmacologically and therapeutically equivalent (*therapeutic* substitution).

NONPROPRIETARY NAMES

The principal reasons for advocating the habitual use of nonproprietary (generic) names in prescribing are:

Clarity: because it gives information of the class of drug e.g. nortriptyline and amitriptyline are plainly related, but their proprietary names Allegron and Lentizol are not. It is not unknown for prescribers, when one drug has failed, unwittingly to add or substitute another drug of the same group (or even the same drug) thinking that different proprietary names must mean different classes of drugs. Such occurrences underline the wisdom of prescribing generically, so group similarities are immediately apparent, but point up the requirement of brand names to be as distinct from each other as possible. Relationships cannot and should not be shown by brand names.

Economy: drugs sold under nonproprietary names are usually, but not always, cheaper than those sold under proprietary names.

Convenience: pharmacists may supply whatever version they stock[5] whereas if a proprietary name is used they are obliged to supply that preparation alone. They may have to buy in the preparation named even though they have an equivalent in stock. Mixtures of drugs are sometimes given nonproprietary names, having the prefix *co-* to indicate more than one active ingredient, e.g. co-amoxiclav for Augmentin, but many are not because they exist for commercial advantage rather than for therapeutic need.[6] No prescriber can be expected to write out

the ingredients, so proprietary names are used in many cases, there being no alternative.

International travellers with chronic illnesses will be grateful for recommended International Nonproprietary Names (above) as proprietary names often differ from country to country. The reasons are linguistic as well as commercial (see below).

PROPRIETARY NAMES

The principal noncommercial reason for advocating the use of propritary names in prescribing is consistency of the product, so that problems of quality, especially of bioavailability, are reduced. There is substance in this argument, though it is often exaggerated.

It is reasonable to use proprietary names when dosage, and therefore pharmaceutical bioavailability, are critical so that small variations in the amount of drug available for absorption can have big effects on the patient, e.g. drugs with low therapeutic ratio, digoxin, hormone replacement therapy, adreno-cortical steroids (oral), antiepileptics, cardiac anti-arrhythmics, warfarin. Also, with the introduction of complex formulations, e.g. sustained-release, it is important clearly to identify these, and use of proprietary names has a role.

The pharmaceutical industry regards freedom to market proprietary names and to advertise or, as it calls the latter, to 'effectively [bring] to the notice of the medical profession', as two of the essentials of the 'process of discovery in a vigorous competitive environment'.[7]

The present situation is that industry spends an enormous amount of money promoting its many names for the same article, and the community, as represented in the UK by the Department of Health, spends a small sum trying to persuade doctors to use nonproprietary names. Ordinary doctors who prescribe for their ordinary patients are the targets of both sides.

This state of affairs is confusing for prescribers. Generic names are intentionally longer than trade names to minimise the risk of confusion, but the use of accepted prefixes and stems for generic names

---

[5] This can result in supply of a formulation of appearance different from that previously used. Patients naturally find this disturbing.
[6] This is a practice largely confined to the UK. It is unknown in Europe, and not widely practised in the USA.

[7] Annual Report, 1963–1964. Association of the British Pharmaceutical Industry.

works well and the average name length is four syllables, which is manageable.

The search for proprietary names is a 'major problem' for pharmaceutical companies, increasing, as they are, their output of new preparations. A company may average 30 new preparations (not new chemical entities) a year, another warning of the urgent necessity for the doctor to cultivate a sceptical habit of mind.

The names that 'look and sound medically seductive' are being picked out. 'Words that survive scrutiny will go into a stock-pile and await inexorable proliferation of new drugs'.[8,9]

One firm (in the USA) commissioned a computer to produce a dictionary of 42 000 nonsense words of an appropriate scientific look and sound. An official said,

> Thinking up names has been driving us cuckoo around here … proper chemical names are hopeless for trade purposes, of course. … Doctors are the market we shoot for. A good trade name carries a lot of weight with doctors … they're more apt to write a prescription for a drug whose name is short, and easy to spell and pronounce, but has an impressive medical ring. … We believe there are enough brand new words in this dictionary to keep us going for years. … We don't yet know what proportion of names is unpronounceable … how many are obscene, either in English or in other languages, and how many are objectionable on grounds of good taste: 'Godamycin' would be a mild example.[9]

For the practising doctor (in the UK) the British National Formulary provides a regularly updated and comprehensive list of drugs in their non-proprietary (generic) and proprietary names. 'The range of drugs prescribed by any individual is remarkably narrow, and once the decision is taken to "think generic" surely the effort required is small'.[10] And, we would add, worthwhile.

Confusing names. The need for both clear thought and clear handwriting is shown by medicines of totally different class that have similar names. Serious events have occurred due to confusion of names and dispensing the wrong drug, e.g. Lasix (frusemide) for Losec (omeprazole) (death); AXT (intending zidovudine) was misinterpreted in the pharmacy and azathiorine was dispensed [do not use abbreviations for drug names]; Daonil (glibenclamide) for De-nol (bismuth chelate) and for Danol (danazol). It will be noted that nonproprietary names are less likely to be confused with other classes of drugs.

GUIDE TO FURTHER READING

Aronson J K 2000 'Where name and image meet' — the argument for 'adrenaline'. British Medical Journal 320: 506–509

Controversies in therapeutics 1988 The cases for and against prescribing genetic drugs. British Medical Journal 297: (Collier J Generic prescribing benefits patients) 1596 (Cruickshank J M Don't take innovative research-based pharmaceutical companies for granted) 1597

Furberg C D, Herrington D M, Psaty B M 1999 Are drugs within a class interchangeable? Lancet 354: 1201–1204 (and correspondence Lancet 2000 355: 316–317

George C F 1996 Naming of drugs: pass the epinephrine please. British Medical Journal 312: 1315 (and correspondence British Medical Journal 1996 313: 688–689)

Jack D B, Soppitt A J 1991 Give a drug a bad name. British Medical Journal 303: 1606

Taussig H B 1963 The evils of camouflage as illustrated by thalidomide. New England Journal of Medicine 180: 92, Editorial, p. 108

---

[8] Pharmaceutical companies increasingly operate worldwide and are liable to find themselves embarrassed by unanticipated verbal associations. For example, names marketed (in some countries) such as Bumaflex, Kriplex, Nokhel and Snootie conjure up in the minds of native English-speakers associations that may inhibit both doctors and patients from using them (see Jack and Soppitt in Guide to Further Reading).

[9] New Yorker, 14 July 1956.

[10] Editorial 1977 British Medical Journal 4: 980 and subsequent correspondence.

FROM PHARMACOLOGY TO TOXICOLOGY

7

General pharmacology

SYNOPSIS

How drugs act and interact, how they enter the body, what happens to them inside the body, how they are eliminated from it; the effects of genetics, age, and disease on drug action — these topics are important for, although they will generally not be in the front of the conscious mind of the prescriber, an understanding of them will enhance rational decision taking.

Knowledge of the requirements for success and the explanations for failure and for adverse events will enable the doctor to maximise the benefits and minimise the risks of drug therapy.

Pharmacodynamics
- Qualitative aspects: Receptors, Enzymes, Selectivity
- Quantitative aspects: Dose response, Potency, Therapeutic efficacy, Tolerance

Pharmacokinetics
- Time course of drug concentration: Drug passage across cell membranes; Order of reaction; Plasma half-life and steady-state concentration; Therapeutic drug monitoring
- Individual processes: Absorption, Distribution, Metabolism, Elimination

SYNOPSIS (CONTINUED)

- Drug dosage: Dosing schedules
- Chronic pharmacology: the consequences of prolonged drug administration and drug discontinuation syndromes
- Individual or biological variation: Variability due to inherited influences, environmental and host influences
- Drug interactions: outside the body, at site of absorption, during distribution, directly on receptors, during metabolism, during excretion

> Pharmacodynamics is what drugs do to the body: pharmacokinetics is what the body does to drugs.

It is self-evident that knowledge of pharmacodynamics is essential to the choice of drug therapy. But the well-chosen drug may fail to produce benefit or may be poisonous because too little or too much is present at the site of action for too short or too long a time. Drug therapy can fail for pharmacokinetic as well as for pharmacodynamic reasons. The practice of drug therapy entails more than remembering an apparently arbitrary list of actions or indications.

Technical incompetence in the modern doctor is inexcusable and technical competence and a humane approach are not incompatible as is sometimes suggested.

Pharmacodynamics

Understanding the mechanisms of drug action is not only an objective of the pharmacologist who seeks to develop new and better drugs, it is also the basis of intelligent use of medicines.

Qualitative aspects

It is appropriate to begin by considering what drugs do and how they do it, i.e. the nature of drug action. Body functions are mediated through control systems that involved chemotransmitters or local hormones, receptors, enzymes, carrier molecules and other specialised macromolecules such as DNA. Most medicinal drugs act by altering the body's control systems; in general they do so by binding to some specialised constituent of the cell selectively to alter its function and consequently that of the physiological or pathological system to which it contributes. Such drugs are structurally specific in that small modifications to their chemical structure may profoundly alter their effect.

MECHANISMS

An overview of the mechanisms of drug action shows that drugs act **on the cell membrane** by:

* Action on *specific receptors*,[1] e.g. agonists and antagonists on adrenoceptors, histamine receptors, acetylcholine receptors
* Interference with selective *passage of ions across membranes*, e.g. calcium entry (or channel) blockers
* Inhibition of membrane bound *enzymes and*

---

[1] A receptor mediates a biological effect, e.g. adrenoceptor; a binding site, e.g. on plasma albumin, does not.

pumps, e.g. membrane bound ATPase by cardiac glycoside; tricyclic antidepressants block the pump by which amines are actively taken up from the exterior to the interior of nerve cells.

Drugs act on **metabolic processes within the cell** by:

* *Enzyme inhibition,* e.g. platelet cyclo-oxygenase by aspirin, cholinesterase by pyridostigmine, xanthine oxidase by allopurinol
* Inhibition of *transport processes* that carry substances across cells, e.g. blockade of anion transport in the renal tubule cell by probenecid can be used to delay excretion of penicillin, and to enhance elimination of urate
* *Incorporation into larger molecules,* e.g. 5-fluorouracil, an anticancer drug, is incorporated into messenger-RNA in place of uracil
* In the case of successful *antimicrobial* agents, altering metabolic processes unique to microorganisms, e.g. penicillin interferes with formation of the bacterial cell wall, or by showing enormous quantitative differences in affecting a process common to both humans and microbes, e.g. inhibition of folic acid synthesis by trimethoprim.

Drugs act **outside the cell** by:

* *Direct chemical interaction,* e.g. chelating agents, antacids
* *Osmosis,* as with purgatives, e.g. magnesium sulphate, and diuretics, e.g. mannitol, which are active because neither they nor the water in which they are dissolved are absorbed by the cells lining the gut and kidney tubules respectively.

RECEPTORS

Most receptors are protein macromolecules. When the agonist binds to the receptor, the proteins undergo an alteration in conformation which induces changes in systems within the cell that in turn bring about the response to the drug. Different types of effector-response exist. (1) The most swift are the *channel-linked receptors,* i.e. receptors coupled directly to membrane ion channels; neurotransmitters act on such receptors in the postsynaptic membrane of a nerve or muscle cell and give a response within milliseconds. (2) Another type of response involves receptors bound to the cell membrane and coupled to intracellular effector systems by a *G-protein*. Catecholamines (the *first messenger*) activate β-adrenoceptors to increase, through a coupled G-protein system, the activity of intracellular adenylate cyclase which raises the rate of formation of cyclic AMP (the *second messenger*), a modulator of the activity of several enzyme systems that cause the cell to act; the process takes seconds. (3) A third type of membrane-bound receptor is the *kinase-linked receptor* (so called because a protein kinase is incorporated within the structure), which is involved in the control of cell growth and differentiation, and the release of inflammatory mediators. (4) Within the cell itself, steroid and thyroid hormones act on nuclear receptors which regulate DNA transcription and, thereby, protein synthesis, a process which takes hours.

Radioligand binding studies[2] have shown that the receptor numbers do not remain constant but change according to circumstances. When tissues are continuously exposed to an agonist, the number of receptors decreases *(down-regulation)* and this may be a cause of tachyphylaxis (loss of efficacy with frequently repeated doses), e.g. in asthmatics who use adrenoceptor agonist bronchodilators excessively. Prolonged contact with an antagonist leads to formation of new receptors *(up-regulation)*. Indeed, one explanation for the worsening of angina pectoris or cardiac ventricular arrhythmia in some patients following abrupt withdrawal of a β-adrenoceptor blocker is that normal concentrations of circulating catecholamines now have access to an increased (up-regulated) population of β-adrenoceptors (see Chronic pharmacology, p. 119).

Agonists. Drugs that activate receptors do so because they resemble the natural transmitter or hormone, but their value in clinical practice often rests on their greater capacity to resist degradation

and so to act for longer than the natural substances (endogenous ligands) they mimic; for this reason bronchodilation produced by salbutamol lasts longer than that induced by adrenaline (epinephrine).

Antagonists (blockers) of receptors are sufficiently similar to the natural agonist to be 'recognised' by the receptor and to occupy it without activating a response, thereby preventing (blocking) the natural agonist from exerting its effect. Drugs that have no activating effect whatever on the receptor are termed *pure antagonists*. A receptor occupied by a low efficacy agonist is inaccessible to a subsequent dose of a high efficacy agonist, so that, in this specific situation, a low efficacy agonist acts as an antagonist. This can happen with opioids.

Partial agonists. Some drugs, in addition to blocking access of the natural agonist to the receptor, are capable of a low degree of activation, i.e. they have both antagonist and agonist action. Such substances are said to show *partial agonist activity* (PAA). The β-adrenoceptor antagonists pindolol and oxprenolol have partial agonist activity (in their case it is often called *intrinsic sympathomimetic activity*) (ISA), whilst propranolol is devoid of agonist activity, i.e. it is a pure antagonist. A patient may be as extensively 'β-blocked' by propranolol as by pindolol, i.e. exercise tachycardia is abolished, but the resting heart rate is lower on propranolol; such differences can have clinical importance.

Inverse agonists. Some substances produce effects that are specifically opposite to those of the agonist. The agonist action of benzodiazepines on the benzodiazepine receptor in the CNS produces sedation, anxiolysis, muscle relaxation and controls convulsions; substances called β-carbolines which also bind to this receptor cause stimulation, anxiety, increased muscle tone and convulsions; they are inverse agonists. Both types of drug act by modulating the effects of the neurotransmitter gamma-aminobutyric acid (GABA).

Receptor binding (and vice versa). If the forces that bind drug to receptor are weak (hydrogen bonds, van der Waals bonds, electrostatic bonds), the binding will be easily and rapidly reversible; if the forces involved are strong (covalent bonds),

---

[2] The extraordinary discrimination of this technique is shown by the calculation that the total β-adrenoceptor protein in a large cow amounts to 1 mg (Maguire ME et al 1977 In: Greengard P, Robison GA (eds) Advances in Cyclic Nucleotide Research. Raven Press, New York: 8:1.)

then binding will be effectively irreversible. An antagonist that binds reversibly to a receptor can by definition be displaced from the receptor by mass action (see p. 99) of the agonist (and vice versa). If the concentration of agonist increases sufficiently above that of the antagonist the response is restored. This phenomenon is commonly seen in clinical practice — patients who are taking a β-adrenoceptor blocker, and whose low resting heart rate can be increased by exercise, are showing that they can raise their sympathetic drive to release enough noradrenaline (agonist) to diminish the prevailing degree of receptor blockade. Increasing the dose of β-adrenoceptor blocker will limit or abolish exercise-induced tachycardia, showing that the degree of blockade is enhanced as more drug becomes available to compete with the endogenous transmitter. Since agonist and antagonist compete to occupy the receptor according to the law of mass action, this type of drug action is termed *competitive antagonism.*

When receptor-mediated responses are studied either in isolated tissues or in intact man, a graph of the logarithm of the dose given (horizontal axis), plotted against the response obtained (vertical axis), commonly gives an S-shaped (sigmoid) curve, the central part of which is a straight line. If the measurements are repeated in the presence of an antagonist, and the curve obtained is parallel to the original but displaced to the **right,** then antagonism is said to be competitive and the agonist to be *surmountable.*

Drugs that bind *irreversibly* to receptors include phenoxybenzamine (to the α-adrenoceptor). Since such a drug cannot be displaced from the receptor, increasing the concentration of agonist does not fully restore the response and antagonism of this type is said to be *insurmountable.*

The log-dose-response curves for the agonist in the absence of and in the presence of a noncompetitive antagonist are not parallel. Some toxins act in this way, e.g. α-bungarotoxin, a constituent of some snake and spider venoms, binds irreversibly to the acetylcholine receptor and is used as a tool to study it. Restoration of the response after irreversible binding requires elimination of the drug from the body and synthesis of new receptor, and for this reason the effect may persist long after drug administration has ceased. Irreversible agents find little place in clinical practice.

Physiological (functional) antagonism

An action on the same receptor is not the only mechanism by which one drug may oppose the effect of another. Extreme bradycardia following overdose of a β-adrenoceptor blocker can be relieved by atropine which accelerates the heart by blockade of the parasympathetic branch of the autonomic nervous system, the cholinergic tone of which (vagal tone) operates continuously to slow it. Bronchoconstriction produced by histamine released from mast cells in anaphylactic shock can be counteracted by adrenaline (epinephrine), which relaxes bronchial smooth muscle (β_2-adrenoceptor effect) or by theophylline. In both cases, a pharmacological effect is overcome by a second drug which acts by a different physiological mechanism, i.e. there is physiological or functional antagonism.

ENZYMES

Interaction between drug and enzyme is in many respects similar to that between drug and receptor. Drugs may alter enzyme activity because they resemble a natural substrate and hence compete with it for the enzyme. For example, enalapril is effective in hypertension because it is structurally similar to that part of angiotensin I which is attacked by angiotensin-converting enzyme (ACE); by occupying the active site of the enzyme and so inhibiting its action enalapril prevents formation of the pressor angiotensin II. Carbidopa competes with levodopa for dopa decarboxylase and the benefit of this combination in Parkinson's disease is reduced metabolism of levodopa to dopamine in the blood (but not in the brain because carbidopa does not cross the blood–brain barrier). Ethanol prevents metabolism of methanol to its toxic metabolite, formic acid, by competing for occupancy of the enzyme alcohol dehydrogenase; this is the rationale for using ethanol in methanol poisoning. The above are examples of competitive **(reversible)** inhibition of enzyme activity.

Irreversible inhibition occurs with organophosphorus insecticides and chemical warfare agents (see p. 437) which combine covalently with the active site of acetylcholinesterase; recovery of cholinesterase activity depends on the formation of new enzyme. Covalent binding of aspirin to cyclo-oxygenase

(COX) inhibits the enzyme in platelets for their entire lifespan because platelets have no system for synthesising new protein and this is why low doses of aspirin are sufficient for antiplatelet action.

SELECTIVITY

The pharmacologist who produces a new drug and the doctor who gives it to a patient share the desire that it should possess a selective action so that additional and unwanted (adverse) effects do not complicate the management of the patient. Approaches to obtaining selectivity of drug action include the following.

Modification of drug structure

Many drugs are designed to have a structural similarity to some natural constituent of the body, e.g. a neurotransmitter, a hormone, a substrate for an enzyme; replacing or competing with that natural constituent achieves selectivity of action. Enormous scientific effort and expertise go into the synthesis and testing of analogues of natural substances in order to create drugs capable of obtaining a specified effect and that alone (see Therapeutic Index p. 94). The approach is the basis of modern drug design and it has led to the production of adrenoceptor antagonists, histamine-receptor antagonists and many other important medicines. But there are biological constraints to selectivity. Anticancer drugs that act against rapidly dividing cells lack selectivity because they also damage other tissues with a high cell replication rate, such as bone marrow and gut epithelium.

Selective delivery (drug targeting)

The objective of target tissue selectivity can sometimes be achieved by simple topical application, e.g. skin and eye, and by special drug delivery systems, as by intrabronchial administration of β_2-adrenoceptor agonists or corticosteroids (inhaled pressurised metered aerosol for asthma). Selective targeting of drugs to less accessible sites of disease offers considerable scope for therapy as technology develops, e.g. attaching drugs to antibodies selective for cancer cells.

Stereoselectivity

Drug molecules are three-dimensional and many drugs contain one or more *asymmetric* or *chiral*[3] centres in their structures, i.e. a single drug can be, in effect, a mixture of two nonidentical mirror images (like a mixture of left- and right-hand gloves). The two forms, which are known as *enantiomorphs,* can exhibit very different pharmacodynamic, pharmacokinetic and toxicological properties. For example, (1) the S form of warfarin is four times more active than the R form,[4] (2) the peak plasma concentration of S fenoprofen is four times that of R fenoprofen after oral administration of RS fenoprofen, and (3) the S, but not the R enantiomorph of thalidomide is metabolised to primary toxins. Many other drugs are available as mixtures of enantiomorphs (racemates). Pharmaceutical development of drugs as single enantiomers rather than as racemic mixtures offers the prospect of greater selectivity of action and lessens risk of toxicity.

Quantitative aspects

That a drug has a desired qualitative action is obviously all-important, but it is not by itself enough. There are also quantitative aspects, i.e. the right amount of action is required and with some drugs the dose has to be very precisely adjusted to deliver this, neither too little nor too much, to escape both inefficacy and toxicity, e.g. digoxin, lithium, gentamicin. Whilst the general correlation between dose and response may evoke no surprise, certain characteristics of the relation are fundamental to the way drugs are used. These are:

DOSE–RESPONSE CURVES

Conventionally dose is plotted on the horizontal and response on the vertical axis. The *slope* of the dose–response curve defines the extent to which a desired response alters as the dose is changed. A

---

[3] Greek: *cheir,* a hand
[4] R (rectus) and S (sinister) refer to the sequential arrangement of the constituent parts of the molecule around the chiral center.

steep-rising and prolonged curve indicates that a small change in dose produces a large change in drug effect over a wide dose range, e.g. with the loop diuretic, frusemide (furosemide) (used in doses from 20 mg to over 250 mg/d). By contrast the dose–response curve for the thiazide diuretics soon reaches a plateau and the clinically useful dose range for bendrofluazide (bendroflumethiazide), for example, extends from 5 mg to 10 mg; increasing the dose beyond this produces no added diuretic effect though it adds to toxicity.

Dose–response curves may be constructed for *wanted* effects, and also for *unwanted* effects (see Fig. 7.1, below).

POTENCY AND PHARMACOLOGICAL EFFICACY

The terms potency and efficacy are often used imprecisely and therefore, confusingly. It is pertinent to make a clear distinction between them, particularly in relation to claims made for usefulness in therapeutics.

Potency is the amount (weight) of drug in relation to its effect, e.g. if weight-for-weight drug A has a greater effect than drug B, then drug A is more potent than drug B, although the maximum therapeutic effect obtainable may be similar with both drugs. The diuretic effect of bumetanide 1 mg is equivalent to frusemide 50 mg, thus bumetanide is more *potent* than frusemide but both drugs achieve about the same maximum effect. The difference in weight of drug that has to be administered is of no clinical significance unless it is great.

Pharmacological efficacy refers to the strength of response induced by occupancy of a receptor by an agonist (intrinsic activity); it is a specialised pharmacological concept. But clinicians are concerned with therapeutic efficacy, as follows.

THERAPEUTIC EFFICACY

Therapeutic efficacy, or effectiveness, is the capacity of a drug to produce an effect and refers to the maximum such effect, e.g. if drug A can produce a therapeutic effect that cannot be obtained with drug B, however much of drug B is given, then drug A has the higher therapeutic efficacy. Differences in therapeutic efficacy are of great clinical importance. Amiloride (*low* efficacy) can at best cause no more than 5% of the sodium load filtered by the glomeruli to be excreted; and there is no point in increasing the dose beyond that which achieves this for no greater diuretic effect can be attained. Bendrofluazide (*moderate* efficacy) can cause no more than 10% of the filtered sodium load to be excreted no matter how much drug is administered. Frusemide (*high* efficacy) can cause 25% and more of filtered sodium to be excreted; hence it is called a high efficacy diuretic.

THERAPEUTIC INDEX

When the dose of a drug is increased progressively, the desired response in the patient usually rises to a maximum beyond which further increases in dose elicit no greater benefit but induce only unwanted effects. This is because a drug does not have a single dose–response curve, but a different curve for *each action*, wanted as well as unwanted. New and unwanted actions are recruited if dose is increased after the maximum therapeutic effect has been achieved.

A sympathomimetic bronchodilator might exhibit one dose–response relation for decreasing airways resistance (wanted) and another for increase in heart rate (unwanted). Clearly the usefulness of any drug is intimately related to the extent to which such dose–response relations can be separated. Ehrlich (p. 201) introduced the concept of the therapeutic index or ratio as the maximum tolerated dose divided by the minimum curative dose but, since such single doses cannot be determined accurately, the index is never calculated in this way in man. More realistically, a dose that has some unwanted effect in 50% of humans, e.g. a specified increase in heart rate (in the case of an adrenoceptor agonist bronchodilator) can be related to that which is therapeutic in 50% (ED_{50}), e.g. a specified decrease in airways resistance (in practice such information is not available for many drugs). Nevertheless the therapeutic index does embody a concept that is fundamental in comparing the usefulness of one drug with another, namely, safety in relation to efficacy. The concept is expressed diagrammatically in Figure 7.1.

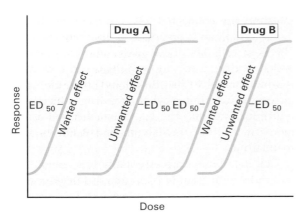

Fig. 7.1 Dose–response curves for two hypothetical drugs. Drug X: the dose that brings about the maximum wanted effect is less than the lowest dose that produces the unwanted effect. The ratio ED50 (unwanted effect)/ED50 (wanted effect) indicates that drug X has a large therapeutic index: it is thus highly selective in its wanted action. Drug Y causes unwanted effects at doses well below those which produce its maximum benefit. The ratio ED50 (unwanted effect)/ED50 (wanted effect) indicates that the drug has a small therapeutic index: it is thus nonselective.

TOLERANCE

Continuous or repeated or administration of a drug is often accompanied by a gradual diminution of the effect it produces. Tolerance is said to have been *acquired* when it becomes necessary to increase the dose of a drug to get an effect previously obtained with a smaller dose, i.e. reduced sensitivity. By contrast, the term *tachyphylaxis* describes the phenomenon of progressive lessening of effect (refractoriness) in response to frequently administered doses (see Receptors, p. 91); it tends to develop more rapidly than tolerance.

Tolerance is readily observed with opioids, as witness the huge doses of morphine that may necessary to maintain pain relief in terminal care; the effect is due to reduced pharmacological efficacy (p. 94) at receptor sites or to down-regulation of receptors. Tolerance is acquired rapidly with nitrates used to prevent angina, possibly mediated by the generation of oxygen free radicals from nitric oxide; it can be avoided by removing transdermal nitrate patches for 4–8 h, e.g. at night, to allow the plasma concentration to fall.

Increased metabolism as a result of enzyme induction (see p. 113) also leads to tolerance, as experience shows with alcohol, taken regularly as opposed to sporadically. There is commonly cross-tolerance between drugs of similar structure.

Failure of certain individuals to respond to normal doses of a drug, e.g. resistance to warfarin, vitamin D, may be said to constitute a form of *natural* tolerance (see Pharmacogenetics p. 122).

BIOASSAY AND STANDARDISATION

Biological assay (bioassay) is the process by which the activity of a substance (identified or unidentified) is measured on living material: e.g. contraction of bronchial, uterine or vascular muscle. It is used only when chemical or physical methods are not practicable as in the case of a mixture of active substances, or of an incompletely purified preparation, or where no chemical method has been developed. The activity of a preparation is expressed relative to that of a standard preparation of the same substance. Biological *standardisation* is a specialised form of bioassay. It involves matching of material of unknown potency with an International or National Standard with the objective of providing a preparation for use in therapeutics and research. The results are expressed as *units* of a substance rather than its weight, e.g. insulin, vaccines.

Pharmacokinetics

To initiate a desired drug action is a qualitative choice but, when the qualitative choice is made, considerations of quantity immediately arise; it is possible to have too much or too little of a good thing. To obtain the right effect at the right intensity, at the right time, for the right duration, with minimum risk of unpleasantness or harm, is what pharmacokinetics is about.

Dosage regimens of long-established drugs were devised by trial and error. Doctors learned by experience the dose, the frequency of dosing and the route of administration that was most likely to benefit and least likely to harm. Apart from being laborious and putting patients at risk, this empirical ('suck it and see') approach left some questions unanswered. It did not explain, for example, why digoxin is effective in a once-daily dose, whereas paracetamol may need to be given six times daily; why the same dose of morphine is more effective if it is given intramuscularly than if is taken by mouth; why insulin is useless unless it is injected. The answers to these questions lie in understanding how drugs cross membranes to enter the body, how they are distributed round it in the blood and other body fluids, how they are bound to plasma proteins and tissues (which act as stores) and how they are eliminated from the body. These processes can now be quantified and allow efficient development of dosing regimens.

> **Pharmacokinetics**[5] is concerned with the rate at which drug molecules cross cell membranes to enter the body, to distribute within it and to leave the body, as well as with the structural changes (metabolism) to which they are subject within it.

The subject will be discussed under the following headings:

* Drug passage across cell membranes
* Order of reaction or process (first- and zero-order)
* Time course of drug concentration and effect
  Plasma half-life and steady-state concentration
  Therapeutic monitoring
* The individual processes
  Absorption
  Distribution
  Metabolism (biotransformation)
  Elimination.

Drug passage across cell membranes

Certain concepts are fundamental to understanding how drug molecules make their way around the body to achieve their effect. The first concerns the modes by which drugs cross cell membranes and cells.

Our bodies are labyrinths of fluid-filled spaces. Some, such as the lumina of the kidney tubules or

intestine, are connected to the outside world; the blood, lymph and cerebrospinal fluid are enclosed. Sheets of cells line these spaces and the extent to which a drug can cross epithelia or endothelia is fundamental to its clinical use. It is the major factor that determines whether a drug can be taken orally for systemic effect and whether within the glomerular filtrate it will be reabsorbed or excreted in the urine.

Cell membranes are essentially bilayers of lipid molecules with 'islands' of protein and they preserve and regulate the internal environment. Lipid-soluble substances diffuse readily into cells and therefore throughout body tissues. So-called tight junctions, some of which are traversed by water-filled channels through which water-soluble substances of small molecular size may filter, link adjacent epithelial or endothelial cells. The jejunum and proximal renal tubule contain many such channels and are called leaky epithelia, whereas the tight junctions in the stomach and urinary bladder do not have these channels and water cannot pass; they are termed tight epithelia. Special protein molecules within the lipid bilayer allow specific substances to enter or leave the cell preferentially (carrier proteins). The natural processes of passive diffusion, filtration and carrier-mediated transport determine the passage of drugs across membranes and cells.

PASSIVE DIFFUSION

This is the most important means by which a drug enters the tissues and is distributed through them. It refers simply to the natural tendency of any substance to move passively from an area of high concentration to one of low concentration. In the context of an individual cell, the drug moves at a rate proportional to the concentration difference across the cell membrane, i.e. it shows first-order kinetics (see p. 99); cellular energy is not required, which means that the process does not become saturated and is not inhibited by other substances.

The extent to which drugs are soluble in water or lipid is central to their capacity to cross cell membranes. Water or lipid solubility is influenced by environmental pH and the structural properties of the molecule.

---

[5] Greek: *pharmacon* drug, *kinein* to move.

The presence of a benzene ring, a hydrocarbon chain, a steroid nucleus or halogen (-Br, -Cl, -F) groups favours lipid solubility. Water solubility is favoured by the possession of alcoholic (-OH), amide (-CO.NH$_2$) or carboxylic (-COOH) groups, and the formation of glucuronide and sulphate conjugates.

It is useful to classify drugs in a physicochemical sense into:

- Those that are variably *ionised* according to environmental pH (electrolytes) (lipid-soluble or water-soluble)
- Those that are *incapable* of becoming ionised whatever the environmental pH (un-ionised, nonpolar substances) (lipid-soluble)
- Those that are *permanently* ionised whatever the environmental pH (ionised, polar substances) (water-soluble).

DRUGS IONISED BY ENVIRONMENTAL pH

Many drugs are weak electrolytes, i.e. their structural groups ionise to a greater or lesser extent, according to environmental pH. Most such molecules are present partly in the ionised and partly in the un-ionised state. The degree of ionisation influences lipid-solubility (and hence diffusibility) and so affects absorption, distribution and elimination.

Ionisable groups in a drug molecule tend either to lose a hydrogen ion (acidic groups) or to add a hydrogen ion (basic groups). The extent to which a molecule has this tendency to ionise is given by the dissociation (or ionisation) constant (Ka). This is usually expressed as the pKa, i.e. the negative logarithm of the Ka (just as pH is the negative logarithm of the hydrogen ion concentration). In an acidic environment, i.e. one already containing many free hydrogen ions, an acidic group tends to retain a hydrogen ion and remains un-ionised; a relative deficit of free hydrogen ions, i.e. a basic environment, favours loss of the hydrogen ion from an acidic group which thus becomes ionised. The opposite is the case for a base. The issue may be summarised:

- Acidic groups become less ionised in an acidic environment

- Basic groups become less ionised in a basic (alkaline) environment and vice versa.

This in turn influences *diffusibility* since:

- Un-ionised drug is lipid-soluble and diffusible
- Ionised drug is lipid-insoluble and nondiffusible.

The profound effect of environmental pH on the degree of ionisation is best shown when the relation between these is quantified. It is convenient to remember that when the pH of the environment is the same as the pKa of a drug within it, then the ratio of un-ionised to ionised molecules is 1:1. But for every unit by which pH is changed, the ratio of un-ionised to ionised molecules changes 10-fold. Thus when the pH is 2 units less than the pKa, molecules of an acid become 100 times more *un-ionised* and when the pH is 2 units more than the pKa, molecules of an acid become 100 more *ionised*. Such pH change profoundly affects drug kinetics.

pH variation and drug kinetics. Studies of the partitioning of a drug across a lipid membrane according to differences in pH have been developed as the *pH partition hypothesis*. There is a wide range of pH in the gut (pH 1.5 in the stomach; 6.8 in the upper and 7.6 in the lower intestine). But the pH inside the body is maintained within a limited range (pH 7.46 ± 0.04) so that only drugs that are substantially un-ionised at this pH will be lipid-soluble, diffuse across tissue boundaries and so be widely distributed, e.g. into the CNS. Urine pH varies between the extremes of 4.6 and 8.2; thus the amount of drug reabsorbed from the renal tubular lumen by passive diffusion can be very much affected by the prevailing urine pH.

Consider the effect of pH changes on the disposition of aspirin (acetylsalicylic acid, pKa 3.5). In the stomach aspirin is un-ionised and thus lipid-soluble and diffusible. When aspirin enters the gastric epithelial cells (pH 7.4) it will ionise, become less diffusible and so will localise there. This *ion trapping* is one mechanism whereby aspirin is concentrated in, and so harms, the gastric mucosa. In the body aspirin is metabolised to salicylic acid (pKa 3.0), which at pH 7.4 is highly ionised and thus remains in the extracellular fluid. Eventually the molecules of salicylic acid in the plasma are filtered by the glomeruli and pass into the tubular fluid, which is generally more acidic than plasma and causes a proportion of salicylic acid to become un-ionised and lipid-soluble so that it diffuses back into the tubular cells. Alkalinising the urine with sodium bicarbonate causes more salicylic acid to become ionised and lipid-insoluble so that it remains in the tubular fluid, and is eliminated in the urine. The effect is sufficiently great for alkalinising the urine to be effective treatment for salicylate (aspirin) overdose. Conversely, acidifying the urine increases the elimination of the base amphetamine (pKa 9.9) (see Acidification of urine, p. 156).

DRUGS INCAPABLE OF BECOMING IONISED

These include digoxin and steroid hormones such as prednisolone. Effectively lacking any ionisable groups, they are unaffected by environmental pH, are lipid-soluble and so diffuse readily across tissue boundaries. These drugs are also referred to as nonpolar.

PERMANENTLY IONISED DRUGS

Drugs that are permanently ionised contain groups which dissociate so strongly that they remain ionised over the range of the body pH. Such compounds are termed polar, for their groups are either negatively charged (acidic, e.g. heparin) or positively charged (basic, e.g. ipratropium, tubocurarine, suxamethonium) and all have a very limited capacity to cross cell membranes. This is a disadvantage in the case of heparin, which is not absorbed by the gut and must be given parenterally. Conversely, heparin is a useful anticoagulant in pregnancy because it does not cross the placenta (which the orally effective warfarin does and is liable to cause fetal haemorrhage as well as being teratogenic). The *clinical relevance* of drug passage across membranes may be illustrated with reference to the following:

Brain and cerebrospinal fluid (CSF). The capillaries of the cerebral circulation differ from those in most other parts of the body in that they lack the filtration channels between endothelial cells through which substances in the blood nominally gain access to the extracellular fluid. Tight junctions between adjacent capillary endothelial cells, together with their basement membrane and a thin covering from the processes of astrocytes, separate the blood from the brain tissue. This barrier places constraints on the passage of substances from the blood to the brain and CSF. Compounds that are lipid-insoluble do not cross it readily, e.g. atenolol, compared with propranolol (lipid-soluble), and CNS side-effects are more prominent with the latter. Therapy with methotrexate (lipid-insoluble) may fail to eliminate leukaemic deposits in the CNS. Conversely lipid-soluble substances enter brain tissue with ease; thus diazepam (lipid-soluble) given intravenously is effective within one minute for status epilepticus, and effects of alcohol (ethanol) by mouth are noted within minutes; the level of general anaesthesia can be controlled closely by altering the concentration of inhaled anaesthetic gas (lipid-soluble).

Placenta. Chorionic villi, consisting of a layer of trophoblastic cells that enclose fetal capillaries, are bathed in maternal blood. The large surface area and blood flow (500 ml/min) are essential for gas exchange, uptake of nutrients and elimination of waste products. A lipid barrier that allows the passage of lipid-soluble substances but excludes water-soluble compounds, especially those with molecular weight exceeding 600,[6] therefore separates the fetal and maternal bloodstreams. This exclusion is of particular importance with short-term use, e.g. tubocurarine (mol. wt 772) (lipid-insoluble) or gallamine (mol. wt 891) used as a muscle relaxant during Caesarian section do not affect the infant; with prolonged use, however, all compounds will eventually enter the fetus to some extent (see: Drugs and the embryo and fetus).

FILTRATION

Aqueous channels in the tight junctions between adjacent epithelial cells allow the passage of some water-soluble substances. Neutral or uncharged, i.e. nonpolar, molecules pass most readily since the pores are electrically charged. Within the alimentary tract, channels are largest and most numerous in jejunal epithelium and filtration allows for rapid

---

[6] Most drugs have a molecular weight of less than 600 (e.g. diazepam 284, morphine 303) but some have more (erythromycin 733, digoxin 780).

equilibration of concentrations and consequently of osmotic pressures across the mucosa. Ions such as sodium enter the body through the aqueous channels, the size of which probably limits passage to substances of low molecular weight, e.g. ethanol (mol. wt 46). Filtration seems to play at most a minor role in drug transfer within the body except for glomerular filtration, which is an important mechanism of drug excretion.

CARRIER-MEDIATED TRANSPORT

Some drugs move into or out of cells against a concentration gradient, i.e. by active transport. These processes involve endogenous molecules, expend cellular energy and are more rapid than transfer by diffusion. The mechanisms show a high degree of specificity for particular compounds because they have evolved from biological needs for the uptake of essential nutrients or elimination of metabolic products. Thus, drugs that are subject to them bear some structural resemblance to natural constituents of the body. Examples of active transport systems are the absorption of iron by the gut, levodopa across the blood–brain barrier and the secretion of many organic acids and bases by renal tubular and biliary duct cells. Carrier-mediated transport that does not require energy is called *facilitated diffusion,* e.g. vitamin B_{12} absorption; carrier-mediated transport is subject to saturation and can be inhibited.

The order of reaction or process

In the body, drug molecules cross cell membranes, are transported across cells, and many are altered by being metabolised. These movements and changes involve interaction with membranes, carrier proteins and enzymes, either as individual chemical reactions or as processes. The *rate* at which these movements or changes can take place is subject to important influences that are referred to as the *order* of reaction or process. In biology generally, two orders of such reactions are recognised, and are summarised as follows:

- First-order processes by which a constant *fraction* of drug is transported/metabolised in unit time.

- Zero-order processes by which a constant *amount* of drug is transported/metabolised in unit time.

FIRST-ORDER (EXPONENTIAL) PROCESSES

In the majority of instances the rates at which absorption, distribution, metabolism and excretion of a drug occur are directly proportional to its concentration in the body. In other words, transfer of drug across a cell membrane or formation of a metabolite is high at high concentrations and falls in direct proportion to be low at low concentrations (an exponential relationship). This is because the processes follow the Law of Mass Action, which states that the rate of reaction is directly proportional to the active masses of reacting substances. In other words, at high concentrations, there are more opportunities for crowded molecules to interact with each other or to cross cell membranes than at low, uncrowded concentrations. Processes for which rate of reaction is proportional to concentration are called *first-order.*

In doses used clinically, most drugs are subject to first-order processes of absorption, distribution, metabolism and elimination. The knowledge that a drug exhibits first-order kinetics is useful. This chapter later illustrates how the rate of elimination of a drug from the plasma falls as the concentration in plasma falls and the time for any plasma concentration to fall by 50% ($t\frac{1}{2}$, the plasma half-life) will always be the same. Thus it becomes possible to quote a constant value for the $t\frac{1}{2}$ of the drug. This occurs because rate and concentration are in proportion, i.e. the process obeys first-order kinetics. The important calculations that depend on knowing $t\frac{1}{2}$, i.e. time to eliminate a drug, time to achieve steady-state plasma concentration, and the construction of dosing schedules, will be correct when the order of reactions involved is known and, in the present case, are first-order.

Zero-order processes (saturation kinetics)

As the amount of drug in the body rises, any metabolic reactions or processes that have limited capacity become saturated. In other words, the rate of the process reaches a maximum amount at which it stays constant, e.g. due to limited activity of an enzyme, and further increase in rate is impossible despite an increase in the dose of drug. Clearly, these are circumstances in which the rate of reaction is no longer proportional to dose, and processes that exhibit this type of kinetics are described as rate-limited or dose-dependent or zero-order or as showing *saturation kinetics*. In practice enzyme-mediated metabolic reactions are the most likely to show rate-limitation because the amount of enzyme present is finite and can become saturated. Passive diffusion does not become saturated. There are some important consequences of zero-order kinetics.

Alcohol (ethanol) (see also p. 178) is a drug whose kinetics has considerable implications for society as well as for the individual, as follows.

Alcohol is subject to first-order kinetics with a $t\frac{1}{2}$ of about one hour at plasma concentrations below 10 mg/dl [attained after drinking about two-thirds of a unit (glass) of wine or beer]. Above this concentration the main enzyme (alcohol dehydrogenase) that converts the alcohol into acetaldehyde approaches and then reaches saturation, at which point alcohol metabolism cannot proceed any faster. Thus if the subject continues to drink, the blood alcohol concentration rises disproportionately, for the rate of metabolism remains the same (at about 10 ml or 8 g/h for a 70 kg man), i.e. a constant amount is metabolised in unit time, and alcohol shows zero-order kinetics.

Consider a man of average size whose life is unhappy to a degree where he drinks about half (375 ml) a standard bottle of whisky (40% alcohol), i.e. 150 ml of alcohol, over a short period, absorbs it and goes very drunk to bed at midnight with a blood alcohol concentration of about 250 mg/dl. If alcohol metabolism were subject to first-order kinetics, with a half-life ($t\frac{1}{2}$) of one hour throughout the whole range of social consumption, the subject would halve his blood alcohol concentration each hour (see Fig. 7.2) and it is easy to calculate that, when he drove his car to work at 08.00 h the next morning, he would have a negligible blood alcohol concentration (less than 1 mg/dl); though, no doubt, a severe hangover might reduce his driving skill.

But at these high concentrations, alcohol is subject to zero-order kinetics and so, metabolising about 10 ml of alcohol per hour, after 8 h the subject will have eliminated 80 ml, leaving 70 ml in his body and giving a blood concentration of about 120 mg/dl. At this level his driving skill would be seriously impaired. The subject could have an accident and be convicted of drunk driving on his way to work despite his indignant protests that the blood or breath alcohol determination must be faulty since he has not touched a drop since midnight. He would be banned from the road, and thus have leisure to reflect on the difference between first-order and zero-order kinetics.

This is an example thought up for this occasion, although no doubt something close to it happens in real life often enough, but an example important in therapeutics is provided by *phenytoin*. At low doses the elimination of phenytoin proceeds as a first-order process and as dose is increased there is a directly proportional increase in the steady-state plasma concentration because elimination increases to match the increase in dose. But gradually the enzymatic elimination process approaches and reaches saturation, attaining a maximum rate beyond which it cannot increase; the process has become constant and zero-order. Since further increases in dose cannot be matched by increase in the rate of metabolism the plasma concentration rises steeply and disproportionately, with danger of toxicity. *Salicylate* metabolism also exhibits saturation kinetics but at high therapeutic doses. Clearly saturation kinetics is a significant factor in delay in recovery from drug overdose, e.g. with aspirin or phenytoin.

When a drug is subject to first-order kinetics and by definition the rate of elimination is proportional to plasma concentration, then the $t\frac{1}{2}$ is a constant characteristic, i.e. a constant value can be quoted throughout the plasma concentration range (accepting that there will be variation in $t\frac{1}{2}$ between individuals), and this is convenient. If the rate of a process, e.g. removal from the plasma by metabolism, is not directly proportional to plasma concentration, then the $t\frac{1}{2}$ cannot be constant. Consequently, when a drug exhibits zero-order elimination kinetics no single value for its $t\frac{1}{2}$ can be quoted for, in fact, $t\frac{1}{2}$ decreases as plasma concentration falls and the calculations on elimination and dosing that are so easy with first-order elimination (see below) become too complicated to be of much practical use.

Zero-order *absorption* processes apply to iron, to depot i.m. formulations and to drug implants, e.g. antipsychotics and sex hormones.

> The $t\frac{1}{2}$ is the single pharmacokinetic characteristic of a drug that it is most useful to know.

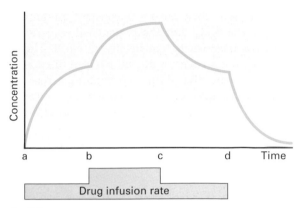

Fig. 7.3

Time course of drug concentration and effect

PLASMA HALF-LIFE AND STEADY-STATE CONCENTRATION

The manner in which plasma drug concentration rises or falls when dosing is begun, altered or ceased follows certain simple rules, which provide a means for rational control of drug effect. Central to understanding these is the concept of **half-life** (**t$\frac{1}{2}$**) or half-time. Consider the time course of a drug in the blood after an i.v. bolus injection, i.e. a single dose injected in a period of seconds as distinct from a continuous infusion. Plasma concentration will rise quickly as drug enters the blood to reach a peak; there will then be a sharp drop as the drug distributes round the body (*distribution phase*), which will be followed by a steady decline as drug is removed from the blood by the liver or kidneys (*elimination phase*). If the elimination processes are first-order, the time taken for any concentration point in the elimination phase to fall to half its value is always the same; in other words, the t$\frac{1}{2}$, which is the time taken for the plasma concentration to fall by half, is a constant, as is illustrated in Figure 7.2. Note that from the peak concentration the drug is virtually eliminated from the plasma in 5 t$\frac{1}{2}$ periods.

The t$\frac{1}{2}$ may be used to predict the manner in which plasma concentration alters in response to starting, altering or ceasing drug administration. These events are illustrated in Figure 7.3 and the subsequent text.

Increases in plasma concentration

When a drug is infused at a constant rate the amount in the body and with it the plasma concentration rise until a state is reached at which the rate of administration of drug to the body is exactly equal to the rate of elimination. This is called the *steady state*: when it is attained the amount of drug in the body remains constant, i.e. the plasma concentration is on a *plateau*, and a stable drug effect can be assumed. Figure 7.3 depicts the smooth changes in plasma concentration that result from a constant i.v. infusion. Clearly if a drug is given by intermittent oral or intravenous dose, the plasma concentration will fluctuate between peaks and troughs, but in time all the peaks will be of equal height and all the troughs will be of equal depth; this is also called a steady-state concentration, since the mean concentration is constant.[7]

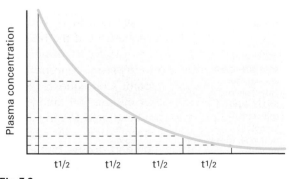

Fig. 7.2

---

[7] The peaks and troughs can be of practical importance with drugs of low therapeutic index, e.g. aminoglycoside antibiotics, and it may be necessary to monitor both for safe and effective therapy.

Time to reach steady state

If a drug is administered by constant-rate i.v. infusion it is important to know *when* steady state has been reached, for maintaining the same dosing schedule will then ensure a constant amount of drug in the body and the patient will experience neither acute toxicity nor decline of effect. The $t\frac{1}{2}$ provides the answer: with the passage of each $t\frac{1}{2}$ period of time, the plasma concentration rises by **half** the difference between the current concentration and the ultimate steady-state (100%) concentration. Thus:

in $1 \times t\frac{1}{2}$, the concentration will reach (100/2) 50%,

in $2 \times t\frac{1}{2}$ (50 + 50/2) 75%,
in $3 \times t\frac{1}{2}$ (75 + 25/2) 87.5%,
in $4 \times t\frac{1}{2}$ (87.5 + 12.5/2) 93.75%
in $5 \times t\frac{1}{2}$ (93.75 + 6.25/2) 96.875% of the ultimate steady state.

> When a drug is given at a constant rate (continuous or intermittent) the *time to reach steady* state depends only on the $t\frac{1}{2}$ and, for all practical purposes, after $5 \times t\frac{1}{2}$ the amount of drug in the body will be constant and the plasma concentration will be at a plateau.

Changes in plasma concentration

The same principle holds for change from any steady-state plasma concentration to a new steady state brought about by increase or decrease in the rate of drug administration, provided the kinetics remain first-order. Thus when the rate of administration is altered to cause either a rise or a fall in plasma concentration, a new steady-state concentration will eventually be reached and it will take a time equal to $5 \times t\frac{1}{2}$ to reach the new steady state.

Note that the actual **level** of any steady-state plasma concentration (as opposed to the **time taken** to reach it) is determined only by the difference between the rate of drug administration (input) and the rate of elimination (output). If drug elimination remains constant and administration is increased by 50%, in time a new steady-state concentration will be reached which will be 50% greater than the original.

Decline in plasma concentration

Since $t\frac{1}{2}$ is the time taken for any plasma concentration to decline by one-half, starting at any steady-state (100%) plasma concentration, in $1 \times t\frac{1}{2}$ the plasma concentration will fall to 50%, in $2 \times t\frac{1}{2}$ to 25%, in $3 \times t\frac{1}{2}$ to 12.5%, in $4 \times t\frac{1}{2}$ to 6.25% and in $5 \times t\frac{1}{2}$ to 3.125% of the original steady-state concentration.

Hence the $t\frac{1}{2}$ can predict the rate and extent of decline in plasma concentration after dosing is discontinued. The relation between $t\frac{1}{2}$ and time to reach steady-state plasma concentration applies to all drugs that obey first-order kinetics, as much to dobutamine ($t\frac{1}{2}$ 2 min) when it is useful to know that an alteration of infusion rate will reach a plateau within 10 min, as to digoxin ($t\frac{1}{2}$ 36 h) when a constant (repeated) dose will give a steady-state plasma concentration only after 7.5 days. Plasma $t\frac{1}{2}$ values are given in the text where they seem particularly relevant. Inevitably, natural variation within the population produces a range in $t\frac{1}{2}$ values for any drug. For clarity only, single average $t\frac{1}{2}$ values are given while recognising that the population range may be as much as 50% from the stated figure in either direction.

A few $t\frac{1}{2}$ values are listed in Table 7.1 so that they can be pondered upon in relation to dosing in clinical practice.

Biological effect $t\frac{1}{2}$ is the time in which the biological effect of a drug declines by one half. With drugs that act competitively on receptors (α- and β-adrenoceptor agonists and antagonists) the biological effect $t\frac{1}{2}$ can be provided with reasonable accuracy.

TABLE 7.1 Plasma $t\frac{1}{2}$ of some drugs

Drug	$t\frac{1}{2}$
adenosine	< 2 sec
dobutamine	2 min
benzylpenicillin	30 min
amoxycillin	1 h
paracetamol	2 h
midazolam	3 h
tolbutamide	6 h
atenolol	7 h
dothiepin (dosulepin)	25 h
diazepam	40 h
piroxicam	45 h
ethosuximide	54 h

Sometimes the biological effect $t\frac{1}{2}$ cannot be provided, e.g. with antimicrobials when the number of infecting organisms and their sensitivity determine the outcome.

THERAPEUTIC MONITORING

The issues that concern the practising doctor are not primarily those of changing drug plasma concentration but relate to drug effect: to the onset, magnitude and duration of action of individual doses. Accurate information about the time course of drug action is less readily obtained than that about plasma concentration. This immediately raises implications about the relation between plasma concentration and drug effect and, particularly, the extent to which useful response may be predicted by measuring the concentration of drug in plasma.

Experience shows that patients differ greatly in the amount of drug required to achieve the same response. The dose of warfarin that maintains a therapeutic concentration may vary as much as 5-fold between individuals, and there are many other examples. This is hardly surprising considering known variation in rates of drug metabolism, in disposition and in tissue responsiveness, and it raises the question of how optimal drug effect can be achieved quickly in each patient, i.e. can drug therapy be individualised? A logical approach is to assume that effect is related to drug concentration at the receptor site in the tissues and that in turn the plasma concentration is likely to be constantly related to, though not necessarily the same as, tissue concentration. Indeed, for many drugs, correlation between plasma concentration and clinical effect is better than that between dose and effect. Yet monitoring therapy by measuring drug in plasma is of practical use only in selected instances. The reasons for this repay some thought.

Plasma concentration may not be worth measuring. This is the case where dose can be titrated against a quickly and easily measured effect such as blood pressure (antihypertensives), body weight (diuretics), INR (oral anticoagulants) or blood sugar (hypoglycaemics).

Plasma concentration has no correlation with effect. This is the case with drugs that act irreversibly and these have been named 'hit and run drugs' because their effect persists long after the drug has left the plasma. Such drugs destroy or inactivate target tissue (enzyme, receptor) and restoration of effect occurs only after days or weeks, when resynthesis takes place, e.g. some monoamine oxidase inhibitors, aspirin (on platelets), some anticholinesterases and anticancer drugs.

Plasma concentration may correlate poorly with effect. Inflammatory states may cause misleading results if only total drug concentration is measured. Many basic drugs, e.g. lidocaine, disopyramide, bind to acute phase proteins, e.g. α_1-acid glycoprotein, which are present in greatly elevated concentration in inflammatory states. The consequent rise in total drug concentration is due to increase in bound (inactive) but not in the free (active) concentration and correlation with effect will be poor if only total drug is measured. The best correlation is likely to be achieved by measurement of free (active) drug in plasma water but this is technically more difficult and total drug in plasma is usually monitored in routine clinical practice.

The assay procedure may not measure metabolites of a drug that are pharmacologically active, e.g. some benzodiazepines, or may measure metabolites that are pharmacologically inactive; in either event correlation between plasma concentration and effect is weakened.

Plasma concentration may correlate well with effect. When this is the case, and when the therapeutic effect is inconvenient to measure, dosage may best be monitored according to the plasma concentration (in relation to a previously defined optimum range).

Plasma concentration monitoring has proved useful in the following situations:

- As a guide to the effectiveness of therapy, e.g. plasma gentamicin and other antimicrobials against sensitive bacteria, plasma theophylline for asthma, blood ciclosporin to avoid transplant rejection
- When the desired effect is suppression of infrequent sporadic events such as epileptic seizures or episodes of cardiac arrhythmia
- To reduce the risk of adverse drug effects, e.g. otic damage with aminoglycoside antibiotics or

adverse CNS effects of lithium, when therapeutic doses are close to toxic doses (low therapeutic index)

- When lack of therapeutic effect and toxicity may be difficult to distinguish. Digoxin is both a treatment for, and sometimes the cause of, cardiac supraventricular tachycardia; a plasma digoxin measurement will help to distinguish whether an arrhythmia is due to too little or too much digoxin
- When there is no quick and reliable assessment of effect, e.g. lithium for mood disorder
- To check patient compliance on a drug regimen, when there is failure of therapeutic effect at a dose that is expected to be effective, e.g. antiepilepsy drugs
- To diagnose and treat drug overdose.

Interpreting plasma concentration measurements

The following points are relevant:

- A target therapeutic concentration range quoted for a drug should be regarded only as a guide to help to optimise dosing and should be evaluated with other clinical indicators of progress.
- Consider whether a patient has been taking a drug for a sufficient time to reach steady-state conditions, i.e. when 5 $t_{\frac{1}{2}}$ periods have elapsed since dosing commenced or since the last change in dose. In the case of drugs that alter their own rates of metabolism by enzyme induction, e.g. carbamazepine and phenytoin, it is best to allow 2–4 weeks to elapse between change in dose and plasma concentration measurement. Sampling when plasma concentrations are still rising or falling towards a steady state is likely to be misleading.
- Consider whether peak or trough concentration should be measured. As a general rule when a drug has a short $t_{\frac{1}{2}}$ it is desirable to know both; monitoring peak (15 min after an i.v. dose) and trough (just before the next dose) concentrations of gentamicin ($t_{\frac{1}{2}}$ 2.5 h) helps to provide efficacy without toxicity. For a drug with a long $t_{\frac{1}{2}}$, it is usually best to sample just before a dose is due; effective immunosuppression with ciclosporin ($t_{\frac{1}{2}}$ 27 h) is obtained with trough concentrations

of 50–200 micrograms/l when the drug is given by mouth.

Recommended plasma concentrations for drugs appear throughout this book where these are relevant.

Individual pharmacokinetic processes

This section considers the processes whereby drugs are absorbed into, distributed around, metabolised by and eliminated from the body.

Absorption

Commonsense considerations of anatomy, physiology, pathology, pharmacology, therapeutics and convenience determine the routes by which drugs are administered. Usually these are:

- *Enteral:* by mouth (swallowed) or by sublingual or buccal absorption; by rectum
- *Parenteral:* by intravenous injection or infusion, intramuscular injection, subcutaneous injection or infusion, inhalation, topical application for local (skin, eye, lung) or for systemic (transdermal) effect
- *Other routes,* e.g. intrathecal, intradermal, intranasal, intratracheal, intrapleural, are used when appropriate.

The features of the various routes, their advantages and disadvantages are relevant.

ABSORPTION FROM THE GASTROINTESTINAL TRACT

The *small intestine* is the principal site for absorption of nutrients and it is also where most orally-administered drugs enter the body. This part of the gut has two important attributes, an enormous surface area due to the intestinal villi, and an epithelium through which fluid readily filters in response to osmotic differences caused by the presence of food. It follows that drug access to the small intestinal mucosa is important and disturbed alimentary motility can reduce absorption, i.e. if gastric emptying is slowed by food, or intestinal transit is accelerated by gut infection. The colon is capable of absorbing drugs and many sustained-release formulations probably depend on absorption there.

Absorption of ionisable drugs from the *buccal mucosa* is influenced by the prevailing pH which is 6.2–7.2. Lipid-soluble drugs are rapidly effective by this route because blood flow through the mucosa is abundant and entry is directly into the systemic circulation, avoiding the possibility of first-pass (presystemic) inactivation in the liver (see below). The stomach does not play a major role in absorbing drugs, even those that are acidic and thus un-ionised and lipid-soluble at gastric pH, because its surface area is much smaller than that of the small intestine and gastric emptying is speedy ($t\frac{1}{2}$ 30 min).

ENTEROHEPATIC CIRCULATION

This system is illustrated by the bile salts, which are conserved by circulating through liver, intestine and portal blood about eight times a day. A number of drugs form conjugates with glucuronic acid in the liver and are excreted in the bile. These glucuronides are too polar (ionised) to be reabsorbed; they therefore remain in the gut, are hydrolysed by intestinal enzymes and bacteria, releasing the parent drug, which is then reabsorbed and reconjugated in the liver. Enterohepatic recycling appears to help sustain the plasma concentration and thus the effect of sulindac, pentaerythritol tetranitrate and ethinyloestradiol (in many oral contraceptives).

SYSTEMIC AVAILABILITY AND BIOAVAILABILITY

When a drug is injected intravenously it enters the systemic circulation and thence gains access to the tissues and to receptors, i.e. 100% is available to exert its therapeutic effect. If the same quantity of the drug is swallowed, it does not follow that the entire amount will reach first the portal blood and then the systemic blood, i.e. its availability for therapeutic effect via the systemic circulation may be less than 100%. The anticipated response to a

drug may not be achieved unless availability to the systemic circulation is taken into account. In a strict sense, considerations of reduced availability apply whenever any drug intended for systemic effect is given by any route other than the intravenous, but in practice the issue concerns enteral admin-istration. The extent of systemic availability is ordinarily calculated by relating the area under the plasma concentration–time curve (AUC) after a single oral dose to that obtained after i.v. admin-istration of the same amount (by which route a drug is 100% systemically available). Different pharmaceutical formulations of the same drug can thus be compared. Factors influencing systemic availability may be thought of in three main ways:

Pharmaceutical factors.[8] The amount of drug that is released from a dose form (and so becomes available for absorption) is referred to as its *bio-availability*. This is highly dependent on its pharma-ceutical formulation. With tablets, for example, particle size (surface area exposed to solution), diluting substances, tablet size and pressure used in the tabletting machine can affect disintegration and dissolution and so the bioavailability of the drug.

Manufacturers are expected to produce a formulation with an unvarying bioavailability so that the same amount of drug is released with the same speed from whatever manufactured batch or brand the patient may be taking. Substantial differences in bioavailability of digoxin tablets from one manufacturer occurred when only the technique and machinery for making the tablets were changed; also tablets containing the same amount

---

[8] Some definitions of enteral dose-forms: *Tablet:* a solid dose form in which the drug is compressed or moulded with pharmacologically inert substances (excipients); variants include sustained-release and coated tablets. *Capsule:* the drug is provided in a gelatin shell or container. *Mixture:* a liquid formulation of a drug for oral administration. *Suppository:* a solid dose-form shaped for insertion into rectum (or vagina, when it may be called a *pessary*); it may be designed to dissolve or it may melt at body temperature (in which case there is a storage problem in countries where the environmental temperature may exceed 37°C); the vehicle in which the drug is carried may be fat, glycerol with gelatin, or macrogols (polycondensation products of ethylene oxide) with gelatin. *Syrup:* the drug is provided in a concentrated sugar (fructose or other) solution. *Linctus:* a viscous liquid formulation, traditional for cough.

of digoxin but made by different companies, were shown to produce different plasma concentrations and therefore different effects, i.e. there was neither *bioequivalence* nor *therapeutic equivalence*. Physicians tend to ignore pharmaceutical formulation as a factor in variable or unexpected responses because they do not understand it and feel entitled to rely on reputable manufacturers and official regulatory authorities to ensure provision of reliable formulations. Good pharmaceutical companies reasonably point out that, having a reputation to lose, they take much trouble to make their preparations consistently reliable. This is a matter of great importance when dosage must be precise (anticoagulants, antidiabetics, adrenal steroids). The following account by Lauder Brunton in 1897 indicates that the phenomenon of variable bioavailability is not recent.

> A very unfortunate case occurred some time ago in a doctor who had prescribed aconitine to a patient and gradually increased the dose. He thought he was quite certain that he knew what he was doing. The druggist's supply of aconitine ran out, and he procured some new aconitine from a different maker. This turned out to be many times stronger than the other, and the patient unfortunately became very ill. The doctor said, 'It cannot be the medicine', and to show that this was true, he drank off a dose himself with the result that he died. So you must remember the difference in the different preparations of aconitine,[9]

i.e. they had different bioavailability and so lacked therapeutic equivalence.

Biological factors. Those related to the gut include destruction of drug by gastric acid, e.g. benzylpenicillin, and impaired absorption due to intestinal hurry which is important for all drugs that are slowly absorbed. Drugs may also bind to food constituents, e.g. tetracyclines to calcium (in milk), and to iron, or to other drugs (e.g. acidic drugs to cholestyramine) and the resulting complex is not absorbed.

Presystemic (first-pass) elimination. Despite the

---

[9] The doctor would have died of cardiac arrhythmia and/or cerebral depression. Aconitine is a plant alkaloid and has no place in medicine.

fact that they readily enter gut mucosal cells, some drugs appear in low concentration in the systemic circulation. The reason lies in the considerable extent to which such drugs are metabolised in a single passage through the gut wall and (principally) the liver. This is a significant feature of the oral route, and as little as 10–20% of the parent drug may reach the systemic circulation unchanged. By contrast, if the drug is given intravenously, 100% becomes systemically available and the patient is exposed to higher concentrations with greater, but more predictable, effect. If a drug produces active metabolites, differences in dose may not be as great as those anticipated on the basis of differences in plasma concentration of the parent drug after intravenous and oral administration. Once a drug is in the systemic circulation, irrespective of which route is used, about 20% is subject to the hepatic metabolic processes in each circulation because that is the proportion of cardiac output that passes to the liver.

As the degree of presystemic elimination differs much between drugs and between individuals, the phenomenon of first-pass elimination adds to variation in systemic plasma concentrations, and thus particularly in initial response to the drugs that are subject to this process. When a drug is taken in overdose, presystemic elimination may be reduced, and bioavailability increased; this may explain rapid onset of toxicity with antipsychotic drugs, many of which undergo first-pass elimination.

Drugs for which **presystemic elimination** is significant include:

Analgesics	Adrenoceptor blockers	Others
dextropropoxyphene	labetalol	clomethiazole
morphine	propranolol	chlorpromazine
pentazocine	metoprolol	isosorbide
pethidine	oxprenolol	dinitrate
		nortriptyline

In severe hepatic cirrhosis with both impaired liver cell function and well-developed channels shunting blood into the systemic circulation without passing through the liver, first-pass elimination is reduced and systemic availability is increased. The result of these changes is an increased likelihood of exaggerated response to normal doses of drugs having high hepatic clearance and, on occasion, frank toxicity.

Drugs that exhibit the hepatic first-pass phenomenon do so because of the rapidity with which they are metabolised. The rate at which drug is delivered to the liver, i.e. blood flow, is then the main determinant of its metabolism. Many other drugs are completely metabolised by the liver but at a slower rate and consequently loss in the first pass through the liver is unimportant. The parenteral dose of these drugs does not need to be reduced to account for presystemic elimination. Such drugs include diazepam, phenytoin, theophylline, warfarin.

ADVANTAGES AND DISADVANTAGES OF ENTERAL ADMINISTRATION

By swallowing

For systemic effect *Advantages* are convenience and acceptability.

Disadvantages are that absorption may be delayed, reduced or even enhanced after food or slow or irregular after drugs that inhibit gut motility (antimuscarinic, opioid). Differences in presystemic elimination are a cause of variation in drug effect between patients. Some drugs are not absorbed (gentamicin) and some drugs are destroyed in the gut (insulin, oxytocin, some penicillins). Tablets taken with too small a quantity of liquid and in the supine position, can lodge in the oesophagus with delayed absorption[10] and may even cause ulceration (sustained-release potassium chloride and doxycycline tablets), especially in the feeble elderly and those with an enlarged left atrium which impinges on the oesophagus.[11]

---

[10] A woman's failure to respond to antihypertensive medication was explained when she was observed to choke on drinking. Investigation revealed a large pharyngeal pouch that was full of tablets and capsules. Her blood pressure became easy to control when the pouch was removed. Birch D J, Dehn T C B 1993 British Medical Journal 306: 1012.

[11] Ideally solid-dose forms should be taken standing up and washed down with 150 ml (tea cup) of water; even sitting (higher intra-abdominal pressure) impairs passage. At least patients should be told to sit and take 3 or 4 mouthfuls of water (a mouthful = 30 ml) or a cupful. Some patients do not even know they should take water.

For effect in the gut *Advantages* are that the drug is placed at the site of action (neomycin, anthelminthics), and with nonabsorbed drugs the local concentration can be higher than would be safe in the blood.

Disadvantages are that drug distribution may be uneven, and in some diseases of the gut the whole thickness of the wall is affected (severe bacillary dysentery, typhoid) and effective blood concentrations (as well as luminal concentrations) may be needed.

Sublingual or buccal for systemic effect

Advantages are that quick effect is obtained, e.g. with glyceryl trinitrate as an aerosol spray, or as sublingual tablets which can be chewed, giving greater surface area for solution. Spitting out the tablet will terminate the effect.

Disadvantages are the inconvenience if use has to be frequent, irritation of the mucous membrane and excessive salivation which promotes swallowing, so losing the advantages of bypassing presystemic elimination.

Rectal administration

For systemic effect (suppositories or solutions).

The rectal mucosa has a rich blood and lymph supply and, in general, dose requirements are either the same or slightly greater than those needed for oral use. Drugs chiefly enter the portal system, but those that are subject to hepatic first-pass elimination may escape this if they are absorbed from the lower rectum which drains directly to the systemic circulation. The degree of presystemic elimination thus depends on distribution within the rectum and this is somewhat unpredictable.

Advantages are that a drug that is irritant to the stomach can be given by suppository (aminophylline, indomethacin); the route is suitable in vomiting, motion sickness, migraine or when a patient cannot swallow, and when cooperation is lacking (sedation in children).

Disadvantages are psychological in that the patient may be embarrassed or may like the route too much; rectal inflammation may occur with repeated use and absorption can be unreliable, especially if the rectum is full of faeces.

For local effect, e.g. in proctitis or colitis, an obvious use.

A survey in the UK showed that a substantial proportion of patients did not remove the wrapper before inserting the suppository.

ADVANTAGES AND DISADVANTAGES OF PARENTERAL ADMINISTRATION

(for systemic and local effect)

Intravenous (bolus or infusion)

An i.v. bolus, i.e. rapid injection, passes round the circulation being progressively diluted each time; it is delivered principally to the organs with high blood flow (brain, liver, heart, lung, kidneys).

Advantages are that the i.v. route gives swift, effective and highly predictable blood concentration and allows rapid modification of dose, i.e. immediate cessation of administration is possible if unwanted effects occur during administration. The route is suitable for administration of drugs that are not absorbed from the gut or are too irritant (anticancer agents) to be given by other routes.

Disadvantages are the hazard if a drug is given too quickly, as plasma concentration may rise at such a rate that normal mechanisms of distribution and elimination are outpaced. Some drugs will act within one arm-to-tongue (brain) circulation time which is 13 ± 3 seconds; with most drugs an injection given over 4 or 5 circulation times seems sufficient to avoid excessive plasma concentrations. Local venous thrombosis is liable to occur with prolonged infusion and with bolus doses of irritant formulations, e.g. diazepam, or microparticulate components of infusion fluids, especially if small veins are used. Infection of the intravenous catheter and the small thrombi on its tip are also a risk during prolonged infusions.

Intramuscular injection

Blood flow is greater in the muscles of the upper arm than in the gluteal mass and thigh, and also increases with physical exercise. (Usually these influences are unimportant but one football-playing patient who was given an intramuscular injection of a sustained-release phenothiazine developed an extrapyramidal disorder towards the end of the game, presumably due to too rapid absorption of the drug.)

Advantages are that the route is reliable, suitable for irritant drugs, and depot preparations (neuroleptics, hormonal contraceptives) can be used at monthly or longer intervals. Absorption is more rapid than following subcutaneous injection (soluble preparations are absorbed within 10–30 min).

Disadvantages are that the route is not acceptable for self-administration, it may be painful, and if any adverse effects occur to a depot formulation, it cannot be removed.

Subcutaneous injection

Advantages are that the route is reliable and is acceptable for self-administration.

Disadvantages are poor absorption in peripheral circulatory failure. Repeated injections at one site can cause lipoatrophy, resulting in erratic absorption (see Insulin).

By inhalation

As a gas, e.g. volatile anaesthetics.

As an aerosol, e.g. β_2-adrenoceptor agonist bronchodilators. Aerosols are particles dispersed in a gas, the particles being small enough to remain in suspension for a long time instead of sedimenting rapidly under the influence of gravity; the particles may be liquid (fog) or solid (smoke).

As a powder, e.g. sodium cromoglicate. Particle size and air flow velocity are important. Most particles above 5 micrometres in diameter impact in the upper respiratory areas; particles of about 2 micrometres reach the terminal bronchioles; a large proportion of particles less than micrometer will be exhaled. Air flow velocity diminishes considerably as the bronchi progressively divide, promoting drug deposition peripherally.

Advantages are that drugs as gases can be rapidly taken up or eliminated, giving the close control that has marked the use of this route in general anaesthesia from its earliest days. Self-administration is practicable. Aerosols and powders provide high local concentration for action on bronchi, minimising systemic effects.

Disadvantages are that special apparatus is needed (some patients find pressurised aerosols difficult to use to best effect) and a drug must be nonirritant if the patient is conscious. Obstructed bronchi (mucus plugs in asthma) may cause therapy to fail.

Topical application

For local effect, e.g. to skin, eye, lung, anal canal, rectum, vagina.

Advantage is the provision of high local concentration without systemic effect (usually[12]).

Disadvantage is that absorption can occur, especially when there is tissue destruction so that systemic effects result, e.g. adrenal steroids and neomycin to the skin, atropine to the eye. Ocular administration of a β-adrenoceptor blocker may cause systemic effects (any first-pass elimination is bypassed) and such eye drops are contraindicated for patients with asthma or chronic lung disease.[13] There is extensive literature on this subject characterised by expressions of astonishment that serious effects, even death, can occur.

For systemic effect. Transdermal delivery systems (TDS) release drug through a rate-controlling membrane into the skin and so into the systemic circulation. Fluctuations in plasma concentration associated with other routes of administration are largely avoided, as is first-pass elimination in the liver. Glyceryl trinitrate and postmenopausal hormone replacement therapy may be given this way, in the form of a sticking plaster attached to the skin[14] or as an ointment (glyceryl trinitrate). A nasal spray containing sumatriptan may be used to treat migraine.

Distribution

If a drug is required to act throughout the body or to reach an organ inaccessible to topical administration, it must be got into the blood and into other body compartments. Most drugs distribute widely, in part dissolved in body water, in part bound to plasma proteins, in part to tissues. Distribution is often uneven, for drugs may bind selectively to plasma or tissue proteins or be localised within particular organs. Clearly, the site of localisation of a drug is likely to influence its action, e.g. whether it crosses the blood–brain barrier to enter the brain; the extent (amount) and strength (tenacity) of protein or tissue binding (stored drug) will affect the time it spends in the body and thereby its duration of action.

Drug distribution, its quantification and its clinical implications are now discussed.

DISTRIBUTION VOLUME

The pattern of distribution from plasma to other body fluids and tissues is a characteristic of each

---

[12] A cautionary tale. A 70-year-old man reported left breast enlargement and underwent mastectomy; histological examination revealed benign gynaecomastia. Ten months later the right breast enlarged. Tests of endocrine function were normal but the patient himself was struck by the fact that his wife had been using a vaginal cream (containing 0.01% dienestrol) initially for atrophic vaginitis but latterly the cream had been used to facilitate sexual intercourse which took place two to three times a week. On the assumption that penile absorption of oestrogen was responsible for the disorder, exposure to the cream was terminated. The gynaecomastia in the remaining breast then resolved (Di Raimondo C V et al 1980 New England Journal of Medicine 302: 1089).

[13] Two drops of 0.5% timolol solution, one to each eye, can equate to 10 mg by mouth.

[14] But TDS may have an unexpected outcome for, not only may the sticking plaster drop off unnoticed, it may find its way onto another person. A hypertensive father rose one morning and noticed that his clonidine plaster was missing from his upper arm. He could not find it and applied a new plaster. His nine-month-old child, who had been taken into the paternal bed during the night because he needed comforting, spent an irritable and hypoactive day, refused food but drank and passed more urine than usual. The missing clonidine patch was discovered on his back when he was being prepared for his bath. No doubt this was accidental, but children also enjoy stick-on decoration and the possibility of poisoning from misused, discarded or new (e.g. strong opioid, used in palliative care) drug plasters means that these should be kept and disposed of as carefully as oral formulations (Reed M T et al 1986 New England Journal of Medicine 314: 1120).

> The distribution volume of a drug is the volume in which it appears to distribute (or which it would require) if the concentration throughout the body were equal to that in plasma, i.e. as if the body were a single compartment.

drug that enters the circulation and it varies between drugs. Precise information on the concentration of drug attained in various tissues and fluids requires biopsy samples and for understandable reasons this is usually not available for humans (although positive emission tomography offers a prospect of obtaining similar information).[15] What can be sampled readily in humans is blood plasma, the drug concentration in which, taking account of the dose, is a measure of whether a drug tends to remain in the circulation or to distribute from the plasma into the tissues. If a drug remains mostly in the plasma, its distribution volume will be small; if it is present mainly in other tissues the distribution volume will be large.

Such information is clinically useful. Consider drug overdose. Removing a drug by haemodialysis is likely to be a beneficial exercise only if a major proportion of the total body load is in the plasma, e.g. with salicylate which has a small distribution volume; but haemodialysis is an inappropriate treatment for overdose with dothiepin which has a large distribution volume. These, however, are generalisations and if the knowledge of distribution volume is to be of practical value it must be quantified more precisely.

The principle for establishing the distribution volume is essentially that of using a dye to find the volume of a container filled with liquid. The weight of dye that is added divided by the concentration of dye once mixing is complete gives the distribution volume of the dye, which is the volume of the container. Similarly, the distribution volume of a drug in the body may be determined after a single intravenous bolus dose by dividing the dose given by the concentration achieved in plasma.[16]

The result of this calculation, the distribution volume, in fact only rarely corresponds with a physiological body space such as extracellular water or total body water, for it is a measure of the volume a drug would apparently occupy knowing the dose given and the plasma concentration achieved and assuming the entire volume is at that concentration. For this reason, it is often referred to as the *apparent distribution volume*. Indeed, for some drugs that bind extensively to extravascular tissues, the apparent distribution volume, which is based on the resulting low plasma concentration, is many times total body volume.

> Distribution volume is the volume of fluid in which the drug appears to distribute with a concentration equal to that in plasma.

The list in Table 7.2 illustrates a range of apparent distribution volumes. The names of those substances that distribute within (and have been used to measure) physiological spaces are printed in italics.

Selective distribution within the body occurs because of special affinity between particular drugs and particular body constituents. Many drugs bind to proteins in the plasma; phenothiazines and chloroquine bind to melanin-containing tissues, including the retina, which may explain the occurrence of retinopathy. Drugs may also concentrate selectively in a particular tissue because of specialised transport mechanisms, e.g. iodine in the thyroid.

---

[15] With positron emission tomography (PET), a positron emitting isotope, e.g. ^{15}O, is substituted for a stable atom without altering the chemical behaviour of the molecule. The radiation dose is very low but can be imaged tomographically using photomultiplier-scintillator detectors. PET can be used to monitor effects of drugs on metabolism in the brain, e.g. 'on' and 'off' phases in parkinsonism. There are many other applications.

[16] Clearly a problem arises in that the plasma concentration is not constant but falls after the bolus has been injected. To get round this, use is made of the fact that the relation between the logarithm of plasma concentration and the time after a single intravenous dose is a straight line. The log concentration-time line extended back to zero time gives the theoretical plasma concentration at the time the drug was given. In effect, the assumption is made that drug distributes instantaneously and uniformly through a single compartment, the distribution volume. This mechanism, although seeming artificial, does usefully characterise drugs according to the extent to which they remain in or distribute out from the circulation.

TABLE 7.2 Apparent distribution volume of some drugs (Figures are in litres for a 70 kg person who would displace about 70 l)[17]

Drug	Distribution volume	Drug	Distribution volume
Evans blue	3 (plasma volume)	atenolol	77
heparin	5	diazepam	140
aspirin	11	pethidine	280
inulin	15 (extracellular water)	digoxin	420
gentamicin	18	nortriptyline	1000
frusemide	21	nortriptyline	1000
amoxycillin	28	dothiepin	4900
antipyrine	43 (total body water)	chloroquine	13000

PLASMA PROTEIN AND TISSUE BINDING

Many natural substances circulate around the body partly free in plasma water and partly bound to plasma proteins; these include cortisol, thyroxine, iron, copper and, in hepatic or renal failure, byproducts of physiological intermediary metabolism. Drugs, too, circulate in the protein-bound and free states, and the significance is that the *free fraction* is pharmacologically active whereas the *protein-bound* component is a reservoir of drug that is inactive because of this binding. Free and bound fractions are in equilibrium and free drug removed from the plasma by metabolism, dialysis or excretion is replaced by drug released from the bound fraction.

Albumin is the main binding protein for many natural substances and drugs. Its complex structure has a net negative charge at blood pH and a high *capacity* but low (weak) *affinity* for many basic drugs, i.e. a lot is bound but it is readily released. Two particular sites on the albumin molecule bind acidic drugs with high affinity (strongly) but these sites have low capacity. Saturation of binding sites on plasma proteins in general is unlikely in the doses in which most drugs are used.

Other binding proteins in the blood include lipoprotein and α_1-acid glycoprotein, both of which carry basic drugs such as quinidine, chlorpromazine and imipramine. Such binding may have implications

for therapeutic drug monitoring according to plasma concentration. Thyroxine and sex hormones are bound in the plasma to specific globulins.

Disease may modify protein binding of drugs to an extent that is clinically relevant as Table 7.3 shows. In *chronic renal failure,* hypoalbuminaemia and retention of products of metabolism that compete for binding sites on protein are both responsible for the decrease in protein binding of drugs. Most affected are acidic drugs that are highly protein bound, e.g. phenytoin, and special care is needed when initiating and modifying the dose of such drugs for patients with renal failure (see also Prescribing in renal disease, p. 541).

Chronic liver disease also leads to hypoalbuminaemia and increase of endogenous substances such as bilirubin that may compete for binding sites on protein. Drugs that are normally extensively protein bound should be used with special caution, for increased free concentration of diazepam, tolbutamide and phenytoin have been demonstrated in patients with this condition (see also Prescribing in liver disease, p. 652).

The free, unbound and therefore pharmacologically active percentages of some drugs are listed in Table 7.3 to illustrate the range and, in some cases, the changes caused by disease.

Drugs may *interact* competitively at plasma protein binding sites as is discussed on page 131.

Tissue binding. Some drugs distribute readily to regions of the body other than plasma, as a glance

TABLE 7.3 Examples of plasma protein binding of drugs and effects of disease

Drug	% unbound (free)
warfarin	1
diazepam	2 (6% in liver disease)
frusemide (furosemide)	2 (6% in nephrotic syndrome)
tolbutamide	2
clofibrate	4 (11% in nephrotic syndrome)
amitriptyline	5
phenytoin	9 (19% in renal disease)
triamterene	19 (40% in renal disease)
trimethoprim	30
theophylline	35 (71% in liver disease)
morphine	65
digoxin	75 (82% in renal disease)
amoxicillin	82
ethosuximide	100

---

[17] Litres per kg are commonly used, but give a less vivid image of the implication of the term 'apparent', e.g. chloroquine.

at Table 7.2 will show. These include many lipid-soluble drugs, which may enter fat stores, e.g. most benzodiazepines, verapamil and lignocaine. Less is known about other tissues, e.g. muscle, than about plasma protein binding because solid tissue samples can be obtained only by invasive biopsy, but extensive binding to tissues delays elimination from the body and accounts for the long $t\frac{1}{2}$ of chloroquine and amiodarone. Displacement from tissue binding sites may be a mechanism for pharmacokinetic interaction (see p. 131).

Metabolism

Most drugs are treated by the body as foreign substances (xenobiotics) and become subject to its various mechanisms for ridding itself of chemical intruders.

Metabolism is a general term for chemical transformations that occur within the body and its processes change drugs in two major ways:

- by reducing lipid solubility
- by altering biological activity.

REDUCING LIPID SOLUBILITY

Metabolic reactions tend to make a drug molecule progressively more water-soluble and so favour its elimination in the urine.

Drug metabolising enzymes were developed during evolution to enable the body to dispose of lipid-soluble substances such as hydrocarbons, steroids and alkaloids, that are ingested with food.[18] Some environmental chemicals may persist indefinitely in our fat deposits, e.g. dicophane (DDT), with consequences that are as yet unknown.

ALTERING BIOLOGICAL ACTIVITY

The end result of metabolism usually is the

[18] Fish lose lipid-soluble substances through the gills. They do not need such effective metabolising enzymes and they have not got them.

abolition of biological activity but various steps in between may have the following consequences:

1. Conversion of a pharmacologically *active* to an *inactive* substance: this applies to most drugs.
2. Conversion of one pharmacologically *active* to another *active* substance: this has the effect of prolonging drug action.

Active drug	Active metabolite
amitriptyline	nortriptyline
codeine	morphine
chloroquine	hydroxychloroquine
diazepam	oxazepam
spironolactone	canrenone

3. Conversion of a pharmacologically *inactive* to an *active* substance, i.e. *prodrugs*; the effect may confer advantage or disadvantage. (The process then follows 1, above.)

Inactive substance	Active metabolite(s)	Comment
benorilate	salicylic acid and paracetamol	possibly reduced gastric toxicity
cholecalciferol	1-α-hydroxy-cholecalciferol	
cyclophosphamide	4-keto-cyclophosphamide	
perindopril	perindoprilat	less risk of first dose hypotension
levodopa	dopamine	levodapa, but not dopamine, can cross the blood–brain barrier possibly reduced gastric toxicity
sulindac	sulindac sulphide	
sulfasalazine	5-aminosalicylic acid	
terfenadine	fexofenadine	life-threatening tachycardia if metabolism is inhibited (see p. 555)
zidovudine	zidovudine triphosphate	

THE METABOLIC PROCESSES

The liver is by far the most important drug metabolising organ, although a number of tissues, including the kidney, gut mucosa, lung and skin also contribute. It is useful to think of drug metabolism in two broad phases:

Phase 1 metabolism brings about a change in the drug molecule by oxidation, reduction or hydrolysis and often introduces a chemically active site into it. The new metabolite may retain biological activity but have different pharmacokinetic properties, e.g. a shorter $t\frac{1}{2}$.

The most important single group of reactions is the oxidations, in particular those undertaken by the so-called *mixed-function* (microsomal) *oxidases* which, as the name indicates, are capable of metabolising a wide variety of compounds. The most important enzyme is a haem protein, *cytochrome P450*, which takes part in a process whereby molecular oxygen is bound and incorporated into the drug molecule, so forming a new hydroxyl group.

The many forms of cytochrome P450 enzymes (called isoenzymes[19]) are grouped into families denoted by the letters CYP (from **cy**tochrome **P**450) followed by numerals. The majority of enzymes concerned with human metabolism belong to familes CYP1, 2 and 3. Within these families, are subdivisions denoted by a capital letter followed by a numeral. The family CYP3A is numerically the most important, being involved in the biotransformation of the majority of all drugs; indeed CYP3A4 is expressed outside the liver and may be an important factor that explains poor oral availability of many drugs. Over 100 drugs are known substrates for CYP2D6, > 60 for CYP2C9 and > 50 for CYP2C19.[20] Another isoenzyme CYP 2E1, catalyses a reaction involved in the metabolism of alcohol, paracetamol, oestradiol and ethynyloestradiol.

In all there may be as many as 200 separate P450 isoenzymes and this is why we do not need to possess new enzymes for every existing or yet-to-be synthesised drug. Each enzyme is encoded by a separate gene and variation in these genes leads to differences between individuals, and sometimes between ethnic groups, in the ability to metabolise drugs. Persons characterised by polymorphisms (see p. 122) inherit diminished ability to metabolise substrate drugs and if inactivation is dependent on the particular isoenzyme, toxicity may result when these drugs accumulate.

Phase I oxidation of some drugs results in the formation of *epoxides* which are short-lived and highly reactive metabolites. Epoxides are important because they can bind irreversibly through covalent bonds to cell constituents; indeed, this is one of the principal ways in which drugs are toxic to body tissues. Glutathione is a tripeptide that combines with epoxides, rendering them inactive, and its presence in the liver is part of an important defence machanism against hepatic damage by halothane and paracetamol.

Phase II metabolism involves union of the drug with one of several polar (water-soluble) endogenous molecules that are products of intermediary metabolism, to form a water-soluble conjugate which is readily eliminated by the kidney or, if the molecular weight exceeds 300, in the bile. Morphine, paracetamol and salicylates form conjugates with *glucuronic acid* (derived from glucose); oral contraceptive steroids form *sulphates*; isoniazid, phenelzine and dapsone are *acetylated*. Conjugation with a more polar molecule is also a mechanism by which natural substances are eliminated, e.g. bilirubin as glucuronide, oestrogens as sulphates. Phase II metabolism almost invariably terminates bilogical activity.

ENZYME INDUCTION

The mechanisms that the body evolved over millions of years to metabolise foreign substances now enable it to meet the modern environmental challenges of tobacco smoke, hydrocarbon pollutants, insecticides and drugs. At times of high exposure, our enzyme systems respond by increasing in amount and so in activity, i.e. they are *induced*; when exposure falls off, enzyme production lessens. For example, a first alcoholic drink taken after a period of abstinence from alcohol may have quite a significant effect on behaviour but the same drink taken at the end of two weeks' regular imbibing may pass almost unnoticed because the individual's liver enzyme activity is increased (induced) so that alcohol is metabolised more rapidly and has less effect, i.e. *tolerance* has been acquired.

Inducing substances in general share some important properties: they tend to be lipid-soluble; they are

---

[19] An isoenzyme is one of a group of enzmes that catalyse the same reaction but differ in protein structure.
[20] Wolf C R, Smith G, Smith R L 2000 Pharmacogenetics. British Medical Journal 320: 987–990.

substrates, though sometimes only minor ones, e.g. DDT, for the enzymes they induce and generally have long $t_{\frac{1}{2}}$. The time for onset and offset of induction depends on the rate of enzyme turnover but significant induction generally occurs within a few days and it passes off over 2 or 3 weeks following withdrawal of the inducer.

It follows that the capacity of the body to metabolise drugs can be altered by certain medicinal drugs themselves and by other substances, especially when these are used long-term; clearly this phenomenon has implications for drug therapy. More than 200 substances have been shown to induce enzymes in animals but the list of proven enzyme inducers in man is much more restricted.

Substances that cause enzyme induction in human	
barbecued meats	griseofulvin
barbiturates	meprobamate
Brussels sprouts	phenobarbital
carbamazepine	phenytoin
DDT (dicophane,	primidone
and other	rifampicin
insecticides)	Saint John's Wort
ethanol (chronic use)	sulphinpyrazone
glutethimide	tobacco smoke

Enzyme induction is relevant to drug therapy for the following reasons:

- Clinically important drug interactions may result, e.g. in failure of oral contraceptives, loss of anticoagulant control, failure of cytotoxic chemotherapy.
- Disease may result. Antiepilepsy drugs increase the breakdown of dietary and endogenously formed vitamin D, producing an inactive metabolite — in effect a vitamin D deficiency state, which can result in osteomalacia. The accompanying hypocalcaemia can increase the tendency to fits and a convulsion may lead to fracture of the demineralised bones.
- Tolerance to drug therapy may result in and provide an explanation for suboptimal treatment, e.g. with an antiepilepsy drug.
- Variability in response to drugs is increased. Enzyme induction caused by heavy alcohol drinking or heavy smoking may be an unrecognised cause for failure of an individual to achieve the expected response to a normal dose of a drug, e.g. warfarin, theophylline.
- Drug toxicity may be more likely. A patient who becomes enzyme-induced by taking rifampicin is more likely to develop liver toxicity after paracetamol overdose by increased production of a hepatotoxic metabolite. (Such a patient will also present with a deceptively low plasma concentration of paracetamol due to accelerated metabolism, see p. 287)

ENZYME INHIBITION

Consequences of inhibiting drug metabolism can be more profound than those of enzyme induction. Effects of enzyme inhibition by drugs also tend to be more selective than those of enzyme induction. Consequently, enzyme inhibition offers more scope for therapy (see Table 7.4).

Enzyme inhibition by drugs is also the basis of a number of clinically important drug interactions (see p. 133).

Elimination

Drugs are eliminated from the body after being partly or wholly converted to water-soluble metabolites or, in some cases, without being metabolised. To avoid repetition the following account refers to drug whereas the processes deal with both drug and its metabolites.

TABLE 7.4 Some drugs that act by enzyme inhibition		
Drug	**Enzyme inhibited**	**Treatment of**
acetazolamide	carbonic anhydrase	glaucoma
allopurinol	xanthine oxidase	gout
benserazide	DOPA decarboxylase	Parkinson's disease
disulfiram	aldehyde dehydrogenase	alcoholism
enalapril	angiotensin converting enzyme	hypertension, cardiac failure
moclobemide	MAO A type	depression
nonsteroidal anti-inflammatory drugs	cyclooxygenase	pain, inflammation
selegiline	MAO B type	Parkinson's disease

RENAL ELIMINATION

The following mechanisms are involved.

Glomerular filtration. The rate at which a drug enters the glomerular filtrate depends on the concentration of free drug in plasma water and on its molecular weight. Substances that have a molecular weight in excess of 50 000 are excluded from the glomerular filtrate while those of molecular weight less than 10 000 (which includes almost all drugs)[21] pass easily through the pores of the glomerular membrane.

Renal tubular excretion. Cells of the proximal renal tubule actively transfer strongly charged molecules from the plasma to the tubular fluid. There are two such systems, one for *acids,* e.g. penicillin, probenecid, frusemide, and another for *bases,* e.g. amiloride, amphetamine.

Renal tubular reabsorption. The glomerular filtrate contains drug at the same concentration as it is free in the plasma, but the fluid is concentrated progressively as it flows down the nephron so that a gradient develops, drug in the tubular fluid becoming more concentrated than in the blood perfusing the nephron. Since the tubular epithelium has the properties of a lipid membrane, the extent to which a drug diffuses back into the blood will depend on its lipid solubility, i.e. on its pKa in the case of an electrolyte, and on the pH of tubular fluid. If the fluid becomes more alkaline, an *acidic* drug ionises, becomes less lipid-soluble and its reabsorption diminishes, but a *basic* drug becomes un-ionised (and therefore more lipid-soluble) and its reabsorption increases. Manipulation of urine pH is given useful expression when sodium bicarbonate is given to alkalinise the urine to treat overdose with aspirin.

FAECAL ELIMINATION

When a drug intended for systemic effect is taken by mouth, a proportion may remain in the bowel and be excreted in the faeces. Sometimes the objective of therapy is that drug should not be absorbed from the gut, e.g. neomycin. Drug in the blood may also diffuse passively into the gut lumen, depending on its pKa and the pH difference between blood and gut contents. The effectiveness of activated charcoal by mouth for drug overdose depends partly on its adsorption of such diffused drug, which is then eliminated in the faeces (see p. 155).

Biliary excretion. In the liver there is one active transport system for acids and one for bases, similar to those in the proximal renal tubule and, in addition, there is a system that transports un-ionised molecules, e.g. digoxin, into the bile. Small molecules tend to be reabsorbed by the bile canaliculi and in general only compounds that have a molecular weight greater than 300 are excreted in bile. (See also, enterohepatic circulation, p. 105)

PULMONARY ELIMINATION

The lungs are the main route of elimination (and of uptake) of volatile anaesthetics. Apart from this, they play only a trivial role in drug elimination. The route however, acquires notable medicolegal significance when ethanol concentration is measured in the air expired by vehicle drivers involved in road traffic accidents (via the breathalyser).

CLEARANCE

Elimination of a drug from the plasma is quantified in terms of its clearance. The term has the same meaning as the familiar renal creatinine clearance, which is a measure of removal of endogenous creatinine from the plasma. Clearance values can provide useful information about the biological fate of a drug. There are pharmacokinetic methods for calculating total body and renal clearance, and the difference between these is commonly taken to represent hepatic clearance. Renal clearance of a drug that is eliminated only by filtration by the kidney obviously cannot exceed the glomerular filtration rate (adult male 124 ml/min, female 109 ml/min). If a drug is found to have a renal clearance in excess of this, then it must in addition be actively secreted by the kidney tubules, e.g. benzylpenicillin (renal clearance 480 ml/min).

---

[21] Most drugs have a molecular weight less than 1000.

BREAST MILK

Most drugs that are present in a mother's plasma appear to some extent in her milk though the amounts are so small that loss of drug in milk is of no significance as a mechanism of elimination.[22] Even small amounts, however, may sometimes be of significance for the suckling child whose drug metabolic and eliminating mechanisms are immature.

Whilst most drugs taken by the mother pose no hazard to the child, there are exceptions, as follows:

DRUGS AND BREAST FEEDING[23]

Alimentary tract. Sulphasalazine may cause adverse effects and mesalazine appears preferable.

Antiasthma. Theophylline and diprophylline are eliminated slowly by the neonate: observe the infant for irritability or disturbed sleep.

Anticancer. Regard as unsafe because of inherent toxicity.

Antidepressants. Avoid doxepin, a metabolite of which may cause respiratory depression.

Antiarrhythmics (cardiac). Amiodarone is present in high and disopyramide in moderate amounts but effects in the infant have not been reported.

Antiepilepsy. General note of caution: observe the infant for sedation and poor suckling. Primidone, ethosuximide and phenobarbital are present in milk in high amounts; phenytoin and sodium valproate less so.

Anti-inflammatory. Regard aspirin (salicylates) as unsafe (possible association with Reye's syndrome).

Antimicrobials. Metronidazole is present in milk in moderate amounts; avoid prolonged exposure. Nalidixic acid and nitrofurantoin should be avoided where glucose-6-phosphate dehydrogenase deficiency is prevalent. Avoid clindamycin, dapsone, lincomycin, sulphonamides. Regard chloramphenicol as unsafe.

Antipsychotics. Phenothiazines, butyrophenones and thioxanthenes are best avoided unless the indications are compelling: amounts in milk are small but animal studies suggest adverse effects on the developing nervous system. In particular,

moderate amounts of sulpiride enter milk. Lithium is probably best avoided.

Anxiolytics and sedatives. Benzodiazepines are safe if use is brief but prolonged use may cause somnolence or poor suckling.

Beta-adrenoceptor blockers. Neonatal hypoglycaemia may occur. Satalol and atenolol are present in the highest amounts.

Hormones. Oestrogens, progestogens and androgens suppress lactation in high dose. Oestrogen/ progestogen oral contraceptives are present in amounts too small to be harmful but may suppress lactation if it is not well established.

Miscellaneous. Bromocriptine suppresses lactation. Caffeine may cause infant irritability in high doses.

Drug dosage

Drug dosage can be of five main kinds:

- **Fixed dose.** The effect that is desired can be obtained at well below the toxic dose (many mydriatics, diuretics, analgesics, oral contraceptives, antimicrobials) and enough drug can be given to render individual variation clinically insignificant.

- **Variable dose**—*with crude adjustments.* Here fine adjustments make comparatively insignificant differences and the therapeutic end-point may be hard to measure (depression, anxiety), may change only slowly (thyrotoxicosis), or may very because of pathophysiological factors (analgesics, adrenal steroids for suppressing disease).

- **Variable dose**—*with fine adjustments.* Here a vital function (blood pressure, blood sugar), that often changes rapidly in response to dose changes and can easily be measured repeatedly, provides the end-point. Adjustment of dose must be accurate. Adrenocortical replacement therapy falls into this group, whereas adrenocortical pharmacotherapy falls into the group above.

- **Maximum tolerated dose** is used when the ideal therapeutic effect cannot be achieved because of the occurrence of unwanted effects (anticancer drugs; some antimicrobials). The usual way of finding this is to increase the dose until

---

[22] But after mercury poisoning breast milk is a major route of elimination.
[23] Bennett P N (ed) 1996 Drugs and human lactation. Elsevier, Amsterdam.

unwanted effects begin to appear and then to reduce it slightly, or to monitor the plasma concentration.

- **Minimum tolerated dose.** This concept is not so common as the one above, but it applies to long-term adrenocortical steroid therapy against inflammatory or immunological conditions, e.g. in asthma and some cases of rheumatoid arthritis, when the dose that provides symptomatic relief may be so high that serious adverse effects are inevitable if it is continued indefinitely. The patient must be persuaded to accept incomplete relief on the grounds of safety. This can be difficult to achieve.

Dosing schedules

Whatever their type, dosing schedules are simply schemes aimed at achieving a desired effect whilst avoiding toxicity. In the discussion that follows it is assumed that drug effect relates closely to plasma concentration, which in turn relates closely to the amount of drug in the body. The objectives of a dosing regimen where continuing effect is required are:

To specify an initial dose that attains the desired effect rapidly without causing toxicity. Often the dose that is capable of initiating drug effect is the same as that which maintains it. On repeated dosing however, it takes $5 \times t_{1/2}$ periods to reach steady-state concentration in the plasma and this lapse of time may be undesirable. The effect may be achieved earlier by giving an inital dose that is larger than the maintenance dose; the initial dose is then called the *priming* or *loading* dose, i.e. the priming dose is that dose which will acheive a therapeutic effect in an individual whose body does not already contain the drug.

To specify a maintenance dose: amount and frequency. Intuitively, the maintenance dose might be half the initial/priming dose at intervals equal to its plasma $t_{1/2}$, for this is the time by which the plasma concentration that achieves the desired effect declines by half. Whether or not this approach is satisfactory or practicable, however, depends very

much on the $t_{1/2}$ itself, as is illustrated by the following cases:

1. *Half-life 6–12 h.* In this instance, replacing half the initial dose at intervals equal to the $t_{1/2}$ can indeed be a satisfactory solution because dosing every 6–12 h is acceptable.
2. *Half-life greater than 24 h.* With once-daily dosing (which is desirable for compliance) giving half the priming dose every day means that more drug is entering the body than is leaving it each day, and the drug will accumulate indefinitely. The solution is to replace only that amount of drug that leaves the body in 24 h. This quantity can be calculated once the inital dose and dose interval have been decided and the $t_{1/2}$ is known.
3. *Half-life less than 3 h.* Dosing at intervals equal to the $t_{1/2}$ would be so frequent as to be unacceptable, and the answer is to use continuous intravenous infusion if the $t_{1/2}$ is very short, e.g. dopamine $t_{1/2}$, 2 min; steady-state plasma concentration will be reached in $5 \times t_{1/2} = 10$ min) or, if the $t_{1/2}$ is longer, e.g. lignocaine ($t_{1/2}$, 90 min) to use a priming dose as an intravenous bolus followed by a constant intravenous infusion. Intermittent adminstration of a drug with short $t_{1/2}$ is nevertheless reasonable provided large fluctuations in plasma concentration are acceptable, i.e. that the drug has a large therapeutic index. Benzylpenicillin has a $t_{1/2}$ of 30 min but is effective in a 6-hourly regimen because the drug is so nontoxic that it is possible safely to give a dose that acheives a plasma concentration many times in excess of the minimum inhibitory concentration for sensitive organisms.

DOSE CALCULATION BY BODY WEIGHT AND SURFACE AREA

There are many circumstances in which a fixed drug dose is likely to be ineffective or toxic in a significant number of individuals, e.g. cytotoxic chemotherapy, aminoglycoside antibiotics. It is usual then to calculate the dose according to body weight. Adjustment according to *body surface area* is also used and may be more appropriate, for this correlates better with many physiological phenomena, e.g. metabolic rate. The relationship between body surface area and weight is curvilinear but a reasonable approximation is that a 70 kg human has a body surface area of 1.8 m². A combination of body weight and height gives a more precise value for surface area (which can be obtained from standard nomograms) and there are several more sophisticated methods.[24]

The issue takes on special significance in the case of children if only the adult drug dose is known; adjustment is then commonly made on the basis of body weight, or body surface area, among other factors (see p. 126).

PROLONGATION OF DRUG ACTION

- A larger dose is the most obvious way to prolong a drug action. As this is not always feasible, other mechanisms are used.
- Vasoconstriction will reduce local blood flow so that distribution of drug away from an injection site is retarded, e.g. local anaesthetic action is prolonged by combination with adrenaline (epinephrine).
- Slowing of metabolism may usefully extend drug action, as when a dopa decarboxylase inhibitor, e.g. carbidopa, is combined with levodopa (as co-careldopa) for parkinsonism.
- Delayed excretion is seldom practicable, the only important example being the use of probenecid to block renal tubular excretion of penicillin, e.g. when the latter is used in single dose to treat gonorrhoea.
- Molecular structure may be altered to prolong effect, e.g. the various benzodiazepines.
- Pharmaceutical formulation. Manipulating the formulation in which a drug is presented by modified-release[25] systems can achieve the objective of an even as well as a prolonged effect.

---

[24] For example: Livingston EH, Lee S 2001 Body surface area prediction in normal-weight and obese patients. American Journal of Physiology Endocrinology and Metabolism 281: 586–591

[25] The term *modified* covers several drug delivery systems. *Delayed-release*: available other than immediately after administration (mesalazine in the colon); *sustained-release*: slow release as governed by the delivery system (iron, potassium); *controlled-release*: at a constant rate to maintain unvarying plasma concentration (nitrate, hormone replacement therapy).

Sustained-release (oral) preparations can reduce the frequency of medication to once a day, and compliance is made easier for the patient. Most long-term medication for the elderly can now be given as a single morning dose. In addition sustained-release preparations may avoid local bowel toxicity due to high local concentrations, e.g. ulceration of the small intestine with potassium chloride tablets, and may also avoid the toxic peak plasma concentrations that can occur when dissolution of the formulation, and so absorption of the drug, are rapid. Some sustained-release formulations also contain an immediate-release component to provide rapid, as well as sustained, effect.

Depot (injectable) preparations are more reliable because the environment in which they are deposited is more constant than can ever be the case in the alimentary tract and medication can be given at longer intervals, even weeks. In general such preparations are pharmaceutical variants, e.g. microcrystals, or the original drug in oil, wax, gelatin or synthetic media. They include phenothiazine neuroleptics, the various insulins and penicillins, preparations of vasopressin, and medroxyprogesterone (i.m., s.c.). Tablets of hormones are sometimes implanted subcutaneously. The advantages of infrequent administration and better patient compliance in a variety of situations are obvious.

REDUCTION OF ABSORPTION TIME

This can be achieved by making a soluble salt of the drug which is rapidly absorbed from the site of administration. In the case of s.c. or i.m. injections the same objective may be obtained with hyaluronidase, an enzyme which deploymerises hyaluronic acid, a constituent of connective tissue that prevents the spread of foreign substances, e.g. bacteria, drugs. Hyaluronidase combined with an i.m. injection e.g. a local anaesthetic, or a subcutaneous infusion, leads to increased permeation with more rapid absorption. Hyaluronidase can also be used to promote resorption of tissue accumulation of blood and fluid.

FIXED-DOSE DRUG COMBINATIONS

This section refers to combinations of drugs in a single pharmaceutical formulation. It does not refer to concomitant drug therapy, e.g. in infections, hypertension and in cancer, when several drugs are given separately.

Fixed-dose drug combinations are **appropriate** for:

- *Convenience,* with improved patient compliance. This is particularly appropriate when two drugs are used at constant dose, long term, for an asymptomatic condition, e.g. a thiazide plus a β-adrenoceptor blocker in mild or moderate hypertension. The fewer tablets the patients have to take, the more reliably will they use them, especially the elderly—who as a group receive more drugs because they have multiple pathology.
- *Enhanced effect.* Single-drug treatment of tuberculosis leads to the emergence of resistant mycobacteria; this effect is prevented or delayed by using two or more drugs simultaneously. Combining isoniazid with rifampicin (Rifinah, Rimactazid) ensures that single drug treament cannot occur; treatment has to be two drugs or no drug at all. Oral contraception (with an oestrogen and progestogen combination) is used for the same reason.
- *Minimisation of unwanted effects.* Combining levodopa with benserazide (Madopar) or with carbidopa (Sinemet) slows its metabolism outside the central nervous system so that smaller amounts of levodopa can be used; this reduces adverse effects.

Fixed-dose drug combinations are **inappropriate:**

- When the dose of one or more of the component drugs may need to be adjusted independently. A drug with a wide dose-range that must be adjusted to suit the patient's response is unsuitable for combination with a drug that has a narrow dose range.
- If the time course of drug action demands different intervals between administration of the components.
- If irregularity of administration, e.g. in response to a symptom such as pain or cough, is desirable for some ingredients but not for others.

CONCLUSIONS

Therapeutic aims should be clear. Combinations should not be prescribed unless there is good reason to

consider that the patient needs all the drugs in the formulation and that the doses are appropriate and will not need to be adjusted separately. Rational combinations can provide advantage, just as inappropriate combinations may be dangerous. Thus a combination of iron with folic acid and cyanocobalamin would be hazardous if it delays the diagnosis of pernicious anaemia. But the fact that iron plus a little folic acid is properly used in pregnancy for routine anaemia prophylaxis simply confirms that combinations can be rationally devised to meet particular needs.

Chronic pharmacology

With many drugs there are differences in pharmaco-dynamics and pharmacokinetics according to whether their use is in a single dose or over a brief period (acute pharmacology) or long term (chronic pharmacology). The proportion of the population taking drugs continuously for large portions of their lives increases as tolerable suppressive and prophylactic remedies for chronic or recurrent conditions are developed; e.g. for arterial hypertension, diabetes mellitus, mental diseases, epilepsies, gout, collagen diseases, thrombosis, allergies and various infections. In some cases long-term treatment introduces significant hazard into patients' lives and the cure can be worse than the disease if it is not skilfully managed. In general the dangers of a drug are not markedly increased if therapy lasts years rather than months; exceptions include renal damage due to analgesic mixtures, and carcinogenicity.

INTERFERENCE WITH SELF-REGULATING SYSTEMS

When self-regulating physiological systems (generally controlled by negative feedback systems, e.g. endocrine, cardiovascular) are subject to interference, their control mechanisms respond to minimise the effects of the interference and to restore the previous steady state or rhythm: this is *homeostasis.* The previous state may be a normal function, e.g. ovulation (a rare example of a positive feedback mechanism), or an abnormal function, e.g.

high blood pressure. If the body successfully restores the previous steady state or rhythm then the subject has become tolerant to the drug, i.e. a higher dose is needed to produce the desired previous effect.

In the case of hormonal contraceptives, persistence of suppression of ovulation occurs and is desired, but persistence of other effects, e.g. on blood coagulation and metabolism, is not desired.

In the case of arterial hypertension, tolerance to a single drug commonly occurs, e.g. reduction of peripheral resistance by a vasodilator is compensated by an increase in blood volume that restores the blood pressure; this is why a diuretic is commonly used together with a vasodilator in therapy.

Feedback systems. The endocrine system serves fluctuating body needs. Glands are therefore capable either of increasing or decreasing their output by means of negative (usually) feedback systems. An administered hormone or hormone analogue activates the receptors of the feedback system so that high doses cause suppression of natural production of the hormone. On withdrawal of the administered hormone restoration of the normal control mechanism takes time; e.g. the hypothalamic/pituitary/adrenal cortex system can take months to recover full sensitivity, and sudden withdrawal of administered corticosteroid can result in an acute deficiency state that may be life-endangering.

Regulation of receptors. The number (density) of receptors on cells (for hormones, autacoids or local hormones, and drugs), the number occupied (receptor occupancy) and the capacity of the receptor to respond (affinity, efficacy) can change in reponse to the concentration of the specific binding molecule or ligand,[26] whether this be agonist or antagonist (blocker). The effects always tend to restore cell function to its normal or usual state. Prolonged high concentrations of agonist (whether administered as a drug or over-produced in the body by a tumour) cause a reduction in the number of receptors available for activation (*down-regulation*); changes in receptor occupancy and affinity and the prolonged occupation of receptors by inert molecules (antagonists) leads to an increase in the number of

receptors (*up-regulation*). At least some of this may be achieved by receptors moving inside the cell and out again (internalisation and externalisation).

Down-regulation and the accompanying receptor changes may explain the tolerant or refractory state seen in severe asthmatics who no longer respond to β-adrenoceptor agonists.

Up-regulation. The occasional exacerbation of ischaemic cardiac disease on sudden withdrawal of a β-adrenoceptor blocker may be explained by up-regulation during its administration, so that on withdrawal, an above-normal number of receptors suddenly becomes accessible to the normal chemotransmitter, i.e. noradrenaline (norepinephrine).

Up-regulation with rebound sympathomimetic effects may be innocuous to a moderately healthy cardiovascular system, but the increased oxygen demand of these effects can have serious consequences where ischaemic disease is present and increased oxygen need cannot be met (angina pectoris, arrhythmia, myocardial infarction). Unmasking of a disease process that has worsened during prolonged suppressive use of the drug, i.e. *resurgence*, may also contribute to such exacerbations.

The rebound phenomenon is plainly a potential hazard and the use of a β-adrenoceptor blocker in the presence of ischaemic heart disease would be safer if rebound could be eliminated. β-adrenoceptor blockers that are not pure antagonists but have some agonist (sympathomimetic ischaemic) activity, i.e. partial agonists, may prevent the generation of additional adrenoceptors (up-regulation). Indeed there is evidence that rebound is less or is absent with pindolol, a partial agonist β-adrenoceptor blocker.

Sometimes a distinction is made between *rebound* (recurrence at intensified degree of the symptoms for which the drug was given) and *withdrawal syndrome* (appearance of new additional symptoms). The distinction is quantitative and does not imply different mechanisms.

Rebound and withdrawal phenomena occur erratically. In general, they are more likely with drugs having a short half-life (abrupt drop in plasma concentration) and pure agonist or antagonist action. They are less likely to occur with drugs

---

[26] 24 Latin: *ligare*, to bind.

having a long half-life and (probably) with those having a mixed agonist/antagonist (partial agonist) action on receptors.

ABRUPT WITHDRAWAL

Clinically important consequences are known, and might occur for a variety of reasons, e.g. a patient interrupting drug therapy to undergo surgery. The following are examples:

- *Cardiovascular system:* β-adrenoceptor blockers, antihypertensives (especially clonidine).
- *Nervous system:* all depressants (hypnotics, sedatives, alcohol, opioids), antiepileptics, antiparkinsonian agents, tricyclic antidepressants.
- *Endocrine system:* adrenal steroids.
- *Immune inflammation:* adrenal steroids.

Resurgence of chronic disease which has progressed in severity although its consequences have been wholly or partly suppressed, i.e. a catching-up phenomenon, is an obvious possible consequence of withdrawal of effective therapy, e.g. levodopa in Parkinson's disease; in corticosteroid withdrawal in autoimmune disease there may be both resurgence and rebound.

Drug discontinuation syndromes, i.e. rebound, withdrawal and resurgence (defined above) are phenomena that are to be expected. In many cases the exact mechanisms remain obscure but clinicians have no reason to be surprised when they occur, and in the case of rebound they may particularly wish to use gradual withdrawal wherever drugs have been used to modify complex self-adjusting systems, and to suppress (without cure) chronic diseases.

OTHER ASPECTS OF CHRONIC DRUG USE

Metabolic changes over a long period may induce disease, e.g. thiazide diuretics (diabetes mellitus), adrenocortical hormones (osteoporosis), phenytoin (osteomalacia). Drugs may also enhance their own metabolism, and that of other drugs (enzyme induction).

Specific cell injury or cell functional disorder occur with individual drugs or drug classes, e.g. tardive dyskinesia (dopamine receptor blockers), retinal damage (chloroquine, phenothiazines), retroperitoneal fibrosis (methysergide), NSAIDs (nephropathy). Cancer may occur, e.g. with oestrogens (endometrium) and with immunosuppressive (anticancer) drugs.

Drug holidays. This term means the deliberate interruption of long-term therapy with the objective of restoring sensitivity (which has been lost) or to reduce the risk of toxicity. Plainly the need for holidays is a substantial disadvantage for any drug. The principal example is methysergide for refractory migraine (see Index). Patients sometimes initiate their own drug holidays (see Patient compliance).

Dangers of intercurrent illness. These are particularly notable with anticoagulants, adrenal steroids and immunosuppressives.

Dangers of interactions with other drugs or food: see index, food, interactions, individual drugs.

CONCLUSIONS

> Drugs not only induce their known listed primary actions, but they:
> - Evoke compensatory responses in the complex inter-related physiological systems they perturb, and these systems need time to recover on withdrawal of the drug (gradual withdrawal can give this time; it is sometimes mandatory and never harmful)
> - Induce metabolic changes that may be trivial in the short term, but serious if they persist for a long time
> - May produce localised effects in specially susceptible tissues and induce serious cell damage or malfunction
> - Increase susceptibility to intercurrent illness and to interaction with other drugs that may be taken for new indications

That such consequences will occur with prolonged drug use is to be expected. With a knowledge of physiology, pathology and pharmacology, combined with an awareness that the unexpected is to be expected ('There are more things in heaven and earth, Horatio, than are dreamt of in your philosophy'[27]) those patients requiring long-term therapy may be managed safely, or at least with minimum risk of harm, and enabled to live happy lives.

Individual or biological variation

Prescribing for special risk groups

That individuals respond differently to drugs, both from time to time and from other individuals, is a matter of everyday experience. Doctors need to accommodate for individual variation, for it may explain both adverse response to a drug and failure of therapy. Sometimes there are obvious physical characteristics such as age, race (genetics) or disease that warn the prescriber to adjust drug dose, but there are no external features that signify, e.g., pseudocholinesterase deficiency, which causes prolonged paralysis after suxamethonium. An understanding of the reasons for individual variation in response to drugs is relevant to all who prescribe. Both pharmacodynamic and pharmacokinetic effects are involved and the issues fall in two general categories: inherited influences and environmental and host influences.

Inherited influences: Pharmacogenetics

Consider how individuals in a population might be expected to respond to a fixed dose of a drug; some would show less than the usual response, most would show the usual response and some would show more than the usual response. This type of variation is described as *continuous* and in a graph the result would appear as a normal or Gaussian (bell-shaped) distribution curve, similar to the

type of curve that describes the distribution of height, weight or metabolic rate in a population. The curve is the result of a multitude of factors, some genetic (multiple genes) and some environmental, that contribute collectively to the response of the individual to the drug; they include race, sex, diet, weight, environmental and body temperature, circadian rhythm, absorption, distribution, metabolism, excretion and receptor density, but no single factor has a predominant effect.

Less commonly, variation is *discontinuous* when differences in response reveal a discrete proportion, large or small, who respond differently from the rest, e.g. poor drug oxidisers or fast and slow acetylators of isoniazid. Discontinuous variation most commonly occurs when response to a drug is controlled by a single gene. The term *genetic polymorphism* refers to the existence in a population of two or more discontinuous forms of a species which are subject to simple inheritance. By convention the frequency of each species is 1% or more.

> **Pharmacogenetics** is concerned with drug responses that are governed by heredity (see also pharmacogenomics p. 42). Inherited factors causing different responses to drugs are commonly biochemical because single genes govern the production of enzymes. Pharmacogenetic polymorphism is often expressed in the form of different drug metabolising capacities, i.e. genetic differences in a single enzymes. Inherited abnormal responses to drugs mediated by single genes are called **idiosyncrasy** and cause increased, decreased and bizarre responses to drugs.

SOME HERITABLE CONDITIONS CAUSING INCREASED OR TOXIC RESPONSES

Defective oxidation. Variation in response to some drugs can be attributed to genetic polymorphisms involving oxidation of their carbon centres (see Metabolism p. 112). The condition was recognised by abnormal metabolism and response to a standard dose of debrisoquine.[28] Individuals may be classed as extensive or poor oxidisers and the latter are at special risk of adverse effects from drugs whose inactivation is strongly dependent on the defective

---

[27] W Shakespeare (1564–1616) Hamlet: IV. 166.

isoenzyme. People who have inherited the 'poor' oxidiser form of CYP 2D6 may show exaggerated or toxic responses to standard doses of a range of drugs that include bufuralol, metoprolol, timolol (increased β-blockade), haloperidol (excessive sedation), flecainide and nortriptyline. The frequency of poor oxidisers ranges from 1% in Asians to 6% in whites (there are over 5 million slow oxidisers in the UK). Additionally, a group of *ultra-rapid* metabolisers is now recognised; they may fail to respond to standard drug doses. A similar but distinct condition is characterised by deficiency in metabolism of the antiepileptic drug mephenytoin (CYP 2C19) and affects 8–23% of Asians and 3–6% of whites. Substrate drugs include diazepam, citalopram, omeprazole and proguanil. A polymorphism of CYP 2C9 affects up to 30% of people and results in slow metabolism (and risk of toxicity) of warfarin, tolbutamide and losartan.

Acetylation is an important route of metabolism for many drugs that possess an amide ($-NH_2$) group. Population studies have shown that most individuals are either rapid or slow acetylators but the proportion of each varies greatly between races. Some 90% of Japanese are rapid acetylators whereas in Western populations the proportion is 50% or less. Global trends are also recognised. Along the Pacific Asian littoral, the frequency of fast acetylators is highest near the Arctic (Inuit 95%) and falls towards the Equator.

Acetylator status is relevant to therapy with certain drugs. Isoniazid may cause peripheral neuropathy in slow acetylators on standard doses and pyridoxine is added to the antituberculosis regimen where there is special risk, e.g. in diabetes, alcoholism, renal failure. Acute hepatocellular necrosis with isoniazid is more common in rapid acetylators, perhaps because they more readily form an hepatotoxic metabolite. Sulphasalazine (salicylazosulphapyridine) (used for rheumatoid arthritis) causes adverse effects more frequently in slow acetylators, probably because of the sulphapyridine component which is inactivated by acetylation. Dapsone appears to cause more red-cell haemolysis in slow acetylators; rapid acetylators may need higher doses to control dermatitis herpetiformis and leprosy. Hydralazine and procainamide may cause antinuclear antibodies to develop in the plasma of slow acetylators, and some proceed to systemic lupus erythematosus.

Glucose-6-phosphate dehydrogenase (G6PD) deficiency. G6PD activity is important to the integrity of the red blood cell through a chain of reactions:

- It is an important source of reduced nicotinamide-adenine dinucleotide phosphate (NADPH) which maintains erythrocyte glultathione in its reduced form.
- Reduced glutathione is necessary to keep haemoglobin in the reduced (ferrous) rather than in its ferric state (methaemoglobin) which is useless for oxygen carriage.
- Build-up of methaemoglobin in erythrocytes impairs the function of sulphydryl groups, especially those associated with the stability of the cell membrane.

Individuals who are G6PD deficient may suffer from acute haemolysis if they are exposed to certain oxidant substances, including drugs. Characteristically there is an acute haemolytic episode 2–3 days after starting the drug. The haemolysis is self-limiting, only older cells with least enzyme being affected. The condition is common in African, Mediterranean, Middle East and South East Asian races and in their descendants and, throughout the world, affects some 100 million people. As deficiency may result from inheritance of any one of numerous variants of G6PD, affected individuals exhibit differing susceptibility to haemolysis, i.e. a substance which affects one G6PD deficient subject

---

[28] The poor oxidiser state was first revealed in the laboratory of R L Smith, Professor of Biochemical Pharmacology, St Mary's Hospital Medical School, London, who was investigating the variable dose requirements of patients receiving the two antihypertensive drugs debrisoquine and bethanidine. He writes: 'I took 40 mg of debrisoquine sulphate; within two hours my blood pressure crashed to 70/50 mmHg and I was unable to stand for four hours due to incapacitating postural hypotension … it was two days until the blood pressure returned to normal. Analysis of my urine revealed that nearly all the dose was excreted as unchanged drug, whereas other subjects who showed little if any cardiovascular response to the same dose of debrisoquine, coverted it to the 4-hydroxy metabolite. However, the drama of the clinical response to a single dose of debrisoquine catalysed a search for its explanation and culminated in the uncovering of the first example of a genetic polymorphism of drug oxidation'.

adversely may be harmless in another. It is usually dose related. The following guidelines apply:[29]

Drugs that carry a **definite** risk of haemolysis in most G6PD deficient subjects include: dapsone (and other sulphones), methylene blue, niridazole, nitrofurantoin, pamaquin, primaquine, quinolone antimicrobials, some sulphonamides.

Drugs that carry a **possible** risk of haemolysis in some G6PD deficient subjects inculde: aspirin (when dose exceeds 1 g/d), menadione, probenecid, quinidine; chloroquine and quinine (both are acceptable in acute malaria).

Affected individuals are also found to be susceptible to exposure to nitrates, anilines and naphthalenes (found in moth balls). Some individuals, particularly children, experience haemolysis after eating the broad bean, *Vicia faba,* and hence the term 'favism'.[30]

Pseudocholinesterase deficiency. The neuromuscular blocking action of suxamethonium is terminated by plasma pseudocholinesterase. 'True' cholinesterase (acetylcholinesterase) hydrolyses acetylcholine released by nerve endings, whereas various tissues and plasma contain other nonspecific, hence 'pseudo', esterases. Affected individuals form so little plasma pseudocholinesterase that metabolism of suxamethonium is seriously reduced. The deficiency characteristically comes to light when a patient fails to breathe spontaneously after a surgical operation, and assisted ventilation may have to be undertaken for hours. Relatives of an affected individual—for this as for other inherited abnormalities carrying avoidable risk—should be sought out, checked to assess their own risk, and told of the result. The prevalence of pseudocholinesterase deficiency in the UK population is about 1 in 2500.

Malignant hyperthermia (p. 427).

Porphyria (p. 139).

Thiopurine methyltransferase (p. 292).

---

[29] Data based on British National Formulary, 2002.
[30] A danger that was recognised by Pythagoras (Greek philosopher, 580–c500 BC). Nebert D W 1999 Clinical Genetics 56: 345–347.

Alcohol (p. 184).

SOME HERITABLE CONDITIONS CAUSING DECREASED DRUG RESPONSES

Resistance to coumarin anticoagulants. Subjects of this rare inherited abnormality possess a variant of the enzyme that coverts vitamin K to its reduced and active form, which enzyme the coumarins normally inhibit; patients require 20 times or more of the usual dose to obtain an adequate clinical response. A similar condition also occurs in rats and has practical importance as warfarin, a coumarin, is used as a rat poison (rats with the gene are dubbed 'super-rats' by the mass media).

Resistance to heparin. Patients with antithrombin deficiency require large doses of heparin therapy for anticoagulant effect. (The action of heparin is dependent on the presence of antithrombin in the plasma.)

Resistance to suxamethonium. This rare condition is characterised by increased pseudocholinesterase activity and failure of normal doses of suxamethonium to cause muscular relaxation (cf Cholinesterase deficiency, above).

Resistance to vitamin D. Individuals develop rickets which responds only to huge doses of vitamin D, i.e. × 1000 the standard dose.

Bacterial resistance to drugs is genetically determined and is of great clinical importance.

CONCLUSION

As the components of the human genome, and their function, are progressively identified, it is certain that many clinically important single gene differences in response to drugs will be discovered. Once a genetic difference, e.g. a metabolic reaction, is understood, it will be possible to predict what will happen when drugs of particular molecular structures are administered. But whether patients should be screened routinely for such differences in drug response is a matter of clinical importance as well as economics and logistics.

Environmental and host influences

A multitude of factors related both to individuals and their environment contribute to differences in drug response. In general, their precise role is less well documented than is the case with genetic factors but their range and complexity are illustrated by the following list of likely candidates: age, sex, pregnancy, lactation, exercise, sunlight, disease, infection, occupational exposures, drugs, circadian and seasonal variations, diet, stress, fever, malnutrition, alcohol intake, tobacco or cannabis smoking and the functioning of the cardiovascular, gastrointestinal, hepatic, immunological and renal systems.[31] Some of the more relevant influences are discussed here.

AGE

The neonate, infant and child[32]

Young human beings differ greatly from adults, not merely in size but also in the proportions and constituents of their bodies and the functioning of their physiological systems. These differences are reflected in the way the body handles and responds to drugs and are relevant to prescribing.

- Rectal absorption is efficient with an appropriate formulation and has been used for diazepam and theophyllines; this route may be preferred with an uncooperative infant.
- The intramuscular or subcutaneous routes tend to give unpredictable plasma concentrations, e.g. of digoxin or gentamicin, because of the relatively low proportion of skeletal muscle and fat. Intravenous administration is preferred in the seriously ill newborn.

---

[31] Vessell E S 1982 Clinical Pharmacology and Therapeutics 31: 1.
[32] A neonate is under 1 month and an infant is 1–12 months of age.

- Drugs or other substances that come in contact with the skin are readily absorbed as the skin is well hydrated and the stratum corneum is thin; overdose toxicity may result, e.g. with hexachlorophane used in dusting powders and emulsions to prevent infection.

An understandable reluctance to test drugs extensively in children means that reliable information is often lacking. Many drugs do not have a licence to be used for children, and their prescription must be 'off licence', a practice that is recognised as necessary, if not actually promoted, by the UK drug regulatory authorities.

Distribution of drugs is influenced by the fact that total body water in the neonate amounts to 80% as compared to 65% in older children. Consequently:

- Weight-related priming doses of aminoglycosides, aminophylline, digoxin and frusemide need to be larger for neonates than for older children.
- Less extensive binding of drugs to plasma proteins is generally without clinical importance but there is a significant risk of elevation of plasma bilirubin (in the neonate) following its displacement from protein binding sites by vitamin K, x-ray contrast media or indomethacin.

Metabolism. Although the enzyme systems that inactivate drugs are present at birth, they are functionally immature, expecially in the preterm baby, and especially for oxidation and for conjugation with glucuronic acid. Inability to conjugate and thus inactivate chloramphenicol causes the fatal 'grey' syndrome in neonates. After the first weeks of life the drug metabolic capacity increases rapidly and young children may require a higher weight-related dose than adults because of their more rapid metabolic rates.

Elimination. Glomerular filtration, tubular secretion and reabsorption are low in the neonate (even lower in preterm babies) only reaching adult values in relation to body surface area at 2–5 months. Therefore drugs that are eliminated by the kidney (e.g. aminoglycosides, penicillins, diuretics) must be given in reduced dose; after about 6 months, body weight- or surface area-related daily doses are the same for all ages.

Dosage in the young. No single rule or formula suffices for all cases. The dose may be established by scaling for body weight but this approach may overdose an obese child, for whom the *ideal* weight should calculated from age and height. Doses based on body surface area are generally more accurate, and preferably should take into account both body weight and height.[33] The fact that the surface area of a 70 kg adult human is 1.8m^2 (see p. 118) may then be used for adjustment, as follows:

$$\text{Approximate dose} = \text{surface area of child (m}^2\text{)} / 1.8 \times \text{adult dose}$$

Information is increased by making pharmacokinetic and pharmacodynamic measurements when opportunities present. General guidance is available from formularies, e.g. the British National Formulary, and specialist publications.[34]

The elderly

The incidence of adverse drug reactions rises with age in the adult, especially after 65 years because of:

- The increasing number of drugs that they need to take because they tend to have multiple diseases
- Poor compliance with dosing regimens
- Bodily changes of aging that require modification of dosage regimens.

Absorption of drugs may be slightly slower because gastrointestinal blood flow and motility are reduced but the effect is rarely important.

Distribution is influenced by the following changes:
- There is a significant decrease in lean body mass so that standard adult doses provide a greater amount of drug per kg.
- Total body water is less and in general the distribution volume of water-soluble drugs is

reduced. Hence standard doses of drugs, especially the priming doses of those that are water-soluble, may exceed the requirement.
- Plasma albumin concentration tends to be well maintained in the healthy elderly but may be reduced by chronic disease, giving scope for a greater proportion of unbound (free) drug; this may be important when priming doses are given.

Metabolism is reduced because liver mass and liver blood flow are decreased. Consequently:
- Metabolic inactivation of drugs is slower.
- Drugs that are normally extensively eliminated in first-pass through the liver appear in higher concentration in the systemic circulation and persist in it for longer. There is thus particular cause initially to use lower doses of most neuroleptics, tricyclic antidepressants and cardiac antiarrhythmic agents.
- Capacity for hepatic enzyme induction appears to be lessened.

Elimination. Renal blood flow, glomerular filtration and tubular secretion decrease with age above 55 years, a decline that is not signalled by raised serum creatinine concentration because production of this metabolite is diminished by the age-associated diminution of muscle mass. Indeed, in the elderly, serum creatinine may be within the concentration range for normal young adults even when the creatinine clearance is 50 ml/min (compared to 127 ml/min in adult male). Particular risk of adverse effects arises with drugs that are eliminated mainly by the kidney and that have a small therapeutic ratio, e.g. aminoglycosides, chlorpropamide, digoxin, lithium.

Pharmacodynamic response may alter with age, to produce either a greater or lesser effect than is anticipated in younger adults, for example:
- Drugs that act on the central nervous system appear to produce an exaggerated response in relation to that expected from the plasma concentration, and sedatives and hypnotics may have a pronounced hangover effect. These drugs are also more likely to depress respiration because vital capacity and maximum breathing capacity are lessened in the elderly.

---

[33] For example: Insley J 1996 A Paediatric Vade-Mecum, 13th Edition, London, Arnold.
[34] Royal College of Paediatrics and Child Health, Neonatal and Paediatric Pharmacists Group. Pocket Medicines for Children. 2001, London.

- Response to β-adrenoceptor agonists and antagonists appears to be blunted in old age partly, it is believed, through reduction in the number of receptors.
- Baroreceptor sensitivity is reduced leading to the potential for orthostatic hypotension with drugs that reduce blood pressure.

These pharmacokinetic and pharmacodynamic differences, together with broader issues particular to the elderly find expression in the choice and use of drugs for this age group, as follows:

Rules of prescribing for the elderly[35]

1. Think about the necessity for drugs. Is the diagnosis correct and complete? Is the drug really necessary? Is there a better alternative?
2. Do not prescribe drugs that are not useful. Think carefully before giving an old person a drug that may have major side-effects, and consider alternatives.
3. Think about the dose. Is it appropriate to possible alterations in the patient's physiological state? Is it appropriate to the patient's renal and hepatic function at the time?
4. Think about drug formulation. Is a tablet the most appropriate form of drug or would an injection, a suppository or a syrup be better? Is the drug suitably packaged for the elderly patient, bearing in mind any disabilities?
5. Assume any new symptoms may be due to drug side-effects, or more rarely, to drug withdrawal. Rarely (if ever) treat a side-effect of one drug with another.
6. Take a careful drug history. Bear in mind the possibility of interaction with substances the patient may be taking without your knowledge, such as herbal or other nonprescribed remedies, old drugs taken from the medicine cabinet or drugs obtained from friends.
7. Use fixed combinations of drugs only when they are logical and well studied and they either aid compliance or improve tolerance or

efficacy. Few fixed combinations meet this standard.
8. When adding a new drug to the therapeutic regimen, see whether another can be withdrawn.
9. Attempt to check whether the patient's compliance is adequate, e.g. by counting remaining tablets. Has the patient (or relatives) been properly instructed?
10. Remember that stopping a drug is as important as starting it.

The old (80+ years) are particulary intolerant of neuroleptics (given for confusion) and of diuretics (given for ankle swelling that is postural and not due to heart failure) which cause adverse electrolyte changes. Both classes of drug may result in admission to hospital of semicomatose 'senior citizens' who deserve better treatment from their juniors.

PREGNANCY

As the pregnancy evolves, profound changes occur in physiology, including fluid and tissue composition.

Absorption. Gastrointestinal motility is decreased but there appears to be no major defect in drug absorption except that reduced gastric emptying delays the appearance in the plasma of orally administered drugs, especially during labour. Absorption from an intramuscular site is likely to be efficient because tissue perfusion is increased due to vasodilatation.

Distribution. Total body water increases by up to 8 litres creating a larger space within which water-soluble drugs may distribute. As a result of haemodilution, plasma albumin (normal 33–55 g/l) declines by some 10 g/l. Thus there is scope for increased free concentration of drugs that bind to albumin. Unbound drug, however, is free to distribute and to be metabolised and excreted; e.g. the free (and pharmacologically active) concentration of phenytoin is unaltered, although the total plasma concentration is reduced.

Therapeutic drug monitoring interpreted by concentrations appropriate for nonpregnant women thus may mislead. A useful general guide during pregnancy is to maintain concentrations at the lower end of the recommended range. Body fat increases

---

[35] By permission from Caird F I (ed) 1985 Drugs for the elderly. WHO (Europe) Copenhagen.

by about 4 kg and provides a reservoir for lipid-soluble drugs.

Hepatic metabolism increases, though not blood flow to the liver. Consequently, there is increased clearance of drugs such as phenytoin and theophylline, whose elimination rate depends on liver enzyme activity. Drugs that are so rapidly metabolised that their elimination rate depends on their delivery to the liver, i.e. on hepatic blood flow, have unaltered clearance, e.g. pethidine.

Elimination. Renal plasma flow almost doubles and there is more rapid loss of drugs that are excreted by the kidney, e.g. amoxicillin, the dose of which should be doubled for systemic infections (but not for urinary tract infections as penicillins are highly concentrated in the urine).

Placenta: see page 98.

DISEASE

Pharmacokinetic changes

Absorption
- Surgery that involves resection and reconstruction of the gut may lead to malabsorption of iron, folic acid and fat-soluble vitamins after partial gastrectomy, and of vitamin B_{12} after ileal resection.
- Delayed gastric emptying and intestinal stasis during an attack of migraine interfere with absorption of drugs.
- Severe low output cardiac failure or shock (with peripheral vasoconstriction) delays absorption from subcutaneous or intramuscular sites; reduced hepatic blood flow prolongs the presence in the plasma of drugs that are so rapidly extracted by the liver that removal depends on their rate of presentation to it, e.g. lignocaine.

Distribution. Hypoalbuminaemia from any cause, e.g. burns, malnutrition, sepsis, allows a higher proportion of free (unbound) drug in plasma. Although free drug is available for metabolism and excretion, there remains a risk of enhanced or adverse responses especially with initial doses of those that are highly protein bound, e.g. phenytoin.

Metabolism. Acute inflammatory disease of the liver (viral, alcoholic) and cirrhosis affect both the functioning of the hepatocytes and blood flow through the liver. Reduced extraction from the plasma of drugs that are normally highly cleared in first pass through the liver results in increased systemic availability of drugs such as metoprolol, labetalol and chlormethiazole. Many other drugs exhibit prolonged $t\frac{1}{2}$ and reduced clearance in patients with chronic liver disease, e.g. diazepam, tolbutamide, rifampicin (see Drugs and the liver, p. 652). Thyroid disease has the expected effects, i.e. drug metabolism is accelerated in hyperthyroidism and diminished in hypothyroidism.

Elimination. Disease of the kidney (p. 541) has profound effects on the pharmacokinetics and thence the actions of drugs that are eliminated by that organ.

Pharmacodynamic changes

- *Asthmatic attacks* can be precipitated by β-adrenoceptor blockers.
- *Malfunctioning of the respiratory centre* (raised intracranial pressure, severe pulmonary insufficiency) causes patients to be intolerant of opioids, and indeed any sedative may precipitate respiratory failure.
- *Myocardial infarction* predisposes to cardiac arrhythmia with digitalis glycosides or sympathomimetics.
- *Myasthenia gravis* is made worse by quinine and quinidine and myasthenics are intolerant of competitive neuromuscular blocking agents and aminoglycoside antibiotics.

FOOD

- The presence of food in the stomach, especially if it is fatty, delays gastric emptying and the absorption of certain drugs; the plasma concentration of ampicillin and rifampicin may be much reduced if they are taken on a full stomach. More specifically, calcium, e.g. in milk, interferes with absorption of tetracyclines and iron (by chelation).
- Substituting protein for fat or carbohydrate in the diet is associated with an increase in drug

oxidation rates. Some specific dietary factors induce drug metabolising enzymes, e.g. alcohol, charcoal grilled (broiled) beef, cabbage and Brussels sprouts.

Protein malnutrition causes changes that are likely to influence pharmacokinetics, e.g. loss of body weight, reduced hepatic metabolising capacity, hypoproteinaemia.

Citrus flavinoids in grapefruit (but not orange) juice decrease hepatic metabolism and may lead to risk of toxicity from amiodarone, terfenadine (cardiac arrhythmia), benzodiazepines (increased sedation), ciclosporin, felodipine (reduced blood pressure).

Alterations in drug action caused by diet are termed *drug–food* interactions

Drug interactions

When a drug is administered, a response occurs; if a second drug is given and the response to the first drug is altered, a drug interaction is said to have occurred.[36] A drug interaction may be *desired* or *undesired*, i.e. *beneficial* or *harmful*. It is deliberately sought in multidrug treatment of tuberculosis and when naloxone is given to treat morphine overdose. It is an embarrassment when a woman taking a combined oestrogen/progestogen oral contraceptive for a desired interaction is prescribed a drug that is a metabolic enzyme inducer, with the result that she becomes pregnant. Although dramatic unintended interactions attract most attention and are the principal subject of this section they should not distract attention from the many therapeutically useful interactions that are the basis of rational polypharmacy. These useful interactions are referred to throughout the book whenever it is relevant to do so.

CLINICAL IMPORTANCE OF DRUG INTERACTIONS

If doctors were to limit their prescribing to the model list of Essential Drugs (WHO) (p. 28) and were to prescribe four drugs for any patient at any

one time, the number of possible combinations would be more than 64 million. There can be no doubt that the number of drug interactions that might occur in this imagined situation would be too large to commit to memory or to paper. But the observation that one drug can be shown measurably to alter the disposition or effect of another drug does not mean that the interaction is necessarily of clinical importance. In this section we highlight the circumstances in which clinically important interactions can occur; we describe their pharmacological basis and provide a schematic framework to identify potential drug interactions during clinical practice.

Clinically important **adverse** drug interactions become likely with the following:

- Drugs that have a steep dose–response curve and a small therapeutic index (p. 94) so that relatively small quantitative changes at the target site, e.g. receptor or enzyme, will lead to substantial changes in effect, as with digoxin or lithium
- Drugs that are known enzyme inducers or inhibitors (pp. 113, 114)
- Drugs that are exhibit saturable metabolism (zero-order kinetics), when small interference with kinetics may lead to large alteration of plasma concentration, e.g. phenytoin, theophylline
- Drugs that are used long-term, where precise plasma concentrations are required, e.g. oral contraceptives, antiepilepsy drugs, cardiac antiarrhythmia drugs, lithium
- When drugs that may interact are used to treat the same disease, for this increases their chance of being given concurrently, e.g. theophylline and salbutamol given for asthma may cause cardiac arrhythmia
- In severely ill patients, for they may be receiving several drugs; signs of iatrogenic disease may be difficult to distinguish from those of existing disease and the patients' condition may be such that they cannot tolerate further adversity
- In patients with significantly impaired liver or kidney function, for these are the principal organs that terminate drug action
- In the elderly, for they tend to have multiple pathology, may receive several drugs concurrently, and are specially susceptible to adverse drug effects (p. 126).

---

[36] The term drug–drug interaction is also used, to make the distinction from drug–food interactions, and interaction with endogenous transmitters and hormones.

PHARMACOLOGICAL BASIS OF DRUG INTERACTIONS

Some knowledge of the pharmacological basis of how one drug may change the action of another is useful in obtaining those interactions that are wanted, as well as in recognising and preventing those that are not.

Drug interactions are of two principal kinds:

1. *Pharmacodynamic interaction:* both drugs act on the target site of clinical effect, exerting synergism (below) or antagonism. The drugs may act on the same or different receptors or processes, mediating similar biological consequences. Examples include: alcohol + benzodiazepine (to produce sedation), morphine + naloxone (to reverse opioid overdose), rifampicin + isoniazid (effective antituberculosis combination).
2. *Pharmacokinetic interaction:* the drugs interact remotely from the target site to alter plasma (and other tissue) concentrations so that the amount of the drug at the target site of clinical effect is altered, e.g. enzyme induction by rifampicin will reduce the plasma concentration of warfarin; enzyme inhibition by ciprofloxacin will elevate the concentration of theophylline.

Interaction may result in antagonism or synergism.

Antagonism occurs when the action of one drug opposes the action of another. The two drugs simply have opposite pharmacodynamic effects, e.g. histamine and adrenaline on the bronchi exhibit physiological or functional antagonism; or they compete reversibly for the same drug receptor, e.g. flumazenil and benzodiazepines exhibit competitive antagonism.

Synergism[37] is of two sorts:
1. *Summation* or addition occurs when the effects of two drugs having the same action are additive, i.e. 2 + 2 = 4 (a β-adrenoceptor blocker plus a thiazide diuretic have an additive antihypertensive effect).
2. *Potentiation* (to make more powerful) occurs when one drug increases the action of another,

i.e. 2 + 2 = 5. Sometimes the two drugs both have the action concerned (trimethoprim plus sulphonamide) and sometimes one drug lacks the action concerned (benserazide plus levodopa), i.e. 0 + 2 = 5.

IDENTIFYING POTENTIAL DRUG INTERACTIONS

Drugs can interact at any stage from when they are mixed with other drugs in a pharmaceutical formulation or by a clinician, e.g. in an i.v. infusion or syringe, to their final excretion either unchanged or as metabolites. When a drug is added to an existing regimen, a doctor can evaluate the possibility of an interaction by logically thinking through the usual sequence of processes to which a drug is subject and which are outlined earlier in this chapter, i.e. interactions may occur:

- outside the body
- at the site of absorption
- during distribution
- on receptors or body systems (pharmacodynamic interactions)
- during metabolism
- during excretion.

INTERACTIONS OUTSIDE THE BODY

Intravenous fluids offer special scope for interactions (incompatibilities) when drugs are added to the reservoir or syringe, for a number of reasons. Drugs commonly are weak organic acids or bases. They are often insoluble and to make them soluble it is necessary to prepare salts. Plainly, the mixing of solutions of salts can result in instability which may or may not be evident from visible change in the solution, i.e. precipitation. Furthermore, the solutions have little buffering capacity and pH readily changes with added drugs. Dilution of a drug in the reservoir fluid may also lead to loss of stability.

A serious loss of potency can result from incompatibility between an infusion fluid and a drug that is added to it. Issues of compatibility are complex but specific sources of information are available in manufacturers' package inserts, formularies or from the hospital pharmacy (where the addition ought to be made). The general rule

---

[37] Greek: *syn*, together; *ergos*, work.

must be to consult these sources before ever adding a drug to an infusion fluid or mixing in a syringe.

Mixing drugs formulated for injection in a syringe may cause interaction, e.g. protamine zinc insulin contains excess of protamine which binds with added soluble insulin and reduces the immediate effect of the dose.

INTERACTIONS AT SITE OF ABSORPTION

In the complex environment of the gut there are opportunities for drugs to interfere with each other both directly and indirectly via alteration of gut physiology. Usually the result is to impair absorption.

Direct chemical interaction in the gut is a significant cause of reduced absorption. Antacids that contain aluminium and magnesium form insoluble complexes with tetracyclines, iron and prednisolone. Milk contains sufficient calcium to warrant its avoidance as a major article of diet when tetracyclines are taken. Colestyramine interferes with absorption of levothyroxine, digoxin and some acidic drugs, e.g. warfarin. Sucralfate reduces the absorption of phenytoin. Interactions of this type depend on both drugs being in the stomach at the same time, and can be prevented if the doses are separated by at least 2 hours.

Gut motility may be altered by drugs. Slowing of gastric emptying, e.g. opioid analgesics, tricyclic antidepressants (antimuscarinic effect), may delay and reduce the absorption of other drugs. Purgatives reduce the time spent in the small intestine and give less opportunity for the absorption of poorly soluble substances such as adrenal steroids and digoxin.

Alterations in gut flora by antimicrobials may potentiate oral anticoagulant by reducing bacterial synthesis of vitamin K (usually only after anti-microbials are given orally in high dose, e.g. to treat *Helicobacter pylori*).

Interactions other than in the gut are exemplified by the use of hyaluronidase to promote dissipation of a s.c. injection, and by the addition of vaso-constrictors, e.g. adrenaline, felypressin, to local anaesthetics to delay absorption and usefully prolong local anaesthesia.

INTERACTIONS DURING DISTRIBUTION

Displacement from plasma protein binding sites may contribute to adverse reaction. A drug that is extensively protein bound can be displaced from its binding site by a competing drug, so raising the free (and pharmacologically active) concentration of the first drug. Unbound drug, however, is available for distribution away from the plasma and for metabolism and excretion. Commonly, the result is that the free concentration of the displaced drug quickly returns close to its original value and any extra effect is transient.

For a displacement interaction to become clinically important, a second mechanism usually operates: sodium valproate can cause phenytoin toxicity because it both displaces phenytoin from its binding site on plasma albumin and inhibits its metabolism. Similarly aspirin and probenecid (and possibly other nonsteroidal anti-inflammatory drugs) displace the folic acid antagonist methotrexate from its protein-binding site and reduce its rate of active secretion by the renal tubules; the result is serious methotrexate toxicity.

Bilirubin is displaced from its binding protein by sulphonamides, vitamin K, X-ray contrast media or indomethacin; in the neonate this may cause a significant risk of kernicterus, for its capacity to metabolise bilirubin is immature.

Direct interaction between drugs may also take place in the plasma, e.g. protamine with heparin; desferrioxamine with iron; dimercaprol with arsenic (all useful).

Displacement from tissue binding may cause unwanted effects. When quinidine is given to patients who are receiving digoxin, the plasma concentration of free digoxin may double because quinidine displaces digoxin from binding sites in tissue (as well as plasma proteins). As with interaction due to displacement from plasma proteins, however, an additional mechanism contributes to the overall effect, for quinidine also impairs renal excretion of digoxin.

INTERACTIONS DIRECTLY ON RECEPTORS OR ON BODY SYSTEMS

This category of pharmacodynamic interactions comprises specific interactions between drugs on the same receptor, and includes less precise interactions involving the same body organ or system; whatever the precise location, the result is altered drug action.

Action on receptors provides numerous examples. Beneficial interactions are sought in overdose, as with the use of naloxone for morphine overdose (opioid receptor), of atropine for anticholinesterase, i.e. insecticide poisoning (acetylcholine receptor), of isoproterolol (isoprenaline) for overdose with a β-adrenoceptor blocker (β-adrenoceptor), of phentolamine for the monoamine oxidase inhibitor–sympathomimetic interaction (α-adrenoceptor).

Unwanted interactions include the loss of the antihypertensive effect of β-blockers when common cold remedies containing ephedrine, phenylpropanolamine or phenylephrine are taken, usually unknown to the doctor; their α-adrenoceptor agonist action is unrestrained in the β-blocked patient.

Actions on body systems provide scope for a variety of interactions. The following list shows something of the range of possibilities; others may be found under accounts of individual drugs:

β-adrenoceptor blockers lose some antihypertensive efficacy when nonsteroidal anti-inflammatory drugs (NSAIDs), especially indomethacin, are co-administered; the effect involves inhibition of production of vasodilator prostaglandins by the kidney leading to sodium retention.

Diuretics, especially of the loop variety, lose efficacy if administered with NSAIDs; the mechanism may involve inhibition of prostaglandin synthesis, as above.

Potassium supplements, given with potassium-retaining diuretics, e.g. amiloride, spironolactone, or with ACE-inhibitors may cause dangerous hyperkalaemia.

Digoxin is more effective, but also more toxic in the presence of hypokalaemia, which may be caused by thiazide or loop diuretics.

Verapamil given i.v. with a β-blocker, e.g. atenolol, for supraventricular tachycardia may cause dangerous bradycardia since both drugs delay atrioventricular conduction.

Theophylline potentiates β-adrenergic effects, e.g. of salbutamol, and cardiac arrhythmia may result during treatment of asthma.

Lithium toxicity may result if a thiazide diuretic is co-administered; when there is sodium depletion, resorption of lithium by the proximal renal tubule is increased and plasma concentrations rise.

Central nervous system depressant drugs including benzodiazepines, several H_1-receptor antihistamines, alcohol, phenothiazines, antiepilepsy drugs interact to augment their sedative effects.

Loop diuretics and *aminoglycoside antibiotics* are both ototoxic in high dose; the chance of an adverse event is greater if they are administered together.

INTERACTIONS DURING METABOLISM

Enzyme induction by drugs and other substances (see p. 113) accelerates metabolism and is a cause of therapeutic failure. The following are examples:

Oral contraceptive steroids are metabolised more rapidly when an enzyme inducer, e.g. phenytoin, is added, and unplanned pregnancy has occured (doctors have been successfully sued for negligence). In this circumstance an oral contraceptive of high oestrogen content may be substituted (or an alternative contraceptive method); if breakthrough bleeding occurs, the oestrogen content is not high enough. The metabolism of progestogens is also increased by enzyme induction.

Anticoagulant control with warfarin is dependent on a steady state of elimination by metabolism. Enzyme induction leads to accelerated metabolism of warfarin, loss of anticoagulant control and danger of thrombosis. Conversely, if a patient's anticoagulant control is stable on warfarin plus an inducing agent, there is a danger of haemorrhage if the inducing agent is discontinued because warfarin will be eliminated at a slower rate.

Chronic alcohol ingestion causing enzyme induction is a likely explanation of the tolerance shown by alcoholics to hydrocarbon anaesthetics and to tolbutamide.

Ciclosporin is extensively metabolised; its concentration in blood may be reduced due to enzyme induction by rifampicin, with danger of inadequate immunosuppression hazarding an organ or marrow transplant.

Enzyme inhibition by drugs (see p. 114) potentiates other drugs that are inactivated by metabolism, causing adverse reactions. Examples appear below, and it will be noted that inhibitors of isoenzymes of microsomal cytochrome P450 figure prominently. The drugs with which they interact are also given but the list is not complete, and there should be a general awareness of the possibility of metabolic inhibition when the following drugs are used.

Cimetidine is an inhibitor of several cytochrome P450 isoenzymes and so potentiates a large number of drugs ordinarily metabolised by that system, notably, theophylline, warfarin, phenytoin and propranolol. Depending on the interacting drug, up to 50% inhibition of metabolism may occur when cimetidine 2000 mg/d is taken.

Erythromycin inhibits a cytochrome P450 isoenzyme and impairs the metabolism of theophylline, warfarin, carbamazepine and methylprednisolone. The mean reduction in drug clearance is 20–25%.

Quinolone antimicrobials inhibit specific isoenzymes of P450 responsible for the metabolism of methylxanthines; thus the clearance of theophylline is reduced by ciprofloxacin.

Monoamine oxidase inhibitors (MAOI) are not completely selective for MAO and impair the metabolism of tricyclic antidepressants, of some sympathomimetics, e.g. phenylpropanolamine, amfetamine, of opioid analgesics, especially pethidine, and of mercaptopurine.

Sodium valproate appears to be a nonspecific inhibitor and impairs the metabolism of phenytoin, phenobarbitone and primidone.

Serotonin specific reuptake inhibitors (see p. 350)

Allopurinol specifically inhibits xanthine oxidase and thus prevents metabolism of azathioprine to mercaptopurine (with potentially dangerous toxicity).

INTERACTIONS DURING EXCRETION

Clinically important interactions, both beneficial and potentially harmful, occur in the kidney.

Interference with passive diffusion (see p. 96). Reabsorption of a drug by the renal tubule can be reduced, and its excretion increased, by altering urine pH (see Drug overdose, p. 155).

Interference with active transport. Organic acids are passed from the blood into the urine by active transport across the renal tubular epithelium. Penicillin is mostly excreted in this way. Probenecid, an organic acid that competes successfully with penicillin for this transport system, may be used to prolong the action of penicillin when repeated administration is impracticable, e.g. in sexually transmitted diseases, where compliance is notoriously poor. Interference with renal excretion of methotrexate by aspirin, of zidovudine by probenecid and of digoxin by quinidine, contribute to the potentially harmful interactions with these combinations.

GUIDE TO FURTHER READING

Chamberlain G 1991 The changing body in pregnancy. British Medical Journal 302: 719–722

Ito S 2000 Drug therapy for breast-feeding women. New England Journal of Medicine 343: 118–126

Koren G, Pastuszak A, Ito S 1998 Drugs in pregnancy. New England Journal of Medicine 338: 1128–1137

Pirmohamed M 2001 Pharmacogenetics and pharmacogenomics. British Journal of Clinical Pharmacology 54: 345–357

Report 1997 Medication for older people. Royal College of Physicians, London

Rolf S, Harper N J N 1995 Ability of hospital doctors to calculate drug doses. British Medical Journal 310: 1173

Roses A D Pharmacogenetics and future drug development and delivery. Lancet 355: 1358–1361

Strauss S E 2001 Geriatric medicine. British Medical Journal 322: 86–88

Tucker G T 2000 Chiral switches. Lancet 355: 1085–1087

8

Unwanted effects and adverse drug reactions

Background

Cur'd yesterday of my disease
I died last night of my physician.[1]

Nature is neutral, i.e. it has no 'intentions' towards humans, though it is often unfavourable to them. It is mankind, in its desire to avoid suffering and death, that decides that some of the biological effects of drugs are desirable (therapeutic) and others are undesirable (adverse). In addition to this arbitrary division, which has no fundamental biological basis, unwanted effects of drugs are promoted, or even caused, by numerous nondrug factors. Because of the variety of these factors, attempts to make a simple account of the unwanted effects of drugs must be imperfect.

There is general agreement that drugs prescribed for disease are themselves the cause of a serious amount of disease (adverse reactions), ranging from mere inconvenience to permanent disability and death.

Since drugs are intended to relieve suffering, patients find it peculiarly offensive that they can also cause disease (especially if they are not forewarned). Therefore it is important to know how much disease they do cause and why they cause it, so that preventive measures can be taken.

It is not enough to measure the incidence of adverse reactions to drugs, their nature and their severity, though accurate data are obviously useful. It is necessary to take, or to try to take, into account which effects are avoidable (by skilled choice and use) and which are unavoidable (inherent in drug or patient). Also, different adverse effects can matter to a different degree to different people.

Since there can be no hope of eliminating all adverse effects of drugs it is necessary to evaluate patterns of adverse reaction against each other. One drug may frequently cause minor ill-effects but pose no threat to life, though patients do not like it and may take it irregularly, to their own detriment. Another drug may be pleasant to take, so that patients take it consistently, with benefit, but it may

---

[1] From, The remedy worse than the disease. Matthew Prior (1664–1721).

rarely kill someone. It is not obvious which drug is to be preferred.

Some patients, e.g. those with a history of allergy or previous reactions to drugs, are up to four times more likely to have another adverse reaction, so that the incidence does not fall evenly. It is also useful to discover the causes of adverse reactions, for such knowledge can be used to render avoidable what are at present unavoidable reactions.

Avoidable adverse effects will be reduced by more skilful prescribing and this means that doctors, amongst all the other claims on their time, must find time better to understand drugs, as well as to understand their patients and their diseases.

Definitions

Many unwanted effects of drugs are medically trivial, and in order to avoid inflating the figures of drug-induced disease, it is convenient to retain the term **side-effects** for minor effects of type A events/effects (p. 139).

The term **adverse reaction** should be confined to: harmful or seriously unpleasant effects occurring at doses intended for therapeutic (including prophylactic or diagnostic) effect and which call for reduction of dose or withdrawal of the drug and/or forecast hazard from future administration; it is effects of this order that are of importance in evaluating drug-induced disease in the community.

Toxicity implies a direct action of the drug, often at high dose, damaging cells, e.g. liver damage from paracetamol overdose, eighth cranial nerve damage from gentamicin. All drugs, for practical purposes, are toxic in overdose and overdose can be absolute or relative; in the latter case an ordinary dose may be administered but may be toxic due to an underlying abnormality in the patient, e.g. disease of the kidney. Mutagenicity, carcinogenicity and teratogenicity (see index) are special cases of toxicity.

Secondary effects are the indirect consequences of a primary drug action. Examples are: vitamin deficiency or opportunistic infection which may occur in patients whose normal bowel flora has been altered by antibiotics; diuretic-induced hypokalaemia causing digoxin intolerance.

Intolerance means a low threshold to the normal pharmacodynamic action of a drug. Individuals vary greatly in their susceptibility to drugs, those at one extreme of the normal distribution curve being intolerant of the drugs, those at the other, tolerant.

Idiosyncrasy (see Pharmacogenetics) implies an inherent qualitative abnormal reaction to a drug, usually due to genetic abnormality, e.g. porphyria.

Causation: degrees of conviction

Reliable attribution of a cause–effect relationship provides the biggest problem in this field. The following degrees of conviction assist in attributing adverse events to drugs:[2]

- *Definite:* time sequence from taking the drug is reasonable; event corresponds to what is known of the drug; event ceases on stopping the drug; event returns on restarting the drug (rarely advisable).
- *Probable:* time sequence is reasonable; event corresponds to what is known of the drug; event ceases on stopping the drug; event not reasonably explained by patient's disease.
- *Possible:* time sequence is reasonable; event corresponds to what is known of the drug; event could readily have been result of the patient's disease or other therapy.
- *Conditional:* time sequence is reasonable; event does not correspond to what is known of the drug; event could not reasonably be explained by the patient's disease.
- *Doubtful:* event not meeting the above criteria.

Recognition of adverse drug reactions. When an unexpected event, for which there is no obvious cause, occurs in a patient already taking a drug, the possibility that it is drug-caused must always

---

[2] Journal of the American Medical Association 1975 234: 1236.

be considered. Distinguishing between natural progression of a disease and drug-induced deterioration is particularly challenging, e.g. sodium in antacid formulations may aggravate cardiac failure, tricyclic antidepressants may provoke epileptic seizures, bronchospasm may be caused by aspirin in some asthmatics.

Pharmacovigilance and pharmacoepidemiology

The principal methods of collecting data on adverse reactions (pharmacovigilance) are:

- *Experimental studies,* i.e. formal therapeutic trials of Phases 1–3. These provide reliable data on only the commoner events as they involve relatively small numbers of patients (hundreds); they detect an incidence of up to about 1:200.
- *Observational studies,* where the drug is observed epidemiologically under conditions of normal use in the community, i.e. pharmaco-epidemiology. Techniques used for post-marketing (Phase 4) studies include the observational cohort study and the case-control study. The systems are described on page 69.

DRUG-INDUCED ILLNESS

The discovery of drug-induced illness can be analysed thus:[3]

- Drug commonly induces an otherwise rare illness: this effect is likely to be discovered by clinical observation in the licensing (premarketing) formal therapeutic trials and the drug will almost always be abandoned; but some patients are normally excluded from such trials, e.g. pregnant women, and detection will then occur later.
- Drug rarely induces an otherwise common illness: this effect is likely to remain undiscovered.
- Drug rarely induces an otherwise rare illness:

this effect is likely to remain undiscovered before the drug is released for general prescribing; the effect should be detected by informal clinical observation or during any special postregistration surveillance and confirmed by a case-control study (see p. 68), e.g. chloramphenicol and aplastic anaemia; practolol and oculomucocutaneous syndrome.
- Drug commonly induces an otherwise common illness: this effect will not be discovered by informal clinical observation. If very common, it may be discovered in formal therapeutic trials and in case-control studies, but if only moderately common it may require observational cohort studies, e.g. proarrhythmic effects of antiarrhythmic drugs.
- Drug adverse effects and illness incidence in intermediate range: both case-control and cohort studies may be needed.

Some impression of the features of drug-induced illness can be gained from the following statistics:

- Adverse reactions cause 2–3% of consultations in general practice.
- Adverse reactions account for 5% of all hospital admissions.
- Overall incidence in hospital inpatients is 10–20%, with possible prolongation of hospital stay in 2–10% of patients in acute medical wards.
- A review of records of a Coroner's Inquests for a district with a population of 1.19 million (UK) during the period 1986–91 found that of 3277 inquests on deaths, 10 were due to errors of prescribing and 36 were caused by adverse drug reactions.[4] Nevertheless, 17 doctors in the UK were charged with manslaughter in the 1990s compared with two in each of the preceding decades, a reflection of 'a greater readiness to call the police or to prosecute'.[5]
- Predisposing factors: age over 60 years or under one month, female, previous history of adverse reaction, hepatic or renal disease.

---

[3] After: Jick H 1977 New England Journal of Medicine 296: 481–485.

[4] Ferner R E, Whittington R M 1994 Journal of the Royal Society of Medicine 87: 145–148.
[5] Ferner R E 2000 Medication errors that have led to manslaughter charges. British Medical Journal 321: 1212–1216.

- Adverse reactions most commonly occur early in therapy (days 1–10).

It is important to avoid alarmist or defeatist extremes of attitude. Many treatments are dangerous, e.g. surgery, electroshock, drugs, and it is irrational to accept the risks of surgery for biliary stones or hernia and refuse to accept any risk at all from drugs for conditions of comparable seriousness.

Many patients whose death is deemed to be partly or wholly caused by drugs are dangerously ill already; justified risks may be taken in the hope of helping them; ill-informed criticism in such cases can act against the interest of the sick. On the other hand there is no doubt that some of these accidents are avoidable. Avoidability is often more obvious when reviewing the conduct of treatment after death, i.e. with hindsight, than it was at the time.

Sir Anthony Carlisle,[6] in the first half of the 19th century, said that 'medicine is an art founded on conjecture and improved by murder'. Although medicine has advanced rapidly, there is still a ring of truth in that statement to anyone who follows the introduction of new drugs and observes how, after the early enthusiasm, the reports of serious toxic effects appear. The challenge is to find and avoid these, and indeed, the present systems for detecting adverse reactions came into being largely in the wake of the thalidomide, practolol and benoxaprofen disasters (see Ch. 5); they are now an increasingly sophisticated and effective part of medicines development.

Another cryptic remark of this therapeutic nihilist was 'digitalis kills people' and this is true. William Withering in 1785 laid down rules for the use of digitalis that would serve today. Neglect of these rules resulted in needless suffering for patients with heart failure for more than a century until the therapeutic criteria were rediscovered. Any drug that is really worth using can do harm.

> It is an absolute obligation on doctors to use only drugs about which they have troubled to inform themselves.

Effective therapy depends not only on the correct choice of drugs but also on their correct use.

This latter is sometimes forgotten and a drug is condemned as useless when it has been used in a dose or way which absolutely precluded a successful result; this can be regarded as a negative adverse effect.

PRACTICALITIES OF DETECTING RARE ADVERSE REACTIONS

For reactions with no background incidence the number of patients required to give a good (95%) chance of detecting the effect is given in Table 8.1. Assuming that three events are required before any regulatory or other action should be taken, it shows the large number of patients that must be monitored to detect even a relatively high incidence adverse effect. The problem can be many orders of magnitude worse if the adverse reactions closely resemble spontaneous disease with a background incidence in the population.

Caution. About 80% of well people not taking any drugs admit on questioning to symptoms (often several) such as are commonly experienced as lesser adverse reactions to drugs. These symptoms are intensified (or diminished) by administration of a placebo. Thus, many (minor) symptoms may be wrongly attributed to drugs.

Classification

It is convenient to classify adverse reactions to drugs under the following headings:

TABLE 8.1 Detecting rare adverse reactions[7]

Expected incidence of adverse reaction	Required number of patients for event		
	1 event	2 events	3 events
1 in 100	300	480	650
1 in 200	600	960	1300
1 in 1000	3000	4800	6500
1 in 2000	6000	9600	13 000
1 in 10 000	30 000	48 000	65 000

---

[6] Noted for his advocacy of the use of 'the simple carpenter's saw' in surgery.

[7] By permission from, Safety requirements for the first use of new drugs and diagnostic agents in man. CIOMS (WHO) 1983. Geneva.

Type A (Augmented) reactions will occur in everyone if enough of the drug is given because they are due to excess of normal, predictable, dose-related, pharmacodynamic effects. They are common and skilled management reduces their incidence, e.g. postural hypotension, hypoglycaemia, hypokalaemia.

Type B (Bizarre) reactions will occur only in some people. They are not part of the normal pharmacology of the drug, are not dose-related and are due to unusual attributes of the patient interacting with the drug. These effects are predictable where the mechanism is known (though predictive tests may be expensive or impracticable), otherwise they are unpredictable for the individual, although the incidence may be known. The class includes unwanted effects due to inherited abnormalities (idiosyncrasy) (see Pharmacogenetics) and immunological processes (see Drug allergy). These account for most drug fatalities.

Type C (Chronic) reactions due to long-term exposure, e.g. analgesic nephropathy, dyskinesias with levodopa.

Type D (Delayed) effects following prolonged exposure, e.g. carcinogenesis or short-term exposure at a critical time, e.g. teratogenesis.

Type E (Ending of use) reactions, where discontinuation of chronic therapy is too abrupt, e.g. of adrenal steroid causing rebound adrenocortical insufficiency, of opioid causing the withdrawal syndrome.

Causes

When an unusual or unexpected event, for which there is no evident natural explanation, occurs in a patient already taking a drug, the possibility that the event is drug-caused must always be considered, and may be categorised as follows:

- **The patient** may be predisposed by age, genetic constitution, tendency to allergy, disease, personality, habits.
- **The drug.** Anticancer agents are by their nature cytotoxic. Some drugs, e.g. digoxin, have steep dose–response curves and small increments of dose are more likely to induce augmented (type A) reactions. Other drugs, e.g. antimicrobials, have a tendency to cause allergy and may lead to bizarre (type B) reactions. Ingredients of a formulation, e.g. colouring, flavouring, sodium content, rather than the active drug may also cause adverse reactions.
- **The prescriber.** Adverse reactions may occur because a drug is used for an inappropriately long time (type C), at a critical phase in pregnancy (type D), is abruptly discontinued (type E) or given with other drugs (interactions).

Aspects of the two sections above, Classification and Causes, appear throughout the book. Selected topics are discussed below.

AGE

The very old and the very young are liable to be intolerant of many drugs, largely because the mechanisms for disposing of them in the body are less efficient. The young, it has been aptly said, are not simply 'small adults' and 'respect for their pharmacokinetic variability should be added to the list of our senior citizens' rights'.[8] The old are also frequently exposed to multiple drug therapy which predisposes to adverse effects (see Prescribing for the elderly, p. 126).

GENETIC CONSTITUTION

Inherited factors that influence response to drugs are discussed in general under Pharmacogenetics (p. 122). It is convenient here to describe the porphyrias, a specific group of disorders for which careful prescribing is vital.

The *porphyrias* comprise a number of rare, genetically determined single enzyme defects in *haem* biosynthesis. Acute porphyrias (acute intermittent porphyria, variegate porphyria and hereditary coproporphyria) are characterised by severe attacks of neurovisceral dysfunction *precipitated principally by a wide variety of drugs* (and also by alcohol, fasting, and infection); nonacute porphyrias (porphyria cutanea tarda, erythropoietic protoporphyria and congenital erythropoietic porphyria) present with cutaneous photosensitivity for which alcohol (and

---

[8] Fogel B S 1983 New England Journal of Medicine 308: 1600.

prescribed oestrogens in women) is the principle provoking agent.

In healthy people, forming haemoglobin for their erythrocytes and haem-dependent enzymes, the rate of haem synthesis is controlled by negative feedback according to the amount of haem present. When more haem is needed there is increased production of the rate-controlling enzyme *delta-aminolaevulinic acid (ALA) synthase* which provides the basis of the formation of *porphyrin* precursors of haem. But in people with porphyria one or other of the enzymes that convert the various porphyrins to haem is deficient and so porphyrins accumulate. A vicious cycle occurs: less haem → more ALA synthase → more porphyrin precursors, the metabolism of which is blocked, and a clinical attack occurs.

It is of interest that those who inherited acute intermittent porphyria and variegate porphyria suffered no biological disadvantage from the natural environment and bred as well as the normal population until the introduction of barbiturates and sulphonamides. They are now at serious disadvantage, for many other drugs can precipitate fatal acute attacks.

The exact precipitating mechanisms are uncertain. Increase in the haem-containing hepatic oxidising enzymes of the cytochrome P450 group causes an increased demand for haem. Therefore drugs that induce these enzymes would be expected to precipitate acute attacks of porphyria and they do so; tobacco smoking may act by this mechanism. Apparently unexplained attacks of porphyria should be an indication for close enquiry into all possible chemical intake. Guaiphenesin, for example, is hazardous; it is included in a multitude of multi-ingredient cough medicines (often nonprescription). Patients must be educated to understand their condition, to possess a list of safe and unsafe drugs, and to protect themselves from themselves and from others, including prescribing doctors.

The greatest care in prescribing for these patients is required if serious illness is to be avoided. Patients (1 in 10 000 UK population) are so highly vulnerable that lists of drugs known or believed to be **unsafe** are available, e.g. in the British National Formulary. Additionally, we provide a table of drugs considered **safe** for use in the acute porphyrias at the time of publication (Table 8.2). The list is revised regularly, mostly with additions made as information becomes available. Updated information can be obtained.[9]

Use of a drug about which there is uncertainty may be justified. Dr M. Badminton writes: 'Essential treatment should never be withheld, especially for a condition that is serious or life-threatening. The clinician should assess the severity of the condition and the activity of the porphyria. If no recognised safe option is available, a reasonable course is to:

1. Measure urine porphyrin and porphobilinogen before starting treatment.
2. Repeat the measurement at regular intervals or if the patient has symptoms in keeping with an acute attack. If there is an increase in the precursor levels, stop the treatment and consider giving haem arginate for acute attack (see below).
3. Contact an expert centre for advice.'

In the treatment of the acute attack it is rational to use any safe means of depressing the formation of ALA-synthase. *Haem arginate* (human haematin) infusion, by replenishing haem and so removing the stimulus to ALA-synthase, is effective if given early, and may prevent chronic neuropathy. Additionally, attention to nutrition, particularly the supply of carbohydrate, relief of pain (with an opioid), and of hypertension and tachycardia (with a β-adrenoceptor blocker) are important. Hyponatraemia is a frequent complication, and plasma electrolytes should be monitored.

In the treatment of the acute attack it would seem rational to use any safe means of depressing the formation of ALA-synthase. Indeed, *haem arginate* (human haematin) infusion, by replenishing haem and so removing the stimulus to ALA-synthase, appears to be effective if given early, and may prevent chronic neuropathy. Additionally, attention to nutrition, particularly the supply of carbohydrate, relief of pain (with opioid), and of hypertension and tachycardia (with propranolol) are important.

THE ENVIRONMENT

Significant environmental factors causing adverse

---

[9] www.uwcm.ac.uk/study/medicine/medical_biochem/porphyria.htm
www.utc.ac.za/depts/liver/porphpts.htm

TABLE 8.2 Drugs that are considered *safe* for use in acute porphyrias

Acetazolamide	Dextran	Ibuprofen	Pirenzepine
Acetylcysteine	Dextromethorphan	Immunisations	Prazosin
Aciclovir	Dextromoramide	Immunoglobulins	Prednisolone
Adrenaline (epinephrine)	Dextropropoxyphene	Indomethacin	Prilocaine
Alfentanil	Dextrose	Insulin	Primaquine
Allopurinol	Diamorphine	Iron	Probucol
Alpha tocopheryl	Diazoxide	Isoflurane	Procainamide
Aluminium salts	Dicyclomine (dicycloverine)	Ispaghula	Procaine
Amantadine	Diflunisal	Ketoprofen	Prochlorperazine
Amethocaine (tetracaine)	Digoxin	Ketotifen	Proguanil
Amiloride	Dihydrocodeine	Lactulose	Promazine
Aminoglycosides	Dimercaprol	Leuproelin	Promethazine
Amitriptyline	Dimeticone	Levothyroxine	Propantheline
Amphotericin	Diphenhydramine	LHRH	Propofol
Ascorbic acid	Diphenoxylate	Lignocaine[2] (lidocaine)	Propylthiouracil
Aspirin	Dipyridamole	Lisinopril[3]	Proxymetacaine
Atropine	Distigmine	Lithium	Pseudoephedrine
Azathioprine	Dobutamine	Lofepramine	Pyridoxine
Beclomethasone	Domperidone	Loperamide	Pyrimethamine
Beta blockers	Dopamine	Loratadine	Quinidine
Bezafibrate	Doxorubicin	Lorazepam	Quinine
Bismuth	Droperidol	Magnesium sulphate	Resorcinol
Bromazepam	Enalapril	Meclozine	Salbutamol
Bumetanide	Enoxaparin	Mefloquine	Senna
Bupivacaine	Epinephrine	Melphalan	Sodium acid phosph
Buprenorphine	Ethambutol	Mequitazine	Sodium bicarbonate
Buserelin	Ether	Mesalazine	Sodium fusidate
Calcitonin	Famciclovir	Metformin	Sodium valproate[4]
Calcium carbonate	Fenbufen	Methadone	Sorbitol
Carbimazole	Fenofibrate	Methotrimeprazine (levomepromazine)	Streptokinase
Chloral hydrate	Fentanyl	Methylphenidate	Streptomycin
Chloroquine	Flucloxacillin[1]	Methylprednisolone	Sucralfate
Chlorothiazide	Flucytosine	Mianserin	Sulindac
Chlorpheniramine (chlorphenamine)	Flumazenil	Midazolam	Suxamethonium
Chlorpromazine	Fluoxetine	Morphine	Temazepam
Colestyramine	Fluphenazine	Naftidrofuryl	Tetracaine
Cisplatin	Flurbiprofen	Nalbuphine	Thiamine
Clobazam	Fructose	Naloxone	Thyroxine (levothyroxine)
Clofibrate	FSH	Naproxen	Tiaprofenic acid
Clomifene	Gabapentin	Neostigmine	Tinzaparin
Clonazepam	Ganciclovir	Nitrous oxide	Tranexamic acid
Co-amoxiclav	Gemfibrozil	Octreotide	Triamterene
Co-codamol	Glipizide	Omeprazole	Triazolam
Co-dydramol	Glucagon	Oxybuprocaine	Trifluoperazine
Codeine phosphate	Glucose	Oxytocin	Trimeprazine
Colchicine	Glycopyrronium	Pancuronium	Urokinase
Colestipol	Gonadorelin	Paracetamol	Vaccines
Corticosteroids	Goserelin	Paraldehyde	Valaciclovir
Corticotrophin	GTN	Penicillamine	Valproate[4]
Cyclizine	Guanethidine	Penicillins	Vancomycin
Cyclopenthiazide	Haloperidol	Pentamidine	Vigabatrin
Cyclopropane	Heparin	Pethidine	Vitamins
Dalteparin	Hetastarch	Phentolamine	Warfarin
Danthron	Hydrochlorothiazide	Phytomenadione	Zalcitabine
Desferrioxamine	Hydrocortisone	Pipothiazine	Zinc preparations

This list is produced jointly by Professor G Elder and Dr M Badminton, the Department of Medical Biochemistry, University Hospital of Wales and the staff of the Welsh Medicines Information Centre (WMIC; fiona.woods@cardiffandvale.wales.nhs.uk). It is based on the best information available at the time of completion. Inclusion of a drug does not guarantee that it will be safe in all circumstances.

[1] Large intravenous doses may be associated with acute attacks (unproven as causative agent).

[2] Intravenous doses should be avoided.

[3] Safety under review; contact WMIC.

[4] Sodium valproate should be used only where other antiepilepsy drugs are ineffective or inappropriate.

reactions to drugs include simple pollution, e.g. penicillin in the air of hospitals or in milk (see below), causing allergy.

Drug metabolism may also be increased by hepatic enzyme induction from insecticide accumulation, e.g. dicophane (DDT) and from alcohol and the tobacco habit, e.g. smokers require a higher dose of theophylline.

Antimicrobials used in feeds of animals for human consumption have given rise to concern in relation to the spread of resistant bacteria that may affect man.

DRUG INTERACTIONS

(see p. 129)

Allergy in response to drugs

Allergic reactions to drugs are the resultant of the interaction of drug or metabolite (or a nondrug element in the formulation) with patient and disease, and subsequent re-exposure.

Lack of previous exposure is not the same as lack of history of previous exposure, and 'first dose reactions' are among the most dramatic. Exposure is not necessarily medical, e.g. penicillins may occur in dairy products following treatment of mastitis in cows (despite laws to prevent this), and penicillin antibodies are commonly present in those who deny ever having received the drug. Immune responses to drugs may be harmful (allergy) or harmless; the fact that antibodies are produced does not mean a patient will necessarily respond to re-exposure with clinical manifestations; most of the UK population has antibodies to penicillins but, fortunately, comparatively few react clinically to penicillin administration.

Whilst macromolecules (proteins, peptides, dextran polysaccharides) can act as complete antigens, most drugs are simple chemicals (mol. wt less than 1000) and act as incomplete antigens or haptens, which become complete antigens in combination with a body protein.

The chief target organs of drug allergy are the skin, respiratory tract, gastrointestinal tract, blood and blood vessels.

Allergic reactions in general may be classified according to four types of hypersensitivity, and drugs can elicit reactions of all types, namely:

Type I reactions: immediate or anaphylactic type. The drug causes formation of tissue-sensitising IgE antibodies that are fixed to mast cells or leucocytes; on subsequent administration the allergen (conjugate of drug or metabolite with tissue protein) reacts with these antibodies, activating but not damaging the cell to which they are fixed and causing release of pharmacologically active substances, e.g. histamine, leukotrienes, prostaglandins, platelet activating factor, and causing effects such as urticaria, anaphylactic shock and asthma. Allergy develops within minutes and lasts 1–2 hours.

Type II reactions: antibody-dependent cytotoxic type. The drug or metabolite combines with a protein in the body so that the body no longer recognises the protein as self, treats it as a foreign protein and forms antibodies (IgG, IgM) that combine with the antigen and activate complement which damages cells, e.g. penicillin- or methyldopa-induced haemolytic anaemia.

Type III reactions: immune complex-mediated type. Antigen and antibody form large complexes and activate complement. Small blood vessels are damaged or blocked. Leucocytes attracted to the site of reaction engulf the immune complexes and release pharmacologically active substances (including lysosomal enzymes), starting an inflammatory process. These reactions include serum sickness, glomerulonephritis, vasculitis and pulmonary disease.

Type IV reactions: lymphocyte-mediated type. Antigen-specific receptors develop on T-lymphocytes. Subsequent administration leads to a local or tissue allergic reaction, e.g. contact dermatitis.

Cross-allergy within a group of drugs is usual, e.g. the penicillins. When allergy to a particular drug is established, a substitute should be selected from a chemically different group. Patients with allergic diseases, e.g. eczema, are more likely to develop allergy to drugs.

The distinctive features of allergic reactions are their:[10]

- Lack of correlation with known pharmacological properties of the drug
- Lack of linear relation with drug dose (very small doses may cause very severe effects)
- Rashes, angioedema, serum sickness syndrome, anaphylaxis or asthma; characteristics of classic protein allergy
- Requirement of an induction period on primary exposure, but not on re-exposure
- Disappearance on cessation of administration and reappearance on re-exposure
- Occurrence in a minority of patients receiving the drug
- Temporary nature in some cases
- Possible response to desensitisation.

PRINCIPAL CLINICAL MANIFESTATIONS AND TREATMENT

1. Urticarial rashes and angioedema (types I, III). These are probably the commonest type of drug allergy. Reactions may be generalised, but frequently are worst in and around the external area of administration of the drug. The eyelids, lips and face are usually most affected. They are usually accompanied by itching. Oedema of the larynx is rare but may be fatal. They respond to adrenaline (epinephrine) (i.m. if urgent), ephedrine, H_1-receptor antihistamine and adrenal steroid.

2a. Nonurticarial rashes (types I, II, IV). These occur in great variety; frequently they are weeping exudative lesions. It is often difficult to be sure when a rash is due to a drug. Apart from stopping the drug, treatment is nonspecific; in severe cases an adrenal steroid should be used. Skin sensitisation to antimicrobials may be very troublesome, especially amongst those who handle them (see Drugs and the Skin, Ch. 16, for more detail).

2b. Diseases of the lymphoid system. Infectious mononucleosis (and lymphoma, leukaemia) is associated with an increased incidence (> 40%) of

characteristic maculopapular, sometimes purpuric, rash which is probably allergic, when an amino-penicillin (ampicillin, amoxycillin) is taken; patients may not be allergic to other penicillins. Erythromycin may cause a similar reaction.

3. Anaphylactic shock (type I) occurs with penicillin, anaesthetics (i.v.), iodine-containing radiocontrast media and a huge variety of other drugs. A severe fall in blood pressure occurs, with bronchoconstriction, angioedema (including larynx) and sometimes death due to loss of fluid from the intravascular compartment. Anaphylactic shock usually occurs suddenly, in less than an hour after the drug, but within minutes if it has been given i.v.

Treatment is urgent, as follows:

- First, 500 micrograms of adrenaline (epinephrine) injection (0.5 ml of the 1 in 1000 solution) should be given i.m. to raise the blood pressure and to dilate the bronchi (vasoconstriction renders the s.c. route less effective). Up to 10% of patients may need a second injection 10–20 min later and subsequent injections may be given until the patient improves. Noradrenaline (norepinephrine) lacks any useful bronchodilator action (β-effect) (see adrenaline, Chapter 23).
- If treatment is delayed and shock has developed, adrenaline 500 micrograms should be given i.v. by slow injection at a rate of 100 micrograms/min (1 ml/min of the Dilute 1 in 10 000 solution over 5 min) with continuous ECG monitoring, stopping when a response has been obtained. For greater control and safety, a further × 10 dilution in dextrose may be preferred (i.e. a solution of 1 in 100 000).
- Note that preventive self-management is feasible where susceptibility to anaphylaxis is known, e.g. in patients with allergy to bee- or wasp-stings. The patient is taught to administer adrenaline i.m. from a prefilled syringe (EpiPen Auto-injector, delivering adrenaline 300 micrograms per dose).
- The adrenaline should be accompanied by an H_1-receptor antihistamine [say chlorpheniramine (chlorphenamine) 10–20 mg by slow i.v. injection] and hydrocortisone (100–300 mg i.m. or i.v.). The adrenal steroid may act by reducing vascular permeability and by suppressing

---

[10] Assem E-S K 1992 In: Davies D M (ed) Textbook of adverse drug reactions. Oxford University Press, London.

further response to the antigen–antibody reaction. Benefit from an adrenal steroid is not immediate; it is unlikely to begin for 30 minutes and takes hours to reach its maximum.

- In severe anaphylaxis, hypotension is due to vasodilation and loss of circulating volume through leaky capillaries. Colloid is more effective at restoring blood volume than crystalloid and 1–2 l of plasma substitute should be infused rapidly. Oxygen and artificial ventilation may be necessary. Advice on the management of anaphylactic shock may be altered from time to time; check the UK Resuscitation Council website (www.resus.org.uk) for current information.

Any hospital ward or other place where anaphylaxis may be anticipated should have all the drugs and equipment necessary to deal with it in one convenient kit, for when they are needed there is little time to think and none to run about from place to place (see also Pseudoallergic reactions, p. 146).

4a. Pulmonary reactions: asthma (type I). Aspirin and other nonsteroidal anti-inflammatory drugs may cause an asthmatic attack. Whether this is an allergic or pseudoallergic reaction or a mixture of the two is uncertain.

4b. Other types of pulmonary reaction (type III) include syndromes resembling acute and chronic lung infections, pneumonitis, fibrosis and eosinophilia.

5. The serum-sickness syndrome (type III). This occurs about 1–3 weeks after administration. Treatment is by an adrenal steroid, and as above if there is urticaria.

6. Blood disorders[11]

6a. Thrombocytopenia (type II, but also pseudo-allergic) may occur after exposure to any of a large number of drugs, including: gold, quinine, quinidine, rifampicin, heparin, thionamide derivatives, thiazide diuretics, sulphonamides, oestrogens, indomethacin. Adrenal steroid may help.

6b. Granulocytopenia (type II, but also pseudo-allergic) sometimes leading to agranulocytosis, is a very serious allergy which may occur with many drugs, e.g. clozapine, carbamazepine, carbimazole, chloramphenicol, sulphonamides (including diuretic and hypoglycaemic derivatives), colchicine, gold.

The value of precautionary leucocyte counts for drugs having special risk remains uncertain.[12] Weekly counts may detect presymptomatic granulocytopenia from antithyroid drugs but onset can be sudden and an alternative view is to monitor only with drugs having special risk, e.g. clozapine. The chief clinical manifestation of agranulocytosis is sore throat or mouth ulcers and patients should be warned to report such events immediately and to stop taking the drug; but they should not be frightened into noncompliance with essential therapy. Treatment of the agranulocytosis involves both stopping the drug responsible and giving a bactericidal drug, e.g. a penicillin, to prevent or treat infection.

6c. Aplastic anaemia (type II, but not always allergic). Causal agents include chloramphenicol, sulphonamides and derivatives (diuretics, antidiabetics), gold, penicillamine, allopurinol, felbamate, phenothiazines and some insecticides, e.g. dicophane (DDT). In the case of chloramphenicol, bone marrow depression is a normal pharmacodynamic effect (type A reaction), although aplastic anaemia may also be due to idiosyncrasy or allergy (type B reaction).

Death occurs in about 50% of cases, and treatment is as for agranulocytosis, with, obviously, blood transfusion.

6d. Haemolysis of all kinds is included here for convenience. There are three principal categories:

- *Allergy (type II)* occurs with methyldopa, levodopa, penicillins, quinine, quinidine,

---

[11] Where cells are being destroyed in the periphery and production is normal, transfusion is useless or nearly so, as the transfused cells will be destroyed, though in an emergency even a short cell life (platelets, erythrocytes) may tip the balance usefully. Where the bone marrow is depressed, transfusion is useful and the transfused cells will survive normally.

---

[12] In contrast to the case of a drug causing bone marrow depression as a pharmacodynamic dose-related effect, when blood counts are part of the essential routine monitoring of therapy, e.g. cytotoxics.

sulfasalazine and organic antimony. It may be that in some of these cases a drug–protein–antigen/antibody interaction involves erythrocytes casually, i.e. a true 'innocent bystander' phenomenon.

- *Dose-related pharmacodynamic action on normal cells* e.g. lead, benzene, phenylhydrazine, chlorates (weed-killer), methyl chloride (refrigerant), some snake venoms.
- *Idiosyncrasy* (see Pharmacogenetics). Precipitation of a haemolytic crisis may also occur with the above drugs in the rare genetic haemoglobinopathies. Treatment is to withdraw the drug, and an adrenal steroid is useful in severe cases if the mechanism is immunological. Blood transfusion may be needed.

7. Fever is common; a mechanism is the release of interleukin-1 by leucocytes into the circulation which acts on receptors in the hypothalamic thermoregulatory centre, releasing prostaglandin E_1.

8. Collagen diseases (type II) and syndromes resembling them, e.g. systemic lupus erythematosus are sometimes caused by drugs, e.g. hydralazine, procainamide, isoniazid, sulphonamides. Adrenal steroid is useful.

9. Hepatitis and cholestatic jaundice are sometimes allergic (type II, see Drugs and the Liver). Adrenal steroid may be useful.

10. Nephropathy of various kinds (types II, III) occurs as does damage to other organs, e.g. myocarditis. Adrenal steroid may be useful.

DIAGNOSIS OF DRUG ALLERGY

This still depends largely on clinical criteria, history, type of reaction, response to withdrawal and systemic rechallenge (if thought safe to do so).

Simple *patch* skin testing is naturally most useful in diagnosing contact dermatitis, but it is unreliable for other allergies. Skin *prick* tests are helpful in specialist hands for diagnosing IgE-dependent drug reactions, notably due to penicillin, cephalosporins, muscle relaxants, thiopental, streptokinase, cisplatin, insulin and latex. They can cause anaphylactic shock. False positive results occur.

Development of reliable in-vitro predictive tests, e.g. employing serum or lymphocytes, is a matter of considerable importance, not merely to remove hazard but to avoid depriving patients of a drug that may be useful. Detection of drug-specific circulating IgE antibodies by the radioallergo-sorbent test (RAST) is best developed for penicillins and succinyl choline.

Drug allergy, once it has occurred, is not necessarily permanent, e.g. less than 50% of patients giving a history of allergy to penicillin have a reaction if it is given again.

DESENSITISATION

Once patients become allergic to a drug, it is better that they should never again come into contact with it. Desensitisation (in hospital) may be considered where a patient has suffered an IgE-mediated reaction to penicillin and requires the drug for serious infection, e.g. meningitis or endocarditis. Such people can be desensitised by giving very small amounts of allergen, which are than gradually increased (usually every few hours) until a normal dose is tolerated. The procedure may necessitate cover with a corticosteroid and a β-adrenoceptor agonist (both of which inhibit mediator synthesis and release), and an H_1-receptor antihistamine may be added if an adverse reaction occurs. A full kit for treating anaphylactic shock should be at hand. Desensitisation may also be carried out for other antimicrobials, e.g. antituberculosis drugs.

The mechanism underlying desensitisation may involve the production by the patient of blocking antibodies that compete successfully for the allergen but whose combination with it is innocuous; or the threshold of cells to the triggering antibodies may be raised. Sometimes allergy is to an ingredient of the preparation other than the essential drug and merely changing the preparation is sufficient. Impurities are sometimes responsible and purified penicillins and insulins reduce the incidence of reactions.

PREVENTION OF ALLERGIC REACTIONS

Prevention is important since these reactions are unpleasant and may be fatal; it provides good reason for taking a drug history. Patients should always be told when they are thought to be allergic to a drug.

> If a patient claims to be allergic to some drug then that drug should not be given without careful enquiry that may include testing (as above); **neglect of this had caused death**

When looking for an alternative drug to avoid an adverse reaction it is important not to select one from the same chemical group, as may inadvertently occur because the proprietary name gives no indication of the nature of the drug. This is another good reason for using the nonproprietary (generic) names as a matter of course.

PSEUDOALLERGIC REACTIONS

These are effects that mimic allergic reactions but have no immunological basis and are largely genetically determined. They are due to release of endogenous, biologically active substances, e.g. histamine and leukotrienes, by the drug. A variety of mechanisms is probably involved, direct and indirect, including complement activation leading to formation of polypeptides that affect mast cells, as in true immunological reactions. Some drugs may produce both allergic and pseudoallergic reactions.

Pseudoallergic effects mimicking type I reactions (above) are called *anaphylactoid* and they occur with aspirin and other nonsteroidal anti-inflammatory drugs (indirect action as above) (see also Pulmonary reactions, above); corticotrophin (direct histamine release); i.v. anaesthetics and a variety of other drugs i.v. (morphine, tubocurarine, dextran, radiographic contrast media) and inhaled (cromoglicate). Severe cases are treated as for true allergic anaphylactic shock (above) from which, at the time, they are not distinguishable.

Type II reactions are mimicked by the haemolysis induced by drugs (some antimalarials, sulphonamides and oxidising agents) and food (broad beans) in subjects with inherited abnormalities of erythrocyte enzymes or haemoglobin (see p. 123).

Type III reactions are mimicked by nitrofurantoin (pneumonitis) and penicillamine (nephropathy). Lupus erythematosus due to drugs (procainamide, isoniazid, phenytoin) may be pseudoallergic.

MISCELLANEOUS ADVERSE REACTIONS

Transient reactions to intravenous injections are fairly common, resulting in hypotension, renal pain, fever or rigors, especially if the injection is very rapid.

Effects of prolonged administration: chronic organ toxicity

While the majority of adverse events occur within days or weeks after a drug is administered, some reactions develop only after months or years of exposure. In general, pharmacovigilance programmes reveal such effects; once recognised, they demand careful monitoring during chronic drug therapy for their occurrence may carry serious consequences for the patient (and the nonvigilant doctor, medicolegally). Descriptions of such (types C and D) reactions appear with the accounts of relevant drugs; some examples are:

Eye. Toxic cataract can be due to chloroquine and related drugs, adrenal steroids (topical and systemic), phenothiazines and alkylating agents. Corneal opacities occur with phenothiazines and chloroquine. Retinal injury occurs with thioridazine (particularly, of the antipsychotics), chloroquine and indomethacin.

Nervous system. Tardive dyskinesias occur with neuroleptics; polyneuritis with metronidazole; optic neuritis with ethambutol.

Lung. Amiodarone may cause pulmonary fibrosis. Sulphasalazine is associated with fibrosing alveolitis.

Kidney. Gold salts may cause nephropathy; see also Analgesic nephropathy (p. 284).

Liver. Methotrexate may cause liver damage and hepatic fibrosis; (see also alcohol p. 184).

Carcinogenesis: see also Preclinical testing (p. 45). Mechanisms of carcinogenesis are complex; prediction from animal tests is uncertain and causal attribution in man has finally to be based on epidemiological studies. The principal mechanisms are:

- *Alteration of DNA* (genotoxicity, mutagenicity). Many chemicals or their metabolites act by causing mutations, activating oncogenes; those substances that are used as medicines include griseofulvin and alkylating cytotoxics. Leukaemias and lymphomas are the most common malignancies.
- *Immunosuppression.*The immune system has a role in suppressing cancers (immune surveillance). A wide range of cancers develop in immunosuppressed patients, e.g after organ transplantation and cancer chemotherapy.
- *Hormonal.* Long-term use of oestrogen replacement in postmenopausal women induces endometrial cancer.

Combined oestrogen/progestogen oral contraceptives may both suppress and enhance cancers (see pp. 719, 723).

Diethylstilbestrol caused vaginal adenosis and cancer in the offspring of mothers who took it during pregnancy in the hope of preventing miscarriage. It was used for this purpose for decades after its introduction in the 1940s, on purely theoretical grounds. Controlled therapeutic trials were not done and there is no valid evidence of therapeutic efficacy. Male fetuses developed nonmalignant genital abnormalities.

Carcinogenesis due to medicines requires that drug exposure be prolonged,[13] i.e. months or years; the cancers develop most commonly over 3–5 years and often years after treatment has ceased.

Incidence of second cancers in patients treated for primary cancer can be as high as 15 times the normal rate. The use of immunosuppression in, e.g. rheumatoid arthritis and organ transplants, also increases the incidence of cancers.

Adverse effects on reproduction

Testing of new drugs on animals for their effects

on reproduction has been mandatory since the thalidomide disaster, even though the extrapolation of the findings to humans is uncertain (see Preclinical testing, p. 47). The placental transfer of drugs from the mother to the fetus is considered on page 98.

Drugs may act on the embryo and fetus:

Directly (thalidomide, cytotoxic drugs, antithyroid drugs, aromatic retinoids, e.g. isotretinoin): any drug affecting cell division, enzymes, protein synthesis or DNA synthesis, is a potential teratogen, e.g. many antimicrobials.

Indirectly:

- on the uterus (vasoconstrictors reduce blood supply and cause fetal anoxia, misoprostol causes uterine contraction leading to abortion)
- on the mother's hormone balance.

Early pregnancy. During the first week after fertilisation, exposure to antimetabolites, misoprostol, ergot alkaloids or stilboesterol can cause abortion which may not be recognised as such. The most vulnerable period for major anatomical abnormality is that of organogenesis which occurs during weeks 2–8 of intrauterine life (4–10 weeks after the first day of the last menstruation). After the organs are formed, abnormalities are less anatomically dramatic. Thus the activity of a teratogen (*teratos:* monster) is most devastating soon after implantation, at doses which may not harm the mother and at a time when she may not know she is pregnant.

Drugs known to be teratogenic include cytotoxics, warfarin, alcohol, lithium, methotrexate, phenytoin, valproate, ACE inhibitors and isotretinoin. Selective interference can produce characteristic anatomical abnormalities, and the phocomelia (flipper-like) limb defect was one factor that caused thalidomide to be so readily recognised. (For an account of thalidomide see p. 81.)

Innumerable drugs have come under suspicion. Those for which evidence of safety was subsequently found include diazepam, oral contraceptives, spermicides, and salicylates. Naturally the subject is a highly emotional one for prospective parents. A definitive list of unsafe drugs is not practicable. Much depends on the dose taken and at what stage

---

[13] Carcinogens that are effective as a single dose in animals are known, e.g. nitrosamines.

of pregnancy. The topic must be followed in the current literature.

Late pregnancy. Because the important organs are already formed, drugs will not cause the gross anatomical defects that can occur when they are given in early pregnancy. Administration of hormones, androgens or progestogens, can cause fetal masculinisation; iodide and antithyroid drugs in high dose can cause fetal goitre, as can lithium; tetracyclines can interfere with tooth and bone development, angiotensin-converting enzyme inhibitors are associated with renal tubular dysgenesis and a skull ossification defect. Tobacco smoking retards fetal growth; it does not cause anatomical abnormalities in man as far as is known.

Inhibitors of prostaglandin synthase (aspirin, indomethacin) may delay onset of labour and, in the fetus, cause closure of the ductus arteriosus, patency of which is dependent on prostaglandins. It is probable that drug allergy in the mother can also occur in the fetus and it is possible that the fetus may be sensitised where the mother shows no effect, e.g. neonatal thrombocytopenia from thiazide diuretics.

The suggestion that congenital cataract (due to denaturation of lens protein) might be due to drugs has some support in man. Chloroquine and chlorpromazine are concentrated in the fetal eye. Since both can cause retinopathy it would seem wise to avoid them in pregnancy if possible.

Anticoagulants in pregnancy: see page 571.

Drugs given to the mother just prior to labour can cause postnatal effects: CNS depressants may persist in and affect the baby for days after birth; vasoconstrictors can cause fetal distress by reducing uterine blood supply; β-adrenoceptor blockers may impair fetal response to hypoxia; sulphonamides displace bilirubin from plasma protein (risk of kernicterus); anticoagulants can cause haemorrhage.

Babies born to mothers dependent on opioids may show a physical withdrawal syndrome.

Drugs given during labour. Any drug that acts to depress respiration in the mother can cause respiratory depression in the newborn; opioid analgesics are notorious in this respect, but there can also be difficulty with any sedatives and general anaesthetics; they may also cause fetal distress by reducing uterine blood flow, and prolong labour by depressing uterine muscle.

Diazepam (and other depressants) in high doses may cause hypotonia in the baby and possibly interfere with suckling. There remains the possibility of later behavioural effects due to impaired development of the central nervous system due to psychotropic drugs used during pregnancy; such effects have been shown in animals, including impaired ability to learn their way around mazes.

Detection of teratogens. Anatomical abnormalities are the easiest to detect. Nonanatomical (functional) effects can also occur, though it is not appropriate to use the term teratogenesis (see definition above). They include effects on brain biochemistry which may have late behavioural consequences.

There is a substantial spontaneous background incidence of birth defect in the community (up to 2%) so that the detection of a low-grade teratogen that increases the incidence of one of the commoner abnormalities presents an intimidating task. Also, most teratogenic effects are probably multifactorial. In this emotionally charged area it is indeed hard for the public and especially for parents of an affected child to grasp that:

> The concept of absolute safety of drugs needs to be demolished … In real life it can never be shown that a drug (or anything else) has no teratogenic activity at all, in the sense of never being a contributory factor in anybody under any circumstances. This concept can neither be tested nor proved.

> Let us suppose for example, that some agent doubles the incidence of a condition that has natural incidence of 1 in 10 000 births. If the hypothesis is true, then studying 20 000 pregnant women who have taken the drug and 20 000 who have not may yield respectively two cases and one case of the abnormality. It does not take a statistician to realise that this signifies nothing, and it may need ten times as many pregnant women (almost half a million) to produce a statistically significant result. This would involve such an extensive multicentre study that hundreds of doctors and hospitals have to participate. The participants then each tend to bend the protocol to

fit in with their clinical customs and in the end it is difficult to assess the validity of the data.

Alternatively, a limited geographical basis may be used, with the trial going on for many years. During this time other things in the environment change, so again the results would not command our confidence. If it were to be suggested that there was something slightly teratogenic in milk, the hypothesis would be virtually untestable.

In practice we have to make up our minds which drugs may reasonably be given to pregnant women. Do we start from a position of presumed guilt or from one of presumed innocence? If the former course is chosen then we cannot give any drugs to pregnant women because we can never prove that they are completely free of teratogenic influence. It therefore seems that we must start from a position of presumed innocence and then take all possible steps to find out if the presumption is correct.

Finally, we must put the matter in perspective by considering the benefit/risk ratio. The problem of prescription in pregnancy cannot be considered from the point of view of only one side of the equation. Drugs are primarily designed to do good, and if a pregnant woman is ill it is in the best interests of her baby and herself that she gets better as quickly as possible. This often means giving her drugs. We can argue about the necessity of giving drugs to prevent vomiting, but there is no argument about the need for treatment of women with meningitis, septicaemia or venereal disease.

What we must try to avoid is medication by the media or prescription by politicians. A public scare about a well-tried drug will lead to wider use of less-tried alternatives. We do not want to be forced to practise the kind of defensive medicine that is primarily designed to avoid litigation.[14]

MALE REPRODUCTIVE FUNCTION

Impotence may occur with drugs affecting autonomic sympathetic function, e.g. some antihypertensives.

Spermatogenesis is reduced by a number of drugs including sulfasalazine and mesalazine (reversible), cytotoxic anticancer drugs (reversible and irreversible) and nitrofurantoin. There has been a global decline in sperm concentration and an environmental cause, e.g. chemicals that possess oestrogenic activity, seems likely.

Causation of birth defects due to abnormal sperm remains uncertain.

GENERAL DISCUSSION

Human toxic effects not predicted from animal experiments are often reversible, but even the most optimistic enthusiasts for drugs must shrink from the thought that their hands wrote prescriptions resulting in deformed, surviving babies.

Clinical data are, at present, inevitably open to doubt, and any list of suspected drugs must become obsolete and misleading very quickly. This topic must, therefore, be followed in the periodical press and manufacturers' up-to-date information.

The medical profession clearly has a grave duty to refrain from all unessential prescribing of drugs with, say, less than 10–15 years widespread use behind them, for all women of childbearing potential. It is not sufficient safeguard merely to ask a woman if she is or may be pregnant, for it is also necessary to consider the possibility of a woman, who is not pregnant at the time of prescribing, may become so whilst taking the drug.

Since morning sickness of pregnancy occurs during the time when the fetus is vulnerable, it is specially important to restrict drug therapy of this symptom to a minimum; but severe vomiting with its accompanying biochemical changes may itself harm the fetus.

Thus, before a drug is condemned as a cause of fetal damage, it is necessary to consider whether the disease for which it was given, or other intercurrent disease, might perhaps be responsible. Since the only way to be certain that a drug causes fetal damage in humans is to test it in humans, it is necessary that doctors should (a) suspect a drug-induced abnormality when it occurs and (b) report it to a central organisation (e.g. UK Committee on Safety of Medicines) or to a national register of all birth defects (such a register ideally should be kept plus a full drug history of the mother from prior to conception). Unfortunately, none of these requirements is easily satisfied. Minor congenital abnor-

---

[14] By permission from Smithells R W 1983 In: Hawkins D F (ed) Drugs and pregnancy. Churchill Livingstone, Edinburgh.

malities are common in the absence of drug therapy and some may be virtually undetectable, e.g. reduced intelligence or learning ability. In addition, the more cautiously a new drug is introduced, the more difficult it is going to be to detect, by epidemiological methods, a capacity to cause fetal abnormality. This is especially so if the abnormality produced is already fairly common. Human frailty also causes any reporting system based on voluntary cooperation to be less than perfect.

The possibility of fetal abnormalities resulting from drugs taken by the father exists but has only begun to be explored.

GUIDE TO FURTHER READING

Edwards I R, Aronson J K 2000 Adverse drug reactions: definitions, diagnosis, and management. Lancet 356: 1255–1259

Ewan P W 1998 Anaphylaxis. British Medical Journal 316: 1442–1445

Gruchalla R S 2000 Clinical assessment of drug-induced disease. Lancet 356: 1505–1511

Herbst A L 1984 Diethylstilboestrol exposure—1984 [effects of exposure during pregnancy on mother and daughters]. New England Journal of Medicine 311: 1433–1435

Kaufman D W, Shapiro S 2000 Epidemiological assessment of drug-induced disease. Lancet 356: 1339–1343

Knowles S R, Uetrecht J, Shear N H 2000 Idiosyncratic drug reactions: the reactive metabolite syndromes. Lancet 356: 1587–1591

Koren D, Pastuszak A, Ito S 1998 Drugs in pregnancy. New England Journal of Medicine 338: 1128–1137 (lists drugs that are safe and unsafe to use in pregnancy)

Meyer U A 2000 Pharmacogenetics and adverse drug reactions. Lancet 356: 1667–1671

Pirmohammed M et al 2000 Adverse drug reactions. British Medical Journal 316: 1295–1298

Scott J L et al 1965 A controlled double-blind study of the haematologic toxicity of chloramphenicol. New England Journal of Medicine 272: 1137

Vervolet D, Durham S 1998 ABC of allergies: adverse reactions to drugs. British Medical Journal 316: 1511–1514

9

Poisoning, overdose, antidotes

SYNOPSIS

- Deliberate and accidental self-poisoning
- Principles of treatment
- Poison-specific measures
- General measures
- Specific poisonings: cyanide, methanol, ethylene glycol, hydrocarbons, volatile solvents, heavy metals, herbicides and pesticides, biological substances (overdose of medicinal drugs is dealt with under individual agents)
- Incapacitating agents: drugs used for torture

drugs, and psychotropic drugs is increasing. Repeated episodes are not rare.[1] Prescribed drugs are used in over 75% of episodes but teenagers tend to favour nonprescribed analgesics available by direct sale, e.g. paracetamol, which is important bearing in mind its potentially serious toxicity. The mortality rate of self-poisoning is very low (less than 1% of acute hospital admissions), but 'completed' suicides by poisoning still number 3500 per annum in England and Wales.

Accidental self-poisoning causing admission to hospital occurs predominantly amongst children under 5 years, usually with medicines left within their reach or with domestic chemicals, e.g. bleach, detergents.

Self-poisoning

Deliberate self-poisoning. A curious by-product of the modern 'drug and prescribing explosion' is the rise in the incidence of nonfatal deliberate self-harm. The majority of people who do this lack serious suicidal intent and are therefore termed parasuicides. In over 90% of instances in the UK, poisoning is the means chosen, usually by medicines taken in overdose and these amount to at least 70 000 hospital admissions per annum in England and Wales (population 51 million). Two or more drugs are taken in over 30% of episodes, not including alcohol which is also taken in over 50% of the instances; the use of hypnotic and sedative

Principles of treatment

Successful treatment of acute poisoning depends on a combination of speed and common sense, as well as on the nature of the poison, the amount taken and the time which has since elapsed. The majority of those admitted to hospital require only observation and medical and nursing supportive measures

---

[1] An extreme example is that of a young man who, over a period of 6 years, was admitted to hospital following 82 episodes of self-poisoning, 31 employing paracetamol; he had had a disturbed, unhappy upbringing and had been expelled from both the Danish Navy and the British Army. Prescott L F et al 1978 British Medical Journal 2: 1399.

while they metabolise and eliminate the poison. Some require a specific antidote or a specific measure to increase elimination. Intensive care facilities are needed by only a few. In the UK the centres of the National Poisons Information Service provide information and advice over the telephone throughout the day and night.[2]

Poison-specific measures

IDENTIFICATION OF THE POISON(S)

The key pieces of information are:

- the identity of the substance(s) taken
- the dose(s)
- the time that has since elapsed. Adults may be sufficiently conscious to give some indication of the poison or may have referred to it in a suicide note, or there may be other circumstantial evidence. Rapid (1–2 h) biochemical 'screens' of plasma or urine are available but are best reserved for seriously ill or unconscious patients in whom the cause of coma is unknown. Analysis of plasma for specific substances is essential in suspected cases of paracetamol or iron poisoning, to indicate which patients should receive antidotes; it is also required for salicylate, lithium and some sedative drugs, e.g. trichloroethanol derivatives, phenobarbitone, when a decision is needed about using urine alkalinisation, haemodialysis or haemoperfusion. Response to a specific antidote may provide a diagnosis, e.g. dilatation of constricted pupils and increased respiratory rate after i.v. naloxone (opioid poisoning) or arousal from unconsciousness in response to i.v. flumazenil (benzodiazepine poisoning).

PREVENTION OF FURTHER ABSORPTION OF THE POISON

From the environment

When a poison has been inhaled or absorbed through the skin, the patient should be taken from the toxic environment, the contaminated clothing removed and the skin cleansed.

From the gut

Oral adsorbents. Activated charcoal (Carbomix, Medicoal) reduces drug absorption better than syrup of ipecacuanha or gastric lavage, is easiest to administer and has fewest adverse effects. It consists of a very fine black powder prepared from vegetable matter, e.g. wood pulp, coconut shell, which is 'activated' by an oxidising gas flow at high temperature to create a network of fine (10–20-nm) pores to give it an enormous surface area in relation to weight ($1000 \text{ m}^2/\text{g}$). This binds to, and thus inactivates, a wide variety of compounds in the gut. Thus it is simpler to list the exceptions, i.e. substances that are **not adsorbed** by charcoal which are: iron, lithium, cyanide, strong acids and alkalis, and organic solvents and corrosive agents.

Indeed, activated charcoal comes nearest to fulfilling the long-sought notion of a 'universal antidote'.[3] It should be given as soon as possible after a potentially toxic amount of a poison has been ingested, and whilst a significant amount remains yet unabsorbed (thus ideally within 1 h). To be most effective, 5–10 times as much charcoal as poison, weight for weight, is needed; in the adult an initial dose of 50–100 g is usual. If the patient is vomiting, the charcoal should be given through a nasogastric tube. Activated charcoal also accelerates elimination of poison that has been absorbed (see p. 155).

Activated charcoal, although unpalatable, appears to be relatively safe but constipation or mechanical bowel obstruction may be caused by repeated use. Aspiration of charcoal into the lungs can cause hypoxia through obstruction and arteriovenous shunting. Charcoal adsorbs and thus inactivates

---

[2] Telephone numbers are to be found in the British National Formulary (BNF).

[3] For centuries it was supposed not only that there could be, but that there actually was, a single antidote to all poisons. This was Theriaca Andromachi, a formulation of 72 (a magical number) ingredients amongst which particular importance was attached to the flesh of a snake (viper). The antidote was devised by Andromachus whose son was physician to the Roman Emperor, Nero (AD 37–68).

ipecacuanha but may be used after successful emesis if this method has been deemed necessary; methionine, used orally for paracetamol poisoning, is also adsorbed.

Other oral adsorbents have specific uses. Fuller's earth and bentonite (both natural forms of aluminium silicate) bind and inactivate the herbicides, paraquat (activated charcoal is superior) and diquat; cholestyramine and colestipol will adsorb warfarin.

Gastric lavage incurs dangers as well as benefits; it is best confined to the hospitalised adult who is believed to have taken a potentially life-threatening amount of a poison within 1 h (or longer in the case of drugs that delay gastric emptying, e.g. aspirin, tricyclic antidepressants, sympathomimetics, theophylline, opioids). Lavage is probably worth undertaking in any unconscious patient who is believed to have ingested poison, and provided the airways are protected by a cuffed endotracheal tube. Paradoxically, lavage may wash an ingested substance into the small intestine, enhancing its absorption. Leaving activated charcoal in the stomach after lavage is appropriate to lessen this risk. Nevertheless, patients who have ingested tricyclic antidepressants or centrally depressant drugs must be subject to continued monitoring after the lavage.

The passing of a gastric tube, naturally, takes second place to emergency resuscitative measures, institution of controlled respiration or suppression of convulsions. Nothing is gained by aspirating the stomach of a corpse.

Emesis has been used for children and also for adults who refuse activated charcoal or gastric lavage, or if the poison is not absorbed by activated charcoal. Its routine use in emergency departments has been abandoned, as there is no clinical trial evidence that the procedure improves outcome for poisoned patients. Emesis is induced, in fully conscious patients only, by Ipecacuanha Emetic Mixture, Pediatric (BNF), 10 ml for a child 6–18 months, 15 ml for an older child and 30 ml for an adult, i.e. all ages may receive the same preparation but in a different dose, which is followed by a tumblerful of water (250 ml). The active constituent of ipecacuanha is emetine; it can cause prolonged vomiting, diarrhoea and drowsiness that may be confused with effects of the ingested poison. Even

fully conscious patients may develop aspiration pneumonia after ipecacuanha.

Both emesis and lavage are contraindicated for corrosive poisons, because there is a risk of perforation of the gut, and for petroleum distillates, as the danger of causing inhalational chemical pneumonia outweighs that of leaving the substance in the stomach.

Cathartics or whole-bowel irrigation[4] have been used for the removal of sustained-release formulations, e.g. theophylline, iron, aspirin. Evidence of benefit is conflicting. Activated charcoal in repeated (10 g) doses is generally preferred. Sustained-release formulations are now common, and patients have died from failure to recognise the danger of continued release of drug from such products, after apparently successful gastric lavage.

SPECIFIC ANTIDOTES[5]

Specific antidotes reduce or abolish the effects of poisons through a variety of mechanisms, which may be categorised as follows:

- receptors, which may be activated, blocked or bypassed
- enzymes, which may be inhibited or reactivated
- displacement from tissue binding sites
- exchanging with the poison
- replenishment of an essential substance
- binding to the poison (including chelation).

---

[4] Irrigation with large volumes of a polyethylene glycol-electrolyte solution, e.g. Klean-Prep, by mouth causes minimal fluid and electrolyte disturbance (it was developed for preparation for colonoscopy). Magnesium sulphate may also be used.

[5] Mithridates the Great (?132–63 BC) king of Pontus (in Asia Minor) was noted for 'ambition, cruelty and artifice'. 'He murdered his own mother … and fortified his constitution by drinking antidotes' to the poisons with which his domestic enemies sought to kill him (Lemprière). When his son also sought to kill him, Mithridates was so disappointed that he compelled his wife to poison herself. He then tried to poison himself, but in vain; the frequent antidotes which he had taken in the early part of his life had so strengthened his constitution that he was immune. He was obliged to stab himself, but had to seek the help of a slave to complete his task. Modern physicians have to be content with less comprehensively effective antidotes, some of which are listed in Table 9.1.

TABLE 9.1 Some specific antidotes, indications and modes of action (see Index for a fuller account of individual drugs)

Antidote	Indication	Mode of action
acetylcysteine	paracetamol, chloroform, carbon tetrachloride	Replenishes depleted glutathione stores
atropine	cholinesterase inhibitors, e.g. organophosphorus insecticides	Blocks muscarinic cholinoceptors
	β-blocker poisoning	Vagal block accelerates heart rate
benzatropine	drug-induced movement disorders	Blocks muscarinic cholinoceptors
calcium gluconate	hydrofluoric acid, fluorides	Binds or precipitates fluoride ions
desferrioxamine	iron	Chelates ferrous ions
dicobalt edetate	cyanide and derivatives, e.g. acrylonitrile	Chelates to form nontoxic cobalti-and cobalto-cyanides
digoxin-specific antibody fragments (FAB)	digitalis glycosides	Binds free glycoside in plasma, complex excreted in urine
dimercaprol (BAL)	arsenic, copper, gold, lead, inorganic mercury	Chelates metal ions
ethanol	ethylene glycol, methanol	Competes for alcohol and acetaldehyde dehydrogenases, preventing formation of toxic metabolites
flumazenil	benzodiazepines	Competes for benzodiazepine receptors
folinic acid	folic acid antagonists e.g. methotrexate, trimethoprim	Bypasses block in folate metabolism
glucagon	β-adrenoceptor antagonists	Bypasses blockade of the β-adrenoceptor; stimulates cyclic AMP formation with positive cardiac inotropic effect
isoprenaline	β-adrenoceptor antagonists	Competes for β-adrenoceptors
methionine	paracetamol	Replenishes depleted glutathione stores
naloxone	opioids	Competes for opioid receptors
neostigmine	antimuscarinic drugs	Inhibits acetylcholinesterase, causing acetylcholine to accumulate at cholinoceptors
oxygen	carbon monoxide	Competitively displaces carbonmonoxide from binding sites on haemoglobin
penicillamine	copper, gold, lead, elemental mercury (vapour), zinc	Chelates metal ions
phenoxybenzamine	hypertension due to α-adrenoceptor agonists, e.g. with MAOI, clonidine, ergotamine	Competes for α-adrenoceptors (long-acting)
phentolamine	as above	Competes for α-adrenoceptors (short-acting)
phytomenadione (vitamine K₁)	coumarin (warfarin) and indandione anticoagulants	Replenishes vitamin K
pralidoxime	cholinesterase inhibitors, e.g. organophosphorus insecticides	Competitively reactivates cholinesterase
propranolol	β-adrenoceptor agonists, ephedrine, theophylline, thyroxine	Blocks β-adrenoceptors
protamine	heparin	Binds ionically to neutralise
Prussian blue (potassium ferric hexacyanoferrate)	thallium (in rodenticides)	Potassium exchanges for thallium
sodium calciumedetate	lead	Chelates lead ions
unithiol	lead, elemental and organic mercury	Chelates metal ions

Table 9.1 illustrates these mechanisms with antidotes that are of therapeutic value.

CHELATING AGENTS

Chelating agents are used for poisoning with heavy metals. They incorporate the metal ions into an inner ring structure in the molecule (Greek: *chele*, claw) by means of structural groups called ligands (Latin: *ligare*, to bind); effective agents form stable, biologically inert complexes that are excreted in the urine.

Dimercaprol (British Anti-Lewisite, BAL). Arsenic and other metal ions are toxic in low concentration because they combine with the SH groups of essential enzymes, thus inactivating them. Dimercaprol provides SH groups which combine with the metal ions to form relatively harmless ring compounds which are excreted, mainly in the urine. As dimercaprol, itself, is oxidised in the body and renally excreted, repeated administration is necessary to ensure that an excess is available until all the metal has been eliminated.

Dimercaprol may be used in cases of poisoning by antimony, arsenic, bismuth, gold and mercury (inorganic, e.g. $HgCl_2$).

Adverse effects are common, particularly with larger doses, and include nausea and vomiting, lachrymation and salivation, paraesthesiae, muscular aches and pains, urticarial rashes, tachycardia and a raised blood pressure. Gross overdosage may cause overbreathing, muscular tremors, convulsions and coma.

Unithiol (dimercaptopropanesulphonate, DMPS) effectively chelates lead and mercury; it is well tolerated.

Sodium calciumedetate is the calcium chelate of the disodium salt of ethylenediaminetetra-acetic acid (calcium EDTA). It is effective in acute lead poisoning because of its capacity to exchange calcium for lead: the lead chelate is excreted in the urine, leaving behind a harmless amount of calcium. Dimercaprol may usefully be combined with sodium calciumedetate when lead poisoning is severe, e.g. with encephalopathy.

Adverse effects are fairly common, and include hypotension, lachrymation, nasal stuffiness, sneezing, muscle pains and chills. Renal damage can occur.

Dicobalt edetate. Cobalt forms stable, nontoxic complexes with cyanide. It is toxic (especially if the wrong diagnosis is made and no cyanide is present), causing hypertension, tachycardia and chest pain; consequent cobalt poisoning is treated by giving sodium calcium edetate and i.v. glucose.

Penicillamine (dimethylcysteine) is a metabolite of penicillin that contains SH groups; it may be used to chelate lead and also copper (see Hepatolenticular degeneration). Its principal use is for rheumatoid arthritis (see Index).

Desferrioxamine: see Iron.

ACCELERATION OF ELIMINATION OF THE POISON

Techniques for eliminating poisons have a role that is limited, but important when applicable.

Each method depends, directly or indirectly, on removing drug from the circulation and successful use requires that:

- The poison should be present in high concentration in the plasma relative to that in the rest of the body, i.e. it should have a small distribution volume
- The poison should dissociate readily from any plasma protein binding sites
- The effects of the poison should relate to its plasma concentration.

Methods used are:

Repeated doses of activated charcoal

Activated charcoal by mouth not only adsorbs ingested drug in the gut, preventing absorption into the body (see above), it also adsorbs drug that diffuses from the blood into the gut lumen when the concentration there is lower; because binding is irreversible the concentration gradient is maintained and drug is continuously removed; this has been called 'intestinal dialysis'. Charcoal may also adsorb drugs that are secreted into the bile, i.e. by interrupting an enterohepatic cycle. Evidence shows that activated charcoal in repeated doses effectively adsorbs (shortens $t_{1/2}$ of) phenobarbital (phenobarbitone), carbamazepine, theophylline, quinine, dapsone and salicylate.[6] Repeated-dose activated charcoal is increasingly preferred to alkalinisation of urine (below) for phenobarbitone and salicylate poisoning. Activated charcoal in an initial dose of 50–100 g should be followed by not less than 12.5 g/h; the regular hourly administration is more effective than larger amounts less often.

Alteration of urine pH and diuresis

By manipulation of the pH of the glomerular filtrate, a drug can be made to ionise, become less lipid-soluble, remain in the renal tubular fluid, and so be eliminated in the urine (see p. 97). Maintenance of a good urine flow (e.g. 100 ml/h) helps this process but it is the alteration of tubular fluid pH that is all important. The practice of forcing

---

[6] Bradberry S M, Vale A J 1995 Journal of Toxicology: Clinical Toxicology 33(5): 407–416.

diuresis with frusemide (furosemide) and large volumes of i.v. fluid does not add significantly to drug clearance but may cause fluid overload; it is obsolete. Alkalinisation may be used for salicylate (> 500 mg/l + metabolic acidosis, or in any case > 750 mg/l), phenobarbital (75–150 mg/l) or phenoxy herbicides, e.g. 2,4-D, mecoprop, dichlorprop. The objective is to maintain a urine pH of 7.5–8.5 by an i.v. infusion of sodium bicarbonate. Available preparations of sodium bicarbonate vary between 1.2 and 8.4% (1 ml of the 8.4% preparation contains 1 mmol of sodium bicarbonate) and the concentration given will depend on the patient's fluid needs.

Acidification may be used for severe, acute amphetamine, dexfenfluramine or phencyclidine poisoning. The objective is to maintain a urine pH of 5.5–6.5 by giving i.v. infusion of arginine hydrochloride (10 g) over 30 min, followed by ammonium chloride (4 g) 2-hourly by mouth. It is rarely necessary. Phenoxybenzamine should be adequate for amphetamine-like drugs (α-adrenoceptor block).

Peritoneal dialysis

Peritoneal dialysis involves instilling appropriate fluid into the peritoneal cavity. Poison in the blood diffuses into the dialysis fluid down the concentration gradient. The fluid is then drained and replaced. The technique requires little equipment but is one-half to one-third as effective as haemodialysis; it may be worth using for lithium and methanol poisoning.

Haemodialysis and haemoperfusion

A temporary extracorporeal circulation is established, usually from an artery to a vein in the arm. In haemodialysis, a semipermeable membrane separates blood from dialysis fluid and the poison passes passively from the blood, where it is present in high concentration. The principle of haemoperfusion is that blood flows over activated charcoal or an appropriate ion-exchange resin which adsorbs the poison. Loss of blood cells and activation of the clotting mechanism are largely overcome by coating the charcoal with an acrylic hydrogel which does not reduce adsorbing capacity, though the patient must be anticoagulated with heparin.

Such artificial methods of removing poison from the body are invasive, demand skill and experience on the part of the operator and are expensive in manpower. Their use should therefore be confined to cases of severe, prolonged or progressive clinical intoxication, when high plasma concentration indicates a dangerous degree of poisoning, and when removal by haemoperfusion or dialysis constitutes a significant addition to natural methods of elimination.

- **Haemodialysis** is effective for: salicylate (> 750 mg/l + renal failure, or in any case > 900 mg/l), isopropanol (present in aftershave lotions and window-cleaning solutions), lithium and methanol.
- **Haemoperfusion** is effective for: phenobarbitone (> 100–150 mg/l, but repeat-dose activated charcoal by mouth appears to be as effective, see above) and other barbiturates, ethchlorvynol, glutethimide, meprobamate, methaqualone, theophylline, trichloroethanol derivatives.

General measures

INITIAL ASSESSMENT AND RESUSCITATION

The initial clinical review should include a search for known consequences of poisoning, which include: impaired consciousness with flaccidity (benzodiazepines, alcohol, trichloroethanol) or with hypertonia (tricyclic antidepressants, antimuscarinic agents), hypotension, shock, cardiac arrhythmia, evidence of convulsions, behavioural disturbances (psychotropic drugs), hypothermia, aspiration pneumonia and cutaneous blisters, burns in the mouth (corrosives).

Maintenance of an adequate oxygen supply is the first priority. A systolic blood pressure of 80 mmHg can be tolerated in a young person but a level below 90 mmHg will imperil the brain or kidney of the elderly. Expansion of the venous capacitance bed is the usual cause of shock in acute poisoning and blood pressure may be restored by placing the patient in the head-down position to encourage venous return to the heart, or by the use of a colloid plasma expander such as gelatin or etherified starch. External cardiac compression may be necessary and should be continued until the cardiac output is self-sustaining, which may be a long time when the patient is hypothermic or poisoned with cardio-depressant drugs, e.g. tricyclic antidepressants, β-adrenoceptor blockers. The airway must be sucked clear of oropharyngeal secretions or regurgitated matter.

Supportive treatment

The salient fact is that patients recover from most poisonings provided they are adequately oxygenated, hydrated and perfused, for, in the majority of cases, the most efficient mechanisms are the patients' own and, given time, they will inactivate and eliminate all the poison. Patients require the standard care of the unconscious, with special attention to the problems introduced by poisoning which are outlined below.

Airway maintenance is essential; some patients require a cuffed endotracheal tube but seldom for more than 24 h.

Ventilation needs should be assessed, if necessary supported by blood gas analysis. A mixed respiratory and metabolic acidosis is common. Hypoxia may be corrected by supplementing the inspired air with oxygen but mechanical ventilation is necessary if the $PaCO_2$ exceeds 6.5 kPa.

Hypotension is common and in addition to the resuscitative measures indicated above, infusion of a combination of dopamine and dobutamine in low dose may be required to maintain renal perfusion.

Convulsions should be treated if they are persistent or protracted. Diazepam i.v. is the first choice.

Cardiac arrhythmia frequently accompanies poisoning, e.g. with tricyclic antidepressants, theophylline, β-adrenoceptor blockers. Acidosis, hypoxia and electrolyte disturbance are often important contributory factors; the emphasis of therapy should be to correct these and to resist the temptation to resort to an antiarrhythmic drug. If arrhythmia leads to persistent peripheral circulatory failure, then an appropriate drug ought to be used, e.g. a β-adrenoceptor blocker for poisoning with a sympathomimetic drug.

Hypothermia may occur if temperature regulation is impaired by CNS depression. Core temperature must be monitored by a low-reading rectal thermometer, while the patient is nursed in a heat retaining 'space blanket'.

Immobility may lead to pressure lesions of peripheral nerves, cutaneous blisters and necrosis over bony prominences.

Rhabdomyolysis may result from prolonged pressure on muscles, from agents that cause muscle spasm or convulsions (phencyclidine, theophylline) or be aggravated by hyperthermia due to muscle contraction, e.g. with MDMA ('ecstasy'). Aggressive volume repletion and correction of acid–base abnormality may be needed, and urine alkalinisation may prevent acute tubular necrosis.

PSYCHIATRIC AND SOCIAL ASSESSMENT

Most cases of self-poisoning are precipitated by interpersonal or social problems, which should be addressed. Major psychiatric illness ought to be identified and treated.

> 'There are said to be occasions when a wise man chooses suicide—but generally speaking it is not in an excess of reasonableness that people kill themselves. Most men and women die defeated...'[7]

Some poisonings

(for medicines: see individual drugs)

Common toxic syndromes[8]

Many substances used in accidental or self-

---

[7] Voltaire (pseudonym of Francios-Marie Arouet, French writer, 1694–1778).
[8] Based on Kulig K 1992 New England Journal of Medicine 326: 1677–1681.

poisoning cause dysfunction of the central or autonomic nervous systems and produce a variety of effects which may be usefully grouped to aid the identification of the agent(s) responsible.

Antimuscarinic syndromes consist of tachycardia, dilated pupils, dry, flushed skin, urinary retention, decreased bowel sounds, mild elevation of body temperature, confusion, cardiac arrhythmias and seizures. They are commonly caused by antipsychotics, tricyclic antidepressants, antihistamines, antispasmodics and many plants (see p. 160).

Cholinergic (muscarinic) syndromes comprise salivation, lachrymation, abdominal cramps, urinary and faecal incontinence, vomiting, sweating, miosis, muscle fasciculation and weakness, bradycardia, pulmonary oedema, confusion, CNS depression and fitting. Common causes include organophosphorus and carbamate insecticides, neostigmine and other anticholinesterase drugs, and some fungi (mushrooms).

Sympathomimetic syndromes include tachycardia, hypertension, hyperthermia, sweating, mydriasis, hyperreflexia, agitation, delusions, paranoia, seizures and cardiac arrhythmias. These are commonly caused by amphetamine and its derivatives, cocaine, proprietary decongestants, e.g. ephedrine, and theophylline (in the latter case, excluding psychiatric effects).

Sedatives, opioids and ethanol cause signs that may include respiratory depression, miosis, hyporeflexia, coma, hypotension and hypothermia.

Poisonings by (nondrug) chemicals

Cyanide causes tissue anoxia by chelating the ferric part of the intracellular respiratory enzyme, cytochrome oxidase. Poisoning may occur as a result of self-administration of hydrocyanic (prussic) acid, by accidental exposure in industry, through inhaling smoke from burning polyurethane foams in furniture, through ingesting amygdalin which is present in the kernels of several fruits including apricots, almonds and peaches (constituents of the unlicensed anticancer agent, laetrile), or from

excessive use of sodium nitroprusside for severe hypertension.[9] The symptoms of acute poisoning are due to tissue anoxia, with dizziness, palpitations, a feeling of chest constriction and anxiety; characteristically the breath smells of bitter almonds. In more severe cases there is acidosis and coma. Inhaled hydrogen cyanide may lead to death within minutes but when it is ingested as the salt several hours may elapse before the patient is seriously ill. Chronic exposure damages the nervous system causing peripheral neuropathy, optic atrophy and nerve deafness.

The principles of specific therapy are as follows:

- *Dicobalt edetate* to chelate the cyanide is the treatment of choice when the diagnosis is certain (see p. 155). The dose is 300 mg given i.v. over one minute (5 min if condition is less serious), followed immediately by a 50 ml i.v. infusion of glucose 50%; a further 300 mg of dicobalt edetate should be given if recovery is not evident within one minute.

- Alternatively, a two-stage procedure may be followed by i.v. administration of:
  (1) *sodium nitrite*, which rapidly converts haemoglobin to methaemoglobin, the ferric ion of which takes up cyanide as cyanmethaemoglobin (up to 40% methaemoglobin can be tolerated);
  (2) *sodium thiosulphate*, which more slowly detoxifies the cyanide by permitting the formation of thiocyanate. When the diagnosis is uncertain, administration of thiosulphate plus oxygen is a safe course.

There is evidence that oxygen, especially if at high pressure (hyperbaric), overcomes the cellular

---

[9] Or in other more bizarre ways. 'A 23-year-old medical student saw his dog (a puppy) suddenly collapse. He started external cardiac massage and a mouth-to-nose ventilation effort. Moments later the dog died, and the student felt nauseated, vomited and lost consciousness. On the victim's arrival at hospital, an alert medical officer detected a bitter almonds odour on his breath and administered the accepted treatment for cyanide poisoning after which he recovered. It turned out that the dog had accidentally swallowed cyanide, and the poison eliminated through the lungs had been inhaled by the master during the mouth-to-nose resuscitation.' Journal of the American Medical Association 1983 249: 353.

anoxia in cyanide poisoning; the mechanism is uncertain, but oxygen should be administered.

Carbon monoxide (CO) is formed when substances containing carbon and hydrogen are incompletely combusted; poisoning results from inhalation. Oxygen transport to cells is impaired and myocardial and neurological injury result; delayed (2–4 weeks) neurological sequelae include parkinsonism and cerebellar signs. The concentration of CO in the blood may confirm exposure (cigarette smoking alone may account for up to 10%) but is no guide to the severity of poisoning. Patients with signs of cardiac ischaemia or neurological defect may be treated with hyperbaric oxygen, although the evidence for its efficacy is conflicting and transport to hyperbaric chambers may present logistic problems.

Lead poisoning arises from a variety of occupational (such as house renovation and stripping old paint), and recreational sources. Environmental exposure had been a matter of great concern, as witness the protective legislation introduced by many countries to reduce pollution, e.g. by removing lead from petrol.

Lead in the body comprises a rapidly exchangeable component in blood (2%, biological $t^1\!/_2$ 35 d) and a stable pool in dentine and the skeleton (95%, biological $t^1\!/_2$ 25 y).

In severe lead poisoning sodium calciumedetate is commonly used to initiate lead excretion. It chelates lead from bone and the extracellular space and urinary lead excretion of diminishes over 5 days thereafter as the extracellular store is exhausted. Subsequently symptoms (colic and encephalopathy) may worsen and this has been attributed to redistribution of lead from bone to brain. Dimercaprol is more effective than sodium calciumedetate at chelating lead from the soft tissues such as brain, which is the rationale for combined therapy with sodium calciumedetate. More recently *succimer* (2,3-dimercaptosuccinic acid, DMSA), a water-soluble analogue of dimercaprol, has been increasingly used instead. Succimer has a high affinity for lead, is suitable for administration by mouth and is better tolerated (has a wider therapeutic index) than dimercaprol. It is licenced for such use in the USA but not the UK.

Methanol is widely available as a solvent and in paints and antifreezes, and may be consumed as a cheap substitute for ethanol. As little as 10 ml may cause permanent blindness and 30 ml may kill, through its toxic metabolites. Methanol, like ethanol, is metabolised by zero-order processes that involve the hepatic alcohol and aldehyde dehydrogenases, but whereas ethanol forms acetaldehyde and acetic acid which are partly responsible for the unpleasant effects of 'hangover', methanol forms formaldehyde and formic acid. Blindness may occur because aldehyde dehydrogenase present in the retina (for the interconversion of retinol and retinene) allows the local formation of formaldehyde. Acidosis is due to the formic acid, which itself enhances pH-dependent hepatic lactate production, so that lactic acidosis is added.

The clinical features are severe malaise, vomiting, abdominal pain and tachypnoea (due to the acidosis). Loss of visual acuity and scotomata indicate ocular damage and, if the pupils are dilated and non-reactive, permanent loss of sight is probable. Coma and circulatory collapse may follow.

Therapy is directed at:

- *Correcting the acidosis.* Achieving this largely determines the outcome; sodium bicarbonate is given i.v. in doses up to 2 mol in a few hours, carrying an excess of sodium which must be managed. Methanol is metabolised slowly and the patient may relapse if bicarbonate administration is discontinued too soon.
- *Inhibiting methanol metabolism. Ethanol*, which occupies the dehydrogenase enzymes in preference to methanol, competitively prevents metabolism of methanol to its toxic products. A single oral dose of ethanol 1 ml/kg (as a 50% solution or as the equivalent in gin or whisky) is followed by 0.25 ml/kg/h orally or i.v., aiming to maintain the blood ethanol at about 100 mg/100 ml until no methanol is detectable in the blood. *Fomepizole* (4-methylpyrazole), also a competitive inhibitor of alcohol dehydrognase, has proved effective in severe methanol poisoning and is less likely to cause cerebral depression.
- *Eliminating methanol* and its metabolites by dialysis. Haemodialysis is 2–3 times more effective than is peritoneal dialysis. Folinic

acid 30 mg i.v. 6-hourly may protect against retinal damage by enhancing formate metabolism.

Ethylene glycol is readily accessible as a constituent of antifreezes for car radiators. It has been used criminally to give 'body' and sweetness to white table wines. Metabolism to glycolate and oxalate causes acidosis and renal damage, and usually the situation is further complicated by lactic acidosis. In the first 12 hours after ingestion the patient appears as though intoxicated with alcohol but does not smell of that; subsequently there is increasing acidosis, pulmonary oedema and cardiac failure, and in 2–3 days renal pain and tubular necrosis develop because calcium oxalate crystals form in the urine. Acidosis is corrected with i.v. sodium bicarbonate and hypocalcaemia with calcium gluconate. As with methanol (above), ethanol or fomepizole is given competitively to inhibit the metabolism of ethylene glycol and haemodialysis is used to eliminate the poison.

Hydrocarbons, e.g. paraffin oil (kerosene), petrol (gasoline), benzene, chiefly cause CNS depression and pulmonary damage from inhalation. It is vital to avoid aspiration into the lungs during attempts to remove the poison or in spontaneous vomiting. Gastric aspiration should be performed only if a cuffed endotracheal tube is effectively in place, if necessary after anaesthetising the subject.

Volatile solvent abuse or 'glue sniffing', is common among teenagers, especially males. The success of the modern chemical industry provides easy access to these substances as adhesives, dry cleaners, air fresheners, deodorants, aerosols and other products. Various techniques of administration are employed: viscous products may be inhaled from a plastic bag, liquids from a handkerchief or plastic bottle. The immediate euphoriant and excitatory effects are replaced by confusion, hallucinations and delusions as the dose is increased. Chronic abusers, notably of toluene, develop peripheral neuropathy, cerebellar disease and dementia; damage to the kidney, liver, heart and lungs also occurs with solvents. Over 50% of deaths from the practice follow cardiac arrhythmia, probably caused by sensitisation of the myocardium to catecholamines and by vagal inhibition

from laryngeal stimulation when aerosol propellants are sprayed into the throat.

Standard cardiorespiratory resuscitation and antiarrhythmia treatment are used for acute solvent poisoning. Toxicity from *carbon tetrachloride* and *chloroform* involves the generation of phosgene (a 1914–18 war gas) which is inactivated by cysteine, and by glutathione which is formed from cysteine; treatment with N-acetylcysteine, as for poisoning with paracetamol, is therefore recommended.

Poisoning by herbicides and pesticides

Organophosphorus pesticides are anticholinesterases; poisoning and its management are described on page 437. Organic carbamates are similar.

Dinitro-compounds. Dinitro-orthocresol (DNOC) and dinitrobutylphenol (DNBP) are used as selective weed killers and insecticides, and cases of poisoning occur accidentally, e.g. when safety precautions are ignored. These substances can be absorbed through the skin and the hands, face or hair are usually stained yellow. Symptoms and signs indicate a very high metabolic rate (due to uncoupling of oxidative phosphorylation); copious sweating and thirst proceed to dehydration and vomiting, weakness, restlessness, tachycardia and deep, rapid breathing, convulsions and coma. Treatment is urgent and consists of cooling the patient and attention to fluid and electrolyte balance. It is essential to differentiate this type of poisoning from that due to anticholinesterases because atropine given to patients poisoned with dinitro-compound will stop sweating and may cause death from hyperthermia.

Phenoxy herbicides (2,4-D, mecoprop, dichlorprop) are used to control broad-leaved weeds. Ingestion causes nausea, vomiting, pyrexia (due to uncoupling of oxidative phosphorylation), hyperventilation, hypoxia and coma. Their elimination is enhanced by urine alkalinisation. Organochlorine pesticides, e.g. dicophane (DDT), may cause convulsions in acute overdose. Treat as for status epilepticus.

Rodenticides include warfarin and thallium (see Table 9.1); for strychnine, which causes convulsions, give diazepam.

Paraquat is a widely used herbicide which is extremely toxic if it is ingested; a mouthful of commercial solution taken and spat out may be enough to kill. Ulceration and sloughing of the oral and oesophageal mucosa are followed 5–10 days later by renal tubular necrosis and subsequently there is pulmonary oedema followed by pulmonary fibrosis; whether the patient lives or dies depends largely on the condition of the lung. Treatment is urgent and includes activated charcoal or aluminium silicate (Fuller's earth) by mouth as adsorbents, gastric lavage, and osmotic purgation (magnesium sulphate). Haemodialysis or haemoperfusion may have a role in the first 24 h, the rationale being that reducing the plasma concentration by using these methods protects the kidney, failure of which allows the slow but relentless accumulation of paraquat in the lung.

Diquat is similar to paraquat but the late pulmonary changes may not occur.

Poisoning by biological substances

Many plants form substances that are important for their survival either by enticing animals which disperse their spores, or by repelling potential predators. Poisoning occurs when children eat berries or chew flowers, attracted by their colour; adults may mistake nonedible for edible varieties of salad plants and fungi (mushrooms) for they may resemble each other closely and some are greatly prized by epicures.

The range of toxic substances that these plants produce is reflected in a diversity of symptoms which may be grouped broadly thus:

- *Atropinic*, e.g. from deadly nightshade (*Atropa belladonna*) and thorn apple (*Datura*), causing dilated pupils, blurred vision, dry mouth, flushed skin, confusion and delirium.
- *Nicotinic*, e.g. from hemlock (*Conium*) and *Laburnum*, causing salivation, dilated pupils, vomiting, convulsions and respiratory paralysis.
- *Muscarinic*, e.g. from *Inocybe* and *Clitocybe* fungi (mushrooms), causing salivation, lachrymation, miosis, perspiration, bradycardia and bronchoconstriction, also hallucinations.
- *Hallucinogenic*, e.g. from psilocybin-containing

mushrooms (liberty cap), which may be taken specifically for this effect ('magic mushrooms').
- *Cardiovascular*, e.g. from foxglove (*Digitalis*), mistletoe *(Viscum album)*) and lily-of-the-valley (*Convallaria*) which contain cardiac glycosides that cause vomiting, diarrhoea and cardiac arrhythmia.
- *Hepatotoxic*, e.g. from *Amanita phalloides* (death cap mushroom), from *Senecio* (ragwort) and *Crotalatia* and from 'bush teas' prepared from these plants in the Caribbean. Aflatoxin, from *Aspergillus flavus*, a fungus which contaminates foods, is probably a cause of primary liver cancer.
- *Convulsant*, e.g. from water dropwort (*Oenanthe*) and cowbane (*Cicuta*), which contain the related and very dangerous substances, oenanthotoxin and cicutoxin.
- *Cutaneous irritation*, e.g. directly with nettle (*Urtica*), or dermatitis following sensitisation with *Primula*.
- *Gastrointestinal symptoms*, nausea, vomiting, diarrhoea and abdominal pain occur with numerous plants.

Treatment of plant poisonings consists mainly of activated charcoal to adsorb toxin in the gastrointestinal tract. Inducing emesis with ipecacuanha may make the diagnosis more difficult for vomiting is often the earliest sign of poisoning. Convulsions should be controlled with diazepam. In 'death cap' mushroom poisoning, penicillin may be used to displace toxin from plasma albumin, provided haemodialysis is being used, which latter may also benefit the renal failure.

Biological agents as weapons

Many natural agents can cause life-threatening infections but their recruitment as biological weapons against communities of people requires particular qualities of infectivity, pathogenicity, stability and ease of production. Among the pathogens that may be considered candidates for this horrific purpose are *Bacillus anthracis* (the causal agent of anthrax), *Brucella* (brucellosis), *Clostridium botulinum* (botulism), *Francisella tularensis* (tularaemia), *Yersinia pestis* (plague), and variola virus (smallpox). Drugs used for the treatment and prophylaxis of some of the bacterial infections appear in Table 11.1 (p. 211). Vaccines are kept in special centres to immunise against anthrax, plague and smallpox, and an antitoxin for botulism. That it has been thought necessary even to make reference to the subject of bioterrorism is surely a sad commentary on the times in which we live.

Incapacitating agents

(harassing, disabling, antiriot agents)

Harassing agents may be defined as chemical substances that are capable when used in field conditions, of rapidly causing a temporary disablement that lasts for little longer than the period of exposure.[10]

The pharmacological requirements for a safe and effective harassing agent must be stringent (it is hardly appropriate to refer to benefit versus risk). As well as potency and rapid onset and offset of effect in open areas under any atmospheric condition, it must be safe in confined spaces where concentration may be very high and may affect an innocent, bedridden invalid should a projectile enter a window.

CS (chlorobenzylidene malononitrile, a tear 'gas') is a favoured substance at present. This is a solid that is disseminated as an aerosol (particles of 1 micron diameter) by including it in a pyrotechnic mixture. The spectacle of its dissemination has been rendered familiar by television. It is not a gas, it is an aerosol or smoke. The particles aggregate and settle to the ground in minutes so that the risk of prolonged exposure out of doors is not great.

According to the concentration of CS to which a person is exposed, the effects vary from a slight pricking or peppery sensation in the eyes and nasal passages up to the maximum symptoms of streaming from the eyes and nose, spasm of the eyelids, profuse lachrymation and salivation, retching and sometimes vomiting, burning of the mouth and throat, cough and gripping pain in the chest.[11]

The onset of symptoms occurs immediately on exposure (an important factor from the point of view of the user) and they disappear dramatically:

At one moment the exposed person is in their grip. Then he either stumbles away, or the smoke plume veers or the discharge from the grenade stops, and, immediately, the symptoms begin to roll away. Within a minute or two, the pain in the chest has gone and his eyes, although still streaming, are open. Five or so minutes later, the excessive salivation and pouring tears stop and a quarter of an hour after exposure, the subject is essentially back to normal.[10]

Exposed subjects absorb small amounts only, and the plasma $t\frac{1}{2}$ is about 5 seconds.

Investigations of the effects of CS are difficult in 'field use', but some have been done and at present there is no evidence that even the most persistent rioter will suffer any permanent effect. The hazard to the infirm or sick seems to be low, but plainly it would be prudent to assume that asthmatics or bronchitics could suffer an exacerbation from high concentrations, though bronchospasm does not occur in healthy people. Vomiting seems to be due to swallowing contaminated saliva. Transient looseness of the bowels may follow exposure. Hazard from CS is probably confined to situations where the missiles are projected into enclosed spaces.

CN (chloroacetophenone, a tear gas) is generally used as a solid aerosol or smoke; solutions (Mace) are used at close quarters.

CR (dibenzoxazepine) was put into production in 1973 after testing on army volunteers. In addition to the usual properties (above) it may induce a transient rise in intraocular pressure. Its solubility allows use in water 'cannons'.

'Authority' is reticent about the properties of all these substances and no further important information is readily available.

This brief account has been included, because, in addition to helping victims, even the most well-conducted and tractable students and doctors

---

[10] Health aspects of chemical and biological weapons. 1970 WHO Geneva.

[11] Home Office Report (1971) of the enquiry into the medical and toxicological aspects of CS. pt II. HMSO, London: Cmnd 4775.

may find themselves exposed to CS smoke in our troubled world; and some may even feel it their duty to incur exposure. The following points are worth making:

- Wear disposable plastic gloves, for the object of treating the sufferer is frustrated if the physician becomes affected.
- Contaminated clothing should be put in plastic bags and skin should be washed with soap and water. Showering or bathing may cause symptoms to return by releasing the agent from contaminated hair. Cutaneous erythema is usual and blistering may occur with high concentrations of CS and CN in warm, moist conditions.
- The eyes should be left to irrigate themselves; raised intraocular pressure may cause acute glaucoma in those over 40 years.

DRUGS USED FOR TORTURE, INTERROGATION AND JUDICIAL EXECUTION

Regrettably, drugs have been and are being used for torture, sometimes disguised as 'interrogation' or 'aversion therapy'. Facts are, not surprisingly, hard to obtain, but it seems that suxamethonium, hallucinogens, thiopentone, neuroleptics, amphetamines, apomorphine and cyclophosphamide have been employed to hurt, frighten, confuse or debilitate in such ways as callous ingenuity can devise. When the definition of criminal activity becomes perverted to include activities in defence of human liberty, the employment of drugs offers inducement to inhuman behaviour. Such use, and any doctors or others who engage in it, or who misguidedly allow themselves to believe that it can be in the interest of victims to monitor the activity by others, must surely be outlawed.

It might be urged that it is justifiable to use drugs to protect society by discovering serious crimes such as murder. There is no such thing as a 'truth drug' in the sense that it guarantees the truth of what the subject says. There always must be uncertainty of the truth of evidence obtained with drugs, e.g.

thiopentone, that cannot be independently confirmed. But accused people, convinced of their own innocence, sometimes volunteer to undergo such tests. The problem of discerning truth from falsehood remains.

In some countries drugs are used for judicial execution, e.g. combinations of thiopentone, potassium, curare, given intravenously.

GUIDE TO FURTHER READING

Dawson A H, Whyte I M 1999 Therapeutic drug monitoring in drug overdose. British Journal of Clinical Pharmacology 48: 278–283

Ernst A, Zibrak J D 1998 Carbon monoxide poisoning. New England Journal of Medicine 339: 1603–1608

Evison D, Hinsley D, Rice P 2002 Chemical weapons. British Medical Journal 324: 332–335

Flanagan R J et al 1990 Alkaline diuresis for acute poisoning with chlorophenoxy herbicides and ioxynil. Lancet 335: 454–458

Fraunfelder F T 2000 Is CS gas dangerous? British Medical Journal 320: 458–459

Hawton K et al 1999 Effects of a drug overdose in a television drama on presentation to hospital for self poisoning: time series and questionnaire study. British Medical Journal 318: 972–977

Henry J A 1992 Ecstasy and the dance of death. British Medical Journal 305: 5–6

Jones A L, Volans G 1999 Management of self poisoning. British Medical Journal 319: 1414–1417

Khan A S, Morse S, Lillibridge S 2000 Public-health preparedness for biological terrorism in the USA. Lancet 356: 1179–1182

Reisman R E 1994 Insect stings. New England Journal of Medicine 331: 523–527

Shannon M 2000 Ingestion of toxic substances by children. New England Journal of Medicine 342: 186–191

Tibbles P M, Edelsberg J S 1996 Hyperbaric-oxygen therapy. New England Journal of Medicine 334: 1642–1648

Yih J-P 1995 CS gas injury to the eye. British Medical Journal 311: 276

Social aspects

The enormous social importance of this subject warrants discussion here.

All the naturally occurring sedatives, narcotics, euphoriants, hallucinogens and excitants were discovered thousands of years ago, before the dawn of civilisation … By the late Stone Age man was systematically poisoning himself. The presence of poppy heads in the kitchen middens of the Swiss Lake Dwellers shows how early in his history man discovered the techniques of self-transcendence through drugs. There were dope addicts long before there were farmers.[1]

The drives that induce a person more or less mentally healthy to resort to drugs to obtain chemical vacations from intolerable selfhood will be briefly considered here, as well as some account of the pharmacological aspects of drug dependence.

The dividing-line between legitimate use of drugs for social purposes and their abuse is indistinct for it is not only a matter of which drug, but of amount of drug and of whether the effect is directed antisocially or not. 'Normal' people seem to be able to use alcohol for their occasional purposes without harm but, given the appropriate personality and/or environmental adversity, many may turn to it for relief and

[1] Huxley A 1957 Annals of the New York Academy of Sciences 67: 677.

become dependent on it, both psychologically and physically. But drug abuse is not primarily a pharmacological problem, it is a social problem with important pharmacological aspects.

A further issue is whether a boundary can be drawn between the therapeutic and nontherapeutic use of a therapeutic drug and, some would argue, if it can be drawn, should it be? The matter has been highlighted by the use of SSRI antidepressants, e.g. fluoxetine (Prozac), not to treat depression but to elevate mood — make a person feel 'better than well' (see nonmedical use, below).

SOME TERMS USED

Abuse potential of a drug is related to its capacity to produce immediate satisfaction, which may be a feature of the drug itself (amfetamine and heroin give rapid effect while tricyclic antidepressants do not) and its route of administration in descending order: inhalation/i.v.; i.m./s.c.; oral.

Drug abuse[2] implies excessive (in terms of social norms) nonmedical or social drug use.

Nonmedical drug use, i.e. all drug use that is not on generally accepted medical grounds, may be a term preferred to 'abuse'. Nonmedical use means the continuous or occasional use of drugs by individuals, whether of their own 'free' choice or under feelings of compulsion, to achieve their own wellbeing, or what they conceive as their own wellbeing (see motives below).

Drugs used for nonmedical purposes are often divided into two groups, hard and soft.

Hard drugs are those that are liable seriously to disable the individual as a functioning member of society by inducing severe psychological and, in the case of cerebral depressants, physical, dependence. The group includes heroin and cocaine.

Soft drugs are less dependence-producing. There

[2] The World Health Organization adopts the definition of the United Nations Convention on Psychotropic Drugs (1971). Drug abuse means the use of psychotropic substances in a way that would 'constitute a public health and social problem'.

may be psychological dependence, but there is little or no physical dependence except with heavy doses of depressants (alcohol). The group includes sedatives and tranquillisers, amphetamines, cannabis, hallucinogens, alcohol, tobacco and caffeine.

This classification fails to recognise individual variation in drug use. Alcohol can be used in heavy doses that are gravely disabling and induce severe physical dependence with convulsions on sudden withdrawal; i.e. for the individual the drug is 'hard'. But there are many people mildly psychologically dependent on it who retain their position in home and society.

Hard-use where the drug is central in the user's life and soft-use where it is merely incidental, are terms of assistance in making this distinction, i.e. what is classified is not the drug but the effect it has on, or the way it is used by, the individual.

Drug dependence (see p. 168).

Addiction. The term 'addict' or 'addiction' has not been completely abandoned in this book because it remains convenient. It refers to the most severe forms of dependence where compulsive craving dominates the subject's daily life. Such cases pose problems as grave as dependence on tea-drinking is trivial. But the use of the term drug dependence is welcome, because it renders irrelevant arguments about whether some drugs are addictive or merely habit-forming. Nonmedical drug use has two principal forms:

- *Continuous use*, when there is a true dependence, e.g. opioids, alcohol, benzodiazepines.
- *Intermittent or occasional use* to obtain a recreational experience, e.g. 'ecstasy' (tenamfetamine), LSD, cocaine, cannabis, solvents, or to relieve stress, e.g. alcohol.

Both uses commonly occur in the same subject, and some drugs, e.g. alcohol, are used in both ways, but others, e.g. 'ecstasy', LSD, cannabis, are virtually confined to the second use.

Drives to nonmedical (or nonprescription) drug use are:

- Relief of anxiety, tension and depression; escape from personal psychological problems; detachment from harsh reality; ease of social intercourse.

- Search for self-knowledge and for meaning in life, including religion. The cult of 'experience' including aestheticism and artistic creation, sex and 'genuine', 'sincere' interpersonal relationships, to obtain a sense of 'belonging'.
- Rebellion against or despair about orthodox social values and the environment. Fear of missing something, and conformity with own social subgroup (the young, especially).
- Fun, amusement, recreation, excitement, curiosity (the young, especially).

Rewards for the individual

It is inherently unlikely that chemicals could be central to a constructive culture and no convincing support for the assertion has yet been produced. (That chemicals might be central to a destructive culture is another matter.) Certainly, like-minded people practising what are often illegal activities will gather into closely knit subgroups for mutual support, and will feel a sense of community, but that is hardly a 'culture'. Even when drug-using subgroups are accepted as representing a subculture, it may be doubted if drugs are sufficiently central to their ideology to justify using 'drug' in the title. But claims for value to the individual and to society of drug experience must surely be tested by the criterion of fruitfulness for both, and the judgement of the individual concerned alone is insufficient; it must be agreed by others. The results of both legal and illegal drug use do not give encouragement to press for a large-scale experiment in this field.

It is claimed that drugs provide *mystical experience* and that this has valid religious content. Mystical experience may be defined as a combination of feelings of unity (oneness with nature and/or God), ineffability (experience beyond the subject's power to express), joy (peace, sacredness), knowledge (insight into truths of life and values, illuminations), and transcendence (of space and time).

When such states do occur there remains the question whether they tell us something about a reality outside the individual or merely something about the mind of the person having the experience. Mystical experience is not a normal dose-related pharmacodynamic effect of any drug, its occurrence depends on many factors such as the subject's personality, mood, environment, conditioning. The drug facilitates rather than induces the experience; and drugs can facilitate unpleasant as well as pleasant experiences. It is not surprising that mystical experience can occur with a wide range of drugs that alter consciousness:

> …I seemed at first in a state of utter blankness … with a keen vision of what was going on in the room around me, but no sensation of touch. I thought that I was near death; when, suddenly, my soul became aware of God, who was manifestly dealing with me, handling me, so to speak, in an intense personal, present reality … I cannot describe the ecstasy I felt.[3]

This experience occurred in the 19th century with chloroform; a general anaesthetic obsolete because of cardiac depression and hepatotoxicity.

There is no good evidence that drugs can produce experience that passes the test of results, i.e. fruitfulness to the individual and to society. Plainly there is a risk of the experience becoming an end in itself rather than a means of development.

CONCLUSIONS

The value of nonmedical use of psychotropic drugs can be summed up thus.

- For relaxation, recreation, protection from and relief of stress and anxiety; relief of depression: moderate use of some 'soft' drugs may be accepted as part of our society.
- For spiritually valuable experience: justification is extremely doubtful.
- As basis for a 'culture' in the sense that drug experience (a) can be, and (b) should be central to an individually or socially constructive way of life: a claim without validity.
- For acute excitement: extremely dangerous.

GENERAL PATTERN OF USE

Divisions are not rigid and they change with fashion.

---

[3] Quoted in James W (1902) Varieties of religious experience. Longmans, Harlow, and many subsequent editions of this classic. See also Leary T (1970). The politics of ecstasy. MacGibbon and Kee, London. Other editions, USA.

- Any age: alcohol; tobacco; mild dependence on hypnotics and tranquillisers; occasional use of LSD and cannabis.
- Aged 16–35 years: hard-use drugs, chiefly heroin, cocaine and amphetamines (including 'ecstasy'). Surviving users tend to reduce or relinquish heavy use as they enter middle age.
- Under 16 years: volatile inhalants, e.g. solvents of glues, aerosol sprays, vaporised (by heat) paints, 'solvent or substance' abuse, 'glue-sniffing'.
- Miscellaneous: any drug or combination of drugs reputed to alter consciousness may have a local vogue, however brief, e.g. drugs used in parkinsonism and metered aerosols for asthma.

Decriminalisation and legalisation

The decision whether any drug is acceptable in medical practice is made after an evaluation of its safety in relation to its efficacy. The same principle should be used for drugs for nonmedical or social use. But the usual scientific criteria for evaluating efficacy are hardly applicable. The reasons why people choose to use drugs for nonmedical purposes are listed above. None of them carries serious weight if the drug is found to have serious risks to the individuals[4] or to society, with either acute or chronic use. Ordinary prudence dictates that any such risks should be carefully defined before a decision on legalisation is made.

There is no doubt that many individuals think, rightly or wrongly, that private use of cannabis, if not of 'harder' drugs, is their own business and that the law should permit this freedom. The likelihood that demand can be extinguished by education or by threats appears to be zero. The autocratic implementation of laws that are not widely accepted in the community leads to violent crime, corruption in the police, and alienation of reasonable people who would otherwise be an important stabilising influence in society.

But though written laws are so often inflexible and combine what would best be separated, informal judicial discretion under present law may be permitting more experimentation than would recurrent legislative debate. It is recognised that this untidy approach, which may be best for the time being, cannot satisfy the extravagant advocates either of licence or of repression.

A suggested intermediate course for cannabis, and perhaps even for heroin, is that penalties for possession of small amounts for personal consumption should be removed (decriminalisation as opposed to legalisation), whilst retaining criminal penalties for suppliers. Such an approach is increasingly and informally being implemented.

Nobody knows what would happen if the production, supply and use of the major drugs, cannabis, heroin and cocaine, were to be legalised, as tobacco and alcohol are legalised (with weak selling restrictions). There are those who, shocked by the evils of illegal trade, consider that legalisation could only make matters better. The debate continues about what kinds of evils affecting the individual and society can be tolerated and how they can be balanced against each other.

Dependence

> **Drug dependence** is a state arising from repeated, periodic or continuous administration of a drug, that results in harm to the individual and sometimes to society. The subject feels a desire, need or compulsion to continue using the drug and feels ill if abruptly deprived of it (abstinence or withdrawal syndrome).

For discussion of abrupt withdrawal of drugs in general see page 119. Drug dependence is characterised by:

- Psychological dependence: the first to appear; there is emotional distress if the drug is withdrawn.
- Physical dependence: accompanies psychological dependence in some cases; there is a physical illness if the drug is withdrawn.
- Tolerance.

---

[4] Hazard to the individual is not a matter for the individual alone if it also has consequences for society.

PSYCHOLOGICAL DEPENDENCE

This may occur with any drug that alters consciousness however bizarre, e.g. muscarine (see p. 436) and to some that, in ordinary doses, do not, e.g. non-narcotic analgesics, purgatives, diuretics; these latter provide problems of psychopathology rather than of psychopharmacology.

Psychological dependence can occur merely on a tablet or injection, regardless of its content, as well as to drug substances. Mild dependence does not require that a drug should have important psychic effects; the subject's beliefs as to what it does are as important, e.g. purgative and diuretic dependence in people obsessed with dread of obesity. We are all physically dependent on food, and some develop a strong emotional dependence and eat too much (or the reverse); sexual activity, with its unique mix of arousal and relaxation, can for some become compulsive or addictive.

PHYSICAL DEPENDENCE AND TOLERANCE

Physical dependence and tolerance imply that adaptive changes have taken place in body tissues so that when the drug is abruptly withdrawn these adaptive changes are left unopposed, resulting generally in a rebound overactivity. The discovery that the CNS employs morphine-like substances (endomorphins, dynorphins) as neurotransmitters offers the explanation that exogenously administered opioid may suppress endogenous production of endorphins by a feedback mechanism. When administration of opioid is suddenly stopped there is an immediate deficiency of endogenous opioid, which thus causes the withdrawal syndrome.

Tolerance may result from a compensatory biochemical cell response to continued exposure to opioid. In short, both physical dependence and tolerance may follow the operation of homeostatic adaptation to continued high occupancy of opioid receptors. Changes of similar type may occur with GABA transmission, involving benzodiazepines.

Tolerance also results from metabolic changes (enzyme induction) and physiological/behavioural adaptation to drug effects, e.g. opioids. Physical dependence develops to a substantial degree with cerebral depressants, but is minor or absent with excitant drugs.

There is commonly cross-tolerance between drugs of similar, and sometimes even of dissimilar, chemical groups, e.g. alcohol and benzodiazepines.

There is danger in personal experimentation; as an American addict has succinctly put it, 'They all think they can take just one joy-pop but it's the first one that hooks you'.[5]

Unfortunately subjects cannot decide for themselves that their dependence will remain mild.

TYPES OF DRUG DEPENDENCE

The World Health Organization recommends that drug dependence be specified by 'type' when under detailed discussion.

Morphine-type:
— psychological dependence severe
— physical dependence severe; develops quickly
— tolerance marked
— cross-tolerance with related drugs
— naloxone induces abstinence syndrome.

Barbiturate-type:
— psychological dependence severe
— physical dependence very severe; develops slowly at high doses
— tolerance less marked than with morphine
— cross-tolerance with alcohol, chloral, meprobamate, glutethimide, chlordiazepoxide, diazepam, etc.

Amfetamine-type:
— psychological dependence severe
— physical dependence slight: psychoses occur during use
— tolerance occurs.

Cannabis-type:
— psychological dependence
— physical dependence dubious (no characteristic abstinence syndrome)
— tolerance occurs.

---

[5] Maurer D W, Vogel V H 1962 Narcotics and narcotic addiction. Thomas, Springfield.

Cocaine-type:
— psychological dependence severe
— physical dependence slight
— tolerance slight (to some actions).

Alcohol-type:
— psychological dependence severe
— physical dependence with prolonged heavy use
— cross-tolerance with other sedatives.

Tobacco-type:
— psychological dependence
— physical dependence.

Drug mixtures: *Barbiturate-amfetamine* mixtures induce a characteristic alteration of mood that does not occur with either drug alone

— psychological dependence strong
— physical dependence occurs
— tolerance occurs.

Heroin-cocaine mixtures: similar characteristics.

ROUTE OF ADMINISTRATION AND EFFECT

With the i.v. route or inhalation much higher peak plasma concentrations can be reached than with oral administration. This accounts for the 'kick' or 'flash' that abusers report and which many seek, likening it to sexual orgasm or better. As an addict said 'The ultimate high is death' and it has been reported that when hearing of someone dying of an overdose, some addicts will seek out the vendor since it is evident he is selling 'really good stuff'.[6] Addicts who rely on illegal sources are inevitably exposed to being supplied diluted or even inert preparations at high prices. North American addicts who have come to the UK believing themselves to be accustomed to high doses of heroin have suffered acute poisoning when given, probably for the first time, pure heroin at an official UK drug dependence clinic.

SUPPLY OF DRUGS TO ADDICTS

In the UK, supply of officially listed drugs (a range of opioids and cocaine) for the purpose of sustaining

---

[6] Bourne P 1976 Acute drug abuse emergencies. Academic Press, New York.

addiction is permitted under strict legal limitations. Addicts must be notified by the physician to the Home Office and in the case of some opioids and cocaine, the physician requires a special licence. By such procedure it is hoped to limit the expansion of the illicit market, and its accompanying crime and dangers to health, e.g. from infected needles and syringes. The object is to sustain young (usually) addicts, who cannot be weaned from drug use, in reasonable health until they relinquish their dependence (often over about 10 years).

When injectable drugs are prescribed there is currently no way of assessing the truth of an addict's statement that he/she needs *x* mg of heroin (or other drug), and the dose has to be assessed intuitively by the doctor. This has resulted in addicts obtaining more than they need and selling it, sometimes to initiate new users. The use of oral methadone or other opioid for maintenance by prescription is devised to mitigate this problem.

TREATMENT OF DEPENDENCE

Withdrawal of the drug. Whilst obviously important, this is only a step on what can be a long and often disappointing journey to psychological and social rehabilitation, e.g. in 'therapeutic communities'. A heroin addict may be given methadone as part of a gradual withdrawal programme (see p. 337) for this drug has a long duration of action and blocks access of injected opioid to the opioid receptor so that if, in a moment of weakness, the subject takes heroin, the 'kick' is blocked. More acutely, the physical features associated with discontinuing high alcohol use may be alleviated by chlordiazepoxide given in decreasing doses for 4–6 days. Sympathetic autonomic overactivity can be treated with a β-adrenoceptor blocker (or clonidine) (see Abrupt withdrawal of drugs).

Maintenance and relapse. Relapsed addicts who live a fairly normal life are sometimes best treated by supplying drugs under supervision. There is no legal objection to doing this in the UK (see above) but naturally this course, which abandons hope of cure, should not be adopted until it is certain that cure is virtually impossible. A less harmful drug by a less harmful route may be substituted, e.g. oral methadone for i.v. heroin. Addicts are often particularly reluctant to abandon the i.v. route, which provides the 'immediate high' that they find, or originally found, so desirable.

Severe pain in an opioid addict presents a special problem. High-efficacy opioid may be ineffective (tolerance) or overdose may result; low-efficacy opioids will not only be ineffective but may induce withdrawal symptoms, especially if they have some antagonist effect, e.g. pentazocine. This leaves as drugs of choice nonsteroidal anti-inflammatory drugs (NSAIDs), e.g. indometacin, and nefopam (which is neither opioid nor NSAID).

Mortality

Young illicit users by i.v. injection (heroin, benzodiazepines, amphetamine) have a high mortality. Either death follows overdose, or septicaemia, endocarditis, hepatitis, AIDS, gas gangrene, tetanus and pulmonary embolism ensue from the contaminated materials used without aseptic precautions (schemes to provide clean equipment mitigate this). Smugglers of illicit cocaine or heroin sometimes carry the drug in plastic bags concealed by swallowing or in the rectum ('body packing'). Leakage of the packages, not surprisingly, may have a fatal result.[7]

Escalation

A variable proportion of subjects who start with cannabis eventually take heroin. This disposition to progress from occasional to frequent soft use of drugs through to hard drug use, when it occurs, is less likely to be due to pharmacological actions, than to psychosocial factors, although increased suggestibility induced by cannabis may contribute.

De-escalation also occurs as users become disillusioned with drugs over about 10 years.

'Designer drugs'

This unhappily chosen term means molecular modifications produced in secret for profit by skilled and criminally minded chemists. Manipulation of fentanyl has resulted in compounds of extraordinary potency.

In 1976 a too-clever 23-year-old addict seeking to manufacture his own pethidine 'took a synthetic shortcut and injected himself with what was later with his help proved to be two closely related byproducts; one was MPTP (methylphenyltetrahydropyridine).[8, 9] Three days later he developed a severe parkinsonian syndrome that responded to levodopa. MPTP selectively destroys melanin-containing cells in the substantia nigra. Further such cases have occurred from use of supposed synthetic heroin. MPTP has since been used in experimental research on parkinsonism. What the future holds for individuals and for society in this area can only be imagined.

Volatile substance abuse

Seekers of the 'self-gratifying high' also inhale any volatile substance that may affect the central nervous system. These include: adhesives ('glue-sniffing'), lacquer-paint solvents, petrol, nail varnish, any pressurised aerosol and butane liquid gas (which latter especially may 'freeze' the larynx, allowing fatal inhalation of food, drink, gastric contents, or even the liquid itself to flood the lungs). Even solids, e.g. paint scrapings, solid shoe polish, may be volatilised over a fire. These substances are particularly abused by the very young (schoolchildren), no doubt largely because they are accessible at home and in ordinary shops and they cannot easily buy alcohol or 'street' drugs (although this latter may be changing as dealers target the youngest). CNS effects include confusion and

---

[7] A 49-year-old man became ill after an international flight. An abdominal radiograph showed a large number of spherical packages in his gastrointestinal tract, and body-packing was suspected. As he had not defaecated, he was given liquid paraffin. He developed ventricular fibrillation and died. Post mortem examination showed that he had ingested more than 150 latex packets, each containing 5 g of cocaine, making a total of almost 1 kg (lethal oral dose 1–3 g). The liquid paraffin may have contributed to his death as the mineral oil dissolves latex. Sorbitol or lactulose with activated charcoal should be used to remove ingested packages, or surgery if there are signs of intoxication. (Visser L et al 1998 Do not give liquid paraffin to packers. Lancet 352: 1352)

[8] Williams A 1984 British Medical Journal 289: 1401–1402.
[9] Davis G C et al 1979 Psychiatry Research 1: 249.

hallucinations, ataxia, dysarthria, coma, convulsions, respiratory failure. Liver, kidney, lung and heart damage occur. Sudden cardiac death may be due to sensitisation of the heart to endogenous catecholamines. If the substance is put in a plastic bag from which the user takes deep inhalations, or is sprayed in a confined space, e.g. cupboard, there is particularly high risk.

> A 17-year-old boy was offered the use of a plastic bag and a can of hair spray at a beach party. The hair spray was released into the plastic bag and the teenager put his mouth to the open end of the bag and inhaled ... he exclaimed, 'God, this stuff hits ya fast!' He got up, ran 100 yards; and died.[10]

Signs of frequent volatile substance abuse include perioral eczema and inflammation of the upper respiratory tract.

Drugs and sport

The rewards of competitive sport, both financial and in personal and national prestige, are the cause of determination to win at (almost) any cost. Drugs are used to enhance performance though efficacy is largely undocumented. Detection can be difficult when the drugs or metabolites are closely related to or identical with endogenous substances, and when the drug can be stopped well before the event without apparent loss of efficacy, e.g. anabolic steroids (but suppression of endogenous trophic hormones can be measured, and can assist).

PERFORMANCE ENHANCEMENT

There follow illustrations of the mechanisms by which drugs can enhance performance in various sports; naturally, these are proscribed by the authorities (International Olympic Committee (IOC) Medical Commission, and the governing bodies of individual sports).

---

[10] Bass M 1970 Sudden sniffing death. Journal of the American Medical Association 212: 2075.

For 'strength sports' in which body weight and brute strength are the principal determinants (weight lifting, rowing, wrestling): anabolic agents, e.g. clenbuterol (β-adrenoceptor agonist), androstenedione, methandienone, nandrolone, stanozolol, testosterone. Taken together with a high-protein diet and exercise, these increase lean body weight (muscle) but not necessarily strength. It is claimed they allow more intensive training regimens (limiting cell injury in muscles). Rarely, there may be episodes of violent behaviour, known amongst athletes as 'roid [steroid] rage'.

High doses are used, with risk of liver damage (cholestatic, tumours) especially if the drug is taken long-term, which is certainly insufficient to deter 'sportsmen'. They may be more inclined to take more seriously the fact that anabolic steroids suppress pituitary gonadotrophin, and so testosterone production.

Growth hormone (somatrem, somatropin) and corticotrophin use may be combined with that of anabolic steroids. *Chorionic gonadotrophin* may be taken to stimulate testosterone production (and prevent testicular atrophy). Similarly, tamoxifen (antioestrogen) may be used to attenuate some of the effects of anabolic steroids.

For events in which **output of energy** is explosive (100 m sprint): stimulants, e.g. amphetamine, bromantan, carphendon, cocaine, ephedrine and caffeine (> 12 mg/1 in urine). Death has probably occured in bicycle racing (continuous hard exercise with short periods of sprint) due to hyperthermia and cardiac arrhythmia in metabolically stimulated and vasoconstricted subjects exercising maximally under a hot sun.

For **endurance sports** to enhance the oxygen carrying capacity of the blood (bicycling, marathon running): *erythropoietin, 'blood doping'* (the athlete has blood withdrawn and stored, then transfused once the deficit had been made up naturally, so raising the plasma haemoglobin above normal).

For events in which **steadiness of hand** is essential (pistol, rifle shooting): *β-adrenoceptor* blockers. Tremor is reduced by the $β_2$-adrenoceptor blocking effect, as are somatic symptoms of anxiety.

For events in which **body pliancy** is a major factor (gymnastics): delaying puberty in child gymnasts by endocrine techniques.

For **weight reduction,** e.g. boxers, jockeys: diuretics. These are also used to flush out other drugs in the hope of escaping detection; severe volume depletion can cause venous thrombosis and pulmonary embolism.

Generally, owing to recognition of natural biological differences most competitive events are sex segregated. In many events men have a natural physical **biological advantage** and the (inevitable) consequence has been that women have been deliberately virilised (by administration of androgens) so that they may outperform their sisters.

It seems safe to assume that anything that can be thought up to gain advantage will be tried by competitors eager for immediate fame. Reliable data are difficult to obtain in these areas. No doubt placebo effects are important, i.e. beliefs as to what has been taken and what effects ought to follow.

The dividing line between what is and what is not acceptable practice is hard to draw. Caffeine can improve physical performance and illustrates the difficulty of deciding what is 'permissible' or 'impermissible'. A cup of coffee is part of a normal diet, but some consider taking the same amount of caffeine in a tablet, injection or suppository to be 'doping'.

For any minor injuries sustained during athletic training NSAIDs and corticosteroids (topical, intra-articular) suppress symptoms and allow the training to proceed maximally. Their use is allowed subject to restrictions about route of administration, but strong opioids are disallowed. Similarly, the IOC Medical Code defines acceptable and unacceptable treatments for relief of cough, hay fever, diarrhoea, vomiting, pain and asthma. Doctors should remember that they may get their athlete patients into trouble with sports authorities by inadvertent prescribing of banned substances.[11]

Some of the isssues seem to be ethical rather than medical as witness the reported competition success of a swimmer who, it is alleged, had been persuaded under hypnosis into the belief that he was being pursued by a shark.

Tobacco

Tobacco was introduced to Europe from South America in the 16th century. Although its potential for harm was early recognised its use was taken up avidly in every society that met it. Current estimates are that there are 1.1 billion smokers worldwide. In 1990 there were 3 million smoking-related deaths per year, projected to rise to 8 million by 2020 (representing 12% of all deaths).[12]

COMPOSITION

The principal components are tar and nicotine, the amounts of which can vary greatly depending on the country in which cigarettes are sold. Regulation and voluntary agreement by manufacturers aspires to achieve a 'global cigarette' containing at most 12 mg of tar and 1 mg of nicotine.

The composition of tobacco smoke is complex (about 500 compounds have been identified) and varies with the type of tobacco and the way it is smoked. The chief pharmacologically active ingredients are nicotine (acute effects) and tars (chronic effects).

Smoke of cigars and pipes is *alkaline* (pH 8.5) and nicotine is relatively un-ionised and lipid-soluble so that it is readily absorbed in the mouth. Cigar and pipe smokers thus obtain nicotine without inhaling (they also have a lower death rate from lung cancer; which is caused by non-nicotine constituents).

Smoke of cigarettes is *acidic* (pH 5.3) and nicotine is relatively ionised and insoluble in lipids. Desired amounts are absorbed only if nicotine is taken into the lungs, where the enormous surface area for absorption compensates for the lower lipid solubility. Cigarette smokers therefore inhale (and have a high rate of death from tar-induced lung cancer). The amount of nicotine absorbed from tobacco smoke varies from 90% in those who inhale to 10% in those who do not.

Tobacco smoke contains 1–5% carbon monoxide and habitual smokers have 3–7% (heavy smokers as much as 15%) of their haemoglobin as carboxy-

---

[11] UK prescribers can find general advice in the British National Formulary.

[12] Editorial 1999 Tobacco money and medical research. Nature Medicine 5: 125

haemoglobin, which cannot carry oxygen. This is sufficient to reduce exercise capacity in patients with angina pectoris. Chronic carboxyhaemoglobinaemia causes polycythaemia (which increases the viscosity of the blood).

Substances *carcinogenic* to animals (polycyclic hydrocarbons and nicotine-derived N-nitrosamines) have been identified in tobacco smoke condensates from cigarettes, cigars and pipes. Polycyclic hydrocarbons are responsible for the hepatic enzyme induction that occurs in smokers.

Tobacco dependence

Psychoanalysts have made a characteristic contribution to the problem. 'Getting something orally', one asserted…, 'is the first great libidinous experience in life'; first the breast, then the bottle, then the comforter, then food and finally the cigarette.[13]

Sigmund Freud, inventor of psychoanalysis, was a lifelong tobacco addict. He suggested that some children may be victims of a 'constitutional intensification of the erotogenic significance of the labial region', which, if it persists, will provide a powerful motive for smoking.[14]

While psychological dependence is strong and accounts for part of the difficulty of stopping smoking, *nicotine* possesses all the characteristics of a drug of dependence and there is powerful reason to regard nicotine addiction as a disease. A report on the subject concludes that most smokers do not do so from choice but because they are addicted to nicotine.[15] The immediate satisfaction of smoking is due to nicotine and also to tars, which provide flavour. Initially the factors are psychosocial; pharmacodynamic effects are unpleasant. But under the psychosocial pressures the subject continues, learns to limit and adjust nicotine intake, so that the pleasant pharmacological effects of nicotine develop

and tolerance to the adverse effects occurs. Thus to the psychosocial pressure is now added pharmacological pleasure.

Tolerance and some physical dependence occur. Transient withdrawal effects include EEG and sleep changes, impaired performance in some psychomotor tests, disturbance of mood, and increased appetite (with weight gain), though it is difficult to disentangle psychological from physical effects in these last.

ACUTE EFFECTS OF SMOKING TOBACCO

- *Increased airways resistance* occurs due to the nonspecific effects of submicronic particles, e.g. carbon particles less than 1 μm across. The effect is reflex; even inert particles of this size cause bronchial narrowing sufficient to double airways resistance; this is insufficient to cause dyspnoea, though it might affect athletic performance. Pure nicotine inhalations of concentration comparable to that reached in smoking do not increase airways resistance.
- *Ciliary activity*, after transient stimulation, is depressed, and particles are removed from the lungs more slowly.
- *Carbon monoxide absorption* may be clinically important in the presence of coronary heart disease (see above) although it is physiologically insignificant in healthy young adults.

Nicotine pharmacology

Pharmacokinetics

Nicotine is absorbed through mucous membranes in a highly pH-dependent fashion. The $t\frac{1}{2}$ is 2 h. It is largely metabolised to inert substances, e.g. cotinine, though some is excreted unchanged in the urine (pH dependent, it is un-ionised at acid pH). Cotinine is used as a marker for nicotine intake in smoking surveys because of its convenient $t\frac{1}{2}$ (20 h).

---

[13] Scott R B 1957 British Medical Journal 1: 67 1.
[14] Quoted in Royal Collage of Physicians 1977 Smoking or health. Pitman, London. In 1929 Freud posed for a photograph holding a large cigar prominently. 'He was always a heavy smoker—twenty cigars a day were his usual allowance and he tolerated abstinence from it with the greatest difficulty'. Jones E 1953 Sigmund Freud: life and work. Hogarth Press, London.

[15] Tobacco Advisory Group, Royal College of Physicians 2000 Nicotine addiction in Britain. London RCP.

Pharmacodynamics

Large doses.[16] Nicotine is an agonist to receptors at the ends of peripheral cholinergic nerves whose cell bodies lie in the central nervous system, i.e. it acts at autonomic ganglia and at the voluntary neuro-muscular junction (see Fig. 21.1). This is what is meant by the term 'nicotine-like' or 'nicotinic' effect. Higher doses paralyse at the same points. The central nervous system is stimulated, including the vomiting centre, both directly and via chemore-ceptors in the carotid body; tremors and convulsions may occur. As with the peripheral actions, depression follows stimulation.

Doses from/with smoking. Nicotine causes release of catecholamines in the CNS, also serotonin, and antidiuretic hormone, corticotrophin and growth hormone. The effects of nicotine on viscera are probably largely reflex, from stimulation of sensory receptors (chemoreceptors) in the carotid and aortic bodies, pulmonary circulation and left ventricle. Some of the results are mutually antagonistic.

The following account tells what generally happens after one cigarette, from which about 1 mg nicotine is absorbed, although much depends on the amount and depth of inhalation and on the duration of end-inspiratory breath-holding.

On the cardiovascular system the effects are those of sympathetic autonomic stimulation. There is vasoconstriction in the skin and vasodilatation in the muscles, tachycardia and a rise in blood pressure of about 15 mmHg systolic and 10 mmHg diastolic, and increased plasma noradrenaline (norepinephrine). Ventricular extrasystoles may occur. Cardiac output, work and oxygen consumption rise. Increased demand for blood flow that is not met because coronary vessels are narrowed by atherosclerosis may be a mechanism of tobacco-induced angina pectoris. Nicotine increases platelet adhesiveness, an effect that may be clinically significant in atheroma and thrombosis.

Metabolic rate. Nicotine increases the metabolic rate, only slightly at rest,[17] but approximately doubles it during light exercise (occupational tasks, house-work). This may be due to increase in autonomic sympathetic activity. The effect declines over 24 h on stopping smoking and accounts for the characteristic weight gain that is so disliked and which is sometimes given as a reason for continuing or resuming smoking. Smokers weigh 2–4 kg less than nonsmokers (not enough to be a health issue).

Tolerance develops to some of the effects of nicotine, taken repeatedly over a few hours; a first experience commonly causes nausea and vomiting, which quickly ceases with repetition of smoking. Tolerance is usually rapidly lost; the first cigarette of the day has a greater effect on the cardiovascular system than do subsequent cigarettes.

Conclusion: the pleasurable effects of smoking are derived from a complex mixture of multiple pharmacological and nonpharmacological factors.

In this account nicotine is represented as being the major (but not the sole) determinant of tobacco dependence after the smoker has adapted to the usual initial unpleasant effects. But there remains some uncertainty as to its role, e.g. nicotine i.v. fails adequately to substitute the effects of smoking. An understanding of the full function of nicotine is important if less harmful alternatives to smoking, such as nicotine chewing gum, are to be exploited.

---

[16] Fatal nicotine poisoning has been reported from smoking, from swallowing tobacco, from tobacco enemas, from topical application to the skin and from accidental drinking of nicotine insecticide preparations. In 1932 a florist sat down on a chair, on the seat of which a 40% free nicotine insecticide solution had been spilled. Fifteen minutes later he felt ill (vomiting, sweating, faintness, and respiratory difficulty, followed by loss of consciousness and cardiac irregularity). He recovered in hospital over about 24 h. On the fourth day he was deemed well enough to leave hospital and was given his clothes which had been kept in a paper bag. He noticed the trousers were still damp. Within one hour of leaving hospital he had to be readmitted suffering again from poisoning due to nicotine absorbed transdermally from his still contaminated trousers. He recovered over three weeks, apart from persistent ventricular extrasystoles [Faulkner J M 1933 JAMA 100: 1663].

---

[17] The metabolic rate at rest accounts for about 70% of daily energy expenditure.

Effects of chronic smoking

SMOKING AND CANCER

Bronchogenic carcinoma

Between 1920 and 1950 an epidemic of bronchogenic carcinoma occurred (rate in men increased 20-fold) which can be attributed to cigarette smoking; lesser causes include exposure to a variety of industrial chemicals and atmospheric pollution. The risk of death from lung cancer is related to the number of cigarettes smoked and the age of starting. Giving up smoking reduces the risk of death progressively from the time of cessation.[18]

Other cancers

The risk of smokers developing cancer of the mouth, throat and oesophagus is 5–10 times greater than that of nonsmokers. It is as great for pipe and cigar smokers as it is for cigarette smokers. Cancer of the pancreas, kidney and urinary tract is also commoner in smokers.

DISEASES OF THE HEART AND BLOOD VESSELS

Coronary heart disease (CHD) is now the leading cause of death in many developed countries. In the UK about 30% of these deaths can be attributed to smoking.

Under the age of 65 years smokers are about twice as likely to die of ischaemic heart disease as are nonsmokers, and heavy smokers about 3.5 times as likely.

Sudden death may be the first manifestation of CHD and, especially in young men, is related to cigarette smoking. Smoking is especially dangerous for people in whom other risk factors (increased blood cholesterol, high blood pressure) are present.

---

[18] Peto R et al 2000 Smoking, smoking cessation, and lung cancer in the UK since 1950: combination of national statistics with two case-control studies. British Medical Journal 321: 323–329.

Atherosclerotic narrowing of the smallest coronary arteries is enormously increased in heavy and even in moderate smokers; the increased platelet adhesiveness caused by smoking increases the readiness with which thrombi form.

Stopping smoking reduces the excess risk of CHD in people under the age of 65, and after about 4 years of abstinence the risk approximates to that of nonsmokers.

Pipe and cigar smokers run little or no excess risk of CHD provided they are not heavy smokers and do not inhale. Heavy cigarette smokers who change over to pipe or cigar smoking often continue to inhale and thereby fail to reduce their risk.

SMOKING AND CHRONIC LUNG DISEASE

The adverse effects of cigarette smoke on the lungs may be separated into two distinct conditions.

- *Chronic mucus hypersecretion,* which causes persistent cough with sputum and fits with the original definition of simple chronic bronchitis. This condition arises chiefly in the large airways, usually clears up when the subject stops smoking and does not on its own carry any substantial risk of death.
- *Chronic obstructive lung disease,* which causes difficulty in breathing due to narrowing of the air passages in the lungs. This condition originates chiefly in the small airways, includes a variable element of destruction of peripheral lung units (emphysema), is progressive and largely irreversible and may ultimately lead to disability and death.

Both conditions can coexist in one person and they predispose to recurrent acute infective illnesses.

The *obstructive syndrome* is as specifically related to smoking as is lung cancer. Despite this, in discussing the health effects of tobacco, there has generally been far more emphasis on lung cancer than on this more disabling, but equally fatal disorder.

INTERACTIONS WITH DRUG THERAPY

Induction of hepatic drug metabolising enzymes by non-nicotine constituents of smoke causes increased metabolism of a range of drugs, including oestrogens, theophylline, warfarin.

WOMEN AND SMOKING

Fertility. Women who smoke are more likely to be infertile or take longer to conceive than women who do not smoke. In addition, smokers are more liable to have an earlier menopause than are nonsmokers. Increased metabolism of oestrogens may not be the whole explanation.

Complications of pregnancy. The risks of spontaneous abortion, stillbirth, and neonatal death are approximately doubled. There are various placental abnormalities. The placenta is heavier in smoking than nonsmoking women and its diameter larger. The enlarged placenta and placental abnormalities may represent adaptations to lack of oxygen due to smoking, secondary to raised concentrations of circulating carboxyhaemoglobin.

The child. The babies of women who smoke are approximately 200 g lighter than those of women who do not smoke. They have an increased risk of death in the perinatal period which is independent of other variables such as social class, level of education, age of mother, race or extent of antenatal care. The increased risk rises two-fold or more in heavy smokers and appears to be entirely accounted for by the placental abnormalities and the consequences of low birthweight. Ex-smokers and women who give up smoking in the first 20 weeks of pregnancy have offspring whose birthweight is similar to that of the children of women who have never smoked.

Starting and stopping use

Contrary to popular belief it is not generally difficult to stop, only 14% finding it 'very difficult'. But ex-smoker status is unstable and the long-term success rate of a smoking withdrawal clinic is rarely above 30%. The situation is summed up by the witticism, 'Giving up smoking is easy, I've done it many times'.

Though they are as aware of the risks of smoking as men, women find it harder to stop; they consistently have lower success rates. This trend crosses every age group and occupation. Women particularly dislike the weight gain.

Aids to giving up. The addictive effects of tobacco smoking are substantially due to *nicotine*, and it is logical to substitute nicotine for tobacco smoke as a pharmacological aid to quitting. Nicotine is available in a number of formulations, including chewing gum, transdermal patch, oral and nasal spray. When used casually without special attention to technique, nicotine formulations have proved no better than other aids but, if used carefully and withdrawn as recommended, the accumulated results are almost two times better than in smokers who try to stop without this assistance.[19] Restlessness during terminal illness may be due to nicotine withdrawal and go unrecognised; a nicotine patch may benefit a (deprived) heavy smoker. Nicotine transdermal patches may cause nightmares and abnormal dreaming, and skin reactions (rash, pruritus and 'burning' at the application site).

Amfebutamone/bupropion may provide an alternative, or addition, to nicotine. When the drug was being investigated as an antidepressant, researchers noticed that patients gave up smoking, and it was developed as an aid to smoking cesation. Amfebutamone selectively inhibits neuronal uptake of noradrenaline (norepinephrine) and dopamine and may reduce nicotine craving by an action on the mesolimbic system. Evidence from a small number of clinical trials suggests that amfebutamone may be at least as effective as the nicotine patch with which it may usefully be combined. It may cause dry mouth and insomnia, and is contraindicated in those with a history of epilepsy.

If the patient is heavily tobacco-dependent and severe anxiety, irritability, headache, insomnia and weight gain (about 3 kg) and tension are concomitants of attempts to stop smoking, an anxiolytic sedative (or β-adrenoceptor blocker) may be useful for a short time, but it is important to avoid substituting one drug-dependence for another.

---

[19] Lancaster T et al 2000 Effectiveness of interventions to help people to stop smoking: findings from the Cochrane Library. British Medical Journal 321: 355–358.

There is ample evidence to warrant strong advice against starting to smoke but over-hasty and unreasonable prohibitions on patients' longstanding pleasures (or vices) do no good. The pliable patient is made wretched, but most are merely alienated.

> My doctor's issued his decree
> That too much wine is killing me,
> And furthermore his ban he hurls
> Against my touching naked girls.
> How then? Must I no longer share
> Good wine or beauties, dark and fair?
> Doctor, goodbye, my sail's unfurled,
> I'm off to try the other world.
> D G Rossetti, poet (1828–82)

Passive (involuntary) smoking

Many nonsmokers are exposed to tobacco smoke, and environmental tobacco smoke has been classified as a known human carcinogen in the USA since 1992.[20] Although the risks are, naturally, smaller, the number of people affected is large. One study estimated that breathing other people's smoke increases a person's risk of ischaemic heart disease by a quarter.[21]

Smoke drawn through the tobacco and taken in by the smoker is known as *mainstream* smoke. Smoke which arises from smouldering tobacco and passes directly into the surrounding air, whence it may be inhaled by smokers and nonsmokers alike, is known as *sidestream* smoke. Mainstream and sidestream smoke differ in composition, partly because of the different temperatures at which they are produced. Substances found in greater concentrations in undiluted sidestream smoke than in undiluted mainstream smoke include: nicotine (× 2.7), carbon monoxide (× 2.5), ammonia (× 73),

and some carcinogens (e.g. benzo-a-pyrene × 3.4). Sidestream smoke constitutes about 85% of smoke generated in an average room during cigarette smoking.

Ethyl alcohol (Ethanol)

> The services rendered by intoxicating substances in the struggle for happiness and in warding off misery rank so highly as a benefit that both individuals and races have given them an established position within their libido-economy. It is not merely the immediate gain in pleasure which one owes to them, but also a measure of that independence of the outer world which is so sorely craved … We are aware that it is just this property which constitutes the danger and injuriousness of intoxicating substances…[22]

Alcohol is chiefly important in medicine because of the consequences of its misuse/abuse. Alcohol misuse is a social problem with pharmacological aspects, which latter are discussed here. The history of alcohol is part of the history of civilisation 'ever since Noah made his epoch-making discovery'.[23]

Pharmacokinetics

Absorption of alcohol taken orally is rapid, for it is highly lipid-soluble and diffusible from the stomach and the small intestine. Solutions above 20% are absorbed more slowly because high concentrations of alcohol inhibit gastric peristalsis, thus delaying the arrival of the alcohol in the small intestine which is the major site of absorption.

Absorption is delayed by food, especially milk, the effect of which is probably due to the fat it contains. Carbohydrate also delays absorption of alcohol.

Distribution of alcohol is rapid and throughout the body water (dist. vol. 0.7 1/kg men: 0.6 1/kg women); it is not selectively stored in any tissue.

---

[20] Environmental Protection Agency (EPA 1992 A/600/6-90/006F).
[21] Law M R, Morris J K, Wald N J 1997 Environmental tobacco smoke exposure and ischaemic heart disease: an evaluation of the evidence. British Medical Journal 315: 973–988.

[22] Freud S 1939 Civilisation, war and death, Psycho-analytic epitomes, No. 4. Hogarth Press, London.
[23] Genesis; 9: 21; Huxley A 1957 Annals of the New York Academy of Sciences 67: 675.

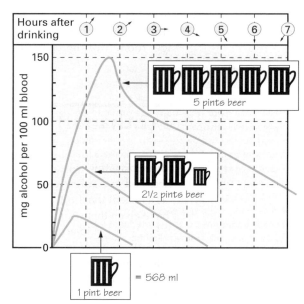

Fig. 10.1 Approximate blood concentrations after three doses of alcohol.

Maximum blood concentrations after oral alcohol therefore depend on numerous factors including the total dose, sex, the strength of the solution, the time over which it is taken, the presence or absence of food, the time relations of taking food and alcohol and the kind of food eaten, as well as on the speed of metabolism and excretion. A single dose of alcohol, say 60 ml (48 g) (equivalent to 145 ml of whisky, 5–6 measures, or units; see Fig. 10.1), taken over a few minutes on an empty stomach will probably produce maximal blood concentration at 30–90 min and will not all be disposed of for 6–8 h or even more. There are very great individual variations.

Metabolism. About 95% of absorbed alcohol is metabolised, the remainder being excreted in the breath, urine and sweat; convenient methods of estimation of alcohol in all these are available.

Alcohol in the systemic circulation is oxidised in the liver; principally (90%) by alcohol dehydrogenase to acetaldehyde and then by aldehyde dehydrogenase to products that enter the citric acid cycle or are utilised in various anabolic reactions. Other alcohol-metabolising enzymes are microsomal cytochrome P450 2E1 (which is also induced by alcohol) and catalase.

Alcohol metabolism by alcohol dehydrogenase follows first-order kinetics after the smallest

doses. Once the blood concentration exceeds about 10 mg/100 ml the enzymatic processes are saturated and elimination rate no longer increases with increasing concentration but becomes steady at 10–15 ml per hour in occasional drinkers. Thus alcohol is subject to dose-dependent kinetics, i.e. saturation or zero-order kinetics, with potentially major consequences for the individual.

Induction of hepatic drug metabolising enzymes occurs with repeated exposure to alcohol and this contributes to tolerance in habitual users, and to toxicity. Increased formation of metabolites causes organ damage in chronic over-consumption (acetaldehyde in the liver and probably fatty ethyl esters in other organs) and increases susceptibility to liver injury when heavy drinkers are exposed to anaesthetics, industrial solvents and to drugs. But chronic use of large amounts reduces hepatic metabolic capacity by causing cellular damage. An acute substantial dose of alcohol (binge drinking) inhibits hepatic drug metabolism.

Inter-ethnic variation is recognised in the ability to metabolise alcohol (see p. 184).

Blood concentration of alcohol (Fig. 10.1) has great medicolegal importance. Alcohol in alveolar air is in equilibrium with that in pulmonary capillary blood and reliable, easily handled measurement devices (breathalyser) are used by police at the roadside on both drivers and pedestrians.[24]

Pharmacodynamics

Alcohol acts on the central nervous system in a manner broadly similar to volatile anaesthetics, exerting on cells a generally depressant effect that is probably mediated through particular membrane ion channels and receptors. Alcohol enhances (inhibitory) GABA-stimulated flux of chloride through receptor-gated membrane ion channels, a receptor subtype

---

[24] An arrested man was told, in a police station, by a doctor, that he was drunk. The man asked, 'Doctor, could a drunk man stand up in the middle of this room, jump into the air, turn a complete somersault, and land down on his feet?' The doctor was injudicious enough to say, "Certainly not"—and was then and there proved wrong. (Worthing C L 1957 British Medical Journal 1: 643.) The introduction of the breathalyser, which has a statutory role only in road traffic situations, has largely eliminated such professional humiliations.

effect that may be involved in the motor impairment caused by alcohol. Other possible modes of action include inhibition of calcium entry via voltage-gated (L type) calcium channels, and inhibition of the (excitatory) NMDA (N-methyl-D-aspartate) receptor. (See page 184 for chronic effects of alcohol on the brain.)

It is not a stimulant; hyperactivity, when it occurs, is due to removal of inhibitory effects. Alcohol in ordinary doses may act chiefly on the arousal mechanisms of the brainstem reticular formation, inhibiting polysynaptic function and enhancing presynaptic inhibition. Direct cortical depression probably only occurs with high doses. With increasing doses the subject passes through all the stages of general anaesthesia and may die of respiratory depression.[25]

Psychic effects are the most important socially (Fig. 10.2), and it is to obtain these that the drug is habitually used in so many societies, to make social intercourse not merely easy but even pleasant. They have been admirably described by Sollmann:

> The first functions to be lost are the finer grades of judgement, reflection, observation and attention— the faculties largely acquired through education, which constitute the elements of the restraint and prudence that man usually imposes on his actions. The orator allows himself to be carried by the impulse of the moment, without reflecting on ultimate consequences, and as his expressions become freer, they acquire an appearance of warmth, of feeling, of inspiration. Not a little of this inspiration is contributed by the audience if they are in a similar condition of increased appreciation ... Another characteristic feature, evidently resulting from paralysis of the higher functions, is the loss of power to control moods.[26]

Environment, personality, mood and dose of alcohol are all relevant to the final effect on the individual. These and other effects that are characteristic of alcohol, have been celebrated in the following couplets:[27]

---

[25] Loss of consciousness occurs at blood concentrations around 300 mg/100 ml; death at about 400 mg/100 ml. But the usual cause of death in acute alcohol poisoning is inhalation of vomit.
[26] Sollmann T 1957 Manual of pharmacology, 8th edn. Saunders, Philadelphia.

> Ho! Ho! Yes! Yes! It's very all well,
> You may drunk I am think, but I tell you I'm not,
> I'm as sound as a fiddle and fit as a bell,
> And stable quite ill to see what's what...
> And I've swallowed, I grant, a beer of lot —
> But I'm not so think as you drunk I am...
> I shall stralk quite weight and not yutter an ell,
> My feech will not spalter the least little jot:
> If you knownly had own!—well, I gave him a dot,
> And I said to him, 'Sergeant, I'll come like a lamb —
> The floor it seems like a storm in a yacht,
> But I'm not so think as you drunk I am.
> I'm sorry, I just chair over a fell —
> A trifle—this chap, on a very day hot —
> If I hadn't consumed that last whisky of tot!
> As I said now, this fellow, called Abraham —
> Ah? One more? Since it's you! just a do me will spot —
> But I'm not so think as you drunk I am.

Innumerable tests of physical and mental performance have been used to demonstrate the effects of alcohol. Results show that alcohol reduces visual acuity and delays recovery from visual dazzle; it impairs taste, smell and hearing, muscular co-ordination and steadiness and prolongs reaction time. It also causes nystagmus and vertigo. At the same time the subjects commonly have an increased confidence in their ability to perform well when tested and underestimate their errors, even after quite low doses. Attentiveness and ability to assimilate, sort and quickly take decisions on con-

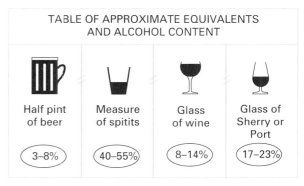

TABLE OF APPROXIMATE EQUIVALENTS AND ALCOHOL CONTENT

Half pint of beer	Measure of spitits	Glass of wine	Glass of Sherry or Port
3–8%	40–55%	8–14%	17–23%

Fig. 10.2 Four standard units of drink (in which social consumption is measured). A unit contains approx. 10 ml (8 g) of alcohol. Knowledge of blood alcohol concentration does not allow a reliable estimate of how much has been consumed.

---

[27] By Sir J C Squire (1884–1958). Quoted, by permission, R H A Squire.

tinuously changing information input, decline. This results particularly in inattentiveness to the periphery of the visual field, which is important in motoring. All these are evidently highly undesirable effects when a person is in a position where failure to perform well may be dangerous.

Car driving and alcohol

The effects of alcohol and psychotropic drugs on motor driving (Fig. 10.3) have been the subject of well-deserved attention, and many countries have made laws designed to prevent motor accidents caused by alcohol. The problem has nowhere been solved. In general it can be said that the weight of evidence points to a steady deterioration of driving skill and an increased liability to accidents beginning with the entry of alcohol into the blood and steadily increasing with blood concentration.

Alcohol plays a huge part in causing motor accidents, being a factor in as many as 50%. For this reason, the compulsory use of a roadside breath test is acknowledged to be in the public interest. In the UK a blood concentration exceeding 80 mg alcohol/ 100 ml blood (17.4 mmol/l)[28] whilst in charge of a car is a statutory offence. At this concentration, the liability to accident is about twice normal. Other countries set lower limits, e.g. Nordic countries,[29] some states of USA, Australia, Greece.

So clearly is it in the public interest that drunken driving be reduced that the privileges normally attaching to freedom of conscience as well as to personal eccentricity must take second place. In one instance, an ingenious driver, having provided a positive breath test, offered a blood sample on the condition it should be taken from his penis; the physician refused to take it; the police demanded a urine sample; the subject refused on the ground that he had offered blood and that his offer had been refused. He was acquitted, but a Court has since decided that the choice of site for blood-taking is for the physician, not for the subject, and that such transparent attempts to evade justice should be treated as unreasonable refusal to supply a specimen under the law. The subject is then treated as though he had provided a specimen that was above the statutory limit. Yet another trick is to take a dose of spirits after the accident and before the police arrive. The police are told it was taken as a remedy for nervous shock. This is known is the 'hip-flask' defence.

Where blood or breath analysis is not immediately available after an accident it may be measured hours later and 'back calculated' to what it would have been at the time of the accident. It is usual to assume that the blood concentration falls at about 15 mg/100 ml/h. Naturally, the validity of such calculations leads to acrimonious disputes in the courts of law.

Prescribed medicines and driving

Ability to drive can be impaired by many prescribed drugs. In road traffic accident fatalities 7.4% of persons had taken a drug 'likely' to affect the CNS (chiefly older subjects). In addition, cannabis was found in 2.6%. Unfortunately, accurate control figures are not available except in the case of epilepsy: 1.3% of fatalities had taken an antiepileptic drug and the incidence of the disease in the general population is 0.4%.[30] Driving may also be influenced by antihistamines (drowsiness, but less commonly with newer nonsedative agents), mydriatics and antimicrobials for topical ocular use (blurred vision), antihypertensives (hypotension) and insulins and oral antidiabetic agents (hypoglycaemia).

FURTHER EFFECTS OF ALCOHOL CONSUMPTION

Peripheral vasodilatation. Alcohol depresses the vasomotor centre and this accounts for the feeling

---

[28] Approximately equivalent to 35 micrograms alcohol in 100 ml expired air (or 107 mg in 100 ml urine). In practice, prosecutions are undertaken only when the concentration is significantly higher to avoid arguments about biological variability and instrumental error. Urine concentrations are little used since the urine is accumulated over time and does not provide the immediacy of blood and breath.

[29] In 1990 Sweden lowered the limit to 20 mg/100 ml, which has been approached by ingestion of glucose which becomes fermented by gut flora—the 'autobrewery' syndrome.

[30] Advice to patients on prescribed medicines is contained in Medical Commission on Accident Prevention 1995 Medical Aspects of Fitness to Drive; HMSO, London.

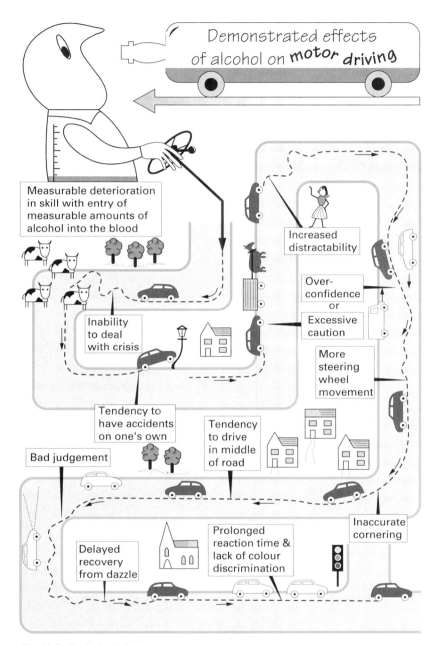

Fig. 10.3 Alcohol and driving.

of warmth that follows taking the drug. Body heat loss is increased so that it is undesirable to take alcohol before going out into severe cold for any length of time, but it may be harmlessly employed on coming into a warm environment from the cold to provide quickly a pleasant feeling of warmth.

Blood pressure. An acute dose of 4–5 units raises the blood pressure which parallels the blood concentration. The mechanism appears to involve centrally mediated sympathetic stimulation.

Diuretic effect. Alcohol acts by inhibiting secretion of antidiuretic hormone by the posterior pituitary gland. The reason it is useless as a diuretic in heart failure is that the diuresis is of water, not of salt.

Gastric mucosa. Injury occurs because alcohol allows back diffusion of acid from the gastric lumen into the mucosa. After an acute binge the mucosa shows erosions and also petechial haemorrhages (recovery may take 3 weeks) and up to 60% of chronic alcoholics show chronic gastritis.

Vomiting. This common accompaniment of acute alcoholism seems to be partly a central effect, for the incidence of vomiting at equivalent blood alcohol concentrations is similar following oral or i.v. administration. This is not to deny that very strong solutions and dietary indiscretions accompanying acute and chronic alcoholism can cause vomiting by local gastric effects. That said, when death occurs, it is commonly due to suffocation from inhaled vomit.

Glucose tolerance. Alcohol initially increases the blood glucose, due to reduced uptake by the tissues. This leads to increased glucose metabolism.

But alcohol also inhibits gluconeogenesis and a person whose hepatic glycogen is already low, e.g. a person who is getting most of his calories from alcohol or who has not eaten adequately for 3 days, can experience hypoglycaemia that can be severe enough to cause irreversible brain damage. Hypoglycaemia can be difficult to recognise clinically in a person who has been drunk, and this adds to the risk.

Hyperuricaemia occurs (with precipitation of gout) due to accelerated degradation of adenine nucleotides resulting in increased production of uric acid and its precursors. Only at high alcohol concentrations does alcohol-induced high blood lactate compete for renal tubular elimination and so diminish excretion of urate.

Effects on sexual function. Nothing really new has been said since William Shakespeare wrote that alcohol 'provokes the desire, but it takes away the performance'. Performance in other forms of athletics is also impaired. Prolonged substantial consumption lowers plasma testosterone concentration at least partly as a result of hepatic enzyme induction;

feminisation may be seen and men have been threatened with genital shrinkage.

Source of energy. Alcohol may be useful as an energy source (rather than a food) in debilitated patients. It is rapidly absorbed from the alimentary tract without requiring digestion and it supplies 7 calories[31] per gram as compared with 9 from fat and 4 from carbohydrate and protein. Heavy doses cause hyperlipidaemia in some people.

Tolerance to alcohol can be acquired and the point has been made that it costs the regular heavy drinker 2.5 times as much to get visibly drunk as it would cost the average abstainer. This is probably due both to enzyme induction and to adaptation of the central nervous system.

Intolerance. Inter-ethnic variation in tolerance to alcohol is well recognised, for Asian persons, particularly Japanese, develop flushing, headache and nausea after what are, by Caucasian standards, small amounts of the substance. Genetic deficiency of aldehyde dehydrogenase with slow metabolism of (toxic) acetaldehyde may explain these features.

Acute alcohol poisoning is a sufficiently familiar condition not to require detailed description. It is notorious that the characteristic behaviour changes, excitement, mental confusion (including 'blackouts'), incoordination and even coma, can be due to numerous other conditions and diagnosis can be extremely difficult if a sick or injured patient happens to have taken alcohol as well. Alcohol can cause severe hypoglycaemia (see above). Measurement of blood alcohol may clarify the situation.

If sedation is essential, diazepam in low dose is least hazardous. Alcohol dialyses well, but dialysis will only be used in extreme cases.

Acute hepatitis, which may be extremely severe, can occur with extraordinarily heavy acute drinking bouts. The serum transaminase rises after alcohol in alcoholics but not in others. The single case-report that after a binge the cerebrospinal fluid tasted of gin remains unconfirmed.

---

[31] 1 calorie = 4.2 joules.

Chronic consumption

For *benefits* of chronic alcohol consumption, see page 187.

Central nervous system. The development of dependence on alcohol appears to involve alterations in central nervous system neurotransmission. The *acute* effect of alcohol is to block NMDA receptors for which the normal agonist is glutamate, the main excitatory transmitter in the brain. *Chronic* exposure increases the number of NMDA receptors and also 'L type' calcium channels, while the action of the (inhibitory) GABA neurotransmitter is reduced. The resulting excitatory effects may explain the anxiety, insomnia and craving that accompanies sudden withdrawal of alcohol (and may explain why resumption of drinking brings about relief, perpetuating dependence).

Malnutrition. With heavy continuous drinking, subjects take all the calories they need from alcohol, cease to eat adequately and develop deficiency of B group vitamins particularly. The malnutrition complicates the long-term effects of alcohol itself.

Organ damage. Chronic heavy alcohol use is associated with: hepatic cirrhosis, deteriorating brain function (psychotic states, dementia, seizures, Wernicke's encephalopathy, episodes of loss of memory); peripheral neuropathy and, separately, myopathy (including cardiomyopathy); cancer of the upper alimentary and respiratory tracts (many alcoholics also smoke heavily, and this contributes), hepatic carcinoma and breast cancer in women; chronic pancreatitis; cardiomyopathy; bone marrow depression, including megaloblastosis (due to the alcohol and to alcohol-induced folate deficiency); deficiency of vitamin K-dependent blood clotting factors (due to liver injury); psoriasis; multiple effects on the hypothalamic/pituitary/endocrine system (endocrine investigations should be interpreted cautiously); Dupuytren's contracture.

Hypertension. Heavy chronic use of alcohol is an important cause of hypertension and this should always be considered in both diagnosis and management. Cessation of use may be sufficient to eliminate or reduce the need for drug therapy. But even social drinking can raise blood pressure, and hypertensives should be told this.

In general, **reversal** of all or most of the above effects is usual in early cases if alcohol is abandoned. In more advanced cases, the disease may be halted (except cancer) but in severe cases it may continue to progress. When wine rationing was introduced in Paris, France, in the 1939–45 war, deaths from hepatic cirrhosis dropped to about one-sixth the previous level; 5 years after the war they had regained their former level.

Blood lipoproteins. Moderate intake of alcoholic drinks may increase high density lipoprotein and diminish low density lipoprotein, which may account for the observed protective effect against ischaemic heart disease (see below).

Alcohol dependence syndrome[32]

General aspects of dependence are discussed earlier in this chapter. Dependence (chronic alcoholism) varies from social drinkers for whom companionship is the principal factor, through individuals who take a drink at the end of a working (or indeed any) day, who feel a need and who would be reluctant to give it up, to the person who is overcome by need, who cannot resist and whose whole life is dominated by the quest for alcohol. The major factors determining physical dependence are dose, frequency of dosing, and duration of abuse.

WITHDRAWAL OF ALCOHOL

Abrupt withdrawal of alcohol from a person who has developed physical dependence, such as may occur when an ill or injured alcoholic is admitted to hospital, can precipitate withdrawal syndrome (agitation, anxiety and excess sympathetic autonomic activity) in 6 h and an acute psychotic attack (delirium tremens) and seizures (at 72 h).

Withdrawal should be supervised in hospital with the patient receiving *chlordiazepoxide* by mouth

---

[32] A World Health Organization report prefers this term to 'alcoholism'.

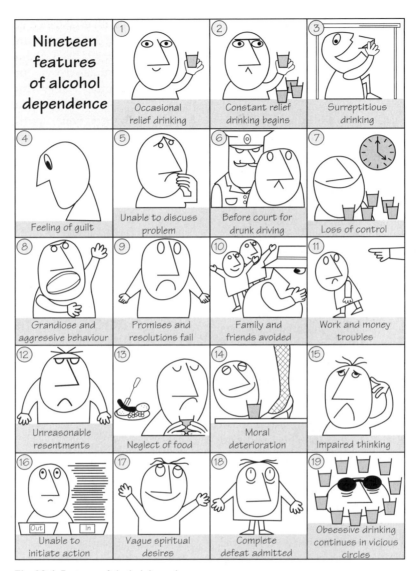

Fig. 10.4 Features of alcohol dependence.

10–50 mg qid, gradually reducing over 7–10 d. Longer exposure to chlordiazepoxide should be avoided as it has the potential to induce dependence. A β-adrenoceptor blocker may be given to attenuate symptoms of sympathetic overactivity. General aspects of care, e.g. attention to fluid and electrolyte balance, are important. It is usual to administer vitamins, especially thiamine, in which alcoholics are commonly deficient, and i.v. glucose unaccompanied by thiamine may precipitate Wernicke's encephalopathy.

Treatment of alcohol dependence

Psychosocial support is more important than drugs, which nevertheless may help.

Acamprosate bears a structural resemblance to both glutamate and GABA and appears to reduce the effect of excitatory amino acids such as glutamate, and modifies GABA neurotransmission. Taken for 1 year (accompanied by counselling and psychosocial support), acamprosate increases the number of alcohol-free days and also the chance of subsequent complete abstinence. The benefit may last for 1 year after stopping treatment. Acamprosate may cause gastrointestinal adverse effects, and cutaneous eruptions.

Disulfiram (Antabuse). In alcoholics who are well and motivated, an attempt may be made to discourage drinking by inducing immediate unpleasantness. Disulfiram inhibits the enzyme aldehyde dehydrogenase so that acetaldehyde (toxic metabolite of alcohol) accumulates. The objective of administering disulfiram is that patients will find the experience so unpleasant that they will avoid alcohol. It should be administered only under specialist supervision.

A typical reaction of medium severity comes on about 5 min after taking alcohol and consists of generalised vasodilatation and fall in blood pressure, sweating, dyspnoea, headache, chest pain, nausea and vomiting. It may result from even small amounts of alcohol (such as may be present in some oral medicines or mouthwashes). Severe reactions include convulsions and circulatory collapse; they may last several hours. Some advocate the use of a test dose of alcohol under supervision (after the fifth day), so that patients can be taught what to expect and also to induce an aversion from alcohol.

SAFE LIMITS FOR CHRONIC CONSUMPTION

These cannot be accurately defined. But both patients and nonpatients justifiably expect some guidance, and doctors and government departments will wish to be helpful. They may reasonably advise as a 'safe' or prudent maximum (there being no particular individual contraindication): men, not more than 21 units per week (and not more than 4 units in any one day), and women, 14 units per week (and not more than 3 units in any one day).[33] Consistent drinking more than these amounts carries a progressive risk to health (see also Alcoholic drinks and mortality, below). In other societies recommended maxima are higher or lower.

Alcoholics with established cirrhosis have usually consumed about 23 units (230 ml; 184 g) daily for 10 years. It has long been thought that total consumption accumulated over time was the crucial factor for cirrhosis. Heavy drinkers may develop hepatic cirrhosis at a rate of about 2% per annum. The type of drink (beer, wine, spirits) is not particularly relevant to the adverse health consequences.

A standard bottle of spirits (750 ml) contains 300 ml (240 g) of alcohol (i.e. 40% by volume). A standard human cannot metabolise more than about 170 g per day. People whose intake is concentrated at the weekend allow their livers time for repair and have a lower risk of liver injury than do those who consume the same total on an even daily basis.

Pregnancy, the fetus and lactation

Pregnancy is unlikely to occur in severely alcoholic women (who have amenorrhoea secondary to liver injury). The spontaneous miscarriage rate in the second trimester is doubled by consumption of 1–2 units/day.

Fetal injury can occur in early pregnancy (fetal alcohol syndrome). It may be due to the metabolite, acetaldehyde, and so acute (binge) consumption is more hazardous than similar total intake on a daily basis. The vulnerable period of pregnancy is at 4–10 weeks. Because of this, prevention cannot be reliably achieved after diagnosis of pregnancy (usually 3–8 weeks).

There is no level of maternal consumption that can be guaranteed safe for the fetus. But it is plainly unrealistic to leave the matter there, and it has been suggested that if the ideal of total abstinence is unachievable then women who are pregnant or are thinking of becoming pregnant should not drink more than 1–2 units of alcohol per week and should avoid periods of intoxication.[34]

In addition to the fetal alcohol syndrome there is general fetal/embryonic growth retardation (1% for

---

[33] Report of an Inter-Departmental Working Group, 1995 Sensible Drinking. Department of Health.

[34] Report of an Inter-Departmental Working Group, 1995 Sensible Drinking. Department of Health.

every 10 g alcohol per day) and this is not 'caught up' later.

Fetal alcohol syndrome includes the following characteristics: microcephaly, mental retardation with irritability in infancy, low body weight and length, poor coordination, hypotonia, small eyeballs and short palpebral fissures, lack of nasal bridge.[35]

Children of about 10% of alcohol abusers may show the syndrome. In women consuming 12 units of alcohol per day the incidence may be as much as 30%.

Lactation. Even small amounts of alcohol taken by the mother delay motor development in the child; an effect on mental development is uncertain.

Alcoholic drinks and mortality

The curve that relates mortality (vertical axis) to alcoholic drink consumption (horizontal axis) is J-shaped; i.e. as consumption rises above zero the all-cause mortality declines, then levels off, and finally rises.

The benefit is largely a reduction of deaths due to cardio- and cerebrovascular disease for regular drinkers of 1–2 units/d for men over 40 years and postmenopausal women. Consumption over 2 units/d does not provide any major additional health benefit. The mechanism may be an improvement in lipoprotein (HDL/LDL) profiles and perhaps a reduction in platelet aggregation.

The effect appears to be due mainly to ethanol itself but nonethanol ingredients (antioxidants, phenols, flavinoids) may contribute (see below).

The rising (adverse) arm of the curve is associated with known harmful effects of alcohol (already described), but also, for example, with pneumonia (which may be secondary to direct alcohol effects, or with the increased smoking of alcohol users).

Whether the cardioprotective effect differs between classes of alcoholic drink remains an open issue. Suggestion that wine confers greater advan-

tage than spirits was not supported by a review of 12 ecological, 3 case-control and 10 prospective cohort studies.[36] The social importance of alcohol combined with the very substantial scientific problems posed by these studies (including the problem of unreliably reported intakes) render the whole matter controversial.

Alcohol and other drugs

All cerebral depressants (hypnotics, tranquillisers, antiepileptics, antihistamines) can either potentiate or synergise with alcohol, and this can be important at ordinary doses in relation to car driving. But, when supplies of hypnotics or tranquillisers are given to patients known to drink heavily, they should be warned to omit the drugs when they have been drinking. Deaths have occurred from these combinations.

Alcohol-dependent people with a physical tolerance are relatively tolerant of some other cerebral depressant drugs (hydrocarbon anaesthetics), but of course the synergism with these drugs still occurs. There is no significant acquired cross-tolerance with opioids.

A disulfiram-like reaction occurs with metronidazole, griseofulvin, cefamandole, chlorpropamide, procarbazine and (possibly) tinidazine.

Oral anticoagulants. Control may be disturbed by alcohol inhibiting hepatic metabolism acutely, or enhancing it by enzyme induction; moderate drinking is unlikely to cause trouble.

Antiepilepsy drugs can be metabolised faster due to enzyme induction and this contributes to its well-known adverse effect on epilepsy.

Monoamine oxidase inhibitors (MAOIs). Some alcoholic (and de-alcoholised) drinks contain tyramine, sufficient to cause a hypertensive crisis in a patient taking a MAOI.

Miscellaneous uses of alcohol. Alcohol precipitates protein and is used to harden the skin in bedridden

---

[35] For pictures see Streissguth A P et al 1985 Lancet 2: 85–91.

[36] Rimm E B et al. 1996 Review of moderate alcohol consumption and reduced risk of coronary heart disease: is the effect due to beer, wine or spirits? British Medical Journal 312: 731–741.

patients. Local application also reduces sweating and may allay itching. As a skin antiseptic 70% by weight (76% by volume) is most effective. Stronger solutions are less effective. Alcohol injections are sometimes used to destroy nervous tissue in cases of intractable pain (trigeminal neuralgia, carcinoma involving nerves).

Psychodysleptics or hallucinogens

These substances produce mental changes that resemble those of some psychotic states. They are used by people seeking a new experience or escape.

Experiences with these drugs vary greatly with the subject's expectations, existing frame of mind and personality and environment. Subjects can be prepared so that they are more likely to have a good 'trip' than a bad one.

Experiences with psychodysleptics

The following brief account of experiences with **LSD** (lysergic acid diethylamide, lysergide) in normal subjects will serve as a model. Experiences with **mescaline** and **psilocybin** are similar:

- Vision may become blurred and there may be hallucinations; these generally do not occur in the blind and are less if the subject is blindfolded. Objects appear distorted, and trivial things, e.g. a mark on a wall, may change shape and acquire special significance.
- Auditory acuity increases, but hallucinations are uncommon. Subjects who do not ordinarily appreciate music may suddenly come to do so.
- Foods may feel coarse and gritty in the mouth.
- Limbs may be left in uncomfortable positions.
- Time may seem to stop or to pass slowly, but usually it gets faster and thousands of years may seem suddenly to go by.
- The subject may feel relaxed and supremely happy, or may become fearful or depressed. Feelings of depersonalisation and dreamy states occur.

The experience lasts a few hours, depending on the dose; intervals of normality then occur and become progressively longer.

Somatic symptoms include nausea, dizziness, paraesthesiae, weakness, drowsiness, tremors, dilated pupils, ataxia. Effects on the cardiovascular system and respiration vary and probably reflect fluctuating anxiety.

There is no shortage of sensational accounts of experience with psychodysleptics, because there has been a vogue amongst intellectuals, begun by Mr Aldous Huxley,[37] for publishing their experiences. Subsequent accounts are tedious to most except their authors and to those who would do the same; they have little pharmacological importance and reveal more about the author's egocentricity than about pharmacology. The same applies to published accounts of what it is like to be a drug addict.

Individual substances

LYSERGIDE (LSD)

Lysergic acid provides the nucleus of the ergot alkaloids and it was during a study of derivatives of this in a search for an analeptic that in 1943 a Swiss worker investigating LSD (which structurally resembles nikethamide) felt peculiar and had visual hallucinations. This led him to take a dose of the substance and so to discover its remarkable potency, an effective oral dose being about 30 microgams. The $t\frac{1}{2}$ is 3 h. (See description of experience, above.) Mechanisms of action are complex and include agonist effect at presynaptic 5-HT receptors in the CNS.

Tachyphylaxis (acute tolerance) occurs to LSD. Psychological dependence may occur; physical dependence does not.

Serious adverse effects include psychotic reactions (which can be delayed in onset) with suicide.

LSD has curious effects in animals: green sunfish become aggressive, Siamese fighting fish float nose up, tail down and goats walk in unaccustomed stereotyped patterns. The elephant exhibits episod-

---

[37] Huxley A 1964 The doors of preception. Chatto and Windus, London.

ically a form of sexual or delinquent behaviour known as 'musth'.

Mescaline is an alkaloid from the Mexican peyote cactus (derived from the Indian word peyotl, meaning 'divine messenger'), the top of which is cut off and dried and used as 'mescal buttons' in religious ceremonies. Mescaline does not induce serious dependence and the drug has little importance except to members of some North and Central American societies and to psychiatrists and biochemists who are interested in the mechanism of induced psychotic states.

Tenamfetamine ('ecstasy', MDMA: methylenedioxy-methamphetamine) is structurally related to mescaline as well as to amphetamine. It was originally patented in 1914 as an appetite suppressant and has recently achieved widespread popularity as a dance drug at 'rave' parties (where it is deemed necessary to keep pace with the beat and duration of the music; popular names reflect the appearance of the tablets and capsules and include White Dove, White Burger, Red and Black, Denis the Menace). Tenamfetamine stimulates central and peripheral α- and β-adrenoceptors; thus the pharmacological effects are compounded by those of physical exertion, dehydration and heat. In susceptible individuals (poor metabolisers who exhibit the CYP450 2D6 polymorphism) a severe and fatal idiosyncratic reaction may occur with fulminant hyperthermia, convulsions, disseminated intravascular coagulation, rhabdomyolysis, and acute renal and hepatic failure. Treatment includes: activated charcoal, diazepam for convulsions, β-blockade (atenolol) for tachycardia, α-blockade (phentolamine) for hypertension, and dantrolene if the rectal temperature exceeds 39°C.

In chronic users, positive emission tomographic (PET) brain scans show selective dysfunction of serotonergic neurones, raising concerns that neuro-degenerative changes accompany long-term use of MDMA.

Phencyclidine ('angel dust') was made in a search for a better intravenous anaesthetic. It is structurally related to pethidine. Phencyclidine was found to induce analgesia without unconsciousness, but with amnesia, in man (dissociative anaesthesia). The postoperative course, however, was complicated by psychiatric disturbance. As the interest of anaesthetists waned, so that of psychiatrists grew and the drug has been used in experimental therapy. Ketamine originated from this work. Overdose can cause agitation, abreactions, hallu-cinations and psychosis, and if severe can result in seizures, coma, hyperthermia, muscular rigidity, and rhabdomyolysis.

Psilocybin is derived from varieties of the fungus *Psilocybe* ('magic mushrooms') that grow in many countries. It is related to LSD.

CANNABIS

Cannabis is obtained from the annual plant *Cannabis sativa* (hemp) and its varieties *Cannabis indica* and *Cannabis americana*. The preparations that are smoked are called marijuana (grass, pot, weed, etc.) and consist of crushed leaves and flowers. There is a wide variety of regional names, e.g. ganja (India, Caribbean), kif (Morocco), dagga (Africa). The resin scraped off the plant is known as hashish (hash). The term cannabis is used to include all the above preparations. Since most preparations are illegally prepared it is not surprising that they are impure and of variable potency. The plant grows wild in the Americas,[38] Africa and Asia. It can also be grown successfully in the open in the warmer southern areas of Britain.

Pharmacokinetics

Of the scores of chemical compounds that the resin contains, the most important are the oily *cannabinoids,* including tetrahydrocannabinol (THC), which is the chief cause of the psychic action. Samples of resin vary greatly in the amounts and proportions of these cannabinoids according to their country of origin; as the sample ages, its THC content declines. As a result, the THC content of samples can vary from almost zero to 8%.

Smoke from a cannabis cigarette (the usual mode of use is to inhale and hold the breath to allow maximum absorption) delivers 25–50% of the THC content to the respiratory tract.

---

[38] The commonest pollen in the air of San Francisco, California is said to be that of the cannabis plant, illegally cultivated.

THC ($t\frac{1}{2}$ 4 d) and other cannabinoids undergo extensive biotransformation in the body, yielding scores of metabolites, several of which are themselves psychoactive. They are extremely lipid-soluble and are stored in body fat from which they are slowly released.[39] Hepatic drug metabolising enzymes are inhibited acutely but may also be induced by chronic use of crude preparations.

Pharmacodynamics

The discovery of cannabinoid CB_1-receptors (expressed by central and peripheral neurones) and CB_2-receptors (expressed by immune cells) and the presence of endogenous agonists will point the way to identifying its mechanisms of action, although these are as yet not well understood.

Psychological reactions are very varied, being much influenced by the behaviour of the group. They commence within minutes of starting to smoke and last 2–3 h. Euphoria is common, though not invariable, with giggling or laughter which can seem pointless to an observer. Sensations become more vivid, especially visual, and contrast and intensity of colour can increase, although no change in acuity occurs. Size of objects and distance are distorted. Sense of time can disappear altogether, leaving a sometimes distressing sense of time-lessness. Recent memory and selective attention are impaired; the beginning of a sentence may be forgotten before it is finished, and the subject is very suggestible and easily distracted. Psychological tests such as mental arithmetic, digit-symbol substitution and pursuit meter tests show impairment. These effects may be accompanied by feelings of deep insight and truth. Memory defect may persist for weeks after abstinence.

Once memory is impaired, concentration becomes less effective, since the object of attention is less well remembered. With this may go an insensitivity to danger or the consequences of actions.

A striking phenomenon is the intermittent wave-like nature of these effects which affects mood, visual impressions, time sense, spatial sense, and other functions.

The desired effects of cannabinoids, as of other psychodysleptics, depend not only on the expectation of the user and the dose, but also on the environmental situation and personality. Genial or revelatory experiences may indeed occur, e.g. 'Haschich Fudge'.[40]

(which anyone can whip up on a rainy day). This is the food of Paradise … euphoria and brilliant storms of laughter, ecstatic reveries and extension of one's personality on several simultaneous planes are to be complacently expected. Almost anything St Teresa[41] did, you can do better…

But this cannot be relied on.

The effects can be unpleasant, especially in inexperienced subjects, particularly timelessness and the feeling of loss of control of mental processes. Feelings of unease, sometimes amounting to anguish and acute panic occur as well as 'flashbacks' of previously experienced hallucinations, e.g. on LSD. There is also, especially in the habitual user, a tendency to paranoid thinking. High or habitual use can be followed by a psychotic state; this is usually reversible, quickly with brief periods of cannabis use, but more slowly after sustained exposures. Evidence suggests that chronic use may precipitate schizophrenia in vulnerable individuals.

The effect of an acute dose usually ends in drowsiness and sleep. It is claimed that death has not occurred.

Tolerance, with continued heavy use, and a withdrawal syndrome occur (depression, anxiety, sleep disturbance, tremor and other symptoms). Many users find it very difficult to abandon cannabis. In studies of self-administration by monkeys, spontaneous use did not occur but, once use was initiated, drug-seeking behaviour developed. Subjects who have become tolerant to LSD or opioids as a result of repeated dosage respond normally to cannabis but

---

[39] When a chronic user discontinues, cannabinoids remain detectable in the urine for an average of 4 weeks and it can be as long as 11 weeks before 10 consecutive daily tests are negative (Ellis G M et al 1986 Clinical Pharmacology and Therapeutics 38: 572).

[40] From The Alice B Toklas cook book 1954 Michael Joseph, London. The author was companion to Gertrude ('rose is a rose is a rose') Stein (1874–1946).

[41] St Teresa of Avila (1515–82) was noted for her power of levitation.

there appears to be cross-tolerance between cannabinoids and alcohol.

'Amotivational syndrome'. This term dignifies an imprecisely characterised state, ranging from a feeling of unease and sense of not being fully effective, up to a gross lethargy, with social passivity and deterioration. It is difficult to assess, when personal traits and intellectual rejection of techno-logical civilisation are also taken into account. Yet the reversibility of the state, its association with cannabinoid use, and its recognition by cannabis users make it impossible to ignore. (Escalation theory, see p. 171.)

Cannabinoids and skilled tasks, e.g. car driving. General performance in both motor and psycho-logical tests deteriorates, more in naive than in experienced subjects. Effects may be similar to alcohol, but experiments in which the subjects are unaware that they are being tested (and so do not compensate voluntarily) are difficult to do, as with alcohol. Some scientists claim the effects are negligible but this view has been 'put in proper perspective' by a commentator[42] who asked how these scientists 'would feel if told that the pilot of their international jet taking them to a psychologists' conference, was just having a reefer or two before opening up the controls'.

Other effects. Cannabis smoked or taken by mouth produces reddening of the eyeballs (probably the forerunner of the general dilatation of blood vessels and fall of blood pressure with higher doses), unsteadiness (particularly for precise movements), and tachycardia. The smoke produces the usual smoker's cough and delivers much more tar than tobacco cigarettes; the tar from reefer cigarettes is as carcinogenic in animal experiments as cigarette tobacco tar. Increase in appetite is commonly experienced.

Cannabinoids are teratogenic in animals, but effect in humans is unproved, although there is impaired fetal growth with repeated use.

A therapeutic role has been suggested for cannabi-noids in a variety of conditions including chronic pain, migraine headaches, muscle spasticity in multiple sclerosis or spinal cord injury, movement disorders, appetite stimulation in AIDS patients and nausea and vomiting. One systematic review concluded that cannabinoids were no more effective that codeine for acute or chronic pain although most of the trials were conducted in the 1970s.[43] A further review concluded that cannabinoids protected against nausea and vomiting induced by chemo-therapy but the studies were conducted mainly in the 1980s, i.e. before the introduction of the (highly effective) serotonin receptor antagonists.[44] Clinical trials now in progress will clarify the value of individual cannabinoids in such conditions, their profile of adverse effects and comparison with other drug and non-drug therapies.

MANAGEMENT OF ADVERSE REACTIONS

Mild and sometimes even severe episodes ('bad trips') can be managed by reassurance including talk, 'talking the patient down', and physical contact, e.g. hand holding (LSD and mescaline). The objective is to help patients relate their experience to reality and to appreciate that the mental experiences are drug-induced and will abate. Because short-term memory is disrupted the treatment can be very time-consuming since therapists cannot absent themselves without risking relapse. But with phencyclidine such intervention may have the opposite effect, i.e. overstimulation. It is therefore appropriate to sedate all anxious or excited subjects with diazepam (or haloperidol). With sedation the 'premorbid ego' may be rapidly re-established.

If the user's 'bad trip' is due to overdose of an antimuscarinic drug, natural or synthetic, then diazepam is specially preferred, or a neuroleptic with no or minimal antimuscarinic effects, e.g. haloperidol. A dose of an anticholinesterase that penetrates the central nervous system (physostig-

---

[42] Dr G Milner.

[43] Campbell FA et al 2001 Are cannabinoids an effective and safe treatment option in the management of pain? A quantitative systematic review. British Medical Journal 323: 13–16.
[44] Tramèr MR et al 2001 Cannabinoids for control of chemotherapy induced nausea and vomiting: quantitative systematic review. British Medical Journal 323: 16–20.

mine, tacrine) is effective in severe reaction to an antimuscarinic.

Stimulants

COCAINE

Cocaine (see also Local anaesthetics, p. 422) use is a widespread and ancient practice amongst South American peasants who chew coca leaves with lime to release the alkaloid. It is claimed to give relief from fatigue and hunger; from altitude sickness in the Andes, experienced even by natives when journeying by car or other 'fast' transportation; and also to induce a pleasant introverted mental state.

Remarkable feats of endurance attributed to chewing coca leaves have been reported, but there is no sound scientific confirmation of them. A United Nations enquiry into coca-leaf chewing reported that there was psychological but no physical dependence. It also reported that its use caused physical exhaustion rather than the reverse, and advocated gradual suppression in the interest of the populations concerned. But what may have been (or even still may be) an acceptable feature of these ancient stable societies has now developed into a massive, criminal business, not for leaf chewing, but for the manufacture and export of purified cocaine to supply an eager and lucrative demand from unhappy but economically richer societies where its use constitutes an intractable social problem. These economically developed societies, which cannot control social demand and importation, seek to eliminate the drug at its source in peasant societies that have come to rely on it for economic subsistence. When coca plantations are destroyed great distress to local populations ensues by a combination of economic deprivation and removal of the coca leaf, which, when used in the traditional way, helps to make tolerable lives of deprivation.

Cocaine (snow) is used as snuff (snorting), swallowed, smoked (below) or injected i.v. It is taken to obtain the immediate characteristic intense euphoria which is often followed in a few minutes by dysphoria. This leads to repeated use (10–45 min) during 'runs' of usually about 12 h. After the 'run'

there follows the 'crash' (dysphoria, irritability, hypersomnia) lasting hours to days. After the 'crash' there may be depression ('cocaine blues') and decreased capacity to experience pleasure (anhedonia) for days to weeks.

Psychological dependence with intense compulsive drug-seeking behaviour is characteristic of even short-term use, but physical dependence is arguably slight or absent. Tachyphylaxis, acute tolerance, occurs.

The psychotropic effects of cocaine are similar to those of amfetamine (euphoria and excitement) but briefer and are due to blockade of the reuptake of dopamine at central nervous system synapses, which increases its concentration at receptors and produces the characteristic 'high'.

Intranasal use causes mucosal vasoconstriction, anosmia and eventually necrosis and perforation of the nasal septum.

Smoking involves converting the nonvolatile HC1 into the volatile 'free base' or 'crack' (by extracting the HC1 with alkali); for use it is vaporised by heat (it pops or cracks) in a special glass 'pipe'; or mixed with tobacco in a cigarette. Inhalation with breath-holding allows pulmonary absorption that is about as rapid as an i.v. injection. It induces an intense euphoric state. The mouth and pharynx become anaesthetised.

Intravenous use gives the expected rapid effect (kick, flash, rush). Cocaine may be mixed with heroin (as 'speedball').

Cocaine is metabolised by plasma esterases; the $t\frac{1}{2}$ is 50 min.

Overdose is common amongst users (up to 22% of heavy users report losing consciousness). The desired euphoria and excitement turns to acute fear, with psychotic symptoms, convulsions, hypertension, haemorrhagic storke, tachycardia, arrhythmias, hyperthermia; coronary vasospasm (sufficient to present as the acute coronary syndrome with chest pain and myocardial infarction) may occur, and acute left ventricular dysfunction. Treatment is chosen according to the clinical picture (and the known mode of action), from amongst, e.g. haloperidol (rather than chlorpromazine) for mental disturbance; diazepam for convulsions; a vasodilator, e.g. a calcium channel blocker, for hypertension; glyceryl trinitrate for myocardial ischaemia (but not a β-blocker which aggravates cocaine-induced coronary vasospasm).

Fetal growth is retarded by maternal use, but teratogenicity is uncertain.

AMFETAMINES

Amfetamine has had multifarious uses. It is now obsolete for depression and as an appetite suppressant, and its use in sport is abuse (see before). There is concern that its illicit use as a psychostimulant is widespread. Amfetamine is a racemic compound: the laevo-form is relatively inactive but dexamphetamine (the dextro- isomer) finds use in medicine. Amfetamine will be described, and structurally-related drugs only in the ways in which they differ.

Mode of action. Amfetamine acts by releasing noradrenaline (norepinephrine) stored in nerve endings in both the CNS and the periphery. As with all drugs acting on the central nervous system, the psychological effects vary with mood, personality and environment, as well as with dose.

Subjects become euphoric and fatigue is postponed. Although physical and mental performance may improve, this cannot be relied on; subjects may be more confident and show more initiative, and be better satisfied with a more speedy performance that has deteriorated in accuracy. On the other hand there may be anxiety and a feeling of nervous and physical tension, especially with large doses, and subjects develop tremors and confusion, and feel dizzy. Time seems to pass with greater rapidity. The sympathomimetic effect on the heart, causing palpitations, may intensify discomfort or alarm. Amfetamine increases the peripheral oxygen consumption and this, together with vasoconstriction and restlessness, leads to hyperthermia in overdose, especially if the subject exercises.

Dependence on amfetamine and similar sympathomimetics occurs; it is chiefly psychological, but there is a withdrawal syndrome, suggesting physical dependence; tolerance occurs.

Mild dependence on prescribed amfetamines became common, particularly amongst people with unstable personalities, depressives and tired, lonely housewives. In the 1960s, adolescents began to turn to amfetamines for occasional use to keep awake to have 'fun' and then as an aid to the challenges normal to that stage of life. Unfortunately, drugs provide only the temporary solution of avoidance and postponement of such challenges, retarding rather than assisting progress to maturity.

As well as oral use, i.v. administration (with the pleasurable 'flash' as with opioids) is employed. Severe dependence induces behaviour disorders, hallucinations and even florid psychosis, which can be controlled by haloperidol. Withdrawal is accompanied by lethargy, sleep, desire for food and sometimes severe depression, which leads to an urge to resume the drug.

Pharmacokinetics. Amfetamine ($t\frac{1}{2}$ 12 h) is readily absorbed by any usual route and is largely eliminated unchanged in the urine. Urinary excretion is pH dependent; being a basic substance, elimination will be greater in an acid urine.

Interactions are as expected from mode of action, e.g. antagonism of antihypertensives; severe hypertension with MAOIs and β-adrenoceptor blocking drugs.

Acute poisoning is manifested by excitement and peripheral sympathomimetic effects; convulsions may occur; also, in acute or chronic overuse, a state resembling hyperactive paranoid schizophrenia with hallucinations develops. Hyperthermia occurs with cardiac arrhythmias, vascular collapse and death. Treatment is chlorpromazine with added antihypertensive, e.g. labetalol, if necessary; these provide sedation and α- and β-adrenoceptor blockade (not a β-blocker alone), rendering unnecessary the enhancement of elimination by urinary acidification.

Chronic overdose can cause a psychotic state mimicking schizophrenia. A vasculitis of the cerebral and/or renal vessels can occur, possibly due to release of vasoconstrictor amines from both platelets and nerve endings. Severe hypertension can result from the renal vasculitis.

Structurally-related drugs include dexamfetamine (used for narcolepsy and in attention deficit hyperactivity disorder (ADHD) see p. 387), methylphenidate (used for ADHD), tenamfetamine (Ecstasy, see p. 189), phentermine, diethylpropion, and pemoline.

METHYLXANTHINES (XANTHINES)

The three xanthines, caffeine, theophylline and theobromine, occur in plants. They are qualitatively similar but differ markedly in potency.

- Tea contains caffeine and theophylline.
- Coffee contains caffeine.
- Cocoa and chocolate contain caffeine and theobromine.
- The cola nut ('cola' drinks) contains caffeine.

Theobromine is weak and is of no clinical importance.

Mode of action. Caffeine and theophylline have complex and incompletely elucidated actions, which include inhibition of phosphodiesterase (the enzyme that breaks down cyclic AMP, see p. 191), effects on intracellular calcium distribution, and noradrenergic function. When theophylline (as aminophylline) is used alongside salbutamol in asthma its action adds up to increased benefit to the bronchi, but increased risk to the heart.

Pharmacokinetics. Absorption of xanthines after oral or rectal administration varies with the preparation used. It is generally extensive (> 95%). Caffeine metabolism varies much between individuals ($t^{1}/_{2}$ 2–12 h). Xanthines are metabolised (more than 90%) by numerous mixed function oxidase enzymes, and xanthine oxidase. (For further details on theophylline, see Asthma.)

Actions on mental performance. Caffeine is more potent than theophylline, but both drugs stimulate mental activity where it is below normal. They do not raise it above normal; thought is more rapid and fatigue is removed or its onset delayed. The effects on mental and physical performance vary according to the mental state and personality of the subject. Reaction-time is decreased. Performance that is inferior because of excessive anxiety may become worse. Caffeine can also improve physical performance both in tasks requiring more physical effort than skill (athletics) and in tasks requiring more skill than physical effort (monitoring instruments and taking corrective action in an aircraft flight simulator). It is uncertain whether the improvement consists only of restoring to normal performance that is impaired by fatigue or boredom, or whether caffeine can also enable subjects to improve their normal maximum performance. The drugs may produce their effects by altering both physical capacity and mental attitude.

There is insufficient information on the effects on learning to be able to give any useful advice to students preparing for examination other than that intellectual performance may be assisted when it has been reduced by fatigue or boredom. Effects on mood vary greatly amongst individuals and according to the environment and the task in hand. In general, caffeine induces feelings of alertness and wellbeing, euphoria or exhilaration. Onset of boredom, fatigue, inattentiveness and sleepiness is postponed.

Overdose will certainly reduce performance (see chronic overdose, below). *Acute* overdose, e.g. aminophylline (see p. 559) i.v., can cause convulsions, hypotension, cardiac arrhythmia and sudden death.

Other effects

Respiratory stimulation occurs with substantial doses.

Sleep. Caffeine affects sleep of older more than it does of younger people and this may be related to the fact that older people show greater catecholamine turnover in the central nervous system than do the young. Onset of sleep (sleep latency) is delayed, bodily movements are increased, total sleep time is reduced, there are increased awakenings. Tolerance to this effect does not occur, as is shown by the provision of decaffeinated coffee.[45]

Skeletal muscle. Metabolism is increased, and this may play a part in the enhanced athletic performance mentioned above. There is significant improvement of diaphragmatic function in chronic obstructive pulmonary disease.

---

[45] The European Union regulations define 'decaffeinated' as coffee (bean) containing 0.3% or less of caffeine (normal content 1–3%).

Cardiovascular system. Both caffeine and theophylline directly stimulate the myocardium and cause increased cardiac output, tachycardia and sometimes ectopic beats and palpitations. This effect occurs almost at once after i.v. injection and lasts half an hour. Theophylline contributes usefully to the relief of acute left ventricular failure. There is peripheral (but not cerebral) vasodilatation due to a direct action of the drugs on the blood vessels, but stimulation of the vasomotor centre tends to counter this. Changes in the blood pressure are therefore somewhat unpredictable, but caffeine 250 mg (single dose) usually causes a transient rise of blood pressure of about 14/10 mmHg in occasional coffee drinkers (but has no additional effect in habitual drinkers); this effect can be used advantageously in patients with autonomic nervous system failure who experience postprandial hypotension (2 cups of coffee with breakfast may suffice for the day). In occasional coffee drinkers 2 cups of coffee (about 160 mg caffeine) per day raise blood pressure by 5/4 mmHg. Increased coronary artery blood flow may occur but increased cardiac work counterbalances this in angina pectoris.

When theophylline (aminophylline) is given i.v., slow injection is essential in order to avoid transient peak concentrations which are equivalent to administering an overdose (below).

Smooth muscle (other than vascular muscle, which is discussed above) is relaxed. The only important clinical use for this action is in reversible airways obstruction (asthma), when the action of theophylline can be a very valuable addition to therapy.

Kidney. Diuresis occurs in normal people chiefly due to reduced tubular reabsorption of Na, similar to thiazide action, but weaker.

Miscellaneous effects. Gastric secretion is increased by caffeine given as coffee (by decaffeinated coffee too) more than by caffeine alone, and the basal metabolic rate may increase slightly (see Skeletal muscle, above).

Preparations and uses of caffeine and theophylline

Aminophylline. The most generally useful preparation is aminophylline which is a soluble, irritant salt of theophylline with ethylenediamine (see Asthma).

Attempts to make nonirritant orally reliable preparations of theophylline have resulted in choline theophyllinate and numerous variants. Sustained-release formulations are convenient for asthmatics, but they cannot be assumed to be bioequivalent and repeat prescriptions should adhere to the formulation of a particular manufacturer. Suppositories are available. *Aminophylline is used in:*

- *Asthma.* In severe asthma (given i.v.) when β-adrenoceptor agonists fail to give adequate response; and for chronic asthma (orally) to provide a background bronchodilator effect.
- *Acute left ventricular failure* (see p. 518).
- *Neonatal apnoea;* caffeine is also effective.

Caffeine is used as an additional ingredient in analgesic tablets; about 60 mg potentiates NSAIDs; also as an aid in hypotension of autonomic failure and to enhance oral ergotamine absorption in migraine

XANTHINE-CONTAINING DRINKS
(see also above)

Coffee, tea and cola drinks in excess can make people tense and anxious. Small children are not usually given tea and coffee because they are thought to be less tolerant of the central nervous system stimulant effect, but cola drinks irrationally escape this prohibition. It is possible to make an imposing list of diseases which may be caused or made worse by caffeine-containing drinks, but there is no conclusive evidence to warrant any general constraints. High doses of caffeine in animals damage chromosomes and cause fetal abnormalities; but studies in man suggest that normal consumption poses no risk. Epidemiological studies are not conclusive but indicate either no, or only slight, increased risk ($\times$ 2–3) of coronary heart disease in heavy (including decaffeinated) coffee consumers (> 4 cups/day) (see Lipids, below).

Tolerance and dependence. The regular, frequent use of caffeine-containing drinks is part of normal social life and mild overdose is common. Slight tolerance to the effects of caffeine (on all systems) occurs. Withdrawal symptoms, attributable to psychological and perhaps mild physical dependence occur in habitual coffee drinkers (5 or more cups/day) 12–16 h after the last cup; they include headache (lasting up to 6 days), irritability, jitteriness; they may occur with transient changes in intake, e.g. high at work, lower at the weekend. Habitual tea and coffee drinkers are seldom willing to recognise that they have a mild drug dependence.

Chronic overdose. Excessive prolonged consumption of caffeine causes anxiety, restlessness, tremors, insomnia; headache, cardiac extrasystoles and confusion; diarrhoea may occur with coffee and constipation with tea. The cause can easily be overlooked if specific enquiry into habits is not made; including children regarding cola drinks. Of coffee drinkers, up to 25% who complain of anxiety may benefit from reduction of caffeine intake. An adult heavy user may be defined as one who takes more than 300 mg caffeine/day, i.e. 4 cups of 150 ml of brewed coffee, each containing 80 ± 20 mg caffeine per cup or 5 cups (60 ± 20) of instant coffee. The equivalent for tea would be 10 cups at approximately 30 mg caffeine per cup; and of cola drinks about 2.0 l. Plainly, caffeine drinks brewed to personal taste of consumer or vendor must have an extremely variable concentration according to source of coffee or tea, amount used, method and duration of brewing. There is also great individual variation in the effect of coffee both between individuals and sometimes in the same individual at different times of life (see Sleep, above).

Decaffeinated coffee contains about 3 mg per cup; cola drinks contain 8–13 mg caffeine/100 ml; cocoa as a drink, 4 mg per cup; chocolate (solid) 6–20 mg per 30 g.

In young people high caffeine intake has been linked to behaviour disorders and a limit of 125 mg/l has been proposed for cola drinks.

Blood lipids. Drinking 5 cups of boiled coffee/day increases serum total cholesterol by up to 10%; this does not occur with coffee made by simple filtration. Cessation of coffee drinking can reduce serum cholesterol concentration in hypercholesterolaemic men.

Breast-fed infants may become sleepless and irritable if there is high maternal intake. Fetal cardiac arrhythmias have been reported with exceptionally high maternal caffeine intake, e.g. 1.5 l cola drinks/day.

Ginseng is the root of 2 plants of the same family (oriental, *Panax ginseng*; Siberian, *Eleutherococcus senticosis*) and contains a range of biologically active substances (ginsenosides).

It has been used as a tonic or stimulant for thousands of years. In animal studies ginseng doubles the time that mice placed in water can swim before becoming exhausted; it appears to have antifatigue effects in various other tests in mice (climbing up a rope that is moving downwards) and it increases sexual activity. In man, ginseng has been claimed to benefit performance of athletes and astronauts (fewer fatigue-caused errors), and to reduce absenteeism due to respiratory illness in mining and steel workers and truck drivers. Oriental soldiers at war have used ginseng. Despite accumulating evidence and wide use by the public, the medical profession in Western countries remains sceptical of the value of this tonic. A range of adverse effects is reported, including oedema, hypertension, rashes, diarrhoea, sleeplessness and oestrogen-like effects

Khat. The leaves of the khat shrub (*Catha edulis*) contain alkaloids (cathinine, cathine, cathidine) which are structurally like amphetamine and produce similar effects. They are chewed fresh (for maximum alkaloid content) so that the habit was confined to geographical areas favourable to the shrub (Arabia, E. Africa) until modern transportation allowed wider distribution. Khat chewers (mostly male) became euphoric, loquacious, excited, hyperactive and even manic. As with some other drug dependencies subjects may give priority to their drug needs above personal, family and other social and economic responsibilities. Cultivation takes up serious amounts of scarce arable land and irrigation water.

Drugs as adjuvants to crime

Since time immemorial drugs have been used to facilitate sexual excess and robbery, e.g. opium and plants containing antimuscarinics, e.g. hyoscine. All such acts constitute a criminal offence. The advent of synthetic drugs widened the scope and ease of administration.

In 19th century Chicago (USA) the proprietor of

the Lone Palm Saloon, Michael J Finn, employed girls to ensure his customers consumed drinks to which he had added chloral hydrate—the 'Mickey Finn'—they were robbed when unconscious.

Recently there has been a vogue for using clonidine for the same purpose (a doctor or pharmacist must surely have been responsible for this curious but, it seems, effective choice). Victims become confused and unresisting from sedation, bradycardia, other cardiac arrhythmias, ataxia, hypothermia, hypo- or hypertension.

GUIDE TO FURTHER READING

Criqui M H, Ringel B L 1994 Does diet explain the French paradox? Lancet 344: 1719–1723 (A study of diet, alcohol and mortality from 21 affluent contries.)

Doll R et al 1994 Mortality in relation to smoking: 40 years' observations on male British doctors. British Medical Journal 309: 901–911

Doll R 1997 One for the heart. British Medical Journal 315: 1664–1668

Gawin F H, Ellinwood E H 1988 Cocaine and other stimulants: actions, abuse, and treatment. New England Journal of Medicine 318: 1173–1182

Green A R, Goodwin G M 1996 Ecstasy and neurodegeneration. British Medical Journal 312: 1493–1494

Hall W, Solowij N 1998 Adverse effects of cannabis. Lancet 352: 1611–1616

Hollander J E 1995 The management of cocaine-associated myocardial ischaemia. New England Journal of Medicine 333: 1267–1272

Lange R A, Hillis L D 2001 Cardiovascular complications of cocaine use. New England Journal of Medicine 345: 351–358

MacAuley D 1996 Drugs in sport. British Medical Journal 313: 211–215

Mendelson J H, Mello N K Management of cocaine abuse and dependence. New England Journal of Medicine 334: 965–972

Ness R B et al Cocaine and tobacco use and the risk of spontaneous abortion. New England Journal of Medicine 340: 333–339

Nutt D J 1996 Addiction: brain mechanisms and their treatment implications. Lancet 457: 31 (see also other articles in this series on pages 97, 162, 237, 301, 373)

Raw M, McNeill A, West R 1999 Smoking cessation: evidence based recommendations for the healthcare system. British Medical Journal 318: 182–185

Strang J, Witton J, Hall W 2000 Improving the quality of the cannabis debate: defining the different domains. British Medical Journal 320: 108–110

Swift R M 1999 Drug therapy for alcohol dependence. New England Journal of Medicine 340: 1482–1490

INFECTION AND INFLAMMATION

11

Chemotherapy of infections

SYNOPSIS

Infection is a major category of human disease and skilled management of antimicrobial drugs is of the first importance. The term *chemotherapy* is used for the drug treatment of parasitic infections in which the parasites (viruses, bacteria, protozoa, fungi, worms) are destroyed or removed without injuring the host. The use of the term to cover all drug or synthetic drug therapy needlessly removes a distinction which is convenient to the clinician and has the sanction of long usage. By convention the term is also used to include therapy of cancer.

- Classification of antimicrobial drugs
- How antimicrobials act
- Principles of optimal antimicrobial therapy
- Use of antimicrobial drugs: choice; combinations; chemoprophylaxis and pre-emptive suppressive therapy
- Problems with antimicrobial drugs: resistance; opportunistic infection; masking of infections
- Antimicrobial drugs of choice (Reference table)

HISTORY

Many substances that we now know to possess therapeutic efficacy were first used in the distant past. The Ancient Greeks used male fern, and the Aztecs chenopodium, as intestinal anthelminthics. The Ancient Hindus treated leprosy with chaulmoogra. For hundreds of years moulds have been applied to wounds, but, despite the introduction of mercury as a treatment for syphilis (16th century), and the use of cinchona bark against malaria (17th century), the history of modern rational chemotherapy did not begin until Ehrlich[1] developed the idea from his observation that aniline dyes selectively stained bacteria in tissue microscopic preparations and could selectively kill them. He invented the word 'chemotherapy' and in 1906 he wrote:

> In order to use chemotherapy successfully, we must search for substances which have an affinity for the cells of the parasites and a power of killing them greater than the damage such substances cause to the organism itself ... This means ... we must learn to aim, learn to aim with chemical substances.

The antimalarials pamaquin and mepacrine were developed from dyes and in 1935 the first sulphonamide, linked with a dye (Prontosil), was introduced as a result of systematic studies by Domagk.[2] The results obtained with sulphonamides

---

[1] Paul Ehrlich (1854–1915), the German scientist who was the pioneer of chemotherapy and discovered the first cure for syphilis (Salvarsan).
[2] Gerhard Domagk (1895–1964), bacteriologist and pathologist, who made his discovery while working in Germany. Awarded the 1939 Nobel prize for Physiology or Medicine, he had to wait until 1947 to receive the gold medal because of Nazi policy at the time.

in puerperal sepsis, pneumonia and meningitis were dramatic and caused a revolution in scientific and medical thinking.

In 1928, Fleming[3] accidentally rediscovered the long-known ability of *Penicillium* fungi to suppress the growth of bacterial cultures but put the finding aside as a curiosity.

In 1939, principally as an academic exercise, Florey[4] and Chain[5] undertook an investigation of antibiotics, i.e. substances produced by microorganisms that are antagonistic to the growth or life of other microorganisms.[6] They prepared penicillin and confirmed its remarkable lack of toxicity.[7]

When the preparation was administered to a policeman with combined staphylococcal and streptococcal septicaemia there was dramatic improvement; unfortunately the manufacture of penicillin (in the local Pathology Laboratory) could not keep pace with the requirements (it was also extracted from the patient's urine and re-injected); it ran out and the patient later succumbed to infection.

---

[3] Alexander Fleming (1881–1955). He researched for years on antibacterial substances that would not be harmful to humans. His findings on penicillin were made at St Mary's Hospital, London.

[4] Howard Walter Florey (1898–1969), Professor of Pathology at Oxford University.

[5] Ernest Boris Chain (1906–79). Biochemist. Fleming, Florey and Chain shared the 1945 Nobel prize for Physiology or Medicine.

[6] Strictly, the definition should refer to substances that are antagonistic in dilute solution because it is necessary to exclude various common metabolic products such as alcohols and hydrogen peroxide. The term antibiotic is now commonly used for antimicrobial drugs in general, and it would be pedantic to object to this. Today, many commonly-used antibiotics are either fully synthetic or are produced by major chemical modification of naturally produced molecules: hence, 'antimicrobial agent' is perhaps a more accurate term, but 'antibiotic' is much the commoner usage.

[7] The importance of this discovery for a nation at war was obvious to these workers but the time, July 1940, was unpropitious, for invasion was feared. The mood of the time is shown by the decision to ensure that, by the time invaders reached Oxford, the essential records and apparatus for making penicillin would have been deliberately destroyed; the productive strain of Penicillium mould was to be secretly preserved by several of the principal workers smearing the spores of the mould into the linings of their ordinary clothes where it could remain dormant but alive for years; any member of the team who escaped (wearing the right clothes) could use it to start the work again (Macfarlane G 1979 Howard Florey, Oxford).

Subsequent development amply demonstrated the remarkable therapeutic efficacy of penicillin.

Classification of antimicrobial drugs

Antimicrobial agents may be classified according to the type of organism against which they are active and in this book follow the sequence:

- Antibacterial drugs
- Antiviral drugs
- Antifungal drugs
- Antiprotozoal drugs
- Anthelminthic drugs.

A few antimicrobials have useful activity across several of these groups. For example, metronidazole inhibits obligate anaerobic bacteria (such as *Clostridium perfringens*) as well as some protozoa that rely on anaerobic metabolic pathways (such as *Trichomonas vaginalis*).

Antimicrobial drugs have also been classified broadly into:

- *bacteriostatic,* i.e. those that act primarily by arresting bacterial multiplication, such as sulphonamides, tetracyclines and chloramphenicol
- *bactericidal,* i.e. those which act primarily by killing bacteria, such as penicillins, cephalosporins, aminoglycosides, isoniazid and rifampicin.

Less used in modern clinical practice, the classification is somewhat arbitrary because most bacteriostatic drugs can be shown to be bactericidal at high concentrations, under certain incubation conditions in vitro and against some bacteria.

Bactericidal drugs act most effectively on rapidly dividing organisms. Thus a bacteriostatic drug, by reducing multiplication, may protect the organism from the killing effect of a bactericidal drug. Such mutual antagonism of antimicrobials may be clinically important, but the matter is complex because of the multiple and changing factors that determine each drug's efficacy at the site of infection. In vitro tests of antibacterial synergy and antagonism may only distantly replicate these conditions.

Probably more important than whether an antibiotic is bacteriostatic or bactericidal in vitro is whether its antimicrobial effect is *concentration-*dependent or *time*-dependent. Examples of the former include the quinolones and aminoglycosides in which the outcome is related to the peak antibiotic concentration achieved at the site of infection in relation to the minimum concentration necessary to inhibit multiplication of the organism (the Minimum Inhibitory Concentration, or MIC). These antimicrobials produce a prolonged inhibitory effect on bacterial multiplication (the Post-Antibiotic Effect, or PAE) which suppresses growth until the next dose is given. In contrast, agents such as the β-lactams and macrolides have more modest PAEs and exhibit time-dependent killing; for optimal efficacy, their concentrations should be kept above the MIC for a high proportion of the time between each dose (Fig. 11.1).

Figure 11.1 shows the results of an experiment in which a culture broth initially containing 10^6 bacteria per ml is exposed to various concentrations of two antibiotics one of which exhibits concentration- and the other time-dependent killing. The 'Control' series contains no antibiotic, and the other series contain progressively higher antibiotic concentrations from $0.5 \times$ to $64 \times$ the MIC. Over 6 hours incubation, the time-dependent antibiotic exhibits killing but there is no difference between the $1 \times$ MIC and $64 \times$ MIC. The additional cidal effect of rising concentrations of the antibiotic which has concentration-dependent killing can be clearly seen.

How antimicrobials act

It should always be remembered that drugs are seldom the sole instruments of cure but act together with the natural defences of the body. Antimicrobials act at different sites in the target organism as follows:

The cell wall. This gives the bacterium its characteristic shape and provides protection against the much lower osmotic pressure of the environment. Bacterial multiplication involves breakdown and extension of the wall; interference with these processes prevents the organism from resisting osmotic pressures, so that it bursts. As the cells of higher, e.g. human, organisms do not possess this type of wall, drugs that act here may be especially selective; obviously, the drugs are effective only against growing cells. They include: penicillins, cephalosporins, vancomycin, bacitracin, cycloserine.

The cytoplasmic membrane inside the cell wall is the site of most of the microbial cell's biochemical activity. Drugs that interfere with its function include: polyenes (nystatin, amphotericin), azoles (fluconazole, itraconazole, miconazole), polymyxins (colistin, polymyxin B).

Protein synthesis. Drugs that interfere at various points with the build-up of peptide chains on the ribosomes of the organism include: chloramphenicol, erythromycin, fusidic acid, tetracyclines, aminoglycosides, quinupristin/dalfopristin, linezolid.

Nucleic acid metabolism. Drugs may interfere

- directly with microbial DNA or its replication or repair, e.g. quinolones, metronidazole, or with RNA, e.g. rifampicin
- indirectly on nucleic acid synthesis, e.g. sulphonamides, trimethoprim.

Principles of antimicrobial chemotherapy

The following principles, many of which apply to drug therapy in general, are a guide to good practice with antimicrobial agents.

Make a diagnosis as precisely as is possible and define the site of infection, the organism(s) responsible and their sensitivity to drugs. This objective will be more readily achieved if all relevant biological samples for the laboratory are taken before treatment is begun. Once antimicrobials have been administered, isolation of the underlying organism may be inhibited and its place in diagnostic samples may be taken by resistant, colonizing bacteria which obscure the true causative pathogen.

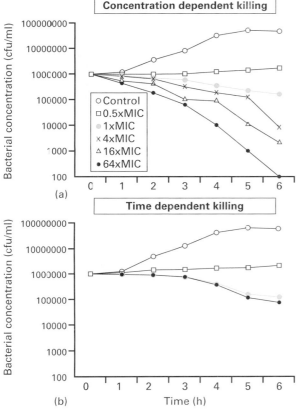

(a) **Concentration dependent killing**

(b) **Time dependent killing**

Fig. 11.1 Efficacy of antimicrobials: examples of concentration-dependent and time-dependent killing (see text) (cfu = colony-forming units).

Remove barriers to cure, e.g. lack of free drainage of abscesses, obstruction in the urinary or respiratory tracts, infected intravenous catheters.

Decide whether chemotherapy is really necessary. As a general rule, acute infections require chemotherapy whilst other measures may be more important for resolution of chronic infections. For example, chronic abscess or empyema respond poorly to antibiotics alone, although chemotherapeutic cover may be essential if surgery is undertaken in order to avoid a flare-up of infection or its dissemination during the breaking down of tissue barriers. Even some of the acute infections are better managed symptomatically than by antimicrobials; thus the risks of adverse drug reactions for previously healthy individuals may outweigh the modest clinical benefits that follow antibiotic therapy

of salmonella gastroenteritis and streptococcal sore throat.

Select the best drug. This involves consideration of:

— *specificity;* ideally the antimicrobial activity of the drug should match that of the infecting organisms. Indiscriminate use of broad-spectrum drugs promotes antimicrobial resistance and encourages opportunistic infections (see p. 210). At the beginning of treatment, empirical 'best guess' chemotherapy of reasonably broad spectrum must often be given because of the absence of precise identification of the responsible microbe. The spectrum of cover should be narrowed once the causative organisms have been identified.
— *pharmacokinetic factors;* to ensure that the chosen drug is capable of reaching the site of infection in adequate amounts, e.g. by crossing the blood–brain barrier.
— *the patient;* who may previously have exhibited allergy to antimicrobials or whose routes of elimination may be impaired, e.g. by renal disease.

Administer the drug in optimum dose and frequency and by the most appropriate route(s). Inadequate dose may encourage the development of microbial resistance. In general, on grounds of practicability, intermittent dosing is preferred to continuous infusion. Plasma concentration monitoring can be performed to optimise therapy and reduce adverse drug reactions (e.g. aminoglycosides, vancomycin, 5-flucytosine).

Continue therapy until apparent cure has been achieved; most acute infections are treated for 5–10 days. There are many exceptions to this, such as typhoid fever, tuberculosis and infective endocarditis, in which relapse is possible long after apparent clinical cure and so the drugs are continued for a longer time, determined by comparative or observational trials. Otherwise, prolonged therapy is to be avoided because it increases costs and the risks of adverse drug reactions.

Test for cure. In some infections, microbiological

proof of cure is desirable because disappearance of symptoms and signs occurs before the organisms are eradicated. This is generally restricted to especially susceptible hosts e.g. urinary tract infection in pregnancy. Microbiological culture must be done, of course, after withdrawal of chemotherapy.

Prophylactic chemotherapy for surgical and dental procedures should be of very limited duration, often only a single large dose being given. It should start at the time of surgery to reduce the risk of selecting resistant organisms prior to surgery (see p. 207).

Carriers of pathogenic or resistant organisms, in general, should not routinely be treated to remove the organisms for it may be better to allow natural re-establishment of a normal flora. The potential benefits of clearing carriage must be weighed carefully against the inevitable risks of adverse drug reactions.

Use of antimicrobial drugs

CHOICE

The general rule is that selection of antimicrobials should be based on identification of the microbe and sensitivity tests. All appropriate specimens (blood, pus, urine, sputum, cerebrospinal fluid) must therefore be taken for examination before administering any antimicrobial.

This process inevitably takes time and therapy at least of the more serious infections must usually be started on the basis of the 'best guess'. With the worldwide rise in prevalence of multiply-resistant bacteria during the past decade, knowledge of local antimicrobial resistance rates is an essential prerequisite to guide the choice of local 'best guess' (or 'empirical') antimicrobial therapy. Publication of these rates (and corresponding guidelines for choice of empirical antibiotic therapy for common infections) is now an important role for clinical diagnostic microbiology laboratories. Such guidelines must be reviewed regularly to keep pace with changing resistance rates.

When considering 'best guess' therapy, infections may be categorised as those in which:

1. Choice of antimicrobial follows automatically from the clinical diagnosis because the causative organism is always the same, and is virtually always sensitive to the same drug, e.g. meningococcal septicaemia (benzylpenicillin), some haemolytic streptococcal infections, e.g. scarlet fever, erysipelas (benzylpenicillin), typhus (tetracycline), leprosy (dapsone with rifampicin).
2. The infecting organism is identified by the clinical diagnosis, but no safe assumption can be made as to its sensitivity to any one antimicrobial, e.g. tuberculosis.
3. The infecting organism is not identified by the clinical diagnosis, e.g. in urinary tract infection or abdominal surgical wound infection.

In the second and third categories particularly, choice of an antimicrobial may be guided by:

Knowledge of the likely pathogens (and their current local susceptibility rates to antimicrobials) in the clinical situation. Thus cephalexin may be a reasonable first choice for lower urinary tract infection (coliform organisms — depending on the prevalence of resistance locally), and benzylpenicillin for meningitis in the adult (meningococcal or pneumococcal).

Rapid diagnostic tests. Use of tests of this type is about to undergo a revolution with the widespread introduction of affordable, sensitive and specific nucleic acid detection assays (especially those based on the Polymerase Chain Reaction, PCR). Classically, antimicrobials were selected in the knowledge that the organism was a Gram-positive or Gram-negative coccus or bacillus, observed by direct staining of body secretions or tissues. It is necessary to know the current local sensitivities to antimicrobial drugs for organisms so classified. Thus flucloxacillin may be indicated when clusters of Gram-positive cocci are found (indicating staphylococci), but vancomycin is preferred in many hospitals with a high prevalence of methicillin-resistant *Staphylococcus aureus* (MRSA). The use of Ziehl-Neelsen staining may reveal acid-fast tubercle bacilli. Light microscopy will remain useful in this way for many years to come, but use of PCR to detect DNA sequences specific for individual microbial species or resistance mechanisms greatly speeds up the institution of definitive, reliable therapy. These methods are already widely used for diagnosing meningitis (detecting *Neisseria meningitidis*, *Streptococcus pneumoniae* and *Haemophilus influenzae*) and tuberculosis (including detection of rifampicin resistance).

Modification of treatment can be made later if necessary, in the light of culture and sensitivity tests. Treatment otherwise should be changed only after adequate trial, usually 2–3 days, for over-hasty alterations cause confusion and encourage the emergence of resistant organisms.

Route of administration. Parenteral therapy (which may be i.m. or i.v.) is preferred for therapy of serious infections because high therapeutic concentrations are achieved reliably and rapidly. Initial parenteral therapy should be switched to the oral route whenever possible once the patient has improved clinically and as long as they are able to absorb the drug i.e. not with vomiting, ileus or diarrhoea. Many antibiotics are, however, well absorbed orally, and the long-held assumption that prolonged parenteral therapy is necessary for adequate therapy of serious infections (such as osteomyelitis) is often not supported by the results of clinical trials.

Although i.v. therapy is usually restricted to hospital patients, continuation parenteral therapy of certain infections, e.g. cellulitis, in patients in the community is sometimes performed by specially-trained nurses. The costs of hospital stays are avoided, but this type of management is suitable only when the patient's clinical state is stable and oral therapy is not suitable.

Oral therapy of infections is usually cheaper and avoids the risks associated with maintenance of intravenous access; on the other hand, it may expose the gastrointestinal tract to higher local concentrations of antibiotic with consequently greater risks of antibiotic-associated diarrhoea. Some antimicrobial agents are available only for topical use to skin, anterior nares, eye or mouth; in general it is better to avoid antibiotics that are also used for systemic therapy because topical use may be especially likely to select for resistant strains. Topical therapy to the conjunctival sac is used for therapy of infections of the conjunctiva and the anterior chamber of the eye.

Other routes used for antibiotics on occasion include inhalational, rectal (as suppositories), intra-ophthalmic, intrathecal (to the CSF), and by direct injection or infusion to infected tissues.

COMBINATIONS

Treatment with a single antimicrobial is sufficient for most infections. The indications for use of two or more antimicrobials are:

- To avoid the development of drug resistance, especially in chronic infections where many bacteria are present (hence the chance of a resistant mutant emerging is high), e.g. tuberculosis.
- To broaden the spectrum of antibacterial activity: (1) in a known mixed infection, e.g. peritonitis following gut perforation or (2) where the infecting organism cannot be predicted but treatment is essential before a diagnosis has been reached, e.g. septicaemia complicating neutropenia or severe community-acquired pneumonia; full doses of each drug are needed.
- To obtain potentiation (or 'synergy'), i.e. an effect unobtainable with either drug alone, e.g. penicillin plus gentamicin for enterococcal endocarditis.
- To enable reduction of the dose of one component and hence reduce the risks of adverse drug reactions, e.g. flucytosine plus amphotericin B for *Cryptococcus neoformans* meningitis.

Selection of agents. A bacteriostatic drug, by reducing multiplication, may protect the organism from a bactericidal drug (see above, Antagonism). When a combination must be used blind, it is theoretically preferable to use two bacteriostatic or two bactericidal drugs, lest there be antagonism.

CHEMOPROPHYLAXIS AND PRE-EMPTIVE SUPPRESSIVE THERAPY

It is sometimes assumed that what a drug can cure it will also prevent, but this is not necessarily so.

The basis of effective, true, chemoprophylaxis is the use of a drug in a healthy person to prevent infection by one organism of virtually uniform susceptibility, e.g. benzylpenicillin against a group A streptococcus. But the term chemoprophylaxis is commonly extended to include suppression of existing infection. To design effective chemoprophylaxis it is essential to know the organisms causing infection and their local resistance patterns, and the period of time the patient is at risk. A narrow-spectrum antibiotic regimen should be administered only during this period — ideally for a few minutes before until a few hours after the risk period. It can be seen that it is much easier to define chemotherapeutic regimens for short-term exposures (e.g. surgical operations) than it is for longer-term and less well defined risks. The main categories of chemoprophylaxis may be summarised as follows:

- *True prevention of primary infection:* rheumatic fever,[8] recurrent urinary tract infection.
- *Prevention of opportunistic infections,* e.g. due to commensals getting into the wrong place (bacterial endocarditis after dentistry and peritonitis after bowel surgery). Note that these are both high-risk situations of short duration; prolonged administration of drugs before surgery would result in the areas concerned (mouth and bowel) being colonised by drug-resistant organisms with potentially disastrous results (see below). Immunocompromised patients can benefit from chemoprophylaxis, e.g. prophylaxis of Gram-negative septicaemia complicating neutropenia with an oral quinolone or of *Pneumocystis carinii* pneumonia with co-trimoxazole.
- *Suppression of existing infection* before it causes overt disease, e.g. tuberculosis, malaria, animal bites, trauma.
- *Prevention of acute exacerbations* of a chronic infection, e.g. bronchitis, in cystic fibrosis.

---

[8] Rheumatic fever is caused by a large number of types of Group A streptococci and immunity is type-specific. Recurrent attacks are commonly due to infection with different strains of these, all of which are sensitive to penicillin and so chemoprophylaxis is effective. Acute glomerulonephritis is also due to group A streptococci. But only a few types cause it, so that natural immunity is more likely to protect and, in fact, second attacks are rare. Therefore, chemoprophylaxis is not used (see also p. 239).

- *Prevention of spread amongst contacts* (in epidemics and/or sporadic cases). Spread of influenza A can be partially prevented by amantadine; in an outbreak of meningococcal meningitis, or when there is a case in the family, rifampicin may be used; very young and fragile nonimmune child contacts of pertussis might benefit from erythromycin

Long-term prophylaxis of bacterial infection can be achieved often by doses that are inadequate for therapy, although prophylaxis of infection associated with surgical procedures should always employ high doses to ensure eradication of the high bacterial numbers that may be introduced to normally sterile sites. Details of the practice of chemoprophylaxis are given in the appropriate sections.

Attempts to use drugs routinely in groups specially at risk to prevent infection by a range of organisms, e.g. pneumonia in the unconscious or in patients with heart failure, in the newborn after prolonged labour, and in patients with long-term urinary catheters, have not only failed but have sometimes encouraged infections with less susceptible organisms. Attempts routinely to prevent bacterial infection secondary to virus infections, e.g. in respiratory tract infections, measles, have not been sufficiently successful to outweigh the disadvantages of drug allergy and infection with drug-resistant bacteria. In these situations it is generally better to be alert for complications and then to treat them vigorously, than to try to prevent them.

CHEMOPROPHYLAXIS IN SURGERY

The principles governing use of antimicrobials in this context are as follows.

Chemoprophylaxis is justified:

— When the risk of infection is high because of the presence of large numbers of bacteria in the viscus which is being operated on, e.g. the large bowel
— when the risk of infection is low but the consequences of infection would be disastrous, e.g. infection of prosthetic joints or prosthetic heart valves, or of abnormal heart valves following the transient bacteraemia of dentistry

— when the risks of infection are low but randomised controlled trials in large numbers of patients have shown the benefits of prophylaxis to outweigh the risks, e.g. single-dose antistaphylococcal prophylaxis for uncomplicated hernia and breast surgery. This indication remains controversial.

Antimicrobials should be selected with a knowledge of the likely pathogens at the sites of surgery and their prevailing antimicrobial susceptibility.

Antimicrobials should be given i.v., i.m. or occasionally rectally at the beginning of anaesthesia and for no more than 48 h. A single preoperative dose, given at the time of induction of anaesthesia, has been shown to give optimal cover for many different operations. Specific instances are:

1. *Colorectal surgery,* because there is a high risk of infection with *Escherichia coli, Clostridium* spp, streptococci and *Bacteroides* spp which inhabit the gut (a cephalosporin plus metronidazole, or benzylpenicillin plus gentamicin plus metronidazole are commonly used)
2. *Gastroduodenal surgery,* because colonisation of the stomach with gut organisms occurs especially when acid secretion is low, e.g. in gastric malignancy, following use of a histamine H_2-receptor antagonist or following previous gastric surgery (usually a cephalosporin will be adequate)
3. *Gynaecological surgery,* because the vagina contains *Bacteroides* spp and other anaerobes, streptococci and coliforms (metronidazole and a cephalosporin are often used).
4. *Leg amputation,* because there is a risk of gas gangrene in an ischaemic limb and the mortality is high (benzylpenicillin, or metronidazole for the patient with allergy to penicillin)
5. *Insertion of prosthetic joints.* Chemoprophylaxis is justified because infection (*Staphylococcus aureus,* coagulase-negative staphylococci and coliforms are commonest) almost invariably means that the artificial joint, valve or vessel must be replaced (various regimens are used, with inclusion of vancomycin when the local MRSA prevalence is high). Single perioperative doses of appropriate antibiotics with plasma

elimination half-lives of several hours (e.g. cefotaxime) are adequate, but if short half-life agents are used (e.g. flucloxacillin) several doses should be given during the first 24 hours.

Problems with antimicrobial drugs

RESISTANCE

Microbial resistance to antimicrobials is a matter of great importance; if sensitive strains are supplanted by resistant ones, then a valuable drug may become useless. Just as:

> Some are born great, some achieve greatness, and some have greatness thrust upon them.[9]

so microorganisms may be naturally ('born') resistant, 'achieve' resistance by mutation or have resistance 'thrust upon them' by transfer of plasmids and other mobile genetic elements.

Resistance may become more prevalent in a human population by spread of microorganisms containing resistance genes, and this may also occur by dissemination of the resistance genes among different microbial species. Because resistant strains are encouraged (selected) at the population level by use of antimicrobial agents, antibiotics are the only group of therapeutic agents which can alter the actual diseases suffered by untreated individuals.

Problems of antimicrobial resistance have burgeoned during the past decade in most countries of the world. Some resistant microbes are currently mainly restricted to patients in the hospital, e.g. MRSA, vancomycin-resistant enterococci (VRE), and coliforms that produce 'extended spectrum β-lactamases'. Others more commonly infect patients in the community, e.g. penicillin-resistant *Streptococcus pneumoniae* and multiply-resistant *Mycobacterium tuberculosis*. Evidence is accruing that the outcomes of infections with antibiotic resistant bacteria are generally poorer than those with

---

[9] Malvolio in Twelfth Night, Act 2 Scene 5, by William Shakespeare (1564–1616).

susceptible strains, and costs of therapy and lengths of hospital stay are greater.

Mechanisms of resistance act as follows:

- *Naturally resistant strains.* Some bacteria are innately resistant to certain classes of antimicrobial agent, e.g. coliforms and many other Gram-negative bacteria possess outer cell membranes which protect their cell walls from the action of certain penicillins and cephalosporins. Facultatively anaerobic bacteria (such as *Escherichia coli*) lack the ability to reduce the nitro group of metronidazole which therefore remains in an inactive form. In the course of therapy, naturally sensitive organisms are eliminated and those naturally resistant proliferate and occupy the biological space newly created by the drug.
- *Spontaneous mutation* brings about organisms with novel antibiotic resistance mechanisms. If these cells are viable, in the presence of the antimicrobial agent selective multiplication of the resistant strain occurs so that it eventually dominates as above.
- *Transmission of genes from other organisms* is the commonest and most important mechanism. Genetic material may be transferred, e.g. in the form of *plasmids* which are circular strands of DNA that lie outwith the chromosomes and contain genes capable of controlling various metabolic processes including formation of β-lactamases (that destroy some penicillins and cephalosporins), and enzymes that inactivate aminoglycosides. Alternatively, genetic transfer may occur through *bacteriophages* (viruses which infect bacteria), particularly in the case of staphylococci.

Resistance is mediated most commonly by the production of enzymes that modify the drug, e.g. aminoglycosides are phosphorylated, β-lactamases hydrolyse penicillins. Other mechanisms include decreasing the passage into or increasing the efflux of drug from the bacterial cell (e.g. imipenem resistance in *Pseudomonas aeruginosa*), modification of the target site so that the antimicrobial binds less effectively (e.g. methicillin resistance in staphylococci), and bypassing of inhibited metabolic pathways (e.g. resistance to trimethoprim in many bacteria).

Limitation of resistance to antimicrobials may be achieved by:

- Avoidance of indiscriminate use by ensuring that the indication for, the dose and duration of treatment are appropriate
- Using antimicrobial combinations in appropriate circumstances, e.g. tuberculosis
- Constant monitoring of resistance patterns in a hospital or community (changing recommended antibiotics used for empirical treatment when the prevalence of resistance becomes high), and good infection control in hospitals (e.g. isolation of carriers, hand hygiene practices for ward staff) to prevent the spread of resistant bacteria
- Restricting drug use, which involves agreement between clinicians and microbiologists, e.g. delaying the emergence of resistance by limiting the use of the newest member of a group of antimicrobials so long as the currently-used drugs are effective; restricting use of a drug may become necessary where it promotes the proliferation of resistant strains.

Although clinical microbiology laboratories report microbial susceptibility test results as 'sensitive' or 'resistant' to a particular antibiotic, this is not an absolute predictor of clinical response. In a given patient's infection, variables such as absorption of the drug, its penetration to the site of infection, and its activity once there (influenced, for example, by protein binding, pH, concentration of oxygen, metabolic state of the pathogen, intracellular location and concentration of microbes) profoundly alter the likelihood that effective therapy will result.

SUPERINFECTION

When any antimicrobial drug is used, there is usually suppression of part of the normal bacterial flora of the patient which is susceptible to the drug. Often, this causes no ill effects, but sometimes a drug-resistant organism, freed from competition, proliferates to an extent which allows an infection to be established. The principal organisms responsible are *Candida albicans* and pseudomonads. But careful clinical assessment of the patient is essential, as the mere presence of such organisms in diagnostic specimens taken from a site in which they may be present as commensals does not necessarily mean they are causing disease.

TABLE 11.1 Reference data on antimicrobial drugs of choice

Infecting organism	Drug(s) of first choice	Alternative drugs
Gram-positive cocci		
*Enterococcus		
endocarditis or other severe infection	benzylpenicillin or amoxicillin + gentamicin, or streptomycin	vancomycin + gentamicin or streptomycin or linezolid
uncomplicated urinary tract infection	amoxicillin	a quinolone
*Staphylococcus aureus or epidermidis		
nonpenicillinase-producing	benzylpenicillin or phenoxymethylpenicillin	a cephalosporin or vancomycin or meropenem or erythromycin
penicillinase-producing	flucloxacillin	a cephalosporin or vancomycin or co-amoxiclav or meropenem or erythromycin
methicillin-resistant	vancomycin ± gentamicin ± rifampicin	co-trimoxazole or a tetracycline or a quinolone or sodium fusidate or rifampicin
Streptococcus pyogenes (Group A) and Groups C and G	benzylpenicillin or phenoxymethypenicillin or amoxicillin	erythromycin or a cephalosporin or vancomycin or clindamycin (the latter for necrotising fasciitis)
Streptococcus Group B	benzylpenicillin or amoxicillin	a cephalosporin or vancomycin or erythromycin
Streptococcus, viridans group (endocarditis)	benzylpenicillin ± gentamicin	vancomycin or a cephalosporin
Streptococcus, anaerobic	benzylpenicillin	metronidazole or a cephalosporin or clindamycin or vancomycin
*Streptococcus pneumoniae (pneumococcus)	benzylpenicillin or phenoxymethylpenicillin or amoxicillin	erythromycin or vancomycin or a cephalosporin or rifampicin or a quinolone (or chloramphenicol for meningitis)
Gram-negative cocci		
Moraxella (Branhamella) catarrhalis)	co-amoxiclav	erythromycin or a tetracycline
*Neisseria gonorrhoeae (gonococcus)	amoxicillin (+ probenecid) or a quinolone or ceftriaxone	spectinomycin or cefixime or cefotaxime
Neisseria meningitidis (meningococcus)	benzylpenicillin	cefotaxime or chloramphenicol
Gram-positive bacilli		
Bacillus anthracis (anthrax)	benzylpenicillin, ciprofloxacin	erythromycin or a tetracycline; prophylaxis, ciprofloxacin orally for 60 d (inhalational form) or 7 d (cutaneous form)
Clostridium difficile (pseudomembraneous colitis)	metronidazole (oral)	vancomycin (oral)
Clostridium perfringens (gas gangrene)	benzylpenicillin	metronidazole or clindamycin
Clostridium tetani (tetanus)	benzylpenicillin	a tetracycline
Corynebacterium diphtheriae (diphtheria)	erythromycin	benzylpenicillin
Listeria monocytogenes (listeriosis)	amoxicillin ± gentamicin	trimethoprim-sulfamethoxazole
Enteric Gram-negative bacilli		
*Bacteroides		
oropharyngeal strains	benzylpenicillin	metronidazole or clindamycin
gastrointestinal strains	metronidazole	co-amoxiclav or clindamycin or meropenem
*Campylobacter jejuni	erythromycin or a quinolone or a quinolone	tetracycline
*Enterobacteriaceae e.g. *Escherichia coli *Klebsiella pneumoniae *Proteus spp. *Enterobacter aerogenes		
lower urinary tract septicaemia	a quinolone or an oral cephalosporin; gentamicin or cefuroxime or cefotaxime	amoxicillin or trimethoprim or meropenem

TABLE 11.1 (continued)

Infecting organism	Drug(s) of first choice	Alternative drugs
Helicobacter pylori	amoxicillin + clarithromycin + metronidazole (with omeprazole)	amoxicillin + metronidazole + bismuth chelate or tetracycline + clarithromycin + bismuth chelate
Salmonella typhi (typhoid fever)	a quinolone	chloramphenicol or co-trimoxazole or amoxicillin or ceftriaxone
*other *Salmonella*	a quinolone	amoxicillin or co-trimoxazole or chloramphenicol or ceftriaxone
Shigella	a quinolone	trimethoprim or ampicillin
Yersinia enterocolitica (yersiniosis)	co-trimoxazole	a quinolone or gentamicin or tetracycline
Yersinia pestis (plague)	streptomycin or gentamicin	tetracycline; for prophylaxis, ciprofloxacin
Other Gram-negative bacilli		
Bordetella pertussis (whooping cough)	erythromycin	ampicillin
Brucella (brucellosis)	a tetracycline + streptomycin	co-trimoxazole or rifampicin + a tetracycline; for prophylaxis, ciprofloxacin
Calymmatobacterium granulomatis (granuloma inguinale)	a tetracycline	steptomycin or gentamicin or co-trimoxazole
Francisella tularensis (tularaemia)	streptomycin or gentamicin	for prophylaxis, ciprofloxacin
Fusobacterium	benzylpenicillin	metronidazole or clindamycin or co-amoxiclav
Gardnerella vaginalis (bacterial vaginosis)	oral metronidazole	topical clindamycin or metronidazole, or oral clindamycin or amoxicillin
Haemophilus ducreyi (chancroid)	erythromycin	a quinolone
Haemophilus influenzae		
meningitis, epiglottitis, arthritis or other serious infections	cefotaxime or ceftriaxone or amoxicillin	cefuroxime (but not for meningitis) or chloramphenicol
upper respiratory infections and bronchitis	amoxicillin	co-amoxiclav or cefuroxime
Legionella pneumophila (Legionnaires' disease)	erythromycin ± rifampicin	a quinolone ± rifampicin
Pasteurella multocida (from animal bites)	benzylpenicillin	co-amoxiclav or a cephalosporin
Pseudomonas aeruginosa		
urinary tract infection	a quinolone	ticarcillin or piperacillin or mezlocillin
other infections	ticarcillin or mezlocillin, or piperacillin or gentamicin or amikacin	ceftazidime or meropenem
Vibrio cholerae (cholera)	tetracycline	a quinolone
Acid-fast bacilli		
Mycobacterium tuberculosis	isoniazid + rifampicin + pyrazinamide + ethambutol or streptomycin	a quinolone or cycloserine or capreomycin or para-aminosalicylic acid or ethionamide
Mycobacterium leprae (leprosy)	dapsone + rifampicin ± clofazimine	ethionamide or cycloserine
Actinomycetes		
Actinomyces israelii (actinomycosis)	benzylpenicillin	a tetracycline
Nocardia	co-trimoxazole	amikacin or minocycline or meropenem
Chlamydiae		
Chlamydia psittaci (psittacosis, ornithosis)	tetracycline	a macrolide or chloramphenicol
Chlamydia trachomatis		
trachoma	azithromycin	tetracycline (topical plus oral) or a sulphonamide (topical plus oral).
inclusion conjunctivitis	erythromycin (oral or i.v.)	a sulphonamide
pneumonia	erythromycin	a sulphonamide
urethritis, cervicitis	azithromycin or doxycycline	erythromycin or ofloxacin
lymphogranuloma venereum	tetracycline	erythromycin
Chlamydia pneumoniae (TWAR strain)	tetracycline	a macrolide erythromycin

TABLE 11.1 (continued)

Infecting organism	Drug(s) of first choice	Alternative drugs
Ehrlichia		
Ehrlichia chaffeensis	doxycycline	
Mycoplasma		
Mycoplasma pneumoniae	erythromycin or tetracycline or clarithromycin or azithromycin	a quinolone
Ureaplasma urealyticum	erythromycin	tetracycline or clarithromycin
Rickettsia		
Q fever, typhus	doxycycline	chloramphenicol or a quinolone
Spirochaetes		
Borrelia burgdorferi (Lyme disease)	doxycycline or amoxicillin or cefuroxime	cefuroxime or ceftriaxone or cefotaxime or benzylpenicillin
Borrelia recurrentis (relapsing fever)	a tetracycline	benzylpenicillin
Leptospira (leptospirosis)	benzylpenicillin	a tetracycline
Treponema pallidum (syphilis)	benzylpenicillin	a tetracycline or ceftriaxone
Treponema pertenue (yaws)	benzylpenicillin	a tetracycline

* Resistance may be a problem; sensitivity tests should be performed.

Antibiotic-associated (or *Clostridium difficile-associated) colitis is an example of a superinfection. It is caused by alteration of the normal bowel flora, which allows multiplication of *Clostridium difficile* which releases several toxins which damage the mucosa of the bowel and promote excretion of fluid. Almost any antimicrobial may initiate this condition, but the drugs most commonly reported today are injectable cephalosporins and amoxi/ampicillin. Clindamycin, not commonly used in routine practice today, had an even greater propensity. It takes the form of an acute, nonspecific colitis (pseudomembranous colitis) with diarrhoeal stools containing blood or mucus, abdominal pain, leucocytosis and dehydration. A history of antibiotic use in the previous 3 weeks, even if the drug therapy has been stopped, should alert the physician to the diagnosis which is confirmed by typical appearances on proctosigmoidoscopy and detection of *Clostridium difficile* toxin in the stools. Mild cases usually respond to discontinuation of the offending antimicrobial allowing re-establishment of the patient's normal bowel flora. More severe cases merit treatment with oral metronidazole.

Opportunistic infection arises in patients whose immune systems are compromised or whose phagocytic cellular defences have been reduced by disease (e.g. AIDS, hypogammaglobulinaemia, leukaemia) or drugs (e.g. cytotoxics, adrenal steroids). Such infections involve organisms that rarely or never cause clinical disease in normal hosts. Treatment of possible infections in such patients should be prompt, initiated before the results of bacteriological tests are known and usually involving combinations of bactericidal drugs administered parenterally. Infections of this type include *Pneumocystis carinii* pneumonia and 'primary' septicaemia with gut organisms such as *Escherichia coli* and *Klebsiella* which cross the mucosa of the gut and invade the bloodstream directly. Local defences may also be compromised and allow opportunistic infection with lowly pathogens in otherwise healthy hosts: the best example is *Staphylococcus epidermidis* infection of intravenous catheters.

MASKING OF INFECTIONS

Masking of infections by chemotherapy is an important possibility. The risk cannot be entirely avoided but it can be minimised by intelligent use of antimicrobials. For example, a course of penicillin adequate to cure gonorrhoea may prevent simultaneously contracted syphilis from showing primary and secondary stages without effecting a cure and a serological test for syphilis should be done 3 months after treatment for gonorrhoea.

Drugs of choice

Table 11.1 is provided for reference. It is a summary of the choice of antimicrobial drugs and owes its form and much of its contents to Medical Letter on Drugs and Therapeutics (USA) (2000). We are grateful to the Chairman of the Editorial Board for permission to use this material which is modified for predominantly UK usage (PNB, MJB).

The table should be used to supplement the general text. Some differences will be noted between text and table for there may be no single correct procedure for each infection. Suggested alternatives do not necessarily comprise all options.

Tables on drugs for viruses, fungi, protozoa and helminths are provided in Chapter 14.

GUIDE TO FURTHER READING

Resources on the World Wide Web

The 'Disease Facts' section of the website of the UK Public Health Laboratory Service (http://www.phls.co.uk/facts/index.htm) is a valuable resource of contemporary background information on the prevalence and epidemiology of infectious diseases and antimicrobial resistance in the UK.

The American FDA website gives background information on resistance with a worldwide perspective:
http://www.fda.gov/fdac/features/795
antibio.html

The Path of Least Resistance: the Report of the Standing Medical Advisory Committee of the UK Department of Health, September 1998:
http://www.open.gov.uk/doh/smac.htm

Printed resources

Ada G 2001 Vaccines and vaccination. New England Journal of Medicine 345: 1042–1053

Antimicrobial resistance: numerous excellent leading articles and reviews on the causes and control of antimicrobial resistance published in: British Medical Journal 1998; 317: 609–616, 645–674

Colebrook L, Kenny M 1939 Treatment with prontosil for puerperal infections. Lancet 2: 1319 (a classic paper)

Fishman J A, Rubin R H 1998 Infection in organ-transplant recipients. New England Journal of Medicine 338: 1741–1751

Fletcher C 1984 First clinical use of penicillin. British Medical Journal 289: 1721–1723 (a classic paper)

Lowy F D 1998 *Staphylococcus aureus* infections. New England Journal of Medicine 339: 520–532

Kwiatkowski D 2000 Susceptibility to infection. British Medical Journal 321: 1061–1065

Leibovici L, Shraga B, Andreassen S et al 1999 How do you choose antibiotic treatment? British Medical Journal 318: 1614–1616

Lambert H P 1999 Don't keep taking the tablets. Lancet 354: 943–945

Loudon I 1987 Puerperal fever, the streptococcus, and the sulphonamides, 1911–1945. British Medical Journal 295: 485–490

Mackowiak P A 1982 The normal microbiological flora. New England Journal of Medicine 307: 83-93

Ryan E T, Wilson M E, Kain K C 2002 Illness after international travel. New England Journal of Medicine 347: 505–516

12

Antibacterial drugs

SYNOPSIS

The range of antibacterial drugs is wide and affords the clinician scope to select with knowledge of the likely or proved pathogen(s) and of factors relevant to the patient, e.g. allergy, renal disease. Antibacterial drugs are here discussed in groups primarily by their site of antibacterial action and secondly by molecular structure, because members of each structural group are usually handled by the body in a similar way and have the same range of adverse effects.

Table 11.1 (p. 211) is a general reference for this chapter.

Classification

INHIBITION OF CELL WALL SYNTHESIS

β-**lactams**, the structure of which contains a β-lactam ring. The major subdivisions are:
(a) *penicillins* whose official names usually include or end in 'cillin'
(b) *cephalosporins* and *cephamycins* which are recognised by the inclusion of 'cef' or 'ceph' in their official names. In the UK recently all these names have been standardised to begin with 'cef'.

Lesser categories of β-lactams include

— carbapenems (e.g. meropenem)
— monobactams (e.g. aztreonam) and
— β-lactamase inhibitors (e.g. clavulanic acid).

Other inhibitors of cell wall synthesis include vancomycin and teicoplanin.

INHIBITION OF PROTEIN SYNTHESIS

Aminoglycosides. The names of those that are derived from streptomyces end in 'mycin', e.g. tobramycin. Others include gentamicin (from *Micromonospora purpurea* which is not a fungus, hence the spelling as 'micin') and semisynthetic drugs, e.g. amikacin.

Tetracyclines as the name suggests are four-ringed structures and their names end in '-cycline'.

Macrolides: e.g. erythromycin. Clindamycin, structurally a lincosamide, has a similar action and overlapping antibacterial activity.
Other drugs that act by inhibiting protein synthesis include quinupristin-dalfopristin, linezolid, chloramphenicol and sodium fusidate.

INHIBITION OF NUCLEIC ACID SYNTHESIS

Sulphonamides. Usually their names contain 'sulpha' or 'sulfa'. These drugs, and trimethoprim, with which they may be combined, inhibit synthesis of nucleic acid precursors.

Quinolones are structurally related to nalidixic acid; the names of the most recently introduced members of the group end in '-oxacin', e.g. ciprofloxacin. They act by preventing DNA replication.

Azoles all contain an azole ring and the names end in '-azole', e.g. metronidazole. They act by the production of short-lived intermediate compounds which are toxic to DNA of sensitive organisms. Rifampicin inhibits bacterial DNA-dependent RNA polymerase.

Antimicrobials that are restricted to certain specific uses, i.e. tuberculosis, urinary tract infections, are described with the treatment of these conditions in Chapter 13.

Inhibition of cell wall synthesis

β-lactams

PENICILLINS

Benzylpenicillin (1942) is produced by growing one of the penicillium moulds in deep tanks. In 1957 the penicillin nucleus (6-amino-penicillanic acid) was synthesised and it became possible to add various side-chains and so to make semisynthetic penicillins with different properties. It is important to recognise that not all penicillins have the same antibacterial spectrum and that it is necessary to choose between a number of penicillins just as it is between antimicrobials of different structural groups, as is shown below.

A general account of the penicillins follows and then of the individual drugs in so far as they differ.

Mode of action. Penicillins act by inhibiting the enzymes (Penicillin Binding Proteins, PBPs) involved in the crosslinking of the peptidoglycan layer of the cell wall which protects the bacterium from its environment; incapable of withstanding

the osmotic gradient between its interior and its environment the cell swells and ruptures. Penicillins are thus bactericidal and are effective only against multiplying organisms because resting organisms are not making new cell wall. The main defence of bacteria against penicillins is to produce enzymes, β-lactamases, which open the β-lactam ring and terminate their activity. Other mechanisms that have been described include modifications to PBPs to render them unable to bind β-lactams, reduced permeability of the outer cell membrane of Gram-negative bacteria, and possession of pumps in the outer membrane which remove β-lactam molecules that manage to enter. Some particularly resistant bacteria may possess several mechanisms that act in concert. The remarkable safety and high therapeutic index of the penicillins is due to the fact that human cells, while bounded by a cell membrane, lack a cell wall. They exhibit time-dependent bacterial killing (see p. 203).

Penicillins		
Narrow spectrum (natural penicillins)	benzylpenicillin, phenoxymethylpenicillin	
Antistaphylococcal penicillins (β-lactamase resistant)	cloxacillin, flucloxacillin	
Broad spectrum	ampicillin, amoxicillin, bacampicillin.	
Mecillinam	pivmecillinam	
Monobactam (active only against Gram-negative bacteria)	aztreonam[1]	
Antipseudomonal		
Carboxypenicillin	ticarcillin	
Ureidopenicillin	piperacillin	
Penicillin-β-lactamase inhibitor combinations	co-amoxiclav, piperacillin-tazobactam, ticarcillin-clavulanate	
Carbapenems	meropenem, imipenem-cilastatin	

Pharmacokinetics. Benzylpenicillin is destroyed by gastric acid and is unsuitable for oral use. Others, e.g. phenoxymethylpenicillin, resist acid and are absorbed in the upper small bowel. The plasma $t_{\frac{1}{2}}$ of penicillins is usually < 2 h. They are distributed mainly in the body water and enter well into the

---

[1] While not strictly a penicillin, it has a similar spectrum of action including some antipseudomonal activity.

CSF if the meninges are inflamed. Penicillins are organic acids and their rapid clearance from plasma is due to secretion into renal tubular fluid by the anion transport mechanism in the kidney. Renal clearance therefore greatly exceeds the glomerular filtration rate (127 ml/min). The excretion of penicillin can be usefully delayed by concurrently giving probenecid which competes successfully for the transport mechanism. Dosage of penicillins may should be reduced for patients with severely impaired renal function.

Adverse effects. The main hazard with the penicillins is *allergic reactions*. These include itching, rashes (eczematous or urticarial), fever and angioedema. Rarely (about 1 in 10 000) there is anaphylactic shock which can be fatal (about 1 in 50 000–100 000 treatment courses). Allergies are least likely when penicillins are given orally and most likely with local application. Metabolic opening of the β-lactam ring creates a highly reactive penicilloyl group which polymerises and binds with tissue proteins to form the major antigenic determinant. The anaphylactic reaction involves specific IgE antibodies which can be detected in the plasma of susceptible persons.

There is *cross-allergy* between all the various forms of penicillin, probably due in part to their common structure, and in part to the degradation products common to them all. *Partial cross-allergy* exists between penicillins and cephalosporins (a maximum of 10%) which is of particular concern when the reaction to either group of antimicrobials has been angioedema or anaphylactic shock. Carbapenems (meropenem and imipenem-cilastatin) and the monobactam aztreonam apparently have a much lower risk of cross-reactivity.

When attempting to predict whether a patient will have an allergic reaction, a reliable history of a previous adverse response to penicillin is valuable. Immediate-type reactions such as urticaria, angiooedema and anaphylactic shock can be taken to indicate allergy, but interpretation of maculopapular rashes is more difficult. Since an alternative drug can usually be found, a penicillin is best avoided if there is suspicion of allergy, although the condition is undoubtedly overdiagnosed and may be transient (see below).

When the history of allergy is not clear-cut and it is necessary to prescribe a penicillin, the presence of IgE antibodies in serum is a useful indicator of reactions mediated by these antibodies, i.e. immediate (type 1) reactions. Additionally, an intradermal test for allergy may be performed using standard amounts of a mixture of a major determinant (metabolite) (benzylpenicilloyl polylysine) and minor determinants (such as benzylpenicillin), of the allergic reaction; appearance of a flare and weal reaction indicates a positive response. The fact that only about 10% of patients with a history of 'penicillin allergy' respond suggests that many who are so labelled are not, or are no longer, allergic to penicillin.

Other (nonallergic) adverse effects include diarrhoea due to alteration in normal intestinal flora which may progress to *Clostridium difficile*-associated diarrhoea. Neutropenia is a risk if penicillins (or other β-lactam antibiotics) are used in high dose and usually for a period of longer than 10 days. Rarely the penicillins cause anaemia, sometimes haemolytic, and thrombocytopenia or interstitial nephritis. Penicillins are presented as their sodium or potassium salts which are inevitably taken in significant amounts if high dose of antimicrobial is used. Physicians should be aware of this unexpected source of sodium or potassium, especially in patients with renal or cardiac disease. Extremely high plasma penicillin concentrations cause convulsions. Co-amoxiclav and flucloxacillin given in high doses for prolonged periods in the elderly may cause hepatic toxicity.

NARROW SPECTRUM PENICILLINS

Benzylpenicillin (penicillin G)

Benzylpenicillin (t½ 0.5 h) is used when high plasma concentrations are required. The short t½ means that reasonably spaced doses have to be large to maintain a therapeutic concentration. Fortunately, the unusually large therapeutic ratio of penicillin allows the resulting fluctuations to be tolerable.[2] Benzylpenicillin is eliminated by the

[2] Is it surprise at the answer that reduces most classes of students to silence when asked the trough:peak ratio for a drug given 6-hourly with a t½ of 0.5 h? (answer: 2^{12} = 4096).

kidney, with about 80% being actively secreted by the renal tubule and this can be blocked by probenecid, e.g. to reduce the frequency of injection for small children or for single dose therapy as in gonorrhoea.

Uses (see Table 11.1, p. 211). Benzylpenicillin is highly active against *Streptococcus pneumoniae* and the Lancefield group A, β-haemolytic streptococcus (*Streptococcus pyogenes*). Viridans streptococci are usually sensitive unless the patient has recently received penicillin. *Enterococcus faecalis* is less susceptible and, especially for endocarditis, penicillin should be combined with an aminoglycoside, usually gentamicin. This combination is synergistic unless the enterococcus is highly resistant to the aminoglycoside; such strains are becoming more frequent in hospital patients and present major difficulties in therapy. Benzylpenicillin used to be active against most strains of *Staphylococcus aureus*, but now over 90% are resistant in hospital and domiciliary practice. Benzylpenicillin is the drug of choice for infections due to *Neisseria meningitidis* (meningococcal meningitis and septicaemia), *Bacillus anthracis* (anthrax), *Clostridium perfringens* (gas gangrene) and *tetani* (tetanus), *Corynebacterium diphtheriae* (diphtheria), *Treponema pallidum* (syphilis), *Leptospira* spp. (leptospirosis) and *Actinomyces israelii* (actinomycosis). It is also the drug of choice for *Borrelia burgdorferi* (Lyme disease) in children. The sensitivity of *Neisseria gonorrhoeae* varies in different parts of the world and, in some, resistance is rife.

Adverse effects are in general uncommon, apart from allergy (above). It is salutary to reflect that the first clinically useful true antibiotic (1942) is still in use and is also amongst the least toxic. Only in patients with bacterial endocarditis, where the requirement for high doses can co-exist with reduced clearance due to immune complex glomerulonephritis, does a risk of dose related toxicity (convulsions) arise.

Preparations and dosage for injection. Benzylpenicillin may be given i.m. or i.v. (by bolus injection or by continuous infusion). For a sensitive infection, benzylpenicillin[3] 600 mg 6-hourly is enough. This is obviously inconvenient in domi-

ciliary practice where a mixture of benzylpenicillin and one of its long-acting variants may be preferred (see below).

For relatively insensitive infections and where sensitive organisms are sequestered within avascular tissue (e.g. infective endocarditis) 7.2 g are given daily i.v. in divided doses. When an infection is controlled, a change may be made to the oral route using phenoxymethylpenicillin, or amoxicillin which is more reliably absorbed in adults.

Procaine penicillin, given i.m. only, is a stable salt and liberates benzylpenicillin over 12–24 h, according to the dose administered. Usually this is 360 mg 12–24-hourly. There is no general agreement on its place in therapy, and it is no longer available in a number of countries. It is best to use benzylpenicillin in the most severe infections, especially at the outset, as procaine penicillin will not give therapeutic blood concentrations for some hours after injection and peak concentrations are much lower.

Preparations and dosage for oral use. Phenoxymethylpenicillin (penicillin V), is resistant to gastric acid and so reaches the small intestine intact where it is moderately well absorbed, sometimes erratically in adults. It is less active than benzylpenicillin against *Neisseria gonorrhoeae* and *meningitidis*, and so is unsuitable for use in gonorrhoea and meningococcal meningitis. It is a satisfactory substitute for benzylpenicillin against *Streptococcus pneumoniae* and *Streptococcus pyogenes*, especially after the acute infection has been brought under initial control by intravenous therapy. The dose is 500 mg 6-hourly.

All oral penicillins are best given on an empty stomach to avoid the absorption delay caused by food.

Antistaphylococcal penicillins

Certain bacteria produce β-lactamases which open the β-lactam ring that is common to all penicillins, and thus terminate the antibacterial activity. β-lactamases vary in their activity against different β-lactams, with side chains attached to the β-lactam

---

[3] 600 mg = 1 000 000 units, 1 mega-unit.

ring being responsible for most of these effects by stearic hindrance of access of the drug to the enzymes' active sites. Drugs that resist the action of staphylococcal β-lactamase do so by possession of an acyl side-chain. The drugs do have activity against other bacteria for which penicillin is indicated, but benzylpenicillin is substantially more active against these organisms — up to 20 times more so in the cases of pneumococci, β-haemolytic streptococci and *Neisseria*. Hence, when infection is mixed, it may be preferable to give benzylpenicillin as well as a β-lactamase-resistant drug in severe cases.

Examples of these agents include:

Flucloxacillin (t$\frac{1}{2}$ 1 h) is better absorbed and so gives higher blood concentrations than does cloxacillin. It may cause cholestatic jaundice, particularly when used for more than 2 weeks or to patients > 55 years.

Cloxacillin (t$\frac{1}{2}$ 0.5 h) resists degradation by gastric acid and is absorbed from the gut, but food markedly interferes with absorption. Recently it has been withdrawn from the market in some countries, including the UK.

Methicillin and *oxacillin*: their use is now confined to laboratory sensitivity tests. Identification of methicillin-resistant *Staphylococcus aureus* (MRSA) in patients indicates the organisms are resistant to flucloxacillin and cloxacillin, all other β-lactam antibiotics and often to other antibacterial drugs, and demands special infection-control measures.

BROAD SPECTRUM PENICILLINS

The activity of these semisynthetic penicillins extends beyond the Gram-positive and Gram-negative cocci which are susceptible to benzylpenicillin, and includes many Gram-negative bacilli. They do not resist β-lactamases and their usefulness has reduced markedly in recent years because of the increased prevalence of organisms that produce these enzymes.

As a general rule these agents are rather less active than benzylpenicillin against Gram-positive cocci, but more active than the β-lactamase-resistant penicillins (above). They have useful activity against *Enterococcus faecalis* and many strains of *Haemophilus influenzae*. *Enterobacteriaceae* are variably sensitive and laboratory testing for sensitivity is important. The differences between the members of this group are pharmacological rather than bacteriological.

Amoxicillin (t$\frac{1}{2}$ 1 h; previously known as amoxycillin) is a structural analogue of ampicillin (below) and is better absorbed from the gut (especially after food), and for the same dose achieves approximately double the plasma concentration. Diarrhoea is less frequent with amoxicillin than with ampicillin. The oral dose is 250 mg 8-hourly; a parenteral form is available but offers no advantage over ampicillin. For oral use, however, amoxicillin is preferred because of its greater bioavailability and fewer adverse effects.

Co-amoxiclav (Augmentin). *Clavulanic acid* is a β-lactam molecule which has little intrinsic antibacterial activity but binds irreversibly to β-lactamases. Thereby it competitively protects the penicillin, so potentiating it against bacteria which owe their resistance to production of β-lactamases, i.e. clavulanic acid acts as a 'suicide' inhibitor. It is formulated in tablets as its potassium salt (equivalent to 125 mg of clavulanic acid) in combination with amoxicillin (250 or 500 mg), as co-amoxiclav, and is a satisfactory oral treatment for infections due to β-lactamase-producing organisms, notably in the respiratory or urogenital tracts. It should be used when β-lactamase-producing amoxicillin resistant organisms are either suspected or proven by culture. These include many strains of *Staphylococcus aureus*, many strains of *Escherichia coli* and an increasing number of strains of *Haemophilus influenzae*. It also has useful activity against β-lactamase-producing *Bacteroides* spp. The t$\frac{1}{2}$ is 1 h and the dose one tablet 8-hourly.

Ampicillin (t$\frac{1}{2}$ 1 h) is acid-stable and is moderately well absorbed when swallowed. The oral dose is 250 mg–1 g 6–8-hourly; or i.m. or i.v. 500 mg 4–6-hourly. Approximately one-third of a dose appears unchanged in the urine. The drug is concentrated in the bile.

Adverse effects. Ampicillin may cause diarrhoea but the incidence (12%) is less with amoxicillin. Ampicillin and amoxicillin are the commonest antibiotics to be associated with *Clostridium difficile* diarrhoea, although this is related to the frequency of their use rather than to their innate risk of causing the disease (this is probably highest for the injectable cephalosporins). Ampicillin and its analogues have a peculiar capacity to cause a macular rash resembling measles or rubella, usually un-accompanied by other signs of allergy. These rashes are very common in patients with disease of the lymphoid system, notably *infectious mononucleosis* and lymphoid leukaemia. A macular rash should not be taken to imply allergy to other penicillins which tend to cause a true urticarial reaction. Patients with renal failure and those taking allopurinol for hyperuricaemia also seem more prone to ampicillin rashes. Cholestatic jaundice has been associated with use of co-amoxiclav even up to 6 weeks after cessation of the drug; the clavulanic acid may be responsible.

MECILLINAM

Pivmecillinam (t$\frac{1}{2}$ 1 h) is an oral agent closely related to the broad spectrum penicillins but with differing antibacterial activity by virtue of having a high affinity for penicillin binding protein. It is active against Gram-negative organisms including β-lactamase-producing *Enterobacteriaceae* but is inactive against *Pseudomonas aeruginosa* and its relatives, and against Gram-positive organisms. *Pivmecillinam* is hydrolysed in vivo to the active form *mecillinam* (which is poorly absorbed by mouth). It has been used to treat urinary tract infection. Diarrhoea and abdominal pain may occur.

MONOBACTAM

Aztreonam (t$\frac{1}{2}$ 2 h) is the first member of this class of β-lactam antibiotic. It is active against Gram-negative organisms including *Pseudomonas aeruginosa*, *Haemophilus influenzae* and *Neisseria meningitidis* and *gonorrhoeae*. Aztreonam is used to treat septicaemia and complicated urinary tract infections, Gram-negative lower urinary tract infections and gonorrhoea.

Adverse effects include reactions at the site of infusion, rashes, gastrointestinal upset, hepatitis, thrombocytopenia and neutropenia. It appears to have a remarkably low risk of causing β-lactam allergy, and may be used with caution in some penicillin-allergic patients.

ANTIPSEUDOMONAL PENICILLINS

Carboxypenicillins

These in general have the same antibacterial spectrum as ampicillin (and are susceptible to β-lactamases), but have the additional capacity to destroy *Pseudomonas aeruginosa* and indole-positive *Proteus* spp.

Ticarcillin (t$\frac{1}{2}$ 1 h) is presented in combination with clavulanic acid (as Timentin), so to provide greater activity against β-lactamase-producing organisms. It is given by i.m. or slow i.v. injection or by rapid i.v. infusion. Note that ticarcillin is presented as its disodium salt and each 1 g delivers about 5.4 mmol of sodium, which should be borne in mind when treating patients with impaired cardiac or renal function. Carboxypenicillins inactivate aminoglycosides if both drugs are administered in the same syringe or intravenous infusion system.

Ureidopenicillins

These are adapted from the ampicillin molecule, with a side-chain derived from urea. Their major advantages over the carboxypenicillins are higher efficacy against *Pseudomonas aeruginosa* and the fact that as monosodium salts they deliver on average about 2 mmol of sodium per gram of antimicrobial (see above) and are thus safer where sodium over-load should particularly be avoided. They are degraded by many β-lactamases. Ureidopenicillins must be administered parenterally and are eliminated mainly in the urine. Accumulation in patients with poor renal function is less than with other penicillins as 25% is excreted in the bile. An unusual feature of their kinetics is that, as the dose is increased, the plasma concentration rises disproportionately, i.e. they exhibit *saturation (zero-order) kinetics.*

For pseudomonas septicaemia, a ureidopenicillin plus an aminoglycoside provides a synergistic effect but the co-administration in the same fluid results in inactivation of the aminoglycoside (as with carboxypenicillins, above).

Azlocillin (t$\frac{1}{2}$ 1 h), highly effective against *Pseudomonas aeruginosa* infections, is less so than other ureidopenicillins against other common Gram-negative organisms and has recently been withdrawn from the market in many countries.

Piperacillin ($t\frac{1}{2}$ 1 h) has the same or slightly greater activity as azlocillin against *Pseudomonas aeruginosa* but is more effective against the common Gram-negative organisms. It is also available as a combination with the β-lactamase inhibitor tazobactam (as tazocin).

Cephalosporins

Cephalosporins were first obtained from a filamentous fungus *Cephalosporium* cultured from the sea near a Sardinian sewage outfall in 1945; their molecular structure is closely related to that of penicillin, and many semisynthetic forms have been introduced. They now comprise a group of antibiotics having a wide range of activity and low toxicity. The term cephalosporins will be used here in a general sense although some are strictly cephamycins, e.g. cefoxitin and cefotetan.

Mode of action is that of the β-lactams, i.e. cephalosporins impair bacterial cell wall synthesis and hence are bactericidal. They exhibit time-dependent bacterial killing (see p. 203).

Addition of various side-chains on the cephalosporin molecule confers variety in pharmacokinetic and antibacterial activities. The β-lactam ring can be protected by such structural manoeuvring, which results in compounds with improved activity against Gram-negative organisms; a common corollary is that such agents lose some anti-Gram-positive activity. The cephalosporins resist attack by β-lactamases but bacteria develop resistance to them by other means. Methicillin-resistant *Staphylococcus aureus* (MRSA) should be considered resistant to all cephalosporins.

Pharmacokinetics. Usually, cephalosporins are excreted unchanged in the urine, but some, including cefotaxime, form a desacetyl metabolite which possesses some antibacterial activity. Many are actively secreted by the renal tubule, a process which can be blocked with probenecid. As a rule, the dose of cephalosporins should be reduced in

patients with poor renal function. Cephalosporins in general have a $t\frac{1}{2}$ of 1–4 h although there are exceptions (e.g. ceftriaxone, $t\frac{1}{2}$ 8 h). Wide distribution in the body allows treatment of infection at most sites, including bone, soft tissue, muscle and (in some cases) CSF. Data on individual cephalosporins appear in Table 12.1.

Classification and uses. The cephalosporins are conventionally categorised by generations having broadly similar antibacterial and pharmacokinetic properties; newer agents have rendered this classification less precise but it retains sufficient usefulness to be presented in Table 12.1.

Adverse effects. Cephalosporins are well tolerated. The most usual unwanted effects are allergic reactions of the penicillin type. There is cross-allergy between penicillins and cephalosporins involving about 7% of patients; if a patient has had a severe or immediate allergic reaction or if serum or skin testing for penicillin allergy is positive (see p. 217), then a cephalosporin should not be used. Pain may be experienced at the sites of i.v. or i.m. injection. If cephalosporins are continued for more than 2 weeks, thrombocytopenia, haemolytic anaemia, neutropenia, interstitial nephritis or abnormal liver function tests may occur especially at high dosage; these reverse on stopping the drug. The broad spectrum of activity of the third generation cephalosporins may predispose to opportunist infection with resistant bacteria or *Candida albicans* and to *Clostridium difficile* diarrhoea. Ceftriaxone achieves high concentrations in bile and, as the calcium salt, may precipitate to cause symptoms resembling cholelithiasis (biliary pseudolithiasis). Cefamandole may cause prothrombin deficiency and a disulfiram-like reaction after ingestion of alcohol.

Other β-lactam antibacterials

CARBAPENEMS

Members of this group have the widest spectrum of all currently available antimicrobials, being

TABLE 12.1 The cephalosporins

Drug	$t^{1/2}$ (h)	Excretion in urine (%)	Comment
First generation			
Parenteral			
Cefazolin	2	90	May be used for staphylococcal infections but generally have been replaced by the newer cephalosporins.
Cefradine (also oral)	1	86	
Oral			
Cefaclor	1	86	All very similar. Effective against the common respiratory pathogens
Cefadroxil	2	88	*Streptococcus pneumoniae* and *Moraxella catarrhalis* but (excepting cefaclor)
Cefalexin	1	88	have poor activity against *Haemophilus influenzae*. Also active against *Escherichia coli* which, increasingly, is demonstrating resistance to amoxicillin and trimethoprim. May be used for uncomplicated upper and lower respiratory tract, urinary tract and soft tissue infections, and also as follow-on treatment once parenteral drugs have brought an infection under control.
Second generation			
Parenteral			
Cefoxitin (a cephamycin) (Cefotetan is similar)	1	90	More resistant to β-lactamases than the first-generation drugs and active against *Staphylococcus aureus*, *Streptococcus pyogenes*, *Streptococcus*
Cefuroxime (also oral)	1	80	*pneumoniae*, *Neisseria* spp., *Haemophilus influenzae* and many
Cefamandole	1	75	*Enterobacteriaceae*. Cefoxitin also kills *Bacteroides fragilis* and is effective in abdominal and pelvic infections. Cefuroxime may be given for community-acquired pneumonia, commonly due to *Strep pneumoniae* (not when causal organism is *Mycoplasma pneumoniae*, *Legionella* or *Chlamydia*). The oral form, *cefuroxime axetil*, is also used for the range of infections listed for the first-generation oral cephalosporins (above)
Third generation			
Parenteral			
Cefodizime	3	80	More effective than the second-generation drugs against Gram-negative
Cefotaxime	1	60	organisms whilst retaining useful activity against Gram-positive bacteria.
Ceftazidime	2	88	Cefotaxime, ceftizoxime and ceftriaxone are used for serious infections
Ceftizoxime	1	90	such as septicaemia, pneumonia, and for meningitis. Ceftriaxone also used
Ceftriaxone	8	56 (44 bile)	for gonorrhoea and Lyme disease.
Oral			
Cefixime	4	23 (77 bile)	Active against a range of Gram-positive and Gram-negative organisms
Ceftibuten	2	65	including *Staphylococcus aureus* (excepting cefixime), *Streptococcus pyogenes*,
Cefpodoxime proxetil	2	80	*Streptococcus pneumoniae*, *Neisseria* spp., *Haemophilus influenzae* and (excepting cefpodoxime) many *Enterobacteriaceae*. Used to treat urinary, upper and lower respiratory tract infections.

bactericidal against most Gram-positive and Gram-negative aerobic and anaerobic pathogenic bacteria. They are resistant to hydrolysis by most β-lactamases. Only occasional pseudomonas relatives are naturally resistant, and acquired resistance is uncommon in all species.

Imipenem

Imipenem ($t^{1/2}$ 1 h) is inactivated by metabolism in the kidney to products that are potentially toxic to renal tubules; combining imipenem with cilastatin (as Primaxin), a specific inhibitor of dihydropeptidase—the enzyme responsible for its renal metabolism—prevents both inactivation and toxicity.

Imipenem is used to treat septicaemia, particularly of renal origin, intra-abdominal infection and nosocomial pneumonia. In terms of imipenem, 1–2 g/d is given by i.v. infusion in 3–4 doses; reduced doses are recommended when renal function is impaired.

Adverse effects. It may cause gastrointestinal upset including nausea, blood disorders, allergic reactions, confusion and convulsions.

Meropenem (t½ 1 h) is similar to imipenem but is stable to renal dihydropeptidase and can therefore be given without cilastatin. It penetrates into the CSF and is not associated with nausea or convulsions.

Other inhibitors of cell wall synthesis

Vancomycin

Vancomycin (t½ 8 h), a 'glycopeptide' or 'peptolide', acts on multiplying organisms by inhibiting cell wall formation at a site different from the β-lactam antibacterials. It is bactericidal against most strains of clostridia (including *Clostridium difficile*), almost all strains of *Staphylococcus aureus* (including those that produce β-lactamase and methicillin-resistant strains), coagulase-negative staphylococci, viridans group streptococci and enterococci, i.e. several organisms that cause endocarditis.

Vancomycin is poorly absorbed from the gut and is given i.v. for systemic infections, as there is no satisfactory i.m. preparation. It distributes effectively into body tissues and is eliminated by the kidney.

Uses. Vancomycin is effective in cases of antibiotic-associated pseudomembranous colitis (caused by *Clostridium difficile* or, less commonly, staphylococci) in a dose of 125 mg 6-hourly by mouth (although oral metronidazole is preferred, being as effective and less costly). Combined with an aminoglycoside, it may be given i.v. for streptococcal endocarditis in patients who are allergic to benzylpenicillin. It may also be used for serious infection with multiply-resistant staphylococci. Dosing is guided by plasma concentration monitoring.

Adverse effects. The main disadvantage to vancomycin is auditory damage. Tinnitus and deafness may improve if the drug is stopped. Nephrotoxicity and allergic reactions also occur. Rapid i.v. infusion may cause a maculopapular rash possibly due to histamine release (the 'red person' syndrome).

Teicoplanin is structurally related to vancomycin and is active against Gram-positive bacteria. The t½ of 50 h allows once daily i.v. or i.m. administration. It is used for serious infection with Gram-positive bacteria including endocarditis, and for peritonitis in patients undergoing chronic ambulatory peritoneal dialysis. It is less likely to cause oto- or nephrotoxicity than vancomycin, but serum monitoring is required for severely ill patients and those with changing renal function to assure adequate serum concentrations are being achieved.

A rising prevalence of clinically-significant resistance and decrease in susceptibility to vancomycin and teicoplanin has become a serious worry recently with the emergence of vancomycin-resistant enterococci (VRE) or glycopeptide-resistant enterococci (GRE) and vancomycin-intermediate resistant *Staphylococcus aureus* (VISA or GISA). Only one naturally occurring strain of vancomycin resistant *Staphylococcus aureus* has been reported, but these will no doubt emerge in time and the appearance of antibiotics active against multiply resistant Gram-positive bacteria, e.g. quinupristin-dalfopristin and linezolid (see p. 229), is welcome.

Cycloserine is used for drug-resistant tuberculosis (see p. 253).

Inhibition of protein synthesis

Aminoglycosides

In the purposeful search that followed the demonstration of the clinical efficacy of penicillin, streptomycin was obtained from *Streptomyces griseus* in 1944, cultured from a heavily manured field, and also from a chicken's throat. Aminoglycosides resemble each other in their mode of action, and their pharmacokinetic, therapeutic and toxic properties. The main differences in usage reflect variation in their range of antibacterial activity; cross-resistance is variable.

Mode of action. The aminoglycosides act inside the cell by binding to the ribosomes in such a way that incorrect amino acid sequences are entered into peptide chains. The abnormal proteins which result are fatal to the microbe, i.e. aminoglycosides are bactericidal and exhibit concentration-dependent bacterial killing (see p. 203).

Pharmacokinetics. Aminoglycosides are water-soluble and do not readily cross cell membranes. Poor absorption from the intestine necessitates their administration i.v. or i.m. for systemic use and they distribute mainly to the extracellular fluid; transfer into the cerebrospinal fluid is poor even when the meninges are inflamed. Their t$\frac{1}{2}$ is 2–5 h.

Aminoglycosides are eliminated unchanged mainly by glomerular filtration, and attain high concentrations in the urine. Significant accumulation occurs in the renal cortex unless there is severe renal parenchymal disease. Plasma concentration should be measured regularly (and frequently in renally-impaired patients) and it is good practice to monitor approximately twice weekly even if renal function is normal. With prolonged therapy, e.g. endocarditis (gentamicin), monitoring must be meticulous. The dose should be reduced to compensate for varying degrees of renal impairment, including that of normal aging. Numerous successful legal actions by patients against doctors for negligence in this area have resulted in large compensation payments, especially for ototoxicity.

Current practice is to administer aminoglycosides as a single daily dose rather than as twice or thrice daily doses. Algorithms are available to guide such dosing according to patients' weight and renal function, and in this case only trough concentrations need to be assayed. Single daily dose therapy is probably less oto- and nephrotoxic than divided dose regimens, and appears to be as effective. The immediate high plasma concentrations that result from single daily dosing are advantageous, e.g. for acutely ill septicaemic patients, as aminoglycosides exhibit concentration-dependent killing (see p. 203).

Antibacterial activity. Aminoglycosides are in general active against staphylococci and aerobic Gram-negative organisms including almost all the *Enterobacteriaceae*; individual differences in activity are given below. Bacterial resistance to aminoglycosides is an increasing but patchily-distributed problem, notably by acquisition of plasmids (see p. 209) which carry genes coding for the formation of drug-destroying enzymes. Gentamicin resistance is rare in community-acquired pathogens in many hospitals in the UK.

Uses include:

- *Gram-negative bacillary infection,* particularly septicaemia, renal, pelvic and abdominal sepsis. Gentamicin remains the drug of choice but tobramycin may be preferred for infections caused by *Pseudomonas aeruginosa*. Amikacin has the widest antibacterial spectrum of the aminoglycosides but is best reserved for infection caused by gentamicin-resistant organisms. As long as local resistance rates are low, an aminoglycoside may be included in the initial best-guess regimen for treatment of serious septicaemia before the causative organism(s) is identified. A potentially less toxic antibiotic may be substituted when culture results are known (48–72 h), and toxicity is very rare after such a short course.
- *Bacterial endocarditis.* An aminoglycoside, usually gentamicin, should comprise part of the antimicrobial combination for enterococcal, streptococcal or staphylococcal infection of the heart valves, and for the therapy of clinical endocarditis which fails to yield a positive blood culture.
- *Other infections:* tuberculosis, tularaemia, plague, brucellosis.
- *Topical uses.* Neomycin and framycetin, whilst too toxic for systemic use, are effective for topical treatment of infections of the conjunctiva or external ear. They are sometimes used in antimicrobial combinations selectively to decontaminate the bowel of patients who are to receive intense immunosuppressive therapy. Tobramycin is given by inhalation for therapy of infective exacerbations of cystic fibrosis. Sufficient systemic absorption may occur to recommend assay of serum concentrations in such patients.

Adverse effects. Aminoglycoside toxicity is a risk when the dose administered is high or of long duration, and the risk is higher if renal clearance is inefficient (because of disease or age), other potentially nephrotoxic drugs are co-administered (e.g.

loop diuretics, amphotericin B) or the patient is dehydrated. It may take the following forms:

- *Ototoxicity.* Both vestibular and auditory damage may occur, causing hearing loss, vertigo and tinnitus which may be permanent (see above). Tinnitus may give warning of auditory nerve damage. Early signs of vestibular toxicity include motion-related headache, dizziness or nausea. Serious ototoxicity can occur with topical application, including ear-drops.
- *Nephrotoxicity.* Dose-related changes, which are usually reversible, occur in renal tubular cells, where aminoglycosides accumulate. Low blood pressure, loop diuretics and advanced age are recognised as added risk factors.
- *Neuromuscular blockade.* Aminoglycosides may impair neuromuscular transmission and aggravate (or reveal) myasthenia gravis, or cause a transient myasthenic syndrome in patients whose neuromuscular transmission is normal.
- *Other reactions* include rashes, and haematological abnormalities, including marrow depression, haemolytic anaemia and bleeding due to antagonism of factor V.

INDIVIDUAL AMINOGLYCOSIDES

Gentamicin is active against aerobic Gram-negative bacilli including *Escherichia coli*, *Enterobacter*, *Klebsiella*, *Proteus* (indole negative and positive) and *Pseudomonas aeruginosa*. In the best-guess treatment of septicaemia, gentamicin should be combined with a β-lactam antibiotic or an antianaerobic agent, e.g. metronidazole, or with both. Gentamicin is a drug of choice for serious Gram-negative septicaemia and it is effective in combination for abdominal and pelvic sepsis. In streptococcal and enterococcal endocarditis gentamicin is combined with benzylpenicillin, in staphylococcal endocarditis with an antistaphylococcal penicillin, and in enterococcal endocarditis with ampicillin (true synergy is seen provided the enterococcus is not highly resistant to gentamicin).

Dose is 3–5 mg/kg body weight per day (the highest dose for more serious infections) either as a single dose or in three equally divided doses. The rationale behind single dose administration is to achieve high peak plasma concentrations (10–14 mg/l, which correlate with therapeutic efficacy) and more time at lower trough concentrations (16 h at < 1 mg/l, which are associated with reduced risk of toxicity). Therapy should rarely exceed 7 days. Patients with cystic fibrosis eliminate gentamicin rapidly and require higher doses. Gentamicin applied to the eye gives effective corneal and aqueous humour concentrations.

Tobramycin is similar to gentamicin; it is more active against most strains of *Pseudomonas aeruginosa* and may be less nephrotoxic. It is commonly administered via a nebulizer for treatment of infective exacerbations of cystic fibrosis caused by pseudomonads or *Enterobacteriaceae*.

Amikacin is mainly of value because it is more resistant to aminoglycoside-inactivating bacterial enzymes than is gentamicin. Since it is more costly, amikacin is reserved for treatment of infections with gentamicin-resistant organisms. Peak plasma concentrations should be kept between 20–30 mg/l and trough concentrations below 10 mg/l.

Netilmicin is a semisynthetic aminoglycoside which is active against some strains of bacteria that resist gentamicin and tobramycin; evidence suggests that it may be less oto- and nephrotoxic.

Neomycin is principally used topically for skin, eye and ear infections and, by some, to reduce the bacterial load in the colon in preparation for bowel surgery, or in hepatic failure. Enough absorption can occur from both oral and topical use to cause eighth cranial nerve damage, especially if there is renal impairment.

Framycetin is similar to neomycin in use and in toxicity.

Streptomycin, superseded as a first-line choice for tuberculosis, may be used to kill resistant strains of the organism.

Spectinomycin is active against Gram-negative organisms but its clinical use is confined to gonorrhoea in patients allergic to penicillin, or to infection with gonococci that are β-lactam drug resistant. The steady growth of resistant gonococci, particularly β-lactamase-producing strains, suggests that spectinomycin will continue to have a significant role in this disease, although resistance to it is reported.

Tetracyclines

Tetracyclines have a broad range of antimicrobial activity and differences between the individual members are in general small.

Mode of action. Tetracyclines interfere with protein synthesis by binding to bacterial ribosomes and their selective action is due to higher uptake by bacterial than by human cells. They are bacteriostatic.

Pharmacokinetics. Most tetracyclines are only partially absorbed from the alimentary tract, enough remaining in the intestine to alter the flora and cause diarrhoea. They are distributed throughout the body and cross the placenta. Tetracyclines in general are excreted mainly unchanged in the urine and should be avoided when renal function is severely impaired. Exceptionally, doxycycline and minocycline are eliminated by nonrenal routes and are preferred for patients with impaired renal function.

Uses. Tetracyclines are active against nearly all Gram-positive and Gram-negative pathogenic bacteria, but increasing bacterial resistance and low innate activity limit their clinical use. They remain drugs of first choice for infection with chlamydiae (psittacosis, trachoma, pelvic inflammatory disease, lymphogranuloma venereum), mycoplasma (pneumonia), rickettsiae (Q fever, typhus), *Vibrio cholerae* (cholera) and borreliae (Lyme disease, relapsing fever) (for use in acne, see p. 313). Their most common other uses are as second line therapy of minor skin and soft tissue infections especially in β-lactam allergic patients; surprisingly, many MRSA strains currently remain susceptible to tetracyclines in the UK.

An unexpected use for a tetracycline is in the treatment of chronic hyponatraemia due to the syndrome of inappropriate antidiuretic hormone secretion (SIADH) when water restriction has failed. Demeclocycline produces a state of unresponsiveness to ADH, probably by inhibiting the formation and action of cyclic AMP in the renal tubule. It is effective and convenient to use in SIADH because this action is both dose-dependent and reversible.

Adverse reactions. Heartburn, nausea and vomiting due to gastric irritation are common, and attempts to reduce this with milk or antacids impair absorption of tetracyclines (see below). Loose bowel movements occur, due to alteration of the bowel flora, and this sometimes develops into diarrhoea and opportunistic infection (antibiotic associated or pseudomembranous colitis) may supervene. Disorders of epithelial surfaces, perhaps due partly to vitamin B complex deficiency and partly due to mild opportunistic infection with yeasts and moulds, lead to sore mouth and throat, black hairy tongue, dysphagia and perianal soreness. Vitamin B preparations may prevent or arrest alimentary tract symptoms.

Tetracyclines are selectively taken up in the teeth and growing bones of the fetus and of children, due to their chelating properties with calcium phosphate. This causes hypoplasia of dental enamel with pitting, cusp malformation, yellow or brown pigmentation and increased susceptibility to caries. After the fourteenth week of pregnancy and in the first few months of life even short courses can be damaging. Prevention of discolouration of the permanent front teeth requires that tetracyclines be avoided from the last 2 months of pregnancy to 4 years, and of other teeth to 8 years of age (or 12 years if the third molars are valued). Prolonged tetracycline therapy can also stain the fingernails at all ages.

The effects on the bones after they are formed in the fetus are of less clinical importance because pigmentation has no cosmetic disadvantage and a short exposure to tetracycline is unlikely significantly to delay growth.

Since tetracyclines act by inhibiting bacterial protein synthesis, the same effect occurring in man causes blood urea to rise (the antianabolic effect). The increased nitrogen load can be clinically important in renal failure and in the elderly.

Tetracyclines induce photosensitisation and other rashes. Liver and pancreatic damage can occur, especially in pregnancy and with renal disease, when the drugs have been given i.v. Rarely tetracyclines cause benign intracranial hypertension, dizziness and other neurological reactions.

Interactions. Dairy products reduce absorption to a degree but antacids and iron preparations do so much more, by chelation to calcium, aluminium and iron.

INDIVIDUAL TETRACYCLINES

Tetracycline may be taken as representative of most tetracyclines. Because of incomplete absorption from the gut i.v. doses need be less than half of the oral dose to be similarly effective. Tetracycline is eliminated by the kidney and in the bile ($t\frac{1}{2}$ 6 h). The dose is 250–500 mg 6-hourly by mouth.

Doxycycline is well absorbed from the gut, even after food. It is excreted in the bile, in the faeces which it re-enters by diffusing across the small intestinal wall and, to some extent, in the urine ($t\frac{1}{2}$ 16 h). These nonrenal mechanisms compensate effectively when renal function is impaired and no reduction of dose is necessary; 200 mg is given on the first day, then 100 mg/d.

Minocycline differs from other tetracyclines in that its antibacterial spectrum includes *Neisseria meningitidis* and it has been used for meningococcal prophylaxis. It is well absorbed from the gut, even after a meal, partly metabolised in the liver and partly excreted in the bile and urine ($t\frac{1}{2}$ 15 h). Dose reduction is not necessary when renal function is impaired; 200 mg initially is followed by 100 mg 12-hourly. Minocycline but not other tetracyclines may cause a reversible vestibular disturbance with dizziness, tinnitus and impaired balance, especially in women.

Other tetracyclines include demeclocycline (see above), lymecycline and oxytetracycline.

Macrolides

Erythromycin

Erythromycin ($t\frac{1}{2}$ 2–4 h) binds to bacterial ribosomes and interferes with protein synthesis; it is bacteriostatic and exhibits time-dependent bacterial killing (see p. 203). It is effective against Gram-positive organisms because these accumulate the drug more efficiently than Gram-negative organisms, and its antibacterial spectrum is similar, but not identical, to that of penicillin.

Absorption after oral administration is best with erythromycin estolate, even if there is food in the stomach. Hydrolysis of the estolate in the body releases the active erythromycin which diffuses readily into most tissues; the $t\frac{1}{2}$ is dose-dependent and elimination is almost exclusively in the bile and faeces.

Uses. Erythromycin is the drug of choice for:

- *Mycoplasma pneumoniae* in children, although in adults a tetracycline may be preferred
- *Legionella* spp. (including Legionnaires' disease), with or without rifampicin
- Diphtheria (including carriers), pertussis and for some chlamydial infections.

In gastroenteritis caused by *Campylobacter jejuni*, erythromycin is effective in eliminating the organism from the faeces, although it does not reduce the duration of the symptoms unless given very early in the course of the illness.

Erythromycin is an effective alternative choice for penicillin-allergic patients infected with *Staphylococcus aureus*, *Streptococcus pyogenes*, *Streptococcus pneumoniae* or *Treponema pallidum*.

Acne; see page 313.

Dose is 250 mg 6-hourly or twice this in serious infection and four times this for Legionnaires' disease. The ethylsuccinate and stearate esters of erythromycin produce lower plasma concentrations of the active drug than does the same dose of the estolate.

Adverse reactions. Erythromycin is remarkably nontoxic, but the estolate can cause cholestatic hepatitis with abdominal pain and fever which may be confused with viral hepatitis, acute cholecystitis or acute pancreatitis. This is probably an allergy, and recovery is usual but the estolate should not be given to a patient with liver disease. Other allergies are rare. Gastrointestinal disturbances occur frequently (up to 28%), particularly diarrhoea and nausea, but, with the antibacterial spectrum being narrower than with tetracycline, opportunistic infection is less troublesome.

Interactions. Erythromycin and the other macrolides are enzyme inhibitors and interfere with the metabolic inactivation of some drugs, e.g. warfarin, carbamazepine, theophylline, disopyramide, increasing their effects. Reduced inactivation of terfenadine may lead to serious cardiac arrhythmias, and of ergot alkaloids may cause ergotism.

Clarithromycin acts like erythromycin and has a similar spectrum of antibacterial activity, i.e. mainly against Gram-positive organisms, although it is usefully more active against *Haemophilus influenzae*. The usual dose is 250 mg 12-hourly or twice that for serious infections. It is rapidly and completely absorbed from the gastrointestinal tract, 60% of a dose is inactivated by metabolism which is saturable (note that the $t\frac{1}{2}$ increases with dose: 3 h after 250 mg, 9 h after 1200 mg) and the remainder is eliminated in the urine. Clarithromycin is used for respiratory tract infections including atypical pneumonias and soft tissue infections. It is concentrated intracellularly, achieving concentrations which allow effective therapy in combination for mycobacterial infections such as *Mycobacterium avium-intracellulare* in patients with AIDS and with pyrimethamine for some *Toxoplasma* infections (see p. 275). It causes fewer gastrointestinal tract adverse effects (7%) than erythromycin. Interactions: see erythromycin (above).

Azithromycin is usefully active against a number of important Gram-negative organisms including *Haemophilus influenzae* and *Neisseria gonorrhoeae*, and also against *Chlamydiae*, but is a little less effective than erythromycin against Gram-positive organisms.

Azithromycin achieves high concentrations in tissues relative to those in plasma. It remains largely unmetabolised and is excreted in the bile and faeces ($t\frac{1}{2}$ 50h). Azithromycin is used to treat respiratory tract and soft tissue infections, and sexually transmitted diseases, especially genital *Chlamydia* infections. Gastrointestinal effects (9%) are less than with erythromycin but diarrhoea, nausea and abdominal pain occur. In view of its high hepatic excretion use in patients with liver disease should be avoided. *Interactions:* see erythromycin (above).

Clindamycin, structurally a lincosamide rather than a macrolide, binds to bacterial ribosomes to inhibit protein synthesis. Its antibacterial spectrum is similar to that of erythromycin (with which there is partial cross-resistance) and benzylpenicillin (but includes penicillin-resistant staphylococci); it has the useful additional property of efficacy against anaerobes such as *Bacteroides fragilis* which are involved in gut-associated sepsis. Clindamycin is well absorbed from the gut and distributes to most body tissues including bone. The drug is metabolised by the liver and enterohepatic cycling occurs with bile concentrations 2–5 times those of plasma ($t\frac{1}{2}$ 3 h). Significant excretion of metabolites occurs via the gut.

Clindamycin is used for staphylococcal bone and joint infections, dental infections and serious intra-abdominal sepsis (in the latter case, it is usually combined with an agent active against Gram-negative pathogens such as gentamicin). It is also a second choice in combination for some *Toxoplasma* infections (see p. 275). Topical preparations are used for therapy of severe acne and non-sexually transmitted infection of the genital tract in women. It is the antibiotic of choice for streptococcal necrotising fasciitis and other serious invasive *Streptococcus pyogenes* infections, although surgical resection of affected tissue plays a prime role.

The most serious **adverse effect** is antibiotic-associated (pseudomembranous) colitis (see p. 210) usually due to opportunistic infection of the bowel with *Clostridium difficile* which produces an enterotoxin; clindamycin should be stopped if any diarrhoea occurs.

Other inhibitors of protein synthesis

Chloramphenicol

Chloramphenicol has a broad spectrum of activity and is primarily bacteriostatic, but may be bactericidal against *Haemophilus influenzae*, *Neisseria meningitidis* and *Streptococcus pneumoniae*.

Pharmacokinetics. For oral use, chloramphenicol is available as the base in capsules to reduce the bitter taste and for i.v. or i.m. use as the succinate ester which is soluble. Chloramphenicol succinate is hydrolysed to the active chloramphenicol and there is much individual variation in the capacity to perform this reaction. Chloramphenicol is inactivated by conjugation with glucuronic acid in the liver (t½ 5 h in adults). In the neonate, the process of glucuronidation is slow, and plasma concentrations are extremely variable especially in premature neonates (see below). Monitoring of plasma concentration is therefore essential if it is ever used in the neonate and infant, and in the adult with serious infection. Chloramphenicol penetrates well into all tissues, including the CSF and brain, even in the absence of meningeal inflammation.

Uses. The decision to use chloramphenicol for systemic infection is influenced by its rare but serious toxic effects (see below). Its role in meningitis and brain abscess has largely been superseded by broad-spectrum cephalosporins such as cefotaxime and ceftriaxone, but it is a second-line agent for these indications, and for haemophilus epiglottitis in children. Chloramphenicol may be used for salmonella infections (typhoid fever, salmonella septicaemia) but ciprofloxacin is now preferred. Topical administration is effective for bacterial conjunctivitis.

Adverse effects include gastrointestinal upset which tends to be mild. Optic and peripheral neuritis occur with prolonged use (which should be avoided) but are uncommon. The systemic use of chloramphenicol is dominated by the fact that it can cause rare (between 1:18 000–100 000 courses) though serious bone marrow damage. This is of two types:

1. a dose-dependent, reversible depression of erythrocyte, platelet and leucocyte formation that occurs early in treatment (type A adverse drug reaction);
2. an idiosyncratic (probably genetically determined), non-dose-related, and usually fatal aplastic anaemia which tends to develop during, or even weeks after, prolonged treatment, and sometimes on re-exposure to the drug ('type B' adverse reaction) (hence avoid repeated courses); this has also occurred, rarely, with eye drops.

Marrow depression may be detected at an early and recoverable stage by frequent checking of the full blood count.

The 'grey baby' syndrome occurs in neonates as circulatory collapse in which the skin develops a cyanotic grey colour. It is caused by high chloramphenicol plasma concentration due to failure of the liver to conjugate, and of the kidney to excrete the drug.

Sodium fusidate

Sodium fusidate is a steroid antimicrobial which is used almost exclusively against β-lactamase producing staphylococci; it has little useful activity against Gram-negative bacteria. Because staphylococci may rapidly become resistant via a one-step genetic mutation, the drug should be combined with another antistaphylococcal drug, e.g. flucloxacillin. Sodium fusidate is readily absorbed from the gut and distributes widely in body tissues including bone. It is metabolised and very little is excreted unchanged in the urine; the t½ is 5 h.

Uses. Sodium fusidate is a valuable drug for treating severe staphylococcal infections, including osteomyelitis and is available as i.v. and oral preparations. In an ointment or gel, sodium fusidate is used topically for staphylococcal skin infection and as a cream is applied to eradicate the staphylococcal nasal carrier state. Another gel preparation is used for topical application to the eye: this contains such a high fusidic acid concentration that it possesses useful activity against most bacteria that cause conjunctivitis, not only staphylococci.

Adverse effects. It is well tolerated, but mild gastrointestinal upset is frequent. Jaundice may develop, particularly with high doses given intravenously, and liver function should be monitored.

Resistance to antimicrobials: quinupristin-dalfopristin and linezolid

These novel antibiotics were developed in response to the emergence of multiply resistant Gram-positive pathogens during the 1990s. Both have clinically useful activity against MRSA (including vancomycin intermediate resistant strains), vancomycin-resistant enterococci and penicillin-resistant *Streptococcus pneumoniae*. They are currently reserved for treatment of infections caused by such bacteria and for use in patients who are allergic to more established antibiotics. Difficult decisions are being faced about how such novel but expensive antimicrobial agents should be used:

> 'No antibiotic should be used recklessly, however difficult it appears to be to select for resistance in vitro. On the other hand, the attitude that "All new antibiotics should be locked away" risks stifling innovation whilst denying life-saving treatments ... Debates on the use of new anti-Gram-positive agents are sure to intensify ... and it is vital that they take place on a basis of science not knee-jerk restrictions or over-zealous marketing.'[4]

They are inactive against most Gram-negative bacteria.

Quinupristin-dalfopristin is a combination of two streptogramin molecules: the dalfopristin component binds first to the 50S bacterial ribosome, inducing a conformational change which allows the additional binding of quinupristin. The combination results in inhibition of both aminoacyl-tRNA attachment and the peptidyl transferase elongation step of protein synthesis resulting in premature release of polypeptide chains from the ribosome. The summative effect is bactericidal. Acquired resistance is currently rare, but a variety of possible mechanisms of resistance have been reported including methylation of the 23S RNA molecule (also involved in erythromycin resistance), enzymatic hydrolysis and phosphorylation and efflux pumps. Most strains of *Enterococcus faecalis* are naturally resistant, but *E. faecium* strains are susceptible. Most Gram-negative bacteria have impermeable membranes and hence are resistant, but the respiratory pathogens *Legionella pneumophila* and *Mycoplasma pneumoniae* are susceptible.

The $t\frac{1}{2}$ is 1.5 h. Quinupristin-dalfopristin is available for administration only by i.v. injection; the usual dose is 7.5 mg/kg × 8 h.

It is licensed in the UK for *Enterococcus faecium* infections, skin and soft tissue infection, and in hospital-acquired pneumonia.

Injection to peripheral veins frequently causes phlebitis, so a central line is required. Arthralgia and myalgia are seen in about 10% patients.

Linezolid, a synthetic oxazolinidone, is the first member of the first totally new class of antibacterial agents to be released to the market for 20 years. It has a unique mode of action, binding to the 50S ribosomal subunit and inhibiting formation of the initiation complex between transfer-RNA, messenger RNA and the ribosomal subunits at the first stage of protein synthesis. It is bacteriostatic against most Gram-positive bacteria, including staphylococci, streptococci and enterococci resistant to other antimicrobial agents, but is bactericidal against pneumococci.

Resistance has been reported so far in only a few enterococci isolated from immunocompromised patients treated with linezolid for long periods. The resistant isolates appeared to possess modified ribosomal RNA genes. Cross-resistance to other antibiotics has not yet been seen. Most Gram-negative bacteria are resistant by virtue of possessing membrane efflux pumps, but many obligate anaerobes are susceptible.

It is eliminated via both renal and hepatic routes ($t\frac{1}{2}$ 6 h) with 30–55% excreted in the urine as the active drug. Oral and parenteral formulations are available, and doses range from 400 to 600 mg 12-hourly by both routes; absorption after oral administration is rapid, little affected by food, and approaches 100%.

Linezolid is licensed in the UK for skin, soft tissue and respiratory tract infections, and it is usually restricted on grounds of cost to those caused by multiply resistant pathogens. The oral formulation may prove useful for follow-on therapy of severe and chronic infections caused by bacteria resistant to other agents, e.g. MRSA osteomyelitis.

Adverse effects include nausea, vomiting and headache with much the same frequency as with penicillin and macrolide therapy; marrow suppression may occur especially where there is pre-

---

[4] Livermore D M. Quinupristin/dalfopristin and linezolid: where, when, which and whether to use? Journal of Antimicrobial Chemotherapy 2000 46: 347–350.

existing renal disease, and full blood counts should be performed weekly on patients receiving linezolid for longer than 2 weeks. Potentiation of the pressor activity of monoamine oxidase inhibitors may occur.

Inhibition of nucleic acid synthesis

Sulphonamides and sulphonamide combinations

Sulphonamides, amongst the first successful chemotherapeutic agents, now have their place in medicine mainly in combination with trimethoprim. Because of the risks of adverse drug reactions associated with their use, this is generally restricted to specific indications where other therapeutic agents have clearly inferior efficacy. Many sulphonamide compounds have been withdrawn from the market. Their individual names are standardised in the UK to begin with 'sulfa-'.

The enzyme dihydrofolic acid (DHF) synthase (see below) converts *p*-aminobenzoic acid (PABA) to DHF which is subsequently converted to tetrahydric folic acid (THF), purines and DNA. The sulphonamides are structurally similar to PABA, successfully compete with it for DHF synthase and thus ultimately impair DNA formation. Most bacteria do not use preformed folate, but humans derive DHF from dietary folate which protects their cells from the metabolic effect of sulphonamides. Trimethoprim acts at the subsequent step by inhibiting DHF reductase, which converts DHF to THF. The drug is relatively safe because bacterial DHF reductase is much more sensitive to trimethoprim than is the human form of the enzyme. Both sulphonamides and trimethoprim are bacteriostatic.

Pharmacokinetics. Sulphonamides for systemic use are absorbed rapidly from the gut. The principal metabolic path is acetylation and the capacity to acetylate is genetically determined in a bimodal form, i.e. there are slow and fast acetylators (see Pharmacogenetics) but the differences are of limited practical importance in therapy. The kidney is the principal route of excretion of drug and acetylate.

CLASSIFICATION AND USES

Sulphonamides may be classified as follows:

Systemic use

Sulphonamide-trimethoprim combination. *Co-trimoxazole* (sulfamethoxazole plus trimethoprim); the optimum synergistic in vitro effect against most susceptible bacteria is achieved with 5:1 ratio of sulfamethoxazole to trimethoprim, although concentrations achieved in the tissues vary considerably. Each drug is well absorbed from the gut, has a $t\frac{1}{2}$ of 10 h and is 80% excreted by the kidney; consequently, the dose of co-trimoxazole should be reduced when renal function is impaired.

Co-trimoxazole, at first, very largely replaced the use of a sulphonamide alone. In turn, trimethoprim on its own is now used in many conditions for which the combination was originally recommended, and it may cause fewer adverse reactions (see below). The combination is, however, retained for:

- Prevention and treatment of pneumonia due to *Pneumocystis carinii,* a life-threatening infection in immunosuppressed patients
- Prevention and treatment of toxoplasmosis, and treatment of nocardiasis

Sulfadiazine ($t\frac{1}{2}$ 10 h), sulfametopyrazine ($t\frac{1}{2}$ 38 h) and sulfadimidine (sulfamethazine) ($t\frac{1}{2}$ approx. 6 h, dose dependent) are available in some countries for urinary tract infections, meningococcal meningitis and other indications, but are not drugs of first choice (resistance rates are high).

Topical application

Silver sulfadiazine is used for prophylaxis and treatment of infected burns, leg ulcers and pressure sores because of its wide antibacterial spectrum (which includes pseudomonads).

Miscellaneous

Sulfasalazine (salicylazosulfapyridine) is used in inflammatory bowel disease (see p. 649); in effect the sulfapyridine component acts as a carrier to release the active 5-aminosalicylic acid in the colon (see also rheumatoid arthritis, p. 292).

Adverse effects of sulphonamides include malaise, diarrhoea, mental depression and rarely cyanosis, which latter is due to methaemoglobinaemia. These may all be transient and are not necessarily indications for stopping the drug. Crystalluria may rarely occur.

Allergic reactions include: rash, fever, hepatitis, agranulocytosis, purpura, aplastic anaemia, peripheral neuritis and polyarteritis nodosa. Rarely, severe skin reactions including erythema multiforme bullosa (Stevens–Johnson syndrome) and toxic epidermal necrolysis (Lyell's syndrome) occur.

Haemolysis may occur in glucose-6-phosphate dehydrogenase deficient subjects. Co-trimoxazole in high dose may cause macrocytic anaemia due to interference with conversion of DHF to THF. Patients with AIDS have a high rate of allergic systemic reactions (fever, rash) to co-trimoxazole used for treatment of *Pneumocystis carinii* pneumonia. Co-trimoxazole should not be used in pregnancy because of the possible teratogenic effects of inducing folate deficiency.

Trimethoprim

Subsequent to its extensive use in combination with sulphonamides, trimethoprim ($t\frac{1}{2}$ 10 h) has emerged as a useful broad spectrum antimicrobial on its own. It is active against many Gram-positive and Gram-negative aerobic organisms excepting the enterococci and *Pseudomonas aeruginosa;* the emergence of resistant organisms is becoming a problem. The drug is rapidly and completely absorbed from the gastrointestinal tract and is largely excreted unchanged in the urine. Trimethoprim is effective as sole therapy in treating urinary and respiratory tract infections due to susceptible organisms and for prophylaxis of urinary tract infections.

Adverse effects are fewer than with co-trimoxazole and include: skin rash, anorexia, nausea, vomiting, abdominal pain and diarrhoea.

Quinolones

(4-quinolones, fluoroquinolones)

The first widely used quinolone, nalidixic acid, was effective for urinary tract infections because it concentrated in the urine, but had little systemic activity. Fluorination of the quinolone structure was subsequently found to produce compounds that were up to 60 times more active than nalidixic acid and killed a wider range of organisms. They act principally by inhibiting bacterial (but not human) DNA gyrase, so preventing the supercoiling of DNA, a process that is necessary for compacting chromosomes into the bacterial cell; they are bactericidal and exhibit concentration-dependent bacterial killing (see p. 203). In general quinolones are extremely active against Gram-negative organisms including *Escherichia coli*, *Salmonella* sp., *Shigella* sp., *Neisseria* sp. and *Haemophilus influenzae* and they have useful activity against *Pseudomonas aeruginosa* and *Legionella pneumophila*. They are less active against Gram-positive organisms (resistance commonly emerges) and currently available examples are not effective against anaerobes.

Pharmacokinetics. Quinolones are well absorbed from the gut, and widely distributed in body tissue. Mechanisms of inactivation (hepatic metabolism, renal and biliary excretion) are detailed below for individual members. There is substantial excretion and re-absorption via the colonic mucosa, and patients with renal failure or intestinal malfunction, e.g. ileus, are prone to accumulate quinolones.

Uses vary between individual drugs (see below).

Adverse effects include gastrointestinal upset and allergic reactions (rash, pruritus, arthralgia, photosensitivity and anaphylaxis). CNS effects may develop with dizziness, headache and confusion, and are sufficient to require cautioning the patient against driving a motor vehicle. Convulsions have occurred during treatment (avoid or use with caution where there is a history of epilepsy or concurrent use of NSAIDs which potentiate this effect). Reversible arthropathy has developed in weight-bearing joints in immature animals exposed to quinolones. While the significance for humans is uncertain quinolones should be used only for serious infections and then with caution in children and adolescents. Rupture of tendons, notably the Achilles tendon, has occurred, more in the elderly and those taking corticosteroids concurrently.

Some of the quinolones are potent liver enzyme inhibitors and impair the metabolic inactivation of other drugs including warfarin, theophylline and sulphonylureas, increasing their effect. Magnesium- and aluminium-containing antacids impair the absorption of quinolones from the gastrointestinal tract probably through forming a chelate complex; ferrous sulphate and sucralfate also reduce quinolone absorption.

Individual members of the group include the following:

Ciprofloxacin ($t\frac{1}{2}$ 3 h) is effective against a range of bacteria but particularly the Gram-negative organisms (see above); it has less activity against Gram-positive bacteria such as *Streptococcus pneumoniae* and *Enterococcus faecalis*. Chlamydia and mycoplasma are sensitive but anaerobes are not. Ciprofloxacin is indicated for use in infections of the urinary, gastrointestinal and respiratory tracts, tissue infections, gonorrhoea and septicaemia caused by sensitive organisms. It has proven especially useful for oral therapy of chronic Gram-negative infections such as osteomyelitis and recurrent cholangitis, and for acute exacerbations of *Pseudomonas* infection in cystic fibrosis. The dose is 250–750 mg 12-hourly by mouth, 200-400 mg 12-hourly i.v. but may be halved when the glomerular filtration rate is < 20 ml/min. Ciprofloxacin impairs the metabolism of theophylline and of warfarin, both of which should be monitored carefully when co-administered.

Acrosoxacin ($t\frac{1}{2}$ 7 h) is effective as a single 300 mg oral dose for gonorrhoea; it is usually reserved for patients who are allergic to penicillin or for organisms that are resistant to that drug.

Cinoxacin ($t\frac{1}{2}$ 2 h) is used for cases of urinary tract infection, but not when renal function is impaired.

Norfloxacin ($t\frac{1}{2}$ 3 h) is used for acute or chronic recurrent urinary tract infections.

Ofloxacin ($t\frac{1}{2}$ 4 h) has modestly greater Gram-positive activity, but less Gram-negative activity than ciprofloxacin. It is indicated for urinary and respiratory tract infections and gonorrhoea.

Nalidixic acid ($t\frac{1}{2}$ 6 h) is now used principally for the prevention of urinary tract infection. It may cause haemolysis in glucose-6-phosphate dehydrogenase deficient subjects.

Others. *Levofloxacin* ($t\frac{1}{2}$ 7 h) has greater activity against *Streptococcus pneumoniae* than ciprofloxacin and is used for respiratory and urinary tract infection. *Moxifloxacin* ($t\frac{1}{2}$ 12 h) has strong anti-Gram-positive activity, and may prove useful for respiratory tract infections including those caused by 'atypical' pathogens and penicillin-resistant *Streptococcus pneumoniae*.

Azoles

This group includes:

- Metronidazole and tinidazole (antibacterial and antiprotozoal) which are described here.
- Fluconazole, itraconazole, clotrimazole, econazole, ketoconazole, isoconazole and miconazole which are described under Antifungal drugs (p. 264).
- Albendazole, mebendazole and thiabendazole which are described under Antihelminthic drugs (p. 276).

Metronidazole

In obligate anaerobic microorganisms (but not in aerobic microorganisms, which it also enters) metronidazole is converted into an active form by reduction of its nitro group: this binds to DNA and prevent nucleic acid formation; it is bacteriostatic.

Pharmacokinetics. Metronidazole is well absorbed after oral or rectal administration and distributed to achieve sufficient concentration to eradicate infection in liver, gut wall and pelvic tissues. It is eliminated in the urine, partly unchanged and partly as metabolites. The $t\frac{1}{2}$ is 8 h.

Uses. Metronidazole is active against a wide range of anaerobic bacteria and also protozoa. Its clinical indications are:

- Treatment of sepsis to which anaerobic organisms, e.g. *Bacteroides* spp. and anaerobic cocci, are contributing, notably postsurgical infection, intra-abdominal infection and septicaemia, but also wound and pelvic infection, osteomyelitis and abscesses of brain or lung
- Antibiotic-associated pseudomembraneous colitis (caused by *Clostridium difficile*)
- Trichomoniasis of the urogenital tract in both sexes
- Amoebiasis *(Entamoeba histolytica)*, including both intestinal and extra-intestinal infection
- Giardiasis *(Giardia lamblia)*
- Acute ulcerative gingivitis and dental infections (*Fusobacterium* spp. and other oral anaerobic flora)
- Anaerobic vaginosis (*Gardnerella vaginalis* and vaginal anaerobes).

Dose. Established anaerobic infection is treated with metronidazole by mouth 400 mg 8-hourly; by rectum 1 g 8-hourly for 3 days followed by 1 g 12-hourly; or by i.v. infusion 500 mg 8-hourly. A topical gel preparation is useful for reducing the odour associated with anaerobic infection of fungating tumours.

Adverse effects include nausea, vomiting, diarrhoea, furred tongue and an unpleasant metallic taste in the mouth; also headache, dizziness and ataxia. Rashes, urticaria and angioedema occur. Peripheral neuropathy occurs if treatment is prolonged and epileptiform seizures if the dose is high. Large doses of metronidazole are carcinogenic in rodents and the drug is mutagenic in bacteria; long-term studies have failed to discover oncogenic effects in humans.

A disulfiram-like effect (see p. 186) occurs with alcohol because metronidazole inhibits alcohol and aldehyde dehydrogenase; patients should be warned appropriately.

Tinidazole is similar to metronidazole but has a longer $t\frac{1}{2}$ (13 h). It is excreted mainly unchanged in the urine. The indications for use and adverse effects are essentially those of metronidazole. The longer duration of action of tinidazole may be an advantage, e.g. in giardiasis, trichomoniasis and acute ulcerative gingivitis, in which tinidazole 2 g by mouth in a single dose is as effective as a course of metronidazole.

MINOR ANTIMICROBIALS

These are included because they are effective topically without serious risk of allergy, although toxicity or chemical instability limits or precludes their systemic use.

Mupirocin is primarily active against Gram-positive organisms including those commonly associated with skin infections. It is available as an ointment for use, e.g. in folliculitis and impetigo, and to eradicate nasual staphylococci, e.g. in carriers of resistant staphylococci. It is rapidly hydrolysed in the tissues.

POLYPEPTIDE ANTIBIOTICS

Colistin is effective against Gram-negative organisms particularly *Pseudomonas aeruginosa*. It is sometimes used for bowel decontamination in neutropenic patients and topically is applied to skin, including external ear infections. It is occasionally used systemically for severe infections with multiply resistant Gram-negative pathogens such as pseudomonads when no alternative agents are available. Adverse effects of systemic administration include nephrotoxicity, neurological symptoms and neuromuscular blockade.

Polymyxin B is also active against Gram-negative organisms, particularly *Pseudomonas aeruginosa*. Its principal use now is topical application for skin, eye and external ear infections.

Gramicidin is used in various topical applications as eye- and ear-drops, combined with neomycin and framycetin.

GUIDE TO FURTHER READING

Alvarez-Elcoro S, Enzler M J 1999 The macrolides: erythromycin, clarithromycin, and azithromycin. Mayo Clinic Proceedings 74: 613–634

Chambers H F 1997 Methicillin resistance in staphylococci: molecular and biochemical basis and clinical implications. Clinical Microbiology Reviews 10: 781–791

Diekema D J, Jones R N 2001 Oxazolidine antibiotics. Lancet 358: 1975–1982

Fisman D N, Kaye K M 2000 Once-daily dosing of aminoglycoside antibiotics. Infectious Disease Clinics of North America 14: 475

Hancock R E W 1997 Peptide antibiotics. Lancet 349: 418–422

Holgate S 1988 Penicillin allergy: how to diagnose and when to treat. British Medical Journal 296: 1213

Johnson A P, Livermore D M 1999 Quinupristin/dalfopristin, a new addition to the antimicrobial arsenal. Lancet 354: 2012–2013

Kelkar P S, Li J T-C 2001 Cephalosporin allergy. New England Journal of Medicine 345: 804–809

Moellering R C 1998 Vancomycin-resistant enterococci. Clinical Infectious Diseases 26: 1196–1199

Piddock L J 1994 New quinolones and Gram-positive bacteria. Antimicrobial Agents & Chemotherapy 38: 163–169

Walker R C 1999 The fluoroquinolones. Mayo Clinic Proceedings 74: 1030–1037

Zopf D, Roth S 1996 Oligosaccharide anti-infective agents. Lancet 347: 1017–1021

13

Chemotherapy of bacterial infections

SYNOPSIS

We live in a world heavily populated by microorganisms of astonishing diversity. Most of these exist in our external environment but certain classes are normally harboured within our bodies, especially colonising mucosal surfaces. Depending on the circumstances, infectious disease can arise from organisms living exogenously or endogenously, and a knowledge of common pathogens at specific sites often provides a good basis for rational initial therapy.

This chapter considers the bacteria that cause disease in individual body systems, the drugs that are used to combat them, and how they are best used. It discusses infection of:

- Blood
- Paransal sinuses and ears
- Throat
- Bronchi, lungs and pleura
- Endocardium
- Meninges
- Intestines
- Urinary tract
- Genital tract
- Bones and joints
- Eye
- Also mycobacteria, that infect many sites

Table 11.1 (p. 211) is a general reference for this chapter.

Infection of the blood

Septicaemia is a medical emergency. Accurate microbiological diagnosis is of the first importance and blood cultures should be taken before starting antimicrobial therapy. Usually, the infecting organism(s) is not known at the time of presentation and treatment must be instituted on the basis of a 'best guess'. The clinical circumstances may provide some clues. Patients who have been in hospital for some time before presenting with septicaemia may need antibiotic regimens that provide more reliable cover for *multiply resistant pathogens,* and examples of suitable choices are given in the list below *in brackets.*

- When septicaemia follows gastrointestinal or genital tract surgery, *Escherichia coli* (or other Gram-negative bacteria), anaerobic bacteria, e.g. *Bacteroides,* streptococci or enterococci are likely pathogens and the following combinations are effective: cefuroxime plus metronidazole or gentamicin plus benzylpenicillin plus metronidazole (meropenem plus vancomycin).
- Septicaemia related to urinary tract infection usually involves *Escherichia coli* (or other Gram-negative bacteria), enterococci: gentamicin plus benzylpenicillin or cefotaxime alone (ciprofloxacin plus vancomycin).
- Neonatal septicaemia is usually due to streptococci or coliforms: benzylpenicillin plus gentamicin.

- Staphylococcal septicaemia may be suspected where there is an abscess, e.g. of bone or lung, or with acute infective endocarditis or infection of intravenous catheters: high dose flucloxacillin is indicated (vancomycin).
- Toxic shock syndrome occurs in circumstances that include healthy women using vaginal tampons, abortion or childbirth, and occasionally with skin and soft tissue infection. The clinical problem is due to systemic effects of toxins produced by staphylococci: while this is not strictly an infection of the blood, flucloxacillin is used to eliminate the source. Elimination of the source by removal of the tampon and drainage of abscesses, and circulatory support are also important.

Antimicrobials should be given i.v. initially in septicaemia.

Infection of paranasal sinuses and ears

SINUSITIS

Acute infection of the paranasal sinuses causes significant morbidity. Since oedema of the mucous membrane hinders the drainage of pus, a logical first step is to open the obstructed passage with a sympathomimetic vasoconstrictor, e.g. ephedrine nasal drops. Antibiotic therapy produces limited additional clinical benefit, but the common infecting organism—*Streptococcus pneumoniae, Haemophilus influenzae, Streptococcus pyogenes, Moraxella (Branhamella) catarrhalis*—usually respond to oral amoxicillin (with or without clavulanic acid) or doxycycline, if the case is serious enough to warrant antibiotic therapy.

In chronic sinusitis, correction of the anatomical abnormalities (polypi, nasal septum deviation) is often important. Very diverse organisms, many of them normal inhabitants of the upper respiratory tract, may be cultured, e.g. anaerobic streptococci, *Bacteroides* spp., and a judgement is required as to whether any particular organism is acting as a pathogen. Choice of antibiotic should be guided by culture and sensitivity testing; therapy may need to be prolonged.

OTITIS MEDIA

Mild cases, characterised by pinkness or infection of the eardrum, often resolve spontaneously and need only analgesia and observation. They are normally viral. A bulging, inflamed eardrum indicates bacterial otitis media usually due to *Streptococcus pneumoniae, Haemophilus influenzae, Moraxella (Branhamella) catarrhalis, Streptococcus pyogenes* (Group A) or *Staphylococcus aureus*. Amoxicillin or co-amoxiclav is satisfactory, but the clinical benefit of antibiotic therapy is very small when tested in controlled trials. Chemotherapy has not removed the need for myringotomy when pain is very severe, and also for later cases, as sterilised pus may not be completely absorbed and may leave adhesions that impair hearing. Chronic infection presents a similar problem to that of chronic sinus infection, above.

Infection of the throat

Pharyngitis is usually viral but the more serious cases may be caused by *Streptococcus pyogenes* (Group A) which is always sensitive to benzylpenicillin. Unfortunately, streptococcal sore throats cannot be clinically differentiated from non-streptococcal with any certainty. Prevention of complications is more important than relief of the symptoms which seldom last long. There is no general agreement whether chemotherapy should be employed in mild sporadic sore throat and expert reviews on the subject reflect the resulting diversity of clinical views.[1,2,3] The disease usually subsides in a few days, septic complications are uncommon and rheumatic fever rarely follows. It is reasonable to withhold penicillin unless streptococci are cultured or the patient develops a high fever. Severe sporadic or epidemic sore throat is likely to be strepto-

[1] Cooper R J, Hoffman J R, Bartlett J G et al 2001 Principles of appropriate antibiotic use for acute pharyngitis in adults: background. Annals of Internal Medicine 134: 506.
[2] Del Mar C B, Glasziou P P, Spinks A B 2001 Antibiotics for sore throat (Cochrane Review). The Cochrane Library 2. Oxford: Update Software.
[3] Thomas M, Del Mar C, Glasziou P 2000 How effective are treatments other than antibiotics for acute sore throat? British Journal of General Practice 50: 817.

coccal and phenoxymethylpenicillin by mouth (or erythromycin/clarithromycin or an oral cephalosporin in the penicillin allergic) should be given to prevent these complications. Ideally, it should be continued for 10 days, but compliance is bad once the symptoms have subsided and 5 days should be the minimum objective. If there is a possibility that the pharyngitis is due to infectious mononucleosis, amoxicillin must not be used as the patient is very likely to develop a rash (see p. 220). In a closed community, chemoprophylaxis of unaffected people to stop an epidemic may be considered, for instance with phenoxymethylpenicillin 125 mg 12-hourly orally, for a period depending on the course of the epidemic.

In *scarlet fever* and *erysipelas,* the infection is invariably streptococcal (Group A) and benzylpenicillin should be used even in mild cases, to prevent rheumatic fever and nephritis.

Chemoprophylaxis

Chemoprophylaxis of streptococcal (Group A) infection with phenoxymethylpenicillin should be undertaken in patients who have had one attack of rheumatic fever. It is continued for at least 5 years, or until aged 20, whichever is the longer period (although some hold that it should continue for life, for histological study of atrial biopsies shows that the cardiac lesions may progress despite absence of clinical activity). Chemoprophylaxis should be continued for life after a second attack of rheumatic fever. A single attack of acute nephritis is not an indication for chemoprophylaxis but in the rare cases of nephritis in which recurrent haematuria occurs after sore throats, chemoprophylaxis should be used. Ideally, chemoprophylaxis should continue throughout the year but, if the patient is unwilling to submit to this, at least the colder months should be covered (see also p. 207).

Adverse effects are uncommon. Patients taking penicillin prophylaxis are liable to have penicillin-resistant viridans type streptococci in the mouth, so that during even minor dentistry, e.g. scaling, there is a risk of bacteraemia and thus of infective endocarditis with a penicillin-resistant organism in those with any residual rheumatic heart lesion. The same risk applies to urinary, abdominal and chest surgery, and patients need special chemoprophylaxis (see Endocarditis). Patients taking penicillins are also liable to be carrying resistant staphylococci and pneumococci.

Other causes of pharyngitis

Vincent's infection (microbiologically complex, includes anaerobes, spirochaetes) responds readily to benzylpenicillin; a single i.m. dose of 600 mg is often enough except in a mouth needing dental treatment, when relapse may follow. Metronidazole 200 mg 8-hourly by mouth for 3 days is also effective.

Diphtheria (*Corynebacterium diphtheriae*). Antitoxin 10 000–100 000 units i.v. in two divided doses 0.5–2 h apart is given to neutralise toxin already formed according to the severity of the disease. Erythromycin or benzylpenicillin is also used, to prevent the production of more toxin by destroying the bacteria.

Whooping-cough (*Bordetella pertussis*). Chemotherapy is needed in children who are weak, have damaged lungs or are under 3 years old. Erythromycin is usually recommended at the catarrhal stage and should be continued for 14 days (also as prophylaxis in cases of special need). It may curtail an attack if given early enough (before paroxysms have begun) but is not dramatically effective; it also reduces infectivity to others. A corticosteroid, salbutamol, and physiotherapy may be helpful for relief of symptoms, but reliable evidence of efficacy is lacking.

Infection of the bronchi, lungs and pleura

BRONCHITIS

Most cases of acute bronchitis are viral; where bacteria are responsible the usual pathogens are *Streptococcus pneumoniae* and/or *Haemophilus influenzae*. It is questionable if there is role for antimicrobials in uncomplicated acute bronchitis but amoxicillin, a tetracycline or trimethoprim are app-ropriate if treatment is considered necessary.

In chronic bronchitis, suppressive chemotherapy, generally needed only during the colder months (in temperate, colder regions), may be considered for patients with symptoms of pulmonary insufficiency, recurrent acute exacerbations or permanently puru-lent sputum. Amoxicillin or trimethoprim is suit-able for treatment.

For intermittent therapy, the patient is given a supply of the drug and is told to take it in full dose at the first sign of a 'chest' cold, e.g. purulent sputum, and to stop it after 3 days if there is rapid improvement. Otherwise, the patient should conti-nue the drug until recovery takes place. If the exacerbation lasts for more than 10 days, there is a need for clinical reassessment.

PNEUMONIAS

The clinical setting is a useful guide to the causal organism and hence to the 'best guess' early choice of antimicrobial, although in seriously ill patients cover for both 'typical' and 'atypical' pathogens should be included from the beginning. It is not possible reliably to differentiate between pneumonias caused by 'typical' and 'atypical' pathogens on clinical grounds alone.

Pneumonia in previously healthy people
(community acquired)

Disease that is segmental or lobar in its distribu-tion is usually caused by *Streptococcus pneumoniae* (pneumococcus). *Haemophilus influenzae* is a rare cause in this group, although it more often leads to exacerbations of chronic bronchitis and does cause pneumonia in patients infected with HIV. Benzyl-penicillin i.v. or amoxicillin p.o. are the treatments of choice if pneumococcal pneumonia is very likely; alternatively, use erythromycin/clarithromycin in a penicillin-allergic patient. Seriously ill patients are best given benzylpenicillin (to cover the pneumo-coccus) plus ciprofloxacin (to cover *Haemophilus* and 'atypical' pathogens). Where penicillin-resistant pneumococci are prevalent, i.v. cefotaxime is a reasonable 'best guess' choice.

Pneumonia following influenza is often caused by *Staphylococcus aureus*, and 'best guess' therapy is usually achieved by adding flucloxacillin to one of the regimens above. When staphylococcal pneumo-nia is proven, sodium fusidate p.o. plus fluclox-acillin i.v. should be used in combination.

'Atypical' cases of pneumonia may be caused by *Mycoplasma pneumoniae* which may be epidemic, or more rarely *Chlamydia pneumoniae* or *psittaci* (psitta-cosis/ornithosis) *Legionella pneumophilia* or *Coxiella burnetii* (Q fever) and a tetracycline or erythromycin/clarithromycin should be given by mouth. Treatment of ornithosis should continue for 10 days after the fever has settled and in mycoplasma pneumonia and Q fever a total of 3 weeks treatment may be needed to prevent relapse.

At the earliest possible stage, once a clinical im-provement has been seen, initial i.v. administration of antibiotics for pneumonia should be switched to the oral route.

Pneumonia acquired in hospital

Pneumonia is usually defined as being nosocomial (Greek: *nosokomeian*, hospital) if it presents after at least 2 days in hospital. It occurs primarily among patients admitted with medical problems or recovering from abdominal or thoracic surgery or on mechanical ventilators. The common pathogens are *Staphylococcus aureus, Enterobacteriaceae, Strepto-coccus pneumoniae, Pseudomonas aeruginosa,* and *Haemophilus influenzae*. It is reasonable to initiate therapy with ciprofloxacin, meropenem or cef-tazidime (plus vancomycin if the local prevalence of MRSA is high) until the results of sputum culture and antimicrobial susceptibility tests are known.

Pneumonia in people with chronic lung disease

Normal commensals of the upper respiratory tract proliferate in damaged lungs especially following viral infections, pulmonary congestion or pulmonary infarction. Mixed infection is therefore common, and since *Haemophilus influenzae* and *Streptococcus pneumoniae* are often the pathogens, amoxicillin or trimethoprim are reasonable choices, but if response is inadequate co-amoxiclav or a quinolone should be substituted.

Klebsiella pneumoniae rarely causes lung infection ('Friedlander's pneumonia') in the alcoholic and debilitated elderly. Abscesses form, particularly in the upper lobes: cefotaxime possibly with an aminoglycoside is recommended.

Moraxella (previously *Branhamella) catarrhalis,* a commensal of the oropharynx, may be a pathogen in patients with chronic bronchitis; because many strains produce β-lactamase, co-amoxiclav or erythromycin/clarithromycin should be used.

Pneumonia in immunocompromised patients

Pneumonia is common, e.g. in acquired immunodeficiency syndrome (AIDS) or in those who are receiving immunosuppressive drugs.

Common pathogenic bacteria may be responsible *(Staphylococcus aureus, Streptococcus pneumoniae)* but often organisms of lower natural virulence *(Enterobacteriaceae,* viruses, fungi) are causal and strenuous efforts should be made to identify the microbe including, if feasible, bronchial washings or lung biopsy.

- Until the pathogen is known the patient should receive broad-spectrum antimicrobial treatment, such as an aminoglycoside plus ceftazidime.
- Aerobic Gram-negative bacilli, e.g. *Enterobacteriaceae, Klebsiella* spp., are pathogens in half of the cases, especially in neutropenic patients, and respond to cefotaxime or ceftazidime. *Pseudomonas aeruginosa* may also cause pneumonia in these patients; for treatment see Reference data on antimicrobial drugs of choice, page 211, Table 11.1.
- An important respiratory pathogen in patients with deficits in cell-mediated immunity is the fungus *Pneumocystis carinii,* which should be treated with co-trimoxazole 120 mg/kg/d by mouth or i.v. in 2–4 divided doses for 14 days, or with pentamidine (see p. 276).

Legionnaires' disease

Legionella pneumophila responds to erythromycin 2–4 g/d i.v. in divided doses but rifampicin may be added in more severe infections. Ciprofloxacin is also effective.

Pneumonia due to anaerobic microorganisms

Pneumonia is often caused by aspiration of material from the oropharynx, or due to the presence of other lung pathology such as pulmonary infarction or bronchogenic carcinoma. As well as conventional microbial causes, the pathogens include anaerobic and aerobic streptococci, *Bacteroides* spp. and *Fusobacterium,* and the diagnosis may be missed unless anaerobic cultures of fresh material are performed. Treatment for several weeks with cefuroxime plus metronidazole may be needed to prevent relapse.

Pulmonary abscess is treated according to the organism identified and with surgery if necessary.

Empyema is treated according to the organism isolated and with aspiration and drainage.

Endocarditis

When suspicion is high enough, three blood cultures should be taken over a few hours and antimicrobial treatment commenced; it can be adjusted later in the light of the results. Delay in treating only exposes the patient to the risk of grave cardiac damage or systemic embolism. Streptococci, enterococci and staphylococci are causal in 80% of cases, with viridans group streptococci the most common pathogens. In intravenous drug users, *Staphylococcus aureus* is the most likely organism. Culture-negative endocarditis (up to 20% of cases) is usually due to prior antimicrobial therapy or to special culture requirements of the microbe; it is best regarded as being due to streptococci and treated accordingly.

PRINCIPLES FOR TREATMENT

- High doses of bactericidal drugs are needed because the organisms are difficult to access in avascular vegetations on valves and the protective host reaction is negligible.
- Drugs should be given parenterally at least

initially and preferably by intravenous bolus injection which achieves the necessary high peak concentration to penetrate the relatively avascular vegetations.

- The infusion site should be examined daily and changed regularly to prevent opportunistic infection, which is usually with coagulase-negative staphylococci or fungi. Alternatively, use may be made of a central subclavian venous catheter sited with meticulous attention to aseptic technique.
- Prolonged therapy is needed, usually 4 weeks, and in the case of infected prosthetic valves at least 6 weeks. The patient should be reviewed one month after completing the antimicrobial treatment. Valve replacement may be needed at any time during and after antibiotic therapy if cardiovascular function deteriorates or if the infection proves impossible to control.
- Dosage must be adjusted according to the sensitivity of the infecting organism. This is established by the Minimum Inhibitory Concentration test (p. 203), rather than by testing dilutions of the patient's serum against the organism (the Serum Bactericidal Titre which was formally recommended, but which has not been proved useful).

DOSE REGIMENS

The following regimens are those commonly recommended:

1. Initial (best guess) treatment should comprise benzylpenicillin 1.2–2.4 g 4-hourly, plus gentamicin in low dose, e.g. 80 mg 12-hourly, by i.v. injection (synergy allows this dose of gentamicin and minimises risk of adverse effects). Regular serum gentamicin assay is vital: trough concentrations should be below 1 mg/l and peak concentrations about 3 mg/l; if *Staphylococcus aureus* is suspected, high-dose flucloxacillin plus either gentamicin or sodium fusidate should be used. Patients allergic to penicillin should be treated with vancomycin.
2. When an organism has been identified and its sensitivity to drugs determined:
   - *Viridans group streptococci:* benzylpenicillin plus gentamicin i.v. for at least 4 weeks or, if the organism is very sensitive, for 2 weeks, followed by amoxicillin p.o. for 2 weeks. Some patients with uncomplicated endocarditis caused by very sensitive strains may be managed as outpatients; for these patients ceftriaxone may be suitable, with its prolonged $t_{\frac{1}{2}}$ allowing convenient once-daily administration.
   - *Enterococcus faecalis (Group D):* benzylpenicillin 1.8–3g 4-hourly plus gentamicin i.v. for 4–6 weeks. The prolonged gentamicin administration carries a significant risk of adverse drug reactions, but is essential to assure eradication of the infection.
   - *Staphylococcus aureus:* flucloxacillin 2 g 4-hourly by i.v. injection for at least 4 weeks plus either gentamicin by i.v. injection or sodium fusidate by mouth for the first 1–2 weeks.
   - *Staphylococcus epidermidis* and other coagulase negative staphylococci infecting native heart valves should be managed as for *Staphylococcus aureus* if the organism is sensitive. These organisms, however, have a predilection for prosthetic valves and such cases should be treated with vancomycin plus rifampicin for at least 6 weeks with gentamicin for the first 2 weeks.
   - *Coxiella* or *Chlamydia:* tetracycline by mouth for at least 4–6 weeks. Valve replacement is advised in most cases, but some may continue indefinitely on tetracycline.
   - *Fungal endocarditis:* amphotericin plus flucytosine are used. Valve replacement is usually essential.
   - *Culture-negative endocarditis:* benzylpenicillin plus gentamicin i.v. are given for 4–6 weeks.

PROPHYLAXIS

Transient bacteraemia is provoked by dental procedures, surgical incision of the skin, instrumentation of the urinary tract, parturition and even seemingly innocent activities such as brushing the teeth or chewing toffee. Experience shows that people with acquired or congenital heart defects are at risk from bacteraemia and may be protected by antimicrobials used prophylactically (although there is no scientific proof of the efficacy of this). The drugs are given as a short course in high dose at the time of the procedure to coincide with the bacteraemia and avoid emergence of resistant organisms. There follow general recommendations[4,5,6] on antimicrobial prophylaxis; not every contingency is covered because prophylaxis may be needed for patients with cardiac defects whenever surgery or instrumentation is undertaken on tissue that is heavily colonised or infected, e.g. in surgery or instrumentation of the upper respiratory or genitourinary tracts, or obstetric, gynaecological or gastrointestinal procedures. Different national Working Parties have recommended differing prophylactic measures,[4,5,6] and the physician should consult special sources and exercise a clinical judgement that relates to individual circumstances. All oral drugs should be taken under supervision.

Dental procedures

Under local or no anaesthesia

- Adults who are *not allergic* to penicillins and who have not taken penicillin more than once in the previous month (including those with a prosthetic valve, but not if they have had endocarditis in the past) should receive amoxicillin 3 g by mouth 1 h before the procedure.
- Patients *allergic* to penicillins or who have taken penicillin more than once in the previous month should receive clindamycin 600 mg by mouth 1 h before the procedure.

Under general anaesthesia

- Patients who are not allergic to penicillins and who have not taken penicillin more than once in the previous month should receive amoxicillin 1 g i.m. or i.v. at induction then 0.5 g by mouth 6 h later. Alternatively amoxicillin 3 g may be taken by mouth together with probenecid 1 g by mouth 4 h before the procedure (probenecid delays renal excretion and thus maintains a high blood concentration of amoxicillin), or amoxicillin 3 g may be followed by another 3 g dose as soon as possible after the procedure.
- **Special risk** patients, i.e. with prosthetic valves or with previous endocarditis, should receive amoxicillin 1 g i.m. or i.v. and gentamicin 120 mg at induction, then amoxicillin 0.5 g by mouth 6 h later. Patients who are penicillin-allergic or have received penicillin more that once in the previous month should receive vancomycin 1 g i.v. over 100 min then gentamicin 120 mg i.v. at induction or 15 min before the procedure; or teicoplanin 400 mg i.v. plus gentamicin 120 mg i.v. at induction or 15 min before the procedure; or clindamycin 300 mg over at least 10 min at induction or 15 min before the procedure then clindamycin 150 mg i.v. or by mouth 6 h later.

Special sources should be consulted for prophylactic regimens recommended for children and for other procedures, such as instrumentation of the urogenital or gastrointestinal tracts.

Meningitis

Speed of initiating treatment and accurate bacteriological diagnosis are the major factors determining the fate of the patient. When meningococcal disease is suspected (and unless the patient has a history of penicillin anaphylaxis) treatment with benzylpenicillin should be started by the general practitioner before transfer to hospital; benefit to the patient outweighs the reduced chance of identifying the causative organism. Newly introduced diagnostic methods such as the Polymerase Chain Reaction (PCR) for bacterial DNA in CSF or blood enable accurate and rapid diagnosis even when the causative organisms have been destroyed by antibiotics.

Drugs must be given i.v. in high dose; the regimens below provide the recommended therapy, with alternatives for patients allergic to first choices. Intrathecal therapy is now considered unnecessary, and can be dangerous, e.g. encephalopathy with penicillin.

[4] Simmons N A 1993 Recommendations for endocarditis prophylaxis. Journal of Antimicrobial Chemotherapy 31: 437.
[5] Littler W A, McGowan D A, Shanson D C 1997 Changes in recommendations about amoxycillin prophylaxis for prevention of endocarditis. Lancet 350: 1100.
[6] Dajani A S, Taubert K A, Wilson W et al 1997 Prevention of bacterial endocarditis. Recommendations by the American Heart Association. Journal of the American Medical Association 277: 1794.

INITIAL THERAPY

Initial therapy should be sufficient to kill all pathogens, which are likely to be:

All ages over 5 years

For *Neisseria meningitidis* and *Streptococcus pneumoniae* benzylpenicillin 2–4 g 4–6-hourly should be given, followed, in the case of *Neisseria meningitidis*, by rifampicin for 2 days prior to discharge from hospital (to eradicate persisting organisms). Some prefer to use cefotaxime 2–3 g 6–8-hourly in all cases until the results of susceptibility tests are known, and this may be the generally preferred choice if penicillin resistance in pneumococci and meningococci rises in prevalence. Optimal therapy for penicillin-resistant pneumococcal meningitis may comprise cefotaxime 2–3 g 6–8-hourly plus vancomycin 1 g 12-hourly plus rifampicin 600 gm 12-hourly.

Children under 5 years

Neisseria meningitidis is now commonest and *Haemophilus influenzae*, formerly a frequent pathogen, is much less often isolated (as a result of immunisation programmes). *Streptococcus pneumoniae* is also less commonly found than in older patients.

Give a cephalosporin, e.g. cefotaxime. When *Haemophilus influenzae* is isolated give rifampicin for 4 days before discharge from hospital to clear naso-pharyngeal carriage.

Neonates

For *Escherichia coli*: give cefotaxime or ceftazidime perhaps with gentamicin. For Group B streptococci: give benzylpenicillin plus gentamicin. Consult a specialist text for details of doses for neonates.

Ampicillin must be added if *Listeria monocytogenes* is suspected.

Dexamethasone given i.v. and early appears to reduce long-term neurological sequelae, especially sensorineural deafness, in infants and children. There is not, however, general agreement about the use of dexamethasone for meningitis in adults.

Chloramphenicol remains a good alternative for 'blind' therapy in patients giving a history of β-lactam anaphylaxis.

SUBSEQUENT THERAPY

When the infecting organism has been identified, specific therapy is chosen as follows. Intravenous administration should continue until the patient is capable of taking drugs by mouth, and whether continuation therapy should be given by mouth or i.v. is a matter of debate. Antimicrobials (except aminoglycosides) enter well into the CSF when the meninges are inflamed; relapse may be due to restoration of the blood–CSF barrier as inflammation is reduced. The following are recommended (adult doses).

Neisseria meniningitidis: benzylpenicillin 2.4 g 4–6-hourly or cefotaxime 2–3 g 6–8-hourly is given. Treatment should continue for a minimum of 5 days.

Streptococcus pneumoniae: cefotaxime 2–3 g 6–8-hourly is given or benzylpenicillin 2.4 g 4–6-hourly if the organism is penicillin-sensitive. Treatment should continue for 10 days after the patient has become afebrile and the physician should be aware of the possibility of relapse.

Haemophilus influenzae: cefotaxime 2–3 g 6–8-hourly or chloramphenicol 100 mg/kg/d is given. Treatment should continue for 10 days after the temperature has settled. Subdural empyema, often presenting as persistent fever, is relatively common after haemophilus meningitis and may require surgical drainage.

Chemoprophylaxis

The three common pathogens (below) are spread by respiratory secretions. Asymptomatic nasopharyngeal carriers seldom develop meningitis but they may transmit the pathogens to close personal contacts. Rifampicin by mouth is effective at reducing carriage rates.

Meningococcal meningitis often occurs in epidemics in closed communities, but also in isolated cases. Close personal contacts should receive oral rifampicin 600 mg 12-hourly for 2 days. Single doses of oral ciprofloxacin (500 mg) or i.m. ceftriaxone (2 g) are alternatives, the latter of particular value for pregnant women.

Haemophilus influenzae type b has an infectivity similar to that of the meningococcus. Rifampicin 600 mg daily should be given for 4 days.

Pneumococcal meningitis tends to occur in isolated cases and chemoprophylaxis of contacts is not recommended.

Infection of the intestines

(For *Helicobacter pylori* see p. 630.) Antimicrobial therapy should be reserved for specific conditions with identified pathogens where benefit has been shown; not all acute diarrhoea is infective for it can be caused by bacterial toxins in food, dietary indiscretions, anxiety and by drugs. Even if diarrhoea is infective, it may be due to viruses; or, if it is bacterial, antimicrobial agents may not reduce the duration of symptoms and may aggravate the condition by permitting opportunistic infection and encouraging *Clostridium difficile* associated diarrhoea. Maintenance of water and electrolyte balance, either by i.v. infusion or orally with a glucose-electrolyte solution together with an antimotility drug (except in small children) are the mainstays of therapy in such cases (see Oral rehydration therapy, p. 643).

Some specific intestinal infections do benefit from chemotherapy:

Campylobacter jejuni. Erythromycin or ciprofloxacin by mouth will eliminate the organism from the stools and a 5-day course is worth giving early in the illness if it is severe.

Shigella. Mild disease requires no specific antimicrobial therapy but toxic shigellosis with high fever should be treated with ciprofloxacin or amoxicillin by mouth.

Salmonella. An antimicrobial should be used for severe salmonella gastroenteritis, or for bacteraemia or salmonella enteritis in an immunocompromised patient. The choice lies between ciprofloxacin, amoxicillin or co-trimoxazole, according to the sensitivity of the pathogen.

Typhoid fever is a generalised infection and requires treatment with ciprofloxacin. Chloramphenicol, amoxicillin or co-trimoxazole are less effective alternatives. The i.v. route should be used at least initially, followed by oral administration. A longer period of treatment may be required for those who develop complications such as osteomyelitis or abscess.

A *carrier state* develops in a few individuals who have no symptoms of disease but who can infect others.[7] Organsims reside in the biliary or urinary tracts. Ciprofloxacin in high dose by mouth for 3–6 months may be successful for what can be a very difficult problem. Cholecystectomy or investigation of urinary tract abnormalities may be needed.

Escherichia coli is a normal inhabitant of the bowel but some enterotoxigenic strains are pathogenic and are frequently a cause of travellers' diarrhoea. A quinolone, e.g. ciprofloxacin, is the drug of choice in most high-risk parts of the world for a severe attack (see Travellers' diarrhoea, p. 644). Antimicrobials are not generally given for prophylaxis but, when it is indicated, a quinolone should be used.

Verotoxic *Escherichia coli* (VTEC; O157) may cause severe bloody diarrhoea and systemic effects such as the haemolytic uraemic syndrome (HUS); antibiotic therapy has been shown in some trials to worsen the prognosis, perhaps by releasing more toxin from dying bacteria. An antimicrobial should generally therefore be avoided for bloody diarrhoea unless the diagnosis has been confirmed bacteriologically not to be VTEC.

Vibrio cholerae. The cause of death in cholera is electrolyte and fluid loss in the stools and this may exceed 1 l/h. The most important aim of treatment is prompt replacement and maintenance of water and electrolytes with oral or intravenous electrolyte solutions. Doxycycline, given early, significantly reduces the amount and duration of diarrhoea and eliminates the organism from the faeces (thus lessening the contamination of the environment). Carriers may be treated by doxycycline by mouth in high dose for 3 days. Ciprofloxacin may be given for resistant organisms.

---

[7] The most famous carrier was Mary Mallon ('Typhoid Mary') who worked as a cook in New York City, USA, using various assumed names and moving through several different households. She caused at least 10 outbreaks with 51 cases of typhoid fever and 3 deaths. To protect the public, she was kept in detention for 23 years.

Suppression of bowel flora is thought by some to be useful in hepatic encephalopathy. Here, absorption of products of bacterial breakdown of protein (ammonium, amines) in the intestine lead to cerebral symptoms and even to coma. In acute coma, neomycin 6 g/d should be given by gastric tube; as prophylaxis, 1–4 g/d may be given to patients with protein intolerance who fail to respond to dietary protein restriction (see also lactulose, p. 640).

Selective decontamination of the gut reduces the risk of nosocomial infection from gut organisms (including fungi) in patients who are immuno-compromised or receiving intensive care (notably mechanical ventilation). The commonest regimen involves combinations of nonabsorbable (framy-cetin, colistin, nystatin and amphotericin) and i.v. (cefotaxime) antimicrobials to reduce the number of Gram-negative bacilli and yeasts while maintaining a normal anaerobic flora. An alternative is to administer oral ciprofloxacin alone.

Peritonitis is usually a mixed infection and anti-microbial choice must take account of coliforms, anaerobes and streptococci; a combination of gentamicin, benzylpenicillin plus metronidazole or of cefuroxime plus metronidazole, or meropenem alone is usually appropriate. Surgical drainage of peritoneal collections and abscesses is usually required as well.

Chemoprophylaxis in surgery: see p. 208.
Antibiotic-associated colitis: see p. 210.

Infection of the urinary tract

(excluding sexually transmitted infections)
Common pathogens include:

- *Escherichia coli (commonest in all patient groups)*
- *Proteus* spp.
- *Klebsiella* spp.
- Other *Enterobacteriaceae*
- *Pseudomonas aeruginosa*
- *Enterococcus* spp.
- *Staphylococcus saprophyticus.*

Patients with abnormal urinary tracts (e.g. renal stones, prostatic hypertrophy, indwelling urinary catheters) are likely to be infected with a more varied and antimicrobial-resistant microbial flora. Identification of the causative organism and of its sensitivity to drugs are important because of the range of organisms and the prevalence of resistant strains.

For infection of the lower urinary tract a low dose may be effective, as many antimicrobials are concentrated in the urine. Infections of the substance of the kidney require the doses needed for any systemic infection. Elimination of infection is hastened by a large urine volume (over 1.5 l/d) and by frequent micturition.

Drug treatment of urinary tract infection falls into several categories:

Lower urinary tract infection

Initial treatment with an oral cephalosporin (e.g. cefalexin), trimethoprim, amoxicillin or co-amoxiclav is usually satisfactory, although current resistance rates of 20–50% among common pathogens for trimethoprim and amoxicillin threaten their value for empirical therapy. Therapy should normally last 3 days and may need to be altered once the results of bacterial sensitivity are known.

Upper urinary tract infection

Acute pyelonephritis may be accompanied by septicaemia and it is advisable to start with genta-micin plus amoxicillin i.v. or alternatively cefotaxime i.v. alone. If oral therapy is considered suitable, ciprofloxacin or norfloxacin is recommended for 2 weeks. This is an infection of the kidney substance and so needs adequate blood as well as urine concentrations.

Recurrent urinary tract infection

Attacks following rapidly with the same organism may be relapses and indicate a failure to eliminate the original infection. Attacks with a longer interval between them and produced by differing bacterial types may be regarded as due to reinfection, most often by ascending infection from the perineal skin. Repeated short courses of antimicrobials should overcome most recurrent infections but, if these fail,

7–14 days of high-dose treatment may be given, following which continuous low-dose prophylaxis may be needed.

Asymptomatic infection ('asymptomatic bacteriuria')

This may be found by routine urine testing of pregnant women or patients with known structural abnormalities of the urinary tract. Such infection may explain micturition frequency or incontinence in the elderly. Appropriate antimicrobial therapy should be given, chosen on the basis of susceptibility tests, and normally for 7–10 days. Amoxicillin or a cephalosporin is preferred in pregnancy, although nitrofurantoin may be used if imminent delivery is not likely (see below).

Prostatitis

The commonest pathogens here are Gram-negative aerobic bacilli, although Chlamydia may also be involved. A quinolone such as ciprofloxacin is commonly used, although trimethoprim or erythromycin are also effective. Being lipid soluble, these drugs penetrate the prostate in adequate concentration; they may usefully be combined. Response to a single, short course is often good, but recurrence is common and a patient can be regarded as cured only if he has been symptom-free without resort to antimicrobials for a year. Four weeks of oral therapy is often given for recurrent attacks.

Chemoprophylaxis

Chemoprophylaxis is sometimes undertaken in patients liable to recurrent attacks or acute exacerbations of ineradicable infection. It may prevent progressive renal damage in children who are found to have asymptomatic bacteriuria on routine screening. Nitrofurantoin (50–100 mg/d), nalidixic acid (0.5–1.0 g/d) or trimethoprim (100 mg/d) are satisfactory. The drugs are best given as a single oral dose at night.

Tuberculosis of the genitourinary tract is treated on the principles described for pulmonary infection (p. 249).

SPECIAL DRUGS FOR URINARY TRACT INFECTIONS

General antimicrobials are used for urinary tract infections and described elsewhere. A few agents are used solely for infection of the urinary tract:

Nitrofurantoin, a synthetic antimicrobial, is active against the majority of urinary pathogens except pseudomonads. It is well absorbed from the gastrointestinal tract and is concentrated in the urine ($t\frac{1}{2}$ 1 h); but plasma concentrations are too low to treat infection of kidney tissue. Excretion is reduced when there is renal insufficiency, rendering the drug both more toxic and less effective. The main use of nitrofurantoin is now for prophylaxis. Adverse effects include nausea and vomiting (much reduced with the macrocrystalline preparation) and diarrhoea. Peripheral neuropathy occurs especially in patients with significant renal impairment, in whom the drug is contraindicated. Allergic reactions include rashes, generalised urticaria and pulmonary infiltration with lung consolidation or pleural effusion. It is safe in pregnancy, except near to term because it may cause neonatal haemolysis, and it must be avoided in patients with glucose-6-phosphate dehydrogenase deficiency (see p. 123).

Nalidixic acid: see page 233.

Genital tract infections

A general account of orthodox literature is given below, but treatment is increasingly the prerogative of specialists, who, as is so often the case, get the best results. Interested readers are referred to specialist texts. Sexually transmitted infections are commonly multiple. Screening of contacts plays a vital part in controlling spread and reducing reinfection.

GONORRHOEA

The problems of β-lactam and quinolone resistance in *Neisseria gonorrhoeae* are increasing, and selection of a particular drug will depend on sensitivity testing and a knowledge of resistance patterns in different geographical locations. Effective treatment requires exposure of the organism briefly to a high concentration of the drug. Single-dose regimens are practicable as well as being obviously desirable for social reasons, including compliance. The following schedules are effective:

Uncomplicated anogenital infections: amoxicillin with probenecid by mouth; spectinomycin i.v., cefotaxime i.m. or ciprofloxacin by mouth may be used for penicillin-allergic patients.

Pharyngeal gonorrhoea responds less reliably, and i.m. cefotaxime is recommended.

Coexistent infection. *Chlamydia trachomatis* is frequently present with *Neisseria gonorrhoeae*; tetracycline by mouth for 7 days or a single oral dose of azithromycin 1g will treat the chlamydial urethritis.

Nongonococcal urethritis

The vast majority of cases of urethritis with pus in which gonococci cannot be identified are due to sexually-transmitted organisms, usually *Chlamydia trachomatis* and sometimes *Ureaplasma urealyticum*. Tetracycline or azithromycin by mouth is effective.

Pelvic inflammatory disease

Several pathogens are involved including *Chlamydia trachomatis*, *Neisseria gonorrhoeae* and *Mycoplasma hominis* and there may be superinfection with bowel and other urogenital tract bacteria. A combination of antimicrobials is usually required, e.g. metronidazole plus doxycycline by mouth.

SYPHILIS

Treponema pallidum is known to be invariably sensitive to penicillin.

Primary and secondary syphilis are effectively treated by benzylpenicillin or procaine penicillin i.m. daily for 10–21 days. Tetracycline or erythromycin orally may be used for penicillin-allergic patients.

Tertiary syphilis should have the same treatment, ensuring that it continues for 3 weeks.

Congenital syphilis in the newborn should be treated with benzylpenicillin for 10 days at least. Some advocate that a pregnant woman with syphilis should be treated as for primary syphilis, in each pregnancy, in order to avoid all danger to children. Therapy is best given between the third and sixth month, as there may be a risk of abortion if it is given earlier.

Results of treatment of syphilis with penicillin are excellent. Follow-up of all cases is essential, for 5 years if possible.

The *Herxheimer* (or Jarisch–Herxheimer) *reaction* is probably caused by cytokine (mainly tumour necrosis factor) release following massive slaughter of spirochaetes. Presenting as pyrexia, it is common during the few hours after the first penicillin injection; other features include tachycardia, headache, myalgia and malaise which last up to a day. It cannot be avoided by giving graduated doses of penicillin. Prednisolone may prevent it and should probably be given if a reaction is specially to be feared, e.g. in a patient with syphilitic aortitis.

CHANCROID

The causal agent, *Haemophilus ducreyi*, normally responds to erythromycin for 7 days or a single dose of ceftriaxone or azithromycin.

GRANULOMA INGUINALE

Calymmatobacterium granulomatis infection is treated with ampicillin or co-trimoxazole or a tetracycline for 2 weeks.

BACTERIAL VAGINOSIS (BACTERIAL VAGINITIS, ANAEROBIC VAGINOSIS)

Bacterial vaginosis is a common form of vaginal discharge in which neither *Trichomonas vaginalis* nor *Candida albicans* can be isolated and inflammatory cells are not present. There is evidence to associate the condition with overgrowth of several normal commensals of the vagina including *Gardnerella vaginalis*, Gram-negative curved bacilli, and anaerobic organisms, especially of the *Bacteroides* genus, the latter being responsible for the characteristic fishy odour of the vaginal discharge. The condition responds well to a single 2 g oral dose of metronidazole, with topical clindamycin offering an alternative.

Candida vaginitis: see page 263.

Trichomonas vaginitis: see page 234.

Infection of bones and joints

Osteomyelitis may be acute or chronic and the causative bacteria arrive in the bloodstream or are implanted directly (through a compound fracture, chronic local infection of local tissue, or surgical operation). *Staphylococcus aureus* is the commonest isolate in all patient groups but *Haemophilus influenzae* is frequently seen in children (much reduced now by the Hib vaccine), and *Salmonella* species in the tropics. Chronic osteomyelitis of the lower limbs (especially when underlying chronic skin infection in the elderly) frequently involves obligate anaerobes (such as *Bacteroides* species) and coliforms.

Strenuous efforts should be made to obtain bone for culture because superficial and sinus cultures are poorly predictive of the underlying flora, and prolonged therapy is required for chronic osteomyelitis (usually 6–8 weeks, sometimes longer). The outcome of chronic osteomyelitis is improved if dead bone can be removed surgically.

Definitive therapy is guided by the results of culture but commonly used regimens include flucloxacillin with or without fusidic acid (for *Staphylococcus aureus*), cefotaxime or co-amoxiclav (in children), and ciprofloxacin (for coliforms). Short courses of therapy (3 weeks) may suffice for acute osteomyelitis.

Septic arthritis is a medical emergency if good joint function is to be retained. *Staphylococcus aureus* is the commonest pathogen, but a very wide range of bacteria may be involved including streptococci coliforms and *Neisseria*. Aspiration of the joint allows specific microbiological diagnosis, differentiation from noninfectious causes such as crystal synovitis, and has therapeutic benefit, e.g. for the hip joint where formal drainage is recommended. Initial therapy is as for chronic osteomyelitis.

Eye infections

Superficial infections, caused by a variety of organisms, are treated by chloramphenicol, fusidic acid, framycetin, gentamicin, ciprofloxacin, ofloxacin or neomycin in drops or ointments. Ciprofloxacin, ofloxacin, gentamicin or tobramycin are used for *Pseudomonas aeruginosa*, and fusidic acid principally for *Staphylococcus aureus*. Preparations often contain hydrocortisone or prednisolone, but the steroid masks the progress of the infection, and should it be applied with an antimicrobial to which the organism is resistant (bacterium or virus) it may make the disease worse by suppressing protective inflammation. Local chemoprophylaxis without corticosteroid is used to prevent secondary bacterial infection in viral conjunctivitis. A variety of antibiotics may be given by direct injection to the chambers of the eye for treatment of bacterial endophthalmitis.

Chlamydial conjunctivitis. In the developed world, the genital (D-K) serotypes of the organism are responsible and the reservoir and transmission is maintained by sexual contact. Endemic trachoma in developing countries is usually caused by serotypes A, B and C. In either case, oral tetracycline is effective. Pregnant or lactating women may receive systemic erythromycin. Neonatal ophthalmia should be treated with systemic erythromycin and topical tetracycline.

Herpes keratitis (see p. 258). It is essential that a corticosteroid should **never** be put on the eye; the disease is exacerbated and permanent blindness can result.

Mycobacterial infections

PULMONARY TUBERCULOSIS

Drug therapy has transformed tuberculosis from a disabling and often fatal disease into one in which almost 100% cure is obtainable, although the recent emergence of multiple drug resistant strains of *Mycobacterium tuberculosis* (MDRTB) in developed countries will disturb this optimistic view. Chemo-therapy was formerly protracted, but a better understanding of the mode of action of antituber-culous drugs has allowed the development of effective short-course regimens.

Principles of antituberculosis therapy

- A large number of actively multiplying bacilli must be killed: *isoniazid* achieves this.
- Treat persisters, i.e. semidormant bacilli that metabolise slowly or intermittently: *rifampicin* and *pyrazinamide* are the most efficacious.
- Prevent the emergence of drug resistance by multiple therapy to suppress single-drug-resistant mutants that may exist de novo or emerge during therapy in all large bacterial populations: *isoniazid* and *rifampicin* are best.
- Combined formulations are used to ensure that poor compliance does not result in monotherapy with consequent drug resistance.

Most contemporary regimens employ an *initial* phase with administration of at least three drugs to reduce the bacterial load as rapidly as possible (usually for 2 months), followed by a *continuation* phase with usually two drugs given for 4 months.

All short-course regimens include isoniazid, pyra-zinamide and rifampicin. After extensive clinical trials, the following three have been found satisfactory:

1. An *unsupervised* regimen of daily dosing comprising isoniazid and rifampicin for 6 months, plus pyrazinamide for the first 2 months.
2. A *supervised* (directly observed) regimen for patients who cannot be relied upon to comply with treatment, comprising thrice-weekly dosing with isoniazid and rifampicin for 6 months, plus pyrazinamide for the first 2 months (isoniazid and pyrazinamide are given in higher dose than in the unsupervised regimen).
   With both the above regimens, ethambutol by mouth or streptomycin i.m. should be added for the first 2 months if there is a likelihood of drug-resistant organisms, or if the patient is severely ill with extensive active lesions.
3. A *less costly*, yet still effective, regimen favoured

by some countries comprises supervised daily administration of isoniazid, rifampicin, pyrazinamide and either ethambutol or streptomycin for 2 months followed by 6 months of unsupervised daily isoniazid and thiacetazone.

All the regimens are highly effective, with relapse rates of 1–2% in those who continue for 6 months; even if patients default after, say, 4 months, tuberculosis can be expected to recur in only 10–15%. Drug resistance seldom develops with any of these regimens.

Although compliance is often a concern with multiple drug therapy given for long periods, espe-cially in the Developing World, directly observed therapy (DOT) has surprisingly not been proven to improve relapse rates in many trials. Combination therapy is assumed to improve compliance: some commonly used combinations include Rifater (rifampicin, isoniazid plus pyrazinamide), and Rifinah or Rimactazid (rifampicin plus isoniazid).

Special problems

Resistant organisms. Initial resistance occurs in about 4% of isolates in the UK, usually to isoniazid. Multiple-drug-resistant tuberculosis, i.e. resistant to rifampicin and isoniazid at least, should be treated with three or four drugs to which the organisms are sensitive and should extend for 12–24 months after cultures become negative. Treatment of such cases requires expert management. Atypical myco-bacteria are often resistant to standard drugs; their virulence is low but they can produce serious infection in immunocompromised patients which may respond, e.g. to clarithromycin or a quinolone, often in combination.

Chemoprophylaxis may be either
- *primary*, i.e. the giving of antituberculosis drugs to uninfected but exposed individuals, which is seldom justified; or
- *secondary*, which is the treatment of infected but symptom-free individuals, e.g. those known to be in contact with the disease and who develop a positive tuberculin reaction. Secondary chemoprophylaxis may be justified in children under the age of 3 because they have a high risk

of disseminated disease; isoniazid alone for 6 months may be used since there is little risk of resistant organisms emerging because the organism load is low.

Pregnancy. Drug treatment should never be interrupted or postponed during pregnancy. On the general principle of limiting exposure of the fetus, the standard three-drug, 6-month course (1 above) is best. Streptomycin should be excluded from any regimen (danger of fetal eighth cranial nerve damage).

Nonrespiratory tuberculosis. The principles of treatment, i.e. multiple therapy and prolonged follow-up, are the same as for respiratory tuberculosis. In only a few cases is surgery now necessary. It should always be preceded and followed by chemotherapy. Many chronic tuberculous lesions may be relatively inaccessible to drugs as a result of avascularity of surrounding tissues; treatment frequently has to be prolonged and dosage high, especially if damaged tissue cannot be removed by surgery, e.g. tuberculosis of bones.

Meningeal tuberculosis. It is essential to use isoniazid and pyrazinamide which penetrate well into the CSF. Rifampicin enters inflamed meninges well but noninflamed meninges less so. An effective regimen is isoniazid, rifampicin, pyrazinamide and streptomycin. Treatment may need to continue for much longer than modern short-course chemotherapy for pulmonary tuberculosis.

Adrenal steroid and tuberculosis. In pulmonary tuberculosis a corticosteroid may be given to severely ill patients. It reduces the injurious reaction of the body to tuberculoprotein and buys time for the chemotherapy to take effect. It also causes the patient to feel better much more quickly. In the absence of effective chemotherapy, an adrenal steroid will cause tuberculosis to extend and it should never be used alone, e.g. for another disease, if tuberculosis is suspected.

Tuberculosis in the immunocompromised. Immunocompromised patients require special measures because they may be infected more readily when exposed, their infections usually involve large numbers of tubercle bacilli (multibacillary disease), and in the case of patients with AIDS, are more likely to be infected with multiply antibiotic resistant strains. Usually at least four drugs are started, and patients are isolated until bacteriological results are obtained and they have shown clinical improvement. If infections are proved to involve antibiotic susceptible mycobacteria, therapy can continue with a conventional 6-month regimen with careful follow-up. Particular problems may occur with multiple drug interactions during antituberculous treatment of patients receiving antiretroviral therapy.

ANTITUBERCULOSIS DRUGS

Isoniazid

Isoniazid (INH, INAH, isonicotinic acid hydrazide) is selectively effective against *Mycobacterium tuberculosis* because it prevents the synthesis of components that are unique to mycobacterial cell walls. Hence it is bactericidal against actively multiplying bacilli (whether within macrophages or at extracellular sites) but is bacteriostatic against nondividing bacilli; it has little or no activity against other bacteria. Isoniazid is well absorbed from the alimentary tract and is distributed throughout the body water, readily crossing tissue barriers and entering cells and cerebrospinal fluid. It should always be given in cases where there is special risk of meningitis (miliary tuberculosis and primary infection). Isoniazid is inactivated by conjugation with an acetyl group and the rate of the reaction is bimodally distributed (see Pharmacogenetics, p. 123). The $t_{\frac{1}{2}}$ is 1 h in fast and 4 h in slow acetylators; steady-state plasma concentration in fast acetylators is less than half that in slow acetylators but standard oral doses (300 mg/d) on daily regimens give adequate tuberculocidal concentrations in both groups.

Adverse effects. Isoniazid is in general well tolerated. The most severe adverse effect is liver damage which may range from moderate elevation of hepatic enzymes to severe hepatitis and death. It is probably caused by a chemically reactive metabolite(s), e.g. acetylhydrazine. Most cases develop within the first 8 weeks of therapy and liver function tests should be monitored monthly during this period at least.

Isoniazid is a structural analogue of pyridoxine and accelerates its excretion, the principal result of which is peripheral neuropathy with numbness and tingling of the feet, motor involvement being less common. Neuropathy is more frequent in slow acetylators, malnourished people, the elderly and those with HIV infection, liver disease and alcoholism. Such patients should receive pyridoxine 10 mg/d by mouth, which prevents neuropathy and does not interfere with the therapeutic effect; some prefer simply to give pyridoxine to all patients. Other adverse effects include mental disturbances, incoordination, optic neuritis and convulsions.

Isoniazid inhibits the metabolism of phenytoin, carbamazepine and ethosuximide, increasing their effect.

Rifampicin

Rifampicin has bactericidal activity against the tubercle bacillus, comparable to that of isoniazid. It is also used in leprosy.

It acts by inhibiting RNA synthesis, bacteria being sensitive to this effect at much lower concentrations than mammalian cells; it is particularly effective against mycobacteria that lie semidormant within cells. Rifampicin has a wide range of antimicrobial activity. Other uses include leprosy, severe Legionnaires' disease (with erythromycin or ciprofloxacin), the chemoprophylaxis of meningococcal meningitis, and severe staphylococcal infection (with flucloxacillin or vancomycin).

Rifampicin is well absorbed from the gastrointestinal tract. It penetrates well into most tissues. Entry into the CSF when meninges are inflamed is sufficient to maintain therapeutic concentrations at normal oral doses but transfer is reduced as inflammation subsides in 1 or 2 months.

Enterohepatic recycling takes place, and eventually about 60% of a single dose is eliminated in the faeces; urinary excretion of unchanged drug also occurs. The $t\frac{1}{2}$ is 4 h after initial doses, but shortens on repeated dosing because rifampicin is a very effective enzyme inducer and increases its own metabolism (as well as that of several other drugs, see below).

Adverse reactions. Rifampicin rarely causes any serious toxicity. Adverse reactions include flushing and itching with or without a rash, and thrombocytopenia. Rises in plasma bilirubin and hepatic enzymes may occur when treatment starts but are often transient and are not necessarily an indication for stopping the drug; fatal hepatitis, however, has occurred. Hepatic function should be checked before starting treatment and at least for the first few months of therapy. Intermittent dosing, i.e. less than twice weekly, either as part of a regimen or through poor compliance, promotes certain effects that probably have an immunological basis, namely, an influenza-like syndrome (malaise, headache and fever, shortness of breath and wheezing), acute haemolytic anaemia and thrombocytopenia and acute renal failure sometimes with haemolysis. Red discolouration of urine, tears and sputum is a useful indication that the patient is taking the drug. Rifampicin also causes an orange discolouration of soft contact lenses.

Interactions. Rifampicin is a powerful enzyme inducer and speeds the metabolism of numerous drugs, including warfarin, steroid contraceptives, narcotic analgesics, oral antidiabetic agents, phenytoin and dapsone. Appropriate increase in dosage, and alternative methods of contraception, are required to compensate for increased drug metabolism (see also paracetamol overdose, p. 287).

Rifabutin ($t\frac{1}{2}$ 36 h) has similar activity and adverse reactions, and is used for prophylaxis of *Mycobacterium avium* infection in patients with AIDS, and for treatment of tuberculous and nontuberculous mycobacterial infection in combination with other drugs.

Pyrazinamide

Pyrazinamide is a derivative of nicotinamide and is included in first-choice combination regimens because of its particular ability to kill intracellular persisters, i.e. mycobacteria that are dividing or semidormant, often within cells. Its action is dependent on the activity of intrabacterial pyrazinamidase which converts pyrazinamide to the active pyrazinoic acid; this enzyme is most effective in an acidic environment such as the interior of cells. It is inactive against *Mycobacterium bovis*. Pyrazinamide is well absorbed from the gastrointestinal tract and metabolised in the liver, very little unchanged drug appearing in the urine ($t\frac{1}{2}$ 9 h). CSF concentrations are almost identical to those in the blood, hence the drug is valuable in tuberculous meningitis. Experience in several countries indicates that pyrazinamide is safe to use in pregnancy.

Adverse effects include hyperuricaemia and arthralgia, which is relatively frequent with daily but less so with intermittent dosing and, unlike gout, affects both large and small joints. Pyrazinoic acid, the principal metabolite of pyrazinamide, inhibits renal tubular secretion of urate. Symptomatic treatment with an NSAID is usually sufficient and it is rarely necessary to discontinue pyrazinamide because of arthralgia. Hepatitis, which was particularly associated with high doses, is not a problem with modern short-course schedules. Sideroblastic anaemia and urticaria also occur.

Ethambutol

Ethambutol, being bacteriostatic, is used in conjunction with other antituberculosis drugs to delay or prevent the emergence of resistant bacilli. It is well absorbed from the gastrointestinal tract and effective concentrations occur in most body tissues including the lung; in tuberculous meningitis, sufficient may reach the CSF to inhibit mycobacterial growth but insignificant amounts cross into the CSF if the meninges are not inflamed. Excretion is mainly by the kidney, by tubular secretion as well as by glomerular filtration ($t\frac{1}{2}$ 4 h); the dose should be reduced when renal function is impaired.

Adverse effects. In recommended oral doses (15 mg/kg per day) (taking account of reduced renal function), ethambutol is relatively nontoxic. The main problem is *optic neuritis* (unilateral or bilateral) causing loss of visual acuity, central scotomata, occasionally also peripheral vision loss and red–green colour blindness. The changes reverse if treatment is stopped promptly; if not, the patient may go blind. It is prudent to note any history of eye disease and to get baseline tests of vision before starting treatment with ethambutol. The drug should not be given to a patient whose vision is much reduced and who may not notice further minor deterioration. Patients should be told to make a point of reading small print in newspapers

(with each eye separately) and if there is any deterioration to stop the drug immediately and seek advice. Patients who cannot understand and comply (especially children) should be given alternative therapy, if possible. The need for repeated specialist ophthalmological monitoring is controversial. Peripheral neuritis occurs but is rare.

Streptomycin: see page 225.

Thiacetazone

Thiacetazone is tuberculostatic and is used with isoniazid to inhibit the emergence of resistance to the latter drug. It is absorbed from the gastrointestinal tract, partly metabolised and partly excreted in the urine ($t\frac{1}{2}$ 13 h).

Adverse reactions include gastrointestinal symptoms, conjunctivitis and vertigo. More serious effects are erythema multiforme, haemolytic anaemia, agranulocytosis, cerebral oedema and hepatitis.

Alternative or reserve drugs are used where there are problems of drug intolerance and bacterial resistance. They are in this class because of either greater toxicity or of lesser efficacy and include: *ethionamide* (gastrointestinal irritation, allergic reactions), *capreomycin* (nephrotoxic), and *cycloserine* (effective but neurotoxic). Quinolone antibiotics such as *ciprofloxacin* and the more recently introduced macrolides such as *clarithromycin* and *azithromycin* also have useful activity against mycobacteria.

LEPROSY

Effective treatment of leprosy is complex and requires much experience to obtain the best results. Problems of resistant leprosy now require that multiple drug therapy be used and involve:

- for *paucibacillary disease:* dapsone and rifampicin for 6 months
- for *multibacillary disease:* dapsone, rifampicin and clofazimine for 2 years. Follow-up for 4–8 years may be necessary.

Dapsone, a bacteriostatic sulphone (related to sulphonamides, and acting by the same mechanism, see p. 231), has for many years been the standard drug for the treatment of all forms of leprosy.

Irregular and inadequate duration of treatment with a single drug have allowed the emergence of resistance, both primary and secondary, to become a major problem. Dapsone is also used to treat dermatitis herpetiformis, and is given for *Pneumocystis carinii* and (with pyrimethamine) malaria prophylaxis. The $t\frac{1}{2}$ is 27 h. Adverse effects range from gastrointestinal symptoms to agranulocytosis, haemolytic anaemia and generalised allergic reactions that include exfoliative dermatitis.

Rifampicin (see above) is bactericidal, and is safe and effective when given once monthly. This long interval renders feasible the directly observed administration of rifampicin which the above regimens require.

Clofazimine has a leprostatic action and an anti-inflammatory effect that prevents erythema nodosum leprosum. It causes gastrointestinal symptoms. Reddish discolouration of the skin and other cutaneous lesions also occur, and may persist for months after the drug has been stopped. The $t\frac{1}{2}$ is 70 days.

Other antileprotics include ethionamide and prothionamide. Thalidomide (see Index), despite its notorious past, still finds a use with corticosteroid in the control of allergic lepromatous reactions.

OTHER BACTERIAL INFECTIONS

Burns. Infection may be reduced by application of silver sulphadiazine cream. Substantial absorption can occur from any raw surface and use of aminoglycoside, e.g. neomycin, preparations can cause ototoxicity.

Gas gangrene. The skin between the waist and the knees is normally contaminated with anaerobic faecal organisms. However assiduous the skin preparation for orthopaedic operations or thigh amputations, this will not kill or remove all the spores. Surgery done for vascular insufficiency where tissue oxygenation may be poor is likely to be followed by infection. Gas gangrene (*Clostridium perfringens*) may occur; it may be prevented by benzylpenicillin or metronidazole prophylaxis.

Wounds. Systemic chemoprophylaxis is necessary for several days at least in dirty wounds where sutures have to be left below the skin, and in penetrating wounds of body cavities. Flucloxacillin is probably best, but in the case of penetrating abdominal wounds, metronidazole should be added, and consideration given to adding an agent active against aerobic Gram-negative bacteria, e.g. gentamicin (see also Tetanus).

Abscesses and infections in bone and serous cavities are treated according to the antimicrobial sensitivity of the organism concerned but require high doses because of poor penetration. Local instillation of the drug may be needed.

Actinomycosis. The anaerobe *Actinomyces israelii* is sensitive to several drugs, but not metronidazole, and access is poor because of granulomatous fibrosis. High doses of benzylpenicillin or amoxicillin are given for several weeks; the infections are often mixed with other anaerobic bacteria so metronidazole is often given in addition to ensure activity against all components of the mixture. Co-amoxiclav may be a convenient alternative. Surgery is likely to be needed.

Leptospirosis. To be maximally effective, chemotherapy should be started within 4 days of the onset of symptoms. Benzylpenicillin is recommended; a Herxheimer reaction may be induced (see Syphilis). General supportive management is important, including attention to fluid balance and observation for signs of hepatic, renal or cardiac failure.

Lyme disease. Keeping the skin covered and use of insect repellants are effective to prevent tick bites and tick removal shortly after attachment (within 24 h) will prevent infection. In most manifestations of the disease, *Borrelia burgdorferi* responds to amoxicillin or doxycycline orally for up to 21 days but when the central nervous system is invaded large doses of cefotaxime should be given i.v. for 14 days.

GUIDE TO FURTHER READING

Adachi J A, Ostrosky-Zeichner L, DuPont H L, Ericsson C D 2000 Empirical antimicrobial therapy for traveler's diarrhea. Clinical Infectious Diseases 31: 1079–1083

Arroll B, Knealy T 2001 Antibiotics for acute bronchitis. British Medical Journal 322: 939–940

Bisno A L 2001 Acute pharyngitis. New England Journal of Medicine 344: 205

Brown P D, Lerner S A 1998 Community-acquired pneumonia. Lancet 352: 1295–1302

Campion E W 1999 Liberty and the control of tuberculosis. New England Journal of Medicine 340: 385–386

Del Mar C et al 1997 Are antibiotics indicated as initial treatment for children with acute otitis media? A meta-analysis. British Medical Journal 314: 1526–1529

Dixon T C et al 1999 Anthrax. New England Journal of Medicine 341: 815–826

Goldenberg D L 1998 Septic arthritis. Lancet 351: 197–202

Gorbach S L 1999 Antibiotics and *Clostridium difficile*. New England Journal of Medicine 341: 1690–1691

Jacobson R R, Krahenbuhl J L 1999 Leprosy. Lancet 353: 655–660

Joint Tuberculosis Committee of the British Thoracic Society 1998 Chemotherapy and management of tuberculosis in the United Kingdom: recommendations. Thorax 53: 536

Lew D P, Waldvogel F A 1997 Osteomyelitis. New England Journal of Medicine 336: 999–1007

Marik P E 2001 Aspiration pneumonitis and aspiration pneumonia. New England Journal of Medicine 344: 665–671

Mead P S, Griffin P M 1998 *Escherichia coli* 0157;H7. Lancet 352: 1207–1212

Mylonakis E, Calderwood S B 2001 Infective endocarditis in adults. New England Journal of Medicine 345: 1318–1330

Nicolle L E 2000 Asymptomatic bacteruria—important or not? New England Journal of Medicine 343: 1037–1039

Rosenstein N E et al 2001 Meningococcal disease. New England Journal of Medicine 344: 1378–1388

Sobel J D 1997 Vaginitis. New England Journal of Medicine 337: 1896–1903

Steere A C 2001 Lyme disease. New England Journal of Medicine 345: 115–125

Whitty C J 1999 Erasmus, syphilis, and the abuse of stigma. Lancet 354: 2147–2148

Working Party 1996 Guidelines for the prevention and treatment of infection in patients with an absent or dysfunctional spleen. British Medical Journal 312: 430

14

Viral, fungal, protozoal and helminthic infections

SYNOPSIS

- **Viruses** present a more difficult problem of chemotherapy than do higher organisms, e.g. bacteria, for they are intracellular parasites that use the metabolism of host cells. Highly selective toxicity is, therefore, harder to achieve. Identification of differences between viral and human metabolism has led to the development of effective antiviral agents, whose roles are increasingly well defined.
- **Fungus infections** range from inconvenient skin conditions to life-threatening systemic diseases; the latter have become more frequent as opportunistic infections in patients immunocompromised by drugs or AIDS, or receiving intensive medical and surgical interventions in ICUs.
- **Protozoal infections.** Malaria is the major transmissible parasitic disease in the world. The life cycle of the plasmodium that is relevant to prophylaxis and therapy is described. Drug resistance is an increasing problem and differs with geographical location, and species of plasmodium.
- **Helminthic infestations** cause considerable morbidity. The drugs that are effective against these organisms are summarised.

Viral infections

Antiviral agents are most active when viruses are replicating. The earlier that treatment is given, therefore, the better the result. An important difficulty is that a substantial amount of viral multiplication has often taken place before symptoms occur. Apart from primary infection, viral illness is often the consequence of reactivation of latent virus in the body. In both cases patients whose immune systems are compromised may suffer particularly severe illness. Viruses are capable of developing resistance to antimicrobial drugs, with similar implications for the individual patient, for the community and for drug development. An overview of drugs that have proved effective against virus diseases appears in Table 14.1.

Herpes simplex and varicella-zoster

ACICLOVIR

Aciclovir inhibits viral DNA synthesis only after phosphorylation by virus-specific thymidine kinase, which accounts for its high therapeutic index.

TABLE 14.1 Drugs of choice for virus infections

Organism	Drug of choice	Alternative
Varicella-zoster		
chickenpox	aciclovir	valaciclovir or
zoster	aciclovir or	famciclovir
	famciclovir	valaciclovir
Herpes simplex		
keratitis	aciclovir(topical)	
labial	aciclovir (topical and/or oral)	valaciclovir
genital	aciclovir (topical and/or oral)	valaciclovir
	famciclovir (oral)	penciclovir
encephalitis	aciclovir	
disseminated	aciclovir	foscarnet
Human immunodeficiency virus (HIV)	zidovudine	zalcitabine
	didanosine	stavudine
	ritonavir	lamivudine
	indinavir	nevirapine
	saquinavir	abacavir
	nelfinavir	efavirenz
Hepatitis B, C or D	interferon alfa-2a and 2b	lamivudine
Influenza A	zanamivir	amantadine
Cytomegalovirus (CMV)	ganciclovir	foscarnet (for retinitis in HIV patients) oidofovir
Respiratory syncytial virus	tribavirin	

Phosphorylated aciclovir inhibits DNA polymerase and so prevents viral DNA being formed. It effectively treats susceptible herpes viruses if started early in the course of infection, but it does not eradicate persistent infection. Taken orally about 20% is absorbed from the gut, but this is sufficient for the systemic treatment of some infections. It distributes widely in the body; the concentration in CSF is approximately half that of plasma, and the brain concentration may be even less. These differences are taken into account in dosing for viral encephalitis (for which aciclovir must be given i.v.). The drug is excreted in the urine ($t\frac{1}{2}$ 3 h). For oral and topical use the drug is given × 5/d.

Indications for aciclovir include:

Herpes simplex virus:

- skin infections, including initial and recurrent labial and genital herpes (as a cream), most effectively when new lesions are forming; skin

and mucous membrane infections (as tablets or oral suspension)
- ocular keratitis (as an ointment)
- prophylaxis and treatment in the immunocompromised (oral, as tablets or suspension)
- encephalitis, disseminated disease (i.v.).

Aciclovir-resistant herpes simplex virus has been reported in patients with AIDS; foscarnet (see p. 262) has been used in these cases.

Varicella-zoster virus:

- chickenpox, particularly in the immunocompromised (i.v.) or in the immunocompetent with pneumonitis or hepatitis (i.v.)
- shingles in immunocompetent persons (as tablets or suspension, and best within 48 h of the appearance of the rash). Immunocompromised persons will often have more severe symptoms and require i.v. administration.

Adverse reactions are remarkably few. The ophthalmic ointment causes a mild transient stinging sensation and a diffuse superficial punctate keratopathy which clears when the drug is stopped. Oral or i.v. use may cause gastrointestinal symptoms, headache and neuropsychiatric reactions. Extravasation with i.v. use causes severe local inflammation.

Valaciclovir is a prodrug (ester) of aciclovir, i.e. after oral administration the parent aciclovir is released. The higher bioavailability of valaciclovir (about 60%) allows dosing only 8-hourly. It is used for treating herpes zoster infections and herpes simplex infections of the skin and mucous membranes.

Famciclovir is a prodrug of penciclovir which is similar to aciclovir; it is used for herpes zoster and genital herpes simplex infections. It need be given only 8-hourly. *Penciclovir* is also available as a cream for treatment of labial herpes simplex.

Idoxuridine was the first widely used antivirus drug. It is superseded by aciclovir and is variably effective topically for ocular and cutaneous herpes simplex with few adverse reactions.

Human immunodeficiency virus (HIV)

GENERAL PRINCIPLES

- No current antiviral agents or combinations eliminate HIV infection, but the most effective combinations (so-called highly-active anti-retroviral therapy, HAART) produce profound suppression of viral replication in many patients which results in useful reconstitution of the immune system. This can be measured by a fall in the plasma viral load and an increase in the numbers of cytotoxic T-cells (CD4 count) in patients' plasma. Rates of opportunistic infections such as *Pneumocystis carinii* pneumonia and CMV retinitis are reduced in patients with restored CD4 counts and their life-expectancy is markedly increased. Efficacy of viral suppression, however, must be balanced against the risks of unwanted effects from the multiple drugs used. Combination therapy reduces the risks of emergence of resistance to antiretroviral drugs, which is increasing in incidence even in patients newly-diagnosed with HIV.
- HAART comprises two nucleoside reverse transcriptase inhibitors used with either a non-nucleoside reverse transcriptase inhibitor or one or two protease inhibitors.
- The decision to begin antiretroviral therapy is based on the CD4 cell count, the plasma viral load and the intensity of the patient's clinical symptoms. Therapy is switched to alternative combinations if these variables deteriorate. Available information about drugs and combinations is accumulating monthly and the choice of agents is best made after reference to contemporary, expert advice.
- Pregnancy and breast-feeding pose especial problems; therapy at this time is aimed to minimise toxicity to the fetus while reducing maternal viral load and the catastrophic results of HIV transmission to the neonate. Prevention of maternal–fetal and maternal–infant transmission is the most cost-effective way of using antiretroviral drugs in less developed countries.
- Combination antiretroviral therapy is associated with redistribution of body fat in some patients ('lipodystrophy syndrome'), and protease inhibitors may disturb lipid and glucose metabolism. Appropriate laboratory tests to monitor these effects should be performed.
- Impaired cell-mediated immunity leaves the host prey to many (opportunistic) infections including: candidiasis, coccidioidomycosis, cryptosporidiosis, cytomegalovirus disease, herpes simplex, histoplasmosis, *Pneumocystis carinii* pneumonia, toxoplasmosis and tuberculosis (with multiply-resistant organisms). Treatment of these conditions is referred to elsewhere in this text; for a comprehensive review of the antimicrobial prophylaxis of opportunistic infections in patients with HIV infection, readers are referred to Kovacs & Masur 2000 New England Journal of Medicine 342: 1416.

Antiretroviral drugs may also be used in combination to reduce the risks of acquisition of HIV from accidental needlestick injuries from HIV-contaminated sharps such as needles. The decision to offer this postexposure prophylaxis (PEP), and the optimal combination of drugs used, should be made by experts and administration must begin rapidly (within a few hours of the injury).

NUCLEOSIDE REVERSE TRANSCRIPTASE INHIBITORS

Zidovudine (Retrovir)

The human immunodeficiency virus replicates by converting its single-standed RNA into double-stranded DNA which is incorporated into host DNA; this crucial conversion, the reverse of the normal cellular transcription of nucleic acids, is accomplished by the enzyme *reverse transcriptase*. Zidovudine, as the triphosphate, was the first anti-HIV drug to be introduced and has a high affinity for reverse transcriptase. It is integrated by it into the viral DNA chain, causing premature chain termination. The drug must be present continuously to prevent viral alteration of the host DNA, which is permanent once it occurs.

Pharmacokinetics. Zidovudine is well absorbed from the gastrointestinal tract (it is available as capsules and syrup) and is rapidly cleared from the plasma ($t\frac{1}{2}$ 1 h); concentrations in CSF are approximately half those in plasma. It is also available i.v. for patients temporarily unable to take oral medications. The drug is mainly metabolically inactivated, but 20% is excreted unchanged by the kidney.

Uses. Zidovudine is indicated for serious manifestations of HIV infection in patients with acquired immunodeficiency syndrome (AIDS) or AIDS-related complex, i.e. those with opportunistic infection, constitutional or neurological symptoms, or with low CD4 counts; treatment reduces the frequency of opportunistic infections and prolongs survival when used in effective combinations. It is also indicated alone for pregnant women and their offspring for prevention of maternal–fetal HIV transmission.

Adverse reactions early in treatment may include anorexia, nausea, vomiting, headache, dizziness, malaise and myalgia, but tolerance develops to these and usually the dose need not be altered. More serious are anaemia and neutropenia which develop more commonly when the dose is high, and with advanced disease. A toxic myopathy (not easily distinguishable from HIV-associated myopathy) may develop with long-term use. Rarely, a syndrome of hepatic necrosis with lactic acidosis may occur with zidovudine (and with other reverse transcriptase inhibitors).

Didanosine (DDI) has a much longer intracellular duration than zidovudine and thus prolonged antiretroviral activity. Didanosine is rapidly but incompletely absorbed from the gastrointestinal tract and is widely distributed in body water; 30–65% is recovered unchanged in the urine which it enters both by glomerular filtration and tubular secretion ($t\frac{1}{2}$ 1 h). Didanosine may cause pancreatitis with an incidence of 7% at a dose of 500 mg/d; a reduced dose may be tolerated after symptoms have resolved. Other adverse effects include peripheral neuropathy, hyperuricaemia and diarrhoea, any of which may give reason to reduce the dose or discontinue the drug. It reduces gastric acidity, which

impairs absorption of a number of drugs frequently used in patients with AIDS including dapsone, ketoconazole, quinolones and indinavir.

Zalcitabine (DDC) ($t\frac{1}{2}$ 1 h) is similar. Adverse effects include peripheral neuropathy, hepatitis and pancreatitis which are reason to discontinue the drug. Oral ulceration, gastrointestinal symptoms and bone marrow suppression have also been reported.

Lamivudine (3TC) is a reverse transcriptase inhibitor with a relatively long intracellular half-life (14 h; plasma $t\frac{1}{2}$ 6 h). In combination with zidovudine, lamivudine appears to reduce viral load effectively and to be well tolerated, although bone marrow suppression may be produced. Rarely, pancreatitis may occur. Lamivudine has also been used for treatment of chronic hepatitis B infection, but resistant strains of virus have been reported.

Abacavir ($t\frac{1}{2}$ 2 h) may be the most potent reverse transcriptase inhibitor. It is usually well-tolerated, but adverse effects may include hypersensitivity reactions especially during the first 6 weeks of therapy.

Stavudine ($t\frac{1}{2}$ 1 h). Hepatic toxicity and pancreatitis have been reported, and a dose-related peripheral neuropathy may occur.

PROTEASE INHIBITORS

Protease inhibitors constitute a new class of agent for HIV infection. In its process of replication, HIV produces protein and also a protease which cleaves the protein into component parts that are subsequently reassembled into virus particles; protease inhibitors disrupt this essential process.

Protease inhibitors have been shown to reduce viral RNA concentration ('viral load'), increase the CD4 count and improve survival when used in combination with other agents and compared against placebo. They are extensively metabolised by isoenzymes of the cytochrome P450 system, notably by CYP 3A4 which is involved in the metabolism of many drugs. Plasma $t\frac{1}{2}$ for each of these is in the range 2–4 h. The drugs have broadly similar therapeutic effects and include:

Amprenavir, indinavir, lopinavir, nelfinavir, ritonavir and saquinavir

Adverse effects. A variety of effects has been associated with these agents, including gastrointestinal disturbance, headache, dizziness, sleep disturbance, raised liver enzymes, neutropenia, pancreatitis, and rashes.

Interactions. Involvement of protease inhibitors with the cytochrome P450 system provides scope for interaction with numerous substances. Agents that induce P450 enzymes (e.g. rifampicin, St John's wort) accelerate their metabolism, and reduce plasma concentration; enzyme inhibitors (e.g. ketoconazole, cimetidine) raise their plasma concentration; competition with other drugs for the cytochrome enzymes can lead to variable results. Ritonavir is itself a powerful inhibitor of CYP 3A4 and CYP 2D6. This effect is utilised when ritonavir in small quantity is combined (in capsules) with lopinavir to inhibit its metabolism and increase its therapeutic efficacy. The present account should be sufficient to warn the physician, and thereby the patient, to take particular heed when seeking to co-administer any drug a with protease inhibitor.

NON-NUCLEOSIDE REVERSE TRANSCRIPTASE INHIBITORS

Efavirenz has a long duration of action and need be taken only once per day (t½ 52 h). Rash is relatively common during the first 2 weeks of therapy, but resolution usually occurs within a further 2 weeks; the drug should be stopped if the rash is severe or if there is blistering, desquamation, mucosal involvement or fever. Neurological adverse reactions occur and may be reduced by taking the drug; gastrointestinal side effects, hepatitis and pancreatitis have also been reported.

Nevirapine is used in combination with at least two other antiretroviral drugs, usually for progressive or advanced HIV infection, although it appears effective also in pregnancy. It penetrates the CSF well, and undergoes hepatic metabolism (t½ 28 h). It is taken once daily, increasing to twice daily if rash is not seen. Rash and hepatitis are the commonest side effects.

Anti-HIV drugs are the subject of intense research and development and several new agents belonging to one or other of the above classes are to be expected.

Influenza A

Amantadine

Amantadine is effective only against influenza A; it acts by interfering with the uncoating and release of viral genome into the host cell. It is well absorbed from the gastrointestinal tract and is eliminated in the urine (t½ 3 h). Amantadine may be used orally for the prevention and treatment of infection with influenza A (but not influenza B) virus. Those most likely to benefit include the debilitated, persons with respiratory disability and people living in crowded conditions, especially during an influenza epidemic.

Adverse reactions include dizziness, nervousness, lightheadedness and insomnia. Drowsiness, hallucinations, delirium and coma may occur in patients with impaired renal function. Convulsions may be induced, and amantadine should be avoided in epileptic patients.

Amantadine for Parkinson's disease: see page 404.

Zanamivir (Relenza)

Zanamivir is a neuraminidase inhibitor which blocks entry of the influenza A and B viruses to target cells and the release of their progeny. It is administered as 5 mg of a dry powder twice daily in 5-day course via a special inhaler. Controlled trials have shown that the duration of symptoms is reduced from about 6 to 5 days, with a smaller reduction in the mean time taken to return to normal activities. In high-risk groups the reduction in duration of symptoms is a little greater, and fewer patients need antibiotics.

Zanamivir was one of the first medicines to be the subject of a technology appraisal by the National Institute for Clinical Excellence (NICE) in the UK. NICE recommends that it be reserved for: at-risk patients (those with chronic respiratory or cardiovascular disease, immunosuppression or diabetes mellitus, or over the age of 65); when virological surveillance in the community indicates that influenza virus is circulating; and only for those who present within 48 h of the onset of influenza-like symptoms.

Unwanted effects are uncommon, but bronchospasm may be precipitated in asthmatics and gastrointestinal disturbance and rash are occasionally seen.

Cytomegalovirus

Ganciclovir

Ganciclovir is similar to aciclovir in its mode of action, but is much more toxic. It is given i.v. or orally and is eliminated in the urine, mainly unchanged ($t\frac{1}{2}$ 4 h). Ganciclovir is active against several types of virus but because of toxicity, its i.v. use is limited to life- or sight-threatening cytomegalovirus (CMV) infection in immunocompromised patients, and (by mouth) for maintenance suppressive treatment of retinitis in patients with AIDS, and to prevent CMV disease in patients receiving immunosuppressive therapy following organ transplantation (especially liver transplants). Ganciclovir-resistant cytomegalovirus isolates have been reported.

Adverse reactions include neutropenia and thrombocytopenia which are usually but not always reversible after withdrawal. Concomitant use of potential marrow-depressant drugs, e.g. cotrimoxazole, amphotericin B, zidovudine, should be avoided. Other reactions are fever, rash, gastrointestinal symptoms, confusion and seizure (the last especially if imipenem is coadministered).

Foscarnet is used i.v. for retinitis due to CMV in patients with HIV infection when ganciclovir is contraindicated; it has also been used to treat aciclovir-resistant herpes simplex virus infection (see p. 258). It causes numerous adverse effects, including renal toxicity, nausea and vomiting, neurological reactions and marrow suppression.

Cidofovir is given by i.v. infusion (usually every 1–2 weeks) for CMV retinitis in patients with AIDS when other drugs are unsuitable. Nephrotoxicity is common, but is reduced by hydration with i.v. fluids before each dose and co-administration with probenecid. A variety of other side effects has been reported, including bone marrow suppression, nausea and vomiting, and iritis and uveitis.

Respiratory syncytial virus (RSV)

Ribavirin (Tribavirin) is a synthetic nucleoside which may be administered by inhalation via a special ventilator for RSV bronchiolitis in infants and children. Efficacy for this indication is controversial, and it is usually reserved for the most severe cases, and those with co-existing illnesses, such as immunosuppression. Systemic absorption by the inhalational route is negligible. It is effective by mouth ($t\frac{1}{2}$ 45 h) in treating Lassa fever and, when combined with interferon alfa-2b, for chronic hepatitis C infection (see below). Systemic ribavirin is an important teratogen, and it may cause cardiac, haematological, gastrointestinal and neurological side effects.

Palivizumab may be given by monthly i.m. injection in the winter and early spring to infants at high risk of suffering RSV infection. Transient fever and local injection site reactions are seen, and rarely gastrointestinal disturbance, rash, leucopenia or disturbed liver function may occur.

Drugs that modulate the host immune system

Interferons

Virus infection stimulates the production of protective glycoproteins (interferons) which act: (1) directly on uninfected cells to induce enzymes that degrade viral RNA; (2) indirectly by stimulating the immune system. Interferons will also modify cell regulatory mechanisms and inhibit neoplastic growth. They are classified as alfa, beta or gamma according to their antigenic and physical properties. Alfa interferons (subclassified -2a, -2b and -N1) are effective against conditions that include hairy cell leukaemia, chronic myelogenous leukaemia, recurrent or metastatic renal cell carcinoma, Kaposi's sarcoma in AIDS patients (an effect that may be partly due to its activity against HIV) and condylomata acuminata (genital warts).

Interferon alfa-2a and -2b also improve the manifestations of viral hepatitis, but responses differ according to the infecting agent (see p. 658). Whereas patients with hepatitis B and C may respond to interferon alfa, those with hepatitis C have a higher rate of relapse and may need prolonged therapy. Interferon alfa-2b has been used in combination with ribavirin for moderate to severe, chronic hepatitis C infection, but not in patients who are heavy imbibers of alcohol because of the risks of liver damage. Successful treatment results in the serum concentration of viral RNA becoming undetectable by polymerase chain reaction (PCR). Hepatitis D requires a much larger dose of interferon to obtain a response and yet relapse may occur if the drug is withdrawn.

Adverse reactions are common and include an influenza-like syndrome (naturally-produced interferon may cause symptoms in natural influenza infection), fatigue and depression which respond to lowering the dose. Other effects are anorexia (sufficient to induce weight loss), convulsions, hypotension, hypertension, cardiac arrhythmias and bone marrow depression. Interferons inhibit the metabolism of theophylline, increasing its effect.

Inosine pranobex

This drug is reported to stimulate the host immune response to virus infection and has been used for mucocutaneous herpes simplex and genital warts (but aciclovir is superior). It is administered by mouth and metabolised to uric acid, so should be used with caution in patients with hyperuricaemia or gout.

Fungal infections

Widespread use of immunosuppressive chemo-

therapy and the emergence of AIDS have contributed to a rise in the incidence of opportunistic infection ranging from comparatively trivial cutaneous infections to systemic disease that demands prolonged treatment with potentially toxic agents. In hospital, candida infections have risen over 10-fold over the past decade, and associated usage of antifungal drugs has risen markedly.

Superficial mycoses

DERMATOPHYTE INFECTIONS
(ringworm, tinea)

Longstanding remedies such as Compound Benzoic Acid Ointment (Whitfield's ointment) are still acceptable for mild infections but a topical imidazole (clotrimazole, econazole, miconazole, sulconazole), which is also effective against candida, is now usually preferred. Tioconazole is effective topically for nail infections. If multiple areas are affected, especially if the scalp or nails are included, and if topical therapy fails, oral itraconazole or terbinafine are used. Griseofulvin has largely been superseded for these indications.

CANDIDA INFECTIONS

Cutaneous infection is generally treated with topical amphotericin, clotrimazole, econazole, miconazole or nystatin. Local hygiene is also important. An underlying explanation should be sought if a patient fails to respond to these measures, e.g. diabetes, the use of a broad-spectrum antibiotic or of immunosuppressive drugs.

Candidiasis of the alimentary tract mucosa responds to amphotericin, fluconazole, ketoconazole, miconazole or nystatin as lozenges (to suck, for oral infection), gel (held in the mouth before swallowing), suspension or tablets.

Vaginal candidiasis is treated by clotrimazole, econazole, isoconazole, ketoconazole, miconazole or nystatin as pessaries or vaginal tablets or cream inserted once or twice a day with cream or ointment on surrounding skin. Failure may be due to a concurrent intestinal infection causing reinfection and nystatin tablets may be given by mouth

8-hourly with the local treatment. Alternatively, oral fluconazole therapy may be used, and this is now available without prescription ('over the counter' medication) in the UK. The male sexual partner may use a similar antifungal ointment for his benefit and for hers (reinfection).

Fluconazole is often given orally or i.v. to heavily immunocompromised patients (e.g. during periods of profound granulocytopenia) and to severely ill patients on intensive care units to reduce the incidence of systemic candidiasis.

Systemic mycoses

The principal treatment options are summarised in Table 14.2.

Pneumocystosis, caused by *Pneumocystis carinii* (now classified as a fungus), is an important cause of potentially fatal pneumonia in the immuno-suppressed. It is treated with co-trimoxazole in high dose (120 mg/kg daily in 2–4 divided doses for 14 days by mouth or i.v. infusion). Intolerant or resistant cases may benefit from pentamidine or, if mild to moderate, from atovaquone, or trimetrexate (given with calcium folinate). Co-trimoxazole by mouth or intermittent inhaled pentamidine are used for prophylaxis in patients with AIDS.

Classification of antifungal agents

- Drugs that disrupt the fungal cell membrane
  polyenes: e.g. amphotericin
  azoles: imidazoles, e.g. ketoconazole triazoles, e.g. fluconazole
  allylamine: terbinafine
- Drug that inhibits mitosis: griseofulvin
- Drug that inhibits DNA synthesis: flucytosine

Drugs that disrupt the fungal cell membrane

POLYENE ANTIBIOTICS

These act by binding tightly to sterols present in cell

TABLE 14.2 Drugs of choice for some fungal infections

Infection	Drug of first choice	Alternative
Aspergillosis	amphotericin	itraconazole
Blastomycosis[1]	itraconazole or amphotericin	ketoconazole[2] or fluconazole
Candidiasis		
mucosal	fluconazole or amphotericin	itraconazole or ketoconazole
systemic	amphotericin or flucytosine	or fluconazole
Coccidiodoidomycosis[1]	fluconazole or amphotericin	itraconazole or ketoconazole[2] or fluconazole
Cryptococcosis	amphotericin + flucytosine	fluconazole or itraconazole
chronic suppression	fluconazole or itraconazole	amphotericin (weekly)
Histoplasmosis	itraconazole or amphotericin	ketoconazole[2]
chronic suppression[3]	itraconazole	amphotericin
Mucormycosis	amphotericin	no dependable alternative
Paracoccidioidomycosis	itraconazole or amphotericin	ketoconazole[2]
Pseudallescheriasis	ketoconazole or itraconazole	
Sporotrichosis		
cutaneous	itraconazole	potassium iodide
deep	amphotericin	Itraconazole or fluconazole

[1] Patients with severe illness, meningitis, AIDS or some other causes of immunosuppression should receive amphotericin.
[2] Continue treatment for 6–12 months.
[3] For patients with AIDS.
This Table is drawn substantially from the Medical Letter on Drugs and Therapeutics (2001, USA). We are grateful to the Chairman of the Editorial Board for permission to publish the material (PNB, MIB).

membranes. The resulting deformity of the membrane allows leakage of intracellular ions and enzymes, causing cell death. Those polyenes that have useful antifungal activity bind selectively to ergosterol, the most important sterol in fungal (but not mammalian) cell walls.

Amphotericin (amphotericin B)

Amphotericin is negligibly absorbed from the gut

and must be given by i.v. infusion for systemic infection; about 10% remains in the blood and the fate of the remainder is not known but it is probably bound to tissues. The $t\frac{1}{2}$ is 15 d, i.e. after stopping treatment, drug persists in the body for several weeks.

Amphotericin is at present the drug of choice for most systemic fungal infections (see Table 14.2). The diagnosis of systemic infection should whenever possible be firmly established because toxicity from conventional amphotericin is significant and the lipid-associated formulations are very expensive; tissue biopsy and culture may be necessary. New molecular diagnostic methods based on the polymerase chain reaction to detect aspergillus DNA may soon revolutionise management of invasive infection. A conventional course of treatment for filamentous fungal infection lasts 6–12 weeks during which at least 2 g of amphotericin is given (usually 1 mg/kg/day), but lower total and daily (e.g. 0.6 mg/kg) doses are used for *Candida* infections with correspondingly lower rates of adverse drug reactions.

Lipid-associated formulations of amphotericin offer the prospect of reduced risk of toxicity while retaining therapeutic efficacy. In an aqueous medium, a lipid with hydrophilic and hydrophobic properties will form vesicles (liposomes) comprising an outer lipid bilayer surrounding an aqueous centre. The AmBisome formulation incorporates amphotericin in a lipid bilayer (diameter 55–75 nm) from which the drug is released. Amphotericin is also formulated as other lipid-associated complexes, e.g. Abelcet ('amphotericin B lipid complex'), and Amphocil ('amphotericin B colloidal dispersion'). Experience with these formulations is growing; AmBisome is the most established, and it is significantly less toxic but much more expensive than conventional amphotericin. It may be more effective for some indications, probably because higher doses may safely be given more quickly (e.g. 3 mg/kg/day). It is the first choice for patients with impaired renal function, but treatment is often begun with the conventional formulation in those with normal kidneys. Therapy can be transferred to AmBisome if the patient's renal function deteriorates. Further clinical trials are needed to establish the best clinically and cost effective ways to use these drugs.

Adverse reactions. Gradual escalation of the dose limits toxic effects but these may have to be accepted in life-threatening infection if conventional amphotericin is used. Renal impairment is invariable, although reduced by adequate hydration and amphotericin need not be stopped until serum creatinine has risen to 180–200 micromol/l; the same dose may then be resumed after 3–5 days. Amphotericin nephrotoxicity is reversible, at least in its early stages. Hypokalaemia (due to distal renal tubular acidosis) may necessitate replacement therapy. Other adverse effects include: anorexia, nausea, vomiting, malaise, abdominal, muscle and joint pains, loss of weight, anaemia, hypomagnesaemia and fever. Aspirin, an antihistamine (H_1 receptor) or an antiemetic may alleviate symptoms. Severe febrile reactions are mitigated by hydrocortisone 25–50 mg before each infusion. Lipid-formulated preparations are much less often associated with adverse reactions, but fever, chills, nausea, vomiting, nephrotoxicity, electrolyte disturbance and occasional hepatotoxicity have been reported.

Nystatin

(named after New York State Health Laboratory)

Nystatin is too toxic for systemic use. It is not absorbed from the alimentary canal and is used to prevent or treat superficial candidiasis of the mouth, oesophagus or intestinal tract (as suspension, tablets or pastilles), for vaginal candidiasis (pessaries) and cutaneous infection (cream, ointment or powder).

AZOLES

The antibacterial, antiprotozoal and anthelminthic members of this group are described in the appropriate sections. Antifungal azoles comprise the following:

- *Imidazoles* (ketoconazole, miconazole, fenticonazole, clotrimazole, isoconazole, tioconazole) interfere with fungal oxidative enzymes to cause lethal accumulation of hydrogen peroxide; they also reduce the formation of ergosterol, an important constituent of the fungal cell wall which thus becomes permeable to intracellular constituents. Lack of selectivity in these actions results in important adverse effects.
- *Triazoles* (fluconazole, itraconazole) damage the

fungal cell membrane by inhibiting a demethylase enzyme; they have greater selectivity against fungi, better penetration of the CNS, resistance to degradation and cause less endocrine disturbance than do the imidazoles.

Ketoconazole

Ketoconazole is well absorbed from the gut (poorly where there is gastric hypoacidity, see below); it is widely distributed in tissues but concentrations in CSF and urine are low; its action is terminated by metabolism by cytochrome P450 3A (CYP 3A) ($t\frac{1}{2}$ 8 h). Ketoconazole is effective by mouth for systemic mycoses (see Table 14.2) but has been superseded by fluconazole and itraconazole for many indications largely on grounds of improved pharmacokinetics, unwanted effect profile and efficacy. Impairment of steroid synthesis by ketoconazole has been put to other uses, e.g. inhibition of testosterone synthesis lessens bone pain in patients with advanced androgen-dependent prostatic cancer.

Adverse reactions include nausea, giddiness, headache, pruritus and photophobia. Impairment of testosterone synthesis may cause gynaecomastia and decreased libido in men. Of particular concern is impairment of liver function, ranging from transient elevation of hepatic transaminases and alkaline phosphatase to severe injury and death.

Interactions. Drugs that lower gastric acidity, e.g. antacids, histamine H_2 receptor antagonists, impair the absorption of ketoconazole from the gastrointestinal tract. Like all imidazoles, ketoconazole binds strongly to several cytochrome P450 isoenzymes and thus inhibits the metabolism (and increases effects of) oral anticoagulants, phenytoin and cyclosporin, and increases the risk of cardiac arrhythmias with terfenadine. A disulfiram-like reaction occurs with alcohol. Concurrent use of rifampicin, by enzyme induction of CYP 3A, markedly reduces the plasma concentration of ketoconazole.

Miconazole is an alternative. *Clotrimazole* is an effective topical agent for dermatophyte, yeast, and other fungal infections (intertrigo, athlete's foot, ringworm, pityriasis versicolor, fungal nappy rash).

Econazole and *sulconazole* are similar. *Tioconazole* is used for fungal nail infections and *isoconazole* and *fenticonazole* for vaginal candidiasis.

Fluconazole

Fluconazole is absorbed from the gastrointestinal tract and is excreted largely unchanged by the kidney ($t\frac{1}{2}$ 30 h). It is effective by mouth for oropharyngeal and oesophageal candidiasis, and i.v. for systemic candidiasis and cryptococcosis (including cryptococcal meningitis; it penetrates the CSF well). It is used prophylactically in a variety of conditions predisposing to systemic *Candida* infections, including at times of profound neutropenia after bone marrow transplantation, and in patients in Intensive Care Units who have intravenous lines in situ, are receiving antibiotic therapy and have undergone bowel surgery. It may cause gastrointestinal discomfort, headaches, elevation of liver enzymes and allergic rash, but is generally very well tolerated. Animal studies demonstrate embryotoxicity and fluconazole ought not to be given to pregnant women. High doses increase the effects of phenytoin, cyclosporin, zidovudine and warfarin.

Itraconazole

Itraconazole is available for oral and i.v. administration. Absorption from the gut is about 55% and is variable. It is improved by ingestion with food, but decreased by fatty meals and therapies that reduce gastric acidity, and is often reduced in patients with AIDS; to assure adequacy of therapy, serum concentrations should be assayed during prolonged use for critical indications. It is heavily protein bound and virtually none is found within the CSF. Itraconazole is almost completely oxidised by the liver (it is a substrate for CYP 3A), and excreted in the bile; little unchanged drug enters the urine ($t\frac{1}{2}$ 25 h, increasing to 40 h with continuous treatment). Itraconazole is used for a variety of superficial mycoses, as a prophylactic agent for aspergillosis and candidiasis in the immunocompromised, and i.v. for treatment of histoplasmosis. It is licensed in the UK as a second line agent for *Candida*, *Aspergillus* and *Cryptococcus* infections, and it may be convenient as 'follow on' therapy after systemic aspergillosis has been brought under control by an amphotericin preparation. It appears to be an effective adjunct treatment for allergic bronchopulmonary aspergillosis.

Adverse effects are uncommon, but include transient hepatitis and hypokalaemia. Prolonged use may lead to cardiac failure, especially in those with pre-existing cardiac disease. Co-administration of a calcium channel blocker adds to the risk.

Interactions. Enzyme induction of CYP 3A, e.g. by rifampicin, reduces the plasma concentration of itraconazole. Additionally, its affinity for several P450 isoforms, notably CYP 3A4, causes it to inhibit the oxidation of a number of drugs, including phenytoin, warfarin, cyclosporine, tacrolimus, midazolam, triazolam, cisapride and terfenidine (see above), increasing their intensity and/or duration of effect.

Voriconazole and *posaconazole* appear to be more active than itraconazole against *Aspergillus*.

ALLYLAMINE

Terbinafine

Terbinafine interferes with ergosterol biosynthesis, and thereby with the formation of the fungal cell membrane. It is absorbed from the gastrointestinal tract and undergoes extensive metabolism in the liver ($t\frac{1}{2}$ 14 h). Terbinafine is used topically for dermatophyte infections of the skin and orally for infections of hair and nails where the site (e.g. hair), severity or extent of the infection render topical use inappropriate (see p. 315). Treatment (250 mg/d) may need to continue for several weeks. It may cause nausea, diarrhoea, dyspepsia, abdominal pain, headaches and cutaneous reactions.

Other antifungal drugs

Griseofulvin

Griseofulvin prevents fungal growth by inhibiting mitosis. The therapeutic efficacy of griseofulvin depends on its capacity to bind to keratin as it is being formed in the cells of the nail bed, hair follicles and skin, for dermatophytes specifically infect keratinous tissues. Griseofulvin does not kill fungus already established, it merely prevents infection of new keratin so that the duration of treatment is governed by the time that it takes for infected keratin to be shed; on average, hair and skin infection should be treated for 4–6 weeks while toenails may need a year or more. Treatment must continue for a few weeks after both visual and microscopic evidence have disappeared. Fat in a meal enhances absorption of griseofulvin; it is metabolised in the liver and induces hepatic enzymes ($t\frac{1}{2}$ 15 h).

Griseofulvin is effective against all superficial ringworm (dermatophyte) infections but is ineffective against pityriasis versicolor, superficial candidiasis and all systemic mycoses.

Adverse reactions include gastrointestinal upset, rashes, photosensitivity, headache, and also various central nervous system disturbances.

Flucytosine

Flucytosine (5-fluorocytosine) is metabolised in the fungal cell to 5-fluorouracil which inhibits nucleic acid synthesis. It is well absorbed from the gut, penetrates effectively into tissues and almost all is excreted unchanged in the urine ($t\frac{1}{2}$ 4 h). The dose should be reduced for patients with impaired renal function, and the plasma concentration should be monitored. The drug is well tolerated when renal function is normal. *Candida albicans* rapidly becomes resistant to flucytosine which ought not to be used alone; it may be combined with amphotericin (see Table 14.2) but this increases the risk of adverse effects (leucopenia, thrombocytopenia, enterocolitis) and it is reserved for serious infections where the risk–benefit balance is favourable (e.g. *Cryptococcus neoformans* meningitis).

Protozoal infections

Malaria

Over 90 million cases of malaria occur each year; in socioeconomic impact, it is the most important of the transmissible parasitic diseases.

Quinine as cinchona bark was introduced into Europe from South America in 1633. It was used for all fevers, amongst them malaria, the occurrence of which was associated with bad air ('mal aria'). Further advance in the chemotherapy of malaria was delayed until 1880, when Laveran[1] finally identified the parasites in the blood.

LIFE CYCLE OF THE MALARIA PARASITE AND SITES OF DRUG ACTION

The incubation period of malaria is 10–35 days. The principal features of the life cycle (Fig. 14.1) of the malaria parasite must be known in order to understand its therapy. Female anopheles mosquitoes require a blood meal for egg production and in the process of feeding they inject salivary fluid containing

---

[1] Charles Louis Alphonse Laveran (1845–1922), Professor of Military Medicine, Paris (France): Nobel prize winner 1907.

sporozoites into humans. Since no drugs are effective against sporozoites, infection with the malaria parasite cannot be prevented.

Hepatic cycle (site 1 in Fig. 14.1)

Sporozoites enter liver cells where they develop into *schizonts* which form large numbers of *merozoites* which, usually after 5–16 days but sometimes after months or years, are released into the circulation. *Plasmodium falciparum* differs in that it has no persistent hepatic cycle.

  Primaquine, proguanil and tetracyclines *(tissue schizontocides)* act at this site and are used for:

- *Radical cure*, i.e. an attack on persisting hepatic forms (*hypnozoites*, i.e. sleeping) once the parasite has been cleared from the blood; this is most effectively accomplished with primaquine; proguanil is only weakly effective

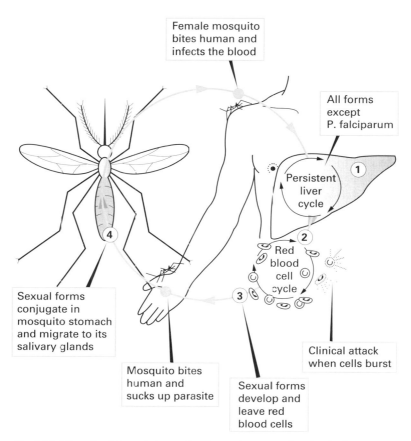

Fig. 14.1 Life cycle of the malaria parasite. The numbers are referred to in the text.

- *Preventing* the *initial* hepatic cycle. This is also called *causal prophylaxis*. Primaquine has long been regarded as too toxic for prolonged use but evidence now suggests it may be used safely, and it is inexpensive; proguanil is weakly effective. Doxycycline may be used short-term.

Erythrocyte cycle (site 2 in Fig. 14.1)

Merozoites enter red cells where they develop into *schizonts* which form more merozoites which are released when the cells burst giving rise to the features of the clinical attack. The merozoites re-enter red cells and the cycle is repeated.

Chloroquine, quinine, mefloquine, halofantrine, proguanil, pyrimethamine, and tetracyclines (*blood schizontocides*) kill these asexual forms. Drugs which act on this stage in the cycle of the parasite may be used for:

- *Treatment* of acute attacks of malaria.
- *Prevention* of attacks by early destruction of the erythrocytic forms. This is called *suppressive prophylaxis* as it does not cure the hepatic cycle (above).

Sexual forms (site 3 in Fig. 14.1)

Some merozoites differentiate into male and female *gametocytes* in the erythrocytes and can develop further only if they are ingested by a mosquito where they form *sporozoites* (site 4 in Fig. 14.1) and complete the transmission cycle.

Quinine, mefloquine, chloroquine, artesunate, artemether and primaquine (*gametocytocides*) act on sexual forms and prevent transmission of the infection because the patient becomes noninfective and the parasite fails to develop in the mosquito (site 4).

In summary, drugs may be selected for:

- treatment of clinical attacks
- prevention of clinical attacks
- radical cure.

Drugs used for malaria, and their principal actions are classified in Table 14.3.

DRUG-RESISTANT MALARIA

Drug-resistant parasites constitute a persistent

TABLE 14.3 Antimalarial drugs and their locus of action

Drug	Biological activity	
	Blood schizontocide	Tissue schizontocide
4-Aminoquinolone		
chloroquine	++	0
Arylaminoalcohols		
quinine	++	0
mefloquine	++	0
Phenanthrene methanol		
halofantrine	++	0
Antimetabolites		
proguanil	+	+
pyrimethamine	+	0
sulfadoxine	+	0
dapsone	+	0
Antibiotics		
tetracycline	+	+
doxycycline	+	+
minocycline	+	+
8-Aminoquinolone		
primaquine	0	+
Sesquiterpenes		
artesunate	+	0
artemether	+	0

problem. *Plasmodium falciparum* is now resistant to chloroquine in many parts of the world and the picture is changing monthly. Areas of high risk for resistant parasites include Sub-Saharan Africa, Latin America, Oceania (Papua New Guinea, Solomon Islands, Vanuatu) and some parts of South-East Asia. Chloroquine-resistant *Plasmodium vivax* is also reported. Any physician who is not familiar with the resistance pattern in the locality from which patients have come or to which they are going, is well advised to check the current position. Because prevalence and resistance rates are so variable, advice on therapy and prophylaxis in this section is given for general guidance only and readers are referred to specialist sources for up-to-date information.

CHEMOTHERAPY OF AN ACUTE ATTACK OF MALARIA[2]

Successful management demands attention to the following points of principle:

---

[2] Treatment regimens vary in detail; those quoted here accord with the recommendations in the British National Formulary 2002, and the BNF is a good source of contact numbers, addresses and websites to obtain expert advice on therapy and prophylaxis of malaria.

- Whenever possible, the diagnosis should be confirmed before treatment by examination of blood smears.
- When the infecting organism is not known or infection is mixed, treatment should begin as for *Plasmodium falciparum* (below).
- Drugs used to treat *Plasmodium falciparum* malaria must always be selected with regard to the prevalence of local patterns of drug resistance.
- Patients not at risk of reinfection should be re-examined several weeks after treatment for signs of recrudescence which may result from inadequate chemotherapy or survival of persistent hepatic forms.

Falciparum ('malignant') malaria

The regimen depends on the condition of the patient; the doses quoted are for adults. Chloroquine resistance is now usual.

If the patient can swallow and there are no serious complications such as impairment of consciousness, treatment options are as follows:

- A quinine salt[3] 600 mg 8-hourly by mouth for 7 days followed by pyrimethamine plus sulfadoxine (Fansidar) 3 tablets as a single dose. Where there is resistance to Fansidar, doxycycline 200 mg, should be given **after** the course of quinine daily for at least 7 days. This additional therapy is necessary as quinine alone tends to be associated with a higher rate of relapse.
- Mefloquine 20–25 mg/kg (base) to a maximum of 1.5 g by mouth may be given as 2–3 divided doses 6–8 h apart.
- Malarone (atovaquone and proguanil hydrochloride) 4 tablets once daily for 3 days.

It is not necessary to add Fansidar or tetracycline after mefloquine or Malarone, but resistance to these agents has been reported from some countries.

Seriously ill patients should be treated with:

- a quinine salt[3] 20 mg/kg as a loading dose[4] (maximum 1.4 g) infused i.v. over 4 h

- followed 8 h later by a maintenance infusion of 10 mg/kg (maximum 700 mg) infused over 4 h
- repeated every 8 h,[5] until the patient can swallow tablets to complete the 7-day course.
- Fansidar or doxycycline should be given subsequently, as above (mefloquine is an alternative, but this must begin at least 12 hours after parenteral quinine has ceased).

Treatment in pregnancy should always be discussed with an expert.

Non-falciparum ('benign') malarias

These are usually due to *Plasmodium vivax* or less commonly to *Plasmodium ovale* or *Plasmodium malariae*; the drug of choice is chloroquine, which should be given by mouth as follows:

- initial dose: 600 mg (base),[6] then 300 mg as a single dose 6–8 h later
- second day, 300 mg as a single dose
- third day, 300 mg as a single dose.

The total dose of chloroquine base over 3 days should be approximately 25 mg/kg base. This is sufficient for *Plasmodium malariae* infection but, for *Plasmodium vivax* and *Plasmodium ovale* eradication of the hepatic parasites is necessary to prevent relapse, by giving:

- primaquine, 15 mg/d for 14–21 days started after the chloroquine course has been completed (30 mg once weekly for 8 weeks will suffice without undue risk of haemolysis). Longer courses may be needed for some *Plasmodium vivax* strains from south-east Asia and the Western Pacific.

---

[3] Acceptable as quinine hydrochloride, dihydrochloride or sulphate, but not quinine bisulphate which contains less quinine.

[4] The loading dose should not be given if the patient has received quinine, quinidine or mefloquine in the previous 24 h; see also warnings about halofantrine (below).
[5] Reduced to 5–7 mg/kg if the infusion lasts for > 72 h.
[6] The active component of many drugs, whether acid or base, is relatively insoluble and may present a problem in formulation. This is overcome by adding an acid to a base or vice versa; the weight of the salt differs according to the acid or base component, i.e. chloroquine base 150 mg = chloroquine sulphate 200 mg = chloroquine phosphate 250 mg (approximately). Where there may be variation, therefore, the amount of drug prescribed is expressed as the weight of the active component, in the case of chloroquine, the base.

CHEMOPROPHYLAXIS OF MALARIA

Geographically variable plasmodial drug resistance has become a major factor in malaria. The World Health Organization gives advice in its annually revised booklet, Vaccination Certificate Requirements and Health Advice for International Travel; and national bodies publish advice (e.g. British National Formulary) that applies particularly to their own residents. These or other appropriate sources ought to be consulted before specific advice is given.

The following general principles apply:

- Chemoprophylaxis is part of a broader regimen and only ever gives relative protection; travellers should protect against bites by using mosquito nets and repellents and wearing well-covering clothing especially during high-risk times of day (after dusk).
- Mefloquine, chloroquine, proguanil, and pyrimethamine plus dapsone (Maloprim), alone or in combination are most commonly advised for prophylaxis regimens; and doxycycline for special cases (drug resistance or intolerance); primaquine is being re-evaluated.
- Effective chemoprophylaxis requires that there be a plasmodicidal concentration of drug in the blood when the first infected mosquito bites, and that it be sustained safely for long periods.
- The progressive rise in plasma concentration to steady state (after $t_{\frac{1}{2}} \times 5$), sometimes attained only after weeks (consider mefloquine $t_{\frac{1}{2}}$ 21 days, chloroquine $t_{\frac{1}{2}}$ 50 days), allows that unwanted effects (that will impair compliance or be unsafe) may occur after a subject has entered a malarial area. Thus it is advised that prophylaxis be begun long enough before travel to reveal acute intolerance and to impress on the subject the importance of compliance (to relate drug-taking to a specific daily or weekly event).
- Prompt achievement of efficacy and safety by one (or two) doses is plainly important for those travellers who cannot wait on dosage schedules to deliver both only when steady-state blood concentrations are attained; the schedules must reflect this need.
- Prophylaxis should continue for at least 4 weeks after leaving an endemic area to kill parasites that are acquired about the time of departure, are still incubating in the liver and will develop into the erythrocyte phase. The traveller should be aware that any illness occurring within a year, and especially within 3 months, of return may be malaria.
- Chloroquine and proguanil may be used for periods of up to 5 years, and mefloquine for up to 1 or 2 years: expert advice should be taken by long-term travellers, especially those going to areas for which other prophylactic drugs are recommended.
- *Naturally acquired immunity* offers the most reliable protection for people living permanently in endemic areas (below). Repeated attacks of malaria confer partial immunity and the disease often becomes no more than an occasional inconvenience. Vaccines to confer active immunity are under development.
- *The partially immune* as a rule should not take a prophylactic. The reasoning is that immunity is sustained by the red cell cycle, loss of which through prophylaxis diminishes their resistance and leaves them highly vulnerable to the disease. There are however exceptions to this general advice and the partially immune may or should use a prophylactic:
  — if it is virtually certain that they will never abandon its use,
  — if they go to another malarial area where the strains of parasite may differ, during the last few months of pregnancy in areas where *Plasmodium falciparum* is prevalent,
  — to avert the risk of miscarriage.

All these factors contribute to conventional advice to travellers.

Examples of standard regimens

- chloroquine 300 mg (base) once weekly (start one week before travel)
- proguanil 200 mg once daily (start 2–3 days before travel)
- chloroquine plus proguanil in the above doses
- mefloquine 250 mg once weekly (start one week, preferably 2–3 weeks, before travel).

For 'last minute' travellers. The standard regimens normally provide immediate protection but for special assurance a priming/loading dose may be considered, e.g. the standard prophylactic dose daily for 2–3 days (this has been suggested for mefloquine).

Drug interactions. Where subjects are already taking other drugs, e.g. antiepileptics, some cardiovascular drugs, it is desirable to start prophylaxis as much as 2–3 weeks in advance to establish safety.

Antimalarial drugs and pregnancy

Women living in endemic areas in which *Plasmodium falciparum* remains sensitive to chloroquine should take chloroquine prophylactically throughout pregnancy. Proguanil (an 'antifol', see below) may be taken for prophylaxis provided it is accompanied by folic acid 5 mg/d. Chloroquine may be used in full dose to treat chloroquine-sensitive infections. Quinine is the only widely available drug that is acceptable as suitable for treating chloroquine-resistant infections during pregnancy. Mefloquine is teratogenic in animals and a woman should avoid pregnancy whilst taking it, and for 3 months after; pyrimethamine plus dapsone (Maloprim) should not be given in the first trimester, but may be given in the second and third trimesters with a folate supplement.

INDIVIDUAL ANTIMALARIAL DRUGS

Chloroquine

Chloroquine ($t\frac{1}{2}$ 50 d) is concentrated within parasitised red cells and forms complexes with plasmodial DNA. It is active against the blood forms and also the gametocytes (formed in the mosquito) of *Plasmodium vivax*, *Plasmodium ovale* and *Plasmodium malariae*; it is ineffective against many strains of *Plasmodium falciparum* and also its immature gametocytes. Chloroquine is readily absorbed from the gastrointestinal tract and is concentrated several-fold in various tissues, e.g. erythrocytes, liver, spleen, heart, kidney, cornea and retina; the long $t\frac{1}{2}$ reflects slow release from these sites. A priming dose is used in order to achieve adequate free plasma concentration (see acute attack, above). Chloroquine is partly inactivated by metabolism and the remainder is excreted unchanged in the urine.

Adverse effects are infrequent at doses normally used for malaria prophylaxis and treatment but are more common with the higher or prolonged doses given for resistant malaria or for rheumatoid arthritis or lupus erythematosus (see p. 293).

Corneal deposits of chloroquine may be asymptomatic or may cause halos around lights or photophobia. These are not a threat to vision and reverse when the drug is stopped. *Retinal toxicity* is more serious, however, and may be irreversible. In the early stage it takes the form of visual field defects; late retinopathy classically gives the picture of macular pigmentation surrounded by a ring of pigment (the 'bull's-eye' macula). The functional defect can take the form of scotomas, photophobia, defective colour vision and decreased visual acuity resulting, in the extreme case, in blindness.

Other reactions include *pruritus*, which may be intolerable and is common in Africans, headaches, gastrointestinal disturbance, precipitation of acute intermittent porphyria in susceptible individuals, mental disturbances and interference with cardiac rhythm, the latter especially if the drug is given intravenously in high dose (it has a quinidine-like action). Long-term use is associated with reversible bleaching of the hair and pigmentation of the hard palate.

Acute overdose may be rapidly fatal without treatment and indeed has even been described as a means of suicide.[7] (Chloroquine may now be bought from pharmacies in the UK without a prescription.) Pulmonary oedema is followed by convulsions, cardiac arrhythmias and coma; as little as 50 mg/kg can be fatal. These effects are principally due to the profound negative inotropic action of chloroquine. Diazepam was found fortuitously to protect the heart and adrenaline (epinephrine) reduces intraventricular conduction time; this combination of drugs, given by separate i.v. infusions, improves survival.

Halofantrine

Halofantrine ($t\frac{1}{2}$ 2.5 d) is active against the erythrocytic forms of all four *Plasmodium* species, especially *Plasmodium falciparum* and *Plasmodium vivax*, and at

---

[7] Report 1993 Chloroquine poisoning. Lancet 307: 49.

the schizont stage. Its mechanism of action is not fully understood. Absorption of halofantrine from the gastrointestinal tract is variable, incomplete and substantially increased (× 6–10) by taking the drug with food (see below). It is metabolised to an active metabolite and no unchanged drug is recovered in the urine. Halofantrine is used for the treatment of uncomplicated chloroquine-resistant *Plasmodium falciparum* and *Plasmodium vivax* malaria. It should not be given for prophylaxis.

Adverse effects. Halofantrine may cause gastro-intestinal symptoms; pruritis occurs but to a lesser extent than with chloroquine which may be reason for it to be preferred. It prolongs the cardiac QT interval and may predispose to hazardous arrhythmia. The drug should therefore not be taken:

* with food
* with other potentially dysrhythmic drugs, e.g. antimalarials, tricyclic antidepressants, antipsychotics, astemizole, terfenadine
* with drugs causing electrolyte disturbance
* by patients with cardiac disease associated with prolonged QT interval.

Mefloquine

Mefloquine (t$\frac{1}{2}$ 21 d) is similar in several respects to quinine although it does not intercalate with plasmodial DNA. It is used for malaria chemo-prophylaxis, to treat uncomplicated *Plasmodium falciparum* (both chloroquine-sensitive and chloroquine resistant) and chloroquine-resistant *Plasmodium vivax* malaria. Mefloquine is rapidly absorbed from the gastrointestinal tract and its action is terminated by metabolism. When used for prophylaxis, 250 mg (base)/week should be taken, commencing 1–3 weeks before entering and continued for 4 weeks after leaving a malarious area. It should not be given to patients with hepatic or renal impairment.

Adverse effects include nausea, dizziness, distur-bance of balance, vomiting, abdominal pain, diar-rhoea and loss of appetite. More rarely, hallucina-tions, seizures and psychoses occur. Mefloquine should be avoided in patients taking β-adrenoceptor and calcium channel antagonists for it causes sinus bradycardia; quinine can potentiate these and other

dose-related effects of mefloquine. Neuropsychiatric events, including seizures and psychoses occur after high-dose therapy in about 1 in 10 000 of those using the drug for prophylaxis. Less severe reactions including headache, dizziness, depression and in-somnia have been reported but there is uncertainty as to whether these can be ascribed to mefloquine. The drug should not be used in travellers with a history of neuropsychiatric disease including convulsions and depression, and in those whose activities require fine coordination or spatial performance, e.g. airline flight-deck crews.

Primaquine

Primaquine (t$\frac{1}{2}$ 6 h) acts at several stages in the development of the plasmodial parasite, possibly by interfering with its mitochondrial function. Its unique effect is to eliminate the hepatic forms of *Plasmodium vivax* and *Plasmodium ovale* after standard chloroquine therapy, but only when the risk of reinfection is absent or slight. Primaquine is well absorbed from the gastrointestinal tract, is only moderately concentrated in the tissues and is rapidly metabolised.

Adverse effects include anorexia, nausea, abdominal cramps, methaemoglobinaemia and haemolytic anae-mia, especially in patients with genetic deficiency of erythrocyte glucose-6-phosphate dehydrogenase (G6PD). Subjects should be tested for G6PD and, in those that are deficient, the risk of haemolytic anaemia is greatly reduced by giving primaquine in reduced dose.

Proguanil (chloroguanide)

Proguanil (t$\frac{1}{2}$ 17 h) inhibits dihydrofolate reductase which converts folic to folinic acid, deficiency of which inhibits plasmodial cell division. Plasmodia, like most bacteria and unlike humans, cannot make use of preformed folic acid. Pyrimethamine and trimethoprim, which share this mode of action, are collectively known as the 'antifols'. Their plasmod-icidal action is markedly enhanced by combination with sulphonamides or sulphones because there is inhibition of sequential steps in folate synthesis (see Sulphonamide combinations, p. 231).

Proguanil is moderately well absorbed from the gut and is excreted in the urine either unchanged or as an active metabolite. Being little stored in the tissues, proguanil must be used daily when given for prophylaxis, its main use, particularly in pregnant women (with folic acid 5 mg/d, which does not antagonise therapeutic efficacy) and nonimmune individuals.

Adverse effects. In prophylactic doses it is well tolerated. Mouth ulcers and stomatitis have been reported. Proguanil should be avoided or used in reduced dose for patients with impaired renal function.

Pyrimethamine

Pyrimethamine (t$\frac{1}{2}$ 4 d) inhibits plasmodial dihydrofolate reductase, for which it has a high affinity. It is well absorbed from the gastrointestinal tract and is extensively metabolised. It is seldom used alone (see below). Pregnant women should receive supplementary folic acid when taking pyrimethamine.

Adverse effects reported include anorexia, abdominal cramps, vomiting, ataxia, tremor, seizures and megaloblastic anaemia.

Pyrimethamine with sulfadoxine

Pyrimethamine acts synergistically with sulfadoxine (as Fansidar) to inhibit folic acid metabolism (see 'antifols', above); sulfadoxine is excreted in the urine. The combination is chiefly used with quinine to treat acute attacks of malaria caused by susceptible strains of *Plasmodium falciparum*; a single dose of pyrimethamine 75 mg plus sulfadoxine 1.5 g (3 tablets) usually suffices.

Adverse effects. Any sulphonamide-induced allergic reactions can be severe, e.g. erythema multiforme, Stevens–Johnson syndrome and toxic epidermal necrolysis. Because of its 'antifol' action the combination should not be used by pregnant women unless they take a folate supplement.

Pyrimethamine with dapsone

Pyrimethamine is combined with dapsone (Maloprim) (see p. 271) for prophylaxis of *Plasmodium falciparum* malaria.

Quinine

Quinine (t$\frac{1}{2}$ 9 h; 18 h in severe malaria) is obtained from the bark of the South American Cinchona tree. It binds to plasmodial DNA to prevent protein synthesis but its exact mode of action remains uncertain. It is used to treat *Plasmodium falciparum* malaria in areas of multiple-drug resistance. Apart from its antiplasmodial effect, quinine is used for myotonia and muscle cramps because it prolongs the muscle refractory period. Quinine is included in dilute concentration in tonics and aperitifs for its desired bitter taste.

Quinine is well absorbed from the gastrointestinal tract and is almost completely metabolised in the liver.

Adverse effects include tinnitus, diminished auditory acuity, headache, blurred vision, nausea and diarrhoea (common to quinine, quinidine, salicylates and called cinchonism). Idiosyncratic reactions include pruritus, urticaria and rashes. Hypoglycaemia may be significant when quinine is given by i.v. infusion and supplementary glucose may be required.

When large amounts are taken, e.g. (unreliably) to induce abortion or in attempted suicide, ocular disturbances, notably constriction of the visual fields, may occur and even complete blindness, the onset of which may be very sudden. Vomiting, abdominal pain and diarrhoea result from local irritation of the gastrointestinal tract. Quinidine-like effects include hypotension, disturbance of atrioventricular conduction and cardiac arrest. Activated charcoal should be given. Supportive measures are employed thereafter as no specific therapy has proven benefit.

Quinidine, the dextrorotatory-isomer of quinine, has antimalarial activity, but is used mainly as a cardiac antiarrhythmic (see p. 500).

Artesunate and **artemether** are soluble derivatives of *artemisinin* which is isolated from the leaves of the Chinese herb qinghao (*Artemisia annua*); they act against the blood, including sexual forms, of plasmodia and may also reduce transmissibility. Artesunate (i.v.) and artemether (i.m.) are rapidly effective in severe and multidrug resistant malaria. They are well tolerated but should be used with caution in patients with chronic cardiac disorders as they prolong the PR and QT interval in some experimental animals. Their place in therapy is being evaluated.

Amoebiasis

Infection occurs when mature cysts are ingested and pass into the colon where they divide into trophozoites; these forms either enter the tissues or reform cysts. Amoebiasis occurs in two forms, both of which need treatment:

- *Bowel lumen amoebiasis* is asymptomatic and trophozoites (noninfective) and cysts (infective) are passed into the faeces. Treatment is directed at eradicating cysts with a luminal amoebicide; *diloxanide furoate* is the drug of choice; *iodoquinol* or *paromomycin* is sometimes used.
- *Tissue-invading amoebiasis* gives rise to dysentery, hepatic amoebiasis and liver abscess. A systemically active drug (tissue amoebicide) effective against trophozoites must be used, e.g. *metronidazole, tinidazole.* Parenteral forms of these are available for patients too ill to take drugs by mouth. In severe cases of amoebic dysentery, *tetracycline* lessens the risk of opportunistic infection, perforation and peritonitis when it is given in addition to the systemic amoebicide.

Treatment with tissue amoebicides should always be followed by a course of a luminal amoebicide to eradicate the source of the infection.

Dehydroemetine (from ipecacuanha), less toxic than the parent emetine, is claimed by some authorities to be the most effective tissue amoebicide. It is reserved for dangerously ill patients, but these are more likely to be vulnerable to its cardiotoxic effects. When dehydroemetine is used to treat amoebic liver abscess, chloroquine should also be given.

The drug treatment of other protozoal infections is summarised in Table 14.4.

TABLE 14.4 Drugs for some protozoal infections

Infection	Drug and comment
Giardiasis	Metronidazole, mepacrine or tinidazole
Leishmaniasis visceral	Sodium stibogluconate or meglumine antimoniate; resistant cases may benefit from combining antimonials with allopurinol, pentamidine, paromomycin or amphotericin (including AmBisome).
cutaneous	Mild lesions heal spontaneously, antimonials may be injected intralesionally.
Toxoplasmosis	Most infections are self-limiting in the immunologically normal patient. Pyrimethamine with sulfadiazine for chorioretinitis, and active toxoplasmosis in immunodeficient patients; folinic acid is used to counteract the inevitable megaloblastic anaemia. Alternatives include pyrimethamine with clindamycin or clarithromycin or azithromycin Spiramycin for primary toxoplasmosis in pregnant women. Expert advice is essential.
Trichomoniasis	Metronidazole or tinidazole is effective
Trypanosomiasis African (sleeping sickness)	Suramin or pentamidine is effective during the early stages but not for the later neurological manifestations for which melarsoprol should be used. Eflornithine is effective for both early and late stages. Expert advice is recommended.
American (Changes disease)	Prolonged (1–3 months) treatment with benznidazole or nifurtimox may be effective.

Notes on drugs for protozoal infections

Atovaquone is a quinone; it may cause gastrointestinal and mild neurological side effects, and rare hepatotoxicity and blood dyscrasias.

Benznidazole is a nitroimidazole that may occasionally cause peripheral neuritis but is generally well tolerated, including by infants.

Dehydroemetine inhibits protein synthesis; it may cause pain at the site of injection, weakness and muscular pain, hypotension, precordial pain and cardiac dysrhythmias.

Diloxanide furoate may cause troublesome flatulence, and pruritus and urticaria may occur.

Eflornithine inhibits protozoal DNA synthesis; it may cause anaemia, leucopenia and thrombocytopenia, and seizures.

Iodoquinol may cause abdominal cramps, nausea and diarrhoea. Skin eruptions, pruritus ani and thyroid gland enlargement have been attributed to its iodine content. The recognition of severe neurotoxicity with the related drug, clioquinol, in Japan in the 1960s, must give cause for caution in its use.

Meglumine antimonate is a pentavalent antimony compound, similar to sodium stibogluconate.

Melarsoprol, a trivalent organic arsenical, acts through its high affinity for sulphydryl groups of enzymes. Adverse effects include encephalopathy, myocardial damage, proteinuria and hypertension.

Mepacrine (quinacrine) was formerly used as an antimalarial. It may cause gastrointestinal upset, occasional acute toxic psychosis, hepatitis and aplastic anaemia.

Nifurtimox is a nitrofuran derivative. Adverse effects include: anorexia, nausea, vomiting, gastric pain, insomnia, headache, vertigo, excitability, myalgia, arthralgia and convulsions. Peripheral neuropathy may necessitate stopping treatment.

Paromomycin, an aminoglycoside, is not absorbed from the gut; it is similar to neomycin.

Pentamidine is a synthetic aromatic amidine; it must be administered parenterally or by inhalation as it is unreliably absorbed from the gastrointestinal tract; it does not enter the CSF. Given systemically it frequently causes nephrotoxicity, which is reversible; acute hypotension and syncope are common especially after rapid i.v. injection. Pancreatic damage may cause hypoglycaemia due to insulin release.

Sodium stibogluconate (Pentostam) is an organic pentavalent antimony compound; it may cause anorexia, vomiting, coughing and substernal pain. Used in mucocutaneous leishmaniasis, it may lead to severe inflammation around pharyngeal or tracheal lesions which may require corticosteroid administration to control. *Meglumine antimoniate* is similar.

Suramin forms stable complexes with plasma protein and is detectable in urine for up to 3 months after the last injection; it does not cross the blood–brain barrier. It may cause tiredness, anorexia, malaise, polyuria, thirst and tenderness of the palms and soles.

Helminthic infections

Helminths have complex life-cycles, special knowledge of which is required by those who treat infections. Table 14.5 will suffice here. Drug resistance has not so far proved to be a clinical problem, though it has occurred in animals on continuous chemoprophylaxis.

Drugs for helminthic infections

Albendazole is similar to mebendazole (below).

Diethylcarbamazine kills both microfilariae and adult worms. Fever, headache, anorexia, malaise, urticaria, vomiting and asthmatic attacks following the first dose are due to products of destruction of the parasite, and reactions are minimised by slow increase in dosage over the first 3 days.

Ivermectin may cause immediate reactions due to the death of the microfilaria (see diethylcarbamazine). It can be effective in a single dose, but is best repeated at 6–12-month intervals.

Levamisole paralyses the musculature of sensitive nematodes which, unable to maintain their anchorage, are expelled by normal peristalsis. It is well tolerated, but may cause abdominal pain, nausea, vomiting, headache and dizziness.

Mebendazole blocks glucose uptake by nematodes. Mild gastrointestinal discomfort may be caused, and it should not be used in pregnancy or in children under the age of 2.

Metriphonate is an organophosphorus anticholinesterase compound that was originally used as an insecticide. Adverse effects include abdominal pain, nausea, vomiting, diarrhoea, headache and vertigo.

Niclosamide blocks glucose uptake by intestinal tapeworms. It may cause some mild gastrointestinal symptoms.

Piperazine may cause hypersensitivity reactions, neurological symptoms (including 'worm wobble') and may precipitate epilepsy.

Praziquantel paralyses both adult worms and larvae. It is extensively metabolised. Praziquantel may cause nausea, headache, dizziness and drowsiness; it cures with a single dose (or divided doses in one day).

Pyrantel depolarises neuromuscular junctions of susceptible nematodes which are expelled in the faeces. It cures with a single dose. It may induce gastrointestinal disturbance, headache, dizziness, drowsiness and insomnia.

TABLE 14.5 Drugs for helminthic infections

Infection	Drug	Comment
Cestodes (tapeworms)		
Beef tapeworm *Taenia saginata*	niclosamide or praziquantel	Praziquantel cures with single dose
Pork tapeworm *Taenia solium*	niclosamide or praziquantel	Praziquantel cures with single dose
Cysticercosis *Taenia solium*	albendazole or praziquantel	Treat in hospital as dying and disintegrating cysts may cause cerebral oedema
Fish tapeworm *Diphyllobothrium latum*	niclosamide or praziquantel	
Hydatid disease *Echinococcus granulosus*	albendazole	Surgery for operable cyst disease
Nematodes (intestinal)		
Ascariasis *Ascaris lumbricoides*	levamisole, mebendazole, pyrantel, piperazine or albendazole	
Hookworm *Ancylostoma duodenale; Necator americanus*	mebendazole, pyrantel, or albendazole	Anaemic patients require iron
Strongyloidiasis *Strongyloides stercoralis*	tiabendazole or ivermectin	Alternatively, albendazole is better tolerated
Threadworm (pinworm) *Enterobius vermicularis*	pyrantel, mebendazole, albendazole or piperazine salts	
Whipworm *Trichuris trichiuria*	mebendazole or albendazole	
Nematodes (tissue)		
Cutaneous larva migrans *Ancylostoma braziliense; Ancylostoma caninum*	tiabendazole (topical for single tracks) invermectin, albendazole or oral tiabendazole (for multiple tracks)	Calamine lotion for symptom relief
Guinea worm *Dracunculus medinensis*	metronidazole, mebendazole	Rapid symptom relief
Trichinellosis *Trichinella spiralis*	mebendazole	Prednisolone may be needed to suppress allergic and inflammatory symptoms
Visceral larva migrans *Toxocara canis; Toxocara cati*	diethylcarbamazine, albendazole or mebendazole	Progressive escalation of dose lessens allergic reactions to dying larvae; prednisolone suppresses inflammatory response in ophthalmic disease
Lymphatic filariasis *Wuchereria bancrofti; Brugia malayi; Brugia timori*	diethylcarbamazine	Destruction of microfilia may cause an immunological reaction (see below)
Onchocerciasis (river blindness) *Onchocerca volvulus*	ivermectin	Cures with single dose. Suppressive treatment; a single annual dose prevents significant complications
Schistosomiasis (intestinal)		
Schistosoma mansoni; Schistosoma japonicum	praziquantel	Oxamniquine only for *Schistosoma mansoni*
Schistosomiasis (urinary)		
Schistosoma haematobium	praziquantel	Metriphonate only for *Schistosoma haematobium*
Flukes (intestinal, lung, liver)		
	praziquantel	Alternatives: niclosamide for intestinal fluke, bithionol for lung fluke

Tiabendazole (formerly known as *thiabendazole*) inhibits cellular enzymes of susceptible helminths. Gastrointestinal, neurological and hypersensitivity reactions, liver damage and crystalluria may be induced.

GUIDE TO FURTHER READING

World Wide Web resources
The American Centers for Disease Control &

Prevention (CDC-P) website includes a comprehensive travel section (http://www.cdc.gov/travel/) which contains high-quality and up to date information about prophylaxis, avoidance, diagnosis and treatment of infectious diseases of travel. Another useful contemporary source is 'Fit for travel', the NHS public access website providing travel health information for people travelling abroad from the UK (http://www.fitfortravel.scot.nhs.uk/).

Printed resources

Balfour H H 1999 Antiviral drugs. New England Journal of Medicine 340: 1255–1268

Bruce-Chwatt L J 1988 Three hundred and fifty years of the Peruvian fever bark. British Medical Journal 296: 1486

Burnham G 1998 Onchocerciasis. Lancet 351: 1341–1346

Carr A, Cooper D A 2000 Adverse effects of antiretroviral therapy. Lancet 356: 1423–1430

Cohen J I 2000 Epstein-Barr virus infection. New England Journal of Medicine 343: 481–492

Couch R B 2000 Prevention and treatment of influenza. New England Journal of Medicine 343: 1778–1787

Croft A 2000 Malaria: prevention in travellers. British Medical Journal 321: 154–160

Flexner C 1998 HIV-protease inhibitors. New England Journal of Medicine 338: 1281–1292

Gilden D H et al 2000 Neurological complications of the reactivation of varicella-zoster virus. New England Journal of Medicine 342: 635–645

Gubareva L V, Kaiser L, Hayden F G 2000 Influenza virus neuraminidase inhibitors. Lancet 355: 827–835

Hall C B 2001 Respiratory syncytial virus and parainfluenza virus. New England Journal of Medicine 344: 1917–1928

Herwaldt B L 1999 Leishmaniasis. Lancet 354: 1191–1199

Hay J, Dutton G N 1995 Toxoplasma and the eye. British Medical Journal 310: 1021–1022

Lipman J, Saadia R 1997 Fungal infections in critically ill patients. British Medical Journal 315: 266–267

Liu L X, Weller P F 1996 Antiparasitic drugs. New England Journal of Medicine 334: 1178–1184

Murray H W et al 2000 Recent advances: tropical medicine. British Medical Journal 320: 490–494

Piscitelli S C, Gallicano K D 2001 Interactions among drugs for HIV and opportunistic infections. New England Journal of Medicine 344: 984–996

Sepkowitz K A 2001 AIDS—the first 20 years. New England Journal of Medicine 344: 1764–1772

Stevens D A 1995 Coccidioidomycosis. New England Journal of Medicine 332: 1077–1082

Weller I V D, Williams I G 2001 ABC of AIDS. Treatment of infections. British Medical Journal 322: 1350–1354

Weller I V D, Williams I G 2001 ABC of AIDS: antiretroviral drugs. British Medical Journal 322: 1410–1412

Whitley R J, Roizman B 2001 Herpes simplex virus infections. Lancet 357: 1513–1518

Winstanley P 1998 Malaria treatment. Journal of the Royal College of Physicians of London 32: 203–207

Zwi K, Soderlund N, Schneider H 2000 Cheaper antiretrovirals to treat AIDS in South Africa. British Medical Journal 320: 1551–1552

15

Inflammation, arthritis and nonsteroidal anti-inflammatory drugs

SYNOPSIS

A third of all general practice consultations are for musculoskeletal complaints. Nonsteroidal anti-inflammatory drugs (NSAIDs) are widely used, and their gastrointestinal effects account for an estimated 1200 deaths per year in the UK. A hitherto unsuspected inflammatory component is now known to accompany conditions such as atherosclerosis. As understanding of the complex mechanisms underlying the inflammatory process increases, new ways of influencing it are developed, as witness therapies directed against specific cytokines, and COX-2 specific NSAIDs (COXIBs).

- Inflammation
- Arthritis
- Nonsteroidal anti-inflammatory drugs
- Disease modifying antirheumatic drugs
- Drug treatment of arthritis
- Gout

Glossary of abbreviations

COX:	cyclo-oxygenase
COXIB:	COX-2 specific NSAIDs
DMARD:	disease modifying antirheumatic drug
FGF:	fibroblast growth factor
GM-CSF:	granulocyte macrophage-colony stimulating factor
M-CSF	macrophage-colony stimulating factor
HPETE:	hydroperoxy-eicosatetraenoic acid
IL:	interleukin
LT:	leukotriene
PG:	prostaglandin
TNF:	tumour necrosis factor
TX:	thromboxane

many different cells and cell products, and only a general account of the current understanding of the inflammatory process is provided here. A normal inflammatory response is essential to fight infections and is part of the repair mechanism and removal of debris following tissue damage. Inflammation can also cause disease, due to damage of healthy tissue. This may occur if the response is over-vigorous, or persists longer than is necessary. Additionally, we now know that some conditions have a previously unrecognised inflammatory component, e.g. atherosclerosis.

Inflammation

The clinical features of inflammation have been recognised since ancient times as swelling, redness, pain and heat. The underlying mechanisms which produce these symptoms are complex, involving

THE INFLAMMATORY RESPONSE

The inflammatory response occurs in vascularised tissues in response to injury; it is part of the innate (nonspecific) immune response. Inflammatory responses require activation of *leukocytes:* neutrophils, eosinophils, basophils, mast cells, monocytes and lymphocytes, although not all cell types need be involved in an inflammatory episode. The cells migrate to the area of tissue damage from the circulation and become activated.

Inflammatory mediators

Activated leukocytes at a site of inflammation release compounds which enhance the inflammatory response. The account below focuses on *cytokines* and *eicosanoids* (arachidonic acid metabolites) because of their therapeutic implications. Nevertheless, the complexity of the response, and its involvement of other systems, is indicated by the *range of mediators*, which include:

Complement products, especially C3b and C5–9 (the membrane attack complex); kinins and the related proteins, bradykinin and the contact system (coagulation factors XI and XII, pre-kallikrein, high molecular weight kininogen); nitric oxide and vasoactive amines (histamine, serotonin and adenosine); activated forms of oxygen; platelet activating factor (PAF); proteinases (collagenses, gelatinases and proteoglycanase).

Cytokines

Cytokines are peptides that regulate cell growth, differentiation and activation, and some have therapeutic value:

- *Interleukins* produced by a variety of cells including T cells, monocytes and macrophages. Recombinant interleukin-2 (aldesleukin) is used to treat metastatic renal cell carcinoma and malignant melanoma. Interleukin-1 may play a part in conditions such as the sepsis syndrome and rheumatoid arthritis, and successful blockade of its receptor offers a therapeutic approach for these conditions.
- *Cytotoxic factors* include tumour necrosis factor (TNF) which is similar to interleukin-1. Biological agents that block TNF, e.g. *etanercept, infliximab* are finding their place amongst drugs that modify the course of rheumatoid disease (and Crohn's disease, see p. 65).
- *Interferons* are so named because they were found to interfere with replication of live virus in

tissue culture. Interferon alfa is used for a variety of neoplastic conditions (see Table 30.3) and for chronic active hepatitis.

- *Colony-stimulating factors* have been developed to treat neutropenic conditions, e.g. *filgrastim* (recombinant human granulocyte colony stimulating factor, G-CSF) and *molgramostim* (recombinant human granulocyte macrophage-colony stimulating factor, GM-CSF) (see Ch. 30).

Eicosanoids

Eicosanoids (prostaglandins, thromboxanes, leukotrienes, lipoxins) is the name given to a group of 20-carbon[1] unsaturated fatty acids derived principally from arachidonic acid in cell walls. They are short-lived, extremely potent and formed in almost every tissue in the body. Eicosanoids are involved in most types of inflammation and it is on manipulation of their biosynthesis that most present anti-inflammatory therapy is based. Their biosynthetic paths appear in Figure 15.1 and are amplified by the following account.

- *Arachidonic acid* is stored mainly in *phospholipids* of cell walls, from which it is mobilised largely by the action of *phospholipase*. Glucocorticoids prevent the formation of arachidonic acid by inducing the synthesis of an inhibitory polypeptide called *lipocortin-1*; the capacity to inhibit the subsequent formation of both prostaglandins and leukotrienes, explains part of the powerful anti-inflammatory effect of glucocorticoids (for other actions, see p. 664).
- Arachidonic acid is further metabolised by *cyclo-oxygenase* (COX, also called PGH synthase), which changes the linear fatty acids into the cyclical structures of the *prostaglandins*. Nonsteroidal anti-inflammatory drugs (NSAIDs) act exert their anti-inflammatory effects by inhibiting COX.
- COX exists as two different types, COX-1 and COX-2. The isoform COX-1 is predominantly constitutive[2] (although activity is increased 2–4-fold by inflammatory stimuli); it is present in

---

[1] The Greek word for 20 is *eicosa*, hence the term eisocanoid.
[2] Constantly produced by the cell regardless of growth conditions.

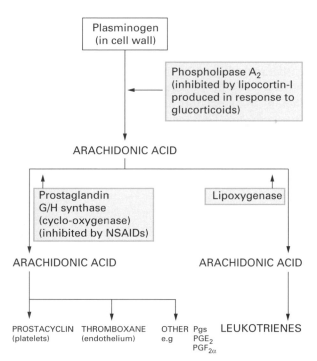

Fig. 15.1 Biosynthetic path of eicosanoids (see text for description). Prostaglandins are found in virtually all tissues of the body.

most tissues, especially stomach, platelets and kidneys. COX-2 is inducible (10–20-fold) by inflammatory stimuli in many cells including macrophages, synoviocytes, chondrocytes, fibroblasts and endothelial cells, and only in low concentration in the gastrointestinal mucosa. Crucially, NSAIDs differ in their relative inhibition of the two isoforms of COX, recognition of which has lead to the development of *selective* COX-2 inhibitors. Such drugs have less adverse effects, especially on the gastrointestinal tract (see below).

- Arachidonic acid is also metabolised by *lipoxygenase* to straight-chain hydroperoxy acids and then to *leukotrienes* which cause increased vascular permeability, vasoconstriction, bronchoconstriction, as well as chemotactic activity for leucocytes (whence their name). Inhibitors of lipoxygenase, e.g. *zileuton*, and leukotriene receptor antagonists, e.g. *montelukast*, *zafirlukast*, have found a place in the therapy of asthma (see p. 559).
- Lipoxins are lipoxygenase-derived eicosanoids that probably down-regulate inflammation in the

gastrointestinal tract and other organs by antagonising effects of TNF-α.

In health, PGs have a number of important physiological roles, namely:

- protection of the gastrointestinal tract (PGE_2 and PGI_2)
- renal homeostasis (PGE_2 and PGI_2)
- vascular homeostasis (PGI_2 and TXA_2)
- uterine function, embryo implantation and labour (PGF_2)
- regulation of the sleep–wake cycle (PGD_2)
- body temperature (PGE_2).

Synthetic analogues of prostaglandins are being used in medicine, namely:

- PGI_2: *epoprostenol* (inhibits platelet aggregation, used for extracorporeal circulation and primary pulmonary hypertension).
- PGE_1: *alprostadil* (used to maintain the patency of the ductus arteriosus in neonates with congenital heart defects, and for erectile dysfunction by injection into the corpus cavernosum of the penis); misoprostol (used for prophylaxis of peptic ulcer associated with NSAIDs); gemeprost (used as pessaries to soften the uterine cervix and dilate the cervical canal prior to vacuum aspiration for termination of pregnancy).
- PGE_2: *dinoprostone* (used as cervical and vaginal gel to induce labour and for late therapeutic abortion).
- PGF_{2a}: *dinoprost* (termination of pregnancy).

CHRONIC INFLAMMATORY DISEASE

In many diseases, the pathological process is *chronic inflammation;* some of these are shown in Table 15.1, together with the predominant inflammatory cell infiltrates. The factors which allow development of a chronic inflammatory state, while not fully known, are thought to include a genetic predisposition and an environmental trigger, perhaps a virus or other infective agent. An imbalance of the inflammatory response occurs in many of these conditions, because proinflammatory mediators are present in excess. This is a feature of rheumatoid arthritis, inflammatory lung disease (fibrosing alveolitis) and inflammatory bowel disease (Crohn's disease). The dominant cell types and some of the key pro-inflammatory cytokines are illustrated in Figure 15.2. Once activated, macrophages may further be upregulated by the cytokines they release (IL8, GM-CSF, M-CSF, called the autocrine loop). TNF-α and IL-1 are potent upregulators of several cell types including fibroblasts and T cells. TNF-α may act earlier in the hierarchy than other cytokines and has proven to be an important target for anticytokine therapy in rheumatoid arthritis and Crohn's disease (see later, anti-TNF therapy). Some small amounts of anti-inflammatory cytokines may also be present (such as IL-10 and interferon-γ), but because the system is not in balance, the end result is inflammation.

Arthritis

The most common types of arthritis in the UK are *osteoarthritis* (UK prevalence 23%) and *rheumatoid arthritis* (1%). The less common types of *inflammatory arthritis* include: juvenile idiopathic arthritis; spondylarthritis (ankylosing spondylitis, Reiter's syndrome, psoriatic arthritis, arthritis associated with inflammatory bowel disease) and reactive arthritis associated with infection. Joint pains (arthralgia) are common in many other diseases, for example the connective tissue diseases (systemic lupus erythematosus, scleroderma), endocrine conditions (hypo- and hyperthyroidism) and malignancies, but in these, joint inflammation and damage do not usually occur.

The *crystal associated conditions*, gout and pseudogout, are considered later in this chapter.

Drugs have an important place in the therapy of all forms of arthritis, to alleviate symptoms, to modifying the course of the disease and, in the case of septic arthritis, to cure. There follows an account of these drugs.

TABLE 15.1 Diseases with a chronic inflammatory component	
Inflammatory disease	**Inflammatory cell infiltrate**
Acute respiratory distress syndrome	Neutrophil
Asthma	Eosinophil, T cell, monocyte, basophil
Atherosclerosis	T cell, monocyte
Glomerulonephritis	Monocyte, T cell, neutrophil
Inflammatory bowel disease	Monocyte, neutrophil, T cell, eosinophil
Osteoarthritis	Monocyte, neutrophil
Psoriasis	T cell, neutrophil
Rheumatoid arthritis	Monocyte, neutrophil
Sarcoidosis	T cell, monocyte

Nonsteroidal anti-inflammatory drugs (NSAIDs)

MODE OF ACTION

The members of this class of drug, although structurally heterogeneous, possess a single common mode of action which is to *block prostaglandin synthesis*. Various NSAIDs have other actions that may contribute to differences between the drugs and these

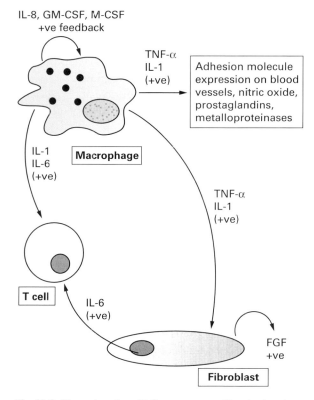

Fig. 15.2 The main cells and inflammatory cytokines in chronic inflammatory disease.

include: the inhibition of lipoxygenases (diclofenac, indomethacin); superoxide radical production and superoxide scavenging; effects on neutrophil aggregation and adhesion, cytokine production and cartilage metabolism. Nevertheless, their key action of inhibiting prostaglandin formation is reflected in the range of effects, beneficial and adverse, which the members exhibit. NSAIDs may be categorised according to their COX specificity as:

- *COX-2 selective* compounds, whose selectivity for inhibiting COX-2 is at least 5 times that for COX-1. The group includes *rofecoxib, celecoxib, meloxicam, etodolac* and *nabumetone.*
- *Non-COX-2 selective* compounds, which comprise all other NSAIDs. These drugs inhibit COX-1 as much as, or even more than, COX-2.

PHARMACOKINETICS

In general, NSAIDs are absorbed almost completely from the gastrointestinal tract, tend not to undergo first-pass (presystemic) elimination, are highly bound to plasma albumin and have small volumes of distribution. Their $t_{\frac{1}{2}}$ values in plasma tend to group into those that are short (1–5 h) or long (10–60 h). Differences in $t_{\frac{1}{2}}$ are not necessarily reflected proportionately in duration of effect, for peak and trough drug concentrations at their intended site of action in synovial (joint) fluid at steady-state dosing, are much less than those in plasma. The vast majority of NSAIDs are weakly acidic drugs that localise preferentially in the synovial tissue of inflamed joints (see pH partition hypothesis, p. 97).

USES

The wide range of recognised uses is expressed below. Some NSAIDs are available 'over the counter' in the UK (without a prescription), an acknowledgement of their general level of safety.

Analgesia: NSAIDs are effective for pain of mild to moderate intensity including musculoskeletal and postoperative pain, and osteo- and inflammatory arthritis; they have the advantage of not causing dependence, unlike opioids (but see analgesic nephropathy, below).

Anti-inflammatory action: this is utilised in all types of arthritis, musculoskeletal conditions and pericarditis.

Antipyretic action: cytokine-induced PG synthesis in the hypothalamus is blocked, thus reducing fever.

Antiplatelet function: aspirin is indicated for the treatment and/or prevention of myocardial infarction, transient ischaemic attacks and embolic strokes.

Prolongation of gestation and labour: inhibition of PG synthesis by the uterus during labour by indomethacin will prolong labour.

Patency of the ductus arteriosus: as PGs maintain the patency, indomethacin given to a new-born child with a patent ductus can result in closure, avoiding the alternative of surgical ligation.

Primary dysmenorrhoea: mefanamic acid is used to reduce the production of PGs by the uterus which cause uterine hypercontractility and pain.

Further areas of potential benefit from NSAIDs are being explored, including the prevention of Alzheimer's dementia and colorectal carcinoma.

ADVERSE REACTIONS

Gastrointestinal effects

Gastric and intestinal mucosal damage is the commonest adverse effect of NSAIDs. The physiological function of mucosal prostaglandins is *cytoprotective,* by inhibiting acid secretion, by promoting the secretion of mucus and by strengthening resistance of the mucosal barrier to back-diffusion of acid from the gastric lumen into the submucosal tissues where it causes damage. Inhibition of prostaglandin biosynthesis removes this protection. Indigestion, gastro-oesophageal reflux, erosions, peptic ulcer, gastrointestinal haemorrhage and perforation, and small and large bowel ulceration occur.

In the UK an estimated 12 000 peptic ulcer complications and 1200 deaths per year are attributable to NSAID use.[3] Toxicity relates to anti-

---

[3] Hawkey C J 1996 Scandinavian Journal of Gastroenterology (Suppl.) 220: 124–127, 221: 23–24.

inflammatory efficacy. A meta-analysis of 12 con-trolled epidemiological studies ranked common NSAIDs according to their propensity for causing gastrointestinal complications.[4] Azapropazone, pir-oxicam, ketoprofen and indomethacin were asso-ciated with high risk (and azapropazone was 9.2 times more likely than low-dose ibuprofen to cause such adverse effects).

Clinical trial evidence in general appears to support the theory that COX-2 selective inhibitors are as effective as, but have fewer adverse effects than, non-COX-2 selective compounds; for example meloxicam is better tolerated than diclofenac or piroxicam.[5,6] The relative risk of serious gastro-intestinal effects (bleeding peptic ulcers) due to rofecoxib (COX-2 selective) was 0.51 compared with conventional NSAIDs.[7] COX-2 selective drugs are yet associated with significant dyspeptic symptoms (indigestion, heartburn), and these effects may result from inhibition of the (protective) constitutively expressed COX-2 in the stomach.

In practice, a minority of patients are intolerant of all NSAIDs. They may benefit from the co-administration of a proton pump inhibitor, a H$_2$-receptor blocker or the prostaglandin analogue, misoprostol. To address this problem, some NSAIDs are presented in combination with misoprostol, e.g. diclofenac with misoprostol (Arthrotec) and nap-roxen with misoprostol (Napratec). Some patients experience abdominal pain and diarrhoea from the misoprostol component.

Ulceration and stricture of the small bowel may also be caused by NSAIDs, and in some patients there is occult blood loss, diarrhoea and malabsorption, i.e. a clinical syndrome indistinguishable from Crohn's disease.

Renal effects

Renal blood flow is reduced because the synthesis of vasodilator renal prostaglandins is inhibited; the result is sodium and fluid retention and arterial blood pressure may rise. Renal failure may occur when glomerular filtration is dependent on the vasodilator action of prostaglandins, e.g. in the elderly, those with pre-existing renal disease, hepatic cirrhosis, cardiac failure, or on diuretic therapy sufficient to reduce intravascular volume.

Analgesic nephropathy. Mixtures of NSAIDs (rather than single agents) taken repeatedly cause grave and often irreversible renal damage, notably chronic interstitial nephritis, renal papillary necrosis and acute renal failure; these effects appear to be due at least in part to ischaemia through inhibition of formation of locally produced vasodilator pro-staglandins. The condition is most common in people who take high doses over years, e.g. for severe chronic rheumatism and patients with personality disorder. Whilst analgesic nephropathy appears to be associated with long-term abuse of NSAID mixtures, the strong evidence that phenacetin was particularly responsible has rendered this drug obsolete.[8]

Cutaneous effects

Urticaria, severe rhinitis and asthma occur in susceptible individuals, e.g. with nasal polyposis, who are exposed to NSAIDs, notably aspirin; the

---

[8] During the influenza pandemic of 1918 a physician to a big factory in a Swedish town prescribed an antipyretic powder containing phenacetin, phenazone (both NSAIDs) and caffeine. Survivors of the epidemic thought they felt fitter and reinvigorated during convalescence if they took the powder and they continued to take it after recovery. Consumption increased and many families 'could not think of beginning the day without a powder. Attractively wrapped packages of powder were often given as birthday presents'. Deaths from renal insufficiency rose in the 'phenacetin town', but not in a similar Swedish town, and in the decade of 1952–61 they were more than 3 times as many. An investigation was resisted by the factory workers to the extent that there was an organised burning of a questionnaire on powder-taking. It was eventually discovered that most of those who used the powders did so, not for pain, but to maintain a high working pace, from 'habit', or to counter fatigue (an effect probably due to the caffeine). Eventually the rising death rate brought home to the consumers the gravity of the matter, something that has yet to be achieved for tobacco smoking or alcohol drinking (Grimlund K 1964 Acta Medica Scandinavica 174: suppl. 405).

---

[4] Henry D et al 1996 British Medical Journal 312: 1563.
[5] Hawkey C J et al 1998 British Journal of Rheumatology 37: 937.
[6] Dequeker J et al 1998 British Journal of Rheumatology 37: 946.
[7] Langman M J et al 1999 Journal of the American Medical Association 282: 1929.

mechanism may involve inhibition of synthesis of bronchodilator prostaglandins, notably PGE2 (see Pseudoallergic reactions, p. 146). Other effects on the skin include photosensitity, erythema multiforme, urticaria, and toxic epidermal necrolysis.

Other general effects include cholestasis, hepatocellular toxicity, thrombocytopenia, neutropenia, red cell aplasia, and haemolytic anaemia. Ovulation may be reduced or delayed (reversibly).

An account of adverse reactions that probably relate to individual chemical classes of NSAID is given later.

INTERACTIONS

NSAIDs give scope for interaction, by differing pharmacodynamic and pharmacokinetic mechanisms, with:

- ACE inhibitors and angiotensin II antagonists: there is risk of renal impairment and hyperkalaemia.
- Quinolone antimicrobials: convulsions may occur if NSAIDs are co-administered.
- Anticoagulant (warfarin) and antiplatelet agents (ticlopidine, clopidogrel): reduced platelet adhesiveness and GI tract damage by NSAIDs increase risk of alimentary bleeding (notably with azapropazone). Phenylbutazone, and probably azapropazone, inhibit the metabolism of warfarin, increasing its effect.
- Antidiabetics: azapropazone and phenylbutazone inhibit the metabolism of sulphonylurea hypoglycaemics, increasing their intensity and duration of action.
- Antiepileptics: azapropazone and phenylbutazone inhibit the metabolism of phenytoin and sodium valproate, increasing their risk of toxicity.
- Antifungal: fluconazole raises the plasma concentration of, and thus risk of toxicity from, celecoxib.
- Antihypertensives: their effect is lessened due to sodium retention by inhibition of renal prostaglandin formation.
- Antivirals: ritonavir may raise plasma concentration of piroxicam; NSAIDs may increase haematological toxicity from zidovudine.

- Ciclosporin: nephrotoxic effect is aggravated by NSAIDs.
- Cytotoxics: renal tubular excretion of methotrexate is reduced by competition with NSAIDs, with risk of methotrexate toxicity (low-dose methotrexate given weekly avoids this hazard).
- Diuretics: NSAIDs cause sodium retention and reduce diuretic and antihypertensive efficacy; risk of hyperkalaemia with potassium-sparing diuretics; increased nephrotoxicity risk (with indomethacin, ketorolac).
- Lithium: NSAIDs delay the excretion of lithium by the kidney and may cause lithium toxicity.

Individual NSAIDs

The currently available NSAIDs exhibit a variety of molecular structures and it is usual to classify these drugs by their chemical class. Clinical trials in rheumatoid arthritis and osteoarthritis, however, rarely find substantial differences in response to average doses of NSAIDs whatever their structure, and this no doubt reflects their common mode of action. Some 60% of patients will respond to any NSAID and many of the remainder will respond to a drug from another group. A structural classification is nevertheless used here as it provides a logical framework; furthermore, specific toxicity profiles tend also to relate to chemical group (see below). Summary data on NSAIDs licenced in the UK are given in Table 15.2.

ADVERSE EFFECTS

A general account of the unwanted effects of NSAIDs is given on page 283. In addition, adverse reactions that feature within particular chemical classes of NSAID appear below, together with comments on some individual drugs.

Paracetamol: see below.

Salicylic acids: see aspirin, below.

Acetic acids. *Indomethacin* may cause prominent salt and fluid retention. Headache is common, often similar to migraine, and is attributed to cerebral oedema; it can be limited by starting at a low dose

TABLE 15.2 Nonsteroidal anti-inflammatory drugs licenced in the UK

Chemical class	Generic name	Compound	Half-life ($t^{1/}_2$)	Usual adult dose
Para-amino phenol	paracetamol	acetaminophen	2 h	I g qid
Salicylic acids	aspirin	acetylsalicylic acid	15 min	300–900 mg q.d.s. maximum 4 g daily
	diflusinal	salicylate	7–15 h	500–1000 mg daily in I or 2 doses
	benorilate	salicylate-paracetamol ester		1.5 g q.d.s.
Acetic acids	indometacin	indole	4 h	initially 50–75 mg daily as I or 2 doses, maximum 200 mg daily
	acemetacin	indole	3 h	60 mg b.d. or t.d.s.
	sulindac	indene	8 h	200 mg b.d.
	diclofenac sodium	phenylacetic acid	2 h	75–150 mg daily in 2 divided doses
	etodolac	pyranocarboxyate	7 h	600 mg o.d.
	ketorolac	ketorolac trometerol	5h	
Fenamic acid	mefanamic acid	fenamate	3 h	500 mg t.i.d.
Propionic acids	ibuprofen	propionic acid	2 h	1.6–2.4 g daily in divided doses
	fenbufen	propionic acid	10 h	300 mg in a.m. and 600 mg nocte, or 450 mg b.d.
	fenoprofen	propionic acid	3 h	300–600 mg t.d.s. or q.d.s., maximum 3 g daily
	flurbiprofen	propionic acid	4 h	150–200 mg daily in divided doses, maximum 300 mg daily
	ketoprofen	propionic acid	I h	100–200 mg in 2–4 divided doses
	naproxen	propionic acid	14 h	250–500 mg b.d.
	tiaprofenic acid	propionic acid	2 h	600 mg in 2–3 divided doses
Enolic acids	piroxicam	oxicam	45 h	20 mg o.d.
	meloxicam	oxicam	20 h	7.5–15 mg o.d.
	tenoxicam	oxicam	72 h	20 mg o.d.
	azapropazone	benzotriazine	18 h	1.2 g daily in 2 or 4 divided doses
	phenylbutazone	pyrazone	72 h	
Non-acid drugs	nabumetone	napthylalkanone	22 h	I g nocte, additional 500 mg — I g o.d. if necessary
	celecoxib	coxib	10 h	200–400 mg daily in divided doses
	aceclofenac	phenylacetoxyacetic acid	4 h	100 mg b.d.
	rofecoxib	coxib	17 h	12.5–25 mg o.d.

and increasing slowly. Vomiting, dizziness and ataxia occur. Allergic reactions occur and there is cross-reactivity with aspirin. Indomethacin may aggravate pre-existing renal disease. Drugs of this group are best avoided where there is gastroduodenal, renal or central nervous system disease or in the presence of infection. Unusually among the NSAIDs, adverse effects of *sulindac* on the kidney may be less likely as the active (sulphide) metabolite of sulindac appears not to inhibit renal prostaglandin synthesis.

Fenamic acid. The principal adverse effects of *mefenamic acid* are diarrhoea, upper abdominal discomfort, peptic ulcer and haemolytic anaemia. Elderly patients who take mefenamic acid may develop nonoliguric renal failure especially if they become dehydrated, e.g. by diarrhoea; the drug should be avoided or used with close supervision in the elderly.

Propionic acids. The main advantage of the

members of this group is a lower incidence of adverse effects particularly in the gastrointestinal tract, and especially with ibuprofen at low dose. Nevertheless epigastric discomfort, activation of peptic ulcer and bleeding may occur. Other effects include headaches, dizziness, fever and rashes.

Enolic acids. Note the generally long $t\frac{1}{2}$ of each member of this group, and in consequence the anticipated time to reach steady state in plasma ($5 \times t\frac{1}{2}$). Adverse effects are those to be expected with NSAIDs in general, gastrointestinal and central nervous system complaints being the commonest. Toxic reactions are relatively frequent with *azapropazone* which should be used only in rheumatoid arthritis, ankylosing spondylitis and acute gout when other drugs have failed. *Phenylbutazone* is also relatively toxic (gastrointestinal, hepatic, renal, bone marrow); it is rarely indicated except in ankylosing spondylitis under specialist supervision.

Nonacidic drugs. COXIBs are associated with fewer gastrointestinal adverse effects, but otherwise the general profile of adverse reactions to NSAIDs applies. The possibility that COXIBs may be associated with increased risk of thrombotic cardiovascular events is the subject of pharmacovigilance studies.

More extensive accounts of *paracetamol* and *aspirin* are given below, because of the importance and widespread use of these drugs.

PARACETAMOL (ACETAMINOPHEN) (PANADOL)

This popular domestic analgesic and antipyretic for adults and children can be bought over the counter in the UK. It is a major metabolite of the now obsolete phenacetin (see p. 284). Its analgesic efficacy is equal to that of aspirin but in therapeutic doses it has only weak anti-inflammatory effects (for this reason it is sometimes deemed not to be an NSAID). Paracetamol inhibits prostaglandin synthesis in the brain but hardly at all in the periphery; it does not affect platelet function. Paracetamol is effective in mild to moderate pain such as that of headache or dysmenorrhoea and it is also useful in patients who should avoid aspirin because of gastric intolerance, a bleeding tendency or allergy, or because they are aged < 12 years.

Pharmacokinetics. Paracetamol ($t\frac{1}{2}$ 2h) is well absorbed from the alimentary tract and is inactivated in the liver principally by conjugation as glucuronide and sulphate. Minor metabolites of paracetamol are also formed of which one oxidation product, N-acetyl-*p*-benzoquinoneimine (NABQI), is highly reactive chemically. This substance is normally rendered harmless by conjugation with glutathione. But the supply of hepatic glutathione is limited and if the amount of NABQI formed is greater than the glutathione available, then the excess metabolite oxidises thiol (SH-) groups of key enzymes, which causes cell death. This explains why a normally safe drug can, in overdose, give rise to hepatic and renal tubular necrosis (the kidneys also contain drug oxidising enzymes).

Dose. The oral dose is 0.5 to 1 g every 4 to 6 h, maximum daily dose 4 g.

Adverse effects. Paracetamol is usually well-tolerated by the stomach because inhibition of prostaglandin synthesis in the periphery is weak; allergic reactions and skin rash sometimes occur. Heavy, long-term daily use may predispose to chronic renal disease.

Acute overdose. Severe hepatocellular damage and renal tubular necrosis can result from taking 150 mg/kg (about 10 or 20 tablets) in one dose, which is only 2.5 times the recommended maximum daily clinical dose. Patients specially at risk are:

- those whose enzymes are induced as a result of taking drugs or alcohol for their livers and kidneys form more NABQI and
- those who are malnourished (chronic alcohol abuse, eating disorder, HIV infection) to the extent that their livers and kidneys are depleted of glutathione to conjugate with NABQI (see above).

The INR (prothrombin time) is preferred to plasma bilirubin and hepatic enzymes as a monitor of liver damage, and renal impairment is better assessed by plasma creatinine than urea (which is metabolised by the liver). The clinical signs (jaundice, abdominal pain, hepatic tenderness) do not become apparent for 24–48 h and liver failure, when it occurs, does so between 2 and 7 days after the overdose. It is vital that this delay be remembered for lives can be saved only by effective anticipatory action (see below). The plasma concentration of paracetamol is of predictive value; if it lies above a semilogarithmic graph joining points between 200 mg/l (1.32 mmol/l) at 4 h after ingestion to 50 mg/l (0.33 mmol/l) at 12 h, then serious hepatic damage is likely. Patients who are enzyme induced or malnourished (see above) are regarded as being at risk at 50% of these plasma concentrations (plasma concentrations measured earlier than 4 h are unreliable because of incomplete absorption).

The general principles for limiting drug absorption apply (Ch. 9) if the patient is seen within 4 h. Activated charcoal by mouth is effective but the decision to use it must take into account its capacity to bind an oral antidote (methionine). Specific therapy is directed at replenishing the store of liver glutathione which combines with and so diminishes the amount of toxic metabolite available to do harm. Glutathione itself cannot be used as it penetrates cells poorly but N-acetylcysteine (NAC) (Parvolex) and methionine are effective as they are precursors for the synthesis of glutathione. NAC is more effective because its conversion into glutathione requires fewer enzymes; also, it is administered by i.v. infusion which is an advantage if the patient is vomiting. Methionine alone may be used to initiate treatment when facilities for infusing NAC are not immediately available.

The earlier such therapy is instituted the better and it should be started if:
- a patient is estimated to have taken > 150 mg/kg, without waiting for the measurement of the plasma concentration
- plasma concentration indicates the likelihood of liver damage (above)
- there is any uncertainty about the amount taken or its timing.

NAC is administered i.v. 150 mg/kg in dextrose 5% (200 ml) over 15 min; then 50 mg/kg in dextrose 5% (500 ml) over 4 h; then 100 mg/kg in dextrose 5% (1000 ml) over 16 h, to a total of about 300 mg/kg in 20 h. While it is most effective if administered within 8 h of the overdose, evidence shows that treatment continuing up to 72 h yet provides benefit.

The INR and serum creatinine should be measured daily. If the INR exceeds 2 there is risk of infection and gastric bleeding, and an antimicrobial plus either sucralfate or a histamine H_2 receptor antagonist should be given prophylactically. The patient should be kept well hydrated and in fluid balance; falling urine output, indicative of acute renal tubular necrosis, will necessitate measures to improve urine flow (see Chapter 23).

A *paracetamol-methionine* combination (co-methiamol; Pameton) has been marketed, the methionine content ensuring that hepatic glutathione concentrations are maintained when the drug is used in therapeutic (and over-) dose. But the problem of ensuring that this is used by the people most likely to benefit from such prophylaxis has not been solved since paracetamol is on direct sale to the public and this proprietary preparation is more expensive than generic paracetamol. A more simple measure, reduction of the pack-size in which paracetamol is sold to the public, appears to have reduced the use of paracetamol as a means of deliberate self-harm.[9]

ASPIRIN (ACETYLSALICYLIC ACID)

Aspirin (acetylsalicylic acid) was introduced in 1899; it is by far the commonest form in which salicylate is taken. The bark of the willow tree *(Salix)* contains salicin from which salicylic acid is derived; it was used for fevers in the 18th century as a cheap substitute for imported cinchona (quinine) bark.

Mode of action. Acetylsalicylic acid is unique among NSAIDs in that it also irreversibly inhibits COX by acylating the active site of the enzyme, so preventing the formation of products including thromboxane, prostacyclin and other prostaglandins, until more COX is synthesised. Acetylsalicylic acid is rapidly hydrolysed to salicylic acid in the plasma. Salicylic acid also has an anti-inflammatory action but additionally exerts important effects on respiration, intermediary metabolism and acid–base balance, and it is highly irritant to the stomach.

The anti-inflammatory, analgesic and antipyretic actions of aspirin are those of NSAIDs in general

---

[9] Hawton K et al 2001 British Medical Journal 322: 1203.

(see before). The following additional actions are relevant.

- Antiplatelet effect is due to permanent inactivation of COX in platelets, preventing synthesis of thromboxane. Being non-nucleated, platelets cannnot regenerate the enzyme as can nucleated cells, and the resumption of thromboxane production is dependent on the entry of new platelets into the circulation (platelet life-span is 8 days). Thus continuous antiplatelet effect is readily achieved with low doses.
- Respiratory stimulation is a characteristic of aspirin intoxication and occurs both directly by stimulation of the respiratory centre and indirectly through increased CO_2 production (see below).
- Metabolic effects including increased O_2 consumption and CO_2 production are relevant when aspirin is taken in overdose.
- Aspirin in high dose reduces renal tubular *reabsorption* of urate (both substances are transported by the same mechanism), but other treatments for hyperuricaemia are preferred. Indeed aspirin should be *avoided in gout* as low doses (< 2 g/day) inhibit urate *secretion,* causing urate retention and on balance its effects on urate elimination are adverse.

Pharmacokinetics. Aspirin ($t\frac{1}{2}$ 15 min) is well absorbed from the stomach and upper intestinal tract. Hydrolysis removes the acetyl group, and the resulting salicylate ion is inactivated largely by conjugation with glycine. At low therapeutic doses this reaction proceeds by first-order kinetics with a $t\frac{1}{2}$ of about 4 h but at higher therapeutic doses and in overdose the process becomes progressively saturated, i.e. kinetics become zero-order, and most of the drug in the body is present as the salicylate. The problem in overdose therefore is to remove salicylate.

A reasonably steady plasma concentration can be maintained if aspirin is given 6-hourly by mouth but if a high dose is given repeatedly there is risk of accumulation to toxic amounts; tinnitus is a useful warning sign.

Salicylate is an organic anion and in addition to undergoing glomerular filtration, is secreted by the proximal renal tubule (see also urate, p. 297).

Doses of 75–150 mg/day are used to prevent thrombotic vascular occlusion; 300 mg as immediate treatment for myocardial infarction; 300–900 mg every 4–6 h for analgesia.

Adverse effects. Gastrointestinal effects are those of NSAIDs in general. Effects particularly associated with aspirin are:

- *Salicylism* (the symptoms of too high dose) is expressed as tinnitus and hearing difficulty, dizziness, headache and confusion.
- *Allergy.* Aspirin is a common cause of allergic or pseudoallergic symptoms and signs. Patients exhibit severe rhinitis, urticaria, angioedema, asthma or shock. Those who already suffer from recurrent urticaria, nasal polyps or asthma are more susceptible.
- *Reye's syndrome.* Epidemiological evidence relates aspirin use to the development of the rare Reye's syndrome (encephalopathy, liver injury) in children recovering from febrile viral infections (respiratory, varicella). Acknowledging this, aspirin should not be given to children under 12 years unless specifically indicated, e.g. for juvenile arthritis, and should be avoided in those up to and including 15 years (paracetamol is preferred). Parents should be educated not to use aspirin as most such administration is on their initiative, not prescribed.

Overdose. A moderate overdose (plasma salicylate 500–750 mg/l) will cause nausea, vomiting, epigastric discomfort, tinnitus, deafness, sweating, pyrexia, restlessness, tachypnoea and hypokalaemia. A large overdose (plasma salicylate > 750 mg/l) may result in pulmonary oedema, convulsions and coma, with severe dehydration and ketosis. Bleeding is unusual, despite the antiplatelet effect of aspirin.

Metabolic changes are important; as the plasma salicylate concentration rises the following occur:

- *Respiratory alkalosis develops,* directly due to stimulation of the respiratory centre, and indirectly by increased CO_2 production (from increased peripheral O_2 consumption due to uncoupling of oxidative phosphorylation).
- *Blood pH thus rises,* and is compensated by renal loss of bicarbonate which is necessarily accompanied by sodium and potassium ions as

well as water; dehydration and hypokalaemia result. The reduction of plasma bicarbonate deprives the body of one of its buffering systems so that it becomes particularly vulnerable to metabolic acidosis.

- *Metabolic acidosis* is the outcome of several factors including accumulation of lactic and pyruvic acids due to toxic interference with citric acid cycle enzymes, and stimulation of lipid metabolism causing increased production of ketone bodies. Late toxic respiratory depression may also cause CO_2 retention.

Adults who have taken a single large quantity usually develop a respiratory alkalosis. Metabolic acidosis suggests severe poisoning. Often, a mixed picture is seen clinically. In children under 4 years, severe metabolic acidosis is more likely than respiratory alkalosis, especially if the drug has been ingested over many hours (mistaken for sweets).

Treatment. Serial measurements of plasma salicylate are necessary to monitor the course of the overdose, for the concentration may rise over the early hours after ingestion. The general management measures described in Chapter 9 apply, but the following are relevant for salicylate overdose.

- *Activated charcoal* 50 g p.o. adsorbs salicylate and prevents its absorption from the alimentary tract; gastric lavage or the use of an emetic is no longer recommended.
- *Correction of dehydration.* Dextrose 5% i.v. with additional potassium is often indicated.
- *Acid–base disturbance.* Alkalosis or mixed alkalosis/acidosis need no specific treatment. Metabolic acidosis is treated with sodium bicarbonate, which alkalinises the urine and accelerates the removal of salicylate in the urine (see p. 97).
- *Haemodialysis* may be necessary, either if renal failure develops or the plasma salicylate concentration exceeds 900 mg/1.

TOPICAL NSAIDS

Several NSAIDs have topical preparations, for example ibuprofen (Ibugel), diclofenac (Voltarol emulgel), piroxicam (Feldene gel) and ketoprofen (Oruvail gel). The objective is to produce therapeutic local concentrations without (undesirable) systemic effects. These should not be used on broken or inflamed skin, or on mucous membranes, and may cause photosensitivity and local skin reactions. Although systemic absorption is less than with oral preparations, there are reports of gastrointestinal and also renal toxicity associated with their use. NSAIDs are also available as suppositories, which some patients prefer. Both local and systemic side effects may occur.

Drug treatment of arthritis

The patient's priority is relief of joint pain, swelling and stiffness. In addition to providing symptomatic relief, the doctor must avoid the long-term effects of inadequately treated joint inflammation, which leads to joint failure requiring multiple orthopaedic operations. There is no cure for arthritis (except septic arthritis), and the available drugs are sometimes poorly tolerated. Many patients with arthritis turn to complementary therapies which may interact with conventional drugs. Successful treatment of arthritis usually requires a multidisciplinary approach with physiotherapy, occupational therapy and adjustment on the part of the patient all being important.

SYMPTOMATIC TREATMENT

NSAIDs provide much symptomatic relief and improve clinical indicators of disease activity such as joint swelling, but do not improve its outcome, i.e. joint destruction. The current strategy for treating rheumatoid arthritis is to start treatment with specific disease-modifying antirheumatic drugs (DMARDs) at an early stage, as these agents have been shown to reduce joint damage (Figure 15.3). Many people with rheumatoid arthritis continue to take NSAIDs even when established on DMARDs. Patients with osteoarthritis make extensive use of NSAIDs.

DISEASE-MODIFYING TREATMENT

In general, disease modifying antirheumatic drugs (DMARDs) are immune modulators that are believed to restore a more normal immune environment

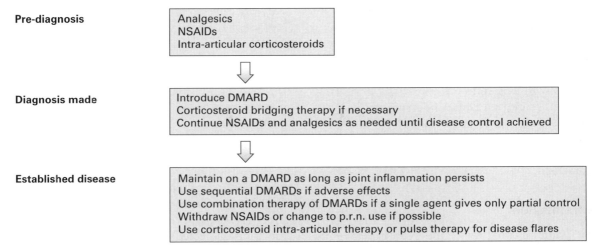

Pre-diagnosis	Analgesics NSAIDs Intra-articular corticosteroids

Diagnosis made	Introduce DMARD Corticosteroid bridging therapy if necessary Continue NSAIDs and analgesics as needed until disease control achieved

Established disease	Maintain on a DMARD as long as joint inflammation persists Use sequential DMARDs if adverse effects Use combination therapy of DMARDs if a single agent gives only partial control Withdraw NSAIDs or change to p.r.n. use if possible Use corticosteroid intra-articular therapy or pulse therapy for disease flares

Fig. 15.3 Flow diagram for the drug treatment of rheumatoid arthritis.

within the joint synovium. DMARDs are used principally for rheumatoid arthritis and in peripheral joint disease associated with spondyloarthropathy.

The benefits are reduced joint pain, swelling and stiffness, and less joint damage in the long term. The principal mechanism which is important in achieving these results is not understood with certainty for any of the DMARDs, although some actions are known, e.g. methotrexate and sulphasalazine are primarily antifolate drugs, whilst ciclosporin affects T-cell function.

The drugs differ in their speed of onset of action, which in general takes weeks to months. Until they work, and often afterwards, most patients will need NSAIDs, and may require bridging therapy with corticosteroid (p.o., i.m., i.v. or intra-articular). As all effect the immune system, *regular monitoring* is required to ensure prompt withdrawal and supportive treatment if, e.g. marrow suppression develops. Most require monitoring of at least one other organ, e.g. kidney or liver. As general rules, patients receiving DMARD should not be given live vaccines, because of their immunosuppressed state, and use of DMARDs during pregnancy and lactation is contraindicated. Management of patients with DMARDs is a matter for specialists, and only a general account of the drugs and their mode of use is provided here.

Methotrexate

Methotrexate acts by competitive inhibition of the enzyme dihydrofolate reductase, but it has actions on other enzymes involved in protein synthesis as well as anti-inflammatory and cytokine-modulating effects. The drug is structurally similar to tetrahydrofolate and enters cells using the active transport system for folate and folinic acid, remaining in the cell for many weeks.

It is absorbed from the gastrointestinal tract by an active process also used by folates. It is eliminated from the plasma by cellular uptake and by renal excretion of the unmetabolised drug ($t_\frac{1}{2}$ 5 h).

Methotrexate is used widely as a DMARD for rheumatoid arthritis, psoriatic arthritis, and for its steroid-sparing effects in many other conditions, especially if azathioprine is not tolerated. In high dose, with folinic acid rescue, methotrexate is used to treat solid and haematological malignancies (see p. 612). Low dose methotrexate slows the progression of rheumatoid arthritis. The evidence for a true disease-modifying effect on psoriatic arthritis is less definite, but methotrexate is often preferred to other DMARDs for its beneficial effect on the skin lesions.

Methotrexate is usually given in a dose of 7.5 mg p.o. per week initially, increasing to the maximum of 20 mg per week.

Adverse reactions. Methotrexate is the best tolerated of the DMARDs and more than half of the patients who commence are still taking the drug more than 5 years later. Nausea and mouth ulcers are reduced or eliminated by the addition of folic acid. Transient elevation of the hepatic transaminases is common (up to 30%) and can be managed by temporary discontinuation. Pancytopenia may occur as an idiosyncratic response at any time, or may be provoked by co-administration of another antifolate drug, e.g. trimethoprim. Hepatic cirrhosis may develop with long-term use (especially in psoriasis patients). Acute interstitial pneumonitis is a rare but potentially fatal complication. Methotrexate is teratogenic and should not be prescribed to premenopausal women unless adequate contraception is practised.

Sulfasalazine

The sulfasalazine molecule comprises sulfapiridine and 5-aminosalicylic acid linked by an azo-bond which is split by colonic bacteria, releasing the component parts. Sulfapiridine, as a sulphonamide, has an antifolate action which is believed to benefit rheumatoid arthritis, while it is the salicylate moiety that is thought to be effective in inflammatory bowel disease; a fuller description appears on page 64. Sulfasalazine is used as a DMARD for rheumatoid arthritis, spondyloarthropathy with peripheral joint involvement, and psoriatic arthritis.

Gold salts

Gold salts modify a variety of cellular and humoral immune responses; their mode of action is not understood but may relate to the formation of aurocyanide in areas of inflammation. *Sodium aurothiomalate* by deep i.m. injection or *auranofin* by mouth are available but oral gold is less effective and is rarely used as initial therapy.

Disposition of gold is complex; it blinds extensively to plasma albumin and is also distributed to inflamed synovium, kidney and liver. Gold is excreted mainly by the kidney and to a lesser extent in the faeces, which it probably enters via the bile. The $t\frac{1}{2}$ of elimination from plasma is 22 days, consistent with which steady-state concentrations are reached only after about 3 months. Retention in deep tissue compartments may persist up to 23 years after therapy has been stopped.

Accumulated experience indicates that gold treatment may be continued indefinitely if it is beneficial and well tolerated.

Adverse effects occur in about one-third of patients and in some gold may have to be discontinued. They include pruritus, dermatitis, glossitis and stomatitis, most commonly, and also leucopenia and thrombocytopenia and marrow failure (which may threaten life), hepatic and renal damage (rarely nephrotic syndrome due to membranous nephritis), peripheral neuritis and encephalopathy. Serious toxicity is rare when observation is careful (monthly blood counts and urinalysis) and the drug stopped at the earliest sign of harm. Any serious effect, or one which does not subside rapidly, should be treated with a chelating agent; dimercaprol is probably preferable to penicillamine. Gold salts are contraindicated in pregnancy and should not be offered to women of child-bearing potential without a careful assessment of the benefits and risks that apply in individual cases. Because of its known toxicity, gold is used less commonly than sulfasalazine or methotrexate as the first choice DMARD.

Azathioprine

Azathoiprine is metabolised to 6-mercaptopurine (see p. 608), which is responsible for many, but not all, of its actions as an inhibitor of purine synthesis. The cellular immune response is impaired, notably the function of both B and T lymphocytes. As a result of a genetic polymorphism, approximately 1 in 300 Caucasian people have very low levels of thiopurine methyltransferase (TPMT) the enzyme that metabolises 6-mercaptopurine; these individuals are at high risk of toxicity to normal doses of azathioprine.

In addition to its use for rheumatoid arthritis, azathoiprine is employed for its steroid-sparing effect in many autoimmune diseases, as an immunosuppressant, e.g. after organ transplant, and to maintain remission in the treatment of vasculitis. Other aspects of azathiopurine are discussed elsewhere in the book (see Index).

Adverse effects include nausea, diarrhoea, rash and hypersensitivity reactions; marrow suppression and hepatotoxicity also occur. Careful monitoring is required.

Allopurinol, a xanthine oxidase inhibitor, potentiates the action of mercaptopurine with danger of toxicity if the drugs are co-administered (see later, gout).

D-Penicillamine

The mode of action of penicillamine in rheumatoid arthritis is unclear but it reduces rheumatoid factor and also the concentration of immune complexes in plasma and synovial fluid. Its action as a chelator of a number of metals (including gold), is valuable in poisoning (see Ch. 9) and hepatolenticular degeneration. Penicillamine is incompletely but adequately absorbed following administration by mouth and undergoes metabolism by the liver, the products being excreted in the urine and faeces. After a single oral dose the $t\frac{1}{2}$ is 3 h.

Adverse effects are frequent. Patients may experience gastrointestinal upset, and dose-related impairment of taste is common. Thrombocytopenia is frequent but resolves when the drug is withdrawn unless it indicates the more serious aplastic anaemia which may also occur. Allergic reactions (rashes, fever) tend to occur during the early stages of treatment. Proteinuria, if it is heavy, is a reason for stopping penicillamine for it may herald the development of the nephrotic syndrome.

Hydroxychloroquine

Hydroxychloroquine (and also chloroquine, see Ch. 14) in addition to their antimalarial actions exert anti-inflammatory and immunomodulating effects that are useful in rheumatoid disease. Hydroxychloroquine accumulates within lymphocytes, macrophages, polymorphs and fibroblasts, and inhibits phagocyte function but its exact mode of action is unknown. Its action is terminated both by metabolism and renal elimination ($t\frac{1}{2}$ 18 days).

Hydroxychloroquine is less effective than other DMARDs but it is also less toxic; it is best used for for arthralgias associated with connective tissue disorders (e.g. SLE) and achieves a useful response in about 50% of patients after 4 weeks. For rheumatoid arthritis hydroxychloroquine is best combined with another DMARD.

Adverse effects. Hydroxychloroquine accumulates in many organs, including the eye where it can cause retinal damage that may be irreversible. In practice this complication is rare in the doses that are used to treat rheumatoid arthritis, even long-term, e.g. below 6.5 mg/kg/d, but it is prudent for patients over 60 years of age to have an ophthalmological examination before starting, and then every 6 months during therapy. Skin discolouration, bleaching of the hair, alopecia, and gastrointestinal upset also occur.

Ciclosporin

See page 619.

Leflunomide

Leflunomide selectively inhibits pyrimidine synthesis and prevents T-cell proliferation, which is thought to be important in the pathogenesis of rheumatoid arthritis. The onset of action is faster than other DMARDs, providing clinical benefit in 4–6 weeks. As the drug is retained in the body for 2 years, elimination therapy with either cholestyramine or activated charcoal may be necessary if a change to another DMARD is planned.

Adverse reactions reported include gastrointestinal upset, mouth ulcers, abdominal pain, deranged liver function tests, hypertension, headache, leucopenia, dizziness, weight loss, erythema multiforme, Stevens–Johnson syndrome, and toxic epidermal necrolysis.

Other treatments

Cyclophosphamide, chlorambucil or mycophenolate are reserved for patients with severe rheumatoid arthritis that is not adequately controlled by standard DMARDs.

BIOLOGICAL AGENTS

Biological compounds, i.e. agents derived from natural substances, and chemically altered, are finding their place in therapy.

Etanercept

Etanercept inhibits the activity of the cytokine, TNF (see p. 280). It is a dimeric fusion protein of two TNF receptors (called p75) joined to the Fc domain (constant region) of a human IgG1 molecule. One molecule of etanercept binds two molecules of TNF-α or TNF-β (lymphotoxin). Unlike infliximab, it is an entirely human molecule. Etanercept has a 50-fold greater affinity for TNF than the naturally occurring soluble TNF receptor, and it has an elimination $t\frac{1}{2}$ (70 h) which is 5-fold longer.

The indications for etanercept will become clarified as evidence grows; at the time of writing its use is reserved for patients with active rheumatoid arthritis who have failed to respond to adequate trials of at least two DMARDs.

Adverse reactions include injection site reactions, infection, headache, dizziness, abdominal pain, dyspepsia, malignancies, rash, cholecystitis, depression, and dyspnoea.

Infliximab

Infliximab is a chimeric antibody consisting of the variable region of a murine (mouse) antibody to TNF-α joined to the Fc (constant) region of a human antibody. It inhibits TNF by binding to it in the circulation or joint cavity. The $t\frac{1}{2}$ following an i.v. infusion is 9 days. No dose adjustment for age or weight need be made.

Infliximab is used in combination with methotrexate (to reduce anti-mouse antibody formation) and, like etanercept, is reserved for patients with severe rheumatoid arthritis who have failed to respond to adequate trials of at least two DMARDs. In the UK it is licensed only for adults with rheumatoid disease (and for nonhealing fistulae associated with Crohn's disease).

Adverse reactions that have been reported include infections, fever, headache, vertigo, hypertension, skin reactions, fatigue, chest pain and worsening congestive cardiac failure, gastrointestinal upset. Active tuberculosis may develop soon after starting treatment with infliximab and patients should be screened for latent infection or disease.

THE ROLE OF ADRENAL CORTICOSTEROIDS

Although symptom relief is dramatic, there is a reluctance to use systemic corticosteroid for rheumatoid disease because of its adverse effects but this course is justified in some circumstances.

- To provide interim relief of inflammatory symptoms during the weeks that it takes DMARDs to act.
- Spaced single enormous doses (pulse treatment), e.g. methylprednisolone (as sodium succinate) up to 1 g i.v. on 3 consecutive days, are sometimes used to suppress highly active inflammatory disease and buy time to change the DMARD or dose.
- In extreme severity, high-dose prednisolone (20–40 mg/d) will very effectively suppress inflammation, e.g. with vasculitis or rheumatoid lung.
- Where DMARDs have failed or have produced intolerable adverse effects. The object is to control inflammation in affected joints whilst minimising adverse effects, e.g. prednisolone 7.5 mg or its equivalent of other steroid given once daily (at 08:00 h to reduce adrenal-pituitary suppression).
- There is evidence that prednisolone 7.5 mg/day added to standard treatment may reduce the rate of joint destruction in moderate or severe disease of less than 2 years duration.[10]

Intra-articular injection of corticosteroid (triamcinolone, hydrocortisone, prednisolone or dexamethasone) is very effective when one joint is more affected than others. Benefit from one injection may last many weeks. Aseptic precautions must be extreme, for any introduced infection may spread dramatically. Too frequent resort to corticosteroid injection may actually promote joint damage by removing the protective limitation conferred by pain; such injections in a single joint would not normally exceed three per year. Other aspects of the treatment of inflammatory arthritis are important but are outside the scope of this book.

DIFFERENT WAYS OF USING DMARDS

DMARDs are administered according to several differing regimens, up to three for any individual patient. The drugs may be administered *in sequence* (to find the most effective), with or without a washout in between each, and using a corticosteroid

---

[10] Kirwan R 1995 New England Journal of Medicine 333: 142.

at each changeover, to cover the time till the new DMARD takes effect. Alternatively, up to three DMARDs may be given *in combination*, with drugs added progressively, or all started at the same time. Patient and physician preference, as well as the course of the disease and response to therapy, determine the strategy adopted in an individual instance and, in fact, there is little hard evidence to base decisions on one or other regimen.

The course of rheumatoid arthritis may be very long (50 years) and drugs may be poorly tolerated, ineffective either in the short or long term, and some patients ultimately 'fail' all the standard treatments. For this group, the advent of biological treatments may be advantageous, as the alternative is long-term maintenance on prednisolone, with its associated problems.

RHEUMATIC FEVER

In the acute stage, joint pains and fever should be controlled by aspirin or possibly a corticosteroid, tailored according to need (but see Reye's syndrome, p. 289).

When there is evidence of carditis (cardiac enlargement or pericarditis), complete bed rest is advised and a corticosteroid should be used instead of aspirin since the latter may precipitate cardiac failure. Prednisolone should be given in a dose sufficient to suppress clinical and laboratory (ESR, plasma viscosity, C-reactive protein) signs of inflammation; 10–15 mg/d is usually adequate in adults, and specific therapy for cardiac failure may also be necessary.

Neither aspirin nor adrenal steroid prevents the development of late cardiac complications.

A 10-day course of benzylpenicillin should be given to kill any streptococci (for prophylaxis see p. 239).

OSTEOARTHRITIS

An NSAID is used, the choice being appropriate to the amount of pain and inflammation experienced by the patient, and on the tolerance of adverse effects. Evidence suggests that use of powerful anti-inflammatory drugs may accelerate destruction of some joints, e.g. the hip, by inhibiting the synthesis of vasodilator prostaglandins which are essential

for adequate perfusion with blood for the natural repair of joint structures. NSAID needs should be regularly reviewed; exposure to other NSAIDs may be limited by use of paracetamol, an opioid-containing compound analgesic or an antidepressant in low dose (see p. 331).

There is no general case for using intra-articular corticosteroid in osteoarthritis but local injection of triamcinolone can provide relief for a single periarticular tender spot or for a knee joint that is acutely inflamed.

Crystal-associated conditions

GOUT AND DRUGS

Gout affects about 0.25% of the population of Europe and North America. Drugs are effective in management and some drugs can precipitate attacks. Patients with gout but no visible tophi have a urate pool that is 2–3 times normal and since this exceeds the amount that can be carried in solution in the extracellular fluid, microcrystalline deposits forming tissues including the joints; patients with tophi have a urate pool that may be 15–26 times normal.

Urate is freely filtered by the glomerulus and then reabsorbed from the tubular fluid. It is also secreted from the blood into the tubular fluid. The urate that appears in the urine represents the net effect of these two transport mechanisms; both are active, energy-requiring processes that can be affected by drugs.

Hyperuricaemia and gout from whatever cause (e.g. metabolic, renal disease, neoplasia) depends essentially on two processes, (1) overproduction and (2) underexcretion of urate. Both mechanisms may operate in the same patient but decreased renal clearance contributes to hyperuricaemia in most patients with gout. Drugs may influence these processes as follows:

Overproduction of urate, due to the excessive cell destruction releasing nucleic acids, occurs when myeloproliferative or lymphoproliferative disorders are treated by drugs.

Underexcretion of urate is caused by all diuretics (except spironolactone), aspirin, ethambutol, pyrazinamide, nicotinic acid, and alcohol (which increases urate synthesis and also causes a rise in blood lactic acid that inhibits tubular secretion of urate). The diagnosis of gout ideally requires the demonstration of negatively birefringent needle-shaped crystals in synovial fluid (monosodium urate monohydrate crystals), not just elevated serum urate.

DRUG MANAGEMENT

The aims are to:

- *suppress the symptoms* (anti-inflammatory drugs) i.e. NSAIDs, colchicine, corticosteroids
- *prevent urate synthesis* i.e. allopurinol
- *promote the elimination of urate* (uricosurics) i.e. sulfinpyrazone.

Colchicine

This is an alkaloid derived from the autumn crocus (*Colchicum*). Colchicine rapidly relieves the pain and inflammation of an acute attack of gout. Such swift relief is considered to confirm the diagnosis because non-gouty arthritis is unaffected, though failure does not prove the patient is free of gout. It is most effective if given within 24 h of onset and is useful in patients in whom NSAIDs are contra-indicated. It is also used in recurrent hereditary polyserositis (Familial Mediterranean Fever) when it may prevent attacks and the development of amyloid. The $t\frac{1}{2}$ is 1 h.

The dose in acute gout is 1 mg by mouth, followed by 500 micrograms 2–3-hourly until either relief or adverse effects develop. The total dose should not exceed 6 mg and the course should not be repeated within 3 days.

Adverse effects may be severe with abdominal pain, vomiting and diarrhoea which may be bloody. Renal damage may result and rarely, blood disorders. Large doses cause muscle paralysis. Many patients are unable to tolerate colchicine and use NSAIDs such as indomethacin or diclofenac for an acute attack of gout; some patients require oral corticosteroid.

Allopurinol

Allopurinol inhibits xanthine oxidase, the enzyme that converts xanthine and hypoxanthine to uric acid. Patients taking allopurinol excrete less uric acid and more xanthine and hypoxanthine in the urine. These compounds are more soluble than uric acid (renal stones are rarely xanthine) and are more readily excreted in renal failure.

Allopurinol ($t\frac{1}{2}$ 2 h) is readily absorbed from the gut, metabolised in the liver to alloxanthine ($t\frac{1}{2}$ 25 h) which is also a xanthine oxidase inhibitor, and is excreted unchanged by the kidney.

Allopurinol is indicated in recurrent gout, when at least three attacks occur per year, in blood diseases where there is spontaneous hyperuricaemia, and during treatment of myeloproliferative disorders where cell destruction creates a high urate load. Allopurinol prevents the hyperuricaemia due to diuretics and may be combined with a uricosuric agent. The dose is usually 300 mg/d by mouth but some patients may need as much as 600 mg daily.

Adverse effects include precipitation of an acute attack of gout (see below), and allergic reactions which are uncommon but may be severe e.g. exfoliative skin rash, arthralgia, fever, lymphadenopathy, vasculitis and hepatitis. Deaths have been reported. For this reason, allopurinol should not be commenced unless the diagnosis is certain, and attacks of gout are frequent despite life-style changes (see below). Allergy to allopurinol can be managed by desensitisation, using very small doses of the drug initially, and continuing over a long period.

Allopurinol prevents the oxidation of mercaptopurine to an inactive metabolite; if an ordinary dose of mercaptopurine is given to a patient whose gout is being treated with allopurinol, dangerous potentiation occurs (see also azathiopurine, p. 292).

Sulfinpyrazone

Sulfinpyrazone competitively inhibits the active transport of organic anions across the kidney tubule, both from the plasma to the tubular fluid and vice versa. The effect is dose-dependent for at low dose sulfinpyrazone prevents secretion of uric acid into tubular fluid, and at high dose, and more powerfully, it prevents reabsorption, increasing its excretion in the urine. A net beneficial uricosuric action is obtained with an initial dose of 100–200 mg/d by mouth with food, increasing over 2–3 weeks to 600 mg/d which should be continued until the serum uric acid level is normal. The dose may then be reduced for maintenance, and may be as little as 200 mg/d.

During initial therapy a fluid intake of at least 2 1/d should be ensured to prevent urate crystalluria. If the uric acid load is high, consider rendering the urine alkaline with Potassium Citrate Mixture 12–24 g/d with water p.o. or sodium bicarbonate powder 5–10 g/d with water p.o., again to prevent uric acid crystal formation in the renal tract. Other adverse effects are mainly gastrointestinal; sulfinpyrazone is contraindicated in peptic ulcer.

Fenofibrate is an antihyperlipidaemic drug with added uricosuric action.

TREATMENT OF GOUT

Acute gout

Acute gout is usually treated with an NSAID in full dose. Any such drug which is tolerated may be used (except aspirin which in low dose promotes urate retention, see below); indomethacin is often chosen because of its strong anti-inflammatory action and efficacy. If treatment is started early, the attack may be terminated in a few hours. Colchicine is useful if NSAIDs are contraindicated. If neither colchicine nor NSAIDs are tolerated, oral prednisolone 40 mg/d and tapered over a week is also effective. It requires only a moment's thought to appreciate that the uricosurics and allopurinol will not relieve an acute attack of gout.

Recurrent gout, tophaceous gout, and gout causing renal damage (gouty nephropathy)

In principle it would seem reasonable that overproducers of urate be treated with allopurinol and underexcreters with a uricosuric drug. In practice most patients respond well to allopurinol, which is the drug of choice, especially if renal function is impaired; a uricosuric may be given in addition.

Treatment is initiated if the serum urate consistently exceeds 0.6 mmol/l and the patient has had three or more attacks of acute gout in a year.

Allopurinol should be started in a quiescent period because it will prolong an attack of gout if started during one, and may precipitate an attack even if started when the joints are quiet. *Rapid lowering of plasma urate* by any means may precipitate acute gout, probably by causing the dissolution of tophi. It is therefore usual to give prophylactic suppressive treatment with indometacin, colchicine or steroid cover during the first 2 months of allopurinol or uricosuric treatment. It can create an unfavourable impression if the patient, who has been told only that the drug will prevent gout, promptly has a severe attack. Aspirin must not be taken concurrently with other uricosurics as it interferes with their action (tell the patient). Colchicine or indometacin may be used if an acute attack is expected, e.g. immediately after surgery. Persuading the patient to avoid chronic dietary excess or acute debauchery is also relevant (see below).

Benefit from the lowered plasma urate will not be noticeable for some weeks. Medication should be adjusted to keep the plasma urate in the normal range. It can seldom be abandoned.

Chronic tophaceous gout. Tophi can sometimes be reduced in size and even removed by the prolonged use of allopurinol and uricosuric agents.

Precipitation of gout by diuretics, and aspirin. Any vigorous diuresis may precipitate acute gout by causing volume depletion which results in increased reabsorption of all substances which are normally only partially reabsorbed in the proximal tubule, including urate. Furthermore, most diuretics are organic acids that may compete with urate for secretion by the renal tubule. Diuretic-induced gout is of special importance in the elderly, in whom the presentation may be atypical. Spironolactone probably alone amongst the diuretics does not induce hyperuricaemia. An episode of gout under these circumstances need not lead to a lifelong prescription for allopurinol.

Aspirin interferes with the balance of urate secretion and reabsorption by renal tubule (see above) in a dose-dependent manner. The result is that aspirin in low dose (1 or 2 g/d) decreases urate

Summary

- Inflammation is an essential part of the normal immune response, but if uncontrolled and persistent, it leads to disease.
- NSAIDs provide symptom relief by their analgesic and anti-inflammatory effects but do not modify the course of inflammatory joint disease.
- Discovery of the isoenzymes COX-1 and COX-2 has led to the development of COX-2 selective drugs, which are less prone to gastrointestinal toxicity.
- DMARDs are used to prevent destruction of inflamed joints; these drugs are potentially toxic and their use demands careful monitoring.
- Identification and understanding of the role of natural mediators has allowed the creation of synthetic agents that can modify inflammatory responses, e.g. the anti-TNF agents, etanercept and infliximab.

excretion and raises plasma concentration; high doses (> 5 g/d) are uricosuric and lower plasma concentration but are too poorly tolerated to be useful.

Diet, alcohol and gout

Dietary purines can be a significant contributory cause of hyperuricaemia and patients should avoid excesses of foods that contain purines, e.g. sweetbread (pancreas, thymus), kidney, sardines, gravies, brain, anchovies, liver. Gouty patients tend also to be overweight and loss of weight lowers the plasma urate. Knowledge that alcohol induces acute gout is of long standing, and has been celebrated in verse:

> A taste for drink, combined with gout,
> Had doubled him up for ever.
> Of that there is no manner of doubt —
> No probable, possible shadow of doubt —
> No possible doubt whatever.[11]

But the author did not know the mechanisms.

ACUTE CALCIFIC PYROPHOSPHATE ARTHROPATHY (PSEUDOGOUT)

Pseudogout (chondrocalcinosis, calcium pyrophosphate dihydrate crystals) is treated in a similar way

---

[11] Don Alhambra's song in Act 1 of the Savoy opera, The Gondoliers or the King of Barataria. W S Gilbert (1836–1911).

to acute gout. NSAIDs are beneficial, whilst allopurinol has no role here. Colchicine may be useful for prophylaxis.

GUIDE TO FURTHER READING

Albert L J, Inman R D 1999 Molecular mimicry and autoimmunity. New England Journal of Medicine 341: 2068–2074

Broe M E, Elseviers M M 1998 Analgesic nephropathy. New England Journal of Medicine 338: 446–452

Choy E H S, Panayi G S 2001 Cytokine pathways and joint inflammation in rheumatoid arthritis. New England Journal of Medicine 344: 907–916

Creamer P, Hochberg M C 1997 Osteoarthritis. Lancet 350: 503–509

Delves P J. Roitt I M 2000 The immune system. New England Journal of Medicine 343: 37–49 (and also subsequent articles in this extensive series on Advances in Immunology)

Emmerson B T 1996 The management of gout. New England Journal of Medicine, 334: 445–451

Fitzgerald G A, Patrono C 2001 The coxibs, selective inhibitors of cyclooxygenase-2. New England Journal of Medicine 345: 433–442

Goodnow C C 2001 Pathways for self-tolerance and the treatment of autoimmune disease. Lancet 357: 2115–2121

Hawkey C J 1999 Cox-2 inhibitors. Lancet 353: 307–314

Lee D M, Weinblatt M E 2001 Rheumatoid arthritis. Lancet 358: 903–911

Lipworth B J 1999 Leukotriene-receptor antagonists. Lancet 353: 57–62

Parkin J, Cohen B 2001 An overview of the immune system. Lancet 357: 1777–1789

Seymour H E, Worsley A, Smith J M, Thomas S H L 2001 Anti-TNF agents for rheumatoid arthritis. British Journal of Clinical Pharmacology 51: 201–208

Sneader W 2000 The discovery of aspirin: a reappraisal. British Medical Journal 321: 1591

Walker-Bone K et al 2000 Medical management of osteoarthritis. British Medical Journal 321: 936–940

Wolfe M M, Lichtenstein D R, Singh G 1999 Gastrointestinal toxicity of nonsteroidal anti-inflammatory drugs. New England Journal of Medicine 340: 1888–1999

16

Drugs and the skin

SYNOPSIS

This account is confined to therapy directed primarily at the skin.
- Pharmacokinetics of the skin
- Topical preparations: Vehicles for presenting drugs to the skin; Emollients, barrier preparations and dusting powders; Topical analgesics; Antipruritics; Adrenocortical steroids; Sunscreens
- Cutaneous adverse drug reactions
- Individual disorders: Psoriasis, Acne, Urticaria, Skin infections

It is easy to do more harm than good with potent drugs, and this is particularly true in skin diseases. Many skin lesions are caused by systemic or topical use of drugs, often taking the form of immediate or delayed hypersensitivity.

Pharmacokinetics

The stratum corneum (superficial keratin layer) is both the principal barrier to penetration of drugs into the skin and a reservoir for drugs; a corticosteroid may be detectable even 4 weeks after a single application.

Drugs are presented in *vehicles*, e.g. cream, ointment, and their entry into the skin is determined by the:

- rate of diffusion of drug from the vehicle to the surface of the skin (this depends on the type of vehicle, see below)
- partitioning of the drug between the vehicle and the stratum corneum (a physicochemical feature of the individual drug) and
- degree of hydration of the stratum corneum (hydration reduces resistance to diffusion of drug).

Vehicles (bases[1]) are designed to vary in the extent to which they increase the hydration of the stratum corneum; e.g. oil-in-water creams promote hydration (see below). Some vehicles also contain substances intended to enhance penetration, e.g. squalane (p. 306).

Absorption through normal skin varies with site; from the sole of the foot and the palm of the hand it is relatively low, it increases progressively on the forearm, the scalp, the face until on the scrotum and vulva absorption is very high.

Where the skin is damaged by inflammation, burn or exfoliation, absorption is further increased.

If an *occlusive dressing* (impermeable plastic membrane) is used, absorption increases by as much as 10-fold (plastic pants for babies are occlusive, and some ointments are partially occlusive). Serious systemic toxicity can result from use of occlusive dressing over large areas.

A drug readily diffuses from the stratum corneum into the epidermis and then into the dermis, where

---

[1] The chief ingredient of a mixture.

it enters the capillary microcirculation of the skin, and thus the systemic circulation. There may be a degree of presystemic (first-pass) metabolism in the epidermis and dermis, a desirable feature to the extent that it limits systemic effects.

Transdermal delivery systems are now used to administer drugs via the skin for systemic effect (see p. 109).

Topical preparations

It is convenient to think of these under the following headings:

- Vehicles for presenting drugs to the skin
- Emollients, barrier preparations and dusting powders
- Topical analgesics
- Antipruritics
- Adrenocortical steroids
- Sunscreens
- Miscellaneous substances.

VEHICLES FOR PRESENTING DRUGS TO THE SKIN

The formulations are described in order of decreasing water content. All water-based formulations must contain preservatives, e.g. chlorocresol, but these rarely cause allergic contact dermatitis.

Lotions or wet dressings

Water is the most important component. Wet dressings are generally used to cleanse, cool and relieve pruritus in acutely inflamed lesions, especially where there is much exudation, e.g. atopic eczema. The frequent reapplication and the cooling effect of evaporation of the water reduce the inflammatory response by inducing superficial vasoconstriction. Sodium chloride solution 0.9%, or solutions of astringent[2] substances, e.g. aluminium acetate lotion, or potassium permanganate soaks or compresses of approx. 0.05%, can be used. The use of lotions or

wet dressings over very large areas can reduce body temperature dangerously in the old or the very ill.

Shake lotions, e.g. calamine lotion, are essentially a convenient way of applying a powder to the skin (see Dusting powders, p. 301) with additional cooling due to evaporation of the water. They are contraindicated when there is much exudate because crusts form. Lotions, after evaporation, sometimes produce excessive drying of the skin, but this can be reduced if oils are included, as in oily calamine lotion.

Creams

These are emulsions either of oil-in-water (washable; cosmetic 'Vanishing' creams) or water-in-oil. The water content allows the cream to rub in well. A cooling effect (cold creams) is obtained with both groups as the water evaporates.

Oil-in-water creams, e.g. aqueous cream (see emulsifying ointment, below), mix with serous discharges and are especially useful as vehicles for water-soluble active drugs. They may contain a wetting (surface tension reducing) agent (cetomacrogol). Aqueous cream is also used as an emollient (see below). Various other ingredients, e.g. calamine, zinc, may be added to it.

Water-in-oil creams, e.g. oily cream, zinc cream, behave like oils in that they do not mix with serous discharges, but their chief advantage over ointments (below) is that the water content makes them easier to spread and they give a better cosmetic effect. They act as lubricants and emollients, and can be used on hairy parts. Water-in-oil creams can be used as vehicles for lipid-soluble substances. A dry skin is mainly short of water, and oily substances are needed to provide a barrier that reduces evaporation of water, i.e. the presence of oils contributes to epidermal hydration.

Ointments

Ointments are greasy and are thicker than creams. Some are both lipophilic and hydrophilic, i.e. by occlusion they promote dermal hydration, but are also water miscible. Other ointment bases are composed largely of lipid; by preventing water loss

---

[2] Astringents are weak protein precipitants, e.g. tannins, salts of aluminium and zinc.

they have a hydrating effect on skin and are used in chronic dry conditions. Ointments contain fewer preservatives and are less likely to sensitise. There are two main kinds:

Water-soluble ointments include mixtures of macrogols and polyethylene glycols; their consistency can be varied readily. They are easily washed off and are used in burn dressings, as lubricants and as vehicles that readily allow passage of drugs into the skin, e.g. hydrocortisone.

Emulsifying ointment is made from emulsifying wax (cetostearyl alcohol and sodium lauryl sulphate) and paraffins. Aqueous cream is an oil-in-water emulsion of emulsifying ointment.

Nonemulsifying ointments do not mix with water. They adhere to the skin to prevent evaporation and heat loss, i.e. they can be considered a form of occlusive dressing (with increased systemic absorption of active ingredients); skin maceration may occur. Nonemulsifying ointments are helpful in chronic dry and scaly conditions, such as atopic eczema, and as vehicles; they are not appropriate where there is significant exudation. They are difficult to remove except with oil or detergents and are messy and inconvenient, especially on hairy skin. Paraffin ointment contains beeswax, paraffins and cetostearyl alcohol.

Collodions

Collodions are preparations of cellulose nitrate (pyroxylin) dissolved in an organic solvent. The solvent evaporates rapidly and the resultant flexible film is used to hold a medicament, e.g. salicylic acid, in contact with the skin. They are irritant and inflammable and are used to treat only small areas of skin.

Pastes

Pastes, e.g. zinc compound paste, are stiff, semi-occlusive ointments containing insoluble powders. They are very adhesive and give good protection to circumscribed lesions, preventing spread of active ingredients to surrounding skin. Their powder content enables them to absorb a moderate amount of discharge. They can be used as vehicles, e.g. coal tar paste, which is zinc compound paste with 7.5% coal tar. Lassar's paste is used as a vehicle for dithranol in the treatment of plaque psoriasis.

EMOLLIENTS, BARRIER PREPARATIONS AND DUSTING POWDERS

Emollients hydrate the skin and soothe and smooth dry scaly conditions. They need to be applied frequently as their effects are short-lived. There is a variety of preparations but aqueous cream in addition to its use as a vehicle (above) is effective when used as a soap substitute. Various other ingredients may be added to emollients, e.g. menthol, camphor or phenol for its mild antipruritic effect and zinc and titanium dioxide as astringents.

Barrier preparations. Many different kinds have been devised for use in medicine, in industry and in the home to reduce dermatitis. They rely on water-repellent substances, e.g. silicones (dimethicone cream), and on soaps, as well as on substances that form an impermeable deposit (titanium, zinc, calamine). The barrier preparations are useful in protecting skin from discharges and secretions (colostomies, napkin rash) but they are ineffective when used under industrial working conditions. Indeed, the irritant properties of some barrier creams can enhance the percutaneous penetration of noxious substances. A simple after-work emollient is more effective.

Silicone sprays and occlusives, e.g. hydrocolloid dressings, may be effective in preventing and treating pressure sores.

Masking creams (camouflaging preparations) for obscuring unpleasant blemishes from view are greatly valued by the victims[3]. They may consist of titanium oxide in an ointment base with colouring appropriate to the site and the patient.

Dusting powders, e.g. zinc starch and talc,[4] may

---

[3] In the UK, the Red Cross offers a free cosmetic camouflage service through hospital dermatology departments.
[4] Talc is magnesium silicate. It must not be used for dusting surgical gloves as it causes granulomas if it gets into wounds or body cavities.

cool by increasing the effective surface area of the skin and they reduce friction between skin surfaces by their lubricating action. Though usefully absorbent, they cause crusting if applied to exudative lesions. They may be used alone or as a vehicle for, e.g. fungicides.

Gels or jellies are semisolid colloidal solutions or suspensions used as lubricants and as vehicles for drugs. They are sometimes useful for treating the scalp.

TOPICAL ANALGESICS

Counterirritants and rubefacients are irritants that stimulate nerve endings in intact skin to relieve pain in skin (e.g. postherpetic), viscera or muscle supplied by the same nerve root. All produce inflammation of the skin which becomes flushed, hence rubefacients. They are often effective though their precise mode of action is unknown.

The best counterirritants are physical agents, especially heat. Many drugs, however, have been used for this purpose and suitable preparations containing salicylates, nicotinates, menthol, camphor and capsaicin (depletes skin substance P) are also available.

Topical NSAIDs (see p. 290) are used to relieve musculoskeletal pain.

Local anaesthetics. Lidocaine and prilocaine are available as gels, ointments and sprays to provide reversible block of conduction along cutaneous nerves (see p. 422). Benzocaine and amethocaine (tetracaine) carry a high risk of sensitisation.

Volatile aerosol sprays, beloved by sportspeople, produce analgesia by cooling and by placebo effect.

ANTIPRURITICS

Mechanisms of itch are both peripheral and central. Impulses pass along the same nerve fibres as those of pain, but the sensation experienced differs qualitatively as well as quantitatively from pain. In the CNS endogenous opioid peptides are released and naloxone can relieve some cases of intractable itch. Local liberation of histamine and other autacoids

in the skin also contributes and may be responsible for much of the itch of urticarial allergic reactions. Histamine release by bile salts may explain some, but not all, of the itch of obstructive jaundice. It is likely that other chemical mediators, e.g. serotonin and prostaglandins, are involved.

Generalised pruritus

In the absence of a primary dermatosis it is important to search for an underlying cause, e.g. iron deficiency, liver or renal failure and lymphoma, but there remain patients in whom the cause either cannot be removed or is not known.

Antihistamines (H_1 receptor), especially chlorphenamine and hydroxyzine orally, are used for their sedative or anxiolytic effect (except in urticaria); they should not be applied topically over a prolonged period for risk of allergy.

In severe pruritus, a sedative antidepressant may also help. The itching of obstructive jaundice may be relieved by androgens but they may increase the jaundice. If obstruction is only partial, colestyramine and phototherapy can be useful. Naltrexone offers short-term relief of the pruritus associated with haemodialysis.

Localised pruritus

Scratching or rubbing seems to give relief by converting the intolerable persistent itch into a more bearable pain. Firm pressure with a finger may relieve the itch. A vicious cycle can be set up in which itching provokes scratching and scratching leads to skin lesions which itch, as in lichenified eczema. Covering the lesion or enclosing it in a medicated bandage so as to prevent any further scratching or rubbing may help.

Topical corticosteroid preparations are used to treat the underlying inflammatory cause of pruritus, e.g. in eczema.

A cooling application such as 0.5–2% menthol in aqueous cream is antipruritic, probably by weak local anaesthetic action.

Calamine and *astringents* (aluminium acetate, tannic acid) may help. Local anaesthetics do not offer any long-term solution and since they are liable to sensitise the skin they are best avoided; lignocaine is least troublesome in this respect. Topical doxepin can be helpful in localised pruritus, but extensive use induces sedation; like other topical antihistamines it induces allergic contact dermatitis.

Crotamiton, an acaricide, is reputed to have a specific but unexplained antipruritic action, although it is irritant.

Pruritus ani is managed by attention to hygiene, emollients, e.g. washing with aqueous cream, and a weak corticosteroid with antiseptic/anticandida application used as briefly as practicable (some cases are a form of neurodermatitis). Secondary contact sensitivity, e.g. to local anaesthetics, is common.

ADRENOCORTICAL STEROIDS

Actions. Adrenal steroids possess a range of actions (see p. 664) of which the following are relevant to topical use:

- Inflammation is suppressed, particularly when there is an allergic factor, and immune responses are reduced
- Antimitotic activity suppresses proliferation of keratinocytes, fibroblasts and lymphocytes (useful in psoriasis, but also causes skin thinning)
- Vasoconstriction reduces ingress of inflammatory cells and humoral factors to the inflamed area; this action (blanching effect on human skin) has been used to measure the potency of individual topical corticosteroids (see below).

Penetration into the skin is governed by the factors outlined at the beginning of this chapter. The vehicle should be appropriate to the condition being treated: an ointment for dry, scaly conditions, a water-based cream for weeping eczema.

Uses. Adrenal steroids should be considered a symptomatic and sometimes curative, but not preventive, treatment. Ideally a potent steroid (see below) should be given only as a short course and reduced as soon as the response allows. Corticosteroids are most useful for eczematous disorders (atopic, discoid, contact) and other inflammatory conditions save those due to infection. Dilute corticosteroids are useful in psoriasis (see p. 309).

Adrenal steroids of highest potency are reserved for recalcitrant dermatoses, e.g. lichen simplex, lichen planus, nodular prurigo and discoid lupus erythematosus.

Topical corticosteroids are of no use for urticarial conditions and are contraindicated in infection, e.g. fungal, herpes, impetigo, scabies, because the infection will exacerbate and spread. Where appropriate, an adrenal steroid formulation may include an antimicrobial, e.g. miconazole, fusidic acid, in infected eczema.

Topical corticosteroids should be applied sparingly ('Marmite rather than marmalade'). The 'finger tip unit'[5] is a useful guide in educating patients (see Table 16.1).

The difficulties and dangers of systemic adrenal steroid therapy are sufficient to restrict such use to serious conditions (such as pemphigus and generalised exfoliative dermatitis) not responsive to other forms of therapy.

Guidelines for the use of topical corticosteroids

- Use for symptom relief and never prophylactically
- Choose the appropriate therapeutic potency (see Table 16.2), i.e. mild for the face. In cases likely to be resistant, use a very potent preparation, e.g. for 3 weeks, to gain control, after which change to a less potent preparation.
- Choose the appropriate vehicle, i.e. a water-based cream for weeping eczema, an ointment for dry scaly conditions.
- Use a combined adrenal steroid/antimicrobial formulation if infection is present.
- Advise the patient to apply the formulation very thinly, just enough to make the skin surface shine slightly.
- Prescribe in small but adequate amounts so that serious overuse is unlikely to occur without the doctor knowing, e.g. weekly quantity by group (Table 16.2): very potent 15 g; potent 30 g; others 50 g.
- Occlusive dressing should be used only briefly. Note that babies' plastic pants are an occlusive dressing as well as being a social amenity.

Choice. Corticosteroids are classified according to their *therapeutic potency* (efficacy), i.e. according to both drug and % concentration (see Table 16.2).

---

[5]The distance from the tip of the adult index finger to the first crease.

TABLE 16.1 Finger tip unit dosimetry for topical corticosteroids

Age	Face/ Neck	Arm/ Hand	Leg/ Foot	Trunk (front)	Trunk (back, including buttocks)
3–6 months	1	1	1.5	1	1.5
1–2 years	1.5	1.5	2	2	3
3–5 years	1.5	2	3	3	3.5
6–10 years	2	2.5	4.5	3.5	5
Adult	2.5	Arm—3 Hand—1	Foot—2 Leg—6	7	7

TABLE 16.2 Topical corticosteroid formulations conventionally ranked according to *therapeutic* potency

Very potent	Clobetasol (0.05%) [also formulations of diflucortolone (0.3%), halcinonide]
Potent	Beclomethasone (0.025%) [also formulations of betamethasone, budesonide, desoxymethasone, diflucortolone (0.1%), fluclorolone, fluocinolone (0.025%), fluocinonide, fluticasone, hydrocortisone butyrate, mometasone (once daily), triamcinolone]
Moderately potent	Clobetasone (0.05%) [also formulations of alclometasone, clobetasone, desoxymethasone, fluocinolone (0.00625%), fluocortolone, fluandrenolone, hydrocortisone plus urea (see p. 307)]
Mildly potent	Hydrocortisone (0.1–1.0%) [also formulations of alclomethasone, fluocinolone (0.0025%), methylprednisolone]

Important note: the ranking is based on agent *and* its concentration: the same drug appears in more than one rank.

Choice of preparation relates both to the disease and the site of intended use. High potency preparations are commonly needed for lichen planus and discoid lupus erythematosus; weaker preparations (hydrocortisone 0.5–2.5%) are usually adequate for eczema, use on the face and in childhood.

When a skin disorder requiring a corticosteroid is already infected, a preparation containing an antimicrobial is added, e.g. fusidic acid or clotrimazole. When the infection is eliminated the corticosteroid may be continued alone.

Intralesional injections are occasionally used to provide high local concentrations without systemic effects in chronic dermatoses, e.g. hypertrophic lichen planus and discoid lupus erythematosus.

Adverse effects. Used with restraint topical corticosteroids are effective and safe. Adverse effects are more likely with formulations ranked therapeutically as very potent or potent in Table 16.2.

- *Short-term use.* Infection may spread.
- *Long-term use.* Skin atrophy can occur within 4 weeks and may or may not be fully reversible. It reflects loss of connective tissue which also causes striae (irreversible) and generally occurs at sites where dermal penetration is high (face, groins, axillae).

Other effects include: local hirsutism; perioral dermatitis (especially in young women) responds to steroid withdrawal and may be mitigated by tetracycline by mouth for 4–6 weeks; depigmentation (local); acne (local). Potent corticosteroids *should not be used on the face* unless this is unavoidable. Systemic absorption can lead to all the adverse effects of systemic corticosteroid use. Fluticasone propionate and mometasone furoate are rapidly metabolised following cutaneous absorption which may reduce the risk of systemic toxicity. Suppression of the hypothalamic/pituitary axis readily occurs with overuse of the very potent agents, and when 20% of the body is under an occlusive dressing with mildly potent agents. Other complications of occlusive dressings include infections (bacterial, candidal) and even heat stroke when large areas are occluded. Antifungal cream containing hydrocortisone and used for vaginal candidiasis may contaminate the urine and misleadingly suggest Cushing's syndrome.[6]

Applications to the eyelids may get into the eye and cause glaucoma.

Rebound exacerbation of the disease can occur after abrupt cessation of therapy. This can lead the patient to reapply the steroid and so create a vicious cycle.

Allergy. Corticosteroids, particularly hydrocortisone and budesonide, or other ingredients in the for-

---

[6] Kelly C J et al 2001 Raised cortisol excretion rate in urine and contamination by topical steroids. British Medical Journal 322: 594.

mulation, may cause allergic contact dermatitis and the possibility of this should be considered where expected benefit fails to occur.

SUNSCREENS
(Sunburn and Photosensitivity)

Ultraviolet (UV) solar radiation consists of:

- UVA (320–400 nanometres): causes skin aging (damage to collagen) and probably skin cancer
- UVB (290–320 nm): is 1000 times more active than UVA, acutely causes sunburn and tanning, and chronically skin cancer and skin aging
- UVC (200–290 nm) is prevented, at present, from reaching the earth at sea level by the stratospheric ozone layer, though it can cause skin injury at high altitude.

Protection of the skin

Protection from UV radiation is effected by:

Absorbent sunscreens. These organic chemicals absorb UVB and UVA at the surface of the skin (generally more effective for UVB).

UVB protection: aminobenzoic acid and aminobenzoates (padimate-O), cinnamates, salicylates, camphors.

UVA protection: benzophenones (mexenone, oxybenzone), dibenzoylmethanes.

Reflectant sunscreens. Inert minerals such as titanium dioxide, zinc oxide and calamine act as a physical barrier to UVB and UVA: they are cosmetically unattractive but the newer micronised preparations are more acceptable.

The performance of a sunscreen is expressed as the *sun protective factor* (SPF) which refers to UVB (UVA is more troublesome to measure and the protection is indicated by a star rating system with 4 stars providing the greatest). A SPF of 10 means that the dose of UVB required to cause erythema must be 10 times greater on protected than on unprotected skin. The SPF should be interpreted only as a rough guide; consumer use is more haphazard and less liberal amounts are applied to the skin in practice. Sunscreens should protect against both UVB and UVA. Absorbent and reflectant

components are combined in some preparations. The washability of the preparation (including removal by sweat and swimming) is also relevant to efficacy and frequency of application; some penetrate the stratum corneum (padimate-O) and are more persistent than others.

Uses. Sun screens are no substitute for light-impermeable clothing and sun avoidance. They are, however, beneficial in protecting those who are photosensitive due to drugs (below) or to disease, i.e. for photodermatoses such as photosensitivity dermatitis, polymorphic light eruption, cutaneous porphyrias and lupus erythematosus. Methodical use of sunscreens appears to reduce the incidence of squamous cell carcinoma in vulnerable individuals.

The lower lip receives a substantial dose of UV but may be neglected when a sunscreen is applied (specific lip-blocks are available). Sunscreens can cause allergic dermatitis or photodermatitis (but not titanium dioxide, though its vehicle may).

Treatment of mild sunburn is usually with a lotion such as oily calamine lotion. Severe cases are helped by topical corticosteroids. NSAIDs, e.g. indometacin, can help if given early, by preventing the formation of prostaglandins.

Photosensitivity

Drug photosensitivity means that an adverse effect occurs as a result of drug plus light, usually UVA; sometimes even the amount of ultraviolet radiation from fluorescent light tubes is sufficient.

Systemically taken drugs that can induce photo-sensitivity are many. Of the drug groups given below, those most commonly reported are:[7]
  antimitotics: dacarbazine, vinblastine
  antimicrobials: demeclocycline, doxycycline, nalidixic acid, sulphonamides
  antipsychotics: chlorpromazine, prochlorperazine
  cardiac arrhythmic: amiodarone
  diuretics: frusemide (furosemide), chlorothiazide, hydrochlorothiazide
  fibric acid derivatives, e.g. fenofibrate
  hypoglycaemic: tolbutamide

---

[7] Data from The Medical Letter 1995 37: 35.

nonsteroidal anti-inflammatory: piroxicam
psoralens (see below).

Topically applied substances that can produce photosensitivity include:
para-aminobenzoic acid and its esters (used as sunscreens)
coal tar derivatives
psoralens from juices of various plants (e.g. bergamot oil)
6-methylcoumarin (used in perfumes, shaving lotions, sunscreens).

There are two forms of photosensitivity:

Phototoxicity, like drug toxicity, is a normal effect of too high a dose of UV in a subject who has been exposed to the drug. The reaction is like severe sunburn. *The threshold returns to normal when the drug is withdrawn.* Some drugs, notably NSAIDs, induce a 'pseudoporphyria', clinically resembling porphyria cutanea tarda and presenting with skin fragility, blisters, and milia on sun-exposed areas, notably the backs of the hands.

Photoallergy, like drug allergy, is a cell-mediated immunological effect that occurs only in some people, and which may be severe with a small dose. Photoallergy due to drugs is the result of a photochemical reaction caused by UVA in which the drug combines with tissue protein to form an antigen. *Reactions may persist for years after the drug is withdrawn;* they are usually eczematous.

Systemic protection, as opposed to application of drug to exposed areas, should be considered when the topical measures fail. Antimalarials such as *hydroxychloroquine* may be effective for short periods in polymorphic light eruption and in cutaneous lupus erythematosus.

Psoralens (obtained from citrus fruits and other plants), e.g. methoxsalen, are used to *induce* photochemical reactions in the skin. After topical or systemic administration of the psoralen and subsequent exposure to UVA there is an erythematous reaction that goes deeper than ordinary sunburn and that may reach its maximum only after 48 h (sunburn maximum is 12–24 h). Melanocytes are activated and pigmentation occurs over the following week. This action is used to repigment areas of disfiguring depigmentation, e.g. vitiligo in black-skinned persons.

In the presence of UVA the psoralen interacts with DNA, forms thymine dimers, and inhibits DNA synthesis. Psoralen plus UVA (PUVA) treatment is used chiefly in severe psoriasis (a disease characterised by increased epidermal proliferation), and cutaneous T cell lymphoma.

Severe adverse reactions can occur with psoralens and ultraviolet radiation, including increased risk of skin cancer (due to mutagenicity inherent in their action), cancer of the male genitalia, cataracts and accelerated skin aging; the treatment is used only by specialists.

Chronic exposure to sunlight induces wrinkling and yellowing due to the changes in the dermal connective tissue. Topical retinoids are widely used in an attempt to reverse some of these tissue changes.

MISCELLANEOUS SUBSTANCES

Keratolytics are used to destroy unwanted tissue, including warts and corns. Great care is obviously necessary to avoid ulceration. They include trichloracetic acid, salicylic acid and many others. Resorcinol and sulphur are mild keratolytics used in acne.

Squalane is a saturated hydrocarbon insoluble in water but soluble in sebum. It therefore penetrates the skin and is a vehicle for delivery of agents; it is water repellent and is used for incontinence and prevention of bed sores. It appears in mixed formulations.

Salicylic acid may enhance the efficacy of a topical steroid in hyperkeratotoic disorders.

Tars are mildly antiseptic, antipruritic and they inhibit keratinisation in an ill-understood way. They are safe in low concentrations and are used in psoriasis. Photosensitivity occurs. There are very many preparations, which usually contain other substances, e.g. coal tar and salicylic acid ointment; it is sometimes useful to add an adrenal steroid.

Ichthammol is a sulphurous tarry distillation product of fossilised fish (obtained in the Austrian Tyrol); it has a weaker effect than coal tar.

Zinc oxide provides mild astringent, barrier and occlusive actions.

Calamine is basic zinc carbonate that owes its pink colour to added ferric oxide. It has a mild astringent action and is used as a dusting powder and in shake and oily lotions. It is of limited value.

Urea is used topically to assist skin hydration, e.g. in ichthyosis.

Insect repellents, e.g. against mosquitoes, ticks, fleas, such as deet (diethyl toluamide), dimethyl phthalate. These are applied to the skin and repel insects principally by vaporisation. They must be applied to all exposed skin, and sometimes also to clothes if their objective is to be achieved (some damage plastic fabrics and spectacle frames). Their duration of effect is limited by the rate at which they vaporise (skin and ambient temperature), by washing off (sweat, rain, immersion) and by mechanical factors causing rubbing (physical activity). They can cause allergic and toxic effects, especially with prolonged use. About 10% is absorbed. Plainly the vehicle in which they are applied is also important, and an acceptable substance achieving persistence of effect beyond a few hours has yet to be developed. But the alternative of spreading an insecticide in the environment causing general pollution and indiscriminate insect kill is unacceptable. Selective environmental measures against some insects, e.g. mosquitoes, are sometimes feasible.

Benzyl benzoate may be used on clothes; it resists one or two washings.

Cutaneous adverse drug reactions

Drugs applied locally or taken systemically often cause rashes. These take many different forms and the same drug may produce different rashes in different people.

Irritant or *allergic contact dermatitis* is eczematous and is often caused by antimicrobials, local anaesthetics, topical antihistamines, and increasingly commonly by topical corticosteroids. It is often due to the vehicle in which the active drug is applied, particularly a cream.

Reactions to *systemically administered drugs* are commonly erythematous, like those of measles, scarlatina or erythema multiforme. They give no useful clue as to the cause. They commonly occur during the first 2 weeks of therapy, but some immunological reactions may be delayed for months.

Patients with the acquired immunodeficiency syndrome (AIDS) have an increased risk of adverse reactions, which are often severe.

> Though drugs may change, the clinical problems remain depressingly the same: a patient develops a rash; he is taking many different tablets; which, if any, of these caused his eruption, and what should be done about it? It is no answer simply to stop all drugs, though the fact that this can often be done casts some doubt on the patient's need for them in the first place. All too often potentially valuable drugs are excluded from further use on totally inadequate grounds. Clearly some guidelines are needed but no simple set of rules exists that can cover this complex subject…[8]

The following questions should be asked in every case:

- Can other skin diseases be excluded?
- Are the skin changes compatible with a drug cause?
- Which drug is most likely to be responsible?
- Are any further tests worthwhile?
- Is any treatment needed?

These questions are deceptively simple but the answers are often difficult.

DRUG-SPECIFIC RASHES

Despite great variability, some hints at drug-specific

---

[8]Hardie R A, Savin J A 1979 British Medical Journal: 1935, to whom we are grateful for this quotation and classification.

or characteristic rashes from drugs taken *systemically,* can be discerned, as follows:

Acne and pustular: e.g. corticosteroids, androgens, ciclosporin, penicillins.

Allergic vasculitis: e.g. sulphonamides, NSAIDs, thiazides, chlorpropamide, phenytoin, penicillin, retinoids

Anaphylaxis: x-ray contrast media, penicillins, ACE inhibitors.

Bullous pemphigoid: frusemide (and other sulphonamide-related drugs), ACE inhibitors, penicillamine, penicillin, PUVA therapy.

Eczema: e.g. penicillins, phenothiazines.

Exanthematic/maculopapular reactions are the most frequent; unlike a viral exanthem the eruption typically starts on the trunk; the face is relatively spared. Continued use of the drug may lead to erythroderma. They commonly occur at about the ninth day of treatment (or day 2–3 in previously exposed patients), although onset may be delayed until after treatment is completed; causes include antimicrobials, especially ampicillin, sulphonamides and derivatives (sulphonylureas, frusemide (furosemide) and thiazide diuretics). Morbilliform (measles-like) eruptions typically recur on rechallenge.

Erythema multiforme: e.g. NSAIDs, sulphonamides, barbiturates, phenytoin.

Erythema nodosum: e.g. sulphonamides, oral contraceptives, prazosin.

Exfoliative dermatitis and erythroderma: gold, phenytoin, carbamazepine, allopurinol, penicillins, neuroleptics, isoniazid.

Fixed eruptions are eruptions that recur at the same site, often circumoral, with each administration of the drug: e.g. phenolphthalein (laxative self-medication), sulphonamides, quinine (in tonic water), tetracycline, barbiturates, naproxen, nifedipine.

Hair loss: e.g. cytotoxic anticancer drugs, acitretin, oral contraceptives, heparin, androgenic steroids (women), sodium valproate, gold.

Hypertrichosis: corticosteroids, ciclosporin, doxasosin, minoxidil.

Lichenoid eruption: e.g. β-adrenoceptor blockers, chloroquine, thiazides, frusemide (furosemide), captopril, gold, phenothiazines.

Lupus erythematosus: e.g. hydralazine, isoniazid, procainamide, phenytoin, oral contraceptives, sulfazaline.

Purpura: e.g. thiazides, sulphonamides, sulphonylureas, phenylbutazone, quinine. Aspirin induces a capillaritis (pigmented purpuric dermatitis).

Photosensitivity: see above.

Pemphigus: e.g. penicillamine, captopril, piroxicam, penicillin, rifampicin.

Pruritus unassociated with rash: e.g. oral contraceptives, phenothiazines, rifampicin (cholestatic reaction).

Pigmentation: e.g. oral contraceptives (chloasma in photosensitive distribution), phenothiazines, heavy metals, amiodarone, chloroquine (pigmentations of nails and palate, depigmentation of the hair), minocycline.

Psoriasis may be aggravated by lithium and antimalarials.

Scleroderma-like: bleomycin, sodium valproate, tryptophan contaminants (eosinophila-myalgia syndrome).

Serum sickness: immunoglobulins and other immunomodulatory blood products.

Stevens–Johnson syndrome and toxic epidermal necrolysis:[9] e.g. anticonvulsants, sulphonamides, aminopenicillins, oxicam NSAIDs, allopurinol, chlormezanone, corticosteroids.

Urticaria and angioedema: e.g. penicillins, ACE inhibitors, gold, NSAIDs, e.g. aspirin, codeine.

Recovery after withdrawal of the causative drug generally begins in a few days, but lichenoid reactions may not improve for weeks.

Diagnosis. The patient's drug history may give clues. Reactions are commoner during early therapy (days) than after the drug has been given for months. Diagnosis by readministration of the drug (challenge) is safe with fixed eruptions, but not with others, particularly those that may be part of a generalised effect, e.g. vasculitis. Patch and photopatch tests are useful in contact dermatitis, for they reproduce the causative process but should be performed only by those with special experience. Fixed drug eruptions can sometimes be reproduced by patch testing with the drug over the previously affected site.

---

[9] Roujeau C-J et al 1995 New England Journal of Medicine 333: 1600

Intradermal tests introduce all the problems of allergy to drugs, e.g. metabolism, combination with protein, fatal anaphylaxis (see p. 143).

Treatment. Remove the cause; use cooling applications and antipruritics; use a histamine H_1 receptor blocker systemically for acute urticaria; give an adrenal steroid for severe cases.

SAFETY MONITORING

Several drugs commonly used in dermatology should be monitored regularly for (principally systemic) adverse effects. These include:

Aciclovir (plasma creatinine)
Azathioprine (blood count and liver function)
Colchicine (blood count, plasma creatinine)
Ciclosporin (plasma creatinine)
Dapsone (liver function, blood count including reticulocytes)
Methotrexate (blood count, liver function)
PUVA (liver function, antinuclear antibodies)
Aromatic retinoids (liver function, plasma lipids).

Individual disorders

> **If it's wet, dry it; if it's dry, wet it.** The traditional advice contains enough truth to be worth repeating. One or two applications a day are all that is usually necessary unless common sense dictates otherwise.

Table 16.3 is not intended to give the complete treatment of even the commoner skin conditions but merely to indicate a reasonable approach.

Secondary infections of ordinarily uninfected lesions may require added topical or systemic antimicrobials.

Analgesics, sedatives or tranquillisers may be needed in painful or uncomfortable conditions, or where the disease is intensified by emotion or anxiety.

Formulations for use on the skin. At the time of writing there are in the UK about 280 preparations for medical prescription (excluding minor variants

and many of those on direct sale to the public). It is not practicable to give other than general guidance on choice. Physicians will select a modest range of products and get to know these well.

PSORIASIS

In psoriasis there is increased ($\times$ 10) epidermal undifferentiated cell proliferation and inflammation of the epidermis and dermis. The consequence of increased numbers of horn cells containing abnormal keratin is that no normal stratum corneum is formed. Drugs are used to

- dissolve keratin (keratolysis)
- inhibit cell division.

An emollient such as aqueous cream will reduce the inflammation. The proliferated cells may be eliminated by a *dithranol* (antimitotic) preparation applied accurately to the lesions (but not on the face) for 1 hour and removed; begin with 0.1% and increase to 1%. Dithranol is available in cream bases or in Lassar's paste (the preparations are not interchangeable). It is used daily until the lesions have disappeared; it is irritant to normal skin and stains skin and fabrics. Tar preparations are less effective alternatives, and are commonly used for psoriasis of the scalp.[10]

Topical adrenal steroid reduces epidermal cell division, and application, especially under occlusive dressings, can be very effective, but increasing the doses (concentrations) becomes necessary and rebound, which may be severe, follows withdrawal. For this reason potent corticosteroid should never be used except for lesions on the scalp, palms and soles. *Systemic* corticosteroid administration should be avoided, for high doses are needed to suppress the disease, which is liable to recur in a more

---

[10] But are not without risk. A 46-year-old man whose psoriasis was treated with topical corticosteroids, UV light and tar was seen in the hospital courtyard bursting into flames. A small ring of fire began several centimeters above the sternal notch and encircled his neck. The patient promptly put out the fire. He admitted to lighting a cigarette just before the fire, the path of which corresponded to the distribution of the tar on his body. Fader D J et al 1994 New England Journal of Medicine 330: 1541.

TABLE 16.3 Summary of treatment for skin disorders

Condition	Treatment	Remarks
Acne	see p. 313	
Alopecia (1) male pattern baldness	(1) Topical minoxidil is worth trying if the patient is embarrassed by baldness. Some hair regrowth can be detected in up to 50% but it is rarely cosmetically significant.	Most patients who take minoxidil orally for hypertension experience some increased hair growth. It may act by a mitogenic effect on hair follicles. The response occurs in 4–12 months: stop treatment if no result in 1 year.
(2) alopecia areata	(2) Finasteride by mouth. (2) Although distressing, the condition is often self-limiting. A few individuals have responded to PUVA or contact sensitistion induced by diphencyprone.	
Dermatitis herpetiformis	Dapsone is typically effective in 24 h, or sulfapyridine. Prolonged therapy necessary, a gluten-free diet can help.	Antipruritics locally as required. Not other sulphonamides; beneficial effect *not* due to antimicrobial action. Methaemoglobinaemia may complicate dapsone therapy.
Eczema Acute weeping	Lotions (aluminium acetate, calamine), wet dressings or soaks (sodium chloride, potassium permanganate); topical corticosteroid cream or lotion with antimicrobial if infected.	Remove the cause where possible. Often exacerbated by soap and water. Antipruritics (not antihistamines or local anaesthetics) may be added to lotions, creams or pastes.
Subacute	Emollients are the mainstay of treatment. Zinc oxide cream or paste, with mild keratolytic if skin thickening present (salicylic acid or coal tar added); topical corticosteroid ointment.	Gamolenic acid (Epogam, evening primrose oil) is of unproven benefit.
Chronic, with dry scaly lesions	Keratolytics and moisturising creams and emollients; topical corticosteroid	For severe chronic dermatitis consider phototherapy (PUVA), azathioprine or ciclosporin in short courses.
Exfoliative dermatitis	Chelating agent if due to a heavy metal. Cooling creams and powders locally. Adrenal steroid systemically when severe.	
Hirsutism in women	*In severe cases:* combined oestrogen/progestogen contraceptive pill: or cyproterone plus ethinyloestradiol (Dianette). Spironolactone, cimetidine have been used.	Local cosmetic approaches: *epilation* by wax or electrolysis: *depilation* (chemical), e.g. thioglycollic acid, barium sulphide. Laser epilation is expensive and the results are transient.
Hyperhidrosis	Astringents reduce sweat production, especially aluminium chloride hexahydrate (20%) in ethyl alcohol (95%). Antimuscarinics (topical or systemic) may help and high local concentrations can be obtained with iontophoresis. Minimally invasive sympathectomy is occasionally necessary; complications include compensatory hyperhidrosis elsewhere. Temporary remission (16 weeks) is achieved by injection of botulinum toxin, most effectively in the axilla.	Treatment better in theory than in practice; the volume of sweat dilutes the topical application; the characteristic smell is produced by bacterial action, so cosmetic deodorants contain antibacterials rather than substances that reduce sweat production.
Ichthyosis vulgaris	Emollients to hydrate and smooth the skin, e.g. emulsifying ointment and urea-based creams, e.g. Calmurid. Very severe variants may need acetretin.	Avoid degreasing skin, e.g. by domestic detergents.

TABLE 16.3 (*continued*)

Condition	Treatment	Remarks
Infections	see p. 314	
Intertrigo	Cleansing lotions, powders. A dilute corticosteroid with anticandidal cream is often helpful.	To cleanse, lubricate and reduce friction.
Larva migrans	Albendazole (single dose) or topical thiabendazole.	
Lichen planus	Antipruritics; potent topical corticosteroid (rarely systemic).	May be drug caused, e.g. a phenothiazine or antimalarial.
Lichen simplex (neurodermatitis)	Antipruritics; topical corticosteroid; explain scratch–itch cycle to patient.	Covering the lesion so as to prevent scratching, e.g. with a medicated bandage, sometimes breaks the vicious cycle.
Lupus erythematosus (affecting the skin)	Photoprotection is essential. Potent adrenal steroid topically or intralesionally. Hydroxychloroquine or mepacrine. Monitor for retinal toxicity when treatment is long-term. Other agents include auranofin, acetretin and in severe chilblain LE, thalidomide.	A systemic disease, but discoid lupus erythematosus typically has no systemic manifestations.
Malignancies	**Actinic keratoses** and **Bowen's disease** can be treated with topical 5-fluorouracil (skin irritation is to be expected) or cryotherapy. Imiquimod is a possible topical alternative. Extensive lesions may respond to photodynamic therapy: the skin is sensitised using a topical haematoporphyrin derivative, e.g. aminolaevulinic acid, and irradiated with a visible light or laser source. **Cutaneous T-cell lymphoma** in its early stages is best treated conservatively; PUVA will often clear lesions for several months or years; alternatives include topical nitrogen mustard, e.g. carmustine. Erythrodermic disease may respond to photopheresis (extracorporeal photochemotherapy).	
Marginal blepharitis (various organisms)	Ointment containing adrenal steroid and an antimicrobial.	Undue persistence can be due to allergy to treatment.
Nappy rash	*Prevention:* rid reusable nappies of soaps, detergents and ammonia by rinsing. Change frequently and use an emollient cream, e.g. aqueous cream, to protect skin. Costly disposable nappies are useful. *Cure:* mild: Zn cream or calamine lotion, plus above measures. Severe: adrenal steroid topically, plus antimicrobial.	
Pediculosis (lice) (head, body, genitals)	Permethrin, phenothrin, carbaryl or malathion; (anticholinesterases, with safety depending on more rapid metabolism in man than in insects, and on low absorption).	Usually two applications 7 days apart to kill lice from eggs that survive the first dose
Pemphigus and pemphigoid	Milder cases of pemphigoid can be treated with dapsone or a combination of nicotinamide and tetracycline. A potent adrenal steroid should be used; other immunosuppressives, e.g. azathioprine, mycophenolate mofetil for adrenal sparing; gold.	Oral hygiene and general nutrition very important.

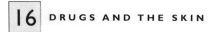
TABLE 16.3 (*continued*)

Condition	Treatment	Remarks
Photosensitivity	see p. 305	
Pityriasis rosea	Antipruritics and emollients as appropriate	The disease is self-limiting
Pruritus	see p. 302	
Psoriasis	see p. 309	
Pyoderma gangrenosum	Systemic corticosteroids are usually effective. Immunosuppressives, e.g. ciclosporin may be used for steroid-sparing effect. Some patients respond to dapsone, minocycline or clofazimine.	
Rosacea	Tetracycline; metronidazole, orally or topically.	Corticosteroid exacerbates. Flushing makes it worse. Oestrogens for menopausal flushing.
Scabies (*Sarcoptes scabiei*)	Permethrin dermal cream. In resistant cases consider monosulfiram or benzyl benzoate. Alternative: ivermectin (single dose) especially for outbreaks in closed communities. Crotamiton or calamine for residual itch.	Apply to all members of the household, immediate family or partner. Change underclothes and bedclothes after application.
Seborrhoeic dermatitis: dandruff (*Pityriasis capitis*)	A proprietary shampoo with pyrithione, selenium sulphide or coal tar; ketoconazole shampoo in more severe cases. Occasionally a corticosteroid lotion may be necessary. Keratolytics, e.g. Cocois are helpful if there is much scaling.	
Urticaria	see p. 314	
Viral warts	All treatments are *destructive* and should be applied with precision. Cryotherapy (liquid nitrogen). Salicylic acid 12% in collodion daily. Many other caustic (keratolytic) preparations exist, e.g. salicylic and lactic acid paint or gel. For plantar warts formaldehyde or glutaraldehyde; podophyllin (antimitotic) for plantar or anogenital warts. Follow the manufacturer's instructions meticulously. If one topical therapy fails it is worth trying a different type. Topical imiquimod is an alternative for genital warts. It is irritant and expensive.	Nonsurgical remedies may act by disrupting the wart so that virus is absorbed, antibodies develop and the wart is rejected immunologically. Warts often disappear spontaneously.
Vitiligo	No safe and reliable treatment. Methoxsalen or other psoralen, topically or systemically, plus daily exposure to UVA (PUVA) is toxic, and ineffective in caucasians. Sunscreens to protect the depigmented areas and reduce pigmentation of surrounding skin.	Probably an autoimmune disease. Note: dose-dependent risk of squamous cell cancer with PUVA.
Xanthelasma palpebrarum	Topical trichloracetic acid applied carefully with an orange stick.	Monitor plasma lipids.
X-ray dermatitis	Emollient and dilute topical corticosteroid.	

unstable form when treatment is withdrawn, as it must be if complications of long-term steroid therapy are to be avoided.

Calcipotriol and *tacalcitol* are analogues of calcitriol, the most active natural form of vitamin D (p. 742). Used topically they appear to be about as effective as dithranol and corticosteroid. They inhibit cell proliferation and encourage cell differentiation. Although they have less effect on calcium metabolism than does calcitriol, excessive use (greater than 100 g/week) can raise the plasma calcium concentration.

Vitamin A (retinols) plays a role in epithelial function and the retinoic acid derivative, acitretin (Neotigason, orally), inhibits psoriatic hyperkeratosis over 4–6 weeks. Acitretin should be used in courses (6–9 months) with intervals (3–4 months). It is **teratogenic,** like the other vitamin A derivatives. Rigorous precautions for use in women of childbearing potential are laid down by the manufacturer and must be followed, including contraception for 2 years after cessation, because the drug is stored in the liver and in fat and released over many months. The plasma t$\frac{1}{2}$ is 3 months. It can cause other serious toxicity (see Vitamin A, p. 739). *Tazarotene,* a topical retinoid, is of some benefit in mild psoriasis, but is irritant.

Ultraviolet B light is effective in guttate psoriasis and potentiates the effects of topical agents such as calcipotriol and dithranol. A *psoralen* followed by ultraviolet light (PUVA) is used in severe cases (see Psoralens, p. 306).

Folic acid antagonists, e.g. methotrexate, can also suppress epidermal activity temporarily, as does ciclosporin, but they are too toxic for use unless the psoriasis or associated arthritis is severely disabling and, preferably, the patients are past their reproductive years.

It is plain from this brief outline that treatment of psoriasis requires considerable judgement and choice will depend on the patient's sex, age and the severity of the condition. The combination of UVB and dithranol is probably the safest. When psoriasis is moderate-to-severe a strategy of rotation of treatments, e.g. UVB plus dithranol → PUVA + acitretin → UVB plus dithranol and so on may help to reduce the unwanted effects of any one therapy.

ACNE

Acne results from disordered function of the pilosebaceous follicle whereby abnormal keratin and sebum (the production of which is androgen driven), form debris which plugs the mouth of the follicle. *Propionibacterium acnes* colonises the debris. Bacterial action releases inflammatory fatty acids from the sebum.

The following measures are used progressively and selectively as the disease is more severe; they may need to be applied for up to 6 months:

- *Mild keratolytic* (exfoliating, peeling) formulations unblock pilosebaceous ducts, e.g. benzoyl peroxide, sulphur, salicylic acid, azelaic acid.
- *Systemic or topical antimicrobial therapy* (tetracycline, minocycline, erythromycin, at low dose) is used over months (response begins after 2 months). Bacterial resistance is not a problem; benefit is due to suppression of bacterial lipolysis of sebum, which generates inflammatory fatty acids. Raised intracranial pressure with loss of vision has occurred with tetracycline used thus.
- *Vitamin A* (retinoic acid) *derivatives* reduce sebum production and keratinisation. Vitamin A is a teratogen.
- *Tretinoin* (Retin-A) is applied topically (not in combination with other keratolytics). It may promote UV-induced skin cancer. Tretinoin should be avoided in sunny weather, and in pregnancy. Benefit is seen in about 10 weeks. *Adapalene,* a synthetic retinoid, may be better tolerated.
- *Isotretinoin* (Roaccutane) (t$\frac{1}{2}$ 15 h) orally is highly effective (in a course of 12–16 weeks), but is known to be a serious teratogen; its use should generally be confined to the more severe cystic and conglobate cases, where other measures have failed. It is available only in specialist centres. Fasting blood lipids should be measured before and during therapy (cholesterol and triglycerides may rise). Women of child-bearing potential should be fully informed on this risk, pregnancy-tested before commencement and use contraception for 4 weeks before, during and for 4 weeks after

cessation.[11] Mood change and severe depression may follow use of isotretinoin.

- *Hormone therapy.* The objective is to reduce androgen production or effect by using, (1) oestrogen, to suppress the hypothalamic/pituitary gonadotrophin production, or (2) an antiandrogen (cyproterone). An oestrogen alone as initial therapy to get the acne under control or, in women, the cyclical use of an oral contraceptive containing 50 micrograms of oestrogen diminishes sebum secretion by 40%. A combination of ethinylestradiol and cyproterone (Dianette) orally is also effective in women (it has a contraceptive effect, which is desirable as the cyproterone may feminise a male fetus).
- Topical corticosteroid should **not** be used.

URTICARIA

Acute urticaria (named after its similarity to the sting of a nettle, *Urtica*) and *angioedema* usually respond well to H$_1$ receptor antihistamines, although severe cases are relieved more quickly with use of adrenaline (epinephrine) (adrenaline injection 1 mg/ml: 0.1–0.3 ml, s.c.). A systemic corticosteroid may be needed in severe cases.

In some individuals, urticarial weals are provoked by physical stimuli, e.g. friction (dermographism), heat or cold. Exercise may induce weals, particularly on the upper trunk (cholinergic urticaria). Physical urticarias may require combined H$_1$- and H$_2$-receptor receptor antagonists fully to block the vascular effects of histamine, which causes flushing and hypotension. Cyproheptadine is usually the preferred choice of H$_1$-antihistamine but causes drowsiness.

Chronic urticaria usually responds to an H$_1$-receptor antihistamine with low sedating properties,

e.g. cetirizine or loratidine. Terfenadine is also effective, but may cause dangerous cardiac arrhythmias if the recommended dose is exceeded or if it is administered with drugs (or grapefruit juice) which inhibit its metabolism.

Hereditary angioedema, with deficiency of C$_1$-esterase inhibitor (a complement inhibitor), may not respond to antihistamines or corticosteroid but only to *fresh frozen plasma* or preferably C$_1$-inhibitor concentrate. Delay in initiating the treatment may lead to death from laryngeal oedema (try adrenaline (epinephrine) i.m. in severe cases). For long-term prophylaxis an androgen (stanozolol, danazol) can be effective.

SKIN INFECTIONS

Superficial bacterial infections, e.g. impetigo, eczema, are commonly staphylococcal or streptococcal. They are treated by a topical antimicrobial for less than 2 weeks and applied twice daily after removal of crusts that prevent access of the drug, e.g. by a povidone-iodine preparation. Very extensive cases need systemic treatment.

Topical *fusidic acid* and *mupirocin* are preferred (as they are not ordinarily used for systemic infections and therefore development of drug resistant strains is less likely to have any serious consequences). Framycetin and polymyxins are also used. Absorption of neomycin from all topical preparations can cause *serious injury* to the eighth cranial nerve. It is also a contact sensitiser.

When prolonged treatment is required, topical antiseptics (e.g. chlorhexidine) are preferred and bacterial resistance is less of a problem.

Combination of antimicrobial with a corticosteroid (to suppress inflammation) can be useful for secondarily infected eczema.

The **disadvantages** of antimicrobials are *contact allergy* and developments of *resistant organisms* (which may cause systemic, as well as local, infection). Failure to respond may be due to development of a contact allergy (which may be masked by corticosteroid).

Infected leg ulcers generally do not benefit from long-term antimicrobials although topical metronidazole is useful when the ulcer is malodorous due to colonisation with Gram-negative organisms. An

---

[11] The risk of birth defect in a child of a woman who has taken isotretinoin when pregnant is estimated at 25%. Thousands of abortions have been done in such women in the USA. It is probable that hundreds of damaged children have been born. There can be no doubt that there has been irresponsible prescribing of this drug, e.g. in less severe cases. The fact that a drug having such a grave effect is yet permitted to be available is attribute to its high efficacy.

antiseptic (plus a protective dressing with compression) is preferred if antimicrobial therapy is needed.

Nasal carriers of staphylococci may be cured (often temporarily) by topical mupirocin or neomycin plus chlorhexidine.

Deep bacterial infections, e.g. boils, generally do not require antimicrobial therapy; but if they do it should be systemic. Cellulitis requires systemic chemotherapy initially with benzylpenicillin and flucloxacillin.

Infected burns are treated with a variety of antimicrobials, including silver-sulphadiazine and mupirocin.

Fungal infections; superficial dermatophyte or candida infections purely involving the skin can be treated with a topical imidazole (e.g. clotrimazole, miconazole). Pityriasis versicolor, a yeast infection, primarily involves the trunk in young adults; it responds poorly to imidazoles but topical terbinafine or selenium sulphide preparations are effective; severe infection may require systemic itraconazole. Invasion of hair or nails by a dermatophyte or a deep mycosis requires systemic therapy; terbinafine is the most effective drug. Terbinafine and griseofulvin are ineffective against yeasts, for which itraconazole is an alternative. Itraconazole can be used in weekly pulses each month for 3–4 months; it is less effective against dermatophytes than terbinafine.

Virus infections. Topical antivirals: aciclovir (acyclovir). (see p. 257). Aciclovir is used systemically for the potentially severe infections, e.g. eczema herpeticum.

Parasite infection. Topical parasiticides (see Table 16.3 for details).

Disinfection and cleansing of the skin. Numerous substances are used according to circumstances:

- *for skin preparation prior to injection:* ethanol or isopropyl alcohol
- *for disinfection:* chlorhexidine salts, cationic surfactant (cetrimide), soft soap, povidone-iodine (iodine complexed with polyvinylpyrrollidone), phenol derivatives (hexachlorophene, triclosan), and hydrogen peroxide.

GUIDE TO FURTHER READING

Brown S K, Shalita A R 1998 Acne vulgaris. Lancet 351: 1871–1876

Callen J P 1998 Pyoderma gangrenosum. Lancet 351: 581–585

Chew A-L, Bashir S T, Maibach H I 2000 Treatment of head lice. Lancet 356: 523–524

Chosidow O 2000 Scabies and pediculosis. Lancet 355: 819–825

Diffey B 2000 Has the sun protection factor had its day? British Medical Journal 320: 176–177

Fine J-D 1999 Management of acquired bullous skin diseases. New England Journal of Medicine 333: 1475–1484

Friedman P S 1998 Allergy and the skin. 11 — Contact and atopic eczema. British Medical Journal 316: 1226–1229

Gibbs S, Harvey I, Sterling J et al 2002 Local treatments for cutaneous warts: systematic review. British Medical Journal 325: 461–464

Greaves M W, Sabroe R A 1998 Allergy and the skin. 1 — Urticaria. British Medical Journal 316: 1147–1150

Greaves M W, Wall P D 1996 Pathophysiology of itching. Lancet 348: 938–940

Gruchalla R S 2000 Clinical assessment of drug-induced disease. Lancet 356: 1505–1511

James M 1996 Isotretinoin for severe acne. (A patient's experience.) Lancet 347: 1749

Kalka K et al 2000 Photodynamic therapy in dermatology. Journal of the American Academy of Dermatology 42: 389–413

Kaplan K P 2002 Chronic urticaria and angioedema. New England Journal of Medicine 346: 175–179

Nousari H C, Anhalt G J 1999 Pemphigus and bullus pemphigoid. Lancet 354: 667–672

Paus R, Cotsarelis G 1999 The biology of hair follicles. New England Journal of Medicine 341: 491–497

Price V H 1999 Treatment of hair loss. New England Journal of Medicine 341: 964–973

Rittmaster H 1997 Hirsutism. Lancet 349: 191–194

Rivers J K 1996 Melanoma. Lancet 347: 803–806

Robert C, Kupper T S 1999 Inflammatory skin

diseases, T cells, and immune surveillance. New England Journal of Medicine 341: 1817–1828

Rudikoff D, Lebwohl M 1998 Atopic dermatitis. Lancet 351: 1715–1720

Roujeau J C, Stern R S 1994 Severe adverse cutaneous reactions to drugs. New England Journal of Medicine 331: 1272–1285

Russell-Jones R 2001 Shedding light on photopheresis. Lancet 357: 820–821

Stern R S 1997 Psoriasis. Lancet 350: 349–353

Williams H 2002 New treatments for atopic dermatitis. British Medical Journal 324: 1533–1534

NERVOUS SYSTEM

17

Pain and analgesics

> But pain is perfect misery, the worst
> Of evils, and, excessive, overturns
> All patience.
> (John Milton, 1608–1674, Paradise Lost)

SYNOPSIS

One of the greatest services doctors can do their patients is to acquire skill in the management of pain.

- Pain: the phenomenon of pain; clinical evaluation of analgesics; choice of analgesics; treatment of pain syndromes; spasm of smooth and striated muscle; neuralgias; migraine
- Drugs in palliative care: symptom control; pain
- Narcotic or opioid analgesics: agonists, partial agonists, antagonists; morphine and other opioids; classification by analgesic efficacy; opioid dependence; opioids used during and after surgery; opioid antagonists;
- Non-narcotic analgesics (NSAIDs): see Ch. 15

tissue damage, or described in terms of such damage.[1] It is mediated by specific nerve fibres to the brain where its conscious appreciation may be modified by various factors.

The word 'unpleasant' comprises the whole range of disagreeable feelings from being merely inconvenienced to misery, anguish, anxiety, depression and desperation, to the ultimate cure of suicide.[2,3]

- **Analgesic drug:** a drug that relieves pain due to multiple causes, e.g. paracetamol, morphine. Drugs that relieve pain due to a single cause or specific pain syndrome only, e.g. ergotamine (migraine), carbamazepine (neuralgias), glyceryl trinitrate (angina pectoris), are not classed as analgesics; nor are adrenocortical steroids that suppress pain of inflammation of any cause.
- **Analgesics** are classed as **narcotic** (which act in the central nervous system and cause drowsiness, i.e. opioids) and **non-narcotic** (which act chiefly peripherally, e.g. diclofenac).
- **Adjuvant drugs** are those used alongside analgesics in the management of pain. They are not themselves analgesics, though they may modify the perception or the concomitants of pain that make it worse (anxiety, fear,

Pain

Pain is an unpleasant sensory and emotional experience associated with actual or potential

---

[1] Merskey H et al 1979 Pain terms: a list with definitions and notes on usage. Pain 6: 249.
[2] Melzack R, Wall P 1982 The challenge of pain. Penguin, London.
[3] Loeser J D, Melzack 1999 Pain: an overview. Lancet 353: 1607.

depression),[4] e.g. psychotropic drugs, or they may modify underlying causes, e.g. spasm of smooth or of voluntary muscle.

The general principle that the best treatment of a symptom is removal of its cause applies. But this is often impossible to achieve and symptom relief of pain by analgesic drug is required.

Pain is the most common symptom for which patients see a doctor. The complaint does not mean that an analgesic is needed. To manage the pain, the doctor needs to know what is happening to the patient in mind and body.

Optimal management of pain requires that the clinician should have a conceptual framework for what is happening to the patient in mind and body.

- *Acute pain* is managed primarily (but not invariably) by analgesic drugs.
- *Chronic pain* often requires adjuvant drugs in addition as well as nondrug measures.

Analgesics are chosen according to the cause of pain and its severity.

Phenomenon of pain

An understanding of the phenomenon of pain ought to accommodate the following points:

- Pain can occur without tissue injury or evident disease and can persist after injury has healed.
- Serious tissue injury can occur without pain.
- Emotion (anxiety, fear, depression) is an inseparable concomitant of pain and can modify both its intensity and the victim's behavioural response.
- There is important processing of afferent nociceptive (see below) and other impulses in the spinal cord and brain.

Appreciation that pain is both a sensory and an emotional (affective) experience has allowed clinicians to realise that to meet a complaint of pain automatically with a prescription alone is not an appropriate response, for 'There is always more to analgesia than analgesics'.[5] Pain that is not the subject of an analysis by the clinician (and explanation to the patient) may be inadequately relieved because of lack of understanding. It is a justified and shaming criticism if doctors do not provide adequate relief of severe pain (postsurgical, palliative care of advanced cancer) by bad choice and by overusing and, also important, underusing drugs, and by defective relations with their patients.

THE VARIOUS ASPECTS OF PAIN

Pain is not simply a perception, it is a complex phenomenon or syndrome, only one component of which is the sensation actually reported as pain.

Pain has four major aspects present to varying extent in any one case:

Nociception[6] is a consequence of tissue injury (trauma, inflammation) causing the release of chemical mediators which activate *nociceptors*, defined as receptors that are capable of distinguishing between noxious and innocuous stimuli in the tissue. That said, it is widely assumed that there is no specific single histological structure that is a nociceptive receptor, but that free unmyelinated terminals in skin, muscle, joints and viscera are activated by noxious stimuli and transmit information by thin myelinated (A-delta) and nonmyelinated (C) fibres to the spinal cord and brain. Thus nociception is not, for example, due to overstimulation of touch or other receptors. A number of receptors, identified by anatomical, electrophysiological and pharmacological means, have been associated with nociceptors, and include acetylcholine, prostaglandin E, adrenergic, 5-hydroxytryptamine, glutamine, bradykinin, opioid and adenosine. The ligands for these receptors may be released in the periphery from neurones or be of non-neuronal origin.

Pain perception is a result of nociceptive input *plus* a pattern of impulses of different frequency and intensity from other peripheral receptors, e.g. heat,

---

[4] Tricyclic antidepressants may reduce morphine requirement in palliative care without noticeably altering mood.

[5] Twycross R G 1984 Journal of the Royal College of Physicians of London 18: 32.
[6] Latin: *noxa*: injury.

and mechanoreceptors whose threshold of response is reduced by the chemical mediators. These are processed in the brain whence modulating inhibitory impulses pass down to regulate the continuing afferent input. But pain can occur without nociception (some neuralgias[7]) and nociception does not invariably cause pain; pain is a psychological state, though most pain has an immediately antecedent physical cause.

Suffering is a consequence of pain and of lack of understanding by patients of the meaning of the pain; it comprises anxiety and fear (particularly in acute pain) and depression (particularly in chronic pain), which will be affected by patients' personalities, and their beliefs about the significance of the pain, e.g. whether merely a postponed holiday, or death, or a future of disability with loss of independence. Depression makes a major contribution to suffering; it is treatable, as are the other affective concomitants of pain.

Pain behaviour comprises consequences of the other three aspects (above); it includes behaviour that is interpreted by others as signifying pain in the victim, e.g. such immediate and obvious aspects as facial expression, restlessness, seeking isolation (or company), medicine-taking, as well as, in chronic pain, the development of querulousness, depression, despair and social withdrawal.

It is thus useful to distinguish between acute pain (an event whose end can be predicted) and chronic pain (a situation whose end is commonly unpredictable, or will only end with life itself).

The clinician's task is to determine the significance of these items for each patient and to direct therapy accordingly. Analgesics may, but not necessarily will, be the mainstay of therapy; adjuvant (nonanalgesic) drugs may be needed, as well as nondrug therapy (radiation, surgery).

TYPES OF PAIN

Acute pain (defined as of < 3 months duration) is transmitted principally by fast conducting A-delta fibres (but to a lesser extent involves slow conducting type C fibres) and has major nociceptive input (physical trauma, pleurisy, myocardial infarct, perforated peptic ulcer). Patients perceive it as a transient, though sometimes severe threat and they react accordingly. It is a symptom that may be dealt with unhesitatingly and effectively with drugs, by injection if necessary, at the same time as the causative disease is addressed. The accompanying anxiety will vary according to the severity of the pain, and particularly according to its meaning for the patient, whether termination with recovery will soon occur, major surgery is threatened, or there is prospect of death or invalidism. The choice of drug will depend on the clinician's assessment of these factors. Morphine by injection has retained a preeminent place for over 100 years because it has highly effective antinociceptive and anti-anxiety effects; modern opioids have not rendered morphine obsolete.

Neuropathic pain follows damage to the nervous system. Acute pain without nociceptive (afferent) input (some neuralgias) is less susceptible to drugs unless consciousness is also depressed, and any frequently recurrent acute pain, e.g. trigeminal neuralgia, poses management problems that are more akin to chronic pain.

Chronic pain is transmitted principally by slow conducting type C fibres (but to a lesser extent by fast conducting A-delta fibres). It is better regarded as a syndrome[8] rather than as a symptom (see above) for it is a collection of disparate pains of long duration, often sharing common emotional and behavioural aspects. It presents a depressing future to the victim who sees no prospect of release from suffering, and poses for that reason long-term management problems that differ from acute pain. Suffering and affective disorders can be of overriding importance and the consequences of poor management may be prolonged and serious for the patient. Analgesics alone are often insufficient and

---

[7] *Neuralgia* is pain felt in the distribution of a peripheral nerve.

[8] A set of symptoms and signs that are characteristic of a condition though they may not always have the same cause (Greek: *syn*: together, *dramein*: to run).

adjuvant drugs as well as nondrug therapy gain increasing importance. Although dependence is less of a problem than might be feared, continuous use of high efficacy opioids, e.g. morphine, pethidine, is generally is best avoided in chronic pain (except that of palliative care). But the lower efficacy opioids (codeine, dextropropoxyphene) may often be needed and used.

Sedation should be avoided and therapy should be oral if possible; regimens should be planned to avoid breakthrough pain. Antidepressants can often be useful. Sedative-hypnotic drugs, e.g. benzodiazepines, may be needed for anxiety but may induce depression.

Chronic pain syndrome is a term used for persistence of pain when detectable disease has disappeared, e.g. after an attack of low back pain. It characteristically does not respond to standard treatment with analgesics. Whether the basis is neurogenic, psychogenic or sociocultural it should not be managed by intensifying drug treatment. Opioid analgesics, which may be producing dependence, should be withdrawan and the use of psychotropic drugs, e.g. antidepressants or neuroleptics, and nondrug therapy, including psychotherapy, should be considered.

Transient pain is provoked by activation of nociceptors in skin or other tissues in the absence of tissue damage. It has evolved to protect humans from physical damage from the environment or excessive stressing of tissues. It is a part of normal life and not a reason to seek medical help. Nevertheless, it is partly through the production of transient pain in physiological experiments that present concepts of pain have evolved.

MECHANISMS OF ANALGESIA

Endogenous opioid neurotransmitters in the spinal cord and brain constitute a *pain inhibitory system;* they are activated by nociceptive and other inputs (including treatments such as transcutaneous nerve stimulation, and acupuncture) and mediate their effects through specific receptors. Activation of opioid receptors prevents the release of substance P (a neurotransmitter and local hormone involved in pain transmission) with the result that pain transmission is inhibited. Several types of receptor have been recognised, principally: μ (mu), δ (delta) and κ (kappa) receptors for which the endogenous ligands respectively are: endomorphins, met-encephalin and dynorphins.

Synthetic opioids produce analgesia by simulating the body's natural opioids and the existence of different types of receptor explains their varying patterns of actions. Definition of these receptors and their subdivisions offers hope for the design of new selective high-efficacy analgesics free from the disadvantages of the existing opioids.

Naloxone, the competitive opioid antagonist, binds to and blocks all opioid receptors but exerts no activating effect. Naloxone has particularly high affinity for the μ-receptor; it worsens (dental) pain, an effect that may be explained by blocking access of endogenous opioids to their receptor(s).[9] It does not induce hyperalgesia or spontaneous pain because the opioid paths are quiescent until activated by nociceptive and other afferent input.

In addition to these opioid mechanisms, non-opioid mediated pathways, e.g. serotonin, are important in pain. There is suggestion that opioid mechanisms are more important in acute severe pain, and nonopioid mechanisms in chronic pain, and that this may be relevant to choice of drugs.

NSAIDs. When a tissue is injured (from any cause), or even merely stimulated, prostaglandin synthesis in that tissue increases. Prostaglandins have two major actions: they are mediators of inflammation and they also sensitise nerve endings, lowering their threshold of response to stimuli, mechanical (the tenderness of inflammation) and chemical, allowing the other mediators of inflammation, e.g. histamine, serotonin, bradykinin, to intensify the activation of the sensory endings.

Plainly, a drug that prevents the synthesis of prostaglandins is likely to be effective in relieving pain due to inflammation of any kind, and this is indeed how aspirin and other nonsteroidal anti-inflammatory drugs (NSAIDs) act. This discovery was made in 1971, aspirin having been extensively

---

[9] Naloxone also appears to cause *pyrovats* (practitioners of religious firewalking ceremonies) to quicken their pace over the hot coals.

used in medicine since 1899.[10] NSAIDs act by inhibiting cyclo-oxygenase (see p. 280). Thus it is evident that NSAIDs will relieve pain when there is some tissue injury with consequent inflammation, as there almost always is with pain. They also act in the central nervous system (prostaglandins, despite their name, are synthesised in all cells except erythrocytes) and there is probably some central component to the analgesic effect of NSAIDs.

But, analgesic and anti-inflammatory effects are not parallel, e.g. aspirin relieves pain rapidly at doses that do not significantly reduce inflammation and the onset of its anti-inflammatory effect at higher doses may be slow. Paracetamol is an effective analgesic for mild pain but has little anti-inflammation effect in arthritis, though substantial effect on post-dental extraction swelling. Other NSAIDs show a different mix of action against pain and inflammation (see Ch. 15).

Corticosteroids diminish inflammation of all kinds by preventing prostaglandin synthesis (the phospholipase A that releases arachidonic acid for such synthesis is inhibited by lipocortin-1 which is produced in response to glucosteroids). Short-term use may be valuable; long-term use poses many problems (see Ch. 34); in general the corticosteroid should be withdrawn after one week if there is no benefit.

The pain threshold is lowered by anxiety, fear, depression, anger, sadness, fatigue, or insomnia, and is raised by relief of these (by drug or nondrug measures) and by successful relief of pain. Since emotion is such an important factor in pain, it is no surprise that placebo tablets or injections alleviate pain but with the added disadvantage that they rapidly lose effect with repetition.

The importance of the meaning of pain to its victim is illustrated by injuries of war and of civilian life:

---

[10] Propagandists for complementary (alternative) medicine allege that conventional scientific medicine will not recognise any therapy, e.g. complementary medicine, unless its mode of action is known. This is untrue. Validated empirical observation, i.e. scientific evidence, is and always has been accepted.

To the wounded soldier who had been under unremitting shell fire for weeks, his wound was a good thing (it meant the end of the war for him) and was associated with far less pain than was the case of the civilians who considered their need for surgery a disaster.[11]

The desire for analgesics has been found to be less amongst victims of battle injuries than amongst comparable civilian injuries. On the other hand, morphine has been found to be relatively ineffective against experimental pain in man, probably because it acts best against pain that has emotional significance for the patient.

New analgesics have been successfully developed by animal testing, possibly because the emotional response to experimental pain in an animal is akin to the human response to disease or accidental injury. This emotional response does not generally occur in a subject who has volunteered to undergo laboratory experiments that can be stopped at any time, and it probably accounts for the fact that a placebo gives relief in only 3% of these cases.

Clinical evaluation of analgesics

Therapeutic trials in acute pain are often conducted on patients who have undergone abdominal surgery or third molar tooth extraction, and in chronic pain on chronic rheumatic conditions. Only the patients can say what they feel and pain is best measured by a questionnaire or by a visual analogue scale; this is a line, 10 cm long, one end of which represents pain 'as bad as it could possibly be' (which patients identify as 'agonising') and the other end 'no pain'; patients mark the line at the point they feel represents their pain between these two extremes. Such techniques are highly reproducible.

Since what is being measured is how patients say they feel, the trial must be double-blind.

---

[11] Beecher H K 1957 Pharmacological Review 9: 59.

Observers who interrogate the patients for relief (intensity and duration) and adverse effects must be constant and trained. If asked by a personable young woman, a higher proportion of patients (of both sexes) admit to pain relief if the same question is put by a man.

Choice of analgesics

RANKED BY CLINICAL EFFICACY[12]

(see also ranking of opioids, p. 338)
Mild pain

- Non-narcotic (nonopioid) analgesics or NSAIDs, e.g. paracetamol, ibuprofen, diclofenac.[13] (Ch. 15) Where these fail after using the full dose range, proceed to drugs for:

Moderate pain

- Narcotic (opioid) analgesics, low-efficacy opioids, e.g. codeine, dihydrocodeine, dextropropoxyphene, pentazocine.
- Combined therapy of NSAIDs plus low-efficacy opioid, either as a fixed-dose formulation, which is convenient for acute pain or separately to find the optimum dose of each, which may be preferable for chronic pain though less convenient.

Where these fail proceed to drugs for:

Severe pain

- High-efficacy opioids, e.g. morphine, diamorphine, pethidine, buprenorphine. An added NSAID is useful if there is an additional tissue injury component, e.g. gout, bone metastasis.

---

[12] Based on Twycross R G 1978 In: Saunders Cicely M (ed) The management of terminal disease. Arnold, London. The work of this author contributes much to this chapter.
[13] Paracetamol is sometimes not classed as an NSAID because its anti-inflammatory pattern differs substantianlly from most, i.e. it is central rather than peripheral, as witness its weak anti-inflammatory efficacy in rheumatoid arthritis.

Where these fail proceed to drugs for:

Overwhelming acute pain

- High efficacy opioid plus a sedative/anxiolytic (diazepam) or a phenothiazine tranquilliser, e.g. chlorpromazine, levomepromazine (methotrimeprazine) (which also has analgesic effect).

Note: adjuvant drugs (p. 331) may be useful in all grades of pain.

COMBINING ANALGESICS

Simultaneous use of two analgesics of different modes of action is rational, but two drugs of the same class/mechanism of action are unlikely to benefit unless there is a difference in emphasis, e.g. analgesia and anti-inflammatory action (paracetamol plus aspirin), or in duration of action; a patient taking an NSAID with a long duration, e.g. naproxen (used once or twice a day), is benefited by an additional drug of shorter duration for an acute exacerbation, e.g. ibuprofen, paracetamol.

A low-efficacy opioid can reduce the effectiveness of a high-efficacy opioid by successfully competing with the latter for receptors. Partial agonist (agonist/antagonist) opioids, e.g. pentazocine, will also antagonise the action of other opioids, e.g. heroin, and may even induce the withdrawal syndrome in dependent subjects.

FIXED-RATIO (COMPOUND) COMBINATIONS

Large numbers of these are offered particularly to bridge the efficacy gap between paracetamol and morphine. Doctors should consider the formulae of these preparations before using them. Caffeine has been shown to enhance the analgesic effect of aspirin and of paracetamol and to accelerate the onset of effect, but at least 30 mg and probably 60 mg are needed (a cup of coffee averages about 80 mg and of tea averages about 30 mg).

Tablets containing paracetamol (325 mg) plus dextropropoxyphene (32.5 mg) (co-proxamol, Distalgesic), in a dose of 1–2 tablets, provide an effective dose of both drugs and have been extremely popular with both prescribers and patients; its popularity may be influenced by a mild euphoriant effect of the opioid, to which dependence can occur. A major concern is that in (deliberate) overdose death may occur within one hour due to the rapid absorption of the dextropropoxyphene, and combination with alcohol appears seriously to add to the hazard. We do not attempt to rank the many preparations available because comparative evidence is lacking.

Pain syndromes and their treatment

In general, pain (acute or chronic) arising from the *somatic structures* (skin, muscles, bones, joints) responds to NSAIDs. Acute pain arising from *viscera*, which is poorly localised, unpleasant, and associated with nausea is best treated with morphine but this induces dependence with prolonged use. This distinction is not, of course, absolute and a high-efficacy opioid is needed for severe somatic pain, e.g. a fractured bone. Mild pain from any source may respond to NSAIDs and these should always be tried first.

SPASM OF VISCERAL SMOOTH MUSCLE

Pain due to spasm of visceral smooth muscle, e.g. biliary, renal colic, when severe, requires a substantial dose of morphine, pethidine or buprenorphine. These drugs themselves cause spasm of visceral smooth muscle and so have a simultaneous action tending to increase the pain. Phenazocine and buprenorphine are less liable to cause spasm. An antimuscarinic drug such as atropine or hyoscine may be given simultaneously to antagonise this effect.

Prostaglandins are involved in control of smooth muscle and colic can be treated with NSAIDs, e.g. diclofenac, indometacin (i.m., suppository or oral).

SPASM OF STRIATED MUSCLE

This is often a cause of pain, including chronic tension headache. Treatment is directed at reduc-

tion of the spasm in a variety of ways, including psychotherapy, sedation and the use of a centrally-acting muscle relaxant as well as non-narcotic analgesics, e.g. baclofen, diazepam; clinical efficacy is variable (see Other muscle relaxants, p. 357). Local infiltration with lignocaine (lidocaine) is sometimes appropriate. Tizanidine is an α_2-adrenoreceptor agonist that may be used to relieve muscle spasticity in multiple sclerosis, spinal cord injury or disease.

NEURALGIAS (NEUROPATHIC PAIN)

These include postherpetic neuralgia, phantom limb pain, peripheral neuropathies of various causes, central pain, e.g. following a stroke, compression neuropathies, and the complex regional pain syndromes (comprising causalgia, when there is nerve damage, and reflex sympathetic dystrophy, when there is tissue but no nerve injury); they present the most challenging problems.

A *tricyclic antidepressant* and/or an *antiepilepsy drug* are commonly used in their management; analgesics play a subsidiary part.

- *Amitriptyline* is most frequently used, starting with 10 mg at night increasing to 75 mg. Nortriptyline is better tolerated by some patients. Their general action is to inhibit noradrenaline (norepinephrine) re-uptake by nerve terminals and benefit in neuropathic pain may follow enhanced activity in noradrenergic pain inhibitory paths in the spinal cord.
- *Gabapentin* is the most commonly used antiepilepsy drug in this setting; *phenytoin* (which raises the threshold of nerve cells to electrical stimulation) or *sodium valproate* are used for resistant neuralgias.
- *Transcutaneous electrical nerve stimulation* (TENS) helps some sufferers; it may act by promoting the release of endorphins. *Ketamine* (see p. 353) or *lidocaine* (lignocaine) (by i.v. infusion) are used in special circumstances. Pain due to nerve compression may be relieved by a corticosteroid injected locally.
- When these measures fail, and an *opioid* appears necessary, methadone, dextroproxyphene, tramadol and oxycodone are preferred; all possess NMDA-receptor antagonist activity as well as being opioid μ-receptor agonists.

Trigeminal neuralgia differs from other peripheral neuropathies in its management. The antiepilepsy drug, carbamazepine (p. 417), was accidentally discovered to be effective, probably by reducing excitability of the trigeminal nucleus. The initial dose should be low, and individuals generally soon learn to alter it themselves during remissions and exacerbations (200–1600 mg/d). It is not used for prophylaxis. Resistant cases may obtain benefit from oxcarbazepine, gabapentin or lamotrigine.

Postherpetic neuralgia. The pain of acute herpes zoster (shingles) is mitigated by NSAIDs and opioids (as well as by oral aciclovir started within 48 h of the rash). Whether the incidence of postherpetic neuralgia is reliably reduced by early treatment with an antivirus drug has yet to be proved. Amitriptyline is an appropriate initial choice, failing which gabapentin may be used. A topical application of capsaicin, derived from *Capsicum* spp (pepper and chilli), may be applied as a counter-iritant, although the initial intense burning sensation may limit its use. Conventional analgesics are ineffective.

HEADACHE

Headache originating inside the skull may be due to traction on or distension of arteries arising from the circle of Willis, or to traction on the dura mater. Headache originating outside the skull may be due to local striated muscle spasm;[14] an anatomical connection, only recently identified, between an extracranial muscle and the cervical dura mater may help to explain headache of cervical origin. Treatment by drugs is directed to relieving the muscle spasm, producing vasoconstriction or simply administering analgesics, beginning, of course, with the non-narcotics, e.g. paracetamol, ibuprofen.

MIGRAINE

The acute migraine attack appears to begin in serotonergic (5-HT) and noradrenergic neurons in the brain. These monoamines affect the cerebral and extracerebral vasculature and also cause release of further vasoactive substances such as histamine, prostaglandins and neuropeptides involved in pain, i.e. there is neurogenic inflammation that can be inhibited by specific antimigraine drugs (below).

The migraine aura of visual or sensory disturbance probably originates in the occipital or sensory cortex; the throbbing headache is due to dilatation of pain-sensitive arteries outside the brain, including scalp arteries.

Identifying and avoiding triggering factors are important. These include stress (exertion, excitement, anxiety, fatigue, anger), food containing vasoactive amines (chocolate, cheese), food allergy, bright lights and loud noise, and also hormonal changes (menstruation and oral contraceptives) and hypoglycaemia. These precipitants may initiate release of vasoactive substances stored in nerve endings and blood platelets. Many attacks, however, have no obvious trigger.

Treatment. A stepped approach to therapy is logical.[15]

- The *acute migraine attack* should be treated as early as possible with an oral dispersible (soluble) analgesic formulation so that it may be absorbed before there is vomiting and accompanying gastric stasis with slow and erratic drug absorption. Aspirin (600 mg) is effective and its antiplatelet action may add to its advantage; paracetamol, ibuprofen and naproxen are alternatives. Metoclopramide or domperidone, dopamine agonists, are useful antiemetics that also promote gastric emptying and enhance absorption of the analgesic. Opioids such as codeine, dihydrocodeine and dextropropoxyphene are not suitable for migraine.
- If the oral route is unsuccessful, a rational alternative is to use suppositories of diclofenac 100 mg for pain and domperidone 30 mg for vomiting, although the diarrhoea that may accompany migraine would compromise their efficacy. Efficient use of an analgesic and an antiemetic is adequate for the majority of acute attacks.

---

[14] As in tension headache or frontal headache from 'eyestrain'.

[15] British Association for the Study of Headache 2001. http://www.bash.org.uk

- *Severe migraine attacks* should be treated with a triptan, e.g. sumatriptan (below). In contrast to symptomatic treatments, triptans are best used during the established headache phase of the acute attack. Headache may return in 6–36 h in about one-third of patients, necessitating a second dose.

- Ergotamine 1–2 mg as a suppository is used if other treatments have failed, but not within 12 h of the last dose of a triptan; similarly a triptan should not be given until 24 h have elapsed after stopping ergotamine.

Sumatriptan

Sumatriptan (Imigran) selectively stimulates a subtype of 5-hydroxytryptamine$_1$-receptors (called 5-HT$_{1B/1D}$-receptors) which are found in cranial blood vessels, causing them to constrict. It is rapidly absorbed after oral administration and undergoes extensive (84%) presystemic metabolism; but bioavailability by the s.c. route is 96%. The t$\frac{1}{2}$ is 2 h.

The oral dose is 50–100 mg, the 24 h total not to exceed 300 mg. The oral route may be avoided by sumatriptan 20 mg given intranasally, repeated once in not less than 2 h, with not more than 40 mg in 24 h. When a rapid response is required, sumatriptan 6 mg is given s.c., the dose to be repeated once if necessary after 1 h but the total should not exceed 12 mg in 24 h.

Sumatriptan is generally well tolerated. Malaise, fatigue, dizziness, vertigo and sedation are associated with oral use. Nausea and vomiting may follow oral or s.c. administration. The most important adverse effects are feelings of chest pressure, tightness and pain in about 5% of cases; these may be accompanied by cardiac arrhythmia and myocardial infarction and appear to be due to coronary artery spasm. Patients with ischaemic heart disease, unstable angina or previous myocardial infarction should not be given sumatriptan; use in relation to ergotamine (see above).

Almotriptan, naratriptan, rizatriptan and zolmitriptan are similar.[16]

---

[16] Ferrari M D et al 2001 Oral triptans (serotonim 5-HT $_{1B/1D}$ agonists) in acute migraine treatment: a meta-analysis of 53 trials. Lancet 358: 1668–1675.

Ergotamine

Ergotamine is a partial agonist at α-adrenoceptors (vasoconstrictor) and also a partial agonist at serotonergic receptors. It must be used with special care.

Ergotamine constricts all peripheral arteries (an effect potentiated by concomitant β-adrenoceptor block), not just those affected by the migraine process. Due to tissue binding, its effect on arteries persists as long as 24 h and repeated doses lead to cumulative effects long outlasting the migraine attack.

It is incompletely absorbed from the gastrointestinal tract; rectal administration may be preferred in the acute attack of migraine. Ergotamine is extensively metabolised in the liver (t$\frac{1}{2}$ 2 h).

Tablets, 1 mg, may be crushed before swallowing with water. Initially 1–2 tablets should be taken and thereafter, not more than 4 tablets should be taken in 24 h, the sequence should not be repeated for 4 days, and not more than 8 tablets should be taken in a week. Suppositories, 2 mg, are now preferred as part of stepped therapy (above); they are subject to the same maximum dose restrictions. Caffeine enhances both the speed of absorption and peak concentration of ergotamine and is often combined with it (though it may prevent sleep).

Paraesthesiae in hands or feet give warning of peripheral ischaemia. Overdose can cause peripheral gangrene. Due to its complex actions on receptors, vasoconstriction is best antagonised by a nonselective vasodilator such as glyceryl trinitrate, nifedipine or sodium nitroprusside (rather than by an α-adrenoceptor blocker). Patients with vascular disease, coronary and peripheral, are particularly at risk.

Ergotamine is a powerful oxytocic and is dangerous in pregnancy. It may precipitate angina pectoris, probably by increasing cardiac pre- and afterload (venous and arterial constriction) rather than by constricting coronary arteries.

Ergotamine should never be used for prophylaxis of migraine.

Drug prophylaxis of migraine

This should be considered when, after adjustment of lifestyle, there are still two or more attacks per month. Benefit may be delayed for several weeks. Options (which may help up to 60% of patients) include:

- *β-adrenoceptor block* by propranolol(dl); (the d-isomer, which lacks β-blocking action though it has membrane stabilising effect, also prevents migraine), as do other pure antagonists (atenolol, metoprolol) but not partial (ant)agonists, see page 474. It seems that β-adrenoceptor block is not the prime therapeutic action. Note that if ergotamine (for an acute attack) is given to a patient taking propranolol for prophylaxis there is risk of additive vasoconstriction (block of β-receptor mediated dilatation with added α-receptor constriction).
- *Calcium entry blockers*, e.g. verapamil, flunarizine, may provide benefit.
- *Pizotifen* and *cyproheptadine* block serotonin (5-HT) receptors as well as having some H_1-antihistamine action; they can be effective.
- *A tricyclic antidepressant*, e.g. amitriptyline in low dose; start with 10 mg at night and increase to 50–75 mg.
- *Methysergide* (an ergot derivative) blocks serotonin receptors but it has a grave rare adverse effect, an inflammatory fibrosis, retroperitoneal (causing obstruction to the ureters), subendocardial, pericardial and pleural. Drug 'holidays', i.e. withdrawal for 1–2 months each 6 months, are a prudent safeguard. Because of this risk, methysergide cannot be a drug of first choice though it may be justified for a patient who is experiencing a sequence of severe attacks.

Cluster headaches may be treated with a $5HT_1$-receptor agonist, e.g. sumatriptan, as for migraine. Since bouts of headache tend to be of limited duration, e.g. a few weeks, short courses of methysergide are justified in intractable cases.

Premenstrual migraine may respond to mefenamic acid or to a diuretic. *After six months* it is worth trying slow withdrawal of the prophylactic drug.

Headache of raised intracranial pressure (cerebral oedema) responds to dexamethasone (10 mg i.v.; 4 mg 6-hourly, 2–10 d) which reduces the pressure; and to nonopioid analgesics (see also Palliative care).

OTHER PAIN SYNDROMES

- Inflammation responds to NSAIDs but may need support from a low-efficacy opioid.
- Arthritis: see Chapter 15.
- Minor trauma, e.g. many sports injuries, is commonly treated by local skin cooling (spray of chlorofluoromethanes), counterirritants (see p. 302) and NSAIDs, e.g. diclofenac, systemically or topically.
- Severe trauma including postsurgical pain (p. 347) usually needs narcotic analgesics.
- Peripheral vascular insufficiency should be treated with non-narcotic analgesics but may eventually require low efficacy opioids; vasodilator drugs may, but equally may not, provide benefit.
- Malignant disease requires the full range of analgesics and adjuvant drugs and procedures (see Palliative care, below).
- Bone pain, including cancer metastases, requires NSAIDs alone and with opioids. Bisphosphonates, e.g. sodium pamidronate, sodium clodronate, relieve pain from osteolytic bone metastases from breast cancer and multiple myeloma.
- Nerve compression can be relieved by local corticosteroid (prednisolone) or nerve block (local anaesthetic); nerve destruction can be achieved by alcohol, phenol.
- Dysmenorrhoea, see page 730.
- Mastalgia may benefit from gamolenic acid (in evening primrose oil), danazol and bromocriptine; or from a combined contraceptive pill.

In sickle cell anaemia crises avoid pethidine as the metabolite norpethidine may accumulate; hydroxyurea reduces the frequency (see p. 599).

PATIENT-CONTROLLED ANALGESIA

The attractions of enabling patients to manage their own analgesics rather than be dependent on others are obvious. In mild and moderate pain it is easy to provide tablets for this purpose, but in severe chronic and acute recurrent pain, e.g. terminal illness, postsurgical, obstetric, other routes are needed to provide speedy relief just when it is needed. Drug delivery systems range from inhalation devices to patient-controlled pumps for i.v., i.m., s.c. and epidural routes.

Despite the obvious problems, e.g. training patients, supervision, preventing overdose, these can achieve the objectives of satisfying the patient while reducing demand on nurses' time, especially when the aim is to allow the patient to die comfortably at home.

Inhalation via a demand valve of nitrous oxide and oxygen, as in obstetrics, may be used temporarily in other situations: e.g. urinary lithiasis, trigeminal neuralgia, during postoperative chest physiotherapy, for changing painful dressings and in emergency ambulances.

Drugs in palliative care

Symptom control

It is a general truth that we are all dying; the difference between individuals is the length and quality of the time that remains.[17] Terminal illness means that period (generally weeks) when active treatment of disease is no longer appropriate and the emphasis of care is palliative, i.e. to provide the maximum quality of life during these final weeks. This means that symptom control becomes the priority because,

> One cannot adequately help a man to come to accept his impending death if he remains in severe pain, one cannot give spiritual counsel to a woman who is vomiting, or help a wife and children say their goodbyes to a father who is so drugged that he cannot respond.[18]

As the scope of life contracts, so the quality of what remains becomes more precious. Symptoms should not be allowed to destroy it. Drugs are preeminent in symptom control. An illustrative instance of success in palliative care is provided here by:

An elderly gentleman with obstructing carcinoma of the oesophagus who was a keen gardener. He remained at home, free from pain, attended a garden show on Saturday, worked in his garden on Sunday, and died on Monday.[19]

He was treated with continuous subcutaneous heroin (diamorphine) infusion. Whilst the randomised controlled trial provides a major basis for therapeutic advance, telling us what generally does happen, the clinical anecdote yet has value, telling us what can happen, and providing examples for us to emulate. With intelligent use of drugs, which follows from informed analyses of objectives, doctors can enable their patients to depart from life in peace[20] and with dignity, i.e. true euthanasia.[21]

Whilst the skilful use of drugs can provide incalculable relief and deserves careful study, this must not hide the fact that the manner, attentiveness and human feeling of the attendants are dominant factors once drugs have controlled any grosser physical and mental aberrations.[22] The needs of the dying have been summarised as security, companionship, symptomatic treatment, and medical nursing

---

[17] Mack R M 1984 Lessons from living with cancer. New England Journal of Medicine 311: 1640. Recommended reading: a personal account by a surgeon who had lung cancer with metastases.

[18] Dr Mary Baines, St Christopher's Hospice, London.

[19] Russell P S B 1984 New England Journal of Medicine 311: 1634.

[20] '...; and for many a time
I have been half in love with easeful Death,
Call'd him soft names in many a mused rhyme,
To take into the air my quiet breath;
 Now more than ever seems it rich to die,
To cease upon the midnight with no pain.'
(John Keats: 1795–1821).

[21] Euthanasia (Greek: *eu*: gentle, easy; *thanatos*: death) is the objective of all. It does not mean deliberately killing people peacefully, which is voluntary euthanasia. That giving increasing doses of opioids and sedative drugs may also shorten life (the 'double effect') 'is not in our view a reason for withholding treatment that would give relief, as long as a doctor acts in accordance with responsible medical practice with the objective of relieving pain or distress, and with no intention to kill'. Report of the select committee on medical ethics. House of Lords, January 1994. HMSO, London.

[22] Give me the doctor partridge plump,
Short in the leg and broad in the rump,
An endomorph with gentle hands,
Who never makes absurd demands
That I abandon all my vices,
Nor pulls a long face in a crisis,
But with a twinkle in his eye
Will tell me that I have to die.

(WH Auden 1907–73)

and domestic care. Nearly half of the deaths in England and Wales occur in the patient's own home.

Pain

The cause of the pain should first be assessed. A tricyclic antidepressant is appropriate for neuropathic pain due to neoplastic extension to peripheral nerves, a corticosteroid for nerve entrapment, an opioid for a liver distended with metastatic disease, a NSAID for bony secondaries.

Analgesics should be given regularly, adjusted to the patient's need to *prevent* pain and not only to suppress it. Suppression of existent pain requires larger doses, particularly where the pain has generated anxiety and fear. When it is certain that pain will return, it is callous to allow it to do so when the means of prevention exist.

A dose of analgesic should be left accessible to the patient, especially at night, when unnecessary suffering may result from reluctance to call a nurse or disturb a relative. In terminal illness, the question of whether or not the patient will become dependent on opioids ceases to be of importance (but see below) and the ordinary precautions against dependence — low, widely-spaced doses — need not be rigorously applied.

Control of severe pain without objectionable sedation can be achieved in palliative care by morphine with adjuvant drugs (given orally) in up to 80% of patients. Oral use preserves patients' independence as well as reducing the unpleasantness of frequent injections.

Full relief can be achieved only by attention to detail. We therefore provide an account of morphine use in this most important area of medical care.

ORAL MORPHINE FOR PAIN IN PALLIATIVE CARE

Oral treatment allows independence and can be provided at home where most patients will prefer to die.

- A simple aqueous solution[23] may be used initially, the strength being adjusted to give a

volume of 5–10 ml per dose, e.g. begin with 1 or 2 mg/ml.

- Alternatively, sustained-release tablets (MST Continus, Oramorph SR) may be preferred.
- The usual oral starting dose to replace a weaker analgesic, e.g. co-proxamol, is 2.5–10 mg 4-hourly (2.5 mg in the frail elderly) of the aqueous solution or 10–30 mg 12-hourly of the sustained-release formulations. Alternatively, use suppositories or buccal (sublingual) formulations (the latter route bypasses the presystemic elimination and does not require such high doses as when swallowed).
- Dose and frequency should be adjusted to meet the patient's need. The interval of sustained-release tablets should remain unaltered, i.e. 12-hourly.
- Breakthrough pain when the patient is taking a sustained-release preparation may be controlled by an additional dose of the aqueous solution; it gives the patient confidence.
- Change to morphine from other high-efficacy opioids; higher starting doses of oral morphine will be needed.
- A larger dose at night (1.5–2 × daytime dose) or an added hypnotic may allow the patient to pass the night without waking in pain (and so to omit one night dose).
- Constipation will occur, see below; it is essential to manage it.
- Initial drowsiness (a few days) and confusion (in the elderly) are common and usually pass off.
- Initial nausea and vomiting are common: an antiemetic, e.g. prochlorperazine, controls it and can generally be withdrawn after 4–5 days.
- Respiratory depression is seldom a problem with morphine dose escalated in this way.
- Dependence need not be feared. Both physical and psychological dependence occurs, but the latter to only a small degree compared with drug abuse or other chronic pain syndromes. The

---

[23] Solutions of morphine deteriorate once they are exposed to air, and if exposed to light (keep in dark) and heat, they lose potency over as few as 2–4 weeks; competent pharmaceutical advice and preparation is required; stable formulations have been developed (Oramorph). The taste of morphine is bitter and patients may choose an accompanying drink to mask it. Tablets may be used.

social, psychological and medical aspects of morphine use in palliative care are so different from that of drug abuse that comparisons are inappropriate. Dose reduction, when required, e.g. after relief of pain by palliative radiotherapy or nerve block, should, of course, be gradual; abrupt withdrawal (accidental) has been found to cause only a mild withdrawal syndrome.

- Acquired tolerance is dealt with by increasing the dose. There is no need for an arbitrary maximum dose.
- Transfer from the oral to the subcutaneous route may become necessary, e.g. due to difficult swallowing, vomiting. Diamorphine (heroin, preferred because it is more soluble than morphine) can be delivered by a portable syringe driver with minimal discomfort. The dose should be one-third the oral dose (4-hourly swallowed).
- A self-adhesive skin patch formulation which releases the opioid fentanyl (25 mg/h for 72 h) transdermally is also available for pain relief in palliative care.

ADJUVANT DRUGS

Phenothiazines are antiemetic, antianxiety and sedative agents and they may change the affective response to pain (particularly methotrimeprazine).

Tricyclic antidepressants (and perhaps others) have a morphine-sparing effect even in the absence of an effect or mood.

In selected cases the full range of techniques of local and regional anaesthesia may be used, including extradural and intrathecal morphine (p. 360).

OTHER SYMPTOMS

- *Anorexia* is common in patients with widespread cancer; prednisolone 15–30 mg daily and/or alcohol (in the patient's preferred form) before meals, many help.
- *Confusion* may not need treatment unless it is accompanied by restlessness. Useful in an emergency is haloperidol, or thioridazine (less sedating) or chlorpromazine (if sedation is desired).
- *Constipation* is usual in dying patients, whether

due to opioid analgesic or to inadequate intake of food and fluid,[24] and physical inactivity. It can be exceedingly troublesome and management should begin early to forestall the need for the major unpleasantness and humiliations of manual removal of faeces and the lesser ones of enemas. Dietary measures should be used where practicable. A stimulant laxative and faecal softener (danthron plus poloxamer: co-danthramer) is commonly effective. Suppositories, e.g. glycerol or bisacodyl, should be used if the bowels have not been opened for three days and the rectum is found to be loaded.

- *Convulsions.* Sodium valproate orally is preferred as it is effective for a wide range of seizure disorders (for status epilepticus see p. 417).
- *Cough*: see page 549.
- *Diarrhoea*: see page 642.
- *Dyspnoea.* Chronic dyspnoea (not due to respiratory failure) may be relieved by an opioid (causing respiratory centre depression and reducing its sensitivity to chemical stimuli) but, when there is respiratory failure due to pulmonary disease, any sedation may be life-threatening. Oxygen is used as appropriate; a benzodiazepine reduces the anxiety of dyspnoea; dexamethasone reduces inflammation around obstructive tumours that cause dyspnoea. Accumulations of mucus that the patient is too weak to expel cause 'death rattle'; this terminal event, often more distressing to others than to the patient, may be eliminated by drying up secretions with an antimuscarinic drug (hyoscine or atropine 4- to 8-hourly).
- *Emergencies* such as major haemorrhage, pulmonary embolus, severe choking, fracture of large bone: give morphine 10 mg plus hyoscine 0.4 mg i.m.; this combination provides acute relief and some desirable short-term retrograde amnesia which may extend to the whole unpleasant episode.

---

[24] It is normal and comfortable to die slightly dehydrated; full hydration leads to full urinary bladder (with discomfort, restlessness, incontinence), salivary drooling and death rattle; it also increases heart failure (with dyspnoea which enhances death rattle); intravenous tubes make final embraces almost impossible (Lamerton R 1991 Lancet 337: 981).

- *Hiccup* (due to diaphragmatic spasm). Where this is intractable and exhausting, chlorpromazine (or other phenothiazine) or metoclopramide may help; also baclofen, nifedipine or sodium valproate.
- *Insomnia*. Use temazepam or zopiclone (which may be less prone to cause confusion in the elderly).
- *Itch*: see page 302.
- *Lymphoedema*, e.g. due to pelvic cancer, that causes pain may be helped by prednisolone (15–30 mg/day).
- Mental distress may be helped by an antidepressant or tranquilliser, according to circumstances. Patients may too easily be drugged into uncomplaining silence, but it does not follow that they are not still in deep distress:

  ...the grief that does not speak
  Whispers the o'er-fraught heart, and bids it break.[25]

  And this unpleasant way of ending life can be avoided by discerning choice and, particularly, careful dosage of drugs.
- *A mouth* that is dry and painful may be due to candidiasis (treat with nystatin), to dehydration (rehydrate the patient judiciously where this can be done orally); the symptom can be managed by frequent small drinks or crushed ice to suck (plus assiduous mouth hygiene to prevent unpleasant infection); if due to antimuscarinic drugs, including some antidepressants, withdraw the drug or adjust its dose.
- *Nausea and vomiting*, whether due to disease or to opioid drug, cause great distress and can be more difficult to manage than pain; two drugs acting by different mechanisms may be needed when a single agent fails, e.g. metoclopramide (dopamine D_2-receptor antagonist) or ondansetron (5-HT_3-receptor antagonist) or hyoscine (antimuscarinic). For vomiting of hypercalcaemia: use an antiemetic and treat the cause (p. 740).
- *Night sweats* can be distressing and cause insomnia: indomethacin helps.
- *Restlessness* in terminal illness that has no obvious cause, e.g. pain, full bladder, may be treated with methotrimeprazine

(levromepromazine; a phenothiazine tranquilliser with analgesic effect) by injection. It may be combined with morphine (or diamorphine), which are tranquillisers as well as being analgesics; diazepam is useful for muscle twitching.
- *Swallowing* of solid-dose forms may be difficult and these may stick in the oesophagus in weak recumbent patients, especially if inadequate fluid is taken with the dose (at least two big gulps or 100 ml with the patient's trunk vertical).
- *Urinary frequency,* urgency and incontinence: flavoxate, tolterodine, oxybutynin (antimuscarinics) may be useful; they may cause retention of urine if there is anatomical obstruction. The pain (with reflex muscle spasm) of an indwelling catheter may be alleviated by diazepam.
- *Raised intracranial pressure* (see p. 328): dexamethasone may be used indefinitely; reduce dose to 5 mg/d if practicable.
- *Fungating tumours* and *ulcers* may smell distressingly due to anaerobic bacterial growth. Benefit may be gained by topical providone-iodine or metronidazole gel.

Narcotic or opioid[26] analgesics

Agonists, partial agonists, antagonists

Among the remedies which it has pleased Almighty God to give to man to relieve his sufferings, none is so universal and so efficacious as opium (Thomas Sydenham, physician, 1680).

Opium (the dried juice of the seed head of the opium poppy) was certainly used in prehistoric times, and medical practice still leans heavily on its

---

[25] William Shakespeare (1564–1616). Macbeth, Act 4, Scene 3.

[26] The term opiate has been used for the natural alkaloids of opium, and opioid for other agents having similar action. The distinction is neither generally observed nor particularly useful. We here use opioid for all receptor-specific substances.

alkaloids, using them as analgesic, tranquilliser, antitussive and in diarrhoea.

The principal active ingredient in crude opium was isolated in 1806 by Friedrich Sertürner, who tested pure morphine on himself and three young men. He observed that the drug caused cerebral depression and relieved toothache, and named it after Morpheus.[27]

Opium contains many alkaloids, but the only important ones are *morphine* (10%) and *codeine; papaverine* is occasionally used as a vasodilator (see p. 546). Purified preparations of mixtures of opium alkaloids, e.g. papaveretum (Omnopon), are available; minus noscapine which is suspected of genotoxicity.

MODE OF ACTION

Endogenous opioid peptides (endorphins, dynorphins, enkephalins), have been termed 'the brain's own morphine'. Their discovery in 1972 explained why the brain has opioid receptors when there were no opioids in the body. These peptides attach to specific opioid receptors, mainly μ (mu), δ (delta) or κ (kappa) located at several spinal and multiple supraspinal sites in the CNS. Opioid receptors are part of the family of G-protein-coupled receptors (see p. 91) and act to open potassium channels and prevent the opening of voltage-gated calcium channels which reduces neuronal excitability and inhibits the release of pain neurotransmitters, including substance P.

The most important is the μ-receptor, of which two subtypes are recognised, the $μ_1$-receptor, associated with analgesia, euphoria and dependence, and the $μ_2$-receptor with respiratory depression and inhibition of gut motility. The κ-receptor is responsible for analgesia at the level of the spinal cord and is also associated with dysphoria. The role of the δ-receptor in humans is less clear.

Pure morphine-like opioid agonists in general act on μ- and κ-receptors.

---

[27] In classical mythology Morpheus was son of Somnus, the infernal deity who presided over sleep. He was generally represented as a corpulent, winged boy holding opium poppies in is hand. His principal function seems to have been to stand by his sleeping father's black-curtained bed of feathers, on watch to prevent his being awakened by noise.

Mixed agonist-antagonists and partial agonists. Opioid drugs may be agonist to one class of opioid receptor, and antagonist to another, which explains the differing patterns of action seen. A single opioid may also have dual agonist/antagonist effect on a single receptor; these are known as partial agonists. Buprenorphine is a partial agonist at the μ- and an antagonist at the κ-receptor. Pentazocine produces analgesia and also dysphoria by activating spinal κ-receptors, and is a weak antagonist of μ-receptors. Partial agonists have a limited ceiling of therapeutic efficacy and by antagonism will precipitate a withdrawal syndrome if given to subjects dependent on morphine or heroin (high-efficacy agonists). In addition, a weak (low-efficacy) agonist (codeine) will compete with a high-efficacy opioid for receptors and so reduce the receptor occupancy, and therefore the therapeutic efficacy of the latter. Thus a weak agonist partially antagonises a strong agonist. It is no surprise that there are differences between opioids in both emphasis and the pattern of their many actions.

Pure competitive opioid antagonists, e.g. naloxone, naltrexone, block all opioid receptors while exerting no activating effect.

Some of the endorphins, dynorphin and enkephalins are about as active as morphine and some have higher efficacy. The discovery of the function of natural opioid mechanisms in physiology and pathology opens up possibilities for major developments in pain management, and indeed, wider, for endogenous opioid mechanisms may play a role, e.g. in shock.

Morphine and other opioids

Morphine will be described in detail and other opioid analgesics principally in so far as they differ. Morphine acts mainly on the opioid $μ_1$-receptor (analgesia, euphoria, dependence) and $μ_2$-receptors (respiratory depression, reduced gut motility). The principal actions of morphine may be summarised:

On the central nervous system:
- *Depression*, leading to: analgesia, respiratory depression, depression of cough reflex, sleep

- *Excitation,* leading to: vomiting, miosis, hyperactive spinal cord reflexes (some only), convulsions (very rare)
- *Changes of mood:* euphoria or dysphoria
- *Dependence;* affects other systems too.

Peripheral nervous system:
- Analgesia, some anti-inflammatory effect

Smooth muscle stimulation:
- Gastrointestinal muscle spasm (delayed passage of contents with constipation)
- Biliary tract spasm
- Bronchospasm

Cardiovascular system:
- Dilatation of resistance (arterioles) and capacitance (veins) vessels.

MORPHINE ON THE CENTRAL NERVOUS SYSTEM

Morphine is the most generally useful high-efficacy opioid analgesic; it eliminates pain and also allows subjects to tolerate pain, i.e. the sensation is felt but is no longer unpleasant. It both stimulates and depresses the central nervous system. It induces a state of relaxation, tranquillity, detachment and well-being (euphoria), or occasionally of unpleasantness (dysphoria), and causes sleepiness, inability to concentrate and lethargy, always supposing that this pleasant state is not destroyed by nausea and vomiting—more common if the patient is ambulant. Excitement can occur but is unusual. Morphine excites cats and horses, though it is illegal to put this to practical use. Generally, morphine has useful hypnotic and tranquillising actions and there should be no hesitation in using it in full dose in appropriate circumstances, e.g. acute pain and fear, as in myocardial infarction or road traffic accidents.

Morphine *depresses respiration,* principally by reducing sensitivity of the respiratory centre to increases in blood $PaCO_2$. With therapeutic doses there is a reduced minute volume first due to diminished rate and then tidal volume. With higher doses carbon dioxide narcosis may develop. In overdose the patient may present with a respiratory rate as low as 2/min.

Morphine is *dangerous* when the respiratory drive is impaired by disease, including CO_2 retention from any cause, e.g. chronic obstructive lung disease, asthma or raised intracranial pressure.

In *asthmatics,* in addition to the effect on the respiratory centre, it may increase viscosity of bronchial secretions, which, with depression of cough and bronchospasm (see below) will increase small airways resistance.

Morphine also suppresses *cough* by a central action. It stimulates the third nerve nucleus causing miosis (pin-point pupils are characteristic of poisoning, acute or chronic; at therapeutic doses the pupil is merely smaller).

The chemoreceptor trigger zone of the *vomiting centre* is stimulated, causing nausea (10%) and vomiting (15%), an effect which, in addition to being unpleasant, can be dangerous to patients soon after abdominal operations or cataract surgery. A preparation of morphine plus an antiemetic, e.g. cyclizine (Cyclimorph) reduces this liability. Some spinal cord reflexes are also stimulated, causing myoclonus and so morphine is unsuitable for use in tetanus and convulsant poisoning; indeed, morphine can itself cause convulsions.

Morphine causes *antidiuresis* by releasing antidiuretic hormone, and this can be clinically important.

Appetite is lost with chronic use.

Peripheral nervous system. The discovery of opioid receptors is sensory nerves and their inhibiting effect on inflammatory mediators may lead to advances in pain control.

MORPHINE ON SMOOTH MUSCLE

Alimentary tract. Morphine activates receptors on the smooth muscle of the stomach (antrum) and of both large and small bowel, causing it to contract. Peristalsis (propulsion) is reduced and segmentation increased. Thus, although morphine 'stimulates' smooth muscle, delayed gastric emptying and constipation occur, with gut muscle in a state of tonic contraction. Delay in the passage of the intestinal contents results in greater absorption of water and increased viscosity of faeces, which contribute to the constipation. The management of such opioid-induced constipation is an important aspect of palliative care.

Morphine increases pressure in the sigmoid colon and colonic diverticula may become obstructed and fail to drain into the colon. Pethidine neither produces these high pressures nor prevents drainage, and so is preferable if the pain of acute diverticulitis is severe enough to demand a narcotic analgesic. Morphine may also endanger anastomoses of the bowel immediately postoperatively and it should not be given in intestinal obstruction (excepting in palliative care).

Intrabiliary pressure may rise substantially after morphine (as much as 10 times in 10 minutes), due to spasm of the sphincter of Oddi. Sometimes biliary colic is made worse by morphine, presumably in a patient in whom the dose happens to be adequate to increase intrabiliary pressure, but insufficient to produce more than slight analgesia. In patients who have had a cholecystectomy this can produce a syndrome sufficiently like a myocardial infarction to cause diagnostic confusion. Naloxone may give dramatic symptomatic relief, as may glyceryl trinitrate. Another result of this action of morphine is to dam back the pancreatic juice and so cause a rise in the serum amylase concentration. Morphine is therefore best avoided in pancreatitis; but buprenorphine has less of this effect.

Bronchial muscle is constricted, partly due to histamine release, but so slightly as to be of no importance, except in asthmatics in whom morphine should be avoided anyway because of its respiratory depressant effect.

Urinary tract. Any contraction of the ureters is probably clinically unimportant. Retention of urine may occur (particularly in prostatic hypertrophy) due to a mix of spasm of the bladder sphincter and to the central sedation causing the patient to ignore afferent messages from a full bladder.

In general, when morphine is used and the smooth muscle effects are objectionable, atropine may be given simultaneously to antagonise spasm. Unfortunately this does not always effectively oppose the rise of pressure induced in the biliary system, nor does it restore bowel peristalsis. Glyceryl trinitrate will relax morphine-induced spasm.

MORPHINE ON THE CARDIOVASCULAR SYSTEM

Morphine, by a central action, impairs sympathetic vascular reflexes (causing veno- and arteriolar dilatation) and stimulates the vagal centre (bradycardia); it also releases histamine (vasodilatation). These effects are ordinarily unimportant, but they can be beneficial in acute left ventricular failure, relieving mental distress by tranquillising, cardiac distress by reduction of sympathetic drive and preload (by venodilatation), and respiratory distress by rendering the centre insensitive to afferent stimuli from the congested lungs.

Other effects of morphine include sweating, histamine release, pruritus and piloerection.

TOLERANCE

Chronic use of morphine and other opioids is marked by acquired tolerance to the depressant agonist effects, e.g. analgesic action and respiratory depression (the fatal dose becomes higher), but not to some stimulant agonist effects, e.g. constipation and miosis, which persist.

Opioids that have mixed agonist/antagonist actions (partial agonists) induce tolerance to the agonist but not to the antagonist effects; naloxone (a pure antagonist) induces no tolerance to itself. There is a cross-tolerance between opioids (for dependence and withdrawal see below).

Acquired tolerance develops over days with continued frequent use and passes off (variably for different actions) over a few days to weeks.

PHARMACOKINETICS

Oral morphine is subject to extensive presystemic metabolism (mainly conjugation in gut wall and liver) and only about 20% of a dose reaches the systemic circulation; the initial oral dose is about twice the injected dose. Given s.c. (particularly) or i.m., morphine is rapidly absorbed when the circulation is normal, but in circulatory shock absorption will be delayed and morphine is best given i.v.

Morphine in the systemic circulation is metabolised by both liver and kidney; the conjugated metabolites include the pharmacologically active morphine-6-glucuronide and morphine-3-glucuronide.[28] Elimination of morphine (10%) and metabolites is largely renal and is prolonged in renal failure, sufficient to warrant care in selecting morphine and deciding its dose and dose interval for such patients. The $t\frac{1}{2}$ is 3 h (active metabolites slightly longer) and the duration of useful analgesia is 3–6 h (shorter in younger than in older subjects).

Morphine crosses the placenta and depresses respiration in the fetus at birth.

Other routes of administration used by specialists are epidural (obstetrics) and intrathecal (see p. 360); very low doses are used.

PRINCIPAL USES OF MORPHINE AND ITS ANALOGUES

- Relief of moderate to severe acute pain (or chronic pain often in terminal illness)
- Brief relief of anxiety in serious and frightening disease accompanied by pain, e.g. trauma
- Relief of dyspnoea in acute left ventricular failure, and in terminal cancer
- Premedication for surgery
- Symptomatic control of acute nonserious diarrhoea, e.g. travellers' diarrhoea (codeine)
- Suppression of cough (codeine)
- Production of euphoria as well as pain relief in the dying.

Opioid-induced nausea, vomiting and dysphoria may interfere with any of the desired effects.

Dose. There is much individual variation: given s.c. or i.m. morphine 10 mg is usually adequate; with 15 mg unwanted effects increase more than does analgesia; i.v. give (slowly) one-quarter to one-half of the i.m. dose. For oral dosage see Palliative care, page 329. Continuous pain suppression can be achieved by morphine orally and s.c. 4-hourly.

---

[28] Metabolites of morphine appear to underlie the curious phenomenon of *allodynia*, when a normally painless stimulus is experienced as painful, *hyperalgesia*, which is the experience of unusually heightened pain from a known painful stimulus, and *myoclonia*. These have been observed in some patients after large and prolonged doses of morphine. The explanation may involve morphine-3-glucuronide which antagonises the analgesic effect of morphine and morphine-6-glucoronide.

Morphine and disease. When intense peripheral vasoconstriction accompanies, e.g. trauma, morphine administered s.c. or i.m. may appear to be ineffective because it fails quickly to enter the systemic circulation; repeating the dose before the first has been absorbed may lead to poisoning when the vasoconstriction passes off. In such circumstances morphine should be given slowly i.v. (2.5 mg every 2–3 min). If the blood volume is low, morphine may cause serious hypotension.

In hepatic failure small doses can cause coma (see p. 656), and it may be dangerous in hypothyroidism (slow metabolism). In an acute asthmatic attack, morphine is dangerous.

Adverse effects (type A) have been discussed. Dependence and overdose are treated below. Opioid use in obstetrics requires special care (p. 362).

Interactions. Morphine (also pethidine and possibly other opioids) is potentiated by monoamine oxidase inhibitors. Any central nervous system depressant (including alcohol) will have additive effects. Patients recently exposed to neuromuscular blocking agents (unless this is adequately reversed, e.g. by neostigmine) are particularly at risk from the respiratory depressant effects of morphine. The effect of diuretic drugs may be reduced by release of antidiuretic hormone by morphine. Useful interactions include the potentiating effect on pain relief of tricyclic antidepressants and of dexamfetamine.

OPIOID DEPENDENCE

Physical dependence begins to occur within 24 h if morphine is given 4-hourly, and after surgery some patients may be unwittingly subjected to a withdrawal syndrome that passes for general postoperative discomfort.

Acquired tolerance may rapidly reach a high degree, and an addict may take morphine 600 mg (heroin equivalent 400 mg) or even more several times a day. An average addict is more likely to take about 300 mg. Duration of tolerance after cessation of administration is variable for different actions, from a few days to weeks. Thus, addicts who have undergone withdrawal and lost tolerance, and who later resume their opioid careers may overdose themselves inadvertently.

Morphine or heroin dependence is more disabling physically and socially than is opium dependence (treatment of pain in opioid dependent subjects, see p. 343). Chronic exposure to opioids leads to adaptive changes in the endogenous opioid system and no doubt in receptor numbers, sensitivity and cellular response. The abrupt withdrawal of administered opioid usually provokes rebound or a withdrawal syndrome. This consists largely of the opposite of the normal actions of opioids. Also, noradrenergic mechanisms are modulated by endogenous opioids and these mechanisms are depressed by continuous opioid administration. Abrupt withdrawal rebound can be described as 'noradrenergic storm'.

ACUTE WITHDRAWAL SYNDROME
(morphine, heroin)

When an addict misses his first shot, he senses mild withdrawal distress ('feels his habit coming on') but this is probably more psychological than physiological, for fear plays a considerable role in the withdrawal syndrome. At this stage a placebo may give relief. During the first 8–16 h of abstinence the addict becomes increasingly nervous, restless and anxious; close confinement tends to intensify these symptoms. Within 14 h (usually less) he will begin to yawn frequently; he sweats profusely and develops running of the eyes and nose comparable to that accompanying a severe head cold.

These symptoms increase in intensity for the first 24 h, after which the pupils dilate and recurring waves of goose-flesh occur. Severe twitching of the muscles (the origin of the term 'kick the habit') occurs within 36 h and painful cramps develop in the backs of the legs and in the abdomen; all the body fluids are released copiously; vomiting and diarrhoea are acute; there is little appetite for food and the subject is unable to sleep. The respiratory rate rises steeply. Both systolic and diastolic blood pressure increase moderately to a maximum between the third and fourth day; temperature rises an average of about 0.5°C, subsiding after the third day; the blood sugar content rises sharply until the third day or after; the basal metabolic rate increases sharply during the first 48 h.

These are the objective signs of withdrawal distress which can be measured; the subjective indications are equally severe and the illness reaches its peak within 48–72 h after the last dose of the opioid, gradually subsiding thereafter for the next 5–10 days. The withdrawal syndrome proper is self-limiting and most addicts will survive it with no medical assistance whatever (this is known as kicking the habit, 'cold turkey'). Abrupt withdrawal is inhumane, but with the use of such drugs as methadone, it is possible to reduce the distress of withdrawal very considerably.[29]

MANAGEMENT OF OPIOID DEPENDENCE

Opioid. *Withdrawal* from dependence[30] is usually managed by substituting another opioid drug. *Methadone* is the treatment of choice; it has an affinity for the μ-receptor that is similar to that of morphine but occupies it for longer (24 h) and its slow offset of effect attenuates withdrawal symptoms. Upward titration of its effect to the dose that prevents withdrawal symptoms is relatively straightforward (initial dose 10–20 mg/day). Thereafter serial reductions in dose are made; in the most rapid regimen this takes 7–21 days but more commonly the process takes many months with more gradual decrements as the dose is lowered. Methadone is also the preferred drug in opioid *maintenance programmes* for addicts who decline to withdraw.

Methadone is less likely to be diverted (traded on the black market) than shorter-acting drugs. In the UK a special Methadone Mixture 1 mg/ml (the concentration is part of the official title) is specially provided for the management of opioid addicts; it is coloured green and formulated to prevent injection.[31]

---

[29] From Maurer D W, Vogel V H 1962 Narcotics and narcotic addiction. Thomas, Springfield, Illinois. Courtesy of the authors and publisher.
[30] For a general account, see: Drug Misuse and Dependence — Guidelines on Clinical Management. HMSO, London, 1999.
[31] It has × 2.5 the strength of Methadone Linctus, for cough (yellow or brown); they must not be confused.

Buprenorphine is an alternative for it also has a long duration of action but it both stimulates and blocks the μ-receptor (i.e. it is a partial agonist) and can provoke withdrawal symptoms in patients taking opioid in high dose. Buprenorphine is appears to have less euphoriant effect than morphine. It is unkind, because it is unnecessary, to use an antagonist as a diagnostic test in suspected addicts but *naltrexone*, a pure antagonist, blocks the opioid euphoriant effect and may be used to prevent relapse in former addicts (see p. 341).

Nonopioid. The withdrawal syndrome is also treatable with nonopioid drugs. *Lofexidine* inhibits sympathetic autonomic outflow by its agonist action on central presynaptic α_2-adrenoceptors and so reduces the effects of noradrenergic hyperactivity (see above). It is similar to clonidine (see p. 482) but less likely to cause hypotension. Evidence indicates that lofexidine is as effective as methadone in withdrawal supervised in residential or community settings; having no 'street value' it is not liable to be traded.

A withdrawal syndrome occurs in the newborn of dependent mothers. It is important not to attempt to reduce the mother's use of opioid late in pregnancy, as a more severe and unpredictable neonatal withdrawal syndrome may result.

OVERDOSE

Death (from all opioids, low and high efficacy; agonist or partial agonist) is due to respiratory failure. Blood pressure is usually well maintained, if the patient is supine, until cerebral anoxia causes circulatory failure. At this stage the (pinpoint) pupils may dilate (also if there is hypothermia). The combination of miosis and bradypnoea gives the diagnosis which is vital, for *naloxone*, a selective competitive antagonist, is life-saving.[32] Naloxone, having none of the agonist effects of morphine (respiratory depression, miosis, coma), is safe to give as a diagnostic test in an unconscious or drowsy patient suspected of opioid overdose. The $t\frac{1}{2}$ of naloxone (1 h) is shorter than most opioids and repeated doses or infusion will be needed. The guide to therapy is the state of respiration, not of consciousness. Patients with opioid overdose should be monitored for recurrence of ventilatory depression, which is an indication for further naloxone (for

details see p. 342). Apart from naloxone the general treatment is the same as for overdose by any cerebral depressant. Addicts often take drug overdoses, whether accidentally or not, and naloxone, as well as reversing the life-endangering respiratory depression, will induce an acute (noradrenergic) withdrawal syndrome. Close cardiovascular monitoring is necessary, with use of peripheral adrenoceptor blocking agents or perhaps lofexidine (see above), according to need.

Classification of opioids by analgesic efficacy

Low efficacy for mild and moderate pain	High efficacy for severe pain
codeine	*buprenorphine
dihydrocodeine	dexromoramide
dextropropoxyphene	diamorphine (heroin)
*nalbuphine	dipipanone
*pentazocine	*meptazinol
	methadone
	morphine
	papaveretum
	pethidine (meperidine)
	phenazocine
	tramadol
*Partial agonist	

Notes:

- The division into two classes is not absolute and some drugs listed for moderate pain can be effective in severe pain by injection.

---

[32] As the following account illustrates: …We saw this guy lying on the ground with two people trying to help him — they were trying to help him breathe by mouth to mouth. When we ran over to them we could tell it was not working. The guy was blue in the face and hardly breathing any more. Right away I gave him one ampoule of naloxone — I didn't think I could find a vein so I just shot it real slow into his upper arm. …Then the guy started to wake up and he started to breathe and shake a little. …When the medics came I told them I had given him naloxone. The medic said 'Wow! So you guys have even got naloxone now?' (Dettmer K, Saunders B, Strang J 2001 British Medical Journal 322: 895–896).

- Fentanyl, alfentanil and remifentanil are high-efficacy opioids used for surgery/anaesthesia.

Partial agonists were developed in the unrealised hope of eliminating the potential for abuse whilst retaining analgesic efficacy. They are indeed less liable to induce dependence and to cause respiratory depression than are the pure agonists but they may induce psychotomimetic reactions. Their antagonist action is chiefly evident against large doses of agonist, e.g. in addicts.

Etorphine is a high-efficacy opioid which, combined with a neuroleptic, is used to immobilise animals in veterinary practice. The doses used in large animals are enough to kill an adult human if, in a struggle, the drug is splashed on skin or mucous membrane, or there is a needle scratch. A competitive antagonist, naloxone (or diprenorphine which accompanies veterinary formulations, and is labelled for use in animals only) should be used at once in man in this urgent situation (do not delay to fetch an official human formulation; death has occurred where this was done). Wash a splashed site copiously *at once*.

Notes on individual opioids

The opioids discussed below are considered in relation to morphine. Note that the $t\frac{1}{2}$ *does not necessarily indicate duration of useful analgesia*, which is also related to affinity of the opioid for receptors; but $t\frac{1}{2}$ gives useful information on accumulation.

CODEINE (methylmorphine)

Codeine is a low-efficacy opioid that binds to μ-receptors; 10% is converted to morphine ($t\frac{1}{2}$ 3 h). It lacks efficacy for severe pain and most of its actions are about one-tenth those of morphine. A qualitative difference from morphine is that large doses cause excitement. Dependence occurs but much less than with morphine.

Its principal uses are for mild and moderate pain and cough (long-term use is accompanied by chronic constipation) and for the short-term symptomatic control of the milder acute diarrhoeas. There are numerous formulations for cough, e.g. Codeine Linctus, and for pain, in which it is commonly combined with paracetamol and/or aspirin.

PETHIDINE (meperidine)

Pethidine attracted attention as a possible analgesic because it caused the tails of laboratory mice to stand erect (Straub phenomenon), a characteristic of morphine-like drugs caused by spasm of the anal sphincter.

Pethidine binds to the μ- and κ-receptors; it is effective for moderate or severe pain but its duration of action is shorter than that of morphine. It is effective against pain beyond the reach of codeine. Despite its substantial structural dissimilarity to morphine, pethidine has many similar properties including that of being antagonised by naloxone.

Pethidine differs from morphine in that it:

- does not usefully suppress cough
- is less likely to constipate; but its effect in the upper small intestine is similar to morphine including contraction of the sphincter of Oddi
- is less likely to cause urinary retention and to prolong childbirth
- has little hypnotic effect
- has a shorter duration of analgesia (2–3 h).

Pethidine is extensively metabolised in the liver and the parent drug and metabolites are excreted in the urine ($t\frac{1}{2}$ 5 h). Norpethidine retains pharmacological activity and may accumulate dangerously when renal function is impaired.

Pethidine causes vomiting about as often as does morphine; it has atropine-like effects, including dry mouth and blurred vision (cycloplegia and sometimes mydriasis, though usually miosis). Overdose or use in renal failure can cause central nervous system stimulation (myoclonus, convulsions) due to norpethidine.

There is disagreement on the extent to which pethidine depresses respiration. It is probable that in equianalgesic doses it is as depressant as morphine.

Pethidine dependence occurs, with some tolerance, especially to the side-effects, but its psychic effects are less constant and less marked than those of morphine. Pethidine has evident advantages over morphine for pain that is not very intense, and it is widely used. It is usually given orally (50–100 mg) s.c. or i.m. (25–100 mg), when its effects last 2–3 h. It is widely used in obstetrics because it does not delay labour like morphine; but it enters the fetus and can depress respiration at birth.

METHADONE

Methadone is a synthetic drug structurally and pharmacologically similar to morphine; it acts mainly at the μ-receptor. Methadone is largely metabolised to products that are excreted in the urine ($t\frac{1}{2}$ 8 h). The principal feature of methadone is its duration of action. Analgesia may last for as long as 24 h. If used for chronic pain in palliative care (12-hourly) an opioid of short $t\frac{1}{2}$ should be provided for breakthrough pain rather than an extra dose of methadone.

The long duration of action also favours its use to cover opioid withdrawal (see before). Occupancy of opioid receptors by methadone reduces the desire for other opioids, and their effects, should any be taken; the slow offset diminishes the severity of the withdrawal. Addicts who are cooperative enough to take oral methadone feel reduced craving and less 'kick/buzz/rush' from i.v. heroin or morphine because their opioid receptors are already occupied by methadone and the i.v. drug must compete. Dependence occurs but this is less severe than with morphine or heroin. Reports of deaths in addicts entering prescribed methadone substitution programmes have been attributed to the cardio-vascular effects of a membrane stabilising action, unlike morphine.

Vomiting is fairly common with methadone (though somewhat less so than with morphine) especially if the patient is ambulant, and sedation is less.

Methadone is also useful for severe cough.

DIAMORPHINE (heroin)

This semisynthetic drug was first made from morphine at St Mary's Hospital, London in 1874. It was introduced in 1898 as a remedy for cough and for morphine addiction; later it was appreciated that it 'cured' morphine addiction by substituting itself as the addicting agent.

Pharmacokinetics. Diamorphine (diacetylmorphine) is converted in the body within minutes to morphine and 6-monoacetylmorphine, a metabolite of both drugs; the effects of diamorphine are principally due to the actions of morphine and 6-monoacetylmorphine on the μ- and, to a lesser extent, the κ-receptors. Diamorphine given parenterally has a $t\frac{1}{2}$ of 3 min. When given orally it is subject to complete presystemic or first-pass metabolism and only morphine ($t\frac{1}{2}$ 3 h) and the metabolites reach the systemic circulation. Thus oral diamorphine is essentially a prodrug. The greater potency of diamorphine (diamorphine 1 mg = morphine 1.5 mg) may be due to the metabolite 6-acetylmorphine and to the common use of morphine as sulphate and diamorphine as hydrochloride.

Use. Diamorphine is used medicinally for acute pain, e.g. myocardial infarction and chronic pain, e.g. in palliative care. Diamorphine provides a more rapid onset of pain relief than morphine because it is more lipid soluble and enters the brain more readily. Its duration of action is about the same and it may cause less nausea and hypotension. Diamorphine is more soluble than morphine to a useful degree.[33] This, together with its greater potency (greater efficacy in relation to weight and therefore requiring a smaller volume) makes dia-morphine suitable to deliver by s.c. infusion through a syringe driver when continuous pain control is required in palliative care and can no longer be achieved by enteral morphine (oral, buccal, sup-pository) (see Patient-controlled analgesia, p. 328).

Diamorphine is also used for severe cough (Diamorphine Linctus).

Abuse. It is commonly stated that diamorphine (heroin) is the 'most potent' of all dependence-producing opioids. Weight-for-weight it is certainly more effective than morphine, and this is of importance in illicit traffic as diamorphine takes up less space, but in so far as efficacy in inducing dependence is concerned, there is doubt.

In almost every country the manufacture of diamorphine, even for use in medicine, is now illegal. The first to try this prohibition as a remedy for widespread drug addiction was the USA, which

---

[33] Solubility in water: morphine sulphate 1 in 21; diamorphine hydrochloride 1 in 1.6.

banned diamorphine manufacture in 1924, provoked by the magnitude of the addiction problem and not yet discouraged by the experience of this type of approach with alcohol prohibition (1919–1933).

An effort was made in 1953 to achieve a worldwide ban on diamorphine in medicine (so that any diamorphine, wherever it was found must be illegal) and many countries agreed. The UK did not agree because legitimate supplies for medicine were not than getting into illicit channels (it has since remained available for medicinal use but is not exported). A ban now would be pointless since illegal diamorphine is readily available worldwide.

PENTAZOCINE

Pentazocine provides a type of analgesia that is different from morphine. Its analgesic effect is probably due to an agonist action at κ-receptors in the spinal cord; it is a weak antagonist of μ-receptors (through which morphine produces analgesia). Thus pentazocine can cause a withdrawal syndrome in addicts (antagonist effect); it can also induce psychological and physical dependence (agonist effect), and this can be severe. It has not proved to be the solution to separating the property of analgesia from that of producing dependence, as was hoped for initially. Its analgesic efficacy approximates to that of morphine, but its potency (weight for weight) is about one-third of morphine. Compared to morphine, pentazocine produces shorter duration of pain relief, less dependence (but this definitely occurs), more psychotomimetic effects, and less sedation and respiratory depression (naloxone can reverse the respiratory depression in overdose).

Pharmacokinetics. Pentazocine is extensively metabolised in the liver and less than 10% is excreted unchanged in the urine ($t^{1/2}$ 5 h).

Uses. Pentazocine is given to relieve moderate to severe pain, and also for chronic pain, for its liability to induce dependence is less than morphine. Its dysphoric effect limits its usefulness.

Adverse effects of this partial agonist include: nausea, vomiting, dizziness, sweating, hypertension, palpitations, tachycardia, central nervous system disturbance (euphoria, dysphoria, psychotomimesis).

Pentazocine has effects on the cardiovascular system, raising systolic blood pressure and pulmonary artery pressure; avoid it in myocardial infarction.

Phenazocine is a high-efficacy agonist used particularly in biliary colic for it has less capacity than other opioids to cause spasm of the sphincter of Oddi. It may be administered sublingually if the patient is vomiting.

Buprenorphine is a high-efficacy partial agonist of the μ-receptor and an antagonist of the κ-receptor. Its high receptor affinity (tenacity of binding) may explain why respiratory depression is only partially reversed by naloxone; a respiratory stimulant (doxapram) may be needed in overdose, or mechanical ventilation. It has less liability to induce dependence and respiratory depression than pure agonists, little effect on the cardiovascular system and may spare the sphincter of Oddi from induced spasm. Its $t^{1/2}$ is 5 h. Because of extensive presystemic elimination when swallowed, buprenorphine is given by the buccal (sublingual) route (200–400 micrograms) or by i.m., or slow i.v., injection (300–600 micrograms). It is a useful analgesic because of the length (about 6 h) and strength of its action, its low liability to cause dependence and the fact that administration by injection can be avoided, e.g. for children, patients with bleeding disorder.

Dextropropoxyphene is structurally similar to methadone and differs in that it is less analgesic, antitussive, and less dependence-producing. Its analgesic usefulness approximates to that of codeine. Dextropropoxyphene is rapidly absorbed from the gastrointestinal tract and its plasma $t^{1/2}$ is 5 h. In overdose the rapidity of absorption is such that respiratory arrest may occur within one hour and also hypotension (probably due to membrane-stabilising or quinidine-like action causing cardiac arrhythmia), so that many subjects die before reaching hospital. Combination with alcohol (common with self-poisoning) enhances respiratory depression. Dextropropoxyphene is commonly combined with paracetamol (co-proxamol, Distalgesic). Dextropropoxyphene interacts with warfarin, enhancing its anticoagulant effect.

Dihydrocodeine (DFI18) is a low-efficacy opioid

with an analgesic efficacy similar to that of codeine. It is used to relieve moderate acute and chronic pain on its own or as a compound tablet (co-dydramol; dihydrocodeine 10 mg plus paracetamol 500 mg). Dihydrocodeine causes histamine release and should not be used in patients with hyper-reactive airways.

Meptazinol is a high-efficacy partial agonist; it also has central cholinergic activity which add to its analgesic effect. It is used to relieve acute or chronic pain of moderate intensity, e.g. postoperatively and in obstetrics. Meptazinol does not cause euphoria and withdrawal effects seem not to occur when it is discontinued. It appears not to induce a withdrawal syndrome in opioid-dependent subjects.

Tramadol is an opioid with additional actions; the basis of its analgesic effects appears to derive from a combination of (relatively weak) agonist action on µ-receptors, inhibition of neuronal noradrenaline uptake and enhanced serotonin release. It is rapidly absorbed from the gastrointestinal tract, 20% of an oral dose undergoes first-pass metabolism and less than 30% dose is excreted unchanged in the urine (t½ 6 h). Tramadol is approximately as effective as pethidine for postoperative pain and as morphine for moderate chronic pain.

Tramadol is claimed to be less likely to constipate, depress respiration and addict. Confusion, convulsions, hallucinations and anaplhylaxis have been reported with its use.

Dipipanone is less sedating and shorter acting than morphine; it is suitable for acute attacks of pain, e.g. breakthrough pain in terminal illness (Diconal is dipipanone plus cyclizine, an antiemetic).

Dextromethorphan, the dextroisomer of the opioid levomethorphan is used as an antitussive, e.g. in Actifed; the latter is sought as a drug of abuse by addicts.

Opioids during and after surgery

Small doses of opioids given with induction can usefully reduce the dose requirements of drugs used during anaesthesia. Those used are:

Fentanyl (t½ 3 h) has higher efficacy than morphine, analgesia lasts 30–60 min (single dose) and is used i.v. Fentanyl is also given for chronic and intractable cancer pain as self-adhesive patches which release the drug at approximately 25 micrograms/h for 72 h. Fentanyl is so potent that discarded patches may yet contain sufficient drug to be dangerous.

Alfentail (t½ 1.5 h), given i.v., provides maximum analgesia in 90 seconds, which lasts about 5–10 min from a single dose; it is used for brief (painful) operations.

Remifentanil is rapidly metabolised, not in the liver but by blood and tissue esterases. Its short duration of action renders it well suited for continuous i.v. infusion without accumulation.

Opioids (nonanalgesic) for an antimotility effect on the gut include loperamide and diphenoxylate (p. 644).

Opioid antagonists

NALOXONE (Narcan)

Naloxone is a pure competitive antagonist at all opioid receptors, notably the µ- and κ- receptors; it has no agonist activity. Naloxone antagonises both agonist and partial agonist opioids (although it may not be sufficient to reverse the effects of buprenorphine in overdose, so tenaciously does the latter drug bind to receptors). It induces an acute withdrawal syndrome in opioid-dependent subjects.

Naloxone undergoes high presystemic elimination when swallowed and is not used by this route; some 70% of a dose appears in the urine as metabolites (t½ 75 min).

Given i.v., it causes reversal of opioid-induced respiratory depression in 1–2 min; reversal of analgesia and depressed consciousness can be slower. A prompt marked improvement in respiration has diagnostic value in opioid overdose, but poor or no response may occur because insufficient has been given, or with burenorphine (above), or due to cerebral hypoxia or severe hyothermia.

Naloxone acts for about one hour after an i.v. injection of 100–200 micrograms, though the peak effect on depressed respiration may be as brief as 10 min. As opioid analgesics in general act for much longer than this, further i.v. boluses of 100 micrograms should be given at 2-min intervals until changes in respiration, pupils or consciousness indicate response; the subsequent doses may be given by i.m. injection. A continuous i.v. infusion commencing with 2.5 micrograms/kg/h may be required for days with opioids having a long $t\frac{1}{2}$ (methadone). Naloxone is also used to counter excess opioid effects after surgical analgesia or childbirth.

Naltrexone ($t\frac{1}{2}$ 4 h: active metabolite 13 h) is similar to naloxone but longer-acting, with duration of effect 1–3 days according to dose. It can be used orally to assist in the rehabilitation of ex-opioid abusers who are fully withdrawn (otherwise it will induce an acute withdrawal syndrome). A patient who then takes an opioid fails to experience the 'kick' or euphoria, although naltrexone does not reduce craving as does the agonist methadone. This use of naltrexone requires careful selection and supervision of subjects.

Pain in opioid addicts

A nonopioid analgesic useful for pain in opioid addicts is *nefopam* (Acupan), being neither an opioid nor an NSAID. Its mode of action is not fully understood but it may involve adrenergic and serotonergic mechanisms. It is effective against moderate pain. Since it lacks the disadvantages of opioids (constipation, respiratory depression) and has greater efficacy than NSAIDs, it provides an alternative. NSAIDs may be used for pain of milder degree (see Ch. 15).

GUIDE TO FURTHER READING

Ashburn M A, Staats P S 1999 Management of chronic pain. Lancet 353: 1865–1869

Besson J M 1999 The neurobiology of pain, Lancet 353: 1610–1615

Billings J A 2000 Palliative care. British Medical Journal 321: 555–558

Carr D B, Goudas L C 1999 Acute pain. Lancet 353: 2051–2058

Cervero F, Laird J M A 1999 Visceral pain. Lancet 353: 2145–2148

Chapman C R, Gavrin J 1999 Suffering: the contribution of persistent pain. Lancet 353: 2233–2237

Goadsby P J, Lipton R B, Ferrari M D 2002 Migraine – current understanding and treatment. New England Journal of Medicine 346: 257–270

McQuay H 1999 Opioids in pain management. Lancet 353: 2229–2232

McQuay H, Moore A, Justins D 1997 Treating acute pain in hospital. British Medical Journal 314: 1531–1535

Nurmikko T J, Nash T P, Wiles J R 1998 Control of pain. British Medical Journal 317: 1438–1441

Portenoy R K, Lesage P 1999 Management of cancer pain. Lancet 353: 1695–1700

Sneader W 1998 The discovery of heroin. Lancet 352: 1697–1699

Woolf C J, Mannion R J 1999 Neuropathic pain: aetiology, symptoms, mechanisms, and management. Lancet 353: 1959–1964

18

Anaesthesia and neuromuscular block

SYNOPSIS

The administration of general anaesthetics and neuromuscular blocking drugs is generally confined to trained specialists. Nevertheless, nonspecialists are involved in perioperative care and will benefit from an understanding of how these drugs act. Doctors from a variety of specialties use local anaesthetics and the pharmacology of these drugs is discussed in detail.

- General anaesthesia
- Pharmacology of anaesthetics
- Inhalation anaesthetics
- Intravenous anaesthetics
- Muscle relaxants: neuromuscular blocking drugs
- Local anaesthetics
- Obstetric analgesia and anaesthesia
- Anaesthesia in patients already taking drugs
- Anaesthesia in the diseased, the elderly and children; sedation in intensive therapy units

General anaesthesia

Until the mid-19th century such surgery as was possible had to be undertaken at tremendous speed. Surgeons did their best for terrified patients by using alcohol, opium, hyoscine,[1] or cannabis. With the introduction of general anaesthesia, surgeons could operate for the first time with careful deliberation. The problem of inducing quick, safe and easily reversible unconsciousness for any desired length of time in man only began to be solved in the 1840s when the long-known substances nitrous oxide, ether, and chloroform were introduced in rapid succession.

The details surrounding the first use of surgical anaesthesia were submerged in bitter disputes on priority following an attempt to take out a patent for ether. The key events around this time were:

- 1842 — W. E. Clarke of Rochester, New York, administered for a dental extraction. However, this event was not made widely known at the time.
- 1844 — Horace Wells, a dentist in Hartford, Connecticut, introduced nitrous oxide to produce anaesthesia during dental extraction.
- 1846 — On October 16 William Morton, a Boston dentist, successfully demonstrated the anaesthetic properties of ether.
- 1846 — On December 21 Robert Liston performed the first surgical operation in England under ether anaesthesia.[2]

---

[1] A Japanese pioneer of about 1800 wished to test the anaesthetic efficacy of a herbal mixture including solanaceous plants (hyoscine-type alkaloids). His elderly mother volunteered as subject since she was anyway expected to die soon. But the pioneer administered it to his wife for, 'as all three agreed, he could find another wife, but could never get another mother' (Journal of the American Medical Association 1966 197: 10).

- 1847 — James Y. Simpson, professor of midwifery at the University of Edinburgh, introduced chloroform for the relief of labour pain.

The next important developments in anaesthesia were in the 20th century when the appearance of new drugs both as primary general anaesthetics and as adjuvants (muscle relaxants), new apparatus, and clinical expertise in rendering prolonged anaesthesia safe, enabled surgeons to increase their range. No longer was the duration and type of surgery determined by patients' capacity to endure pain.

STAGES OF GENERAL ANAESTHESIA

Surgical anaesthesia is classically divided into four stages: analgesia, delirium, surgical anaesthesia (subdivided into four planes), and medullary paralysis (overdose). This gradual procession of stages was described when ether was given to un-premedicated patients, a slow unpleasant process. Ether is obsolete and the speed of induction with modern inhalational agents or intravenous anaesthesia drugs makes a detailed description of these separate stages superfluous.

Balanced surgical anaesthesia (hypnosis with analgesia and muscular relaxation) with a single drug requires high doses that will cause adverse effects such as slow and unpleasant recovery, and depression of cardiovascular and respiratory function. In modern practice, different drugs are used to attain each objective so that adverse effects are minimised.

DRUGS USED

The perioperative period may be divided into three phases and in each of these a variety of factors will determine the choice of drugs given:

---

[2] Frederick Churchill, a butler from Harley Street, had his leg amputated at University College Hospital, London. After removing the leg in 28 seconds, a skill necessary to compensate for the previous lack of anaesthetics, Robert Liston turned to the watching students, and said "this Yankee dodge, gentlemen, beats mesmerism hollow". That night he anaesthetised his house surgeon in the presence of two ladies. Merrington W R 1976 University College Hospital and its Medical School: A History. Heinemann, London.

Before surgery, an assessment is made of:
- the patient's physical and psychological condition
- any intercurrent illness
- the relevance of any existing drug therapy.

All of these may influence the choice of anaesthetic drugs.

During surgery, drugs will be required to provide:
- unconsciousness
- analgesia
- muscular relaxation when necessary
- control of blood pressure, heart rate, and respiration.

After surgery, drugs will play a part in:
- reversal of neuromuscular block
- relief of pain, and nausea and vomiting
- other aspects of postoperative care, including intensive care.

Patients are often already taking drugs affecting the central nervous and cardiovascular systems and there is considerable potential for interaction with anaesthetic drugs.

The techniques for giving anaesthetic drugs and the control of ventilation and oxygenation are of great importance, but are outside the scope of this book.

Before surgery (premedication)

The principal aims are to provide:

Anxiolysis and amnesia. A patient who is going to have a surgical operation is naturally apprehensive and this anxiety is reduced by reassurance and a clear explanation of what to expect. Very anxious patients will secrete a lot of adrenaline (epinephrine) from the suprarenal medulla and this may make them more liable to cardiac arrhythmias with some anaesthetics. In the past, sedative premedication was given to virtually all patients undergoing surgery. This practice has changed dramatically because of the increasing proportion of operations undertaken as 'day cases' and the recognition that sedative premedication prolongs recovery. Sedative premedication is now reserved for those who are particularly anxious or those undergoing major surgery.

Benzodiazepines, such as temazepam (10–30 mg for an adult), provide anxiolysis and amnesia for the immediate presurgical period.

Analgesia is indicated if the patient is in pain preoperatively or it can be given pre-emptively to prevent postoperative pain. Severe preoperative pain is treated with a parenteral opioid such as morphine. Nonsteroidal anti-inflammatory drugs and paracetamol are commonly given orally pre-operatively to prevent postoperative pain after minor surgery. For moderate or major surgery, these drugs are supplemented with an opioid towards the end of the procedure.

Drying of bronchial and salivary secretions using antimuscarinic drugs to inhibit the parasympathetic autonomic system is rarely undertaken these days. The exceptions include those patients who are expected to require an awake fibreoptic intubation or those undergoing bronchoscopy. Glycopyrronium is the antimuscarinic of choice for this purpose and atropine and hyoscine are alternatives.

Timing. Premedication is given about an hour before surgery.

Gastric contents. Pulmonary aspiration of gastric contents can cause severe pneumonitis. Patients at risk of aspiration are those with full stomachs, e.g., bowel obstruction, recently consumed food and drink, third trimester of pregnancy, and those with incompetent gastro-oesophageal sphincters, e.g. hiatus hernia. A single dose of an antacid, e.g. sodium citrate, may be given before a general anaesthetic to neutralise gastric acid in high-risk patients. Alternatively or additionally, a histamine H_2-receptor blocker, e.g. ranitidine, or proton-pump inhibitor, e.g. omeprazole, will reduce gastric secretion volume as well as acidity. Metoclopramide usefully hastens gastric emptying, increases the tone of the lower oesophageal sphincter and is an antiemetic.

During surgery

The aim is to induce unconsciousness, analgesia and muscular relaxation. Total muscular relaxation (paralysis) is required for some surgical procedures, e.g., intra-abdominal surgery, but most surgery can be undertaken without neuromuscular blockade.

A typical general anaesthetic consists of:

- *Induction:*
  1. Usually intravenous: pre-oxygenation followed by a small dose of an opioid, e.g., fentanyl or alfentanil to provide analgesia and sedation, followed by propofol or, less commonly, thiopental or etomidate to induce anaesthesia. Airway patency is maintained with an oral airway and face-mask, a laryngeal mask airway (LMA), or a tracheal tube. Insertion of a tracheal tube usually requires paralysis with a neuromuscular blocker and is undertaken if there is a risk of pulmonary aspiration from regurgitated gastric contents or from blood.
  2. Inhalational induction, usually with sevo-flurane, is undertaken taken less commonly. It is used in children, particularly if intravenous access is difficult, and in patients at risk from upper airway obstruction.

- *Maintenance:*
  1. Most commonly with nitrous oxide and oxygen, or oxygen and air, plus a volatile agent, e.g., isoflurane or sevoflurane. Additional doses of a neuromuscular blocker or opioid are given as required.
  2. A continuous intravenous infusion of propofol can be used to maintain anaesthesia. This technique of *total intravenous anaesthesia* is becoming more popular because the quality of recovery may be better than after inhalational anaesthesia.

When appropriate, peripheral nerve block with a local anaesthetic, or neural axis block, e.g., spinal or epidural, provides intraoperative analgesia and muscle relaxation. These local anaesthetic techniques provide excellent postoperative analgesia.

After surgery

The anaesthetist ensures that the effects of neuro-muscular blocking agents and opioid-induced respiratory depression have either worn off or have been adequately reversed by an antagonist; the patient is not left alone until conscious, with protective reflexes restored, and a stable circulation.

Relief of pain after surgery can be achieved with a variety of techniques. An epidural infusion of a mixture of local anaesthetic and opioid provides excellent pain relief after major surgery such as laparotomy. Parenteral morphine, given intermittently by a nurse or by a patient-controlled system, will also relieve moderate or severe pain but has the attendant risk of nausea, vomiting, sedation and respiratory depression. The addition of regular paracetamol and a NSAID, given orally or rectally, will provide additional pain relief and reduce the requirement for morphine. NSAIDs are contra-indicated if there is a history of gastrointestinal ulceration of if renal blood flow is compromised.

Postoperative nausea and vomiting (PONV) is common after laparotomy and major gynaecological surgery, e.g., abdominal hysterectomy. The use of propofol, particularly when given to maintain anaesthesia, has dramatically reduced the incidence of PONV. Antiemetics, such as cyclizine, metoclopramide, and ondansetron, may be helpful.

SOME SPECIAL TECHNIQUES

Dissociative anaesthesia is a state of profound analgesia and anterograde amnesia with minimal hypnosis during which the eyes may remain open (see ketamine, p. 353). It is particularly useful where modern equipment is lacking or where access to the patient is limited, e.g. at major accidents or on battlefields.

Sedation and amnesia without analgesia are provided by midazolam i.v. or, less commonly nowadays, diazepam. These drugs can be used alone for procedures causing mild discomfort, e.g. endoscopy, and with a local anaesthetic where more pain is expected, e.g., removal of impacted wisdom teeth. Benzodiazepines produce anterograde, but not retrograde, amnesia. By definition, the sedated patient remains responsive and cooperative. (For a general account of benzodiazepines and the competitive antagonist flumazenil, see Ch. 19.)

Benzodiazepines can cause respiratory depression and apnoea especially in the elderly and in patients with respiratory insufficiency. The combination of an opioid and a benzodiazepine is particularly dangerous. Benzodiazepines depress laryngeal reflexes and place the patient at risk of inhalation of oral secretions or dental debris.

Entonox, a 50:50 mixture of nitrous oxide and oxygen, is breathed by the patient using a demand valve. It is particularly useful in the prehospital environment and for brief procedures, such as splinting limbs.

Pharmacology of anaesthetics

All successful general anaesthetics are given intravenously or by inhalation because these routes allow closest control over blood concentrations and so of effect on the brain.

MODE OF ACTION

General anaesthetics act on the brain, primarily on the midbrain reticular activating system. Many anaesthetics are lipid soluble and there is good correlation between this and anaesthetic effectiveness (the Overton–Meyer hypothesis); the more lipid soluble tend to be the more potent anaesthetics, but such a correlation is not invariable. Some anaesthetic agents are not lipid soluble and many lipid soluble substances are not anaesthetics. Until recently it was thought that the principal site of action of general anaesthetics was the neuronal lipid bilayer membrane. The current view is that their anaesthetic activity is caused by interaction with protein receptors. It is likely that there are several modes of action, but the central mechanism of action of volatile anaesthetics is thought to be facilitation at the inhibitory γ-aminobutyric acid ($GABA_A$) and glycine receptors. Agonists at these receptors open chloride ion channels and the influx of chloride ions into the neuron results in hyper-polarisation. This prevents propagation of nerve impulses and renders the patient unconscious. Some general anaesthetics increase the time that the chloride channels are open while others increase the frequency of chloride channel opening.

ASSESSMENT OF ANAESTHETIC AGENTS

Comparison of the efficacy of inhalational agents is made by measuring the minimum alveolar concentration (MAC) in oxygen required to prevent movement in response to a standard surgical skin incision in 50% of subjects. The MAC of the volatile agent is reduced by the co-administration of nitrous oxide.

Inhalation anaesthetics

PREFERRED ANAESTHETICS

The preferred inhalation agents are those that are minimally irritant and nonflammable, and comprise nitrous oxide and the fluorinated hydrocarbons, e.g., isoflurane.

PHARMACOKINETICS (VOLATILE LIQUIDS, GASES)

The level of anaesthesia is correlated with the tension (partial pressure) of anaesthetic drug in the brain tissue and this is dependent on the development of a series of tension gradients from the high partial pressure delivered to the alveoli and decreasing through the blood to the brain and other tissues. These gradients are dependent on the blood/gas and tissue/gas solubility coefficients, as well as on alveolar ventilation and organ blood flow.

An anaesthetic that has high solubility in blood, i.e., a high blood/gas partition coefficient, will provide a slow induction and adjustment of the depth of anaesthesia. This is because the blood acts as a reservoir (store) for the drug so that it does not enter the brain easily until the blood reservoir has been filled. A rapid induction can be obtained by increasing the concentration of drug inhaled initially and by hyperventilating the patient.

Agents that have low solubility in blood, i.e., a low blood/gas partition coefficient (nitrous oxide, sevoflurane), provide a rapid induction of anaesthesia because the blood reservoir is small and agent is available to pass into the brain sooner.

During induction of anaesthesia the blood is taking up anaesthetic agent selectively and rapidly and the resulting loss of volume in the alveoli leads to a flow of agent into the lungs that is independent of respiratory activity. When the anaesthetic is discontinued the reverse occurs and it moves from the blood into the alveoli. In the case of nitrous oxide, this can account for as much as 10% of the expired volume and so can significantly lower the alveolar oxygen concentration. Thus mild hypoxia occurs and lasts for as long as 10 minutes. Though harmless to most, it may be a factor in cardiac arrest in patients with reduced pulmonary and cardiac reserve, especially when administration of the gas has been at high concentration and prolonged, when the outflow is especially copious. Oxygen should therefore be given to such patients during the last few minutes of anaesthesia and the early postanaesthetic period. This phenomenon, *diffusion hypoxia,* occurs with all gaseous anaesthetics, but is most prominent with gases that are relatively insoluble in blood, for they will diffuse out most rapidly when the drug is no longer inhaled, i.e. just as induction is faster, so is elimination. Nitrous oxide is especially powerful in this respect because it is used at concentrations of up to 70%. Highly blood-soluble agents will diffuse out more slowly, so that recovery will be slower just as induction is slower, and with them diffusion hypoxia is insignificant.

NITROUS OXIDE

Nitrous oxide (1844) is a gas with a slightly sweetish smell. It is neither flammable nor explosive. It produces light anaesthesia without demonstrably depressing the respiratory or vasomotor centre provided that normal oxygen tension is maintained.

Advantages. Nitrous oxide reduces the requirement for other more potent and intrinsically more toxic anaesthetic agents. It has a strong analgesic action; inhalation of 50% nitrous oxide in oxygen (Entonox) may have similar effects to standard doses of morphine. Induction is rapid and not unpleasant although transient excitement may occur, as with all agents. Recovery time rarely exceeds 4 min even after prolonged administration.

Disadvantages. Nitrous oxide is expensive to buy and to transport. It must be used in conjuction with more potent anaesthetics to produce full surgical anaesthesia.

Uses. Nitrous oxide is used to maintain surgical anaesthesia in combination with other anaesthetic agents, e.g., isoflurane or propofol, and, if required, muscle relaxants. Entonox provides analgesia for obstetric practice, for emergency management of injuries, and during postoperative physiotherapy.

Dosage and administration. For the maintenance of anaesthesia, nitrous oxide must always be mixed with at least 30% oxygen. For analgesia, a concentration of 50% nitrous oxide with 50% oxygen usually suffices.

Contraindications. Any closed, distendable air-filled space expands during administration of nitrous oxide, which moves into it from the blood. It is therefore contraindicated in patients with: demonstrable collections of air in the pleural, pericardial or peritoneal spaces; intestinal obstruction; arterial air embolism; decompression sickness; severe chronic obstructive airway disease; emphysema. Nitrous oxide will cause pressure changes in closed, noncompliant spaces such as the middle ear, nasal sinuses, and the eye.

Precautions. Continued administration of oxygen may be necessary during recovery, especially in elderly patients (see diffusion hypoxia, above).

Adverse effects. The incidence of nausea and vomiting increases with the duration of anaesthesia. Nitrous oxide interferes with the synthesis of methionine, deoxythymidine and DNA. Exposure of to nitrous oxide for more than 4 hours can cause megaloblastic changes in the bone marrow. Because prolonged and repeated exposure of staff as well as of patients may be associated with bone-marrow depression and teratogenic risk, scavenging systems are used to minimise ambient concentrations in operating theatres.

Drug interactions. Addition of 50% nitrous oxide/oxygen mixture to another inhalational anaesthetic reduces the required dosage (minimum alveolar concentration, MAC) of the latter by about 50%.

Storage. Nitrous oxide is supplied under pressure in cylinders, which must be maintained below 25°C. Cylinders containing premixed oxygen 50% and nitrous oxide 50% (Entonox) are available for analgesia. The constituents separate out at –7°C, in which case adequate mixing must be assured before use.

HALOGENATED ANAESTHETICS

Halothane was the first halogenated agent to be used widely, but in the developed world it has been largely superseded by isoflurane and sevoflurane. We provide a detailed description of isoflurane, and of the others in so far as they differ. The MAC of some volatile agents is:

- Isoflurane   1.2%
- Enflurane   1.7%
- Sevoflurane   2.0%
- Halothane   0.74%.

Isoflurane

Isoflurane is a volatile colourless liquid, which is not flammable at normal anaesthetic concentrations. It is relatively insoluble, and has a lower blood/gas coefficient than halothane or enflurane, which allows rapid adjustment of the depth of anaesthesia. It has a pungent odour and can cause bronchial irritation, which makes inhalational induction unpleasant. Isoflurane is minimally metabolised (0.2%), and none of the breakdown products has been related to anaesthetic toxicity.

Respiratory effects. Isoflurane causes respiratory depression: the respiratory rate increases, tidal volume decreases, and the minute volume is reduced. The ventilatory response to carbon dioxide is diminished. Although it irritates the upper airway it is a bronchodilator.

Cardiovascular effects. Anaesthetic concentrations of isoflurane, i.e. 1–1.5 MAC, cause only a slight impairment of myocardial contractility and stroke volume and cardiac output is usually maintained by a reflex increase in heart rate. Isoflurane causes peripheral vasodilatation and reduces blood pressure. It does not affect atrioventricular conduction and does not sensitise the heart to catecholamines. Low concentrations of isoflurane (< 1 MAC) do not increase cerebral blood flow or intracranial pressure, and cerebral autoregulation is maintained. Isoflurane is a potent coronary vasodilator and in the presence of a coronary artery stenosis it may cause redistribution of blood away from an area of inadequate perfusion to one of normal perfusion. This phenomenon of 'coronary steal' may cause regional myocardial ischaemia.

Other effects. Isoflurane relaxes voluntary muscles and potentiates the effects of nondepolarising muscle relaxants. Isoflurane depresses cortical EEG activity and does not induce abnormal electrical activity or convulsions.

Sevoflurane is a chemical analogue of isoflurane. It is less chemically stable than the other volatile anaesthetics in current use. About 3% is metabolised in the body and it is degraded by contact with carbon dioxide absorbents, such as soda lime. The reaction with soda lime causes the formation of a vinyl ether (Compound A), which may be nephrotoxic. Sevoflurane is less soluble than isoflurane and is very pleasant to breathe, which makes it an excellent choice for inhalational induction of anaesthesia, particularly in children. The respiratory and cardiovascular effects of sevoflurane are very similar to isoflurane.

Enflurane is a structural isomer of isoflurane. It is more soluble than isoflurane. It causes more respiratory depression than the other volatile anaesthetics and hypercapnia is almost inevitable in patients breathing spontaneously. It causes more cardiovascular depression than isoflurane and is occasionally associated with cardiac arrythmias. Two percent of enflurane is metabolised and prolonged administration or use in enzyme-induced patients generates sufficient free inorganic fluoride from the drug molecule to cause polyuric renal failure. There have been a few cases of jaundice and heptatoxicity associated with enflurane but the incidence of about one in 1–2 million anaesthetics is lower than with halothane.

Desflurane has the lowest blood/gas partition coefficient of any inhaled anaesthetic agent and thus gives particularly rapid onset and offset of effect. As it undergoes negligible metabolism (0.03%), any release of free inorganic fluoride is minimised; this characteristic favours its use for prolonged anaesthesia. Desflurane is extremely volatile and cannot be administered with conventional vaporisers. It has a very pungent odour and causes airway irritation to an extent that limits its rate of induction of anaesthesia.

Halothane has the highest blood/gas partition coefficient of the volatile anaesthetic agents and recovery from halothane anaesthesia is comparatively slow. It is pleasant to breathe and is second choice to sevoflurane for inhalational induction of anaesthesia. Halothane reduces cardiac output more than any of the other volatile anaesthetics. It sensitises the heart to the arrhythmic effects of catecholamines and hypercapnia; arrhythmias are common, in particular atrioventricular dissociation, nodal rhythm and ventricular extrasystoles. Halothane can trigger malignant hyperthermia in those who are genetically predisposed (see p. 363).

About 20% of halothane is metabolised and it induces hepatic enzymes, including those of anaesthetists and operating theatre staff. Hepatic damage occurs in a small proportion of exposed patients. Typically fever develops 2 or 3 days after anaesthesia accompanied by anorexia, nausea and vomiting. In more severe cases this is followed by transient jaundice or, very rarely, fatal hepatic necrosis. Severe hepatitis is a complication of repeatedly administered halothane anaesthesia and has an incidence of 1:50 000. It follows immune sensitisation to an oxidative metabolite of halothane in susceptible individuals. This serious complication, along with the other disadvantages of halothane and the popularity of sevoflurane for inhalational induction, has almost eliminated its use in the developed world. It remains in common use other parts of the world because it is comparatively inexpensive.

OXYGEN IN ANAESTHESIA

Supplemental oxygen is always used with inhalational agents to prevent hypoxia, even when air is used as the carrier gas. The concentration of oxygen in inspired anaesthetic gases is usually at least 30%, but oxygen should not be used for prolonged periods at a greater concentration than is necessary to prevent hypoxaemia. After prolonged administration, concentrations greater than 80% have a toxic effect on the lungs, which presents initially as a mild substernal irritation progressing to pulmonary congestion, exudation and atelectasis. Use of unnecessarily high concentrations of oxygen in incubators causes retrolental fibroplasia and permanent blindness in premature infants.

Oxygen is supplied under pressure in cylinders, when it remains in the gaseous state. In most hospitals a vacuum insulated evaporator is used to store oxygen in liquid form. This provides for huge volumes of gaseous oxygen and will supply all the piped oxygen outlets in the hospital.

ATMOSPHERIC POLLUTION OF OPERATING THEATRES

Pollution by inhalation anaesthetics has been suspected of being harmful to theatre personnel. Epidemiological studies have raised questions relating to excess of fetal malformations and miscarriages, hepatitis and cancer in operating theatre personnel. Sensible use of preventive measures renders the risks negligible, e.g. use of circle systems that allow low fresh gas flows, scavenging systems, and improved ventilation of theatres. The increasing use of total intravenous anaesthesia (TIVA) and regional anaesthesia will also reduce pollution.

Intravenous anaesthetics

Intravenous anaesthetics should be given only by those fully trained in their use and who are experienced with a full range of techniques of managing the airway, including tracheal intubation.

PHARMACOKINETICS

Intravenous anaesthetics allow an extremely rapid induction because the blood concentration can be raised rapidly, establishing a steep concentration gradient and expediting diffusion into the brain.

The rate of transfer depends on the lipid solubility and arterial concentration of the unbound, non-ionised fraction of the drug. After a single, induction dose of an intravenous anaesthetic recovery occurs quite rapidly as the drug is redistributed around the body and the plasma concentration reduces. Recovery from a single dose of intravenous anaesthetic is not related to its rate of metabolic breakdown. With the exception of propofol, repeated doses or infusions of intravenous anaesthetics will result in considerable accumulation and prolonged recovery. Attempts to use thiopental as the sole anaesthetic in war casualties led to its being described as an ideal form of euthanasia.[3] It is common practice to induce anaesthesia intravenously and then to use a volatile anaesthetic for maintenance. When administration of a volatile anaesthetic is stopped, it is eliminated quickly through the lungs and the patient regains consciousness. The recovery from propofol is rapid, even after repeat doses or an infusion. This advantage, and others, has resulted in propofol displacing thiopental as the most popular intravenous anaesthetic.

Propofol

Propofol (2,6-diisopropylphenol) is available as a 1% or 2% emulsion, which contains soya bean oil and purified egg phosphatide. Induction of anaesthesia with 1.5–2.5 mg/kg occurs within 30 seconds and is smooth and pleasant with a low incidence of excitatory movements. It causes pain on injection but adding lidocaine 20 mg to an ampoule of propofol eliminates this. The recovery from propofol is rapid and the incidence of nausea and vomiting is extremely low, particularly when propofol is used as the sole anaesthetic. Recovery from a continuous infusion of propofol is relatively rapid. On stopping the infusion the plasma concentration decreases rapidly as a result of both redistribution and clearance of the drug. Special syringe pumps incorporating pharmacokinetic algorithms allow the anaesthetist to select a target plasma propofol concentration (e.g. 6 micrograms/ml for induction of anaesthesia) once details of the patient's age and weight have been entered. This technique of target-

---

[3] Halford J J 1943 A critique of intravenous anaesthesia in war surgery. Anesthesiology 4: 67.

controlled infusion (TCI) provides a convenient method for giving a continuous infusion of propofol.

Central nervous system. Propofol causes dose-dependent cortical depression and is an anticonvulsant. It depresses laryngeal reflexes more than barbiturates, which is an advantage when inserting a laryngeal mask airway.

Cardiovascular system. Propofol reduces vascular tone, which lowers systemic vascular resistance and central venous pressure. The heart rate remains unchanged and the result is a fall in blood pressure to about 70–80% of the preinduction level and a small reduction in cardiac output.

Respiratory system. Unless it is undertaken very slowly, induction with propofol causes transient apnoea. On resumption of respiration there is a reduction in tidal volume and increase in rate.

Metabolism. Propofol is conjugated in the liver by glucuronidation making it more water soluble; 88% then appears in the urine and 2% in the faeces.

Thiopental (thiopentone)

Thiopental is a very short-acting barbiturate, which induces anaesthesia smoothly, within one arm-to-brain circulation time. The typical induction dose is 3–5 mg/kg. Rapid distribution (initial $t_{\frac{1}{2}}$ 4 min) allows swift recovery after a single dose. The terminal $t_{\frac{1}{2}}$ of thiopental is 11 h and repeated doses or continuous infusion lead to significant accumulation in fat and very prolonged recovery. Thiopental is metabolised in the liver. The incidence of nausea and vomiting after thiopental is slightly higher than after propofol. The pH of thiopental is 11 and considerable local damage results if it extravasates. Accidental intra-arterial injection will also cause serious injury distal to the injection site.

Central nervous system. Thiopental has no analgesic activity and may be antanalgesic. It is a potent anticonvulsant. Cerebral metabolic rate of oxygen consumption ($CMRO_2$) is reduced, which leads to cerebral vasoconstriction with a concomitant reduction in cerebral blood flow and intracranial pressure.

Cardiovascular system. Thiopental reduces vascular tone, causing hypotension and a slight compensatory increase in heart rate. Antihypertensives or diuretics may augment the hypotensive effect.

Respiratory system. Thiopental reduces respiratory rate and tidal volume.

Methohexitone is a barbiturate similar to thiopental but its terminal $t_{\frac{1}{2}}$ is considerably shorter. Since the introduction of propofol, its use is almost entirely confined to inducing anaesthesia for electroconvulsive therapy (ECT). Propofol shortens seizure duration and may reduce the efficacy of ECT.

Etomidate is a carboxylated imidazole, which is formulated in a mixture of water and propylene glycol. It causes pain on injection and excitatory muscle movements are common on induction of anaesthesia. It is associated with a 20% incidence of nausea and vomiting. Etomidate causes adrenocortical suppression by inhibiting 11 β- and 17 β-hydroxylase and for this reason is not used for prolonged infusion; single bolus doses cause short-lived, clinically insignificant adrenocortical suppression. Despite all these disadvantages it remains in common use, particularly for emergency anaesthesia, because it causes less cardiovascular depression and hypotension than thiopental or propofol.

Ketamine

Ketamine is a phencyclidine (hallucinogen) derivative and an antagonist of the NMDA-receptor.[4] In anaesthetic doses it produces a trance-like state known as *dissociative anaesthesia* (sedation, amnesia, dissociation, analgesia).

Advantages. Anaesthesia persists for up to 15 min after a single intravenous injection and is characterised by profound analgesia. Ketamine may be used as the sole analgesic agent for diagnostic and minor surgical interventions. In contrast to most other anaesthetic drugs, ketamine usually produces a tachycardia and increases blood pressure and cardiac output. This effect makes it a popular choice for inducing anaesthesia in shocked patients. The

---

[4] *N*-methyl-D-aspartate.

cardiovascular effects of ketamine are accompanied by an increase in plasma noradrenaline (norepinephrine) concentration. Because pharyngeal and laryngeal reflexes are only slightly impaired, the airway may be less at risk than with other general anaesthetic techniques. It is a potent bronchodilator and is sometimes used to treat severe bronchospasm in those asthmatics requiring mechanical ventilation. (See also Dissociative anaesthesia, p. 348.)

Disadvantages. Ketamine produces no muscular relaxation. It increases intracranial and intraocular pressure. Hallucinations can occur during recovery (the emergence reaction), but they are minimised if ketamine is used solely as an induction agent and followed by a conventional inhalational anaesthetic. Their incidence is reduced by administration of a benzodiazepine both as a premedication and after the procedure.

Uses. Subanaesthetic doses of ketamine can be used to provide analgesia for painful procedures of short duration such as the dressing of burns, radiotherapeutic procedures, marrow sampling and minor orthopaedic procedures. Ketamine can be used for induction of anaesthesia prior to administration of inhalational anaesthetics, or for both induction and maintenance of anaesthesia for short-lasting diagnostic and surgical interventions, including dental procedures that do not require skeletal muscle relaxation. It is of particular value for children requiring frequent repeated anaesthetics.

Dosage and administration. Premedication with atropine will reduce the salivary secretions produced by ketamine and a benzodiazepine will reduce the incidence of hallucinations.

Induction. *Intravenous route:* 1–2 mg/kg by slow intravenous injection over a period of 60 seconds. A dose of 2 mg/kg produces surgical anaesthesia within 1–2 min, which will last 5–10 min. *Intramuscular route:* 5–10 mg/kg by deep intramuscular injection. This dose produces surgical anaesthesia within 3–5 min and may be expected to last up to 25 min.

Maintenance. Following induction, serial doses of 50% of the original intravenous dose or 25% of the

intramuscular dose is given to prevent movement in response to surgical stimuli. Tonic and clonic movements resembling seizures occur in some patients. These do not indicate a light plane of anaesthesia or a need for additional doses of the anaesthetic.

A dose of 0.5 mg/kg i.m. or i.v. provides excellent analgesia and may be supplemented by further doses of 0.25 mg/kg.

Recovery. Return to consciousness is gradual. Emergence reactions with delirium may occur. Their incidence is reduced by benzodiazepine premedication and by avoiding unnecessary disturbance of the patient during recovery.

Contraindications include: moderate to severe hypertension, congestive cardiac failure or a history of stroke; acute or chronic alcohol intoxication, cerebral trauma, intracerebral mass or haemorrhage or other causes of raised intracranial pressure; eye injury and increased intraocular pressure; psychiatric disorders such as a schizophrenia and acute psychoses.

Precautions. Ketamine should be used under the supervision of a clinician experienced in tracheal intubation, should this become necessary. Pulse and blood pressure must be monitored closely. Supplementary opioid analgesia is often required in surgical procedures causing visceral pain.

Use in pregnancy. Ketamine is contraindicated in pregnancy before term, since it has oxytocic activity. It is also contraindicated in patients with eclampsia or pre-eclampsia. It may be used for assisted vaginal delivery by an experienced anaesthetist. Ketamine is better suited for use during caesarean section; it causes less fetal and neonatal depression than other anaesthetics.

Muscle relaxants

NEUROMUSCULAR BLOCKING DRUGS

A lot of surgery, especially of the abdomen, requires

that voluntary muscle tone and reflex contraction be inhibited. This can be attained by deep general anaesthesia, regional nerve blockade, or by using neuromuscular blocking drugs. Deep general anaesthesia causes cardiovascular depression, respiratory complications, and slow recovery. Regional nerve blocks may be difficult to do or contraindicated, for example if there is a haemostatic defect. Selective relaxation of voluntary muscle with neuromuscular blocking drugs allows surgery under light general anaesthesia with analgesia; it also facilitates tracheal intubation, quick induction and quick recovery. But it requires mechanical ventilation and technical skill. Neuromuscular blocking agents should be given only after induction of anaesthesia.

Neuromuscular blocking agents first attracted scientific notice because of their use as arrow poisons by the natives of South America, who used the most famous of all, curare, for killing food animals[5] as well as enemies. In 1811 Sir Benjamin Brodie smeared 'woorara paste' on wounds of guinea-pigs and noted that death could be delayed by inflating the lungs through a tube introduced into the trachea. Though he did not continue until complete recovery, he did suggest that the drug might be of use in tetanus.

Despite attempts to use curare for a variety of diseases including epilepsy, chorea and rabies, the lack of pure and accurately standardised preparations, as well as the absence of convenient techniques of mechanical ventilation if overdose occurred, prevented it from gaining any firm place in medical practice until 1942, when these difficulties were removed.

Drugs acting at the myoneural junction produce complete paralysis of all voluntary muscle so that movement is impossible and mechanical ventilation is needed. It is plainly important that a paralysed patient should be in a state of full analgesia and unconscious during surgery.[6] Using modern anaes-

thetic techniques and monitoring, awareness while paralysed for a surgical procedure is extremely rare. In the UK, general anaesthesia using volatile agents should always be monitored with agent analysers, which measure and display the end-tidal concentration of volatile agent. In the past, misguided concerns about the effect of volatile anaesthetics on the newborn led many anaesthetists to use little, if any, volatile agent when giving general anaesthesia for caesarean section. Under these conditions some mothers were conscious and experienced pain while paralysed and therefore unable to move. Despite its extreme rarity nowadays, fear of awareness under anaesthesia is still a leading cause of anxiety in patients awaiting surgery.

Mechanisms

When an impulse passes down a motor nerve to voluntary muscle it causes release of acetylcholine from the nerve endings into the synaptic cleft. This activates receptors on the membrane of the motor endplate, a specialised area on the muscle fibre, opening ion channels for momentary passage of sodium which depolarises the endplate and initiates muscle contraction.

---

[5] Curare was obtained from several sources but most commonly from the vine *Chondrodenron tomentosum*. The explorers Humboldt and Bonpland in South America (1799–1804) reported that an extract of its bark was concentrated as a tar-like mass and used to coat arrows. The potency was designated 'one tree' if a monkey, struck by a coated arrow, could only make one leap before dying. A more dilute ('three tree') from was used to paralyse animals so that they could be captured alive – an early example of a dose–response relationship.

[6] The introduction of tubocurarine into surgery made it desirable to decide once and for all whether the drug altered consciousness. Doubts were resolved in a single experiment.

A normal subject was slowly paralysed (curarised) after arranging a detailed and complicated system of communication. Twelve minutes after beginning the slow infusion of curare, the subject, having artificial respiration, could move only his head. He indicated that the experience was not unpleasant, that he was mentally clear and did not want an endotracheal tube inserted. After 22 min, communication was possible only by slight movement of the left eyebrow and after 35 min paralysis was complete and direct communication lost. An airway was inserted. The subject's eyelids were then lifted for him and the resulting inhibition of alpha rhythm of the electroencephalogram suggested that vision and consciousness were normal. After recovery, aided by neostigmine, the subject reported that he had been mentally 'clear as a bell' throughout, and confirmed this by recalling what he had heard and seen. The insertion of the endotracheal airway had caused only minor discomfort, perhaps because of the prevention of reflex muscle spasm. During artificial respiration he had 'felt that (he) would give anything to be able to take one deep breath' despite adequate oxygenation. Smith S M et al 1947 Anesthesiology 8: 1. Note: a randomised controlled trial is not required for this kind of investigation.

Neuromuscular blocking agents used in clinical practice interfere with this process. Natural substances that prevent the release of acetylcholine at nerve endings exist, e.g. *Clostridium botulinum* toxin (see p. 429) and some venoms.

There are two principal mechanisms by which drugs used clinically interfere with neuromuscular transmission:

1. **By competition** with acetylcholine (atracurium, cisatracurium, mivacurium, pancuronium, rocuronium, vecuronium). These drugs are competitive antagonists of acetylcholine. They do not cause depolarisation themselves but protect the endplate from depolarisation by acetylcholine. The result is a flaccid paralysis.

Reversal of this type of neuromuscular block can be achieved with anticholinesterase drugs, such as neostigmine, which prevent the destruction by cholinesterase of acetylcholine released at nerve endings, allow the concentration to build up and so reduce the competitive effect of a blocking agent.

2. **By depolarisation** of the motor endplate (suxamethonium). Such agonist drugs activate the acetylcholine receptor on the motor endplate and at their first application voluntary muscle contracts but, as they are not destroyed immediately, like acetylcholine, the depolarisation persists.

It might be expected that this prolonged depolarisation would result in muscles remaining contracted but this is not so (except in chickens). With prolonged administration a depolarisation block changes to a competitive block (dual block). Because of the uncertainty of this situation a competitive blocking agent is preferred for anything other than short procedures.

COMPETITIVE ANTAGONISTS

Atracurium is unique in that it is altered spontaneously in the body to an inactive form ($t\frac{1}{2}$ 30 min) by a passive chemical process (Hofmann elimination). The duration of action (15–35 min) is thus uninfluenced by the state of the circulation, the liver or the kidneys, a significant advantage in patients with hepatic or renal disease and in the aged. It has very little direct effect on the cardiovascular system

but at doses of greater than 0.5–0.6 mg/kg histamine release may cause hypotension and bronchospasm.

Cisatracurium is a stereoisomer of atracurium; it is less prone to cause histamine release.

Vecuronium is a synthetic steroid derivative that produces full neuromuscular blockade about 3 minutes after a dose of 0.1 mg/kg. After this dose, its duration of action is 20–30 minutes. It has no cardiovascular side-effects and does not cause histamine release.

Rocuronium is another steroid derivative that has the advantage of a rapid onset of action. After a dose of 0.6 mg/kg tracheal intubation can be achieved after 60 seconds. It has negligible cardiovascular effects and has a similar duration of action to vecuronium.

Mivacurium belongs to the same chemical family as atracurium. It is the only nondepolarisng neuromuscular blocker that is metabolised by plasma cholinesterase. It is comparatively short acting (10–15 minutes), depending on the initial dose. Mivacurium can cause some hypotension because of histamine release.

Pancuronium was the first steroid-derived neuromuscular blocker in clinical use. It is longer acting than vecuronium and causes a slight tachycardia.

Tubocurarine is obsolete and is no longer available in the UK. It is a potent antagonist at autonomic ganglia and causes significant hypotension.

Antagonism of competitive neuromuscular block: neostigmine

The action of competitive acetylcholine blockers is antagonised by anticholinesterase drugs, which allow accumulation of acetylcholine. Neostigmine (p. 437) is given intravenously, mixed with glycopyrronium to prevent bradycardia caused by the parasympathetic autonomic effects of the neostigmine. It acts in 4 minutes and lasts for about 30 minutes. Too much neostigmine can cause neuromuscular block by depolarisation, which will cause confusion unless there have been some signs of recovery before neostigmine is given. Progress can be monitored with a nerve stimulator.

DEPOLARISING NEUROMUSCULAR BLOCKER

Suxamethonium (succinylcholine)

Paralysis is preceded by muscular fasciculation, and this may be the cause of the muscle pain experienced commonly after its use. The pain may last 1–3 days and can be minimised by preceding the suxamethonium with a small dose of a competitive blocking agent. Suxamethonium is the neuromuscular blocker with the most rapid onset and the shortest duration of action. Tracheal intubation is possible in less than 60 seconds and total paralysis lasts up to 4 min with 50% recovery in about 10 min (t½ for effect). It is particularly indicated for rapid sequence induction of anaesthesia in patients who are at risk of aspiration — the ability to secure the airway rapidly with a tracheal tube is of the utmost importance. If intubation proves impossible, recovery from suxamethonium and resumption of spontaneous respiration is relatively rapid. Unfortunately, if it is impossible to ventilate the paralysed patient's lungs, recovery may not be rapid enough to prevent the onset of hypoxia.

Suxamethonium is destroyed by plasma pseudo-cholinesterase and so its persistence in the body is increased by neostigmine, which inactivates that enzyme, and in patients with hepatic disease or severe malnutrition whose plasma enzyme concentrations are lower than normal. Approximately 1 in 3000 of the European population have hereditary defects in amount or kind of enzyme, and cannot destroy the drug as rapidly as normal individuals.[7] Paralysis can then last for hours and the individual requires ventilatory support and sedation until recovery occurs spontaneously.

Repeated injections of suxamethonium can cause bradycardia, extrasystoles, and even ventricular arrest. These are probably due to activation of cholinoceptors in the heart and are prevented by atropine. It can be used in caesarian section as it does not readily cross the placenta. Suxamethonium de-polarisation causes a release of *potassium* from muscle, which in normal patients will increase the plasma potassium by 0.5 mmol/l. This is a problem only if the patient's plasma potassium was already high, for example in acute renal failure. In patients with spinal cord injuries and those with major burns, suxamethonium may cause a grossly exaggerated release of potassium from muscle, sufficient to cause cardiac arrest.

USES OF NEUROMUSCULAR BLOCKING DRUGS

Only those who can undertake tracheal intubation and ventilation of the patient's lungs should use these drugs.

- They are used to provide muscular relaxation during surgery and occasionally to assist mechanical ventilation in intensive therapy units.
- They are used during electroconvulsive therapy to prevent injury to the patient due to excessive muscular contraction.

OTHER MUSCLE RELAXANTS

Drugs that provide muscle relaxation by an action on the central nervous system or on the muscle itself are not useful for this purpose in surgery; they are insufficiently selective and full relaxation, even if achievable, is accompanied by general cerebral depression. But there is a place for drugs that reduce spasm of the voluntary muscles without impairing voluntary movement. Such drugs can be useful in spastic states, low back syndrome, and rheumatism with muscle spasm.

Baclofen is structurally related to gamma-ami-nobutyric acid (GABA), an inhibitory central nervous system transmitter; it inhibits reflex activity mainly in the spinal cord. Baclofen reduces spasticity and flexor spasms, but as it has no action on voluntary muscle power, function is commonly not improved. Ambulant patients may need their leg spasticity to provide support and reduction of spasticity may expose the weakness of the limb. It benefits some cases of trigeminal neuralgia. Baclofen is given orally (t½ 3 h).

---

[7] There are wide inter-ethnic differences. When cases are discovered the family should be investigated for low plasma cholinesterase activity and affected individuals warned.

Dantrolene acts directly on muscle and prevents the release of calcium from sarcoplasm stores (see Malignant hyperthermia, p. 427).

ANAPHYLAXIS

Anaphylactic reactions result from the interaction of antigens with specific IgE antibodies, which have been formed by previous exposure to the antigen. *Anaphylactoid* reactions are clinically indistinguishable from anaphylaxis but do not result from prior exposure to a triggering agent and do not involve IgE. Intravenous anaesthetics and muscle relaxants can cause anaphylactic or anaphylactoid reactions and, rarely, they are fatal. Muscle relaxants are responsible for 70% of anaphylactic reactions during anaesthesia and suxamethonium accounts for almost half of these.

Local anaesthetics

Cocaine had been suggested as a local anaesthetic for clinical use when Sigmund Freud investigated the alkaloid in Vienna in 1884 with Carl Koller. The latter had long been interested in the problem of local anaesthesia in the eye, for general anaesthesia has disadvantages in ophthalmology. Observing that numbness of the mouth occurred after taking cocaine orally he realised that this was a local anaesthetic effect. He tried cocaine on animals' eyes and introduced it into clinical ophthalmological practice, whilst Freud was on holiday. Freud had already thought of this use and discussed it but, appreciating that sex was of greater importance than surgery, he had gone to see his fiancée. The use of cocaine spread rapidly and it was soon being used to block nerve trunks. Chemists then began to search for less toxic substitutes, with the result that procaine was introduced in 1905.

Desired properties. Innumerable compounds have local anaesthetic properties, but few are suitable for clinical use. Useful substances must be water-soluble, sterilisable by heat, have a rapid onset of effect, a duration of action appropriate to the operation to be performed, be nontoxic, both locally

and when absorbed into the circulation, and leave no local after-effects.

Mode of action. Local anaesthetics prevent the initiation and propagation of the nerve impulse (action potential). By reducing the passage of sodium through voltage-gated sodium ion channels they raise the threshold of excitability; in consequence, conduction is blocked at afferent nerve endings, and by sensory and motor nerve fibres. The fibres in nerve trunks are affected in order of size, the smallest (autonomic, sensory) first, probably because they have a proportionately greater surface area, and then the larger (motor) fibres. Paradoxically the effect in the central nervous system is stimulation (see below).

Pharmacokinetics. The distribution rate of a single dose of a local anaesthetic is determined by diffusion into tissues with concentrations approximately in relation to blood flow (plasma $t\frac{1}{2}$ only a few minutes). By injection or infiltration, local anaesthetics are usually effective within 5 min and have a useful duration of effect of 1–1.5 h, which in some cases may be doubled by adding a vasoconstrictor (below).

Most local anaesthetics are used in the form of the acid salts, as these are both soluble and stable. The acid salt (usually HCl) dissociates in the tissues to liberate the free base, which is biologically active. This dissociation is delayed in abnormally acid, e.g. inflamed, tissues; but the risk of spreading infection makes local anaesthesia undesirable in infected areas.

Absorption from mucous membranes on topical application varies according to the compound. Those that are well absorbed are used as surface anaesthetics (cocaine, lidocaine, prilocaine). Absorption of topically applied local anaesthetic can be extremely rapid and give plasma concentrations comparable to those obtained by injection. This has led to deaths from overdosage, especially via the urethra.

For topical effect on intact skin for needling procedures a eutectic[8] mixture of bases of prilocaine or lidocaine is used (EMLA — eutectic mixture of

---

[8] A mixture of two solids that becomes a liquid because the mixture has a lower melting point than either of its components.

local anaesthetics). Absorption is very slow and a cream is applied under an occlusive dressing for at least 1 h. Tetracaine gel 4% (Ametop) is more effective than EMLA cream and allows pain free venepuncture 30 minutes after application.

Ester compounds (cocaine, procaine, tetracaine, benzocaine) are hydrolysed by liver and plasma esterases and their effects may be prolonged where there is genetic enzyme deficiency.

Amide compounds [lignocaine (lidocaine), prilocaine, bupivacaine, levobupivacaine, ropivacaine] are dealkylated in the liver.

Impaired liver function, whether due to primary cellular insufficiency or to low liver blood flow as in cardiac failure, may both delay elimination and allow higher peak plasma concentrations of both types of local anaesthetic. This is likely to be important only with large or repeated doses or infusions. These considerations are important in the management of cardiac arrhythmias by i.v. infusion of lignocaine (lidocaine) (see p. 502).

PROLONGATION OF ACTION BY VASOCONSTRICTORS

The effect of a local anaesthetic is terminated by its removal from the site of application. Anything that delays its absorption into the circulation will prolong its local action and can reduce its systemic toxicity where large doses are used. Most local anaesthetics, with the exception of cocaine, cause vascular dilation. The addition of a vasoconstrictor such as adrenaline (epinephrine) reduces local blood flow, slows the rate of absorption of the local anaesthetic, and prolongs its effect; the duration of action of lidocaine is doubled from one to two hours. Normally, the final concentration of adrenaline (epinephrine) should be 1 in 200 000, although dentists use up to 1 in 80 000.

A vasoconstrictor should not be used for nerve block of an extremity (finger, toe, nose, penis). For obvious anatomical reasons, the whole blood supply may be cut off by intense vasoconstriction so that the organ may be damaged or even lost. Enough adrenaline (epinephrine) can be absorbed to affect the heart and circulation and reduce the plasma potassium. This can be dangerous in cardiovascular disease, and with co-administered tricyclic antidepressants and potassium-losing diuretics. An alternative vasoconstrictor is *felypressin* (synthetic vasopressin), which, in the concentrations used, does not affect the heart rate or blood pressure and may be preferable in patients with cardiovascular disease.

OTHER EFFECTS

Local anaesthetics also have the following clinically important effects in varying degree:

- Excitation of parts of the central nervous system, which may manifest as anxiety, restlessness, tremors, euphoria, agitation and even convulsions, which are followed by depression.
- Quinidine-like actions on the heart.

USES

Local anaesthesia is generally used when loss of consciousness is neither necessary nor desirable and also as an adjunct to major surgery to avoid high-dose general anaesthesia. It can be used for major surgery, with sedation, though many patients prefer to be unconsciousness. It is invaluable when the operator must also be the anaesthetist, which is often the case in some parts of the developing world.

Local anaesthetics may be used in several ways to provide:

- Surface anaesthesia, as solution, jelly, cream or lozenge.
- Infiltration anaesthesia, to paralyse the sensory nerve endings and small cutaneous nerves
- Regional anaesthesia.

Regional anaesthesia

Regional anaesthesia requires considerable knowledge of anatomy and attention to detail for both success and safety.

Nerve block means to anaesthetise a region, which may be small or large, by injecting the drug around, not into, the appropriate nerves, usually either a peripheral nerve or a plexus. Nerve block provides its own muscular relaxation as motor fibres are blocked as well as sensory fibres, although with care differential block, affecting sensory more than motor fibres, can be achieved. There are various specialised forms: brachial plexus, paravertebral, paracervical, pudendal block. Sympathetic nerve blocks may be used in vascular disease to induce vasodilatation.

Intravenous. A double cuff is applied to the arm, inflated above arterial pressure after elevating the limb to drain the venous system, and the veins filled with local anaesthetic, e.g. 0.5–1% lidocaine *without* adrenaline (epinephrine). The arm is anaesthetised in 6–8 min, and the effect lasts for up to 40 min if the cuff remains inflated. The cuff must not be deflated for at least 20 minutes. The technique is useful in providing anaesthesia for the treatment of injuries speedily and conveniently, and many patients can leave hospital soon after the procedure. The technique must be meticulously conducted, for if the full dose of local anaesthetic is accidentally suddenly released into the general circulation severe toxicity and even cardiac arrest may result. Bupivacaine is no longer used for intravenous regional anaesthesia as cardiac arrest caused by it is particularly resistant to treatment. Patients should be fasted and someone skilled in resuscitation must be present.

Extradural (epidural) anaesthesia is used in the thoracic, lumbar and sacral (caudal) regions. Lumbar epidurals are used widely in obstetrics and low thoracic epidurals provide excellent analgesia after laparotomy. The drug is injected into the extradural space where it acts on the nerve roots. This technique is less likely to cause hypotension than spinal anaesthesia. Continuous analgesia is achieved if a local anaesthetic, often mixed with an opioid, is infused through an epidural catheter.

Subarachnoid (intrathecal) block (spinal anaesthesia). By using a solution of appropriate specific gravity and tilting the patient the drug can be kept at an appropriate level. Sympathetic nerve blockade causes hypotension. Headache due to CSF leakage is virtually eliminated by using very narrow atraumatic 'pencil point' needles.

Serious local neurological complications, for example infection and nerve injury, are extremely rare.

Opioid analgesics are used intrathecally and extradurally. They diffuse into the spinal cord and act on its opioid receptors (see p. 333); they are highly effective in skilled hands for postsurgical and intractable pain. Respiratory depression may occur. The effect begins in 20 min and lasts about 5 h. Diamorphine or other more lipid-soluble opioids, such as fentanyl, may be used.

ADVERSE REACTIONS

Excessive absorption results in paraesthesiae (face and tongue), anxiety, tremors and even convulsions. The latter are very dangerous, are followed by respiratory depression and may require diazepam or thiopental for control. Cardiovascular collapse and respiratory failure occur with higher plasma concentrations of the local anaesthetic and is caused by direct myocardial depression compounded by hypoxia associated with convulsions. Cardiopulmonary resuscitation must be started immediately.

Anaphylactoid reactions are very rare with amide local anaesthetics and some of those reported have been due to preservatives. Most reported reactions to amide local anaesthetics are due to co-administration of adrenaline (epinephrine), intravascular injection or psychological effects (vasovagal episodes). Reactions with ester local anaesthetics are more common.

INDIVIDUAL LOCAL ANAESTHETICS
(Table 18.1)

Amides

Lignocaine (lidocaine) is a first choice drug for surface use as well as for injection, combining efficacy with comparative lack of toxicity; the $t\frac{1}{2}$ is 1.5 h. It is also useful in cardiac arrhythmias although it is being replaced by amiodarone for this purpose.

Prilocaine is used similarly to lidocaine ($t\frac{1}{2}$ 1.5 h), but it is slightly less toxic. It used to be the preferred drug for intravenous regional anaesthesia but it is

TABLE 18.1 Licenced doses for three widely used amide local anaesthetics

		Solution	Dose by vol. (adult)	Duration of effect
Lidocaine	infiltration	0.25–0.5% + adrenaline (epinephrine)	up to 60 ml	
	nerve block (peripheral)	1% + adrenaline (epinephrine)	up to 50 ml	
		2% + adrenaline (epinephrine)	up to 25 ml	1.5 h
	surface	2%	up to 20 ml	
	anaesthesia	4%	up to 5 ml	
Bupivacaine	infiltration	0.25%	up to 60 ml	
	nerve block (peripheral)	0.25%	up to 60 ml	3–4 h
		0.5%	up to 30 ml	
Prilocaine	infiltration	0.5%	up to 80 ml	
	nerve block (peripheral)	1%	up to 40 ml	1.5–3 h
		2%	up to 20 ml	
		3% + felypressin (dental use)	up to 20 m	

Notes:
1. Time to peak effect is about 5 min, except bupivacaine (see text).
2. Maximum doses of local anaesthetic plus vasoconstrictor are toxic in absence of the vasoconstrictor and so substantially less should be used. All doses are approximate only; larger amounts may be safe, but deaths have occurred with smaller amounts, so that the minimum dose that will suffice should be used.
3. Maximum dose of adrenaline (epinephrine) is 500 micrograms (see below).
4. Concentrations of solutions and dose of drug: errors of calculation occur with sometimes fatal results. We provide these figures becuse experience of conducting examinations with medical students has taught us that they frequently lack the facility of calculating the dose of a drug in a given volume of known concentration.
   1% means one gram in 100 ml = 1000 mg in 100 ml = 10 mg per ml: 2% = 20 mg per ml, and so on.
   It is traditional to express adrenaline (epinephrine) concentrations as 1 in 200 000, or 1 in 80 000, or 1 in 1000.
   1 in 1000 means 1000 mg (1.0 g) in 1000 ml = 1 mg per ml.
   1 in 200 000 means 1000 mg (1.0 g) in 200 000 ml = 5 micrograms per ml.
   Thus the maximum dose of adrenaline (epinephrine), 500 micrograms (see above), is contained in 100 ml of 1 in 200 000 solution.

no longer available as a preservative-free solution and most clinicians now use lidocaine instead. Crystals of prilocaine and lidocaine base, when mixed, dissolve in one another to form a eutectic emulsion that penetrates skin and is used for dermal anaesthesia (EMLA, see p. 358), e.g., before venepuncture in children.

Bupivacaine is long-acting ($t\frac{1}{2}$ 3 h) (see Table 18.1) and is used for peripheral nerve blocks, and epidural and spinal anaesthesia. Whilst onset of effect is comparable to lidocaine, peak effect occurs later (30 min).

Levobupivacaine is the S-enantiomer of racemic bupivacaine. The relative therapeutic ratio (levobupivacaine:racemic bupivacaine) for CNS toxicity is 1.03, indicating that levobupivacaine is marginally less toxic.

Ropivacaine may provide better separation of motor and sensory nerve blockade; effective sensory blockade can be achieved without causing motor weakness. The rate of onset of ropivacaine is similar to bupivacaine, but its absolute potency and duration of effect is slightly less. The indications for ropivacaine are similar to those of bupivacaine.

Ester

Cocaine (alkaloid) is used medicinally solely as a surface anaesthetic (for abuse toxicity, see p. 192) usually as a 4% solution, because adverse effects are both common and dangerous when it is injected. Even as a surface anaesthetic sufficient absorption may take place to cause serious adverse effects and cases continue to be reported; only specialists should use it and the dose must be checked and restricted. Cocaine prevents the uptake of catecholamines [adrenaline (epinephrine), noradrenaline (norepinephrine)] into sympathetic nerve endings, thus increasing their concentration at receptor sites, so that cocaine has a built-in vasoconstrictor action, which is why it retains a (declining) place as a surface anaesthetic for surgery involving mucous membranes, e.g. nose. Other local anaesthetics do not have this action, indeed most are vasodilators and added adrenaline (epinephrine) is not so efficient.

Obstetric analgesia and anaesthesia

Although this soon ceased to be considered immoral on religious grounds, it has been a technically controversial topic since 1853 when it was announced that Queen Victoria had inhaled chloroform during the birth of her eighth child. The *Lancet* recorded 'intense astonishment … throughout the profession' at this use of chloroform, 'an agent which has unquestionably caused instantaneous death in a considerable number of cases'. But the Queen (perhaps ignorant of these risks) took a different view, writing in her private journal of 'that blessed chloroform' and adding that 'the effect was soothing, quieting and delightful beyond measure'.

The ideal drug must relieve labour pain without making the patient confused or uncooperative. It must not interfere with uterine activity nor must it influence the fetus, e.g. to cause respiratory depression by a direct action, by prolonging labour or by reducing uterine blood supply. It should also be suitable for use by a midwife without supervision.

Pethidine is widely used. There is little difference between the effects of equipotent doses of morphine and pethidine with regard to analgesia, respiratory depression, and nausea and vomiting (but it may delay labour less). All opioids have the potential to cause respiratory depression of the newborn but this can be reversed with naloxone if necessary. The popular choice of pethidine for analgesia during labour in the UK is not because of any clear pharmacological advantage, but because it remains the only opioid licensed for use by midwives.

Nitrous oxide and oxygen (50% of each: Entonox) may be administered for each contraction from a machine the patient works herself or supervised by a midwife (about 10 good breaths are needed for maximal analgesia).

Epidural local anaesthesia provides the most effective pain relief, but the technique should only be undertaken after adequate training. In the UK, only anaesthetists insert epidural anaesthetics.

Spinal anaesthesia is now used more commonly then epidural anaesthesia for Caesarean section. The vast majority of Caesarean sections are now undertaken with regional rather than general anaesthesia.

General anaesthesia during labour presents special problems. Gastric regurgitation and aspiration are a particular risk (see p. 347). The safety of the fetus must be considered; all anaesthetics and analgesics in general use cross the placenta in varying amounts and, apart from respiratory depression, produce no important effects except that high doses interfere with uterine retraction and may be followed by uterine haemorrhage. Neuromuscular blocking agents can be used safely.

Anaesthesia in patients already taking medication

Anaesthetists are in an unenviable position. They are expected to provide safe service to patients in any condition, taking any drugs. Sometimes there is opportunity to modify drug therapy before surgery but often there is not. Anaesthetists require a particularly detailed drug history from the patient.

DRUGS THAT AFFECT ANAESTHESIA

Adrenal steroids: chronic corticosteroid therapy with the equivalent of prednisolone 10 mg daily within the previous 3 months suppresses the hypothalamic-pituitary-adrenal system. Without steroid supplementation perioperatively the patient may fail to respond appropriately to the stress of surgery and become hypotensive (see Ch. 34). A single dose of *etomidate* depresses the hypothalamic-pituitary-adrenal axis for a few hours but this is not associated with an adverse outcome.

Antibiotics: aminoglycosides, e.g. neomycin, gentamicin, potentiate neuromuscular blocking drugs.

Anticholinesterases: can potentiate suxamethonium.

Antiepilepsy drugs: continued medication is essential to avoid status epilepticus. Drugs must be given parenterally (e.g. phenytoin, sodium valproate) or by rectum (e.g. carbamazepine) until the patient can absorb enterally.

Antihypertensives of all kinds: hypotension may complicate anaesthesia, but it is best to continue therapy. Hypertensive patients are particularly liable to excessive rise in blood pressure and heart rate during intubation, which can be dangerous if there is ischaemic heart disease. Postoperatively, parenteral therapy may be needed for a time.

β-adrenoceptor blocking drugs: can prevent the homeostatic sympathetic cardiac response to cardiac depressant anaesthetics and to blood loss.

Diuretics: hypokalaemia, if present, will potentiate neuromuscular blocking agents and perhaps general anaesthetics.

Oral contraceptives containing oestrogen and postmenopausal hormone replacement therapy: predispose to thromboembolism (see p. 724).

Psychotropic drugs: neuroleptics potentiate or synergise with opioids, hypnotics and general anaesthetics.

Antidepressants: monoamine oxidase inhibitors can cause hypertension when combined with certain amines, e.g. pethidine, or indirect-acting sympathomimetics, e.g. ephedrine. Tricyclics potentiate catecholamines and some other adrenergic drugs.

Anaesthesia in the diseased, and in particular patient groups

The normal response to anaesthesia may be greatly modified by disease. Some of the more important aspects include:

Respiratory disease and smoking predispose the patient to postoperative pulmonary complications, principally infective. The site of operation, e.g. upper abdomen, chest, and the severity of pain influence the impairment to ventilation and coughing.

Cardiac disease. The aim is to avoid the circulatory stress (with increased cardiac work which can compromise the myocardial oxygen supply) caused by hypertension and tachycardia. Intravenous drugs are normally given slowly to reduce the risk of overdosage and hypotension.

Patients with fixed cardiac output, e.g. with aortic stenosis or constrictive pericarditis, are at special risk from reduced cardiac output with drugs that depress the myocardium and vasomotor centre, for they cannot compensate. Induction with propofol or thiopental is particularly liable to cause hypotension in these patients. Hypoxia is obviously harmful. Skilled technique rather than choice of drugs on pharmacological grounds is the important factor.

Hepatic or renal disease is generally liable to increase drug effects and should be taken into account when selecting drugs and their doses.

Malignant hyperthermia (MH) is a rare pharmacogenetic syndrome with an incidence of between 1:15 000 and 1:150 000 in North America, exhibiting autosomal dominant inheritance with variable penetrance. The condition occurs during or immediately after anaesthesia and may be precipitated by potent inhalation agents (enflurane, halothane, isoflurane), or suxamethonium. The patient may have experienced an uncomplicated general anaesthetic previously. The mechanism involves a sudden rise in release of bound (stored) calcium of the sarcoplasm, stimulating contraction, rhabdomyolysis, and a hypermetabolic state. Malignant hyperthermia is a life-threatening medical emergency. Oxygen consumption increases by up to three times normal, and body temperature may rise as fast as 1°C every 5 min, reaching as high as 43°C. Rigidity of voluntary muscles may not be evident at the outset or in mild cases.

Dantrolene 1 mg/kg i.v., is given immediately. Further doses are given at 10-min intervals until the patients responds, to a maximum dose of 10 mg/kg. Dantrolene probably acts by preventing the release of calcium from the sarcoplasm store that ordinarily follows depolarisation of the muscle membrane. The $t\frac{1}{2}$ is 9 h.

Nonspecific treatment is needed for the hyperthermia (cooling, oxygen), and insulin and dextrose are given for hyperkalaemia due to potassium release from contracted muscle. Hyperkalaemia and acidosis may trigger severe cardiac arrhythmias.

Once the immediate crisis has resolved, the patient and all immediate relatives should undergo investigation for MH. This involves a muscle biopsy, which is tested for sensitivity to initiating agents.

Anaesthesia in MH-susceptible patients is achieved safely with total intravenous anaesthesia using propofol and opioids. Dantrolene for intravenous use must be available in every surgical theatre. The relation of malignant hyperthermia syndrome with neuroleptic malignant syndrome (for which dantrolene may be used as adjunctive treatment, see p. 388) is uncertain.

Diabetes mellitus: see page 695.

Thyroid disease: see page 705.

Porphyria: see page 141.

Muscle diseases. Patients with myasthenia gravis are very sensitive to (intolerant of) competitive but not to depolarising neuromuscular blocking drugs. Those with myotonic dystrophy may recover less rapidly than normal from central respiratory depression and neuromuscular block; they may fail to relax with suxamethonium.

Sickle-cell disease. Hypoxia and dehydration can precipitate a crisis.

Atypical (deficient) pseudocholinesterase. There is a delay in the metabolism of suxamethonium and mivacurium. The duration of neuromuscular block depends on the type of pseudocholinesterase.

Raised intracranial pressure will be made worse by high expired concentration inhalation agents, e.g. > 1% isoflurane, by hypoxia or hypercapnia, and in response to intubation if anaesthesia is inadequate. Without support from a mechanical ventilator, excessive doses of opioids will cause hypercapnia and increase intracranial pressure.

The elderly (see p. 126) are liable to become confused by cerebral depressants, especially by hyoscine. Atropine also crosses the blood–brain barrier and can cause confusion in the elderly; glycopyrronium is preferable. In general, elderly patients require smaller doses of all drugs than the young. The elderly tolerate hypotension poorly; they are prone to cerebral and coronary ischaemia.

Children (see p. 125). The problems with children are more technical, physiological and psychological than pharmacological.

Sedation in critical care units is used to reduce patient anxiety and improve tolerance to tracheal tubes and mechanical ventilation. Whenever possible, patients are sedated only to a level that allows them to open their eyes to verbal command; oversedation is harmful. Commonly used drugs include propofol and midazolam, and opioids such as fentanyl, alfentanil, or morphine.

Neuromuscular blockers are only rarely required to assist mechanical ventilation. If pain is treated properly and patient-triggered modes of ventilation are used, many patients in the critical care unit will not require sedation. Reassurance from sympathetic nursing staff is extremely important and far more effective than drugs.

GUIDE TO FURTHER READING

Bovill J G 2000 Mechanisms of anaesthesia: time to say farewell to the Meyer–Overton rule. Current Opinion in Anaesthesiology 13: 433–436

Carter A J 1999 Dwale: an anaesthetic from old England. British Medical Journal 319: 1623–1626 (use of medicinal herbs to render a patient unconscious for surgery, before modern general anaesthesia)

Columb M O 2001 Local anaesthetic agents. Anaesthesia and Intensive Care Medicine 2: 288–291

Fryer J M 2001 Intravenous induction agents. Anaesthesia and Intensive Care Medicine 2: 277–280

Gepts E 1998 Pharmacokinetic concepts for TCI anaesthesia. Anaesthesia 53 (S1): 4–12

Harper N 2001 Inhalational anaesthetics. Anaesthesia and intensive care medicine 2: 241–244

Pollard B J 2001 Neuromuscular blocking agents. Anaesthesia and Intensive Care Medicine 2: 281–285

Sandin R H et al 2000 Awareness during anaesthesia: a prospective case study. Lancet 355: 707–711

Whiteside J B, Wildsmith J A W 2001 Developments in local anaesthetic drugs. British Journal of Anaesthesia 87: 27–35

19

Psychotropic drugs

SYNOPSIS

Advances in drug treatment have revolutionised the practice of psychiatry over the past six decades. Drugs provide a degree of stability and control in the lives of those suffering from schizophrenia, a chronic debilitating illness with impact so profound that it accounts for 2–3% of UK national health spending. Similarly, the impact of medication in alleviating the burden on individuals, their families and society of depression, which has a lifetime prevalence of up to 1 in 6 of the population, is substantial. Psychotropic drugs greatly improve the prognosis of other common conditions such as anxiety disorders, attention deficit/hyperactivity disorder and bipolar affective disorder.

In this chapter the following drug groups are considered

- Antidepressants
- Antipsychotics ('neuroleptics')
- Mood stabilisers
- Drugs for anxiety and sleep disorders
- Drugs for Alzheimer's dementia
- Drugs for attention deficit/hyperactivity disorder

Writing prescriptions is easy, understanding people is hard. (Franz Kafka, 1883–1924)

In 1940 psychotropic medication was limited to chloral hydrate, barbiturates and amphetamine. By contrast, the modern-day formulary lists almost 100 psychotropic drugs, with efficacious treatment available for the vast majority of psychiatric diagnoses and in all phases of life. Psychotropic medication has been a key factor in accelerating the closure of Victorian 'asylums' such that the psychiatric inpatient population is now a tiny fraction of its 1954 peak of 148,000 in England and Wales.

DIAGNOSTIC ISSUES

Older classifications of psychiatric disorder divided diseases into 'psychoses' and 'neuroses'. The term 'psychosis' is still widely used to describe a severe mental illness with the presence of hallucinations, delusions or extreme abnormalities of behaviour including marked overactivity, retardation and catatonia, usually accompanied by a lack of insight. Psychotic disorders therefore include schizophrenia, severe forms of depression and mania. Psychosis may also be due to illicit substances or organic conditions. Clinical features of schizophrenia may be subdivided into 'positive symptoms', which include hallucinations, delusions and thought disorder and 'negative symptoms' such as apathy, flattening of affect and poverty of speech.

Disorders that would formerly have been grouped under 'neuroses' include depression in the absence of psychotic symptoms, anxiety disorders (e.g. panic disorder, generalised anxiety disorder, obsessive-compulsive disorder, phobias and post-traumatic stress disorder), eating disorders (e.g. anorexia nervosa and bulimia nervosa) and sleep disorders.

Also falling within the scope of modern psychiatric diagnostic systems are organic mental disorders (e.g. dementia in Alzheimer's disease), disorders due to substance misuse (e.g. alcohol and opiate dependence—see Chapter 10), personality disorders, disorders of childhood and adolescence (e.g. attention deficit/hyperactivity disorder, Tourette's syndrome) and mental retardation (learning disabilities).

DRUG THERAPY IN RELATION TO PSYCHOLOGICAL TREATMENT

No account of drug treatment strategies for psychiatric illness would be complete without consideration of psychological therapies. Psychotherapy is broad in content, ranging from simple counselling and 'supportive psychotherapy' sessions through ongoing formal psychoanalysis to newer techniques such as cognitive behavioural therapy.

As a general rule, psychotic illnesses (e.g. schizophrenia, mania and depressive psychosis) require drugs as first-line treatment, with psychotherapeutic approaches limited to an adjunctive role, for instance in promoting drug compliance, improving family relationships and helping individuals cope with distressing symptoms. By contrast, for non-psychotic depression and anxiety disorders such as panic disorder and obsessive-compulsive disorder, forms of psychotherapy are available which provide alternative first-line treatment to medication. The choice between drugs and psychotherapy depends on treatment availability, previous history of response, patient preference and the ability of the patient to work appropriately with the chosen therapy. In many cases there is scope to use drugs and psychotherapy in combination.

Taking depression as an example, an extensive evidence base exists for the efficacy of several forms of psychotherapy. These include cognitive therapy (in which individuals identify faulty views and negative automatic thoughts and attempt to replace them with ways of thinking less likely to lead to depression), interpersonal therapy (which focuses on relationships, roles and losses), brief dynamic psychotherapy (a time-limited version of traditional psychoanalysis) and cognitive analytical therapy (another well structured time-limited therapy which combines the best points of cognitive therapy and traditional analysis).

Finally, it must be stressed that all doctors who prescribe psychotropic drugs engage in a 'therapeutic relationship' with their patients. A depressed person whose doctor is empathic, supportive and appears to believe in the efficacy of the drug prescribed is more likely both to take the medication and to adopt a mindset that might actually make him or her feel better than if the doctor seemed aloof and ambivalent about the value of psychotropic drugs. Remembering that placebo response rates of 30–40% are common in double-blind trials of antidepressants, we should never underestimate the importance of our 'therapeutic relationship' with the patient in enhancing the pharmacological efficacy of the drugs we use.

Antidepressant drugs

Antidepressants can be broadly divided into four main classes (Table 19.1), *tricyclics* (TCA, named after their three ring structure), *selective serotonin reuptake* inhibitors (SSRIs), *monoamine oxidase inhibitors* (MAOIs), and *novel compounds* some of which are related to TCAs or SSRIs. Clinicians who wish to have a working knowledge of antidepressants would be advised to be familiar with the use of at least one drug from each of the four main categories tabulated. A more thorough knowledge base would demand awareness of differences between individual TCAs and of the distinct characteristics of the novel compounds. Since antidepressants are largely similar in their therapeutic efficacy, awareness of profiles of unwanted effects is of particular importance.

An alternative categorisation of antidepressants is based solely on mechanism of action (Fig. 19.1). The majority of antidepressants, including TCAs, SSRIs and related compounds are *reuptake inhibitors*. Certain novel agents including trazodone and mirtazapine are *receptor blockers* while MAOIs are *enzyme inhibitors*.

The first TCAs (imipramine and amitriptyline) and MAOIs appeared between 1957 and 1961 (Fig. 19.1). The MAOIs were developed from antituberculosis agents which had been noted to elevate mood. Independently, imipramine was synthesised from the antipsychotic drug chlorpromazine and found to have antidepressant rather than antipsychotic properties. Over the next 25

TABLE 19.1 Classification of antidepressants

Tricyclics	Selective serotonin reuptake inhibitors	Monoamine oxidase inhibitors
Dothiepin (dosulepin)	Fluoxetine	Phenelzine
Amitriptyline	Paroxetine	Isocarboxazid
Lofepramine	Sertraline	Tranylcypromine
Clomipramine	Citalopram*	
Imipramine	Fluvoxamine	Moclobemide (RIMA)
Trimipramine		
Doxepin		
Nortriptyline		
Protriptyline		
Desipramine		

Novel compounds

Mainly noradrenergic
Reboxetine (NaRI)

Mainly serotonergic
Trazodone †
Nefazodone †

Mixed
Venlafaxine (SNRI)
Mirtazapine (NaSSA) †
Milnacipran (SNRI) ¶

Within each class or subclass drugs are listed in order of frequency of prescription in the United Kingdom (1997 data). Abbreviations; RIMA—reversible inhibitor of monoamine oxidase; NaRI—noradrenaline reuptake inhibitor; SNRI—serotonin and noradrenaline reuptake inhibitor; NaSSA—noradrenaline and specific serotonergic antidepressant.
* Citalopram is a racemic mixture of S and R isomers. The antidepressant activity of citalopram appears to reside in the S-isomer. Escitalopram the pure S-isomer, may offer clinical benefits over existing preparations.
† Trazodone, nefazodone and mirtazapine have been classed as 'receptor blocking' antidepressants based on their antagonism of postsynaptic serotonin receptors (trazodone, nefazodone) and presynaptic α_2-receptors (trazodone, mirtazapine). Nefazodone has additional weak SSRI activity.
¶ Not available in the United Kingdom.

years the TCA class enlarged to more than 10 agents with heterogeneous pharmacological profiles and further modifications of the original three ring structure gave rise to the related (but pharmacologically distinct) antidepressant trazodone.

In the 1980s an entirely new class of antidepressant arrived with the SSRIs, firstly fluvoxamine immediately followed by fluoxetine (Prozac). Within 10 years, the SSRI class accounted for half of antidepressant prescriptions in the United Kingdom. Further developments in the evolution of the antidepressants have been novel compounds such as venlafaxine, reboxetine, nefazodone and mirtazapine, and a reversible monoamine oxidase inhibitor, moclobemide.

Mechanism of action

The monoamine hypothesis proposes that, in depression, there is deficiency of the neurotransmitters *noradrenaline* and *serotonin* in the brain which can be altered by antidepressants. Drugs that affect depression can modify amine storage, release, or uptake (Fig. 19.2). Thus the concentration of amines

in nerve endings and/or at postsynaptic receptors is enhanced. In support of the monoamine hypothesis are the findings that amfetamines, which release presynaptic noradrenaline and dopamine from stores and prevent their reuptake, have a weak antidepressant effect, whilst the antihypertensive agent reserpine, which prevents normal noradrenaline storage, causes depression, as does experimental depletion of the serotonin precursor tryptophan. The importance of serotonin is further illustrated by the finding that depressed patients may exhibit down-regulation of some postsynaptic serotonin receptors.

Specific serotonin reuptake inhibitors, as the class name implies, act predominantly by preventing serotonin reuptake and have more limited effects on noradrenaline reuptake. Tricyclic antidepressants in general inhibit noradrenaline reuptake, but effects on serotonin reuptake vary widely; desipramine and protriptyline have minimal potential for raising serotonin concentrations, whereas clomipramine possesses a greater propensity for blocking serotonin reuptake than for noradrenaline. The

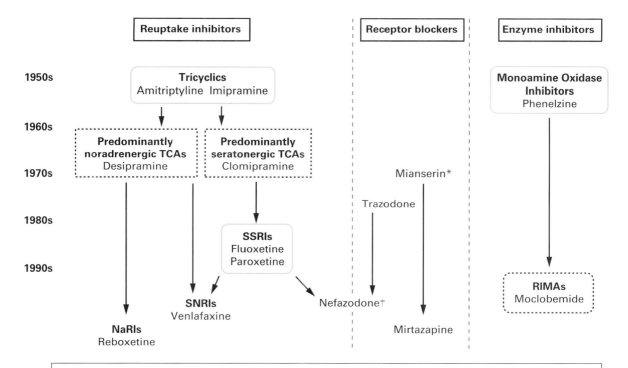

Fig. 19.1 Flow chart of the evolution of antidepressant drugs and classification by mechanism of action.

novel compound venlafaxine is capable of exerting powerful inhibition of reuptake of both transmitters, noradrenergic activity appearing at doses greater than 200 mg/day. Mirtazapine also achieves an increase in noradrenergic and serotonergic neurotransmission, but through antagonism of presynaptic α₂-autoreceptors (receptors that mediate negative feedback for transmitter release, i.e. an autoinhibitory feedback system). Nefazodone has properties of weak serotonin reuptake inhibition but additionally has complex but principally antagonist effects on postsynaptic serotonin receptors, a property it shares with trazodone.

MAOIs increase the availability of noradrenaline and serotonin by preventing their destruction by the monoamine oxidase type A enzyme in the presynaptic terminal. The older MAOIs, phenelzine,

tranylcypromine and isocarboxazid, bind irreversibly to monamine oxidase enzyme by forming strong (covalent) bonds. The enzyme is thus rendered permanently ineffective such that amine metabolising activity can be restored only by production of fresh enzyme, which takes weeks. These MAOI are thus called *hit and run* drugs as their effects greatly outlast their detectable presence in the body.

But how do changes in monoamine transmitter levels produce an eventual elevation of mood? Raised neurotransmitter concentrations produce immediate alterations in postsynaptic receptor activation, leading to changes in second messenger (intracellular) systems and to gradual modifications in cellular protein expression. Antidepressants increase a **c**yclic AMP **r**esponse-**e**lement **b**inding (CREB) protein which in turn is involved in

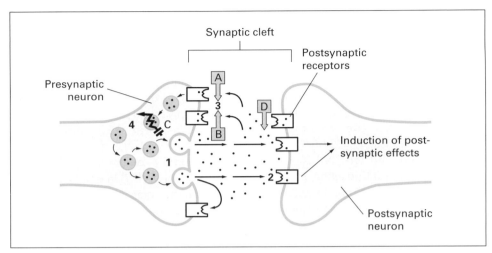

Physiological processes at the synapse:
1. When an electrical signal reaches the presynaptic terminal, presynaptic amine vesicles fuse with the neuronal membrane and release their contents into the synaptic cleft.
2. Amines in the synaptic cleft bind to postsynaptic receptors to produce a post synaptic response.
3. Amines may be removed from the synaptic cleft by reuptake into the presynaptic neuron.
4. The monoamine oxidase enzyme breaks down presynaptic amines.

Effects of antidepressants:
A. Tricyclics prevent presynaptic reuptake of the amines nonadrenaline and serotonin
B. SSRIs predominantly block reuptake of serotonin.
C. MAOIs reduce the activity of monoamine oxidase in breaking down presynaptic amines (leaving more available for release into the presynaptic cleft).
D. Some antidepressants (e.g. nefazodone) block postsynaptic receptors directly.

Fig. 19.2 Mechanism of action of antidepressant drugs at the synapse.

regulating the transcription of genes that influence survival of other proteins including **b**rain **d**erived **n**eurotrophic **f**actor (BDNF) which exerts effects on neuronal growth. The role of BDNF in depression is supported by the observation that stress both reduces its expression and impairs neurogenesis.

While the monoamine hypothesis of depression is conceptually straightforward, it is in reality it is an oversimplification of a complicated picture. Other systems that are implicated in the aetiology of depression (and which provide potential targets for drug therapy) include the hypothalamopituitary-thyroid axis and the hypothalamopituitary-adrenal axis (HPA). The finding that 50% of depressed patients have elevated plasma cortisol concentrations constitutes evidence that depression may be associated with increased HPA drive.

Drugs with similar modes of action to antidepressants find other uses in medicine. Amfebutamone/ buproprion inhibits reuptake of both dopamine and noradrenaline and was originally developed and used as an antidepressant; it is now used to assist smoking cessation (see p. 178). Sibutramine, licenced as an anorectic agent, is a serotonin and noradrenaline reuptake inhibitor (see p. 697). Despite its similarity of action to venlafaxine and evidence of an anti-depressant effect from animal studies, sibutramine has yet to be recognised as effective for depression.

PHARMACOKINETICS

The antidepressants listed in Table 19.1 are generally well absorbed after oral administration. Steady-state plasma concentrations of TCAs show great individual variation but correlate with thera-peutic effect. Measurement of plasma concentration can be useful especially where there is apparent failure of response (though it is often not available).

Antidepressants in general are inactivated principally by metabolism by hepatic cytochrome P450 enzymes (see p. 112). Of the many isoenzymes identified, the most important in antidepressant metabolism are Cytochrome P450 (CYP) 2D6 (Table 19.2a) and CYP 3A4 (Table 19.2b). Other important P450 enzymes are CYP 1A2 (inhibited by the SSRI fluvoxamine, induced by cigarette smoking, substrates include caffeine and the atypical antipsychotics clozapine and olanzapine) and the CYP 2C group (inhibition by fluvoxamine and fluoxetine, involved in breakdown of moclobemide). Sometimes several CYP enzymes are capable of mediating the same metabolic step. For example at least six isoenzymes, including CYP 2D6, 3A4 and 2C9 can mediate the desmethylation of the SSRI sertraline to its major metabolite.

Several of these drugs produce active metabolites which prolong their action (e.g. fluoxetine is metabolised to norfluoxetine, $t\frac{1}{2}$ 200 h). The metabolic products of certain TCAs are antidepressants in their own right, e.g. nortriptyline (from amitriptyline), desipramine (from lofepramine) and imipramine (from clomipramine).

Half-lives of TCAs lie generally in the range of 15 h (imipramine) to 100 h (protriptyline) and those for SSRIs from 15 h (fluvoxamine) to 72 h (fluoxetine).

Around 7% of the Caucasian population have very limited CYP 2D6 enzyme activity. Such 'poor metabolisers' may find standard doses of tricyclic antidepressants intolerable and it is often worth starting at a very low dose. If the drug is then tolerated, plasma concentration assay may to confirm the suspicion that the patient is a poor metaboliser.

TABLE 19.2A Psychotropic (and selected other) drugs known to be CYP 2D6 substrates and inhibitors

CYP 2D6 inhibitors
Antidepressants
Paroxetine
Fluoxetine

CYP 2D6 substrates

Antidepressants	*Antipsychotics*	*Miscellaneous*
Paroxetine	Chlorpromazine	Dexfenfluramine
Fluoxetine	Haloperidol	Opioids
Citalopram	Thioridazine	Codeine
Sertraline	Zuclopenthixol	Hydrocodeine
Venlafaxine*	Perphenazine	Dihydrocodeine
Amitriptyline	Risperidone	Tramadolol
Clomipramine		Ethyl Morphine
Desipramine		Tenamfetamine
Imipramine		('Ecstasy')
Nortriptyline		Bupropion
		β-blockers
		Propanolol
		Metoprolol
		Timolol
		Bufaralol

A *substrate* is a substance that is acted upon and changed by an enzyme. An enzyme *inducer* accelerates metabolism of co-prescribed drugs which are substrates of the same enzyme, reducing their effect. An enzyme *inhibitor* retards metabolism of co-prescribed drugs, increasing their effects (see Chapter 7, Metabolism). Competition between drugs that are substrates for the same enzyme may retard their metabolism, increase plasma concentration and lead to enhanced therapeutic or adverse effects.
*CYP 2D6 is involved only in the breakdown of venlafaxine to its active metabolite and implications of 2D6 interactions are of limited significance.

TABLE 19.2B Psychotropic (and selected other) drugs known to be CYP 3A4 substrates, inhibitors and inducers

CYP 3A4 inhibitors

Antidepressants	*Other drugs*
Nefazodone	Cimetidine
Fluoxetine	Erythromycin
	Ketoconazole
	(and grapefruit juice)

CYP 3A4 substrates

Antidepressants	*Anxiolytics, hypnotics and antipsychotics*	*Miscellaneous*
Fluoxetine	Alprazolam	Buprenorphine
Sertraline	Buspirone	Carbamazepine
Amitriptyline	Diazepam	Cortisol
Imipramine	Midazolam	Dexamethasone
Nortriptyline	Triazolam	Methadone
Trazodone*	Zopiclone	Testosterone
	Haloperidol	Calcium channel blockers
	Quetiapine	Diltiazem
	Sertindole	Nifedipine
		Amlodipine
		Other drugs
		Amiodarone
		Omeprazole
		Oral contraceptives
		Simvastatin

CYP 3A4 inducers

Antidepressant	*Miscellaneous*
St. John's Wort	Carbamazepine
	Phenobarbital
	Phenytoin

* mCPP, the active metabolite of trazodone, is a CYP 2D6 substrate; observe for unwanted effects when trazodone is co-administered with the 2D6 inhibitors fluoxetine or paroxetine.

THERAPEUTIC EFFICACY

Provided antidepressant drugs are prescribed at an adequate dose and taken regularly, 60–70% of patients with moderate or severe depression should respond within 3–4 weeks. Meta-analyses have shown little evidence that any particular drug or class of antidepressant is more efficacious than others, but there are four possible exceptions to this general statement.

- Small trials have suggested that the SNRI agent *venlafaxine*, in high dose (> 150 mg/day) may have greater efficacy than other antidepressants.
- *Amitriptyline* appears to be slightly more effective than other TCAs and also SSRIs but this advantage is compromised by its poor tolerability relative to more modern agents.
- The older MAOIs (e.g. *phenelzine*) may be more effective than other classes in 'atypical' depression, a form of depressive illness where mood reactivity is preserved, lack of energy may be extreme and biological features are the opposite of the normal syndrome i.e. excess sleep and appetite with weight gain.
- Evidence suggests that in patients hospitalised with *severe* depression, TCAs as a class (also venlafaxine) may be slightly more effective than either SSRIs or MAOIs.

SELECTION

An antidepressant should be selected to match individual patients' requirements, such as the need or otherwise for a sedative effect or the avoidance of antimuscarinic effects (especially in the elderly). In the absence of special factors the choice rests on tolerability, safety in overdose and likelihood of an effective dose being reached. *SSRIs, lofepramine, mirtazapine, nefazodone, reboxetine* and *venlafaxine* are highlighted as best fulfilling these needs.

MODE OF USE

The action of *TCAs* in ameliorating mood is usually absent in the first 2 weeks of therapy and at least 4 weeks must elapse to constitute an adequate trial. Where a minimal response is noted in this period, it is reasonable to extend the trial to 6 weeks to see if further benefit is achieved. By contrast, patients may experience unwanted drug effects immediately on starting treatment (and they should be warned), but such symptoms often diminish with time. Titrating from a generally tolerable starting dose, e.g. amitriptyline 30–75 mg/day (25–50 mg/day for imipramine), with weekly increments to a recognised 'minimum therapeutic' dose, usually around 125 mg/day (140 mg/day for lofepramine) lessens the impact of adverse symptoms before a degree of tolerance (and therapeutic benefit) develops. Low starting doses are particularly important for elderly patients. Only when the drug has reached the minimum therapeutic dose and been taken for at least 4 weeks can the test of response or nonresponse be considered adequate.

Some patients do achieve response or remission at subtherapeutic doses, for reasons of drug kinetics and individual metabolism, the self-limiting nature of depression or by a placebo effect (reinforced by the experience of side effects suggesting that the drug must be having some action).

TCAs are given either in divided doses or, for the more sedative compounds, as a single evening dose.

SSRIs have advantages over tricyclics in simplicity of introduction and use. Dose titration is often unnecessary since the minimum therapeutic dose can usually be tolerated as a starting dose. Divided doses are not required and administration is by a single morning or evening dose. Evidence suggests that patients commencing treatment on SSRIs are more likely to reach an effective dose than those starting on TCAs.

The novel compounds nefazodone and trazodone usually require titration to a minimum therapeutic dose of at least 200 mg/day. Response to reboxetine, venlafaxine and mirtazapine may occur at the starting dose but some dose titration is commonly required. Venlafaxine is licensed for treatment-resistant depression by gradual titration from 75 to 375 mg/day. There is some need for dose titration when using MAOIs although recommended starting doses (e.g. phenelzine 15 mg t.d.s.) may be effective. Unlike other drug classes, reduction to a lower maintenance dose is recommended after a response is achieved.

CHANGING AND STOPPING ANTIDEPRESSANTS

When an antidepressant fails through lack of efficacy despite an adequate trial or due to unacceptable side effects, it is generally advisable to change to a drug of a different class. For a patient who does not respond to an SSRI it is logical to try a TCA or a novel compound such as venlafaxine, reboxetine or mirtazapine. Any of these options may offer a greater increase in synaptic noradrenaline than the ineffective SSRI. There is also evidence to suggest that patients failing on one SSRI may respond to a different drug within the class, an approach which is particularly useful where other antidepressant classes have been unsuccessful previously, are contraindicated, or have characteristics which the patient or doctor feel are undesirable. For example, a patient who is keen to avoid putting on weight may prefer to try a second SSRI after an initial failure than to switch to a TCA or MAOI since both of these classes commonly cause weight gain. Awareness of differences between drugs within a class may also be helpful, e.g. the greater serotonergic enhancing effects of clomipramine compared to other tricyclics may be advantageous in a patient who cannot tolerate any other drug class.

When changing between SSRIs and/or TCAs doses should be reduced progressively over 2–4 weeks. Where a new drug is to be introduced it should be 'cross-tapered' i.e. the dose gradually increased as that of the substituted drug is reduced. Changes to or from MAOIs must be handled with great caution due to the dangers of interactions between antidepressant classes (see below). Therefore MAOIs cannot safely be introduced within 2 weeks of stopping paroxetine, sertraline or tricyclics (3 weeks for imipramine and clomipramine; combination of the latter with tranylcypramine is particularly dangerous), and not until 5 weeks after stopping fluoxetine, the active metabolite of which has a very long $t_\frac{1}{2}$ (9 days). Similarly, TCAs and SSRIs should not be introduced until 2–3 weeks have elapsed from discontinuation of MAOI (as these are irreversible inhibitors, see p. 370). No washout period is required when using the reversible monoamine oxidase inhibitor moclobemide.

When a patient achieves remission, the antidepressant should be continued for at least 9 months at the dose which returned mood to normal. Premature dose reduction or withdrawal is associated with increased risk of relapse. In cases where three or more depressive episodes have occurred, evidence suggests that long-term continuation of an antidepressant offers protection, as further relapse is almost inevitable in the next three years.

When ceasing use of an antidepressant, the dose should be reduced over at least 6 weeks to avoid a discontinuation syndrome (symptoms include anxiety, agitation, nausea and mood swings). Discontinuation of SSRIs and venlafaxine are associated additionally with dizziness, electric shock-like sensations and paraesthesia. Short-acting drugs that do not produce active metabolites are most likely to cause such problems. Paroxetine in particular is associated with severe withdrawal symptoms including bad dreams, paraesthesia and dizziness (which can be misdiagnosed as labyrinthitis).

AUGMENTATION

Augmentation, i.e. the addition of another drug, is used to enhance the effects of standard antidepressants when two or more have successively failed to alleviate depressive symptoms despite treatment at an adequate dose for an adequate time. The therapeutic efficacy of new agents, e.g. venlafaxine, has provided clinicians with further options which now tend to be employed before augmentation but the following may be used.

The most common is augmentation is with the mood stabiliser *lithium carbonate*. Indeed, lithium may be effective as monotherapy for depression but is not preferred because of its adverse effect profile and need for plasma concentration monitoring. Its prescription in combination with antidepressants that have failed to produce remission is more usual and evidence suggests that up to 50% of patients who have not responded to standard antidepressants can respond after lithium augmentation. Addition of lithium requires careful titration of the plasma concentration up to the therapeutic range, with periodic checks thereafter and monitoring for toxicity (see p. 389).

Thyroid hormones also aid antidepressant action. Guidance points to the combination of *tri-iodotyronine* (T_3) and TCAs as being most effective (but effects of lofepramine may be augmented by levothyroxine to the extent that co-administration should be avoided). The amino acid isomer *L-tryptophan*, a precursor of serotonin, may also augment but such use is restricted to hospital specialists who must monitor haematological function (it is associated with an eosinophilia/myalgia syndrome though this may have been due to an impurity rather than the L-tryptophan itself). The β-adrenoceptor blocker *pindolol* can augment the action of SSRIs. Pindolol may act by binding to a serotonin autoreceptor and thus interfere with a homeostatic mechanism which acts to reduce serotonin concentrations after the initial elevation by SSRI action.

None of these augmentation strategies is ideal, since they either require plasma monitoring (lithium, tryptophan, tri-iodothyronine), expose the patient to potential toxicity (lithium, tryptophan) or have only a moderate evidence base for efficacy (tri-iodothyronine, pindolol).

OTHER INDICATIONS FOR ANTIDEPRESSANTS

Antidepressants may benefit most forms of *anxiety disorder,* including panic disorder, generalised anxiety disorder, post-traumatic stress disorder, obsessive-compulsive disorder and social phobia (see p. 393).

SSRIs are effective in milder cases of the eating disorder *bulimia nervosa,* particularly fluoxetine (in higher doses than are required for depression). This effect is independent of that on depression (which may co-exist) and may therefore involve action on transmitter systems other than those involved in modulating depression. Antidepressants appear to be ineffective in anorexia nervosa.

ADVERSE EFFECTS

As most antidepressants have similar therapeutic efficacy, the decision regarding which drug to select often rests on adverse effect profiles and potential to cause toxicity.

Tricyclic antidepressants

The commonest unwanted effects are those of the antimuscarinic action, i.e. dry mouth (predisposing to tooth decay), blurred vision and difficulty with accommodation, raised intraocular pressure (glaucoma may be precipitated), bladder neck obstruction (may lead to urinary retention in older males).

Patients may also experience: postural hypotension (through inhibition of α-adrenoceptors) which is often a limiting factor in their utility in the elderly, interference with sexual function, weight gain (through blockade of histamine H_1 receptors), prolongation of the QT interval of the ECG which predisposes to cardiac arrhythmias especially in overdose (use of TCAs after myocardial infarction is contraindicated).

Some TCAs (especially trimipramine and amitriptyline) are heavily sedating through a combination of antihistaminergic and α-adrenergic blocking actions. This presents special problems to those whose lives involve driving vehicles or performing skilled tasks. In selected patients, sedation may be beneficial, e.g. a severely depressed person who has a disrupted sleep pattern or marked agitation.

It is essential to remember that there is great heterogeneity in adverse effect profiles between TCAs. Imipramine and lofepramine cause relatively little sedation and lofepramine is associated with milder antimuscarinic effects (but is contraindicated in patients with severe liver disease).

Overdose. Depression is a risk factor for both parasuicide and completed suicide, and TCAs are commonly taken by those who deliberately self-harm. *Dothiepin (dosulepin)* and *amitriptyline* are particularly toxic in overdose, being responsible for up to 300 deaths per year in the UK despite the many alternative antidepressants that are available. Lofepramine is at least 15 times less likely to cause death from overdose; clomipramine and imipramine occupy intermediate positions.

Clinical features of overdose reflect the pharmacology of TCAs. Antimuscarinic effects result in warm, dry skin from vasodilatation and inhibition of sweating, blurred vision from paralysis of accommodation, pupillary dilatation and urinary retention.

Consciousness is commonly dulled and respiration depression and hypothermia may develop. Neurological signs include hyperreflexia, myoclonus and divergent strabismus. Extensor plantar responses may accompany lesser degrees of impaired consciousness and provide scope for diagnostic confusion, e.g. with structural brain damage. Convulsions occur in a proportion of patients. Hallucinations and delirium occur during recovery of consciousness, often accompanied by a characteristic plucking at bedclothes.

Sinus tachycardia (due to vagal blockade) is a common feature but abnormalities of cardiac conduction accompany moderate to severe intoxication and may proceed to dangerous tachy- or bradyarrhythmias. Hypotension may result from a combination of cardiac arrhythmia, reduced myocardial contractility and dilatation of venous capacitance vessels.

Supportive treatment suffices for the majority of cases. Activated charcoal by mouth is indicated to prevent further absorption from the alimentary tract and may be given to the conscious patient in the home prior to transfer to hospital. Convulsions are less likely if unnecessary stimuli are avoided but severe or frequent seizures often preceed cardiac arrhythmias and arrest, and their suppression with diazepam is important. The temptation to treat cardiac arrhythmias ought to be resisted if cardiac output and tissue perfusion are adequate. Correction of hypoxia with oxygen and acidosis by i.v. infusion of sodium bicarbonate are reasonable first measures and usually suffice.

Reboxetine is not structurally related to tricyclic agents and acts predominantly by noradrenergic reuptake inhibition. Antimuscarinic effects trouble only a minority of patients, postural hypotension may occur and impotence in males. It is relatively safe in overdose.

Selective serotonin reuptake inhibitors

SSRIs have a range of unwanted effects including nausea, anorexia, dizziness, gastrointestinal disturbance, agitation, akathisia (motor restlessness) and anorgasmia (failure to experience an orgasm). They lack direct sedative effect, an advantage in patients who need to drive vehicles. SSRIs can disrupt the pattern of sleep with increased awakenings, transient reduction in the amount of REM and increased REM latency but eventually sleep improves due to elevation of mood. This class of antidepressant does not cause the problems of postural hypo-

tension, antimuscarinic or antihistaminergic effects seen with TCAs. Their use is not associated with weight gain and conversely they may induce weight loss through their anorectic effects. SSRIs are relatively safe in overdose.

The serotonin syndrome is a rare but dangerous complication of SSRIs and features restlessness, tremor, shivering and myoclonus possibly leading on to convulsions, coma and death. Risk is increased by co-administration with drugs that enhance serotonin transmission, especially MAOIs, the antimigraine drug sumatriptan and St. John's Wort.

Note. When SSRIs are compared with TCAs for patients who discontinue therapy (a surrogate endpoint for tolerability), most meta-analyses show a slight benefit in favour of SSRIs. Comparisons which exclude TCAs with the most prominent antimuscarinic effects (amitriptyline and imipramine) show either marginal benefits in favour of SSRIs or no difference between the groups. It is noteworthy that despite their pronounced adverse effects, amitriptyline and imipramine tend to be selected as 'standard' TCAs against which SSRIs are compared. Lofepramine, the second most prescribed TCA in the UK and the one TCA which causes little sedation, has few antimuscarinic effects and is as safe as SSRIs in overdose is; it under-represented in meta-analyses

Novel compounds

Venlafaxine produces some unwanted effects that resemble those of SSRIs with a higher incidence of nausea. Sustained hypertension (due to blockade of noradrenaline reuptake) is a problem in a small percentage of patients at high dose and blood pressure should be monitored when > 200 mg/day is taken.

Nefazodone lacks antimuscarinic effects but may cause postural hypotension and abdominal discomfort. It appears to improve sleep quality and seems not to interfere with sexual function.

Mirtazapine also has benefits in rarely being associated with sexual dysfunction and in improving sleep independent of mood but like TCAs it may cause unwanted sedation and weight gain.

Trazodone has structural similarities with TCAs but probably acts by antagonism of postsynaptic serotonin receptors and presynaptic α-adrenoceptors. It is an option for depressed patients where heavy sedation is required. Trazodone also has the advantages of lacking antimuscarinic effects and being relatively safe in overdose. Males should be warned of the possibility of priapism (painful penile erections), attributable to the drug's blockade of α_1-adrenoceptors.

Monoamine oxidase inhibitors

Adverse effects include postural hypotension (especially in the elderly) and dizziness. Less common are headache, irritability, apathy, insomnia, fatigue, ataxia, gastrointestinal disturbances including dry mouth and constipation, sexual dysfunction (especially anorgasmia), blurred vision, difficult micturition, sweating, peripheral oedema, tremulousness, restlessness and hyperthermia. Appetite may increase inappropriately, causing weight gain.

INTERACTIONS

Antidepressant use offers considerable scope for an adverse interaction with other drugs through both pharmacodynamic and pharmakokinetic mechanisms. It is therefore prudent always to check specific sources for a possibly unwanted outcome whenever a new drug is added or removed to a prescription list that includes an antidepressant.

TCAs and SSRIs

Pharmacodynamic interactions. Many TCAs cause sedation and therefore co-prescription with other sedative agents such as opioid analgesics, antihistamines, anxiolytics, hypnotics and alcohol may lead to excessive drowsiness and daytime somnolence. The majority of TCAs can have undesirable cardiovascular effects, in particular prolongation of the QT interval. A similar risk of QT prolongation arises with many other cardiovascular drugs including amiodarone, disopyramide, procainamide, propafenone, quinidine, terfenadine, also psychotropic agents such as pimozide, sertindole and thioridazine. Their use in combination with TCAs known to prolong QT enhances the risk of ventricular arrhythmias (for further discussion see p. 509). The combination of thioridazine with any such TCA is thought to be particularly dangerous and is formally contraindicated. TCAs potentiate the effects of catecholamines and other sympathomimetics but not β_2-receptor agonists used in asthma. Even the small amounts of adrenaline or noradrenaline in dental local anaesthetics may produce a serious rise in blood pressure.

Both TCAs and SSRIs may cause central nervous system toxicity if co-prescribed with the dopaminergic drugs entacapone and selegiline (for Parkinson's disease). SSRIs increase the risk of toxicity (the serotonin syndrome) when combined with other drugs which upregulate serotonin transmission, e.g. the $5HT_1$ antagonist sumatriptan (antimigraine) and the anti-obesity drug sibutramine (see p. 697).

Tricyclics and SSRIs can lower the convulsion threshold making epilepsy more difficult to control by anti-epilepsy drugs and lengthening seizure time in electroconvulsive therapy. The situation is further complicated by the ability of carbamazepine to accelerate (induce) the metabolism of antidepressants and inhibition of carbamazepine metabolism by certain antidepressants (below).

Pharmacokinetic interactions. TCAs and SSRIs are metabolised extensively by cytochrome P450 enzymes and adding, changing or stopping antidepressants to a drug regimen can have important consequences.

Potential interactions through the cytochrome P450 CYP 2D6 and CYP 3A4 enzymes can be noted from Tables 19.2a and 19.2b. The combination of drugs that are substrates of the same enzyme creates potential for competitive inhibition of their metabolism with unexpected elevation of plasma concentration. Similarly, potent inhibitors, e.g. fluoxetine and paroxetine (CYP 2D6), fluoxetine and nefazodone (CYP 3A4) and fluvoxamine (CYP 1A2), may cause adverse effects by reducing metabolic breakdown of co-prescribed drugs that are used in standard doses. Antidepressants are commonly prescribed with antipsychotics in a depressive psychosis. Some combinations may have an un-expected adverse outcome unless anticipatory dose adjustment is made, e.g. paroxetine + thioridazine (CYP 2D6), fluoxetine + sertindole (CYP 3A4) and fluvoxamine + olanzapine (CYP 1A2) but others, e.g. fluoxetine + quetiapine (CYP 3A4) appear to be of less significance. An interaction of particular importance involves zuclopenthixol acetate used rapidly to tranquillise psychotic patients who are also receiving fluoxetine or paroxetine and an oral antipsychotic (see p. 363). Inhibition of zuclopenthixol metabolism (CYP 2D6) by fluoxetine or paroxetine, and exacerbated by competition from another anti-psychotic CYP 2D6 substrate, can provoke serious over-sedation and respiratory depression.

Epilepsy is a common co-morbid illness in patients who have both psychiatric illness and learning disabilities. The necessary combination of the anti-epilepsy drug carbamazepine, a CYP 3A4 enzyme inducer, with a CYP 3A4 inhibiting SSRI antidepressant then calls for particularly careful increment in drug doses supported by monitoring of plasma carbamazepine concentration.

Depression and hypertension are both common conditions such that some co-morbidity is inevitable, and panic disorder is epidemiologically associated with hypertension. Co-prescription of an enzyme-inhibiting antidepressant with a β-adrenoceptor blocker (metoprolol, CYP 2D6) or with a calcium antagonist (diltiazem, amlodipine, CYP 3A4) may exaggerate antihypertensive effects.

P450 enzyme inhibition by SSRIs may also augment effects of alcohol, tramadol, methadone, terfenadine (danger of cardiac arrhythmia), -caine anaesthetics and theophylline.

Monoamine oxidase inhibitors

Hypertensive reactions. Many sympathomimetic substances can cause highly dangerous hypertensive reactions if taken by patients using MAO inhibitors. Patients taking MAOIs are vulnerable for two reasons. Firstly, since MAOIs cause an increase in catecholamine stores in adrenergic and dopaminer-gic nerve endings, there is potentiation of sympa-thomimetics that act indirectly by releasing stored noradrenaline. Secondly, patients taking a mono-amine oxidase inhibitor are deprived of the protec-tion of the MAO enzyme present in large quantities in the gut wall and liver. Thus orally administered sympathomimetics that would normally be inacti-vated by this enzyme can be absorbed in much greater quantities. Note that potentiation of admin-istered adrenaline, noradrenaline and isoprenaline is not to be expected since these substances are chiefly destroyed by catechol-O-methyltransferase in the blood and liver.

Symptoms and treatment of hypertensive crisis. Symptoms include a severe, sudden throbbing headache with slow palpitation, flushing, visual disturbance, nausea, vomiting and severe hyper-tension. If headache occurs without hypertension it may be due to histamine release. The hypertension is due both to vasoconstriction from activation of α-adrenoceptors and to increased cardiac output consequent on activation of cardiac β-adrenoceptors. The mechanism is thus similar to that of the episodic hypertension in a patient with phaeochro-mocytoma. The rational and effective treatment is an α-adrenoceptor blocker (phentolamine, 5 mg i.v.) and a β-blocker may be later added in case of excessive tachycadia.

Patient education. It is essential to warn patients taking MAOIs not to use over-the-counter med-ication, as many simple remedies sold direct to the public, such as those for nasal congestion, coughs and colds, will contain sympathomimetics (ephedrine, phenylpropanolamine). Patients must receive detailed instructions about their diet and be made aware of the need to avoid the many foods containing substantial amounts of sympathomime-tics, most commonly tyramine, which acts by releasing tissue-stored noradrenaline. For example, degradation of the protein 'casein' by resident bacteria in well matured cheese can produce tyramine from the amino acid tyrosine, hence use of the term 'cheese reaction' to describe provocation of a hypertensive crisis by orally administered sympathomimetics. Stale foods also present a danger, since any food subjected to autolysis or microbial decomposition during preparation or storage may contain pressor amines resulting from decarboxylation of amino acids.

Moclobemide offers the dual advantages of selective MAO-A inhibition which theoretically

Foods likely to produce hypertensive crises

The following foods are capable of producing dangerous hypertensive effects:

- cheese, especially if well matured
- red wines (especially Chianti) and some white wines; and some beer (non- or low-alcohol varieties contain variable but generally low amounts of tyramine)
- yeast extracts (Marmite, Oxo, Bovril)
- some pickled herrings
- broad bean pods (contain dopa, a precursor of adrenaline)
- over-ripe bananas, avocados, figs
- game
- stale foods
- fermented bean curds including soy sauce
- fermented sausage (e.g. salami), shrimp paste
- flavoured textured vegetable protein (Vegemite).

This list may be incomplete and any partially decomposed food may cause a reaction. Milk and yoghurt appear safe.

should avoid the 'cheese' reaction by sparing the intestinal MAO, which is mainly MAO-B, and by being a competitive, reversible inhibitor. Whereas the irreversible inhibitors inactivate the MAO enzyme and can therefore continue to cause dangerous interactions in the 2–5 weeks after withdrawal, until more enzyme can be synthesised, reversible MAO inhibition is incomplete except during peak plasma concentrations. Since the inhibition is competitive, tyramine can then displace the inhibitor from the active site of the MAO enzyme. Consequently there are less dietary restrictions for patients using moclobemide but hypertensive reactions have been reported.

Interactions with other drugs. The mechanisms of many of the following interactions are obscure and some are probably due to inhibition of drug metabolising enzymes other than MAO as MAOIs are not entirely selective in their action. Effects last for weeks after stopping a MAOI. Reactions can be very severe and even fatal.

Antidepressants: Combination with tricyclic antidepressants has the potential to precipiate hypertensive crisis complicated by hyperreflexia, rigidity and hyperpyrexia. MAOI-SSRI combinations may provoke the life-threatening 'serotonin syndrome' (p. 376). Strict rules apply regarding washout periods when switching between MAOIs and other

drugs (see 'Changing antidepressants', above). Very occasionally, MAOIs are co-prescribed with other antidepressants but since many combinations are highly dangerous, such practice should be reserved for specialists only and then as a last resort.

Narcotic analgesics: with co-prescribed pethidine respiratory depression, restlessness, even coma, and hypo- or hypertension may result (probably due to inhibition of its hepatic demethylation). Interaction with other opioids occurs but is milder. Other drugs which cause minor interactions with MAOIs include antiepileptics (convulsion threshold lowered), dopaminergic drugs (e.g. selegeline [MAO B inhibitor] may cause dyskinesias), antihypertensives and antidiabetes drugs (metformin and sulponylureas potentiated). Concomitant use with amfebutanone/bupropion (smoking cessation), sibutramine (weight reduction), and $5HT_1$-agonists (migraine) should be avoided. Because of the use of numerous drugs during and around surgery, an MAOI is best withdrawn 2 weeks before, if practicable.

Overdose with MAOIs can cause hypomania, coma and hypotension or hypertension. General measures are used as appropriate with minimal administration of drugs: chlorpromazine for restlessness and excitement; phentolamine for hypertension, no vasopressor drugs for hypotension, because of risk of hypertension (use posture and plasma volume expansion).

ST JOHN'S WORT

Many patients with mild to moderate depression are aware of the potential benefits of the herbal remedy St. John's Wort (*Hypericum perforatum*). The active ingredients in the hypericum extract have yet to be identified and their mode of action is unclear, although it has been postulated that several of the known mechanisms of existing antidepressants are incorporated (inhibition of monoamine reuptake and the monoamine oxidase enzyme, as well as a stimulation of GABA receptors). Much of the original research into the efficacy of St. John's Wort was performed in Germany where its use is well established. Several direct comparisons with tricyclic antidepressants have shown equivalent rates of response but these studies should be interpreted with caution since many trials failed to use standardised ratings for depressive symptoms, patients tended to receive tricyclic regimes below the minimum therapeutic dose and sometimes received hypericum in doses above the maximum recommended in commercially available preparations. A large multicentre trial found only limited evidence of benefit for St. John's Wort over placebo in significant major depression.[1]

Despite these reservations, there is certainly a small proportion of patients who when presented with all the available facts, express a strong desire to take only St. John's Wort, perhaps from a preference for herbally derived compounds over conventional medicine. For patients with mild depression, it is reasonable on existing evidence to go along with this preference rather than to destroy the therapeutic alliance and risk prescribing a standard antidepressant which will not be taken.

Use of St. John's Wort is complicated by the lack of standardisation of the ingredients. Those who wish to take St. John's Wort should be made aware that it may cause dry mouth, dizziness, sedation, gastrointestinal disturbance and confusion. Importantly also, it induces hepatic P450 enzymes (CYP 1A2 and CYP 3A4) with the result that the plasma concentration and therapeutic efficacy of warfarin, oral contraceptives, some anticonvulsants, antipsychotics and HIV protease/reverse transcriptase inhibitors are reduced. Concomitant use of tryptophan and St John's Wort may cause serotonergic effects including nausea and agitation.

ELECTROCONVULSIVE THERAPY

Electroconvulsive therapy (ECT) involves the passage of a small electric charge across the brain by electrodes applied to the frontotemporal aspects of the scalp with the aim of inducing a tonic-clonic seizure. Reference to it is made here principally to indicate its place in therapy. ECT requires the patient to be receiving a general anaesthetic, carrying the small risks equivalent to those associated with general anaesthesia in minor surgical operations. It may cause memory deficits although this is generally transient. For these reasons as well as the

relative ease of use of antidepressant drugs, ECT is usually reserved for psychiatric illness where pharmacological treatments have been unsuccessful or where the potential for rapid improvement characteristic of ECT treatment is important. This may arise where patients are in acute danger from their mental state, for instance the severely depressed patient who has stopped eating or drinking. Modern-day ECT is a safe and effective alternative to pharmacological treatment and remains a first-line option in clinical circumstances where rapid response is desired, when it can be life-saving.

Antipsychotics

CLASSIFICATION

Originally tested as an antihistamine and then proposed as a drug for combating helminth infections, *chlorpromazine* emerged as an effective treatment for psychotic illness in the 1950s. Chlorpromazine-like drugs were originally termed 'neuroleptics' or 'major tranquillisers' but the class adopted the name 'antipsychotics' as over 20 compounds were brought to market during the next 30 years. Classification is by chemical structure (e.g. phenothiazines, butyrophenones). Within the large phenothiazine group, compounds are divided into three types on the basis of the side chain since these tend to predict adverse effect profiles (Table 19.3).

The continuing search for greater efficacy and better tolerability led researchers and clinicians to reinvestigate *clozapine,* a drug which was originally licenced in the 1960s but subsequently withdrawn because of serious haematological effects. Clozapine appeared to offer greater effectiveness in treatment-resistant schizophrenia, to have efficacy against negative in addition to positive psychiatric symptoms (see Table 19.4), and to be less likely to cause extra-pyramidal motor symptoms. It regained its licence in the early 1990s with strict requirements on dose titration and haematological monitoring. The renewed interest in clozapine and its unusual efficacy and tolerability stimulated researchers to examine similar 'atypical' antipsychotic drugs.

Thus the most important distinction in modern-day classification of antipsychotic drugs is between

---

[1] Shelton R C et al 2001 Effectiveness of St. John's Wort in major depression. A randomised control trial. Journal of the American Medical Association 285: 1978–1986

the *classical* (typical) agents such as chlorpromazine, haloperidol and zuclopenthixol, and the *atypical* antipsychotics, which include clozapine, and now risperidone, olanzapine and quetiapine. These latter are 'atypical' in their mode of action, effects on experimental animals (lack of extrapyramidal motor symptoms in rats) and adverse effect profiles. Categorisation of atypical agents by their chemical structure is of limited value clinically as they are very heterogenous. A classification by receptor binding profiles is likely to emerge with growing evidence on the clinical importance of their actions on inter-related transmitter systems.

INDICATIONS

Antipsychotic drugs are used for the prophylaxis and acute treatment of psychotic illnesses including *schizophrenia* and *psychoses associated with depression and mania.* They also have an important role as an alternative or adjunct to benzodiazepines in the management of the *acutely disturbed patient,* both for tranquillisation and sedation. Antipsychotics have been used short-term in severe anxiety but are now given only as a last resort. Certain antipsychotics have an antidepressant effect which is distinct from their ability to treat the psychosis associated with depression but use as antidepressants is difficult to justify given the many pharmacological options now available for treating depression. Antipsychotics have also proved useful in the tic disorder Tourette's syndrome and for recurrent self-harming behaviour.

The threshold for seeking specialist involvement in starting antipsychotics is much lower than that when initiating antidepressant drugs. This reflects the complexity of diagnosis of psychotic illness, its chronicity, the increased likelihood of poor compliance without appropriate support and the potential toxicity of antipsychotic agents.

MECHANISM OF ACTION

Historically the beneficial effects of classical antipsychotic agents were explained by their action on brain pathways in which *dopamine* is the neurotransmitter. Dopaminergic pathways include the tuberoinfunibular pathway (moderating prolactin release from the hypothalamus), the nigrostriatal pathway (involved in motor control and deficient in Parkinson's Disease) and the mesolimbic pathway, which runs from the ventrotegmental area via the nucleus accumbens to the prefrontal cortex (Fig. 19.3) (and is overactive in psychotic illness according to the dopamine hypothesis of schizophrenia). Five dopamine receptor types are identified. D_1- and D_5-receptor activation increases intracellular cyclic AMP concentrations whereas activation of D_2, D_3 and D_4 subtypes has the opposite effect. Since all classical antipsychotic agents shared an ability substantially to block D_2-receptors, their effects in ameliorating psychosis were ascribed to preventing activation of these receptors. Thus it was postulated that the key deficit in schizophrenia was *increased dopaminergic activity,* brought about by a rise in the number of brain dopamine D_2-receptors, or receptor supersensitivity, or excess availability of dopamine for D_2-receptor activation from overproduction or reduced destruction through enzyme deficiency.

TABLE 19.3	Antipsychotic drugs	
Atypical antipsychotics*	**Classical antipsychotics**	
Clozapine	*Phenothiazines*	
Olanzapine	Type I	Chlorpromazine
Quetiapine		Promazine
Risperidone	Type 2	Thioridazine † ¶
Ziprasidone		Pericyazine
Amisulpride**	Type 3	Trifluoperazine
Zotepine		Prochlorperazine
Sertindole***		Fluphenazine
	Butyrophenones	Haloperidol
		Benperidol
	Substituted benzamide	Sulpiride** ¶
	Thioxanthines	Flupentixol
		Zuclopenthixol
	Others	Pimozide
		Loxapine

* No recognised classification system exists for atypical antipsychotics. Tentative terms based on receptor binding profiles have been applied to certain drug groupings, for example 'broad spectrum atypicals' for clozapine, olanzapine and quetiapine, whilst risperidone and ziprasidone have been described as 'high affinity serotonin-dopamine antagonists'.
** Amisulpride and sulpiride are structurally related.
*** Sertindole is available only on a named patient basis.
† Licenced indications for thioridazine were severely restricted in 2000 after evidence emerged of cardiovascular toxicity.
¶ In some classifications thioridazine and sulpiride are considered to be 'atypical' due to their low propensity to cause extrapyramidal adverse effects.

The reality is more complex since the receptor binding profile of clozapine and the newer atypical antipsychotic agents suggests that D$_2$-receptor blockade is not essential for antipsychotic effect. The atypical drugs act on numerous receptors and modulate several interacting transmitter systems. Clozapine is a highly effective antipsychotic. It has little affinity for the D$_2$-receptor compared with classical drugs but binds more avidly to other dopamine subtypes (e.g. D$_1$, D$_3$ and D$_4$). It blocks muscarinic acetylcholine receptors, as do certain classical agents (e.g. thioridazine), a property which may reduce the experience of extrapyramidal effects. Clozapine binds more readily as an antagonist at α$_2$-adrenoceptors than the classical drugs and also blocks histamine and serotonin receptors (5HT$_2$ and others).

The newer atypical psychotropics vary widely in their receptor binding profiles. Olanzapine and quetiapine bear resemblance to the profile of clozapine in that their therapeutic effects appear to derive from action on different receptors and transmitter systems. All atypicals (except amisulpride) exhibit greater antagonism of 5HT$_2$-receptors than D$_2$-receptors compared with the classical agents. Atypical drugs that do antagonise dopamine D$_2$-receptors appear to have affinity for those in the mesolimbic system (producing antipsychotic effect) rather than the nigrostriatal system (associated with unwanted motor effects). In contrast to classical antipsychotics, risperidone shares with clozapine an ability antagonise α$_2$-adrenoceptors, a property which may have utility in the treatment of schizophrenia and is seen as an area of interest for developing new drugs.

PHARMACOKINETICS

Like antidepressants, antipsychotics are well absorbed and distributed after oral administration. In situations where very rapid relief of symptoms or disturbed behaviour is required, faster uptake into plasma can be achieved through the intramuscular route. Again in common with antidepressants, antipsychotics are mainly metabolised by cytochrome P450 isoenzymes in the liver, e.g. CYP 2D6 (zuclopenthixol, risperidone [Table 19.2a]), CYP 3A4 (sertindole [Table 19.2b]), CYP 1A2 (olanzapine, clozapine). Metabolism of some compounds is particularly complex (e.g. chlorpromazine, haloperidol), involving more than one main pathway, utilising several P450 enzymes or resulting in the production of many inactive metabolites. Antipsychotic plasma levels can be increased or decreased by co-prescription of drugs which are inhibitors, inducers or substrates of the same isozyme. Amisulpride is an exception to the general rule as it is eliminated by the kidneys without hepatic metabolism.

Examples of plasma half-lives for antipsychotics include quetiapine 7 h, clozapine 12 h, haloperidol 18 h and olazapine 33 h. Depot intramuscular injections are available from which drug is released over 2–4 weeks.

EFFICACY

Symptoms in schizophrenia are defined as *positive* and *negative* (Table 19.4). Whilst a classical antipsychotic drug should provide adequate treatment of positive symptoms including hallucinations and delusions in at least 60% of cases, patients are often left with unresolved negative symptoms such as apathy, flattening of affect and alogia. Evidence suggests that clozapine and the newer atypicals have a significant advantage over classical drugs against negative symptoms. Clozapine has a

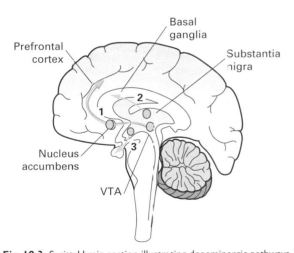

Fig. 19.3 Sagittal brain section illustrating dopaminergic pathways. 1. *Mesolimbic pathway* (overactive in psychotic illness according to the dopamine hypothesis of schizophrenia). VTA= ventrotegmental area. 2. *Nigrostriatal pathway* (involved in motor control, underactive in Parkinson's Disease and associated with extrapyramidal motor symptoms). 3. *Tuberoinfundibular pathway* (inhibits prolactin release from the hypothalamus).

further advantage over all other antipsychotics, whether classical or atypical, in that it may be effective when other antipsychotics prescribed at adequate doses have failed or are not tolerated.

Schizophrenia often runs a chronic relapsing and remitting course. Less than one-quarter of patients who experience a psychotic episode and are diagnosed as having schizophrenia succeed in avoiding further episodes. Nevertheless, taking antipsychotics as prophylaxis significantly reduces the likelihood of relapse.

MODE OF USE

Since the potency (therapeutic efficacy in relation to weight) of antipsychotic agents varies markedly between compounds, it is useful to think of the effective antipsychotic dose of classical agents in terms of 'chlorpromazine equivalents' (see Table 19.5). For example, haloperidol has a relatively high antipsychotic potency, such that 2–3 mg is equivalent to chlorpromazine 100 mg, whereas sulpiride 200 mg (low potency) is required for the same antipsychotic effect.

Patients who are 'neuroleptic naïve' (i.e. have never previously taken any antipsychotic agent) should start at the lowest available dosage, such as haloperidol 0.5 mg/day or chlorpromazine 25 mg/day, in case the patient is particularly susceptible to adverse effects, especially extrapyramidal motor symptoms. Conservative starting doses are also recommended in the elderly and for patients with learning disabilities who may require antipsychotics for psychosis or severe behavioural disturbance. The dose can be titrated up at intervals, until the desired effect in treating psychotic symptoms, calming disturbed behaviour or effecting sedation is achieved. The interval depends on the context, with the urgency of the situation and previous use of antipsychotics being factors which would accelerate the upward titration. An important issue is that the longer a psychosis is left untreated the less favourable is the outcome; thus drug treatment should be instigated as soon as an adequate period of assessment has allowed a provisional diagnosis to be established.

For each antipsychotic agent there is a licensed maximum dose; for example up to 1000 mg of chlorpromazine/day may be given under the United Kingdom licence. Prescribing beyond the licensed maximum dose requires specialist consent. When two antipsychotics are co-prescribed, the maximum antipsychotic dose should not exceed 1000 mg of chlorpromazine equivalents/day except under specialist supervision. For some antipsychotics the licenced maximum dose is considerably less than 1000 mg of chlorpromazine equivalents/day. For instance, the licenced maximum dose of thioridazine was reduced to 600 mg/day following concerns about its cardiovascular toxicity. Note

---

TABLE 19.4 Symptoms of schizophrenia

Positive symptoms	Negative symptoms
Hallucinations, most commonly auditory (i.e. voices) in the 3rd person, which patients may find threatening. The voices may also give commands. Visual hallucinations are rare.	*Affective flattening* manifest by unchanging facial expression with lack of communication through expression, poor eye contact, lack of responsiveness, psychomotor slowing
Delusions, most commonly persecutory. 'Passivity phenomena' include delusions of thought broadcasting, thought insertion or thought withdrawal, made actions, impulses or feelings.	*Alogia* (literally 'absence of words' manifesting clinically as a lack of spontaneous speech (poverty of speech).
Bizarre behaviours including agitation, sexual disinhibition, repetitive behaviour, wearing of striking but inappropriate clothing.	*Anhedonia* (inability to derive pleasure from any activity) and *Associality* (narrowing of repertoire of interests and impaired relationships)
Thought disorder manifest by failure in the organisation of speech such that it drifts away from the point (tangentiality), never reaches the point (circumstantiality), moves from one topic to the next illogically (loosened associations, knight's move thinking), breaks off abruptly only to continue on an unrelated topic (derailment) or moves from one topic to the next on the basis of a pun or words which sound similar (clang association).	*Apathy/Avolution* involving lack of energy, lack of motivation to work, participate in activities or initiate any goal-directed behaviour, and poor personal hygiene. *Attention problems* involving an inability to focus on any one issue or engage fully with communication.

that plasma electrolytes and an ECG should be checked on introducing or increasing the dose of thioridazine and that an ECG should be seen before prescribing pimozide and sertindole.

Prescription of atypical antipsychotics follows similar rules to those for classical drugs, starting at low doses in neuroleptic naïve patients. Whereas there is a wide range of effective doses for many classical agents (e.g. chlorpromazine 25–1000 mg/day), much narrower ranges have been defined for atypical agents (Table 19.5). While classical antipsychotics are licenced for the management of acutely disturbed behaviour as well as for schizophrenia, atypical agents are generally licenced only for the latter indication, although that for risperidone is broader. For most atypical agents used in schizophrenia, a brief period of dose titration by protocol up to a stated lowest therapeutic dose is usual, e.g. risperidone 4 mg/day, quetiapine 300 mg/day. Dose increases are indicated where there is no response after 2 weeks and these may be repeated until the maximum licenced dose is achieved.

Clozapine may be initiated only under specialist supervision and only after two other antipsychotic agents have failed through lack of efficacy or adverse effects. Additionally, leucocyte count monitoring is mandatory (danger of agranulocytosis) and blood pressure checking is required (for hypotensive effect). Patients are most vulnerable to agranulocytosis on initiation of therapy with 75% of cases occurring in the first 18 weeks. The dose titration schedule must be followed strictly, starting with clozapine 12.5 mg nocte and working up over a period of four weeks to a target therapeutic dose of 450 mg/day.

Alternative administration strategies in acute use of antipsychotics

Some of the antipsychotics are available as intramuscular injections for patients who are unable or unwilling to swallow tablets (as is common in psychosis or severe behavioural disturbance). *Haloperidol* is most often used for these indications on psychiatric inpatient wards (chlorpromazine i.m. being restricted due to hypotension and skin nodule formation). Olanzapine may be given i.m.

for acute behavioural disturbance in schizophrenia. This drug is also presented as a 'velotab' which dissolves rapidly on contact with the tongue allowing drug to be absorbed despite lack of cooperation from a disturbed patient.

Long-acting (depot) injections

Haloperidol, zuclopenthixol, fluphenazine, flupentixol and *pipothiazine* are available as depot intramuscular injections for maintenance treatment of patients with schizophrenia and other chronic psychotic disorders. Provided the patient is willing to agree to have depot injections, usually by a community psychiatric nurse at intervals of 2–4 weeks, the need to take tablets two or three times a day is removed. Poor compliance with oral medication is the most common cause of admission to hospital with a relapse of schizophrenia. A reduced initial dose of the depot medication should be given, with a review for unwanted effects after 5–10 days.

Rapid tranquillisation

Rapid tranquillisation protocols have been devised for patients who are severely disturbed and violent or potentially violent and have not responded to nonpharmacological approaches. The risks from administering psychotropic drugs (e.g. cardiac arrhythmia with high-dose antipsychotics) may greatly outweigh the risk of leaving the patient untreated, including physical trauma and the consequences of over-stressing the cardiovascular system.

A benzodiazepine, e.g. *lorazepam* 1–2 mg i.v. (into a large vein) failing which i.m. (dilute with an equal volume of water or physiological saline) is the first option if the patient is not already receiving an antipsychotic drug. Patients requiring rapid tranquillisation are commonly taking antipsychotics for established illness and an additional antipsychotic may then be used if the patient has not received an adequate dose; otherwise a benzodiazepine should given. *Haloperidol* 2–10 mg i.m. is currently preferred for rapid tranquillisation, but new protocols may evolve with the development of atypical antipsychotics that can be given i.m. When i.m. antipsychotic or benzodiazepine tranquilliser is given as an emergency, pulse, blood pressure, temperature and respiration should be monitored, and pulse oximetry (oxygen saturation) if consciousness is lost.

When at least two doses of haloperidol i.m. fail to produce the desired result, zuclopenthixol acetate i.m. is an alternative. This heavily sedating drug usually produces a calming effect within 2 h, persisting for 2–3 days if used at appropriate dose. Zuclopenthixol acetate should never be prescribed to the neuroleptic naïve. Patients must be observed with the utmost care following administration. Some will require a second dose within 1–2 days.

Amylobarbitone and paraldehyde have a role in emergencies when antipsychotic and benzodiazepine options have been exhausted.

ADVERSE EFFECTS (see Table 19.5)

Active psychotic illnesses often cause patients to have poor insight into their condition; unwanted drug effects can compromise already fragile compliance and lead to avoidable relapse.

Classical antipsychotics

It is rare for any patient taking classical antipsychotic agents completely to escape their adverse effects. Thus it is essential to discuss with patients the possibility of unwanted effects and regularly to review this aspect of their care.

Extrapyramidal symptoms. All classical antipsychotics are capable of producing these effects because they act by blocking dopamine receptors in the nigrostriatal pathway. The result is that some 75% of patients experience extrapyramidal symptoms which may appear shortly after starting the drug or increasing its dose (acute effects), or some time after a particular dose level has been established (tardive effects, see p. 387).

Acute extrapyramidal symptoms. *Dystonias* are manifest as abnormal movements of the tongue and facial muscles with fixed postures and spasm, including torticollis and bizarre eye movements ('oculogyric crisis'). *Parkinsonian symptoms* result in the classical triad of bradykinesia, rigidity and tremor. Both dystonias and parkinsonian symptoms

are believed to result from a shift in favour of cholinergic rather than dopaminergic neurotransmission in the nigrostriatal pathway (see p. 422). Anticholinergic agents, e.g. procyclidine, orphenadrine or benztropine, restore the balance in favour of dopaminergic transmission but are liable to provoke antimuscarinic effects (dry mouth, urine retention, constipation, exacerbation of glaucoma and confusion) and they offer no relief for tardive dyskinesia, which may even worsen. They should be used only in response to clear dystonic or parkinsonian symptoms rather than for prophylaxis. Benzodiazepines, with their general inhibitory effects, are an alternative. *Thioridazine* and related Type 2 phenothiazines are less likely to provoke extrapyramidal effects as they also block cholinergic transmission (but patients may suffer antimuscarinic effects). Note that confusion from anticholinergic effects may mimic or complicate schizophrenic thought disorder.

Akathisia is a state of motor and psychological restlessness, in which patients exhibit persistent foot tapping, moving of legs repetitively and being unable to settle or relax. A strong association has been noted between its presence in treated schizophrenics and subsequent suicide. A β-adrenoceptor blocker is the best treatment, although anticholinergic agents may be effective where akathisia coexists with dystonias and parkinsonian symptoms. Differentiating symptoms of psychotic illness from adverse drug effects is often difficult: drug-induced akathisia may be mistaken for agitation induced by psychosis.

Tardive dyskinesia affects about 25% of patients taking classical antipsychotic drugs, the risk increasing with length of exposure. It was formerly thought to be a consequence of up-regulation or supersensitivity of dopamine receptors. A preferred explanation is that tardive dyskinesia is a consequence of oxidative damage after neuroleptic-induced increases in glutamate transmission. Patients display a spectrum of abnormal movements from minor tongue protusion, lip-smacking, rotational tongue movements and facial grimacing, choreoathetoid movements of the head and neck and even to twisting and gyrating of the whole body. It is less likely to remit on stopping the causative agent than

TABLE 19.5 Relative frequency of selected adverse effects of antipsychotic drugs

Drug	CPZ Equiv Dose	Max dose (/day)	Structure	Extrapyramidal effects	Anticholinergic effects	Hyperprolactinaemia	Weight gain	Cardiotoxicity	Blood dyscrasias	Sedation
Classical										
Chlorpromazine	100 mg	1000 mg	Type 1 Phenothiazine	++	++	+++	++	+	+	+++
Thioridazine	50 mg	300 mg*	Type 2 Phenothiazine	+	+++	+++	+++	+++	+	+++
Trifluoperazine	5 mg	50 mg	Type 3 Phenothiazine	+++	+	+++	++	+	+	+
Haloperidol	3 mg	30 mg	Butyrophenone	+++	+	+++	++	+	+	+
Sulpiride	200 mg	2400 mg	Substituted benzamide	+	+	+++	+	−	+	−
Zuclopenthixol	25 mg	150 mg	Thioxanthene	++	++	+++	++	+	+	++
	Min eff. dose (/day)	**Max dose (/day)**								
Atypical										
Clozapine**	300 mg	900 mg	Dibenzodiazepine	−	+++	−	+++	+	+++	+++
Olanzapine	5–10 mg	20 mg	Theinobenzodiazepine	−	++	+	+++	−	+	++
Quetiapine	300 mg	750 mg	Dibenzothiazepine	−	+	−	+	−	+	+++
Risperidone	4mg	16 mg	Benzisoxazole	+	+	++	+	−	+	+
Amisulpride	800 mg¶	1200 mg	Substituted benzamide	+	−	++	+	−	+	−

Key: CPZ equiv dose = Chlorpromazine equivalent dose. This concept is of value in comparing the potency of classical antipsychotics. Dose ranges are not specified as they are extremely wide and drugs are normally titrated up from low starting doses (e.g. chlorpromazine 25 mg or equivalent) until an adequate antipsychotic effect is achieved or the maximum dose reached. The chlorpromazine equivalent dose concept is of less value for atypical antipsychotics since minimum effective doses (Min. eff. dose) and narrower therapeutic ranges have been defined. Maximum dose (Max. dose) can be exceeded only under specialist supervision.
* The maximum recommended dose of thioradazine was reduced to 300 mg/day (or 600 mg/day in hospitalised patients) following concerns about QT prolongation and risk of fatal cardiac arrhythmias at higher doses.
** A dose of clozapine 50 mg is considered equivalent to chlorpromazine 100 mg.
¶ Lower doses of amisulpride (e.g. 100 mg/day) are indicated for patients with negative symptoms of schizophrenia only.

are simple dystonias and parkinsonian symptoms. Any anticholinergic agent should be withdrawn immediately. Reduction of the dose of classical antipsychotic is often advised but psychotic symptoms may then worsen or be 'unmasked'. Alternatively, an atypical antipsychotic can provide rapid improvement whilst retaining control of psychotic symptoms.

Atypical drugs, particularly at high doses, can yet cause extrapyramidal effects and this strategy is not always helpful. If the classical antipsychotic is simply continued, tardive dyskinesia remits spontaneously in around 30% of patients within a year but since the condition is difficult to tolerate, patients may be keen to try other medications, even where evidence suggests that the success rates for remission are limited. These include vitamin E, benzodiazepines, β-blockers, bromocriptine and

tetrabenazine. Clozapine, which does not appear to cause tardive dyskinesia, may be used in severe cases where continuing antipsychotic treatment is required and symptoms have not responded to other medication strategies.

Cardiovascular effects. Postural hypotension may result from blockade of α-adrenoceptors; it is dose-related. Prolongation of the QT interval in the cardiac cycle may rarely lead to ventricular arrhythmias and sudden death (but particular warnings and constraints apply to the use of thioridazine and pimozide).

Prolactin elevation. Classical antipsychotics raise plasma prolactin concentrations by their blocking action on dopamine receptors in the tuberoinfundibular pathway (Fig. 19.3 and p. 711) and can cause gynaecomastia and galactorrhoea in both sexes, and menstrual disturbances. A change to an atypical agent such as quetiapine or olanzapine (but not risperidone or amisulpride) should minimise these effects. If continuation of the existing classical antipsychotic is obligatory, a dopamine agonist such as bromocriptine or amantadine may be beneficial.

Sedation. In the acute treatment of psychotic illness this may be a highly desirable property but it may be unwelcome as the patient seeks to resume work, study or relationships.

Classical antipsychotics may also be associated with:

- *weight gain* (a problem with almost all classical antipsychotics with the exception of loxapine, most pronounced with fluphenazine and flupentixol)
- *seizures* (chlorpromazine and thioridazine are especially likely to lower the convulsion threshold)
- *interference with temperature regulation* (hypothermia or hyperthermia, especially in the elderly)
- *skin problems* (phenothiazines, particularly chlorpromazine, may provoke photosensitivity necessitating advice about limiting exposure to sunlight. Rashes and urticaria may also occur)
- *sexual dysfunction* (ejaculatory problems through α-adrenoceptor blockade)
- *retinal pigmentation* (chlorpromazine, thioridazine, vision is affected if dose is prolonged and high)
- *corneal and lens opacities*
- *blood dyscrasias* (agranulocytosis and leucopenia)
- *osteoporosis* (associated with prolactin elevation)
- *jaundice* (including cholestatic).

Atypical antipsychotics

Atypical drugs can provoke a range of adverse effects that is similar to that of the classical antipsychotics but is generally lesser in degree (with exceptions). The following are the main differences.

Atypical antpipsychotics provoke *fewer extrapyramidal effects* (less blockade of dopamine D_2-receptors in the nigrostriatal pathway). Nevertheless, extrapyramidal effects are seen, notably with high dose of risperidone (8–12 mg per day) and olanzapine (> 20 mg/day).

Clozapine and olanzapine are the most likely of the atypical agents to cause *anticholinergic (antimuscarinic) effects.* They are more likely than other atypicals to cause *weight gain* (glucose tolerance may be impaired and should be monitored in susceptible individuals) and are second only to quetiapine in their *sedative effects*. Sexual dysfunction and skin problems are rare with atypical antipsychotics. Risperidone and amisulpride are as likely as classical antipsychotics to raise prolactin concentrations and cause *galactorrhoea.*

Clozapine warrants further mention, given its value for patients with treatment-resistant schizophrenia or severe treatment-related extrapyramidal symptoms. It may cause postural hypotension and tachycardia, and provoke seizures in 3–5% of patients at doses above 600 mg/day. Most important is the risk of *agranulocytosis* in up to 2% of patients (compared with 0.2% in classical antipsychotics). When clozapine was first licenced without requirements for regular white count monitoring, the haematological problems caused appreciable mortality. Thanks to strict monitoring, there have been no recorded deaths from agranulocytosis since clozapine was reintroduced in the United Kingdom, and internationally the death rate among the small minority who develop agranulocytosis is now less than 1 in 1000.

Neuroleptic malignant syndrome

The syndrome may develop in up to 1% of patients using antipsychotics and is more prevalent at high doses. The elderly, and those with organic brain disease, hyperthyroidism or dehydration are thought to be most susceptible. Clinical features include:

- fever
- confusion or fluctuating consciousness
- rigidity of muscles which may become severe
- autonomic instability manifest by labile blood pressure
- tachycardia
- urinary incontinence or retention.

Raised plasma creatine kinase concentration and white cell count are suggestive (but not conclusive) of neuroleptic malignant syndrome. There is some clinical overlap with the 'serotonin syndrome' (see

p. 376) and concomitant use of SSRI antidepressants (or possibly TCAs) with antipsychotics may increase risk.

It is essential to discontinue the antipsychotic when the syndrome is suspected and to be ready to transfer the patient to a medical ward for rehydration. Benzodiazepines are indicated for sedation and their transquillising effect may be useful where active psychosis has to be left untreated. Dopamine agonists (bromocriptine, dantrolene) are beneficial in some cases. There is also evidence to support a role for electroconvulsive therapy in treatment of neuroleptic malignant syndrome. Even when recognised and treated, the condition carries a mortality of 12–15%, through cardiac arrhythmia, rhabdomyolysis or respiratory failure. The condition usually lasts for 5–7 days after the antipsychotic is stopped but may continue longer when a depot preparation has been used. Fortunately those who survive tend to have no long lasting physical effects from their ordeal.

CLASSICAL VERSUS ATYPICAL ANTIPSYCHOTICS

As atypical antipsychotics have become established as alternatives to classical agents, clinicians are presented with the dilemma as to which should be their first choice in patients with schizophrenia and psychotic illnesses, and indeed whether there is sufficient justification to transfer a patient stabilised on a classical agent over to an atypical.

Atypical antipsychotics may have advantages in three areas. First, they appear to be better tolerated,[2] in particular being less likely than classical agents to induce extrapyramidal effects and hyperprolac-

tinaemia (with gynaecomastia and galactorrhoea), although these latter remain common with risperidone and amisulpride. Improved tolerance is reflected in better compliance with taking atypical agents, so lessening the chance of psychosis being untreated with the likelihood of relapse once remission has been achieved. Secondly, atypical antipsychotics are more efficacious against the negative symptoms of schizophrenia which are particularly debilitating in chronic illness.

Thirdly, clozapine (but not the newer atypicals) is more effective than classical agents for resistant schizophrenia.

Atypical antipsychotics are significantly more expensive than classical drugs. In some countries this will be the overriding argument for retaining classical agents as first choice drugs in schizophrenia. Additionally, if a patient is successfully maintained on a classical antipsychotic, transfer to an atypical agent is difficult to justify. Where a classical antipsychotic is not achieving optimal results or causes unwanted effects, a more persuasive case for change to an atypical can be made.

But economic analysis must take into account factors beyond the crude cost of drugs. If atypical antipsychotics truly cause fewer distressing extrapyramidal symptoms and improve compliance, they may prevent relapse of psychotic illness and protect patients against lasting damage from periods of untreated psychosis. Greater effectiveness in treating negative symptoms would afford patients with schizophrenia more opportunity of re-integrating into the community and to make positive contributions to society rather than the alternative of long-term institutionalisation. Such factors alleviate the cost burden of psychotic illness on society, and must form part of the overall accounting between classical and atypical drugs as first line treatment.

---

[2] Whilst the advantages of atypicals over classical antipsychotics may seem clear cut, one analysis using only trials where doses of classical antipsychotics were at or below a dose of haloperidol 12 mg/day or equivalent (now regarded as the upper limit for optimised use of these agents) produced rather different results. Although the atypicals retained their advantage in causing extrapyramidal side effects less frequently, overall tolerability and efficacy appeared to be similar. Geddes J et al 2000 Atypical antipsychotics in the treatment of schizophrenia: systematic overview and meta-regression analysis. British Medical Journal 321: 1371–1376.

Mood stabilisers

In bipolar affective disorder patients suffer episodes of mania, hypomania and depression, classically with periods of normal mood in between. *Manic episodes* involve greatly elevated mood, often interspersed with periods of irritability or undue excitement, accompanied by biological symptoms (increased energy, restlessness, decreased need for sleep, increased sex drive), loss of social inhibitions, irresponsible behaviour and grandiosity. Psychotic features may be present, particularly disordered thinking manifested by grandiose delusions and 'flight of ideas' (acceleration of the pattern of thought with rapid speech). *Hypomania* is a less dramatic and dangerous presentation but retains the features of elation or irritability and the biological symptoms, abnormalities in speech being limited to increased talkativeness and in social conduct to overfamiliarity and mild recklessness. *Depressive episodes* may include any of the depressive symptoms described before and may include psychotic features.

Lithium salts were known anecdotally to have beneficial psychotropic effects as long ago as the middle of the 19th century but scientific evidence of their efficacy followed a serendipitous discovery. In 1949, during a search for biologically active substances in mania, urine from manic patients was injected into guinea pigs. The animals appeared to be affected by the accompanying large amounts of urea and it was postulated that administration of urate would exacerbate manic effects. Lithium urate, which is highly soluble, was selected to conduct investigations into urate toxicity. It was found to be sedative and to protect against manic urine toxicity. Lithium carbonate was tried in manic patients, was found to be effective in the acute state and, later, to prevent recurrent attacks.[3]

Lithium salts are ineffective for prophylaxis of bipolar affective disorder in around 35% of patients and cause several unwanted effects. The search for alternatives has produced drugs that are more familiar as anticonvulsants, notably carbamazepine and sodium valproate, and possibly lamotrigine.

LITHIUM

The mode of action is not fully understood. The main effect of lithium is probably to inhibit hydrolysis of inositol phosphate, so reducing the recycling of free inositol for synthesis of phosphatidylinositides. These intracellular molecules are part of the transmembrane signalling system that is important in regulating intracellullar calcium ion concentration, which subsequently affects neurotransmitter release. Other putative mechanisms involve the cyclic AMP 'second messenger' system and monoaminergic and cholinergic neurotransmitters.

Pharmacokinetics. Knowledge of pharmacokinetics of lithium is important for successful use since the therapeutic plasma concentration is close to the toxic concentration (low therapeutic index). Lithium is a small ion that, given orally, is rapidly absorbed throughout the gut. High peak plasma concentrations are avoided by using sustained-release formulations which deliver the peak plasma lithium concentrations in about 5 h. At first lithium is distributed throughout the extracellular water but with continued administration it enters the cells and is eventually distributed throughout the total body water with a somewhat higher concentration in brain, bones and thyroid gland. The apparent volume of distribution is about 50 1 in a 70 kg person (whose total body water is about 40 1) which is compatible with the above. Lithium is easily dialysable from the blood but the concentration gradient from cell to blood is not great and the intracellular concentration (which determines toxicity) falls slowly. Lithium enters cells about as readily as does sodium but does not leave as readily (mechanism uncertain). Being a metallic ion it is not metabolised, nor is it bound to plasma proteins.

Only the kidneys eliminate lithium. Like sodium, it is filtered by the glomerulus and 80% is reabsorbed by the proximal tubule but it is not reabsorbed by the distal tubule. Intake of sodium and water are the principal determinants of its elimination. In sodium deficiency lithium is retained in the body, thus concomitant use of a diuretic can reduce lithium clearance by as much as 50% and precipitate toxicity. Sodium chloride and water are used to treat lithium toxicity.

With chronic use the plasma $t_{1/2}$ of lithium is 15–30 h. Lithium is usually given 12-hourly to avoid unnecessary fluctuation (peak and trough concentrations) and maintain a plasma concentration just below the toxic level. A steady-state plasma concentration will be attained after about 5–6 days (i.e. $5 \times t_{1/2}$) in patients with normal renal

---

[3] Cade J F. 1970 The story of lithium. In: Ayd F J, Blackwell B (eds) Biological psychiatry. Lippincott, Philadelphia.

function. Old people and patients with impaired renal function will have a longer t½ so that steady state will be reached later and dose increments must be adjusted accordingly.

Indications and use. Lithium carbonate is effective *treatment* in > 75% of episodes of acute mania or hypomania. Because its therapeutic action takes 2–3 weeks to develop, lithium is generally used in combination with a benzodiazepine such as lorazepam or diazepam (or with an antipsychotic agent where there are also psychotic features).

For *prophylaxis,* lithium is indicated when there have been two episodes of mood disturbance in two years, although in some cases it is advisable to continue with prophylactic use after one severe episode. When an adequate dose of lithium is taken consistently, around 65% of patients achieve improved control of their illness.

Patients who start lithium only to discontinue it within two years have a significantly poorer outcome than matched patients who are not given any pharmacological prophylaxis. The existence of this 'rebound effect' dictates that persistence with long-term treatment is of great importance.

Lithium is also used to augment the action of antidepressants in treatment-resistant depression (see p. 375).

Pharmaceutics. It is important for any patient to adhere to the same pharmaceutical brand, as the dose of lithium ion (Li⁺) delivered by each tablet depends on the pharmaceutical preparation. For example, each *Camcolit* 250 mg tablet contains 6.8 mmol, each *Liskonium* 450 mg tablet contains 12.2 mmol and each *Priadel* 200 mg tablet contains 5.4 mmol of Li⁺. Thus the proprietary name must be stated on the prescription. Some patients cannot tolerate slow-release preparations because release of lithium ions distally in the intestine causes diarrhoea; they may be better served by the liquid preparation, lithium citrate, which is absorbed proximally. Patients who are naïve to lithium should be started at the lowest dose of the preparation selected. Any change in preparation demands the same precautions as does initiation of therapy.

Monitoring. The difference between therapeutic and toxic doses is narrow and therapy must be guided by monitoring of the plasma concentration once a steady state is reached. Increments are made at weekly intervals until the concentration lies within the required range of 0.4–1 mmol/l (maintenance at the lower level is preferred for elderly patients). The timing of blood sampling is important. By convention a blood sample is taken prior to the morning dose, as close as possible to 12 h after the evening dose. When the therapeutic range is reached, the plasma concentration should be checked every three months. Likewise, for toxicity monitoring, thyroid function (especially in women) and renal function (plasma creatinine and electrolytes) should be measured before initiation and every 3 months during therapy.

Patient education about the role of lithium in the prophylaxis of bipolar affective disorder and discussion of the pros and cons of taking the drug are particularly important to encourage compliance with therapy; treatment cards, information leaflets and where appropriate, video material are used.

Adverse effects. Lithium is associated with three categories of adverse effects.

- Those experienced at plasma concentrations within the *therapeutic range* (see above) include fine tremor (especially involving the fingers; if this is difficult to tolerate a β-blocker may benefit), constipation, polyuria and polydipsia (due to loss of concentrating ability by the distal renal tubules), metallic taste in the mouth, weight gain, oedema, goitre, hypothyroidism, acne, rash, diabetes insipidus and cardiac arrhythmias. There can also be mild cognitive and memory impairment.
- Signs of *intoxication,* associated with plasma concentrations greater than 1.5 mmol/l are mainly gastrointestinal (diarrhoea, anorexia, vomiting) and neurological (blurred vision, muscle weakness, drowsiness, sluggishness and coarse tremor, leading on to giddiness, ataxia and dysarthria).
- Frank *toxicity,* due to severe overdosage or rapid reduction in renal clearance, usually associated with plasma concentration greater than 2 mmol/l, constitutes an acute medical emergency. Hyperreflexia, hyperextension of

limbs, convulsions, toxic psychoses, syncope, oliguria, coma and even death may result if treatment is not instigated urgently.

Overdose is treated by use of i.v. fluid to maintain a good urine output guided by frequent measurement of plasma electrolytes and osmolality. Hypernatraemia indicates probable diabetes insipidus and isotonic dextrose should then be used until plasma sodium concentration and osmolality become normal. Isotonic saline forms part of the fluid regimen (but overuse may result in hypernatraemia) and potassium supplement will be required. Haemodialysis is effective but may have to be repeated frequently as plasma concentration rises after acute reduction (due to equilibration as lithium leaves cells and also by continued absorption from sustained-release formulations).

Interactions. Several types of drug interfere with lithium excretion by the renal tubules, causing the plasma concentration to rise. These include diuretics (thiazides more than loop type), ACE inhibitors and angiotensin-11 antagonists, and non-steroidal anti-inflammatory analgesics. Theophylline and sodium-containing antacids reduce plasma lithium concentration. The effects can be important because lithium has such a low therapeutic ratio. Diltiazem, verapamil, carbamazepine and phenytoin may cause neurotoxicity without affecting the plasma lithium. Concomitant use of thioridazine should be avoided as ventricular arrhythmias may result.

Carbamazepine

Carbamazepine is licenced as an alternative to lithium for prophylaxis of bipolar affective disorder, although clinical trial evidence is actually stronger to support its use in the treatment of acute mania. Carbamazepine appears to be more effective than lithium for rapidly cycling bipolar disorders, i.e. with recurrent swift transitions from mania to depression. It is also effective in combination with lithium. Its mode of action is thought to involve agonism of inhibitory GABA transmission at the GABA-benzodiazepine receptor complex (see also Epilepsy, p. 417).

Valproic acid

Valproic acid is the drug of first choice for prophylaxis of bipolar affective disorder in the United States, despite the lack of robust clinical trial evidence in support of this indication. But treatment with valproic acid is easy to initiate (especially compared to lithium), it is well tolerated and its use appears likely to extend if the evidence-base expands. As the *semisodium salt,* valproic acid is licenced for use in the treatment of acute mania unresponsive to lithium. (Note: *sodium valproate,* see p. 420, is unlicenced for this indication.)

Treatment with carbamazepine or valproic acid appears not to be associated with the 'rebound effect' of relapse into manic symptoms that may accompany early withdrawal of lithium therapy.

Other drugs

Evidence is emerging regarding the efficacy of lamotrigine in prophylaxis of bipolar affective disorder and treatment of bipolar depression. Other drugs which have been used in augmentation of existing agents include the anticonvulsant gabapentin, the benzodiazepine clonazepam, and the calcium channel blocking agents verapamil and nimodipine.

Drugs used in anxiety and sleep disorders

The disability and health costs caused by anxiety disorders are comparable to those of other common medical conditions such as diabetes, arthritis or hypertension. People with anxiety disorders experience impaired physical and role functioning, more work days lost due to illness, increased impairment at work and high use of health services. Our understanding of the nature of anxiety has increased greatly from advances in research in psychology and neuroscience. It is now possible to distinguish different types of anxiety with distinct biological and cognitive symptoms. Clear criteria have been accepted for the diagnosis of various anxiety disorders. The last decade has seen developments in both drug and psychological therapies such that a range of treatment options can be tailored to individual patients and their condition.

The GABA$_A$-benzodiazepine receptor complex

This subject is central to any discussion of anxiety and its treatment. *Gamma aminobutyric acid* (GABA) is probably the most important inhibitory transmitter in the central nervous system. GABAergic neurones are distributed widely in the CNS but are virtually absent outside the brain and the spinal cord. GABA controls the state of excitability in all brain areas and the balance between excitatory inputs (mostly glutamatergic) and the inhibitory GABAergic activity determines the prevailing level of neuronal activity. If the balance swings in favour of GABA, then sedation, amnesia, muscle relaxation and ataxia appear and nervousness and anxiety are reduced. The mildest reduction of GABAergic activity elicits arousal, anxiety, restlessness, insomnia and exaggerated reactivity.

When GABA binds with the GABA$_A$-benzodiazepine receptor complex, the permeability of the central pore of the receptor to chloride ions increases, allowing more ions into the neurone and decreasing excitability. Classical benzodiazepines (BDZs) in clinical use enhance the effectiveness of GABA by lowering the concentration of GABA required for opening the channel, so enabling the GABAergic circuits to produce a larger inhibitory effect (Fig. 19.4). These drugs are *agonists* at the receptor and there is an *antagonist* (flumazenil) which prevents agonists from binding at the receptor site and enhancing GABA function.

Drugs that act as agonists at this receptor are used mostly but not exclusively in sleep and anxiety disorders. Benzodiazepines (see later) have hypnotic, sedative, anxiolytic, anticonvulsant and (central) muscle relaxant actions. They form a significant but not the only part of available pharmacological treatments, as the following account will illustrate.

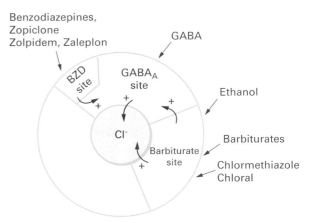

Fig. 19.4 Schematic representation of the GABA$_A$-benzodiazepine (B2D) receptor complex. Note that drugs that bind to the benzodiazepine (B2D) receptor site do not open the chloride channel directly but rather augment the capacity of GABA to do so. Conversely agents such as the barbiturates at lower doses enhance GABA action but at higher doses act directly to open the chloride channel.

Classification of anxiety disorders

The diagnostic criteria of DSM-IV (Diagnostic and Statistical Manual) or ICD 10 (International Classification of Disease) are generally used. Both divide anxiety into a series of sub-syndromes with clear operational criteria to assist in distinguishing them. At any one time many patients may have symptoms of more than one syndrome but making the primary diagnosis is important as this markedly influences the choice of treatment.

The key features of each anxiety disorder are given below, with a practical description of the preferred choice of medication, its dose and duration.

PANIC DISORDER

The main feature is recurrent, unexpected panic attacks. These are discrete periods of intense fear accompanied by characteristic physical symptoms such as skipping or pounding heart, sweating, hot flushes or chills, trembling/shaking, breathing difficulties, chest pain, nausea, diarrhoea and other gastrointestinal symptoms, dizziness or light-headedness. The first panic attack often occurs without warning but may subsequently become associated with specific situations e.g. in a crowded shop, driving. Anticipatory anxiety and avoidance behaviour develop in response to this chain of events. The condition must be distinguished from alcohol withdrawal, caffeinism, hyperthyroidism and (rarely) phaeochromocytoma.

Patients experiencing panic attacks often do not know what is happening to them, and because the symptoms are similar to those of cardiovascular, respiratory or neurological conditions, often present to nonpsychiatric services e.g. casualty departments, family doctors, medical specialists, where they may either be extensively investigated or given reassurance that there is nothing wrong. A carefully taken history reduces the likelihood of this occurrence.

Treatment. The choice lies between a fast-acting benzodiazepine such as *alprazolam* (1–3 mg/day p.o.) and a drug with delayed efficacy but fewer problems of withdrawal such as a TCA, e.g. *clomipramine* (100–250 mg/day p.o.) or an SSRI, e.g. *paroxetine* (20–50 mg/day p.o.). The different time course of these two classes of agent in panic disorder is depicted in Fig. 19.5 (see also Tables 19.5 and 19.6).

Benzodiazepines rapidly reduce panic frequency and severity and continue to be effective for months; significant tolerance to the therapeutic action is uncommon. On withdrawal of the benzodiazepine, even when it is gradual, increased symptoms of anxiety and panic attacks may occur, reaching a maximum when the final dose is stopped. Indeed, about 20% of patients find they are unable to withdraw and remain long-term on a benzodiazepine.

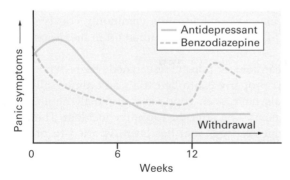

Fig. 19.5 Schematic representation of the time course of panic treatments.

Antidepressants (both SSRIs and TCAs) have a slower onset of action and, indeed, may induce an initial increase in both anxiety and panic frequency, such that a patient may discontinue medication, even after a single dose. This provoking reaction usually lasts for only 2–3 weeks after which panic frequency and severity improve but patients need help to stay on treatment over this period. The doctor needs to give a clear explanation of the likely course of events and the antidepressant should be started at half the usual initial dose to reduce the likelihood of exacerbation. Where the exacerbation is particularly of anxiety, a short course of a long-acting benzodiazepine can provide benefit. The dose of antidepressant required to treat panic disorder is generally as high or higher than that for depression and maximal benefit may not emerge for 8–12 weeks. Patients should therefore receive as high a dose as can be tolerated for this length of time.

If there is no response to adequate trial of an SSRI, followed by a TCA, the MAOI, *phenelzine* should be used at doses of up to 90 mg/d. MAOIs tend to produce less exacerbation at the beginning of treatment than the other antidepressants but can increase anxiety and panics in more sensitive individuals.

SOCIAL ANXIETY DISORDER

The essential feature of social phobia is a marked and persistent fear of performance situations when patients feel they will be the centre of attention and will do something humiliating or embarrassing. The situations that provoke this fear can be quite specific, for example public speaking, or be of a much more generalised nature involving fear of most social interactions, for example initiating or maintaining conversations, participating in small groups, dating, speaking to anyone in authority. Exposure to the feared situation almost invariably provokes anxiety with similar symptoms to those experienced by patients with panic attacks but some seem to be particularly prominent and difficult i.e. blushing, tremor, sweating and a feeling of 'drying up' when speaking.

Treatment. The drugs with established efficacy are the SSRI, *paroxetine,* the MAOI, *phenelzine* and

TABLE 19.5 Relative effectiveness of pharmacological treatments for anxiety disorders

	Benzodiazepine	SSRI	TCA	Other
Panic disorder	++	+++	+++	MAOI ++
Social phobia (social anxiety disorder)	+	++	+	MAOI++
Generalised anxiety disorder	++	++	++	Venlafaxine++ MAOI+ Buspirone++
Obsessive-compulsive disorder	–/+	++	++ (Clomipramine)	Addition of antipsychotics
Post-traumatic stress disorder	+	++	+	
Acute stress reaction	++			

TABLE 19.6 Properties of anti-anxiety drugs

	Benzodiazepines	Buspirone	Antidepressants SSRIs	TCAs
Onset	fast	slow	slow	slow
Initial worsening of symptoms	no	rarely	sometimes (especially panic)	
Withdrawal symptoms				
Acute	yes (~30%)	no	sometimes	sometimes
Chronic	?yes (~10%)	no	no	no
Abuse potential	low	zero	zero	zero
Interactions with alcohol	marked	slight		
Adverse effects				
Sedation	yes	no	no	some TCAs
Amnesia	yes	no	no	mild
Cardiovascular	no	no	no	yes
Gastrointestinal	no	slight	yes	no
Sexual	no	no	yes	no
Depression	sometimes	no	no	no
Relative safety in overdose	yes	yes	yes	no

the RIMA, *moclobemide* in the same doses as for depression. These achieve equivalent degrees of improvement; phenelzine has a slightly faster onset of action but produces more adverse effects. Some benzodiazepines and other SSRIs are reported to provide benefit but evidence for their therapeutic efficacy is less conclusive. β-adrenoceptor blockers continue to be widely used despite their having no proven efficacy in social phobia. But they have a place in the treatment of specific performance anxiety in, e.g. musicians, when management of the tremor is crucial.

The duration of treatment is as for depression or longer, for this can be a lifelong condition.

POST-TRAUMATIC STRESS DISORDER (PTSD)

Symptoms characteristically follow exposure to an extreme traumatic stressor event. These include persistent re-experiencing of the traumatic event, persistent avoidance of stimuli associated with the trauma and numbing of general responsiveness, and persistent symptoms of increased arousal. In taking a history the association with the event is usually obvious. PTSD is differentiated from acute stress disorder (below) by its persistence—the symptoms of the latter resolve within about 4 weeks. Depression quite commonly coexists with PTSD and should be enquired for in the history.

Treatment is poorly researched; there have been few properly controlled trials and almost all open trials have been conducted on small numbers of patients long after the causative incident. The wide range of drugs that has been reported to provide some benefit includes benzodiazepines, TCAs and MAOIs; *paroxetine* (SSRI) (20–50 mg/day p.o.) is now licenced for this indication in the UK. The preferred treatment immediately following the incident should probably be a short course of a benzodiazepine to promote sleep and help minimise mental rehearsal of the trauma that may lead to its perpetuation. Long-term therapy appears to be indicated at doses in the same range as for other anxiety disorders.

ACUTE STRESS DISORDER/ ADJUSTMENT DISORDER

Acute stress disorder is anxiety in response to a recent extreme stress. Although in some respects it is a normal and understandable reaction to an event, the problems associated with it are not only the severe distress the anxiety causes but also the risk that it may evolve into a more persistent state.

Treatment. A benzodiazepine used for a short time is the preferred approach for treating overwhelming anxiety that needs to be brought rapidly under control. It particularly relieves the accompanying anxiety and sleep disturbance. A drug with a slow onset of action such as *oxazepam* (60–120 mg/day p.o.) causes less dependence and withdrawal, and is preferred to those that enter the brain rapidly, e.g. diazepam, lorazepam. Some patients find it hard to discontinue the benzodiazepine, so its use should be reserved for those in whom extreme distress disrupts normal coping strategies.

GENERALISED ANXIETY DISORDER (GAD)

The essential feature of this condition is chronic anxiety and worry. To the nonsufferer the focus of the worry often seems to be trivial, e.g. getting the housework done or being late for appointments, but to the patient it is insurmountable. The anxiety is often associated with other symptoms, which include restlessness, difficulty in concentrating, irritability, muscle tension and sleep disturbance. The course of the disorder is typically chronic with exacerbations at times of stress and is often associated with depression. Its chronic nature with worsening at times of stress helps to distinguish GAD from anxiety in the form of episodic panic attacks with associated anticipatory anxiety (panic disorder). Hyperthyroidism and caffeinism should also be excluded.

Treatment. Historically *benzodiazepines* have been seen as the most effective treatment for GAD for they rapidly reduce anxiety and improve sleep and somatic symptoms. Consequently patients like taking them but the chronic nature of GAD raises issues of duration of treatment, tolerance, dependence and withdrawal reactions.

Buspirone is structurally unrelated to other anxiolytics and was the first nonbenzodiazepine to demonstrate efficacy in GAD. Its mode of action is unclear, although we know it suppresses 5HT neurotransmission through a selective activation of the inhibitory presynaptic 5HT1$_A$-reactor. Buspirone has a t$\frac{1}{2}$ of 7 h, and is metabolised in the liver; it has an active metabolite that may accumulate over weeks. Twice daily dosing is suitable, with the usual range being 15–30 mg/d p.o., maximum 45 mg/d.

Buspirone is generally less effective and slower in action than benzodiazepines and does not improve sleep; it does not benefit benzodiazepine withdrawal symptoms. The advantages are that it does not seem to cause dependence or withdrawal reactions and does not interact with alcohol. It appears to be less effective in patients who have previously received benzodiazepines and is therefore probably best used in benzodiazepine naïve patients. A disadvantage is that useful anxiolytic effect is delayed for 2 or more weeks.

Adverse effects can include dizziness, headache, nervousness, excitement, nausea, tachycardia and drowsiness.

Paroxetine (SSRI) and venlafaxine (SNRI) are effective (and are licenced for GAD in the UK), and TCAs have also been shown to give benefit. These drugs have a slower onset of action than benzodiazepines, are less well tolerated but cause fewer problems of dependence and on withdrawal.

A delayed response in GAD is not as critical as with acute situational anxiety. A sensible approach (especially in benzodiazepine naïve patients) is to start with buspirone for 6–8 weeks, at least 30 mg day increasing over 2–3 weeks to minimise unwanted actions; patients should be warned not to expect an immediate benefit. Those who do not respond should receive an antidepressant (SSRI or venlafaxine) for 6–8 weeks at full therapeutic dose. There remain some patients, including those with a long history of benzodiazepine use, who yet fail to respond. A benzodiazepine may be the only medication that provides relief for such resistant cases, and can be used as the sole treatment.

The duration of therapy depends on the nature of the underlying illness. If symptoms are intermittent, i.e. triggered by anxiety-provoking situations, then intermittent use of a benzodiazepine (for a few weeks) may be sufficient. More typically GAD requires treatment over 6–8 months with gradual withdrawal of medication thereafter. This may suffice but some patients experience severe, unremitting anxiety and the best resort is to chronic maintenance treatment with a benzodiazepine (analogous to long-term drug use in epilepsy). Such clinically supervised benzodiazepine use is justified because, without treatment, patients often derive comfort from the most widely accessible, easily available anxiolytic, alcohol.

Specific phobia

A specific phobia is a fear of a circumscribed object or situation, for instance fear of spiders, fear of flying. The diagnosis is not usually in doubt. A course of treatment by a trained therapist, involving graded exposure to the feared stimulus is the treatment of choice and can be very effective. By its nature such therapy generates severe anxiety and a *benzodiazepine* may permit patients fully to engage in therapy.

Obsessive-compulsive disorder (OCD)

Obsessive-compulsive disorder has two main components:

- the repetition of acts or thoughts which are involuntary, recognised by the sufferer to be generated by their own brain but are not in keeping with their usual thought processes, morals or values, and are therefore very distressing and

- anxiety provoked by the occurrence of such acts or thoughts.

OCD on its own often starts in late adolescence and has a chronic and pervasive course unless treated. OCD starting later on in life is often associated with affective or anxiety disorders. Symptoms often abate briefly if the individual is taken to a new environment.

Treatments are cognitive behavioural therapy and an *SSRI* or *clomipramine* (i.e. an antidepressant that enhances serotonergic function), used at higher doses and for much longer periods than for depressive disorders. Neuroleptics, atypical antipsychotics in low dose and benzodiazepines can be used successfully to augment the SSRIs if they are not wholly effective, especially in patients with tics (habitual, repeated contraction of certain muscles). Psychosurgery is still occasionally used for severe and treatment resistant cases. Interestingly, the brain pathways targeted by the surgeon are those that show abnormalities in neuroimaging (PET) studies of OCD, i.e. the basal ganglia/orbitofrontal pathways.

GENERAL COMMENTS ON DRUG TREATMENT FOR ANXIETY DISORDERS

The *effective dose* of antidepressant for anxiety is generally *higher* than that for antidepressant effect and takes *longer* for improvements to be seen (at least 4–8 weeks compared to 2–3 weeks for depression). The patient should be maintained on as high a dose as can be tolerated for at least 8 weeks before changing a medication. Educating the patient is crucial to obtaining cooperation.

The *duration of treatment* is often a controversial issue. Anxiety disorders (apart from the self-limiting acute stress reaction) are chronic conditions and may require treatment for as long as that used in depression. In a first episode, patients may need medication for at least 6 months, withdrawing over a further 4–8 weeks if they are well. Those with recurrent illness may need treatment for 1–2 years to enable them to learn and put into place psychological approaches to their problems. In many cases the illnesses are lifelong and chronic maintenance treatment is justified if it has significantly improved their wellbeing and function. A combination of medication with psychological techniques is likely to be most beneficial, especially for resistant cases.

Sleep disorders

NORMAL SLEEP

Humans spend about a third of the time asleep but why we sleep is not yet fully understood. Sleep is a state of inactivity accompanied by loss of awareness and a markedly reduced responsiveness to environmental stimuli. When a recording is made of the electroencephalogram (EEG) and other physiological variables such as muscle activity and eye movements during sleep (a technique called polysomnography), a pattern of sleep emerges, consisting of five different stages. This pattern varies from person to person, but usually consists of four or five cycles of *quiet* sleep alternating with *paradoxical*, or active, rapid eye movement (REM) sleep, with longer periods of paradoxical sleep in the latter half of the night. A representation of these stages and cycles over time is known as a *hypnogram*, and one derived from a normal subject appears in Figure 19.6, with paradoxical sleep depicted as the shaded areas.

Quiet sleep is further divided into four stages, each with a characteristic EEG appearance, during which there is progressive relaxation of the muscles and slower, more regular breathing as the deeper stages are reached. Most sleep in these deeper stages occurs in the first half of the night.

During paradoxical sleep, the EEG appearance is similar to that of waking or drowsiness. There is irregular breathing, complete loss of tone of the skeletal muscles, and frequent phasic movements particularly of the eyes, consisting of conjugate movements which are mostly lateral but can also be vertical (hence the term *rapid eye movement* sleep); most dreaming takes place in this stage.

The length of total sleep in a day varies between 3 and 10 hours in normal subjects with an average in the 20–45 year age group of 7–8 h. Sleep time is decreased in older subjects, to about 6 h in the over 70 year age group, with increased daytime napping reducing the actual night time sleep even more. The amount of time spent in each of the five stages varies between subjects and particularly with age, with much less slow wave sleep in older people. The number of awakenings after the onset of sleep also increases with advancing age. A normal subject has several short awakenings during the night, most of which are not perceived as awakenings unless they last more than about 2 minutes. Probably there will not be clear consciousness but subject may have occasional brief thoughts of how comfortable

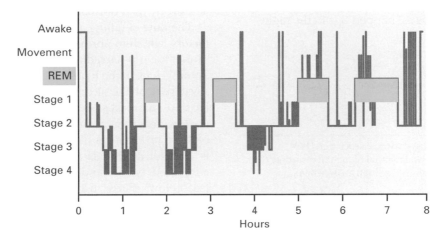

Fig. 19.6 Normal hypnogram

they feel or how pleased that it's not time to get up yet, with an immediate return to sleep. If during the short period of waking some factor causes anxiety or anger, e.g. aircraft noise, partner's snores or dread of being awake, progress to full awakening and being remembered is much more likely. The more times this happens the more subjects complain of an unrefreshing sleep. The time spent asleep as a percentage of the time in bed is used as a measure of *sleep efficiency* (96% in the case shown in Figure 19.6).

One of the most common ways in which insomnia develops is by 'clock watching'; subjects check the time on awakening, remember it and repeat this cycle many times during the night. Remembering the time of a transient awakening reinforces the subject's perception of sleeping poorly (periods of sleep in between are neglected) and also produces anger and frustration which in turn delay their return to sleep and may promote subsequent awakenings.

TYPES OF SLEEP DISORDER

Several types of sleep disorder are recognised and their differentiation is important; a simplified summary is given below but reference to DSM, ICD or ICD[4] will clarify the exact diagnostic criteria

- *insomnia:* not enough sleep or sleep of poor quality; problems of falling asleep (initial insomnia) or staying asleep (maintenance insomnia), or waking too early
- *hypersomnia:* excessive daytime sleepiness
- *parasomnia:* unusual happenings in the night
    nightmares
    night terrors
    sleep walking
    REM behaviour disorder

- *other*
    sleep scheduling disorders (circadian rhythm disorder)
    restless legs syndrome
    periodic leg movements of sleep.

Insomnia

Insomnia is characterised by the complaint of poor sleep, with difficulty either in initiating sleep or maintaining sleep throughout the night. It can occur exclusively in the course of another physical disorder such as pain, mental disorder, e.g. depression, or sleep disorder, e.g. sleep apnoea. In a large proportion of patients it is a primary sleep disorder and causes significant impairment in social, occupational or other important areas of functioning. One survey showed similar deficits in quality of life in insomniacs as in patients with long-term disorders such as diabetes.

About 60% of patients with insomnia have abnormal sleep when measured objectively but the rest have no sleep abnormality which can be measured at present, yet are as disabled by their perceived symptoms as those with measurable sleep.

Insomnia may or may not be accompanied by daytime fatigue but is not usually accompanied by subjective sleepiness during the day. When sleep propensity in the daytime is measured by objective means (time to EEG sleep) these patients are in fact less sleepy than normal subjects.

The time of falling asleep is determined by three factors, which in normal sleepers occur at bedtime. These are (a) circadian rhythm, i.e. the body's natural clock in the hypothalamus triggers the rest/sleep part of the sleep-wake cycle, (b) 'tiredness', i.e. time since last sleep, usually about 16 hours and (c) lowered mental and physical arousal. If one of these processes is disrupted then sleep initiation is difficult, and it is these three factors that are addressed by a standard sleep hygiene program (see below). Early in the course of insomnia rigorous adherence to sleep hygiene principles alone may restore the premorbid sleep pattern but in some patients the circadian process is less stable and they are less susceptible to these measures.

---

[4] DSM-IV American Psychiatric Association (1994) Diagnostic and statistical manual of mental disorders (DSM IV), 1st edition. American Psychiatric Association, Washington DC.
ICSD American Sleep Disorders Association (1992) International Classification of Sleep Disorders: Diagnostic and Coding Manual.
ICD-10 WHO (1994) Classification of Mental and Behavioural Disorders.

A summary of precipitating factors for insomnia is shown in Table 19.7.

TREATMENT OF INSOMNIA

Timely treatment of short-term insomnia is valuable, as it may prevent progression to a chronic condition, which is much harder to alleviate. Psychological treatments are effective and pharmacotherapy may be either unnecessary or used as a short-term adjunct. The approaches are to:

- treat any precipitating cause (above)
- educate about trigger factors for sleep and reassure that sleep will improve
- establish good sleep hygiene
- consider hypnotic medication.

Sleep hygiene

- keep regular bedtimes and rising times
- reduce daytime napping
- daytime (but not evening) exercise and exposure to daylight
- avoid stimulants, alcohol and cigarettes in evening
- establish bedtime routine — 'wind down' — milk drink may be helpful
- avoid dwelling on problems in bed
- bed should be comfortable and not too warm or too cold.

In the treatment of *long-term* insomnia the most important factor is *anxiety about sleep,* arising from conditioning behaviours that predispose to heightened arousal and tension at bedtime. Thus the

---

TABLE 19.7   Precipitating factors for insomnia

Pharmacological
- nonprescription drugs such as *caffeine* or *alcohol*. Alcohol reduces the time to onset of sleep but disrupts sleep later in the night. Regular and excessive consumption disrupts sleep continuity; insomnia is a key feature of alcohol withdrawal. Excessive intake of caffeine and theophylline, either in tea, coffee or cola drinks, also contributes to sleeplessness.
- starting treatment with certain *antidepressants,* especially seroton in reuptake inhibitors (e.g. fluoxetine, fluvoxamine), or monoamine uptake inhibitors; sleep disruption is likely to resolve after 3–4 weeks.
- other drugs which increase central noradrenergic and serotonergic activity include *stimulants* such as amphetamine, cocaine and methylphenidate and *sympathomimetics* such as the β-adrenergic agonist salbutamol and associated compounds.
- *withdrawal* from hypnotic drugs: this is usually short-lived.
- treatment with *β-adrenoceptor blockers* may disrupt sleep, perhaps because of their serotonergic action; a β-blocking drug which crosses blood–brain barrier less readily is preferred, e.g. atenolol.

Psychological: hyperarousal due to
- *stress*
- the need to be *vigilant* at night e.g. because of sick relatives or young children
- being *'on-call'*.

Physical
- *pain,* in which case adequate analgesia will improve sleep
- *pregnancy*
- *coughing* or wheezing: adequate control of asthma with stimulating drugs as above, may paradoxically improve sleep by reducing waking due to breathlessness
- *respiratory and cardiovascular disorders*
- *need to urinate;* this may be affected by timing of diuretic medication
- *neurological disorders,* e.g. stroke, movement disorders
- *periodic leg movements of sleep* (frequent jerks or twitches during the descent into deeper sleep), rarely reduce subjective sleep quality but are more likely to cause them in the subject's sleeping partner.

Psychiatric
- Patients with *depressive illnesses* often have difficulty falling asleep at night and complain of restless, disturbed and unrefreshing sleep, and early morning waking. When their sleep is analysed by polysomnography, time to sleep onset is indeed prolonged, and there is a tendency for more REM sleep to occur in the first part of the night, with reduced deep quiet sleep in the first hour or so after sleep onset and increased awakenings during the night. They may wake early in the morning and fail to get back to sleep again.
- *Anxiety* disorders may cause patients to complain about their sleep, either because there is a reduction in sleep continuity or because normal periods of nocturnal waking are somehow less well tolerated. Nocturnal panic attacks can make patients fearful of going off to sleep.
- *Bipolar* patients in the hypomanic or manic phase will sleep less than usual and sometimes changes in sleep pattern can be an early warning that an episode is imminent.

Disruption of circadian rhythm
Shift work, jet lag and *irregular routine* can cause insomnia, in that patients cannot sleep when they wish to.

bedroom is associated with not sleeping and automatic negative thoughts about the sleeping process occur in the evening. *Cognitive behavioural therapy* is helpful in dealing with 'psychophysiological' insomnia and together with education and sleep hygiene measures as above is the treatment of choice for long-term primary insomnia. Cognitive behavioural therapists are specially trained in changing behaviour and thoughts about sleep, particularly concentrating on learned sleep-incompatible behaviours and automatic negative thoughts at bedtime. The availability of these therapies is often limited and some patients are unwilling or unable to engage with them.

Drug therapy may:

• relieve short-term insomnia when precipitating causes cannot be improved
• prevent progression to a long-term problem by establishing a sleep habit
• interrupt the vicious cycle of anxiety about sleep itself.

DRUGS FOR INSOMNIA

Most drugs used in insomnia act as *agonists* (see GABA receptor above) at the $GABA_A$-benzodiazepine receptor and have effects other than their direct sedating action, including muscle relaxation, memory impairment, and ataxia, which can impair performance of skills such as driving. Clearly those drugs with onset and duration of action confined to the night period will be most effective in insomnia and less prone to unwanted effects during the day. Those with longer duration of action are likely to affect psychomotor performance, memory and concentration; they will also have enduring anxiolytic and muscle-relaxing effects.

Benzodiazepines

A general account of the benzodiazepines is appropriate here, although their indications clearly extend beyond use as hypnotics.

All benzodiazepines and newer benzodiazepine-like drugs are safe and effective for insomnia, if the compound with the right timing of onset of action and elimination is chosen. However, care should be taken in prescribing them to patients with co-morbid sleep-related breathing disorders such as obstructive sleep apnoea syndrome (see below) which is exacerbated by benzodiazepines. Objective measures of sleep show that benzodiazepines decrease time to sleep onset and waking during the night; subjective effects of improved sleep are usually greater than the objective changes, probably because of their anxiolytic effects (selectivity between anxiolytic and sedative effect is low). Other changes in sleep architecture are to some extent dependent on duration of action, with the very short-acting compounds having the least effect. Most commonly very light (stage 1) sleep is decreased, and stage 2 sleep is increased. Higher doses of longer-acting drugs partially suppress slow wave sleep.

Occasionally the agonist (sedative) compounds in current use cause *paradoxical effects*, e.g. excitement, aggression and antisocial acts. Alteration of dose, up or down, may eliminate these (as may chlorpromazine in an acute severe situation).

Pharmacokinetics. Benzodiazepines are effective after administration by mouth but enter the circulation at very different rates that are reflected in the speed of onset of action, e.g. alprazolam is rapid, oxazepam is slow (Table 19.8). The liver metabolises them, usually to inactive metabolites but some compounds produce active metabolites, some with long $t\frac{1}{2}$ which greatly extends drug action, e.g. chlordiazepoxide, clorazepate and diazepam all form desmethyldiazepam ($t\frac{1}{2}$ 80 h).

Uses. Benzodiazepines are used for: insomnia, anxiety, alcohol withdrawal states, muscle spasm due to a variety of causes, including tetanus and cerebral spasticity, epilepsy (clonazepam, see p. 421), anaesthesia and sedation for endoscopies and cardioversion.

The choice of drug as hypnotic and anxiolytic is determined by pharmacokinetic properties (see before, and Table 19.8).

Doses. Oral doses as anxiolytics are given with their indications (see before) and those for hypnotics appear in Table 19.8. Injectable preparations:

• Intravenous formulations, e.g. diazepam 10–20 mg, given at 5 mg/min into a large vein (antecubital fossa) to minimise thrombosis: the

TABLE 19.8   Properties of drugs used for insomnia

	Works selectively to enhance GABA	Rapid onset	$t\frac{1}{2}$ (hours)	Usual dose (p.o.)	Daytime (hangover) effects	Safety
Zopiclone	✓	+	3.5–6	7.5 mg	?Yes	✓
Zolpidem	✓	++	1.5–3	10 mg	No	✓
Zaleplon*	✓	++	1–2	10 mg	No	✓
Temazepam	✓		5–12	20 mg	?Yes	✓
Loprazolam	✓		5–13	1 mg	?Yes	✓
Lormetazepam	✓	+	8–10	1 mg	?Yes	✓
Nitrazepam	✓	+	20–48	5–10 mg	Yes	✓
Lorazepam	✓	+	10–20	0.5–1 mg	Yes	✓
Diazepam	✓	+	20–60	5–10 mg	Yes	✓
Oxazepam	✓		5–20	15–30 mg	Yes	✓
Alprazolam	✓	+	9–20	0.5 mg	Yes	✓
Clonazepam	✓	+	18–50	0.5–1 mg	Yes	✓
Chloral hydrate/chloral betaine	✗	+	8–12	0.7–1 g	?Yes	✗
Clomethiazole	✗	+	4–8	192 mg	?Yes	✗
Barbiturates	✗	+			Yes	✗
Promethazine	✗		7–14	25 mg	?Yes	✗/✓

* Can be taken during the night, up to 5 h before vehicle driving.

dose may be repeated once in 10 min for status epilepticus or in 4 h for severe acute anxiety or agitation: midazolam is a shorter-acting alternative, e.g. for endoscopies. The dose should be titrated according to response, e.g. drooping eyelids, speech, response to commands.

• Intramuscular injection of diazepam is absorbed erratically and may be slower in acting than an oral dose: lorazepam and midazolam i.m. are absorbed rapidly.

Tolerance to the *anxiolytic* effects does not seem to be a problem. In *sleep disorders* the situation is not so clear; studies of subjective sleep quality show enduring efficacy but about half of the objective (EEG) studies indicate decreased effects after 4–8 weeks, implying that some tolerance develops. That said, the necessity for dose escalation in sleep disorders is rare.

Dependence. Both animal and human research has shown that brain receptors do change in character in response to chronic treatment with benzodiazepines and therefore will take time to return to premedication levels after cessation of medication. Features of withdrawal and dependence vary. Commonly there is a kind of psychological dependence based on the fact that the treatment works to

reduce patients' anxiety or sleep disturbance and therefore they are unwilling to stop. If they do stop, there can be *relapse*, where original symptoms return. There can be a *rebound* of symptoms, particularly after stopping hypnotics, where there is a worsening of sleep disturbance for one or two nights, with longer sleep onset latency and increased waking during sleep—this is common. In anxiety disorders there may be a few days of increased anxiety and edginess which then resolves, probably in 10–20% of patients. More rarely, there is a *longer withdrawal syndrome* characterised by the emergence of symptoms not previously experienced, e.g. agitation, headache, dizziness, dysphoria, irritability, fatigue, depersonalisation, hypersensitivity to noise and visual stimuli. Physical symptoms include nausea, vomiting, muscle cramps, sweating, weakness, muscle pain or twitching and ataxia. After prolonged high doses abrupt withdrawal may cause confusion, delirium, psychosis and convulsions. The syndrome is ameliorated by resuming medication but resolves in weeks; in a very few patients it persists, and these people have been the subject of much research, mainly focusing on their personality and cognitive factors.

Withdrawal of benzodiazepines should be gradual after as little as 3 weeks' use but for long-term users it should be very slow, e.g. about 0.125 (1/8) of the dose every 2 weeks, aiming to complete it in 6–12 weeks. Withdrawal should be slowed if marked symptoms occur and it may be useful to substitute a long $t\frac{1}{2}$ drug (diazepam) to minimise rapid fluctuations in plasma concentrations. Abandonment of the final dose may be particularly distressing. In difficult cases withdrawal may be assisted by concomitant use of an antidepressant.

Adverse effects. In addition to those given above, benzodiazepines can affect memory and balance. Hazards with car driving or operating any machinery can arise from amnesia and impaired psychomotor function, in addition to sleepiness (warn the patient). Amnesia for events subsequent to administration occurs with i.v. high doses, for endoscopy, dental surgery (with local anaesthetic), cardioversion, and in these situations it can be regarded as a blessing.[5]

Women, perhaps as many as 1 in 200, may experience sexual fantasies, including sexual assault, after large doses of benzodiazepine as used in some dental surgery, and have brought charges in law against male staff. Plainly a court of law has, in the absence of a witness, great difficulty in deciding whom to believe. No such charges have yet been brought, it seems, by a man against a woman.

Paradoxical behaviour effects (see above) and perceptual disorders, e.g. hallucinations, occur occasionally. Headache, giddiness, alimentary tract upset, skin rashes and reduced libido can occur. Extrapyramidal reactions, reversible by flumazenil, are rare.

Benzodiazepines in pregnancy. The drugs are not certainly known to be safe and indeed diazepam is teratogenic in mice. The drugs should be avoided in early pregnancy as far as possible. It should be remembered that safety in pregnancy is not only a matter of avoiding prescription after a pregnancy has occurred but that individuals on long-term therapy may become pregnant. Benzodiazepines cross the placenta and can cause fetal cardiac arrhythmia, and muscular hypotonia, poor suckling, hypothermia and respiratory depression in the newborn.

Interactions. All potentiate the effects of alcohol and other central depressants, and all are likely to exacerbate breathing difficulties where this is already compromised, e.g. in obstructive sleep apnoea.

Overdose. Benzodiazepines are remarkably safe in acute overdose and the therapeutic dose × 10 induces sleep from which the subject is easily aroused. It is said that there is no reliably recorded case of death from a benzodiazepine taken alone by a person in good physical (particularly respiratory) health, which is a remarkable tribute to their safety (high therapeutic index); even if the statement is not absolutely true, death must be extremely rare. But deaths have occurred in combination with alcohol (which combination is quite usual in those seeking to end their own lives) and from complications of prolonged unconsciousness. Flumazenil selectively reverses benzodiazepine effects and is useful in diagnosis and in treatment (see below).

Temazepam is a benzodiazepine that was until recently the most popular hypnotic in the form of a soft gel liquid-filled capsule but, being readily injected, it was widely also abused and the formulation was withdrawn. Temazepam is now classed as a controlled drug; it is available as a tablet, with a much longer absorption time and duration of action making daytime hangover effect more likely. Consequently it is much less often prescribed.

Benzodiazepine antagonist: flumazenil is a competitive antagonist at benzodiazepine receptors and it may have some agonist actions, i.e. it is a partial agonist. Clinical uses include reversal of benzodiazepine sedation after endoscopies, dentistry and in intensive care. Heavily sedated patients become alert within 5 minutes. The $t\frac{1}{2}$ of 1 h is much shorter than that of most benzodiazepines (see Table 19.8), so that repeated i.v. administration may be needed. Thus the recovery period needs supervision lest sedation recurs; if used in day surgery it is im-

---

[5] Although one patient, normally a gentle man, believed he was being lied to when told his endoscopy had been performed. 'He assaulted his physician and was calmed only by a second endoscopy.' Later he was very embarrassed and apologised repeatedly (Lurie Y et al 1990 Lancet 336: 576). Another post-dental surgery patient purchased a bone china teaset and later condemned his wife for extravagance.

portant to tell patients that they may not drive a car home. The dose is 200 micrograms by i.v. injection given over 15 seconds, followed by 100 micrograms over 60 seconds if necessary, to a maximum of 300–600 micrograms. Flumazemil is useful for diagnosis of self-poisoning and also for treatment, when 100–400 micrograms are given by continuous i.v. infusion and adjusted to the degree of wakefulness.

Adverse effects of flumazenil can include brief anxiety, seizures in epileptics treated with a benzodiazepine and precipitation of withdrawal syndrome in dependent subjects. Rarely, vomiting is induced.

Buspirone (see p. 396).

Nonbenzodiazepine hypnotics that act at the GABA$_A$-benzodiazepine receptor

Although structurally unrelated to the benzodiazepines, these drugs act on the same macromolecular receptor complex but at different sites from the benzodiazepines; their effects can be blocked by flumazenil, the receptor antagonist. Those described below are all effective in insomnia, have low propensity for tolerance, rebound insomnia, withdrawal symptoms and abuse potential but there are few data of their effects in long-term studies.

Zopiclone is a cyclopyrrolone in structure. It has a fairly fast (about 1 hour) onset of action which lasts for 6–8 hours, making it an effective drug both for initial and maintenance insomnia. It may cause fewer problems on withdrawal than benzodiazepines. Its duration of action is prolonged in the elderly and in hepatic insufficiency. About 40% of patients experience a metallic aftertaste. Care should be taken with concomitant medication that affects its metabolic pathway (see Table 19.2a). The dose is 3.75–7.5 mg p.o.

Zolpidem is an imidazopyridine in structure and has a fast onset (30–60 min) and short duration of action. Patients over 80 years have slower clearance of this drug.

Zaleplon is a pyrazolopyrimidine. It has a fast onset and short duration of action. Studies of psychomotor performance in volunteers have shown that it has no effect on psychomotor skills, including driving skills, when taken at least 5 hours before testing. This means that it can be taken during the night (either when patients have tried getting off to sleep for a long time, or if they wake during the night and cannot return to sleep) without hangover effect.

OTHER DRUGS THAT ACT ON THE GABA$_A$-BENZODIAZEPINE RECEPTOR

Chloral hydrate, clomethiazole and barbiturates also enhance GABA function but at high doses have the additional capacity directly to open the membrane chloride channel (see Figure 19.4); this may lead to potentially lethal respiratory depression and explains their low therapeutic ratio. These drugs also have a propensity for abuse/misuse and are very much second-line treatments.

Chloral hydrate has a fast (30–60 min) onset of action and duration of action 6–8 h. It is a prodrug, being rapidly metabolised by alcohol dehydrogenase into the active hypnotic trichloroethanol (t$\frac{1}{2}$ 8h). Chloral is dangerous in serious hepatic or renal failure and aggravates peptic ulcer. Interaction with ethanol is to be expected since both are metabolised by alcohol dehydrogenase. Ethanol also appears to induce the formation of trichloroethanol which attains higher plasma concentrations if alcohol is co-administered, increasing sedation. Triclofos (Tricloryl) and cloral betaine (Welldorm) are related compounds.

Clomethiazole is structurally related to vitamin B 1 (thiamine) and is a hypnotic, sedative and anticonvulsant. It is comparatively free from hangover; it can cause nasal irritation and sneezing. Dependence occurs and use should always be brief. When taken orally, it is subject to extensive hepatic first-pass metabolism (which is defective in the elderly and in liver damaged alcoholics who get higher peak plasma concentrations), and the usual t$\frac{1}{2}$ is 4 h (with more variation in the old than the young); it may also be given i.v.

Barbiturates have a low therapeutic index, i.e. relatively small overdose may endanger life; they also cause dependence and have been popular drugs of abuse. The use of intermediate-acting drugs (amylobarbital, butobarbital, secobarbital) is now limited to severe intractable insomnia in patients *already taking* barbiturates (they should be avoided in the elderly). The long-acting phenobarbital is used for epilepsy (see Chapter 20), and very short-acting thiopental for anaesthesia (see p. 353). Overdose following self-poisoning by hypnotic barbiturates may have severe features including hypotension (may lead to renal failure), hypothermia, respiratory depression and coma. Supportive measures may suffice with i.v. fluid to restore central venous pressure and so cardiac output and, if that fails, using a drug with cardiac inotropic effect (see p. 457). A good urine volume (e.g. 200 ml/h) promotes elimination of the drug. Urine alkalinisation accelerates removal of phenobarbital (an acid, pKa 7.2) as do repeated doses of activated charcoal. Active elimination by haemoperfusion or dialysis may be needed in particularly severe and complicated cases.

Other drugs used in insomnia

Antihistamines. Most proprietary (over the counter) sleep remedies contain antihistamines. Promethazine (Phenergan) has a slow (1–2 h) onset and long (t½ 12 h) duration of action. It reduces sleep onset latency and awakenings during the night after a single dose but there have been no studies showing enduring action. It is sometimes used as a hypnotic in children. There are no controlled studies showing improvements in sleep after other antihistamines. Trimeprazine (alimemazine) is used for short-term sedation in children. Most antihistamine sedatives have a relatively long action and may cause daytime sedation.

Antidepressants. In the depressed patient, improvement in mood is almost always accompanied by improvement in subjective sleep and therefore choice of antidepressant should not usually involve additional consideration of sleep effects. Nevertheless, some patients are more likely to continue with medication if there is a short-term improvement, in which case mirtazapine or nefazodone provide an effective antidepressant together with sleep-promoting effects.

Antidepressant drugs, particularly those with 5HT$_2$-blocking effects, may occasionally be effective in long-term insomnia (but see Table 19.6).

Antipsychotics have been used to promote sleep in resistant insomnia occurring as part of another psychiatric disorder, probably due to a combination of 5HT$_2$-receptor, α_1-adrenoceptor and histamine H$_1$-receptor antagonism, in addition to their primary dopamine antagonist effects. Their long action leads to daytime sedation and extrapyramidal movement disorders may result from dopamine receptor blockade (see p. 380, Antipsychotics). Nevertheless, modern antipsychotics, e.g. quetiapine, have been occasionally used for intractable insomnia.

Melatonin, the hormone produced by the pineal gland during darkness, has been investigated for insomnia but it appears to be ineffective. The impressive nature of the diurnal rhythm in melatonin secretion has stimulated interest in its use therapeutically to reset circadian rhythm to prevent jet-lag on long-haul flights and for blind or partially sighted people who cannot use daylight to synchronise their natural rhythm. There is controversy about dose and timing of treatment and in most countries pharmaceutical preparations are not generally available.

Herbal preparations. Randomised clinical trials have shown some effect of valerian in mild to moderate insomnia, and hops, lavender and other herbal compounds show promise in pilot studies that are presently being pursued more fully.

Summary of pharmacotherapy for insomnia

- Drug treatment may be effective for a short period (2–4 weeks).
- Some patients may need long-term medication.
- Intermittent medication, i.e. taken only on nights that symptoms occur, is preferable and may often be possible with modern, short-acting, compounds.
- Discontinuing hypnotic drugs is usually not a problem if the patient knows what to expect. There will be a short period (usually 1–2 nights) of rebound insomnia on stopping hypnotic drugs which can be ameliorated by phased withdrawal.

HYPERSOMNIA

Sleep-related breathing disorders causing excessive daytime sleepiness are rarely treated with drugs. Sleepiness caused by the night-time disruption of *obstructive sleep apnoea syndrome* is sometimes not completely abolished by the standard treatment of continuous positive airway pressure overnight, and the use of wake-promoting drugs, e.g. modafinil, is being evaluated in these patients.

Narcolepsy is a chronic neurological disorder and is characterised by excessive daytime sleepiness (EDS), usually accompanied by *cataplexy* (attacks of weakness on emotional arousal). These symptoms are often associated with the intrusion into wakefulness of other elements of rapid eye movement (REM) sleep, such as sleep paralysis and hypnagogic hallucinations, i.e. in a transient state preceding sleep.

Stimulants are effective in the treatment of EDS due to narcolepsy. Suitable agents include dexamfetamine, methylphenidate, and modafinil.

Amfetamines release stored neurotransmitters, primarily dopamine and noradrenaline, in the brain. This causes a behavioural excitation, with increased alertness, elevation of mood, increase in physical activity.

Dexamfetamine, the dextrorotatory isomer of amfetamine, is about twice as active in humans as the laevo isomer and is the main prescribed amfetamine. It is rapidly absorbed and its duration of action varies among individuals; most people with narcolepsy find twice daily dosing optimal to maintain alertness during the day.

About 40% of narcoleptic patients find it necessary to increase their dose, indicating tolerance. Although physical dependence does not occur, there is mental and physical depression on withdrawal.

Unwanted effects include edginess, restlessness, insomnia and appetite suppression, weight loss, and increase in blood pressure and heart rate. Amphetamines are commonly abused because of their stimulant effect but this is rare in narcolepsy.

Methylphenidate releases stored dopamine but most of its action is to inhibit uptake of central neurotransmitters. Its effects and adverse effects are very similar to amphetamines. Methylphenidate has a low systemic availability and slow onset of action, making it less liable to abuse. Its duration of effect is quite short (3–4 h) so patients with narcolepsy need to plan the timing of their tablets to fit with daily activities. It is also used in attention deficit/hyperactivity disorder (see below).

Modafinil is a wake-promoting agent whose specific biochemical mechanism of action is obscure. It increases brain concentrations of dopamine after chronic administration in animals but has no overtly stimulant effect like amphetamines. It appears to have a slow onset and its action lasts 8–12 h; abuse potential is very low. Modafinil is used in narcolepsy and other hypersomnias and has also been studied in normal people who need to stay awake for long periods and function well.

In narcolepsy, patients usually need a stimulant for their hypersomnia and a TCA or SSRI for their cataplexy, so care should be taken when combining these. Dexamfetamine and methylphenidate must not be given with MAOIs. There is potential for interaction between methylphenidate and TCAs (hypertension) and SSRI antidepressants. It appears that modafinil, methylphenidate and dexamfetamine may themselves be combined without adverse outcome (modafinil is occasionally used regularly and dexamfetamine added intermittently when peak alertness is particularly critical). Modafinil accelerates the metabolism of oral contraceptives, reducing their efficacy.

Cataplexy is most effectively treated with 5HT uptake-blocking drugs such as *clomipramine* or *fluoxetine,* or some other antidepressant drugs, e.g. *reboxetine.*

PARASOMNIAS

Nightmares arise out of REM sleep and are reported by the patient as structured, often stereotyped dreams that are very distressing. Usually the patient wakes up fully and remembers the dream. Psychological methods of treatment may be appropriate, e.g. a program of rehearsing the dream, inventing different endings. In a small number of cases where adverse events such as angina have been provoked by recurrent nightmares it may be appropriate to consider drug treatment with an antidepressant with a marked suppressing effect on REM sleep, such as the MAOI, phenelzine. Nightmares of a particularly distressing kind are a feature of post-traumatic stress disorder. Case reports indicate benefit from various pharmacological agents but no particular drug emerges as superior. Many prefer to use a 5HT-blocker such as trazodone or nefazodone.

Night terrors and sleep-walking arise from slow wave sleep and they are often coexistent. There is usually a history dating from childhood and often a family history. Exacerbations commonly coincide with periods of stress and alcohol will increase their likelihood. In a night terror patients usually sit or jump up from deep sleep (mostly early in the night) with a loud cry, look terrified and move violently, sometimes injuring themselves or others. They appear asleep and uncommunicative, often returning to sleep without being aware of the event. These terrors are thought to be a welling-up of anxiety from deep centres in the brain which is normally inhibited by cortical mechanisms. They can occur in up to 30% of normal children but become troublesome and often dangerous in adults. They can be successfully treated with the benzodiazepine, clonazepam or the SSRI, paroxetine.

Nocturnal panic attacks may be distinguished from night terrors by the fact that the patient will wake fully before panic symptoms have reached a peak and is fully aware.

REM behaviour disorder, first described by in 1988, consists of lack of paralysis during REM sleep which results in acting out of dreams, often vigorously with injury to self or others. It can occur acutely as a result of drug or alcohol withdrawal but its chronic manifestation can be idiopathic or associated with neurological disorder (about 50% of each). It is much commoner among older patients. Successful treatment has been described with clonazepam or clonidine which decrease REM sleep without increasing awakenings.

OTHER SLEEP DISORDERS

Restless legs syndrome (RLS) is a disorder that usually occurs prior to sleep onset and is characterised by disagreeable sensations, that cause an almost irresistible urge to move the legs. The sensation is described as 'crawling', 'aching', 'tingling' and is partially or completely relieved with leg motion, returning after movement ceases. Most if not all patients with this complaint also have periodic limb movements disorder (PLMD), which may occur independently of RLS. These periodic limb movements consist of highly stereotyped movements, usually of the legs, that occur repeatedly (typically every 20–40 seconds) during the night. They may wake the patient, in which case there may be a complaint of daytime sleepiness or occasionally insomnia, but often only awaken the sleeping partner, who is usually kicked. RLS and PLMS are considered to be movement disorders and may respond to formulations of levodopa but dopamine agonists, e.g. ropinirole, and other treatments such as gabapentin are under investigation

Sleep scheduling disorders. Circadian rhythm disorders are often confused with insomnia and both can be present in the same patient. With such sleep scheduling disorders, sleep occurs at the 'wrong' time, i.e. at a time that does not fit with work, social or family commitments. A typical pattern may be a difficulty in initiating sleep for a few nights due to stress, whereupon once asleep the subject continues sleeping well into the morning to 'catch up' the lost sleep. Thereafter the 'time since last sleep' cue for sleep initiation is delayed and the sleep period gradually becomes more delayed until the subject is sleeping in the day instead of at night. A behavioural program with strategic light exposure is appropriate, with pharmacological treatment as an adjunct, e.g. melatonin, to help reset the sleep–wake schedule.

Drugs for Alzheimer's[6] disease (dementia)

Dementia is described as a syndrome 'due to disease of the brain, usually of chronic or progressive nature in which there is disturbance of multiple higher cortical functions, including memory, thinking, orientation, comprehension, calculation, learning capacity, language and judgement, without clouding of consciousness.'[7] Deterioration in emotional control, social behaviour or motivation may accompany or precede cognitive impairment. Alzheimer's and vascular (multi-infarct) disease are the two most common forms of dementia, accounting for about 80% of presentations. Alzheimer's disease is associated with deposition of beta-amyloid in brain tissue and abnormal phosphorylation of the intracellular tau proteins, causing abnormalities of microtubule assembly and collapse of the cytoskeleton. Pyramidal cells of the cortex and subcortex are particularly affected.

In Western countries, the prevalence of dementia is below 1% in those aged 60–64 years, but it doubles with each 5-year cohort to a figure of around 16% in those aged 80–84 years. The emotional impact of dementia on relatives and carers and the cost to society in social support and care facilities are great. Hence the impetus for an effective form of treatment is compelling.

Evidence indicates that *cholinergic transmission* is diminished in Alzheimer's disease. All agents that benefit the condition act to enhance *acetylcholine* activity by inhibition of the acetylcholinesterase which metabolises and inactivates synaptically-released acetylcholine. Consequently acetylcholine remains usable for longer. Individual drugs are categorised by the type of enzyme inhibition they cause. *Donepezil* is classed as a 'reversible' agent as binding to the acetylcholinesterase enzymes lasts only minutes, whereas *rivastigmine* is considered 'pseudo-irreversible' since inhibition lasts several hours. *Galantamine* is associated both with reversible inhibition and with enhanced acetylcholine action on nicotinic receptors.[8] Clinical trials show that these agents produce an initial increase in patients' cognitive ability. There may be associated global benefits, including improvements in non-cognitive aspects such as depressive symptoms. But the drugs do not alter the underlying process, and the relentless advance of the disease is paralleled by reduction in acetylcholine production with decline in cognition.

The beneficial effects of drugs are therefore to:

- *stabilise* the condition initially and sometimes improve cognitive function,
- *delay* the overall pace of decline (and therefore the escalating levels of support required),
- *postpone* the onset of severe dementia.

The severity of cognitive deficits in patients suffering from, or suspected of having, dementia can be quantified by a simple 30-point schedule, the mini mental-state examination (MMSE) of Folstein. A score of 21–26 denotes mild, 10–20 moderate and less than 12 severe Alzheimer's disease. The MMSE can also be used to monitor progress.

Given the limited evidence of overall benefit in relation to cost, the use of these drugs is the subject of debate but there follows a practical position.

The UK National Institute for Clinical Excellence (NICE) recommends that donepezil, galantamine and rivastigmine should be available as adjuvant therapy for those with a MMSE score above 12 points, subject to the following conditions:

- Alzheimer's disease must be diagnosed and assessed in a specialist clinic; the clinic should also assess cognitive, global and behavioural functioning, activities of daily living, and the likelihood of compliance with treatment
- treatment should be initiated by specialists but may be continued by general practitioners under a shared-care protocol
- the carers' views of the condition should be sought before and during drug treatment
- the patient should be assessed 2–4 months after maintenance dose is established; drug treatment should continue only if MMSE score has improved or has not deteriorated *and* behavioural and functional assessment shows improvement
- the patient should be assessed every 6 months and drug treatment should normally continue only if MMSE score remains above 12 points and if treatment is considered to have a worthwhile effect on the global functional and behavioural condition.

---

[6] Alois Alzheimer (1864–1915) German psychiatrist who studied the brains of demented and senile patients and correlated hisological findings with clinical features.

[7] ICD-10 diagnostic system.

[8] Irreversible antagonists exist but, not surprisingly, have no place in therapeutics (sarin nerve gas is an example).

Doses p.o. are:

donepezil 5–10 mg nocte increasing to 10 mg nocte after one month,

galantamine 4 mg b.d. increasing to 8–12 mg b.d. at
    4 weekly intervals,
rivastigmine 1.5 mg b.d. increasing to 3–6 mg b.d.
    at intervals of 2 weeks.

Adverse effects inevitably include cholinergic
symptoms with nausea, diarrhoea and abdominal
cramps appearing commonly. There may also
be bradycardia, sinoatrial or atrioventricular block.
Urinary incontinence, syncope, convulsions, and
psychiatric disturbances also occur. Rapid dose
increase appears to make symptoms more pronounced. Hepatotoxicity is a rare association with
donepezil.

The deterioration of function in dementia of
Alzheimer's disease is often accompanied by
acute behavioural disturbance and the development of a range of psychotic symptoms. Therapy
with atypical drugs is then preferred because they
provoke fewer adverse effects than classical
antipsychotics.

Other substances that are being evaluated in
Alzheimer's disease include the antioxidant vitamin E, the monoamine oxidase type B inhibitor,
selegeline (see p. 425) and the plant extract *gingko
biloba,* which is though to have antioxidant and
cholinergic activity. Oestrogens and nonsteroidal
anti-inflammatory agents may also have protective
effects.

Drugs in attention deficit/ hyperactivity disorder

Attention deficit hyperactivity disorder (ADHD) is
characterised by inattention, impulsivity and motor
overactivity, present before the age of 7 years, and
causing pervasive impairment across situations as
opposed to occurring only at school or within the
home. Some diagnostic systems use the narrower
definition of *hyperkinetic disorder* rather than ADHD.
Hyperkinetic disorder is reported to affect 1–2% of
school-aged children in the United Kingdom and
ADHD 5%.

Methylphenidate (see above) is effective in children
with ADHD and hyperkinetic disorder, reducing

each of the three principal symptoms. It should be
initiated only by a specialist in these conditions and
should form part of a comprehensive treatment
programme of psychological, educational and social
measures. Periodic breaks in treatment once symptoms have been stabilised ('drug holidays') are
recommended to allow expected improvement in
function to be quantified.

Unwanted effects include anxiety, anorexia and
difficulty sleeping, which usually subside. Methylphenidate reduces expected weight gain and has
been associated with slight growth retardation.
Monitoring of therapy should include height and
weight, also blood pressure and blood counts
(thrombocytopenia and leucopenia occur).

Methylphenidate should be avoided in children
with Tourette's syndrome or where there is a family
history of this disorder. Thyroid disease is also a
contraindication.

Dexamfetamine is an alternative for it has similar
efficacy in ADHD. Unwanted effects and contraindications are broadly similar to those of methylphenidate. Dexamfetamine is the preferred drug in
children who also have epilepsy. It has a greater
potential for abuse.

Clonidine, tricyclic antidepressants and *antipsychotic agents* (e.g. risperidone, sulpiride) may have a
role in ADHD where methylphenidate and dexamfetamine are contraindicated or have failed to
produce benefit.

Drugs and skilled tasks

Drugs can affect skilled tasks and car driving, and
it is convenient to consider the implications of this
broad issue.

Many medicines affect performance, not only
psychotropic drugs[9] (amongst which sedative antidepressants, benzodiazepines, hypnotics and antipsychotics are the most obvious examples) but also
antihistamines, antimuscarinics, analgesics including
some NSAIDs, (e.g. indomethacin), antiepileptics,
antidiabetics (hypoglycaemia) and some antihypertensives. Alcohol and cannabis are discussed on
pages 178 and 190.

TABLE 19.9 Summary of indications for psychotropic drug

	Antidepressants	Lithium and mood stabilisers	Antipsychotics	Benzodiazepines	Other hypnotic and anxiolytic drugs	Other drug groups
Depressive disorders	*	*1				
Depressive disorders with psychotic symptoms	*	*1	*			
Bipolar affective disorder (prophylaxis)		*				
Bipolar affective disorder (acute manic episode)		*	*	*		
Generalised anxiety disorder	*2		*3	*	*4	
Panic disorder	*			*		
Social phobia	*5				*5	
Obsessive-compulsive disorder	*6		*7			
Post-traumatic stress disorder	*8					
Schizophrenia			*			
Acute behavioural disturbance			*	*		
Alcohol withdrawal				*	*9	*10
Insomnia	*11			*	*	
Eating disorders	*12					
Dementia of Alzheimer's disease						*13
Attention deficit/hyperactivity disorder			*14			*14

Key: *recognised indication; where numbers appear in the table, see notes below.
Notes:
(1) Lithium augmentation may be used in depression (p. 375). Lithium is given in combination with a TCA, SSRI or novel antidepressant, usually when the symptoms have proved resistant to adequate trials of two or more antidepressants.
(2) Formerly, antidepressants were thought to be less effective in generalised anxiety disorder than in panic disorder. Evidence now suggests that the SSRI, paroxetine and the SNRI, venlafaxine are beneficial.
(3) Antipsychotics may be used short-term for management of severe anxiety, but only where other drug options have failed (due to adverse effect).
(4) Buspirone may be used in generalised anxiety disorder as an alternative to a benzodiazepine.
(5) SSRIs and MAOIs are effective in social phobia. β-adrenoceptor blockers may also be helpful, particularly in performance anxiety, combating tremor and other symptoms of autonomic overactivity.
(6) Serotonergic antidepressants, including the tricyclic clomipramine and the SSRIs are effective in the treatment of obsessive-compulsive disorder.
(7) Augmentation with classical or atypical antipsychotics may be attempted when obsessive-compulsive disorder is resistant to antidepressant treatment.
(8) TCAs (especially imipramine and amitriptyline) and SSRIs may be effective in post-traumatic stress disorder.
(9) Clomethiazole was an alternative to a benzodiazepine for alcohol withdrawal but is now rarely used due to concerns over respiratory depression and abuse potential.
(10) Drugs for alcohol dependence and withdrawal are discussed in Chapter 10.
(11) When a patient complaining of insomnia also has depression, a sedative antidepressant such as trazodone, nefazodone or mirtazapine should be considered. SSRIs do not provide direct sedation in such patients but may improve the quality of sleep over a longer period as mood improves.
(12) Fluoxetine is licenced in the UK for the treatment of bulimia nervosa.
(13) Acetylcholinesterase inhibitors provide transient improvement in cognitive and global functioning in mild to moderate dementia of Alzheimer's disease. They delay the onset of severe illness but cannot ultimately halt or change the course of the disease.
(14) The CNS stimulants methylphenidate and dexamfetamine are drugs of choice for attention deficit/hyperactivity disorder. Second line treatment options include clonidine and the antipsychotic agents risperidone, haloperidol and sulpiride.

It is plain that prescribers have a major responsibility here, both to warn patients and, in the case of those who need to drive for their work, to choose medicines having minimal liability to cause impairment. Patients who must drive when taking a drug of known risk (e.g. benzodiazepine) should be specially warned of times of peak impairment.

A patient who has an accident and who was not warned of drug hazard, whether orally or by labelling, may successfully sue the doctor in law. It is also necessary that patients be advised of the additive effect of alcohol with prescribed medicines.[10]

Car driving is a complex multifunction task that includes:[11]

- visual search and recognition
- vigilance
- information processing under variable demand
- decision-making and risk-taking
- sensorimotor control.

How the patient feels is not a reliable guide to recovery of skills and drivers may be more than usually accident prone without any subjective feeling of sedation or dysphoria: the fact that they feel OK does not mean that they are OK.

The criteria for safety in air-crew are more stringent than those for car drivers.

Resumption of car driving or other skilled activity after anaesthesia is a special case, and an extremely variable one, but where a sedative (e.g. i.v. benzodiazepine, opioid or neuroleptic), or any general anaesthetic has been used it seems reasonable not to drive for 24 h at least.

The emphasis on psychomotor and physical aspects (injury) should not distract from the possibility that those who live by their intellect and imagination (politicians and even journalists may be included here) may suffer cognitive disability from thoughtless prescribing.

Summary

Table 19.9 summarises indications of the major groups of psychotropic drugs. Psychiatric illnesses are often associated with co-morbid conditions which may require treatment, e.g. schizophrenia may be associated with depression.

GUIDE TO FURTHER READING

Anderson I M, Nutt D J et al 2000 Evidence-based guidelines for treating depressive disorders with antidepressants: a revision of the 1993 British Association for Psychopharmacology guidelines. Journal of Psychopharmacology 14: 3–20

Ballenger J C et al 1998 Consensus statement on panic disorder from the International Consensus Group on Depression and Anxiety. Journal of Clinical Psychiatry 59: 47–54

Ballenger J C et al 1998 Consensus statement on social anxiety disorder from the International Consensus Group on Depression and Anxiety. Journal of Clinical Psychiatry 59: 54–60

Ballenger J C et al 2000 Consensus statement on posttraumatic stress disorder from the International Consensus Group on Depression and Anxiety. Journal of Clinical Psychiatry 61: 60–66

Ballenger J C et al 2001 Consensus statement on generalized anxiety disorder. Journal of Clinical Psychiatry 62: 53–58

Davies S J C et al 1999 Association of panic disorder and panic attacks with hypertension. American Journal of Medicine 107: 310–316

Ferrier I N 2001 Developments in mood stabilisers. British Medical Bulletin 57: 179–192

Fink M 2001 Convulsive therapy: a review of the first 55 years. Journal of Affective Disorders 63: 1–15

---

[9] A dose–response relationship was found between benzodiazepine use and road-traffic accidents. Barbone F et al 1998 Lancet 352: 1331–1336

[10] Nordic countries require that medicines liable to impair ability to drive or to operate machinery be labelled with a red triangle on a white background. The scheme covers antidepressants, benzodiazepines, hypnotics, drugs for motion sickness and allergy, cerebral stimulants, antiepileptics and antihypertensive agents. In the UK there are some standard labels that pharmacists are recommended to apply. e.g. 'Warning. May cause drowsiness. If affected do not drive or operate machinery. Avoid alcoholic drink'. They are offered as 'a carefully considered balance between the unintelligibly short and the inconveniently long' (see BNF).

[11] In: Willett R E et al (eds) 1983 Drugs, driving and traffic safety. WHO, Geneva.

Glassman A H, Bigger J T 2001 Antipsychotic drugs: Prolonged QTc interval, Torsade de pointes, and sudden death. American Journal of Psychiatry 158: 1774–1782

Kent J M 2000 SNaRIs, NaSSAs, and NaRIs: new agents for the treatment of depression. Lancet 355: 911–918

Kryger M H et al (eds) 2000 Principles And Practice Of Sleep Medicine, Third Edition. Philadelphia: W B Saunders

Kuperberg G R, Murray R 1996 Advances in the treatment of schizophrenia. British Journal of Clinical Practice 50: 315–323

Mayeux R, Sano M 1999 Treatment of Alzheimer's disease. New England Journal of Medicine 341: 1670–1679

Nelson J C 1997. Treatment of refractory depression. Depression and Anxiety 5: 165–174

Nutt D J, Malizia A L 2001. New insights into the role of the GABA-A benzodiazepine receptor. British Journal of Psychiatry 179: 390–396

Paykel E S 2001 Continuation and maintenance therapy in depression. British Medical Bulletin 57: 145–159

Preskorn S H 1998 Debate resolved: there are differential effects of serotonin selective reuptake inhibitors on cytochrome P450 enzymes. Journal of Psychopharmacology 12: Supp B S89–S97

Roth T et al 2001 Consensus for the pharmacological management of insomnia in the new millennium. International Journal of Clinical Practice 55: 42–52

Sack R L et al 1997 Sleep-promoting effects of melatonin: at what dose, in whom, under what conditions and by what mechanisms? Sleep 20: 908–915

Schultz S K, Andreasen N C 1999 Schizophrenia. Lancet 353: 1425–1430

Shiloh R, Nutt D J, Weizman A 1999 *Atlas of Psychiatric Pharmacotherapy.* London: Martin Dunitz

Whooley M A, Simon G E 2000 Managing depression in medical outpatients. New England Journal of Medicine 343: 1942–1950

Wilson S J et al 1997 Adult night terrors and paroxetine. Lancet 350: 185

Yehuda R 2002 Post-traumatic stress disorder. New England Journal of Medicine 346: 108–114

Zametkin A J, Ernst M 1999 Problems in the management of attention deficit hyperactivity disorder. New England Journal of Medicine 340: 40–45

20

Epilepsy, parkinsonism and allied conditions

Antiepilepsy drugs

Epilepsy affects 5–10 per 1000 of the general population.[1] It is due to sudden, excessive depolarisation of some or all cerebral neurons. This may remain localised (focal seizure) or may spread to cause a secondary generalised seizure, or affect all cortical neurons simultaneously (primary generalised seizure).

Bromide (1857) was the first drug to be used for the treatment of epilepsy, but it is now obsolete. Phenobarbital, introduced in 1912, controlled patients resistant to bromides. The next success was the discovery in 1938 of phenytoin (a hydantoin) which is structurally related to the barbiturates. Since then many other drugs have been discovered, but phenytoin still remains a drug of choice in the treatment of major epilepsy. Over the past ten years there has been a dramatic increase in the number of new anticonvulsant drugs (vigabatrin, gabapentin, lamotrigine, topiramate, oxcarbazepine, levetiracetam), but none has been shown to be superior to the major standard anticonvulsants (phenytoin, carbamazepine and sodium valproate).

MODE OF ACTION

Antiepilepsy (anticonvulsant) drugs inhibit the neuronal discharge or its spread, and do so in one or more of three ways:

1. Reducing cell membrane permeability to ions, particularly the voltage-dependent sodium channels which are responsible for the inward current that generates an action potential. Cells that are firing repetitively at high frequency are blocked preferentially, which permits discrimination between epileptic and physiological activity.
2. Enhancing the activity of gamma-aminobutyric

---

[1] Some people with epilepsy make pilgrimages to Terni (Italy) to seek intercession from Saint Valentine to relieve their condition. There was more than one Saint Valentine and it is unclear if he was also the patron saint of lovers.

acid (GABA) the principal inhibitory transmitter of the brain; the result is increased membrane permeability to chloride ion, which reduces cell excitability.

3. Inhibiting excitatory neurotransmitters, e.g. glutamate.

CLASSIFICATION OF EPILEPSIES

A generally accepted classification is given in Table 20.2 (p. 418), together with drugs of choice for the various seizure disorders.

Principles of management

These call for attention to nondrug as well as drug measures, as set out below:

- Any causative factor must, of course, be treated, e.g. cerebral neoplasm.
- Educate the patient about the disease, duration of treatment and need for compliance.
- Avoid precipitating factors, e.g. alcohol, sleep deprivation, emotional stress.
- Anticipate natural variation, e.g. fits may occur particularly or exclusively around periods in women (catamenial[2] epilepsy).
- Give antiepilepsy drugs only if seizure type and frequency require it, i.e. more than one fit every 6–12 months.

GENERAL GUIDE TO ANTIEPILEPSY DRUG THERAPY

The decision whether or not to initiate drug therapy after a single seizure remains controversial since approximately 25% of patients may not have another seizure. Some advocate treatment on the basis that early initiation may improve prognosis but the matter has not yet been resolved.

1. Therapy should start with a *single* well-tried and safe drug. The majority of patients (70%) can be controlled on one drug (monotherapy).
2. Anticonvulsant drug treatment should be

appropriate to the *type* of seizure disorder. Although some drugs have a wide spectrum of action against different seizure types, some are more specific and may even aggravate certain seizure types. Carbamazepine is a drug of first choice for focal and secondary generalised epilepsy but aggravates myoclonic and absence seizures. Sodium valproate and lamotrigine have a wide spectrum of action and are active against both primary and secondary generalised epilepsy.

3. Choice of drug is also determined by the patient's *age* and *sex*. This is particularly true for women who prefer to avoid drugs associated with teratogenesis or that have adverse effects on their appearance, e.g. hirsutism from phenytoin.

4. If the attempt to control a patient's epilepsy by use of a single drug is unsuccessful, it should be withdrawn and replaced by a *second line* drug, though these are effective in only about 10% of patients. There is little evidence that three drugs are better than two, and not much that two are better than one. More drugs often mean more adverse effects.

5. *Abrupt withdrawal.* Effective therapy must never be stopped suddenly either by the doctor (carelessness) or by the patient (carelessness, intercurrent illness or ignorance), or status epilepticus may occur. But if rapid withdrawal is required by the occurrence of toxicity, a substantial dose of another antiepilepsy drug should be given at once.

6. In cases where fits are liable to occur at a particular *time,* e.g. the menstrual period, dosage should be adjusted to achieve maximal drug effect at that time or drug treatment can be confined to this time. For example, in catamenial epilepsy, clobazam can be useful given only at period time.

Dosage and administration

Generally drugs are best given as a *single* or *twice daily* dose to increase compliance. Many patients dislike taking medication to work or school and being seen to take it but, necessarily, drugs with short duration of action may require to be taken three or even four times a day.

---

[2] Greek *katamenios,* monthly

Regimens for *initial dosing* tend to vary with different drugs. In general, drugs are started in a small dose and increased at two-weekly intervals to the minimum effective dose. The patient's seizures are then monitored and further increases in dose only made if seizures continue. The time interval for dosage increases should therefore be sufficiently wide apart to allow changes in the seizure frequency due to changes in drug therapy to be accurately determined. These issues are particularly important for a doctor, e.g. in an emergency department, who has never seen the patient with a fit or series of fits. It is important then to consider the cause, whether it is noncompliance (which can be due to intercurrent disease), an inadequate drug regimen or an increase in the severity of the disease.

MONITORING BLOOD CONCENTRATIONS OF ANTICONVULSANTS

Many biochemistry laboratories no longer undertake routine measurement of the plasma concentration for most anticonvulsant drugs because plasma concentrations are insufficiently stable to serve as a useful guide to change of dose. The exception is phenytoin, where a small increase in dose may lead to a disproportionate rise in the plasma drug concentration (see zero-order pharmacokinetics, p. 99) and plasma monitoring is essential. With other drugs the dose is increased to the maximum tolerated level and, if seizures continue, it is replaced by another.

DRUG WITHDRAWAL

After a period of at least 2–3 years free from seizures, withdrawal of antiepilepsy drug therapy can be considered. The prognosis of a seizure disorder is determined by a number of factors. Some are known to remit spontaneously e.g. benign rolandic epilepsy and petit mal, whereas others never remit e.g. juvenile myoclonic epilepsy. In many types of epilepsy the outlook is less certain and only general indicators are available. The following factors can be important:

- The *type* of seizure disorder — major seizures are more easily controlled.

- The *time* to remission — early remission carries a better outlook.
- The *number* of drugs required to induce remission — rapid remission on a single drug is a favourable indicator for successful withdrawal.
- The presence of an *underlying lesion* — control is often difficult.
- The presence of an associated *neurological deficit* or learning difficulty — control is often difficult.

In general, if a patient with a major epilepsy has no neurological deficit or structural lesion and is of normal intelligence, there is a reasonable chance of continued remission, particularly if this is rapidly achieved with a single drug. In general, in adult epilepsy, discontinuing the antiepilepsy drug is associated with about 20% relapse during withdrawal and a further 20% relapse over the following 5 years; after this period relapse is unusual. It is generally recommended that the antiepilepsy drug be withdrawn over a period of 6 months. If a fit occurs during this time, full therapy must be resumed again until the patient has been free from seizures for a further 2–3 years.

DRIVING REGULATIONS AND EPILEPSY

The UK allows patients to drive a car (but not a truck or bus) if they have not had a daytime fit for 1 year (or after 3 years if they continue to be subject to fits only whilst asleep). Any fit that occurs during or after drug withdrawal incurs loss of the driving licence for a year. Because losing the right to drive is perceived to be a significant social disability, most patients prefer to remain on medication.

PREGNANCY AND EPILEPSY

Pregnancy can affect seizure disorder which worsens in about a third, improves in a third, and remains unchanged in the remainder. Ideally, patients should have their seizure disorder properly investigated and treated before pregnancy with the best control achieved on the lowest dose of the least teratogenic drug. *Major* seizures are harmful to the developing fetus because of the possibility of anoxia and metabolic disorder. *Minor* seizures are probably harmless and therefore need not be eradicated. Patients should be advised of the necessity of taking folic acid supplements, since some antiepilepsy drugs affect folic acid metabolism and folic acid deficiency is a risk factor for neural tube defects. Hepatic enzyme inducing antiepilepsy drugs lower the mother's concentration of vitamin K, which can aggravate any postpartum haemorrhage. Pregnant mothers should therefore be given an oral vitamin K for the last two weeks of pregnancy.

Pharmacokinetics in pregnancy

The total plasma concentration of drug falls, especially towards the end of pregnancy, due to *haemodilution*, but the therapeutically important *free (unbound) fraction* in plasma is less affected. In practice, the patient's clinical state is observed closely and the dose of drug is increased if seizures occur more often than expected. Hepatic drug metabolism tends to increase during pregnancy. After delivery, the pharmacokinetics revert to the prepregnancy state over a few days.

Breast feeding

Antiepilepsy drugs pass into breast milk (see p. 116), phenobarbital, primidone and ethosuximide in significant quantities, phenytoin and sodium valproate less so. There is a risk that the baby will become sedated or suckle poorly but, provided a watch is maintained for these effects, the balance of advantage favours breast feeding whilst taking antiepilepsy drugs.

Teratogenic effects

Children of mothers taking antiepilepsy drugs have an approximately 2–3 × increased frequency of malformations at birth. In a case-control study of pregnant women, the frequency of malformation was 20.6% in infants whose mothers took one anticonvulsant drug and 28.0% with two or more such drugs, compared to 8.5% in matched controls.[3] Infants of mothers who gave a history of epilepsy but did not take antiepilepsy drugs did not have a higher frequency than the controls, indicating that malformations are largely due to the antiepilepsy

drugs themselves (rather than to factors related to the mother or her epilepsy).

The features of what has collectively become known as *anticonvulsant embryopathy* comprise: major malformations (often cardiac), microcephaly, growth retardation, and hypoplasia of the midface and fingers. The frequency of most malformations was increased in infants exposed to phenytoin alone or phenobarbital alone. Carbamazepine was associated with major malformations, microcephaly and growth retardation but not hypoplasia of the midface and fingers. In general, the major malformations were not distinct from those occurring among infants whose mothers had not taken antiepilepsy drugs, with two exceptions: marked hypoplasia of the nails and stiff joints were strongly associated with phenytoin with or without phenobarbitone, and lumbosacral spina bifida was commoner in infants exposed to carbamazepine or sodium valproate.

With current information, *carbamazepine* seems to be the safest drug for use during pregnancy. Data on lamotrigine (more recently introduced) are increasing but it has not been shown to be strongly associated with malformations.

When counselling whether or not to treat, and with which drug, factors such as the severity and type of seizure disorder also need to be taken in to account since control of major seizures is of fundamental importance.

EPILEPSY AND ORAL CONTRACEPTIVES

Some antiepilepsy drugs (carbamazepine, phenytoin, barbituates, topiramate, oxcarbazepine) induce steroid metabolising enzymes and can cause hormonal contraception to fail. Patients who are taking these drugs need a higher dose of oestrogen (least 50 micrograms/day) if they wish to continue on the pill, although this does not guarantee complete protection from pregnancy with the associated risks to the fetus. Lamotrigine and sodium valproate are not enzyme inducers and their use is not reason to alter the dose of oral contraceptive.

EPILEPSY IN CHILDREN

Fits in children are treated as in adults, but children

---

[3] Holmes LB et al 2001 New England Journal of Medicine 344: 1132–1138.

may respond differently and become irritable, e.g. with *sodium valproate* or *phenobarbitone*. Whether antiepilepsy drugs interfere with later mental and physical development remains uncertain, and it is unwise to assume they do not. The sensible course is to control the epilepsy with monotherapy in minimal doses and with special attention to precipitating factors, and to attempt drug withdrawal when it is deemed safe (see above).

When a child has *febrile convulsions* the decision to embark on continuous prophylaxis is serious for the child, and depends on an assessment of risk factors, e.g. age, nature and duration of the fits. Most children who have febrile convulsions do not develop epilepsy. Prolonged drug therapy, e.g. with phenytoin or phenobarbitone, has been shown to interfere with cognitive[4] development, the effect persisting for months after the drug is withdrawn. Parents may be supplied with a specially formulated solution of diazepam for rectal administration (absorption from a suppository is too slow) for easy and early administration, and advised on managing fever, e.g. use paracetamol at the first hint of fever, and tepid sponging.

STATUS EPILEPTICUS

Status epilepticus is a medical emergency. *Lorazepam* i.v. is now the preferred initial choice. *Clonazepam* is an alternative. *Diazepam* i.v. was widely used as the first line drug, but it is more likely to cause hypotension and respiratory depression, and its antiepilepsy effect wears off after about 20 minutes, so that phenytoin i.v must also be given at the same time to suppress further fitting (with ECG and blood pressure monitoring, since cardiac arrhythmias and further hypotension may result). For this reason some consider *phenobarbitone* to be safer. If resuscitation facilities are not immediately available, diazepam can be given by rectal solution. *Midazolam* (nasally) may be preferred in institutions, e.g. mental hospitals, rather than diazepam rectally because patient and carer compliance are better. *Clomethiazole* is often given in status epilepticus since it is easy to administer, but it has no prolonged anticonvulsant effect and is prone

TABLE 20.1	Treatment of status epilepticus in adults
Early status	Lorazepam 4 mg i.v.; repeat once after 10 minutes if necessary or Clonazepam 1 mg i.v. over 30 seconds, repeat if necessary or Diazepam 10–20 mg over 2–4 min; repeat once after 30 minutes if necessary.
Established status	Phenytoin 15–18 mg/kg i.v. at a rate of 50 mg/minute and/or Phenobarbitone 10–20 mg/kg i.v. at a rate of 100 mg/minute or
Refractory status	Thiopental or Propofol or Midazolam with full intensive care support

to cause respiratory depression and hypotension. Details of further management appear in Table 20.1.

Once the emergency is over, exploration of the reason for the episode and reinstitution of normal therapy are essential. Magnesium sulphate may be better than phenytoin for the treatment of the seizure disorder of eclampsia (see also p. 493).[5]

Paraldehyde is now rarely used. It smells and tastes unpleasant and is partly excreted unchanged via the lungs (75% is metabolised; $t\frac{1}{2}$ 5 h); it is an irritant (avoid in peptic ulcer) and causes painful muscle necrosis when injected i.m. It dissolves plastic syringes.

Pharmacology of individual drugs

The drugs used in the treatment of epilepsy are given in Table 20.2.

CARBAMAZEPINE

Carbamazepine (Tegretol) has a range of actions, of which the most important probably is blockade of voltage-dependent sodium ion channels, reducing membrane excitability.

---

[4] Activities associated with thinking, learning and memory.

[5] Eclampsia Trial Collaborative Group 1995 Lancet 345: 1455–1463.

TABLE 20.2 Drugs of choice for the treatment of epilepsy

Seizure disorder	Drug	Usual daily oral dose	
		Adult	**Child**
Generalised seizures Primary generalised tonic-clonic (grand mal)			
	Drugs of choice		
	Sodium valproate	1–2 g	15–40 mg/kg
	Lamotrigine	(a)	(a)
	Alternatives		
	Clonazepam	2–6 mg	< 1 y 0.5–1 mg
			1–5 y 1–3 mg
			5–12 y 3–6 mg
	Topiramate	200–400 mg	5–9 mg/kg (2–16 y)
	Carbamazepine (b)	0.8–1.2 g	< 1 y 100–200 mg
			1–5 y 200–400 mg
			5–10 y 400–600 mg
			10–15 y 0.6–1 g
	Phenytoin	200–400 mg	4–8 mg/kg
Absence (petit mal)			
	Drugs of choice		
	Ethosuximide	1–1.5 g	> 6 y 1–1.5 g
	Sodium valproate	(as above)	(as above)
	Alternatives		
	Clonazepam	(as above)	(as above)
	Lamotrigine	(a)	(a)
Atypical absence, myotonic, atonic			
	Drugs of choice		
	Sodium valproate	(as above)	(as above)
	Clonazepam	(as above)	(as above)
	Lamotrigine (c)	(a)	(a)
	Phenytoin	(as above)	(as above)
	Ethosuximide	(as above)	(as above)
	Phenobarbital	60–90 mg	5–8 mg/kg
Myoclonic			
	Drug of choice		
	Sodium valproate (d)	(as above)	(as above)
	Clonazepam	(as above)	(as above)
	Alternatives		
	Lamotrigine	(a)	
Partial and/or secondary generalised seizures			
	Drugs of choice		
	Carbamazepine	(as above)	(as above)
	Sodium valproate	(as above)	(as above)
	Alternatives		
	Phenytoin	(as above)	(as above)
	Lamotrigine	(a)	(a)
	Gabapentin	0.9–1.2 g	0.9 g (26–36 kg b. wt.)
			1.2 g (37–50 kg b. wt.)
	Vigabatrin (e)	2–3 g	0.5–1 g (10–15 kg b. wt.)
			1–1.5 g (15–30 kg b. wt.)
			1.5–3 g (30–50 kg b. wt.)
			2–3 g (> 50 kg b. wt.)
	Topiramate	(as above)	(as above)
	Oxcarbazepine	0.6–2.4 g	
	Levetiracetam	1–3 g	

(a) Varies with mono- or adjunctive therapy; see manufacturer's recommendations.
(b) Avoid if major seizures are accompanied by absence seizures or myoclonic jerks.
(c) Lamotrigine may be effective, particularly if used with sodium valproate.
(d) Alone or in combination with clonazepam, which may be synergistic.
(e) In adults, used as a last resort; in children, used for infantile spasms (West's syndrome). Regular visual field monitoring is mandatory.

Pharmacokinetics. Carbamazepine is extensively metabolised; one of the main products, an epoxide (a chemically reactive form), has anticonvulsant activity similar to that of the parent drug but may also cause some of its adverse effects. The $t_{1/2}$ of carbamazepine falls from 35 h to 20 h over the first few weeks of therapy due to induction of hepatic enzymes that metabolise it as well as other drugs, including corticosteroids (adrenal and contraceptive), theophylline and warfarin. Cimetidine and valproate inhibit its metabolism. There are complex interactions with other antiepilepsy drugs, which constitute a reason for monodrug therapy.

Standard tablets are taken twice a day, but with higher doses a three or four times a day regimen may be necessary. Rectal and liquid formulations are available, but there is no i.v. preparation.

Uses. Carbamazepine is used for secondary generalised and partial seizures, and primary generalised seizures. Because another antiepilepsy drug (phenytoin) was sometimes beneficial in *trigeminal neuralgia*, carbamazepine was tried in this condition, for which it is now the drug of choice

Adverse effects include CNS symptoms (reversible blurring of vision, diplopia, dizziness and ataxia) and depression of cardiac AV conduction. Alimentary symptoms, skin rashes, blood disorders and liver and kidney dysfunction also occur. Osteomalacia by enhanced metabolism of vitamin D (enzyme induction) occurs over years; so also does folate deficiency. Enzyme induction reduces the efficacy of combined and progestogen-only contraceptives. Carbamazepine impairs cognitive function less than phenytoin.

Oxcarbazepine, like its analogue carbamazepine, acts by blocking voltage-sensitive sodium channels. It is rapidly and extensively metabolised in the liver; the $t_{1/2}$ of the parent drug is 2 h but that of its principal metabolite (which also has therapeutic activity) is 11 h. Unlike carbamazepine, it does not form an epoxide which may explain why oxcarbazepine has fewer unwanted effects. Oxcarbazepine is a selective inducer of a cytochrome isoenzyme that metabolises the oral contraceptive and a 50 microgram oestrogen preparation is necessary for

contraception. It does not induce hepatic enzymes in general.

Oxcarbazepine is as effective as carbamazepine, sodium valproate and phenytoin in the treatment of partial and secondary generalised seizures, for which it is used either as monotherapy or add on therapy.

The most common chronic adverse effect is hyponatraemia, but this is usually mild, asymptomatic and of no clinical significance. Routine serum monitoring of the plasma sodium is indicated only where there is special risk, e.g. patients taking diuretics or the elderly.

PHENYTOIN

Phenytoin (diphenylhydantoin, Epanutin, Dilantin) alters ionic fluxes but principally the voltage-dependent sodium ion channels in the neuronal membrane; this action is described as membrane stabilising, and discourages the spread (rather than the initiation) of seizure discharges.

Pharmacokinetics. Phenytoin provides a good example of the application of pharmacokinetics for successful prescribing. The important aspects are:

- Saturation (zero-order) kinetics
- Hepatic enzyme induction and enzyme inhibition
- Opportunities for clinically important unwanted interactions are extensive.

Saturation kinetics. Phenytoin is extensively hydroxylated in the liver and this process becomes saturated at about the doses needed for therapeutic effect. Thus phenytoin at low doses exhibits first-order kinetics but saturation or zero-order kinetics develop as the therapeutic plasma concentration range (10–20 mg/l) is approached, i.e. the dose increments of equal size produce *disproportional rise in steady-state plasma concentration.*

A clinically meaningful single half-life can be quoted where a drug is subject only to first-order kinetics. At low doses, giving subtherapeutic plasma concentrations, the $t_{1/2}$ of phenytoin is 6–24 h. But at doses giving therapeutic plasma concentrations, when metabolism is becoming saturated, elimination of the drug is relatively slower. This has significant implications for patient care, e.g. the time taken to reach a steady-state plasma concentration after a dose increment (about $5 \times t\frac{1}{2}$) is 2–3 days at low dose and about 2 weeks at high doses. Thus dose increments should become smaller as the dose increases (which is why there is a 25-mg capsule). Plainly, monitoring serial plasma concentration measurement will help.

Enzyme induction and inhibition. Phenytoin is a potent inducer of hepatic metabolising enzymes affecting itself, other drugs and dietary and endogenous substances (including vitamin D and folate). The consequences of this are: a slight fall of steady state phenytoin level over the first few weeks of therapy, though this may not be noticeable if dose increments are being given; enhanced metabolism of other drugs, e.g. carbamazepine, warfarin, steroids (adrenal and gonadal), thyroxine, tricyclic antidepressants, doxycycline. Naturally this can also work in reverse, and other enzyme inducers, e.g. rifampicin, ethanol, may lower phenytoin concentrations when there is capacity for increase in enzyme induction.

Drugs that inhibit phenytoin metabolism (causing its plasma concentration to rise) include: sodium valproate, cimetidine, co-trimoxazole, isoniazid, chloramphenicol, some NSAIDs, disulfiram. There is a considerable body of mediocre and contradictory data, the lesson of which is that possible interaction should be borne in mind wherever other drugs are prescribed to a patient taking phenytoin.

Phenytoin is 90% bound to plasma albumin so that quite small changes in binding, e.g. a drop to 80%, will result in a higher concentration of free, active, drug. Since free drug is also available to be metabolised, the effect of such changes is probably short-lived. Phenytoin orally is well absorbed but there have been pharmaceutical bioavailability problems in relation to the nature of the diluent in the capsule; patients should always use the same formulation. Phenytoin should not be given i.m. since it precipitates and is poorly absorbed. It may be diluted and given by i.v. infusion over 1 hour but care should be taken to follow the manufacturer's instructions including the use of an in-line filter, because phenytoin may also precipitate in infusion fluids, particularly dextrose.

Uses. Phenytoin is used to prevent all types of partial epilepsy, whether or not the seizures thereafter become generalised, and to treat generalised seizures and status epiepticus. It is not used for absence attacks.

Other uses. The membrane-stabilising effect of phenytoin has been used in cardiac arrhythmias and, rarely, in cases of resistant pain, e.g. trigeminal neuralgia.

Adverse effects of phenytoin, many of which can be very slow to develop, include impairment of cognitive function, which has led many physicians to prefer carbamazepine and valproate. Other nervous system effects range from sedation to delirium to acute cerebellar disorder to convulsions. Peripheral neuropathy also occurs. Cutaneous reactions include rashes (dose related), coarsening of facial features and hirsutism. Gum hyperplasia (due to inhibition of collagen catabolism) may develop and is more marked in children and when there is poor gum hygiene.

Other effects include Dupuytren's contracture and pseudolymphoma. Some degree of macrocytosis is common but anaemia probably occurs only when dietary folate is inadequate. This responds to folate supplement (the requirement for folate is increased, as it is a cofactor in some hydroxylation reactions that are accelerated by enzyme induction by phenytoin). Osteomalacia due to increased metabolism of vitamin D occurs after years of therapy.

Overdose (causing cerebellar symptoms and signs, coma, apnoea) is treated according to general principles. The patient may remain unconscious for a long time because of saturation kinetics, but will recover if respiration and circulation are sustained.

Fosphenytoin, a prodrug of phenytoin, is soluble in water, easier and safer to administer; its conversion in the blood to phenytoin is rapid and it may be used as an alternative to phenytoin for status epilepticus (Table 20.1).

SODIUM VALPROATE

Sodium valproate (valproic acid) (Epilim) acts by inhibiting GABA transaminase, the enzyme responsible for the breakdown of the inhibitory neurotransmitter, GABA, so increasing its concentration at GABA receptors.

Sodium valproate is extensively metabolised in the liver and has a $t\frac{1}{2}$ of 13 h. It is 90% bound to plasma albumin. Sodium valproate is a nonspecific inhibitor of metabolism, and indeed inhibits its own metabolism, and that of lamotrigine, phenobarbitone, phenytoin and carbamazepine. Sodium valproate does not induce drug metabolising enzymes but its metabolism is enhanced by induction due to other drugs, including antiepileptics.

Sodium valproate is effective for a wide range of seizure disorders, including generalised and partial epilepsy, and the prophylaxis of febrile convulsions and post-traumatic epilepsy.

Adverse effects can be troublesome. The main ones of concern, particularly to women, are weight gain, teratogenicity (see p. 416), polycystic ovary syndrome, and loss of hair which grows back curly.[6] Nausea may be a problem. Some patients exhibit a rise in liver enzymes which is usually transient and without sinister import, but they should be closely monitored until the biochemical tests return to normal as, rarely, liver failure occurs (risk maximal at 2–12 weeks); this is often indicated by anorexia, malaise and a recurrence of seizures. Other reactions include pancreatitis, and coagulation disorder due to inhibition of platelet aggregation (coagulation should be assessed before surgery).

Ketone metabolites may cause confusion in uring testing in diabetes.

Metabolic inhibition by valproate prolongs the action of co-administered antiepilepsy drugs (see above). The effect is significant and the dose of lamotrigine, for example, should be halved in patients who are also taking sodium valproate.

BARBITURATES

Antiepilepsy members include *phenobarbital* (phenobarbitone) ($t\frac{1}{2}$ 100 h), methylphenobarbital and *primidone* (Mysoline), which is largely metabolised to phenobarbital, i.e. it is a prodrug. They are still used for generalised seizures; sedation is usual.

CLONAZEPAM

Clonazepam (Rivotril) ($t\frac{1}{2}$ 25 h) is a benzodiazepine used as a second line drug for treatment of primary generalised epilepsy and for status epilepticus (see Table 20.1).

Vigabatrin (Sabril) ($t\frac{1}{2}$ 6 h) is structurally related to the inhibitory CNS neurotransmitter GABA and it acts by irreversibly inhibiting GABA-transaminase so that GABA accumulates. GABA-transaminase is resynthesised over 6 days. Vigabatrin is not metabolised and does not induce hepatic drug metabolising enzymes.

Vigabatrin is effective in partial, secondary generalised seizures which are not satisfactorily controlled by other anticonvulsants, and in infantile spasms, as monotherapy. It worsens absence and myoclonic seizures

Unwanted effects from drugs sometimes become apparant only following prolonged use, and vigabatrin is a case in point. Vigabatrin had been licenced for a number of years, before it was found to cause visual field constriction in up to 40% of patients, an effect that is insidious and leads to irreversible tunnel vision.[7] Its discovery emphasises the value of postmarketing drug surveillance programmes.[8] Vigabatrin is now indicated only for patients with the specific seizure disorders responsive to the drug (above), and no other. Patients should undergo visual field monitoring at six-monthly intervals whilst taking the drug. Other adverse effects on the CNS are similar to those of antiepilepsy drugs in general but include confusion and psychosis. Increase in weight also occurs in up to 40% of patients during the first 6 months of treatment.

Lamotrigine acts to stabilise presynaptic neuronal membranes by blocking voltage-dependent sodium channels (a property it shares with carbamazepine and phenytoin) and it reduces the release of excitatory amino acids, such as glutamate and aspartate. The $t\frac{1}{2}$ of 24 h allows for a single daily dose.

---

[6] 'We thought the change might be welcomed by the patients, but one girl preferred her hair to be long and straight, and one boy was mortified by his curls and insisted on a short hair cut.' Jeavons P M 1977 Lancet 1: 359.

[7] Eke T, Talbot J F et al. 1997 British Medical Journal 314: 180–181.
[8] Wilton L V, Stephens M D B, Mann R D 1999 British Medical Journal 319: 1165–1166.

Lamotrigine is effective as monotherapy and adjunctive therapy for partial and primary and secondarily generalised tonic-clonic seizures. It is generally well tolerated but may cause serious adverse effects on the skin, including Stevens–Johnson syndrome and toxic epidermal necrolysis (fatally, on rare occasions). The risk of cutaneous effects can be lessened if treatment is begun with a low dose and is escalated slowly. Concomitant use of valproate, which inhibits the metabolism and thus the inactivation of lamotrigine, adds to the hazard. Carbamazepine, phenytoin or primidone accelerate the metabolic breakdown of lamotrigine which must be given in higher dose when combined.

Gabapentin is an analogue of GABA that is sufficiently lipid soluble to cross the blood–brain barrier but its mode of action is uncertain. It is excreted unchanged and, unlike other antiepilepsy agents, does not induce or inhibit hepatic metabolism of other drugs.

Gabapentin is effective only for partial seizures and secondary generalised epilepsy (not absence or myoclonic epilepsy), in combination with established agents. It is also used for *neuropathic pain.* Gabapentin may cause somnolence, unsteadiness, dizziness and fatigue.

Topiramate possesses a range of actions that include blockade of voltage-sensitive sodium channels, enhancement of GABA activity and possibly weak blockade of glutamate receptors. The $t\frac{1}{2}$ of 21 h allows once daily dosing; it is excreted in the urine mainly as unchanged drug.

Topiramate is used as adjunctive treatment for partial seizures, with or without secondary generalisation. It use is limited by its unwanted effects, particularly sedation, naming difficulty and weight loss. Acute myopia and raised intraocular pressure may occur.

Levetiracetam acts in a manner different to other antiepilepsy drugs. It has a potentially broad spectrum of use but is currently indicated for adjunctive treatment in partial seizures with or without secondary generalisation. It is rapidly and completely absorbed after oral administration, and is effective with twice-daily dosing. Its therapeutic index appears to be high and the commonest of the adverse effects are asthenia, dizziness and drowsiness.

Succinimides. *Ethosuximide* (Zarontin) ($t\frac{1}{2}$ 55 h) differs from other antiepilepsy drugs in that it blocks a particular type of calcium channel that is active in absence seizures (petit mal), and it is used specifically for this condition. Adverse effects include gastric upset, CNS effects and allergic reactions including eosinophilia and other blood disorders, and lupus erythematosus.

Parkinsonism

A NOTE ON PATHOPHYSIOLOGY

Parkinson's disease[9] affects about 1 in 200 of the elderly population. In broad terms, it is caused by degeneration of the substantia nigra[10] in the midbrain, and consequent loss of dopamine-containing neurons in the nigrostriatal pathway (see Fig. 19.3, p. 382). There is no known cure but drug treatment can, if properly managed, dramatically improve quality of life in this progressive disease.

Two balanced systems are important in the extrapyramidal control of motor activity at the level of the corpus striatum and substantia nigra: in one the neurotransmitter is *acetylcholine;* in the other it is a *dopamine.* In Parkinson's disease there is degenerative loss of nigrostriatal dopaminergic neurons and the symptoms and signs of the disease are due to *dopamine depletion.*

Certain drugs also produce the features of Parkinson's disease (see below) and the general term 'parkinsonism' is used to cover both the disease and the drug-induced states. The *symptom triad* of the disease is *bradykinesia, rigidity* and *tremor.* Patients who have received levodopa for a long time may exhibit the 'on-off' phenomenon in which, abruptly and distressingly, dyskinesia (the 'on' phase) alternates with hypokinesia (the 'off' phase). One sufferer, a physician, wrote about his condition:

---

[9] James Parkinson (1755–1824), physician; he described *paralysis agitans* in 1817.
[10] *Substantia nigra* is (Latin) black substance. A coronal section at this point in the brain shows the distinctive black areas, visible with the naked eye in the normal brain, but absent from the brains of patients with Parkinson's disease.

'One of its most trying aspects is the extent to which it interferes with the trivial events in daily life. Nothing is easy in Parkinson's disease. There is no feature of any task that is not potentially out of control. A cuff-link refuses to find its way into a tuxedo shirt, my wife is out of town, and I miss the annual dinner. I am unable to stuff change from a $5 bill into my wallet, and the patrons in line behind the cash register fume. Bow ties won't tie and shoelaces won't lace. A cube of beef obstructs the glottis. In Parkinson's disease one must expect the unexpected … About five years ago, my disease began to close in on me, becoming more aggressive and difficult to handle. I had increasing discomfort from hyperkinesias. My voice was almost inaudible, and periods when my feet felt frozen to the floor became commonplace. I lost the advantage I had previously enjoyed of a comfortable margin between the effective dose and the dose with intolerable side effects. I had an "off" spell … in a telephone booth…'[11]

Objectives of therapy

The dopaminergic/cholinergic balance may be restored by the following mechanisms.

1. **Enhancement of dopaminergic activity** by drugs which may:
   (a) *replenish* neuronal dopamine by supplying levodopa, which is its natural precursor; administration of dopamine itself is ineffective as it does not cross the blood–brain barrier
   (b) act as *dopamine agonists* (bromocriptine, pergolide, cabergoline, apomorphine);
   (c) *prolong* the action of dopamine through selective inhibition of its metabolism (selegiline).
   (d) *release* dopamine from stores and inhibit re-uptake (amantadine) or
2. **Reduction of cholinergic activity** by antimuscarinic (anticholinergic[12]) drugs; this

---

[11] Saltzman E W 1996 Living with Parkinson's disease. New England Journal of Medicine 334: 114–116.
[12] The term *antimuscarinic* is now preferred (see p. 435).

approach is most effective against tremor and rigidity, and less effective in the treatment of bradykinesia (including iatrogenic, caused by dopamine receptor antagonists).

Both approaches are effective in therapy and may usefully be combined. It therefore comes as no surprise that drugs which prolong the action of acetylcholine (anticholinesterases) or drugs which deplete dopamine stores (reserpine) or block dopamine receptors (antipsychotics, e.g. chlorpromazine) will exacerbate the symptoms of parkinsonism or induce a parkinson-like state.

Other parts of the brain in which dopaminergic systems are involved include the medulla (induction of vomiting), the hypothalamus (suppression of prolactin secretion) and certain paths to the cerebral cortex. Different effects of dopaminergic drugs can be explained by activation of these systems, namely emesis, suppression of lactation (mainly direct dopamine agonists) and occasionally psychotic illness. Classical antipsychotics (see p. 381) used to manage psychotic behaviour act by blockade of dopamine D_2 receptors and, as is to be expected, they are also antinauseant, may sometimes cause galactorrhoea, and can induce parkinsonism. Drug-induced parkinsonism is alleviated by anti-muscarinics, but not by levodopa or dopamine agonists, because the antipsychotics block dopamine receptors by which these drugs act. Since many antipsychotics also have some antimuscarinic activity, those with greatest efficacy in this respect, e.g. thioridazine, are the least likely to cause parkinsonism.

Drugs for Parkinson's disease

DOPAMINERGIC DRUGS

Levodopa and dopa-decarboxylase inhibitors

Levodopa ('dopa' stands for dihydroxyphenyl-alanine) is a natural amino acid precursor of dopamine. The latter cannot be used because it is rapidly metabolised in the gut, blood and liver by monoamine oxidase and catechol-*O*-methyltransferase; even intravenously administered dopamine, or dopamine formed in peripheral tissues, is insufficiently lipid-soluble to penetrate the CNS. But levodopa is readily absorbed from the upper small intestine by active amino acid transport and has a $t\frac{1}{2}$ of 1.5 h. It can traverse the blood–brain barrier by a similar active transport, and within the brain it is decarboxylated (by dopa decarboxylase) to the neurotransmitter *dopamine.*

But a major disadvantage is that levodopa is also extensively decarboxylated to dopamine in peripheral tissues so that only 1–5% of an oral dose of levodopa reaches the brain. Thus large quantities of levodopa would have to be given. These inhibit gastric emptying, delivery to the absorption site is erratic and fluctuations in plasma concentration occur. The drug and its metabolites cause significant adverse effects by peripheral actions, notably nausea, but also cardiac arrhythmia and postural hypotension. This problem has been largely circumvented by the development of *decarboxylase inhibitors,* which do not enter the central nervous system, so that they prevent only the *extracerebral* metabolism of levodopa. The inhibitors are given in combination with levodopa and there is a range of formulations comprising a decarboxylase inhibitor with levodopa:

- *co-careldopa* (carbidopa + levodopa in proportions 12.5/50 mg, 10/100, 25/100, 25/250) (Sinemet)
- *co-beneldopa* (benserazide + levodopa in proportions 12.5 mg/50 mg, 25/100, 50/200) (Madopar).

The combinations produce the same brain concentrations as with levodopa alone, but only 25% of the dose of levodopa is required, which smooths the action of levodopa and reduces the incidence of adverse effects, especially nausea, from about 80% to less than 15%.

Dose management

Levodopa alone and in combination (see above) is introduced gradually and titrated according to response, the dose being altered every 2 weeks. The dose is increased to provide sufficient benefit for each individual patient, not to a standard dose since this is very variable.

Compliance is important. Abrupt discontinuation of therapy leads to dramatic relapse.

Adverse effects. *Postural hypotension* occurs. *Nausea* may be a limiting factor if the dose is increased too rapidly; it may be helped by cyclizine 50 mg taken 30 min before food or by domperidone (little of which enters the brain). Levodopa-induced *dyskinesias* take the form of involuntary limb jerking or head, lip or tongue movements and constitute a major constraint on how the drug is used (see later). *Mental changes* may be seen: these include depression, which is common (best controlled with a tricyclic antidepressant), dreams, and hallucinations and delusions (clozapine may help). *Agitation and confusion* occur but it may be difficult to decide whether these are due to drug or to disease. In these circumstances, the drugs most likely to be the cause of a toxic confusional state (antimuscarinics and direct dopamine agonists) are withdrawn.

Interactions. With nonselective monoamine oxidase inhibitors (MAOI), the monoamine dopamine formed from levodopa is protected from destruction; it accumulates and also follows the normal path of conversion to noradrenaline (norepinephrine), by dopamine β-hydroxylase; *severe hypertension results.* The interaction with the selective MAO-B inhibitor, selegiline, is possibly therapeutic (see below). Tricyclic antidepressants are safe. Levodopa antagonises the effects of antipsychotics (dopamine receptor blockers). Some antihypertensives enhance hypotensive effects of levodopa. Metabolites of dopamine in the urine interfere with some tests for phaeochromocytoma, and in such patients it is best to measure the plasma catecholamines directly.

Dopa-decarboxylase is a pyridoxine-dependent enzyme and concomitant use of pyridoxine, e.g. in self-medication with a multivitamin preparation, can enhance peripheral conversion of levodopa to dopamine so that less is available to enter the CNS, and benefit is lost. This effect does not occur, of course, with the now usual levodopa-decarboxylase inhibitor combinations.

Dopamine agonists

These mimic the effects of dopamine, the endogenous agonist, which stimulates both the main two types of dopamine receptor, D_1 and D_2 (coupled respectively to adenylyl cyclase stimulation and inhibition). The D_2-receptor is the principal target in Parkinson's disease; chronic D_1 stimulation appears to potentiate the response to D_2 stimulation despite acutely having an inhibitory action on adenylyl cyclase. The main problems with dopamine (i.e. the prodrug, levodopa) are its short $t^1/_2$ and, possibly, the consequences of delivering large amounts of substrate to an oxidative pathway, MAO (see below). On the other hand, the problems of developing synthetic alternatives are:

- reproducing the right balance of D_1 and D_2 stimulation (dopamine itself is slightly D_1 selective, in test systems, but its net effect in vivo is determined also by the relative amounts and locations of receptors — which differ in Parkinsonian patients from normal)
- avoiding the undesired effects of peripheral, mainly gastric, D_2-receptors
- synthesising a full, not partial, agonist.

Bromocriptine (a derivative of ergot) is a D_2-receptor agonist, but also a weak α-adrenoreceptor antagonist. It is commonly used with levodopa. The drug is rapidly absorbed after administration by mouth; the $t^1/_2$ is 5 h, so that its action is smoother than that of levodopa, which can be an advantage in patients who develop end-of-dose deterioration with levodopa. Dosing should start very low (1–1.25 mg p.o. at night), increasing at approximately weekly intervals and according to clinical response.

Nausea and vomiting are the commonest adverse effects; these may respond to domperidone but tend to become less marked as treatment continues. Postural hypotension may cause dizziness or syncope. In high dose confusion, delusions or hallucinations may occur and, after prolonged use, pleural effusion and retroperitoneal fibrosis.

Lisuride ($t^1/_2$ 2 h) and **pergolide** ($t^1/_2$ 6 h) are similar to bromocriptine, though the latter also stimulates D_1-receptors. *Cabergoline*, also an ergot derivative, has a $t^1/_2$ of more than 80 h. This long duration of action allows it to be used in a single daily (or even twice weekly) dose, which is appreciated by patients who are often taking other drugs every

2–3 hours; it is also valuable for night-time problems due to lack of levodopa. *Pramipexole* is a non-ergot dopamine D_2-receptor agonist that is more effective against tremor than the others. *Ropinirole* is a direct D_2-receptor agonist, which is also a non-ergot derivate. There are insufficient data to allow an informed choice between these drugs.

Apomorphine is a derivative of morphine having structural similarities to dopamine; it is a full agonist at D_1- and D_2-receptors. Its main use is in young patients with severe motor fluctuations and dyskinesias (the 'on-off' phenomenon, see above) when it is given by s.c. injection or infusion for patients with levodopa resistant 'off'. The rapid onset of action by the s.c. route (self-administration can be taught) enables the 'off' component to be aborted without the patient waiting 45–60 minutes to absorb another oral dose of levodopa. Apomorphine may need to be accompanied by an antiemetic, e.g. domperidone (which does not cross the blood–brain barrier as does metoclopramide), to prevent its characteristic emetic action. Overdose causes respiratory depression; it is antagonised by naloxone. Apomorphine can induce penile erection (without causing sexual excitement) and it enhances the penile response to visual erotic stimulation.

Inhibition of dopamine metabolism

Monoamine oxidase (MAO) enzymes have an important function in modulating the intraneuronal content of neurotransmitter. The enzymes exist in two principal forms, A and B, defined by specific substrates some of which cannot be metabolised by the other form (Table 20.3). The therapeutic importance of recognising these two forms arises because they are to some extent present in different tissues, and the enzyme at these different locations can be selectively inhibited by the individual inhibitors: moclobemide for MAO-A (used for depression, p. 379) and selegiline for MAO-B (Table 20.3).

Selegiline is a selective, irreversible inhibitor of MAO type B. The problem with nonselective MAO inhibitors is that they prevent degradation of dietary amines, especially tyramine, which is then able to act systemically as a sympathomimetic: the

TABLE 20.3 Isoforms of monoamine oxidase: MAO-A and MAO-B: an explanation
The table shows the definition of the isoforms by their specific substrates, and then their selectivity (or nonselectivity) towards a number of other substrates and inhibitors. Determination of therapeutic and adverse effects is a function of selectivity of the inhibitor and the tissue location of the enzyme.

Enzyme	MAO-A	MAO-A and B	MAO-B
Substrate	Serotonin (see below)	Noradrenaline (norepinephrine) (see below) Adrenaline (epinephrine) Dopamine Tyramine	Phenylethylamine
Inhibitors	Moclobemide	Tranylcypromine Phenelzine Iproniazid	Selegiline
Tissues	Liver CNS (neurons) Sympathetic neurons	See MAO-A, MAO-B	Gut CNS (glial cells)

Explanation: the specific substrate for MAO-A is serotonin, whilst for MAO-B it is the nonendogenous amine, phenylethylamine (present in many brands of chocolate). Noradrenaline, tyramine and dopamine can be metabolised by both isoforms of MAO. MAO-A is the major form in liver and in neurons (both CNS and peripheral sympathetic); MAO-B is the major form in gut, but is also present in the liver, lungs and glial cells of the CNS.

hypertensive 'cheese reaction'. As will be apparent from Table 20.3, selegiline does not cause the cheese reaction, because MAO-A is still present in the liver to metabolise tyramine. MAO-A also metabolises tyramine in the sympathetic nerve endings, so providing a further line of protection (tyramine is an indirect acting amine which displaces noradrenaline from the nerve endings). In the CNS selegiline protects dopamine from intraneuronal degradation. It has no effect on synaptic cleft concentrations of those amines like serotonin and noradrenaline, which are normally potentiated by the MAOI used in depression; therefore selegiline has no antidepressant action.

Selegiline was originally introduced in the belief that it would delay end-of-dose deterioration by prolonging the action of levodopa; subsequently it was held that this action might be protective of dopaminergic neurons and so allow later initiation of therapy with levodopa. It became one of the most widely prescribed drugs for Parkinson's disease. Later clinical trials, however, failed to confirm these effects and indeed, combined treatment with levodopa and selegiline was associated with excess mortality;[13] many patients discontinued selegiline without worsening of their condition. A minority deteriorated acutely and they have continued to

receive selegiline although the reason for this benefit is not clear.

Entacapone inhibits catechol-*O*-methyltransferase (COMT), one of the principal enzymes responsible for the metabolism of dopamine; the action of levodopa is thus prolonged. It is most effective for patients with early end-of-dose deterioration, and allows them to take levodopa at 3- or 4-hourly intervals, giving a more predictable and useful response. Entacapone is preferred to long-acting preparations of levodopa whose main disadvantage is their slow onset of action. It can increase the dyskinesias seen in the late stages of Parkinson's disease.

Dopamine release

Amantadine antedates the discovery of dopamine receptor subtypes, and its discovery as an antiparkinsonian drug was an example of serendipity. It is an antivirus drug which, given for influenza to a parkinsonian patient, was noticed to be beneficial. The two effects are probably unrelated. It appears to act by increasing synthesis and release of dopamine, and by diminishing neuronal reuptake. It also has slight antimuscarinic effect. The drug is much less effective than levodopa, whose action it will slightly enhance. It is more effective than the standard antimuscarinic drugs, with which it has an additive effect. Amantadine is relatively free from adverse effects, which, however, include ankle

[13] Ben-Sholomo Y, Churchyard A, Head J, Hurwitz B, Overstall P, Ockelford J, Lees A J 1998 British Medical Journal 316: 1191–1196.

oedema (probably a local effect on blood vessels), postural hypotension, livedo reticularis and central nervous system disturbances: insomnia, hallucinations and, rarely, fits.

ANTIMUSCARINIC (ANTICHOLINERGIC) DRUGS
(see also p. 441)

Antimuscarinic drugs benefit parkinsonism by blocking acetylcholine receptors in the central nervous system, thereby partially redressing the imbalance created by decreased dopaminergic activity. Their use originated when hyoscine was given to parkinsonian patients in an attempt to reduce sialorrhoea by peripheral effect, and it then became apparent that they had other beneficial effects in this disease. Synthetic derivatives are now used orally. These include benzhexol (trihexyphenidyl), orphenadrine, benzatropine, procyclidine, biperiden. There is little to choose between these. Antimuscarinics produce modest improvements in tremor, rigidity, sialorrhoea, muscular stiffness and leg cramps, but little in bradykinesia, the most disabling symptom of Parkinson's disease. They are also effective i.m. or i.v. in acute drug-induced dystonias.

Unwanted effects include dry mouth, blurred vision, constipation, urine retention, glaucoma, hallucinations, memory defects, toxic confusional states and psychoses (which should be distinguished from presenile dementia).

Treatment of Parkinson's disease

The main features that require alleviation are *tremor*, *rigidity* and *bradykinesia*.

General measures are important and include the encouragement of regular physical activity and specific help such as physiotherapy, speech therapy and occupational therapy.

DRUG THERAPY

Drugs play the most important role in symptom relief. No agent has yet been found to alter the progressive course of the disease.

Initial treatment

Treatment should begin only when it is judged necessary in each individual case. For example, a young man with a physically demanding job will require treatment before an older retired person. Two conflicting objectives have to be balanced: the desire for satisfactory relief of current symptoms and the avoidance of adverse effects as a result of long-continued treatment. There is debate as to whether the treatment should commence with levodopa or a synthetic dopamine agonist. *Levodopa* provides the biggest improvement in motor symptoms but its use is associated with the development dyskinesias, which are inevitable after some 5–10 years, and sometimes sooner. *Dopamine agonists* have a much less powerful motor effect but are less likely to produce dyskinesias. Some neurologists therefore prefer a dopamine agonist alone as the initial choice. Unfortunately, only about 30% of patients obtain a satisfactory motor response. An alternative, therefore, is to begin treatment with levodopa in low dose to get a good motor response, and to add a dopamine agonist when the initial benefit begins to wane. With either approach, it seems likely that the position after 5 years treatment may well be the same, but that by starting with levodopa the patient will have had the benefit of a earlier motor response.

Antimuscarinic drugs are suitable only for younger patients predominantly troubled with tremor and rigidity. They do not benefit bradykinesia, the main disabling symptom. The unwanted effects of acute angle glaucoma, retention of urine, constipation and psychiatric disturbance are general contraindications to the use of antimuscarinics in the elderly.

Amantadine or *selegiline* can delay the use of either levodopa or a synthetic dopamine agonist in the early stages of the disease if mild symptomatic benefit is required, but this approach is seldom necessary.

A typical course is that for about 2–4 years on treatment with levodopa or a dopamine agonist, the patient's disability and motor performance remains near normal despite progression of the underlying disease. After some 5 years, about 50% of patients exhibit the problems of long-term treatment, namely, dyskinesia and end-of-dose deterioration with the 'on-off' phenomenon. After 10 years virtually 100% of patients are affected.

Dyskinesia comprises involuntary writhing movement of the face and limbs that may be biphasic (occurring at the start and end of motor response) or develop at the time of the maximum plasma levodopa concentration. They respond initially to reducing the dose of levodopa but at the cost of bradykinesia and as time passes there is progressively less scope to obtain benefit without unwanted effects.

End-of-dose deterioration is managed by increasing the frequency of dosing with levodopa (e.g. to 2–3-hourly), but this tends to result in the appearance, or worsening of the dyskinesia. The motor response then becomes more brittle with abrupt swings between hyper- and hypomobility (the on-off phenomenon). Despite their unpredicatable nature over the course of a single day, these changes are in fact dose-related, an effect that becomes apparent only when the response is related to total medication taken over a week.

Various strategies have been devised to overcome these problems. Controlled release preparations of levodopa tend to be associated with an inadequate initial response and disabling dyskinesia at the end of the dose. A more effective approach appears to be the use of a *COMT inhibitor,* e.g. entacapone, which can sometimes allay early end-of-dose deterioration without causing dyskinesia. This is now the main indication for its use. In any event, many patients with Parkinson's disease take at least two and sometimes more drugs at frequent intervals each day, an outcome that tends to rule their lives.

Continuous subcutaneous infusion of *apomorphine* can transform the quality of life of younger patients with severe motor fluctuations and dyskinesia, but this may lead to neuropsychiatric effects. If drug treatment fails in young non-demented patients, stereotactic subthalamotomy or bilateral stereotactic subthalamic stimulation can be very successful with only a small risk of surgical complications in experienced hands. Some 20% of patients with Parkinson's disease, notable the older ones, develop impairment of memory and speech with a fluctuating confusional state and hallucinations. As these symptoms are often aggravated by medication, it is preferable gradually to reduce the antiparkinsonian treatment, even at the expense of lessened mobility.

DRUG-INDUCED PARKINSONISM

The classical antipsychotic (see p. 380) drugs block dopamine receptors and their antipsychotic activity relates closely to this action, which notably involves the D_2-receptor, the principal target in Parkinson's disease. It comes as no surprise, therefore, that these drugs can induce a state whose clinical features are very similar to those of idiopathic Parkinson's disease. The piperazine phenothiazines, e.g. trifluoperazine, and the butyrophenones, e.g. haloperidol, are most commonly involved. In one series[14] of 95 new cases of parkinsonism referred to a department of geriatric medicine, 51% were associated with prescribed drugs and half of these required hospital admission. After withdrawal of the offending drug most cases resolved completely in 7 weeks. But

> One old lady who had received trifluoperazine (for a minor fright and anxiety) for 5 weeks, took 36 weeks to recover from the drug-induced parkinsonism but never managed to get home again.

When drug-induced parkinsonism is troublesome, an antimuscarinic drug, e.g. benzhexol, is beneficial. Atypical antipsychotics provoke fewer extrapyrimidal effects (see p. 387).

Other movement disorders

Essential tremor is often, and with justice, called benign, but a few individuals may be incapacitated by it. Alcohol, through a central action, helps about 50% of patients but is plainly unsuitable for long-term use and a nonselective β-adrenoceptor blocker, e.g. propranolol 120 mg/day, will benefit about 50%; clonazepam or primidone are sometimes beneficial.

---

14 Stephen P J, Williamson J 1984 Lancet 2: 1082.

Drug-induced dystonic reactions are seen:

- as an acute reaction, often of the torsion type, and occur following administration of dopamine receptor blocking antipsychotics, e.g. haloperidol, and antiemetics, e.g. metoclopramide. An antimuscarinic drug, e.g. biperiden or benzatropine, given i.m. or i.v. and repeated as necessary, provides relief
- in some patients who are receiving levodopa for Parkinson's disease
- in younger patients on long-term antipsychotic treatment, who develop tardive dyskinesia (see p. 387).

Hepatolenticular degeneration (Wilson's disease) is caused by a genetic failure to eliminate copper absorbed from food so that it accumulates in the liver, brain, cornea and kidneys. Chelating copper in the gut with penicillamine (p. 293) or trientine can establish a negative copper balance (with some clinical improvement if treatment is started early). The patients may also develop cirrhosis, and the best treatment for both may be orthotopic liver transplantation.

Chorea of any cause may be alleviated by dopamine receptor blocking antipsychotics, and also by tetrabenazine, which inhibits neuronal storage of dopamine and serotonin.

Involuntary muscle spasm: blepharospasm, hemifacial spasm, spasmodic torticollis, and indeed the spasm of chronic anal fissure, are treated with botulinum toxin. This irreversibly blocks release of acetylcholine from cholinergic nerve endings and is injected locally. Its effect lasts about 3 months. Botulinum toxin is at least partially effective in up to 90% of patients with these conditions. Mild dysphagia occurs in ~30% of patients receiving injections into their neck for torticollis due to spread of the toxin in to the pharyngeal muscles.

Spasticity results from lesions at various sites within the central nervous system and spinal cord. Drugs used include the GABA agonist baclofen, diazepam and tizanidine (an α_2-adrenoceptor agonist).

Myotonia in which voluntary muscle fails to relax after contraction may be symptomatically benefitted by drugs that increase muscle refractory period, e.g. procainamide, phenytoin, quinidine.

Multiple sclerosis

Drugs are used to alleviate chronic muscle spasm or spasticity (see above) but until recently, there has been no disease-modifying treatment in this relapsing and remitting condition, where the placebo effect of most drugs can appear quite powerful. Although its cause remains unknown, it is now held to be an autoimmune disorder. This has led to the testing of both old and new forms of drugs, which might modify the immune response, and release of cytokines.

Interferon beta is set to test the resilience of patients, doctors, health economists and administrators. In placebo-controlled trials, it is the first treatment to show a reduction in the number of relapses. Interferon beta may also have a modest effect in delaying disability by 12–18 months in relapsing/remitting disease. In a clinical trial 372 patients with relapsing-remitting disease, able to walk 100 metres without aid or rest, were randomised to receive 8 million IU or 1.6 million IU of interferon beta or placebo by s.c. injection on alternate days. After 2 years there was a reduction in the relapse rate from 1.27 per year in the placebo group to 0.84 per year in the patients receiving the higher dose.[15]

Interferon beta is not indicated in patients with progressive forms of disease, or in severely disabled patients. The high cost per patient treated in relation to the benefit gained has prevented widespread access to this drug. In the UK, only designated neurologists can prescribe interferon beta.

Motor-neuron disease

The cause of the progressive destruction of upper and lower motor neurons is unknown. The only drug available, *riluzole,* may act by inhibiting accumulation of the neurotransmitter, glutamate. In 959 patients, riluzole prolonged median survival time from 13 to 16 months, with no effect on motor function.[16] It may cause neutropenia.

---

[15] The IFNB Multiple Sclerosis Study Group and the University of British Columbia MS/MRI Analysis Group 1995. Neurology 45: 1277–1285

[16] Lacomblez L et al 1996 Lancet 347: 1425–1431.

Tetanus

Objectives of management are to:

- immediately neutralise with globulin any toxin that has not yet become attached irreversibly to the central nervous system
- destroy tetanus bacteria by chemotherapy, thus stopping toxin production
- control convulsions whilst maintaining respiratory and cardiovascular function, which may be disordered by the toxin
- prevent intercurrent infection (usually pulmonary)
- prevent electrolyte disturbances and maintain nutrition.

TREATMENT

Human tetanus immunoglobulin 150 units/kg should be given intramuscularly at multiple sites to neutralise unbound toxin. Where present, wounds should be debrided. Metronidazole is an antibiotic of choice for *Clostridium tetani*, but penicillin, erythromycin, tetracycline, chloramphenicol and clindamycin are acceptable alternatives (see p. 211).

Avoid unnecessary stimulation, which may induce rigidity and spasms. The primary treatment for spasms and rigidity is sedation with a benzodiazepine, such as midazolam or diazepam. Additional sedation may be provided with propofol or a phenothiazine, usually chlorpromazine. In severe disease prolonged spasms and respiratory dysfunction will necessitate tracheal intubation and mechanical ventilation will be required. If the patient has been intubated and sedation alone is inadequate to control spasms, a neuromuscular blocking drug, e.g., intermittent doses of pancuronium or a continuous infusion of atracurium, will be required.

Tetanus toxin often causes disturbances in autonomic control, resulting in sympathetic overactivity and high plasma catecholamine concentrations. The first-line treatment for autonomic dysfunction is by sedation with a benzodiazepine and opioid. Infusion of the short-acting β-blocker esmolol, or the α_2-adrenergic agonist clonidine, helps to control episodes of hypertension. Intravenous magnesium sulphate is also used to reduce autonomic disturbance.

Severe cases of tetanus generally require admission to an intensive care unit for 3–5 weeks. Weight loss is universal in tetanus and these patients require enteral nutrition. Other important measures include: close control of fluid balance, chest physiotherapy to prevent pneumonia, prophylaxis of thromboembolism and intensive nursing care to prevent pressure sores.

GUIDE TO FURTHER READING

Brodie M J, French J A 2000 Management of epilepsy in adolescents and adults. Lancet 356: 323–328

Browne T R, Holmes G L 2001 Epilepsy. New England Journal of Medicine 344: 1145–1151

Cook T M, Protheroe R T, Handel J M 2001 Tetanus: a review of the literature. British Journal of Anaesthesia 87: 477–487

Compston A, Coles A 2002 Multiple sclerosis. Lancet 359: 1221–1231

Delanty N, Vaughn C J, French J A 1998 Medical causes of seizures. Lancet 532: 383–390

Harten P N van, Hoek H W, Kahn R S 1999 Acute dystonia induced by drug treatment. British Medical Journal 319: 623–626

Heafield M T E 2000 Managing status epilepticus. British Medical Journal 320: 953–954

Kapoor W N 2000 Syncope. New England Journal of Medicine 343: 1856–1862

Kwan P, Brodie M J 2001 Neuropsychological effects of epilepsy and antiepileptic drugs. Lancet 357: 216–222

Martin J B 1999 Molecular basis of the neurodegenerative disorders. New England Journal of Medicine 340: 1970–1980

Münchau A, Bhatia K P 2000 Uses of botulinum toxin injection in medicine today. British Medical Journal 320: 161–165

Polman C H, Uitdehaag B M J 2000 Drug treatment of multiple sclerosis. British Medical Journal 2000: 490–494

Shaw P J 1999 Motor neuron disease. British Medical Journal 318: 1118–1121

Stephen L J, Brodie M J 2000 Epilepsy in elderly people. Lancet 355: 1441–1446

Schapira A H V 1999 Parkinson's disease. British Medical Journal 318: 311–314

SECTION 5

CARDIO-RESPIRATORY AND RENAL SYSTEMS

21

Cholinergic and antimuscarinic (anticholinergic) mechanisms and drugs

SYNOPSIS

Acetylcholine is a widespread chemotransmitter in the body, mediating a broad range of physiological effects. There are two distinct classes of receptor for acetylcholine defined on the basis of their preferential activation by the alkaloids, nicotine (from tobacco) and muscarine (from a fungus, *Amanita muscaria*).

Cholinergic drugs (acetylcholine agonists) mimic acetylcholine at all sites although the balance of nicotinic and muscarinic effects is variable.

Acetylcholine antagonists (blockers) that block the nicotine-like effects (neuromuscular blockers and autonomic ganglion blockers) are described elsewhere (see Ch. 18).

Acetylcholine antagonists that block the muscarine-like effects, e.g. atropine, are often imprecisely called anticholinergics. The more precise term antimuscarinic is preferred here.

- Cholinergic drugs
  — Classification
  — Sites of action
  — Pharmacology
  — Choline esters
  — Alkaloids with cholinergic effects
  — Anticholinesterases; organophosphate poisoning
  — Disorders of neuromuscular transmission: myasthenia gravis
- Drugs which oppose acetylcholine
  — Antimuscarinic drugs

Cholinergic drugs (cholinomimetics)

These drugs act on postsynaptic acetylcholine receptors (cholinoceptors) at all the sites in the body where acetylcholine is the effective neurotransmitter. They initially stimulate and usually later block transmission. In addition, like acetylcholine, they act on the noninnervated receptors that relax vascular smooth muscle in peripheral blood vessels.

Uses of cholinergic drugs

- For myasthenia gravis, both to diagnose (edrophonium) and to treat (neostigmine, pyridostigmine, distigmine)
- To stimulate the bladder and bowel after surgery (bethanechol, carbachol, distigmine)
- To lower intraocular pressure in chronic simple glaucoma (pilocarpine)
- To bronchodilate patients with airflow obstruction (ipratropium, oxitropium)
- To improve cognitive function in Alzheimer's disease (rivastigmine, donepezil)

CLASSIFICATION

Direct-acting (receptor agonists)

- Choline esters (carbachol, bethanechol) which act at all sites like acetylcholine. They are resistant to degradation by cholinesterases. Muscarinic effects are much more prominent than nicotinic (see p. 435).

- Alkaloids (pilocarpine, muscarine) which act selectively on end-organs of postganglionic, cholinergic neurons.

Indirect-acting

- Cholinesterase inhibitors, or anticholinesterases (physostigmine, neostigmine, pyridostigmine, distigmine, rivastigmine, donepezil), which inhibit the enzyme that destroys acetylcholine, allowing the endogenous transmitter to persist and produce intensified effects.

SITES OF ACTION

- Autonomic nervous system
  (1) *Parasympathetic* division: ganglia; postganglionic endings (all)
  (2) *Sympathetic* division: ganglia; a minority of postganglionic endings, e.g. sweat glands
- Neuromuscular junction
- Central nervous system
- Noninnervated sites: blood vessels, chiefly arterioles.

Acetylcholine is the neurotransmitter at all these sites, acting on a postsynaptic receptor, except on most blood vessels in which the action of cholinergic drugs is unrelated to cholinergic 'vasodilator' nerves. It is also produced in tissues unrelated to nerve endings, e.g. placenta and ciliated epithelial cells, where it acts as a local hormone (autacoid) on local receptors.

A list of principal effects is given below. Not all occur with every drug and not all are noticeable at therapeutic doses. For example, central nervous system effects of cholinergic drugs are best seen in cases of anticholinesterase poisoning. Atropine antagonises all the effects of cholinergic drugs except nicotinic actions on autonomic ganglia and the neuromuscular junction; i.e. it has antimuscarinic but not antinicotinic effects (see below).

PHARMACOLOGY

Autonomic nervous system

Parasympathetic division. Stimulation of cholino-ceptors in autonomic ganglia and at the post-ganglionic endings affects chiefly the following organs:

Eye: miosis and spasm of the ciliary muscle occur so that the eye is accommodated for near vision. Intraocular pressure falls due, perhaps, to dilation of vessels at the point where intraocular fluids pass into the blood.

Exocrine glands: there is increased secretion most noticeably of the salivary, lachrymal, bronchial and sweat glands. The last are cholinergic, although anatomically part of the sympathetic system; some sweat glands, e.g. axillary, may be adrenergic.

Heart: bradycardia occurs with atrioventricular block and eventually cardiac arrest.

Bronchi: there is bronchoconstriction and mucosal hypersecretion that may be clinically serious in asthmatic subjects, in whom cholinergic drugs should be avoided, as far as possible.

Gut: motor activity is increased and may cause colicky pain. Exocrine secretion is also increased. Tone in sphincters falls which may cause defaecation (anal sphincter) or acid reflux/regurgitation (oeso-phageal sphincter).

Bladder and ureters contract and the drugs promote micturition.

Sympathetic division. The ganglia only are stimulated, also the cholinergic nerves to the adrenal medulla. These effects are overshadowed by effects on the parasympathetic system and are commonly evident only if atropine has been given to block the latter, when tachycardia, vasoconstriction and hypertension occur.

Neuromuscular (voluntary) junction

The neuromuscular junction has a cholinergic nerve ending and so is activated by anticholinesterases which allow acetylcholine to persist, causing muscle fasciculation. Prolonged activation leads to a secondary depolarising neuromuscular block.

Central nervous system

There is usually stimulation followed by depression but variation between drugs is great, possibly due to differences in CNS penetration. In overdose, mental excitement occurs, with confusion and rest-lessness, insomnia (with nightmares when sleep does come), tremors and dysarthria and sometimes even convulsions and coma.

Blood vessels

There is stimulation of cholinergic vasodilator nerve endings in addition to the more important dilating action on arterioles and capillaries mediated through noninnervated receptors. Anticholinesterases potentiate acetylcholine that exists in the vessel walls independently of nerves.

Nicotinic and muscarinic effects

It was Henry Dale, in 1914, who first made this functional division which remains a robust and useful way of classifying cholinergic drug effects. He noted that the actions of acetylcholine and substances acting like it at autonomic ganglia and the neuromuscular junction (i.e. at the end of cholinergic nerves arising within the central nervous system) mimic the stimulant effects of nicotine (hence nicotinic). In contrast, the actions at postganglionic cholinergic endings (parasympathetic endings plus the cholinergic sympathetic nerves to the sweat glands) and noninnervated receptors on blood vessels resembled the alkaloid, muscarine (hence muscarinic).

CHOLINE ESTERS

Acetylcholine

Since acetylcholine has such great importance in the body it is not surprising that attempts have been made to use it in therapeutics. But a substance with such a huge variety of effects and so rapidly destroyed in the body is unlikely to be useful when given systemically, as its history in psychiatry illustrates.

Acetylcholine was first injected intravenously as a therapeutic convulsant in 1939, in the justified expectation that the fits would be less liable to cause fractures than those following therapeutic leptazol convulsions. Recovery rates of up to 80% were claimed in various psychotic conditions. Enthusiasm began to wane however when it was shown that the fits were due to anoxia resulting from cardiac arrest and not to pharmacological effects on the brain.[1]

The following description is illustrative:

A few seconds after the injection (which was given as rapidly as possible, to avoid total destruction in the blood) the patient sat up 'with knees drawn up to the chest, the arms flexed and the head bent forward. There were repeated violent coughs, sometimes with flushing. Forced swallowing and loud peristaltic rumblings could be heard'. Respiration was laboured and irregular. 'The coughing abated as the patient sank back in the bed. Forty seconds after the injection the radial and apical pulse were zero and the patient became comatose.' The pupils dilated, and deep reflexes were hyperactive. In 45 seconds the patient went into opisthotonos with brief apnoea. Lachrymation, sweating and borborygmi were prominent. The deep reflexes became diminished. The patient then relaxed and 'lay quietly in bed — cold moist and gray. In about 90 seconds, flushing of the face marked the return of the pulse'. The respiratory rate rose and consciousness returned in about 125 seconds. The patients sometimes micturated but did not defaecate. They 'tended to lie quietly in bed after the treatment'. 'Most of the patients were reluctant to be retreated'.[2]

OTHER CHOLINE ESTERS

Carbachol is not destroyed by cholinesterase, its actions are most pronounced on the bladder and gastrointestinal tract, so that the drug has been used to stimulate these organs, e.g. after surgery. This use (also of bethanecol, below) is now much diminished and, for example, catheterisation is preferred for bladder atony. Carbachol is stable in the gut, hence it can be given orally; it is extremely dangerous if given i.v., but can be safely administered s.c.

Bethanechol resembles carbachol in its actions but is some 10-fold less potent (it differs by a single β-methyl group) and has no significant nicotinic effects at clinical doses.

---

[1] Harris M et al 1943 Archives of Neurology and Psychiatry 50: 304.
[2] Cohen L H et al 1944 Archives of Neurology and Psychiatry 51: 171.

ALKALOIDS WITH CHOLINERGIC EFFECTS

Nicotine (see also p. 173) is a social drug that lends its medicinal use as an adjunct to stopping its own abuse as tobacco. It is available as either gum to chew, as dermal patches or as an inhalation. These deliver a lower dose of nicotine than cigarettes and appear to be safe in patients with ischaemic heart disease. The patches are slightly better tolerated than the gum, which releases nicotine in a more variable fashion depending on the rate at which it is chewed and the salivary pH, which is influenced by drinking coffee and carbonated drinks. Nicotine treatment is reported to be nearly twice as effective as placebo in achieving sustained withdrawal from smoking (18% vs. 11% in one review).[3] Treatment is much more likely to be successful if it is used as an aid to, not a substitute for, continued counselling. Bupropion is possibly more effective than the nicotine patch[4] (see also p. 177).

Pilocarpine, from a South American plant (*Pilocarpus* spp.), acts directly on end-organs innervated by postganglionic nerves (parasympathetic system plus sweat glands); it also stimulates and then depresses the central nervous system. The chief clinical use of pilocarpine is to lower intraocular pressure in chronic simple glaucoma, as an adjunct to a topical beta-blocker; it produces miosis, opens drainage channels in the trabecular network and improves the outflow of aqueous humour. Oral pilocarpine is available for the treatment of xerostomia (dry mouth) in Sjogren's syndrome, or following irradiation of head and neck tumours. The commonest adverse effect is sweating; adverse cardiac effects have not been reported.

Arecoline is an alkaloid in the betel nut, which is chewed extensively throughout India and southeast Asia. Presumably the lime mix in the 'chews' provides the necessary alkaline pH to maximise its buccal absorption. It produces a mild euphoric effect like many cholinomimetic alkaloids.

Muscarine is of no therapeutic use but it has pharmacological interest. It is present in small amounts in the fungus *Amanita muscaria* (Fly agaric), named after its capacity to kill the domestic fly (*Musca domestica*); muscarine was so named because it was thought to be the insecticidal principle, but it is relatively nontoxic to flies (orally administered). The fungus may contain other antimuscarinic substances and GABA-receptor agonists (such as muscimol) in amounts sufficient to be psychoactive in man.

Poisoning with these fungi may present with antimuscarinic, with cholinergic or with GABAergic effects. All have CNS actions. Happily, poisoning by *Amanita muscaria* is seldom serious. Species of *Inocybe* contain substantially larger amounts of muscarine (see Ch. 9). The lengths to which man is prepared to go in taking 'chemical vacations' when life is hard, are shown by the inhabitants of Eastern Siberia who used *Amanita muscaria* recreationally, for its cerebral stimulant effects. They were apparently prepared to put up with the autonomic actions to escape briefly from reality. The fungus was scarce in winter and the frugal devotees discovered that by drinking their own urine they could prolong the intoxication. Sometimes, in generous mood, the intoxicated person would offer his urine to others as a treat.

ANTICHOLINESTERASES

At cholinergic nerve endings and in erythrocytes there is an enzyme that specifically destroys acetylcholine, *true cholinesterase* or acetylcholinesterase. In various tissues, especially plasma, there are other esterases which are not specific for acetylcholine but which also destroy other esters, e.g. suxamethonium, procaine (and cocaine) and bambuterol (a pro-drug that is hydrolysed to terbutaline). These are called nonspecific or *pseudocholinesterases*. Chemicals which inactivate these esterases (anticholinesterases) are used in medicine and in agriculture as pesticides. They act by allowing naturally synthesised acetylcholine to accumulate instead of being destroyed. Their effects are almost entirely due to this accumulation in the central nervous system, neuromuscular junction, autonomic ganglia, postganglionic cholinergic nerve endings (which are principally in the parasympathetic nervous

---

[3] Drug and Therapeutics Bulletin 1999; 37 (July issue).
[4] Jorenby D E et al 1999 New England Journal of Medicine 340: 685–692.

system) and in the walls of blood vessels, where acetylcholine has a paracrine role not necessarily associated with nerve endings. Some of these effects oppose each other, e.g. the effect of anticholinesterase on the heart will be the resultant of stimulation at sympathetic ganglia and the opposing effect of stimulation at parasympathetic (vagal) ganglia and at postganglionic nerve endings.

Physostigmine is an alkaloid, obtained from the seeds of the West African Calabar bean (spp. Physostigma), which has long been used both as a weapon and as an ordeal poison.[5] It acts for a few hours. Physostigmine is used synergistically with pilocarpine to reduce intraocular pressure. It has been shown to have some efficacy in improving cognitive function in Alzheimer-type dementia.

Neostigmine (t$\frac{1}{2}$ 2 h) is a synthetic reversible anticholinesterase whose actions are more prominent on the neuromuscular junction and the alimentary tract on the cardiovascular system and eye. It is therefore principally used in myasthenia gravis, to stimulate the bowels and bladder after surgery,[6] and as an antidote to competitive neuromuscular blocking agents. Neostigmine is effective orally, and by injection (usually s.c.). But higher doses may be used in myasthenia gravis, often combined with atropine to reduce the unwanted muscarinic effects.

Pyridostigmine is similar to neostigmine but has a less powerful action that is slower in onset and slightly longer in duration, and perhaps fewer visceral effects. It is used in myasthenia gravis.

Distigmine is a variant of pyridostigmine (two linked molecules as the name implies).

Edrophonium is structurally related to neostigmine but its action is brief and autonomic effects are minimal except at high doses. The drug is used to diagnose myasthenia gravis and to differentiate a myasthenic crisis (weakness due to inadequate anticholinesterase treatment or severe disease) from a cholinergic crisis (weakness caused by overtreatment with an anticholinesterase). Myasthenic weakness is substantially improved by edrophonium whereas cholinergic weakness is aggravated but the effect is transient; the action of 3 mg i.v. is lost in 5 minutes.

Carbaryl (carbaril) is another reversible carbamoylating anticholinesterase that closely resembles physostigmine in its actions. It is widely used as a garden insecticide and, clinically, to kill head and body lice. Sensitive insects lack cholinesterase-rich erythrocytes and succumb to the accumulation of acetylcholine in the synaptic junctions of their nervous system. Effective and safe use in humans is possible because we possess cholinesterase, and absorption of carbaryl is very limited after topical application. The anticholinesterase *malathion* is effective against scabies, head and crab lice.

A more recent use of anticholinesterase drugs has been to improve cognitive function in patients with Alzheimer's disease, where both the degree of dementia and amyloid plaque density correlate with the impairment of brain cholinergic function. *Donepezil* and *rivastigmine*[7] are licensed in the UK for this indication. Both are orally active and cross the blood–brain barrier readily (see p. 408).

Anticholinesterase poisoning

The anticholinesterases used in therapeutics are generally of the *carbamate* type that reversibly inactivate cholinesterase only for a few hours. This contrasts markedly with the very long-lived inhibition caused by inhibitors of the *organophosphate* (OP) type. In practice, the inhibition is so long that clinical recovery from organophosphate exposure is usually dependent on synthesis of new enzyme. This process may take weeks to complete although clinical recovery is usually evident in days. Cases of acute poisoning are usually met outside therapeutic practice, e.g. after agricultural, industrial or transport accidents. Substances of this type have also been developed and used in war, especially the

---

[5] To demonstrate guilt or innocence according to whether the accused died or lived after the judicial dose. The practice had the advantage that the demonstration of guilt provided simultaneous punishment.

[6] Ponec R J et al 1999 New England Journal of Medicine 341: 137–141.

[7] Report. Drug and Therapeutics Bulletin 1998 38: 15–16.

three G agents, GA (tabun), GB (sarin) and GD (soman). Although called nerve 'gas', they are actually volatile liquids, which facilitates their use.[8] Where there is known risk of exposure, prior use of pyridostigmine, which occupies cholinesterases reversibly for a few hours (the lesser evil), competitively protects them from access by the irreversible warfare agent (the greater evil); soldiers expecting attack have been provided with preloaded syringes (of the same design as the Epipen for delivering adrenaline) as antidote therapy (see below). Organophosphate agents are absorbed through the skin, the gastrointestinal tract and by inhalation. Diagnosis depends on observing a substantial part of the list of actions below.

Typical features of *acute poisoning* involve the gastrointestinal tract (salivation, vomiting, abdominal cramps, diarrhoea, involuntary defaecation), the respiratory system (bronchorrhoea, bronchoconstriction, cough, wheezing, dyspnoea), the cardiovascular system (bradycardia), the genitourinary system (involuntary micturition), the skin (sweating), the skeletal system (muscle weakness, twitching) and the nervous system (miosis, anxiety, headache, convulsions, respiratory failure). Death is due to a combination of the actions in the central nervous system, to paralysis of the respiratory muscles by peripheral depolarising neuromuscular block, and to excessive bronchial secretions and constriction causing respiratory failure. At autopsy, ileal intussusceptions are commonly found.

Quite frequently, and typically 1–4 days after resolution of symptoms of acute exposure, the *intermediate syndrome* may develop, characterised by a proximal flaccid limb paralysis which may reflect muscle necrosis. Even later, after a gap of 2–4 weeks, some exposed persons exhibit the *delayed polyneuropathy*, with sensory and motor impairment usually of the lower limbs. Claims of chronic effects (subtle cognitive defects, peripheral neuropathy) following recurrent, low-dose exposure, as with organophosphate used as sheep dip, continues to be the subject of investigation but, as yet, no conclusive proof.

---

[8] In recent times, there have been major instances of use against populations by both military and terrorist bodies (in the field and in an underground transport system).

Treatment. Since the most common circumstance of accidental poisoning is exposure to pesticide spray or spillage, contaminated clothing should be removed and the skin washed. Gastric lavage is needed if any of the substance has been ingested. Attendants should take care to ensure that they themselves do not become contaminated.

- *Atropine* is the mainstay of treatment; 2 mg is given i.m. or i.v. as soon as possible and repeated every 15–60 min until dryness of the mouth and a heart rate in excess of 70 beats per minute indicate that its effect is adequate. A poisoned patient may require 100 mg or more for a single episode. Atropine antagonises the muscarinic parasympathomimetic effects of the poison, i.e. due to the accumulated acetylcholine stimulating postganglionic nerve endings (excessive secretion and vasodilatation), but has no effect on the neuromuscular block, which is nicotinic.
- *Mechanical ventilation* may therefore be needed to assist the respiratory muscles; special attention to the airway is vital because of bronchial constriction and excessive secretion.
- *Diazepam* may be needed for convulsions.
- *Atropine eyedrops* may relieve the headache caused by miosis.
- *Enzyme reactivation.* The organophosphate (OP) pesticides inactivate cholinesterase by irreversibly phosphorylating the active centre of the enzyme. Substances that reactivate the enzyme hasten the destruction of the accumulated acetylcholine and, unlike atropine, they have both antinicotinic and antimuscarinic effects. The principal agent is *pralidoxime,* 1 g of which should be given 4-hourly i.m. or (diluted) by slow i.v. infusion, as indicated by the patient's condition; its efficacy is greatest if administered within 12 hours of poisoning then falls of steadily as the phosphorylated enzyme is further stabilised by 'aging'. If significant reactivation occurs, muscle power improves within 30 min.

Poisoning with *reversible* anticholinesterases is appropriately treated by atropine and the necessary general support; it lasts only hours.

In poisoning with *irreversible* agents, erythrocyte or plasma cholinesterase content should be measured if possible, both for diagnosis and to determine when a poisoned worker may return to the task (should he or she be willing to do so). Return should not be allowed until the cholinesterase exceeds 70% of normal, which may take several weeks. Recovery from the intermediate syndrome and delayed polyneuropathy is slow and is dependent on muscle and nerve regeneration.

DISORDERS OF NEUROMUSCULAR TRANSMISSION

Myasthenia gravis

In myasthenia gravis synaptic transmission at the neuromuscular junction is impaired; most cases have an autoimmune basis and some 85% of patients have a raised titre of autoantibodies to the muscle acetylcholine receptor. The condition is probably heterogeneous, however, as about 15% do not have receptor antibodies, or have antibodies to another neuromuscular junction protein (muscle specific kinase) and rarely it occurs with penicillamine used for rheumatoid arthritis.

Neostigmine was introduced in 1931 for its stimulant effects on intestinal activity. In 1934 it occurred to Dr Mary Walker that since the paralysis of myasthenia had been (erroneously) attributed to a curare-like substance in the blood, physostigmine (eserine), an anticholinesterase drug known to antagonise curare, might be beneficial. It was, and she reported this important observation in a short letter.[9] Soon after this she used neostigmine by mouth with greater benefit. The sudden appearance of an effective treatment for an hitherto untreatable chronic disease must always be a dramatic event for its victims. One patient described the impact of the discovery of the action of neostigmine, as follows.

My myasthenia started in 1925, when I was 18. For several months it consisted of double vision and fatigue … An ophthalmic surgeon … prescribed glasses with a prism. However, soon more alarming symptoms began. [Her limbs became weak and she] 'was sent to an eminent neurologist. This was a horrible experience. He … could find no physical signs … declared me to be suffering from hysteria and asked me what was on my mind.

When I answered truthfully, that nothing except anxiety over my symptoms, he replied 'my dear child, I am not a perfect fool…', and showed me out. [She became worse and at times she was unable to turn over in bed. Eating and even speaking were difficult. Eventually, her fiancé, a medical student, read about myasthenia gravis and she was correctly diagnosed in 1927.] There was at that time no known treatment and therefore many things to try. [She had gold injections, thyroid, suprarenal extract, lecithin, glycine and ephedrine. The last had a slight effect.] Then in February 1935, came the day that I shall always remember. I was living alone with a nurse … It was one of my better days, and I was lying on the sofa after tea … My fiancé came in rather late saying that he had something new for me to try. My first thought was 'Oh bother! Another injection, and another false hope'. I submitted to the injection with complete indifference and within a few minutes began to feel very strange … when I lifted my arms, exerting the effort to which I had become accustomed, they shot into the air, every movement I attempted was grotesquely magnified until I learnt to make less effort … it was strange, wonderful and at first, very frightening … we danced twice round the carpet. That was my first meeting with neostigmine, and we have never since been separated.[10]

Pathogenesis. The clinical features of myasthenia gravis are caused by specific autoantibodies to the nicotinic acetylcholine receptor. These antibodies accelerate receptor turnover shortening their typical lifetime in the skeletal muscle membrane from around 7 days to 1 day in a myasthenic. This process results in marked depletion of receptors from myasthenic skeletal muscle (about 90%) explaining its fatigability. The frequent finding of a specific haplotype (A1-B8-Dw3 HLA) in myasthenics and concurrent hyperplasia or tumours of the thymus support the autoimmune basis for the disease.

Diagnosis. Edrophonium dramatically and transiently (5 min) relieves myasthenic muscular weakness. A syringe is loaded with edrophonium 10 mg;

---

[9] Walker M B 1934 Lancet 1: 1200.

[10] Disabilities and how to live with them. Lancet Publications (1952), London.

2 mg are given i.v. and if there is no improvement in weakness in 30 s the remaining 8 mg are injected. A syringe loaded with atropine should be at hand to block severe cholinergic autonomic (muscarinic) effects, e.g. bradycardia, should they occur. Acetylcholine receptor antibodies should also be measured in the plasma, for an elevated titre confirms the diagnosis.

Treatment involves immunosuppression, thymectomy (unless contraindicated) and symptom relief with drugs.

- *Immunosuppressive treatment* is directed at eliminating the acetylcholine receptor autoantibody. Prednisolone induces improvement or remission in 80% of cases. The dose should be increased slowly using an alternate day regimen until the minimum effective amount is attained; an immunosuppressive improvement may take several weeks. Azathioprine may be used as a steroid-sparing agent. Prednisolone is effective for ocular myasthenia, which is fortunate, for this variant of the disease responds poorly to thymectomy or anticholinesterase drugs. Some acute and severe cases respond poorly to prednisolone with azathioprine and, for these, intermittent plasmapheresis or immunoglobulin i.v. (to remove circulating antireceptor antibody) can provide dramatic short-term relief.
- *Thymectomy* should be offered to those with generalised myasthenia gravis under 40 years of age, once the clinical state allows and unless there are powerful contraindications to surgery. Most cases benefit and about 25% can discontinue drug treatment. Thymectomy should also be undertaken in all myasthenic patients who have a thymoma, but the main reason is to prevent local infiltration for the procedure is less likely to relieve the myasthenia.
- *Symptomatic* drug treatment is decreasingly used. Its aim is to increase the concentration of acetylcholine at the neuromuscular junction with anticholinesterase drugs. The mainstay is usually *pyridostigmine*, starting with 60 mg by mouth 4-hourly. It is preferred because its action is smoother than that of neostigmine, but the latter is more rapid in onset and can with advantage be given in the mornings to get the patient mobile.

Either drug can be given parenterally if bulbar paralysis makes swallowing difficult. An antimuscarinic drug, e.g. propantheline (15–30 mg tid), should be added if muscarinic effects are troublesome.

Excessive dosing with an anticholinesterase can actually worsen the muscle weakness in myasthenics if the accumulation of acetylcholine at the neuromuscular junction is sufficient to cause depolarising blockade (*cholinergic* crisis). It is important to distinguish this type of muscle weakness from an exacerbation of the disease itself (*myasthenic* crisis). The dilemma can be resolved with a test dose of edrophonium, which relieves a myasthenic crisis but worsens a cholinergic one. The latter may be severe enough to precipitate respiratory failure and should be attempted only with full resuscitation facilities, including mechanical ventilation, at hand.

A cholinergic crisis should be treated by withdrawing all anticholinesterase medication, mechanical ventilation if required, and atropine i.v. for muscarinic effects of the overdose. The neuromuscular block is a nicotinic effect and will be unchanged by atropine. A resistant myasthenic crisis may be treated by withdrawal of drugs and mechanical ventilation for a few days. Plasmapheresis or immunoglobulin i.v. may be beneficial by removing antireceptor antibodies (see above).

Lambert-Eaton syndrome

Separate from myasthenia gravis is the Lambert-Eaton syndrome, where symptoms similar to those in myasthenia gravis occur in association with a carcinoma: in 60% of patients this is a small-cell lung cancer. The defect here is *pre*synaptic with a deficiency of acetylcholine release due to an autoantibody directed against L-type voltage-gated calcium channels.

Patients with the Lambert-Eaton syndrome do not usually respond well to anticholinesterases. The drug 3,4-diaminopyridine (3,4-DAP) increases neurotransmitter release and also the action potential (by blocking potassium conductance); these actions lead to a nonspecific excitatory effect on the cholinergic system, and provide benefit. It should be taken orally, 4–5 times per day. Adverse effects due to CNS excitation (insomnia, seizures) can occur. 3,4-DAP is an example of an orphan drug without product licence, available in the UK for 'named patient' use from specialist pharmacies.

Drug-induced disorders of neuromuscular transmission

Quite apart from the neuromuscular blocking agents used in anaesthesia, a number of drugs possess actions that impair neuromuscular transmission and, in appropriate circumstances, give rise to:

• Postoperative respiratory depression in people whose neuromuscular transmission is otherwise normal
• Aggravation or unmasking of myasthenia gravis
• A drug-induced myasthenic syndrome.

These drugs include:

Antimicrobials. Aminoglycosides (neomycin, streptomycin, gentamicin), polypeptides (colistimethate sodium, polymyxin B) and perhaps the quinolones (e.g. ciprofloxacin) may cause postoperative breathing difficulty if they are instilled into the peritoneal or pleural cavities. It appears that the antibiotics both interfere with the release of acetylcholine and also have a competitive curare-like effect on the acetylcholine receptor.

Cardiovascular drugs. Those that possess local anaesthetic properties [quinidine, procainamide, lignocaine (lidocaine)] and certain β-blockers (propranolol, oxprenolol) interfere with acetylcholine release and may aggravate or reveal myasthenia gravis.

Other drugs. *Penicillamine* causes some patients, especially those with rheumatoid arthritis, to form antibodies to the acetylcholine receptor and a syndrome indistinguishable from myasthenia gravis results. Spontaneous recovery occurs in about two-thirds of cases when penicillamine is withdrawn. *Phenytoin* may rarely induce or aggravate myasthenia gravis, or induce a myasthenic syndrome, possibly by depressing release of acetylcholine. *Lithium* may impair presynaptic neurotransmission by substituting for sodium ions in the nerve terminal.

Drugs which oppose acetylcholine

These may be divided into:

Antimuscarinic drugs which act principally at postganglionic cholinergic (parasympathetic) nerve endings, i.e. atropine-related drugs (see Fig. 21.1, site 2). Muscarinic receptors can be subdivided according to their principal sites, namely in the brain and gastric parietal cells (M_1), heart (M_2) and glandular and smooth muscle cells (M_3). As with many receptors, the molecular basis of the subtypes has been defined together with two further cloned subtypes (M_4 and M_5) for which no functional counterpart has yet been described.

Antinicotinic drugs
Ganglion-blocking drugs (Fig. 21.1, site 1) (see Ch. 24).
Neuromuscular blocking drugs (Fig. 21.1, site 5) (see Ch. 18).

ANTIMUSCARINIC DRUGS

Atropine is the prototype drug of this group and will be described first. Other named agents will be mentioned only in so far as they differ from atropine. All act as non-selective and competitive antagonists of the various muscarinic receptor subtypes (M1–3). Atropine is a simple tertiary amine; certain others (see Summary) are quaternary nitrogen compounds, a modification that is important as it intensifies antimuscarinic potency in the gut, imparts ganglion-blocking effects and reduces CNS penetration.

Atropine

Atropine is an alkaloid from the deadly nightshade *(Atropa belladonna).*[11] In general, the effects of

---

[11] The first name commemorates its success as a homicidal poison, for it is derived from the senior of three legendary Fates, Atropos, who cuts with shears the web of life spun and woven by her sisters Clothos and Lachesis (there is a minor synthetic atropine-like drug called lachesine). The term belladonna (Italian: beautiful woman) refers to the once fashionable female practice of using an extract of the plant to dilate the pupils (incidentally blocking ocular accommodation) as part of the process of making herself attractive.

- **For their central actions**, some [benzhexol (trihexyphenidyl) and orphenadrine] are used against the rigidity and tremor of *parkinsonism,* especially drug-induced parkinsonism, where doses higher than the usual therapeutic amounts are often needed and tolerated.

  They are used as *antiemetics* (principally hyoscine, promethazine). Their *sedative* action is used in anaesthetic premedication (hyoscine).

- **For their peripheral actions**, atropine, homatropine and cyclopentolate are used in *ophthalmology* to dilate the pupil and to paralyse ocular accommodation. Patients should be warned of a transient, but unpleasant stinging sensation, and that they cannot read or drive (at least without dark glasses) for at least 3–4 hours. Tropicamide is the shortest acting of the mydriatics. If it is desired to dilate the pupil and to spare accommodation, a sympathomimetic, e.g. phenylephrine, is useful.

  In *anaesthesic premedication,* atropine, and hyoscine* block the vagus and reduce mucosal secretions; hyoscine also has useful sedative effects. Glycopyrronium* is frequently used during anaesthetic recovery to block the muscarinic effects of neostigmine given to reverse a nondepolarising neuromuscular blockade.

  In the *respiratory tract,* ipratropium* is a useful bronchodilator in chronic obstructive pulmonary disease and acute asthma.

- **For their actions on the gut**, against muscle spasm and hypermotility, e.g. against colic (pain due to spasm of smooth muscle) and to reduce morphine-induced smooth muscle spasm when the analgesic is used against acute colic.

- **In the urinary tract**, flavoxate, oxybutynin, propiverine, tolterodine, trospium and propantheline* are used to relieve muscle spasm accompanying infection in cystitis, and for detrusor instability.

- **In disorders of the cardiovascular system**, atropine is useful in bradycardia following myocardial infarction.

- **In cholinergic poisoning**, atropine is an important antagonist of both central nervous, para-sympathomimetic and vasodilator effects, though it has no effect at the neuromuscular junction and will not prevent voluntary muscle paralysis. It is also used to block muscarinic effects when cholinergic drugs, such as neostigmine, are used for their effect on the neuromuscular junction in myasthenia gravis.

Disadvantages of the antimuscarinics include glaucoma, and urinary retention where there is prostatic hypertrophy.

*Quaternary ammonium compounds (see text).

atropine are inhibitory but in large doses it stimulates the CNS (see poisoning, below). Atropine also blocks the muscarinic effects of injected cholinergic drugs both peripherally and on the central nervous system. The clinically important actions of atropine at parasympathetic postganglionic nerve endings are listed below; they are mostly the opposite of the activating effects on the parasympathetic system produced by cholinergic drugs.

Exocrine glands. All secretions except milk are diminished. Dry mouth and dry eye are common. Gastric acid secretion is reduced but so also is the total volume of gastric secretion so that pH may be little altered. *Sweating* is inhibited (sympathetic innervation but releasing acetylcholine). *Bronchial* secretions are reduced and may become viscid, which can be a disadvantage, as removal of secretion by cough and ciliary action is rendered less effective.

Smooth muscle is relaxed. In the gastrointestinal tract there is reduction of tone and peristalsis. Muscle spasm of the intestinal tract induced by morphine is reduced, but such spasm in the biliary tract is not significantly affected. Atropine relaxes bronchial muscle, an effect that is useful in some asthmatics. Micturition is slowed and urinary retention may be induced especially when there is pre-existing prostatic enlargement.

Ocular effects. Mydriasis occurs with a rise in intraocular pressure in eyes predisposed to narrow-angle glaucoma. This is due to the dilated iris blocking drainage of the intraocular fluids from the angle of the anterior chamber. An attack of glaucoma may be induced. There is no significant effect on pressure in normal eyes. The ciliary muscle is paralysed and so the eye is accommodated for distant vision. After atropinisation, normal pupillary reflexes may not be regained for 2 weeks. Atropine use is a cause of unequal sized and unresponsive pupils.[12]

Cardiovascular system. Atropine reduces vagal tone thus increasing the heart rate, and enhancing conduction in the bundle of His, effects that are less marked in the elderly in whom vagal tone is low. Full atropinisation may increase rate by 30 beats/min in the young, but has little effect in the old.

Transient vagal stimulation, probably in the CNS, may cause bradycardia, e.g. if atropine is given i.v. with neostigmine and the effects of the two drugs summate.

Atropine has no significant effect on peripheral blood vessels in therapeutic doses but, in poisoning, there is marked vasodilatation.

Central nervous system. Atropine is effective against both tremor and rigidity of *parkinsonism*. It prevents or abates motion sickness.

Antagonism to cholinergic drugs. Atropine opposes the effects of all cholinergic drugs on the CNS, at postganglionic cholinergic nerve endings and on the peripheral blood vessels. It does not oppose cholinergic effects at the neuromuscular junction or significantly at the autonomic ganglia, i.e. atropine opposes the muscarine-like but not the nicotine-like effects of acetylcholine.

Pharmacokinetics. Atropine is readily absorbed from the gastrointestinal tract and may also be injected by the usual routes. The occasional cases of atropine poisoning following use of eye drops are due to the solution running down the lacrimal ducts into the nose and being swallowed. Atropine is in part destroyed in the liver and in part excreted unchanged by the kidney ($t \frac{1}{2}$ 2 h).

Dose. 0.6–1.2 mg by mouth at night or 0.6 mg i.v. and repeated as necessary to a maximum of 3 mg per day; for chronic use it has largely been replaced by other antimuscarinic drugs.

Poisoning with atropine (and other antimuscarinic drugs) presents with the more obvious peripheral

---

[12] A doctor, after working in his garden greenhouse, was alarmed to find that the vision in his left eye was blurred and the pupil was grossly dilated. Physical examination failed to reveal a cause and the pupil gradually and spontaneously returned to normal, suggesting that the explanation was exposure to some exogenous agent. The doctor then recalled that his greenhouse contained flowering plants called 'angels' trumpet' (sp. *Brugmansia,* of the nightshade family), and he may have brushed against them. Angels' trumpet is noted for its content of scopolamine (hyoscine), and is very toxic if ingested. The plant is evidently less angelic than the name suggests. Merrick J, Barnett S 2000 British Medical Journal 321: 219.

effects: dry mouth (with dysphagia), mydriasis, blurred vision, hot, flushed, dry skin, and, in addition, hyperthermia (CNS action plus absence of sweating), restlessness, anxiety, excitement, hallucinations, delirium, mania. The cerebral excitation is followed by depression and coma or, as it has been described with characteristic American verbal felicity, 'hot as a hare, blind as a bat, dry as a bone, red as a beet and mad as a hen'.[13] It may occur in children who have eaten berries of solanaceous plants, e.g. deadly nightshade and henbane. When the diagnosis is doubtful, it is said to be worth putting a drop of the patient's urine in one eye of a cat. Mydriasis, if it results, confirms the diagnosis, but absence of effect proves nothing. Treatment involves giving activated charcoal to adsorb the drug, and diazepam for excitement.

Other antimuscarinic drugs

In the following accounts of drugs, the principal peripheral atropine-like effects of the drugs may be assumed; differences from atropine are described.

Atropine is also a racemate (dl-hyoscyamine), and almost all of its antimuscarinic effects are attributable to the l-isomer alone. It is, however, more stable chemically as the racemate which is the preferred formulation.

Hyoscine (scopolamine) is structurally related to atropine. It differs chiefly in being a central nervous system depressant, although it may sometimes cause excitement. Elderly patients are often confused by hyoscine and so it is avoided in their anaesthetic premedication. Mydriasis is also briefer than with atropine.

Hyoscine butylbromide (strictly N-butylhyoscine bromide, Buscopan) also blocks autonomic ganglia. If injected, it is an effective relaxant of smooth muscle, including the cardia in achalasia, the pyloric antral region and the colon, which properties are utilised by radiologists and endoscopists. It may sometimes be useful for colic.

Homatropine is used for its ocular effects (1% and 2% solutions as eye drops). Its action is shorter than atropine and therefore less likely to cause serious rises of intraocular pressure; the effect wears off in a

day or two. Complete cycloplegia cannot always be obtained unless repeated instillations are made every 15 min for 1–2 h. It is especially unreliable in children, in whom cyclopentolate or atropine is preferred. The pupillary dilation may be reversed by physostigmine eyedrops.

Tropicamide (Mydriacyl) and *cyclopentolate* (Mydrilate) are useful (as 0.5% or 1% solutions) for mydriasis and cycloplegia. They are quicker and shorter-acting than homatropine. Both cause mydriasis in 10–20 min and cycloplegia shortly after. The duration of action is 4–12 h.

Ipratropium (Atrovent) is used by inhalation as a bronchodilator, and can be useful when cough is a pronounced symptom in an asthmatic patient.

Flavoxate (Urispas) is used for urinary frequency, tenesmus and urgency incontinence because it increases bladder capacity and reduces unstable detrusor contractions (see p. 543).

Oxybutynin is also used for detrusor instability, but antimuscarinic adverse effects may limit its value.

Glycopyrronium is used in anaesthetic premedication to reduce salivary secretion; given i.v. it causes less tachycardia than does atropine.

Propantheline (Pro-Banthine) also has ganglion-blocking properties. It may be used as a smooth

---

- Acetylcholine is the most important receptor agonist neurotransmitter in both the brain and peripheral nervous system.
- It acts on neurons in the CNS and at autonomic ganglia, on skeletal muscle at the neuromuscular junction, and at a variety of other effector cell types, mainly glandular or smooth muscle.
- The effector response is rapidly terminated through enzymatic destruction by acetylcholinesterase.
- Outside the CNS, acetylcholine has two main classes of receptor: those on autonomic ganglia and skeletal muscle responding to stimulation by nicotine and the rest that respond to stimulation by muscarine.
- Drugs that mimic or oppose acetylcholine have a wide variety of uses. For instance, the muscarinic agonist pilocarpine lowers intraocular pressure and antagonist atropine reverses vagal slowing of the heart.
- The main use of drugs at the neuromuscular junction is to relax muscle in anaesthesia, or to inhibit acetylcholinesterase in diseases where nicotinic receptor activation is reduced, e.g. myasthenia gravis.

---

[13] Cohen H L et al 1944 Archives of Neurology and Psychiatry 51: 171.

muscle relaxant, e.g. for irritable bowel syndrome and diagnostic procedures.

Dicyclomine (Merbentyl) is an alternative.

Benzhexol (trihexyphenidyl) and *orphenadrine:* see parkinsonism.

Promethazine: see p. 555.

Propiverine, tolterodine and *trospium* diminish unstable detrusor contractions and are used to reduce urinary frequency, urgency and incontinence.

Oral antimuscarinics have occasional use in the treatment of hyperhidrosis.

GUIDE TO FURTHER READING

Cohen H L et al 1944 Acetylcholine treatment of schizophrenia. Archives of Neurology and Psychiatry 51: 171

Hawkins J R et al 1956 Intravenous acetylcholine therapy in neurosis. A controlled trial (p. 43); Carbon dioxide inhalation therapy in neurosis. A controlled clinical trial (p. 52); The placebo response (p. 60). Journal of Mental Science 102: 43

HMSO 1987 Medical manual of defence against chemical agents. (No. 0117725692) JSP: 312

Lambert D 1981 (personal paper) Myasthenia gravis. Lancet 1:937

Morita H et al 1996 Sarin poisoning in Matsumoto, Japan. Lancet 346: 290–293

Morton H G et al 1939 Atropine intoxication. Journal of Pediatrics 14: 755

Report 1998 Organophosphate sheep dip. Clinical aspects of long-term low-dose exposure. Royal College of Physicians (London) and Royal College of Psychiatrists

Steenland K 1996 Chronic neurological effects of organophosphate pesticides. British Medical Journal 312: 1312–1313

Vincent A et al 2001 Myasthenia gravis. Lancet 357: 2122–2128

22

Adrenergic mechanisms and drugs

SYNOPSIS

Anyone who administers drugs acting on cardiovascular adrenergic mechanisms requires an understanding of how they act in order to use them to the best advantage and with safety.

- Adrenergic mechanisms
- Classification of sympathomimetics: by mode of action and selectivity for adrenoceptors
- Individual sympathomimetics
- Mucosal decongestants
- Shock
- Chronic orthostatic hypotension

Adrenergic mechanisms

The discovery in 1895 of the hypertensive effect of adrenaline (epinephrine) was initiated by Dr Oliver, a physician in practice, who conducted a series of experiments on his young son into whom he injected an extract of bovine suprarenal. The effect was confirmed in animals and led eventually to the isolation and synthesis of adrenaline in the early 1900s. Many related compounds were examined and, in 1910, Barger and Dale invented the word sympathomimetic[1] and also pointed out that noradrenaline (norepinephrine) mimicked the action of the sympathetic nervous system more closely than did adrenaline.

Adrenaline, noradrenaline and dopamine are formed in the body and are used in therapeutics. The natural synthetic path is:

tyrosine → dopa → dopamine → noradrenaline → adrenaline.

Classification of sympathomimetics

BY MODE OF ACTION

Noradrenaline is synthesised and stored in adrenergic nerve terminals and can be released from these stores by stimulating the nerve or by drugs (ephedrine, amfetamine). These noradrenaline stores may be replenished by i.v. infusion of noradrenaline, and abolished by reserpine or by cutting the sympathetic neuron.

Sympathomimetics may be classified as those that act:

1. **directly:** *adrenoceptor agonists*, e.g. adrenaline,

---

[1] 'Compounds which … simulate the effects of sympathetic nerves not only with varying intensity but with varying precision … a term … seems needed to indicate the types of action common to these bases. We propose to call it "sympathomimetic". A term which indicates the relation of the action to innervation by the sympathetic system, without involving any theoretical preconception as to the meaning of that relation or the precise mechanism of the action.' Barger G, Dale H H 1910 Journal of Physiology XLI: 19–50.

noradrenaline, isoprenaline (isoproterenol), methoxamine, xylometazoline, oxymetazoline, metaraminol (entirely); and dopamine and phenylephrine (mainly)

2. **indirectly:** by causing a *release of noradrenaline* from stores at nerve endings, e.g. amphetamines, tyramine; and ephedrine (largely)

3. **by both mechanisms** (1 and 2, though often with a preponderance of one or other): *other synthetic agents.*

Tachyphylaxis (rapidly diminishing response to repeated administration) is a particular feature of group 2 drugs. It reflects depletion of the 'releasable' pool of noradrenaline from adrenergic nerve terminals that makes these agents less suitable as, for example, pressor agents than drugs of group 1. Longer-term *tolerance* (see p. 95) to the effects direct sympathomimetics is much less of a clinical problem and reflects an alteration in adrenergic receptor density or coupling to second messenger systems.

Interactions of sympathomimetics with other vasoactive drugs are complex. Some drugs block the reuptake mechanism for noradrenaline in adrenergic nerve terminals and potentiate the pressor effects of noradrenaline e.g. cocaine, tricyclic antidepressants or highly noradrenaline-selective reuptake inhibitors such as roboxetine. Others deplete or destroy the intracellular stores within adrenergic nerve terminals (e.g. reserpine and guanethidine) and thus block the action of indirect sympathomimetics.

Sympathomimetics are also generally optically active drugs, with only one stereoisomer conferring most of the clinical efficacy of the racemate: for instance laevo-noradrenaline is at least 50 times as active as the dextro- form. Noradrenaline, adrenaline and phenylephrine are all used clinically as their laevo-isomers.

History. Up to 1948 it was known that the peripheral motor (vasoconstriction) effects of adrenaline were preventable and that the peripheral inhibitory (vasodilatation) and the cardiac stimulant actions were not preventable by the then available antagonists (ergot alkaloids, phenoxybenzamine). That same year, Ahlquist hypothesised that this was due to two different sorts of adrenoceptors (α and β). For a further 10 years, only antagonists of α-receptor effects (α-adrenoceptor block) were known, but in 1958 the first substance selectively and competitively to prevent β-receptor effects (β-adrenoceptor block), dichloroisoprenaline, was synthesised. It was, however, unsuitable for clinical use because it behaved as a partial agonist, and it was not until 1962 that pronethalol (an isoprenaline analogue) became the first β-adrenoceptor blocker to be used clinically. Unfortunately it had a low therapeutic index and was carcinogenic in mice, and was soon replaced by propranolol (Inderal).

It is evident that the site of action has an important role in selectivity, e.g. drugs that act on end-organ receptors *directly* and stereospecifically may be highly selective, whereas drugs that act *indirectly* by discharging noradrenaline indiscriminately from nerve endings, e.g. amfetamine, will have a wider range of effects.

Subclassification of adrenoceptors is shown in Table 22.1.

Consequences of adrenoceptor activation

All adrenoceptors are members of the G-coupled family of receptor proteins i.e. the receptor is coupled to its effector protein through special transduction proteins called G-proteins (themselves a large protein family). The effector protein differs amongst adrenoceptor subtypes. In the case of β-adrenoceptors, the effector is adenylyl cyclase and hence cyclic AMP is the second messenger molecule. For α-adrenoceptors, phospholipase C is the commonest effector protein and the second messenger here is IP_3. It is the cascade of events initiated by the second messenger molecules that produces the variety of tissue effects as shown in Table 22.1 It should be clear that specificity is provided by the receptor subtype, not the messengers.

Complexity of adrenergic mechanisms

Drugs may mimic or impair adrenergic mechanisms:

- *directly,* by binding on adrenoceptors: as agonists (adrenaline) or antagonists (propranolol)

TABLE 22.1 Clinically relevant aspects of adrenoceptor functions and actions of agonists

α_1-adrenoceptor effects[1]	β-adrenoceptor effects
Eye:[2] mydriasis	**Heart** (β_1, β_2)[3] increased rate (SA node) increased automaticity (AV node and muscle) increased velocity in conducting tissue increased contractility of myocardium increased O_2 consumption decreased refractory period of all tissues
Arterioles: constriction (only slight in coronary and cerebral)	**Arterioles:** dilatation (β_2) **Bronchi** (β_2): relaxation **Anti-inflammatory effect:** inhibition of release of autacoids (histamine, leukotrienses) from mast cells, e.g. asthma in type I allergy
Uterus: contraction (pregnant) **Skin:** sweat, pilomotor **Male ejaculation** **Blood platelet:** aggregation **Metabolic effect:** hyperkalaemia	**Uterus** (β_2): relaxation (pregnant) **Skeletal muscle:** tremor (β_2) **Metabolic effects:** hypokalaemia (β_2) hepatic glycogenolysis (β_2) lipolysis (β_1, β_2)
Bladder sphincter: contraction	**Bladder detrusor:** relaxation
Intestinal smooth muscle relaxation is mediated by α- and β-adrenoceptors. α_2-**adrenoceptor effects:**[1] α_2-receptors on the nerve ending i.e. presynaptic autoreceptors mediate negative feedback which inhibits noradrenaline release.	

[1] For the role of subtypes (α_1 and α_2) see prazosin.
[2] Effects on intraocular pressure involve both α- and β-adrenoceptors as well as cholinoceptors.
[3] Cardiac β_1-receptors mediate effects of sympathetic nerve stimulation. Cardiac β_2-receptors mediate effects of circulating adrenaline, when this is secreted at a sufficient rate, e.g. following a myocardial infarction or in heart failure. Both receptors are coupled to the same intracellular signalling pathway (cyclic AMP production) and mediate the same biological effects.

The use of the term cardioselective to mean β_1-receptor selective only, especially in the case of β-receptor blocking drugs, is no longer appropriate. Although in most species the β_1-receptor is the only cardiac β-receptor, this is not the case in humans. What is not generally appreciated is that the endogenous sympathetic neurotransmitter, noradrenaline, has about a 20-fold selectivity for the β_1-receptor — similar to that of the antagonist, atenolol — with the consequence that under most circumstances, in most tissues, there is little or no β_2-receptor stimulation to be affected by a nonselective β-blocker. Why asthmatics should be so sensitive to β-blockade is paradoxical: all the bronchial β-receptors are β_2, and the bronchi themselves are not innervated by adrenergic fibres; the circulating adrenaline levels are, if anything, low in asthma.

- *indirectly,* by discharging noradrenaline stored in nerve endings[2] (amfetamine)
- *by preventing reuptake* into the adrenergic nerve ending of released noradrenaline (and dopamine) (cocaine, tricyclic antidepressants and noradrenaline-selective reuptake inhibitors such as roboxetine)

- *by preventing the destruction* of noradrenaline (and dopamine) in the nerve ending (monoamine oxidase inhibitors)
- *by depleting the stores of noradrenaline* in nerve endings (reserpine)
- *by preventing the release of noradrenaline* from nerve endings in response to a nerve impulse (guanethidine)
- *by activation of adrenoceptors on adrenergic nerve endings* that inhibit release of

---

[2] Fatal hypertension can occur when this class of agent is taken by a patient treated with monoamine oxidase inhibitor.

noradrenaline (α_2-autoreceptors) (clonidine)

- *by blocking sympathetic autonomic ganglia* (trimetaphan).

All the above mechanisms operate in both the central and peripheral nervous systems. This discussion is chiefly concerned with agents that influence peripheral adrenergic mechanisms.

SELECTIVITY FOR ADRENOCEPTORS

The following classification of sympathomimetics and antagonists is based on selectivity for receptors and on use. But selectivity is relative, not absolute; some agonists act on both α- and β-receptors, some are partial agonists and, if enough is administered, many will extend their range. The same applies to selective antagonists (receptor blockers), e.g. a β_1-selective adrenoceptor blocker can cause severe exacerbation of asthma (a β_2 effect) even at low dose. It is important to remember this because patients have died in the hands of doctors who have forgotten or been ignorant of it.[3]

Adrenoceptor agonists (Table 22.1)

$\alpha + \beta$ **effects, nonselective:** *adrenaline* is used as a vasoconstrictor (a) with local anaesthetics, as a mydriatic and in the emergency treatment of anaphylactic shock, for which condition it has the right mix of effects (bronchodilator, positive cardiac inotropic, vasoconstriction at high dose).

α_1 **effects:** *noradrenaline* (with slight β effect on heart) is selectively released physiologically where it is wanted; as therapeutic agents for hypotensive states (excepting septic shock) dopamine and dobutamine are preferred (for their cardiac inotropic effect). Also having predominantly α_1 effects are imidazolines (xylometazoline, oxymeta-

zoline), metaraminol, phenylephrine, phenylpropanolamine, ephedrine, pseudoephedrine: some are used solely for topical vasoconstriction (nasal decongestants).

α_2 **effects in the central nervous system:** *clonidine.*

β **effects, nonselective** (i.e. $\beta_1 + \beta_1$): *isoprenaline* (isoproterenol). Its uses as bronchodilator (β_2), for positive cardiac inotropic effect and to enhance conduction in heart block (β_1, β_2) have been largely superseded by agents with a more appropriately selective profile of effects. Other agents with nonselective β effects, ephedrine, orciprenaline, are also obsolete for asthma.

β_1 **effects, with some α effects:** *dopamine*, used in cardiogenic shock.

β_1 **effects:** *dobutamine*, used for cardiac inotropic effect.

β_2 **effects**, used in *asthma,* or to relax the *uterus,* include: salbutamol, terbutaline, fenoterol, pirbuterol, reproterol, rimiterol, isoxsuprine, orciprenaline, ritodrine.

Adrenoceptor antagonists (blockers)

See page 474.

Effects of a sympathomimetic

The *overall effect* of a sympathomimetic depends on the site of action (receptor agonist or indirect action), on *receptor specificity* and on *dose;* for instance adrenaline ordinarily dilates muscle blood vessels (β_2; mainly arterioles, but veins also) but in very large doses constricts them (α). The end results are often complex and unpredictable, partly because of the variability of homeostatic reflex responses and partly because what is observed, e.g. a change in blood pressure, is the result of many factors, e.g. vasodilatation (β) in some areas, vasoconstriction (α) in others, and cardiac stimulation (β).

To block all the effects of adrenaline and noradrenaline, antagonists for both α- and β-receptors must be used. This can be a matter of practical importance, e.g. in phaeochromocytoma (see p. 495).

---

[3] While it is simplest to regard the selectivity of a drug as relative, being lost at higher doses, strictly speaking it is the *benefits* of the receptor selectivity of an agonist or antagonist, which are dose-dependent. A 10-fold selectivity of an agonist at the β_1-receptor, for instance, is a property of the agonist that is independent of dose, and means simply that 10 times less of the agonist is required to activate this receptor compared to the β_2-subtype.

Physiological note. The termination of action of noradrenaline released at nerve endings is by:

- reuptake into nerve endings where it is stored and also subject to MAO degradation
- diffusion away from the area of the nerve ending and the receptor (junctional cleft)
- metabolism (by extraneuronal MAO and COMT).

These processes are slower than the very swift destruction of acetylcholine at the neuromuscular junction by extracellular acetylcholinesterase seated alongside the receptors. This difference reflects the differing signalling requirements: almost instantaneous (millisecond) responses for voluntary muscle movement versus the much more leisurely contraction of arteriolar muscle to control vascular resistance.

Synthetic noncatecholamines in clinical use have $t\frac{1}{2}$ of hours, e.g. salbutamol 4 h, because they are more resistant to enzymatic degradation and conjugation. They may be given orally although much higher doses are required. They penetrate the central nervous system and may have prominent effects, e.g. amphetamine. Substantial amounts appear in the urine.

Pharmacokinetics

Catecholamines (adrenaline, noradrenaline, dopamine, dobutamine, isoprenaline) (plasma $t\frac{1}{2}$ approx. 2 min) are metabolised by two enzymes, monoamine oxidase (MAO) and catechol-O-methyltransferase (COMT). These enzymes are present in large amounts in the liver and kidney and account for most of the metabolism of injected catecholamines. MAO is also present in the intestinal mucosa (and in nerve endings, peripheral and central). Because of these enzymes catecholamines are ineffective when swallowed, but noncatecholamines, e.g. salbutamol, amphetamine, are effective orally.

Adverse effects

These may be deduced from their actions (Table 22.1, Fig. 22.1). Tissue necrosis due to intense vasoconstriction (α) around injection sites occurs as a result of leakage from i.v. infusions. The effects on the heart (β_1) include tachycardia, palpitations, cardiac arrhythmias including ventricular tachycardia and fibrillation, and muscle tremor (β_2). Sympathomimetic drugs should be used with great caution in patients with heart disease.

The effect of the sympathomimetic drugs on the pregnant uterus is variable and difficult to predict, but serious fetal distress can occur, due to reduced placental blood flow as a result both of contraction of the uterine muscle (α) and arterial constriction (α). β_2-agonists are used to relax the uterus in premature labour, but unwanted cardiovascular actions can be troublesome. Sympathomimetics were particularly likely to cause cardiac arrhythmias (β_1 effect) in patients who received halothane anaesthesia (now much less used).

Sympathomimetics and plasma potassium. Adrenergic mechanisms have a role in the physiological control of plasma potassium concentration. The biochemical pump that shifts potassium into cells is activated by the β_2-adrenoceptor agonists (adrenaline, salbutamol, isoprenaline) and can cause hypokalaemia. β_2-adrenoceptor antagonists block the effect.

The hypokalaemia effects of administered (β_2) sympathomimetics may be clinically important, particularly in patients having pre-existing hypokalaemia, e.g. due to intense adrenergic activity such as occurs in myocardial infarction,[4] in fright (admission to hospital is accompanied by transient hypokalaemia), or with previous diuretic therapy, and taking digoxin. In such subjects the use of a sympathomimetic infusion or of an adrenaline-containing local anaesthetic may precipitate a cardiac arrhythmia. Hypokalaemia may occur during treatment of severe asthma, particularly where the β_2-receptor agonist is combined with theophylline.

β-adrenoceptor blockers, as expected, enhance the hyperkalaemia of muscular exercise; and one of their benefits in preventing cardiac arrhythmias

---

[4] Normal subjects, infused i.v. with adrenaline in amounts that approximate to those found in the plasma after severe myocardial infarction, show a fall in plasma K of about 0.8 mmol/l (Brown M J 1983 New England Journal of Medicine 309: 1414).

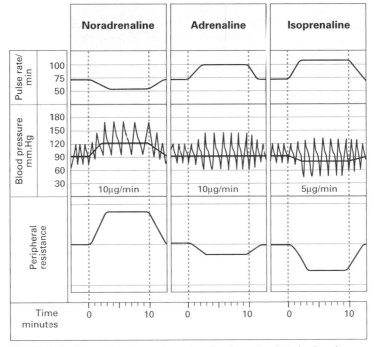

Fig. 22.1 Cardiovascular effects of noradrenaline (norepinephrine), adrenaline (epinephrine) and isoprenaline (isoproterenol): pulse rate/min, blood pressure in mmHg (dotted line is mean pressure), peripheral resistance in arbitrary units. The differences are due to the differential α and β agonist selectivities of these agents (see text). (By permission, after Ginsburg J, Cobbold A F 1960 In: Vane J R et al (eds) Adrenergic mechanism. Churchill, London)

after myocardial infarction may be due to block of β_2-receptor-induced hypokalaemia.

Overdose of sympathomimetics is treated according to rational consideration of mode and site of action (see Adrenaline, below).

Individual sympathomimetics

The actions are summarised in Table 22.1. The classic, mainly endogenous substances will be described first despite their limited role in therapeutics, and then the more selective analogues that have largely replaced them.

CATECHOLAMINES[5]

For pharmacokinetics, see above.

Adrenaline (epinephrine)

Adrenaline (α- and β-adrenoceptor effects) is used:

- as a vasoconstrictor with local anaesthetics (1:80 000 or weaker) to prolong their effects (about 2-fold)
- as a topical mydriatic (sparing accommodation; it also lowers intraocular pressure)
- for severe allergic reactions, i.m., i.v. (or s.c.). The route must be chosen with care. For adults, adrenaline 500 micrograms (i.e. 0.5 ml of the 1 in 1000 solution) may be given i.m. and repeated

---

[5] Traditionally catecholamines have had a dual nomenclature (as a consequence of a company patenting the name Adrenalin), broadly European and N. American. The latter has been chosen by the World Health Organization as International Nonproprietary Names (INN) (see Ch. 6), and the European Union has directed member states to use INN. Because uniformity has not yet been achieved and because of the scientific literature, we use both.
For pharmacokinetics, see above.

at 5-min intervals according to the response (see Ch. 8, p. 143). If the circulation is compromised to a degree that is immediately life-threatening, adrenaline 500 micrograms may be given by **slow** i.v. injection at a rate of 100 micrograms/min (i.e. 1 ml/min of the dilute 1 in 10 000 solution) with continuous monitoring of the ECG. This course requires extreme caution and use of a further × 10 dilution (i.e. a 1 in 100 000 solution) may be preferred as providing finer control and greater safety. The s.c. route is generally not recommended as there is intense vasoconstriction, which slows absorption.

Adrenaline is used in anaphylactic shock because its mix of actions, cardiovascular and bronchial, provide the best compromise for speed and simplicity of use in an emergency; it may also stabilise mast cell membranes and reduce release of vasoactive autacoids (see p. 280). Patients who are taking nonselective β-blockers may not respond to adrenaline (use salbutamol i.v.) and indeed may develop severe hypertension (see below).

Adrenaline (topical) decreases intraocular pressure in chronic open-angle glaucoma, as does dipivefrine, an adrenaline ester prodrug. They are contraindicated in closed-angle glaucoma because they are mydriatics. Hyperthyroid patients are intolerant of adrenaline.

Accidental overdose with adrenaline occurs occasionally. It is rationally treated by propranolol to block the cardiac β effects (cardiac arrhythmia) and phentolamine or chlorpromazine to control the α effects on the peripheral circulation that will be prominent when the β effects are abolished. Labetalol (α + β block) would be an alternative. β-adrenoceptor block alone is hazardous as the then unopposed α-receptor vasoconstriction causes (severe) hypertension (see Phaeochromocytoma, p. 494). Use of antihypertensives of most other kinds is irrational and some may also potentiate the adrenaline.

Noradrenaline (norepinephrine) (chiefly α and β₁ effects)

The main effect of administered noradrenaline is to raise the blood pressure by constricting the arterioles

and so raising the total peripheral resistance, with reduced blood flow (except in coronary arteries which have few α_1-receptors). Though it does have some cardiac stimulant (β_1) effect, the tachycardia of this is masked by the profound reflex bradycardia caused by the hypertension. Noradrenaline is given by i.v. infusion to obtain a gradual sustained response; the effect of a single i.v. injection would last only a minute or so. It is used where peripheral vasoconstriction is specifically desired, e.g. vasodilation of septic shock. Adverse effects include peripheral gangrene and local necrosis; tachyphylaxis occurs and withdrawal must be gradual.

Isoprenaline (isoproterenol)

Isoprenaline (isopropylnoradrenaline) is a nonselective β-receptor agonist, i.e. it activates both β_1- and β_2-receptors. It relaxes smooth muscle, including that of the blood vessels, has negligible metabolic or vasoconstrictor effects, but a vigorous stimulant effect on the heart. This latter is its main disadvantage in the treatment of bronchial asthma. Its principal uses are in complete heart block and occasionally in cardiogenic shock (hypotension).

Dopamine

Dopamine activates different receptors depending on the dose used. At the lowest effective dose it stimulates specific dopamine (D_1) receptors in the CNS and the renal and other vascular beds (dilator); it also activates presynaptic autoreceptors (D_2) which suppress release of noradrenaline. As dose is raised, dopamine acts as an agonist on β_1-adrenoceptors in the heart (increasing contractility and rate); at high doses it activates α-adrenoceptors (vasoconstrictor). It is given by continuous i.v. infusion because, like all catecholamines, its $t\frac{1}{2}$ is short (2 min). An i.v. infusion (2–5 micrograms/kg/min) increases renal blood flow (partly through an effect on cardiac output). As the dose rises the heart is stimulated, resulting in tachycardia and increased cardiac output. At these higher doses, dopamine is referred to as an 'inoconstrictor'.

Dopamine is stable for about 24 h in sodium chloride or dextrose. Subcutaneous leakage causes vasoconstriction and necrosis and should be treated by local injection of an α-adrenoceptor blocking agent (phentolamine 5 mg, diluted).

It may be mixed with dobutamine.

For CNS aspects of dopamine, agonists and antagonists: see Neuroleptics, Parkinsonism.

Dobutamine

Dobutamine is a racemic mixture of d- and l-dobutamine. The racemate behaves primarily a β_1-adrenoceptor agonist with greater inotropic than chronotropic effects on the heart; it has some α-agonist effect, but less than dopamine. It is useful in shock (with dopamine) and in low output heart failure (in the absence of severe hypertension).

Dopexamine

Dopexamine is a synthetic catecholamine whose principal action is as an agonist for the cardiac β_2-adrenoceptors (positive inotropic effect). It is also a weak dopamine agonist (thus causing renal vasodilatation) and inhibitor of noradrenaline uptake thereby enhancing stimulation of cardiac β_1-receptors by noradrenaline. It is used occasionally to optimise the cardiac output, particularly perioperatively.

NONCATECHOLAMINES

Salbutamol, fenoterol, rimiterol, reproterol, pir-buterol, salmeterol, ritodrine and terbutaline are β-adrenoceptor agonists that are relatively selective for β_2-receptors, so that cardiac (chiefly β_1-receptor) effects are less prominent. Tachycardia still occurs because of atrial (sinus node) β_2-receptor stimulation; the β_2-adrenoceptors are less numerous in the ventricle and there is probably less risk of serious ventricular arrhythmias than with the use of nonselective catecholamines. The synthetic agonists are also longer-acting than isoprenaline because they are not substrates for catechol-O-methyltransferase, which methylates catecholamines in the liver. They are used principally in asthma, and to reduce uterine contractions in premature labour.

Salbutamol (see also Asthma)

Salbutamol (Ventolin) ($t\frac{1}{2}$ 4 h) is taken orally, 2–4 mg up to 4 times/day; it also acts quickly by inhalation and the effect can last as long as 4 h,

which makes it suitable for both prevention and treatment of asthma. Of an inhaled dose < 20% is absorbed and can cause cardiovascular effects. It can also be given by injection, e.g. in asthma, premature labour (β_2-receptor) and for cardiac inotropic (β_1) effect in heart failure (where the β_2 vasodilator action is also useful). Clinically important hypokalaemia can also occur (the shift of potassium into cells). The other drugs above are similar.

Salmeterol (Serevent) is a variant of salbutamol that has additional binding property to a site adjacent to the β_2-adrenoceptor, which results in slow onset and long duration of action (about 12 h) (see p. 560).

Ephedrine

Ephedrine ($t\frac{1}{2}$ approx. 4 h) is a plant alkaloid with indirect sympathomimetic actions that resemble adrenaline peripherally. Centrally (in adults) it produces increased alertness, anxiety, insomnia, tremor and nausea; children may be sleepy when taking it. In practice central effects limit its use as a sympathomimetic in asthma.

Ephedrine is well absorbed when given orally and, unlike most other sympathomimetics, undergoes relatively little first-pass metabolism in the liver; it is largely excreted unchanged by the kidney. It is usually given by mouth but can be injected. It differs from adrenaline principally in that its effects come on more slowly and last longer. Tachyphylaxis occurs on repeated dosing. Ephedrine can be used as a bronchodilator, in heart block, as a mydriatic and as a mucosal vasoconstrictor, but newer drugs, which are often better for these purposes, are displacing it. It is sometimes useful in myasthenia gravis (adrenergic agents enhance cholinergic neuromuscular transmission). *Pseudoephedrine* is similar.

Phenylpropanolamine (norephedrine) is similar but with less CNS effect. Prolonged administration of phenylpropanolamine to women as an anorectic has been associated with pulmonary valve abnormalities and led to its withdrawal in some countries.

Amfetamine (Benzedrine) and *dexamphetamine* (Dexedrine) act indirectly. They are seldom used for their peripheral effects, which are similar to those of ephedrine, but usually for their effects on the central nervous system (narcolepsy, attention deficit in children). (For a general account of amphetamine, see p. 193)

Phenylephrine has actions qualitatively similar to noradrenaline but a longer duration of action, up to an hour or so. It can be used as a nasal decongestant (0.25–0.5% solution), but sometimes irritates. In the doses usually given, the central nervous effects are minimal, as are the direct effects on the heart. It is also used as a mydriatic and briefly lowers intraocular pressure.

Mucosal decongestants

Nasal and bronchial decongestants (vasoconstrictors) are widely used in allergic rhinitis, colds, coughs and sinusitis, and to prevent otitic barotrauma, as nasal drops or nasal sprays. All the sympathomimetic vasoconstrictors, i.e. with α effects, have been used for the purpose, with or without an antihistamine (H$_1$-receptor), and there is little to choose between them. Ischaemic damage to the mucosa is possible if they are used excessively (more often than 3-hourly) or for prolonged periods (> 3 weeks). The occurrence of rebound congestion is also liable to lead to overuse. The least objectionable drugs are ephedrine 0.5% and phenylephrine 0.5%. Xylometazoline 0.1% (Otrivine) should be used, if at all, for only a few days since longer application reduces the ciliary activity and will lead to rebound congestion. Naphazoline and adrenaline should not be used, and nor should blunderbuss mixtures of vasoconstrictor antihistamine, adrenal steroid and antibiotics. Oily drops and sprays, used frequently and long-term, may enter the lungs and eventually cause lipoid pneumonia.

It may sometimes be better to give the drugs orally rather than up the nose. They interact with antihypertensives and can be a cause of unexplained failure of therapy unless enquiry into patient self-medication is made. Fatal hypertensive crises have occurred when patients treated for depression with a monoamine oxidase inhibitor have taken these preparations.

Shock

Definition. Shock is a state of inadequate capillary perfusion (oxygen deficiency) of vital tissues to an extent that adversely affects cellular metabolism (capillary endothelium and organs) causing malfunction, including release of enzymes and vasoactive substances,[6] i.e. it is a *low flow* or *hypoperfusion* state.

The cardiac output and blood pressure are low in fully developed cases. But a maldistribution of blood (due to constriction, dilatation, shunting) can be sufficient to produce tissue injury even in the presence of high cardiac output and arterial blood pressure (warm shock), e.g. some cases of septic shock.

The essential element, hypoperfusion of vital organs, is present whatever the cause, whether pump failure (myocardial infarction), maldistribution of blood (septic shock) or loss of total intravascular volume (bleeding or increased permeability of vessels damaged by bacterial cell products, burns or anoxia). Function of vital organs, brain (consciousness, respiration) and kidney (urine formation) are clinical indicators of adequacy of perfusion of these organs.

Treatment may be summarised:
- *Treatment of the cause:* bleeding, infection, adrenocortical deficiency
- *Replacement of any fluid lost* from the circulation
- *Perfusion of vital organs* (brain, heart, kidneys) and maintenance of the mean blood pressure.

Blood flow (oxygen delivery) rather than blood pressure is of the greatest immediate importance for the function of vital organs. A reasonable blood pressure is needed to ensure organ perfusion but peripheral vasoconstriction may maintain a normal mean arterial pressure despite a very low cardiac output. Under these circumstances, blood flow to vital organs will be inadequate and multiple organ

---

[6] In fact, a medley of substances (autacoids), kinins, prostaglandins, leukotrienes, histamine, endorphins, serotonin, vasopressin, has been implicated. In endotoxic shock, the toxin also induces synthesis of nitric oxide, the endogenous vasodilator, in several types of cells other than the endothelial cells which are normally its main source.

failure will ensue unless the patient is resuscitated adequately.

The decision how to treat shock depends on assessment of the pathophysiology:

- whether cardiac output, and so peripheral blood flow, is inadequate (low pulse volume, cold-constricted periphery)
- whether cardiac output is normal or high and peripheral blood flow is adequate (good pulse volume and warm dilated periphery), but there is maldistribution of blood
- whether the patient is hypovolaemic or not, or needs a cardiac inotropic agent, a vasoconstrictor or a vasodilator.

Types of shock

In poisoning by a cerebral depressant or after spinal cord trauma, the principal cause of hypotension is low peripheral resistance due to reduced vascular tone. The cardiac output can be restored by simply tilting the patient head-down and by increasing the venous filling pressure by infusing fluid. Vasoactive drugs (noradrenaline, dobutamine) may be beneficial.

In central circulatory failure (cardiogenic shock, e.g. after myocardial infarction) the cardiac output and blood pressure are low due to pump failure; myocardial perfusion is dependent on aortic pressure. Venous return (central venous pressure) is normal or high. The low blood pressure may trigger the sympathoadrenal mechanisms of peripheral circulatory failure summarised below.

Not surprisingly, the use of drugs in low output failure due to acute myocardial damage is disappointing. Vasoconstriction (by an α-adrenoceptor agonist), by increasing peripheral resistance, may raise the blood pressure by increasing afterload, but this additional burden on the damaged heart can further reduce the cardiac output. Cardiac stimulation with a β_1-adrenoceptor agonist may fail; it increases myocardial oxygen consumption and may cause an arrhythmia. Dobutamine, dopexamine or dopamine offer a reasonable choice if a drug is judged necessary; dobutamine is preferred as it tends to vasodilate, i.e. it is an 'inodilator'. A selective phosphodiesterase inhibitor such as enoximone may also be effective, unless its use is limited by hypotension.

If there is bradycardia (as sometimes complicates myocardial infarction), cardiac output can be increased by vagal block with atropine, which accelerates the heart rate.

Septic shock is severe sepsis with hypotension that is not corrected by adequate intravascular volume replacement. It is caused by lipopolysaccharide (LPS) endotoxins from Gram-negative organisms and other cell products from Gram-positive organisms; these initiate host inflammatory and procoagulant responses through the release of cytokines, e.g. interleukins, and the resulting diffuse endothelial damage is responsible for many of the adverse manifestations of shock, including multi-organ failure. First, there is a peripheral vasodilatation from activation of nitric oxide by LPS and cytokines, with eventual fall in arterial pressure. This initiates a vigorous sympathetic discharge that causes constriction of arterioles and venules; the cardiac output may be high or low according to the balance of these influences. There is a progressive peripheral anoxia of vital organs and acidosis. The veins (venules) dilate and venous pooling occurs so that blood is sequestered in the periphery and effective circulatory volume falls because of this, and of fluid loss into the extravascular space from endothelial damage caused by bacterial products.

When septic shock is recognised, appropriate antimicrobials should be given in high dose immediately after the taking of blood cultures (see p. 237). Beyond that, the prime aim of treatment is to restore cardiac output and vital organ perfusion by accelerating venous return to the heart and to reverse the maldistribution of blood. Increasing intravascular volume will achieve this, guided by the central venous pressure to avoid overloading the heart. Oxygen is essential as there is often uneven pulmonary perfusion.

After adequate fluid resuscitation has been established, inotropic support is usually required. *Noradrenaline* is the inotrope of choice for septic shock: its potent α-adrenergic effect increases the mean arterial pressure and its modest β_1 effect may raise cardiac output, or at least maintain it as the peripheral vascular resistance increases. *Dobutamine* may be added further to augment cardiac output.

Some clinicians use *adrenaline,* in preference to noradrenaline plus dobutamine, on the basis that its powerful α and β effects are appropriate in the setting of septic shock; it may exacerbate splanchnic ischaemia and lactic acidosis.

Hypotension in (atherosclerotic) occlusive vascular disease is particularly serious, for these patients are dependent on pressure to provide the necessary blood flow in vital organs whose supplying vessels are less able to dilate. It is important to maintain an adequate mean arterial pressure, whichever inotrope is selected.

CHOICE OF DRUG IN SHOCK

On present knowledge the best drug would be one that both stimulates the myocardium and selectively modifies peripheral resistance to increase flow to vital organs.

- *Dobutamine* is used when cardiac inotropic effect is the primary requirement.
- *Adrenaline* is used when a more potent inotrope than dobutamine is required, e.g. when the vasodilating action of dobutamine compromises mean arterial pressure.
- *Noradrenaline* is used when vasoconstriction is the first priority, plus some slight cardiac inotropic effect, e.g. septic shock.

Monitoring drug use

Modern monitoring by both invasive and non-invasive techniques is complex and is undertaken in units dedicated to and, equipped for, this activity. The present comment is an overview. Monitoring will normally require close attention to heart rate and rhythm, blood pressure, fluid balance and urine flow, pulmonary gas exchange and central venous pressure. The use of drugs in shock is secondary to accurate assessment of cardiovascular state (especially of peripheral flow) and to other essential management, treatment of infection and maintenance of intravascular volume.

Restoration of intravascular volume[7]

In an emergency, speed of replacement is more important than its nature. *Crystalloid* solutions, e.g.

isotonic saline, Hartmann's, Plasma-Lyte, are immediately effective, but they leave the circulation quickly. (Note that dextrose solutions are completely ineffective because they distribute across both the extracellular and intracellular compartments.) Macro-molecules (*colloids*) remain in the circulation longer. The two classes (crystalloids and colloids) may be used together.

The choice of crystalloid or colloid for fluid resuscitation remains controversial. There have been no prospective, randomised trials of sufficient power in either sepsis or trauma, to detect a significant difference in mortality. Albumin is relatively expensive and offers no advantage over cheaper, synthetic colloids such as etherified starch.

Colloidal isotonic solutions of macromolecules include: dextrans (glucose polymer), gelatin (hydrolysed collagen) and hydroxyethyl starch.

Dextran 70 (mol. wt. 70 000) has a plasma restoring effect lasting 5–6 h. Dextran 40 is used to decrease blood sludging and so to improve peripheral blood flow.

Gelatin products (Haemaccel, Gelofusine) have a plasma restoring effect of 2–3 h (at best).

Etherified starch. Several hydroxyethyl starch solutions are available, with widely differing effects on plasma volume. The high molecular weight (450 000) solutions have a volume restoring effect for 6–12 h, while that of medium molecular weight (200 000) starches last 4–6 h.

Adverse effects include anaphylactoid reactions; dextran and hetastarch can impair haemostatic mechanisms.

Chronic orthostatic hypotension

Chronic orthostatic hypotension occurs most commonly with increasing age, in primary progressive

---

[7] Nolan J 2001 Fluid resuscitation for the trauma patient. Resuscitation 48: 57–69.

autonomic failure and secondary to parkinsonism and diabetes. The clinical features can be mimicked by saline depletion. The two conditions are clearly separated by measurement of plasma levels of noradrenaline (supine and erect) and renin. These are elevated in saline depletion, but depressed in most causes of hypotension due to autonomic failure.

Since blood pressure can be considered a product of 'volume' and 'vasoconstriction', the logical initial treatment of orthostatic hypotension is to expand blood volume using a sodium-retaining adrenocortical steroid (fludrocortisone[8]) or desmopressin (p. 716) — plus elastic support stocking to reduce venous pooling of blood when erect.

It is more difficult to reproduce the actions of the endogenous vasoconstrictors, and especially their selective release on standing, in order to achieve erect normotension without supine hypertension. Because of the risk of hypertension when the patient is supine, only a modest increase in erect blood pressure should be sought; fortunately a systolic blood pressure of 85–90 mmHg is usually adequate to maintain cerebral perfusion in these patients. Few drugs have been formally tested or can be recommended with confidence. Clonidine and pindolol are partial agonists at, respectively, α and β receptors, and may therefore be more effective agonists in the absence of the endogenous agonist, noradrenaline, than in normal subjects. Midodrine, an α-adrenoceptor agonist, is the only vasoconstrictor drug to receive UK regulatory approval for the treatment of postural hypotension. It should be given at doses of 5–15 mg t.i.d.

Postprandial fall in blood pressure (probably due to redistribution of blood to the splanchnic area) is characteristic of this condition; it especially occurs after breakfast (blood volume is lower in the morning). Substantial doses of caffeine (two large cups of coffee) can mitigate this, but they need to be taken before or early in the meal. The action may be due to block of splanchnic vasodilator adenosine receptors. Administration of the somatostatin analogue, octreotide, prevents postprandial hypotension, but the requirement for twice daily subcutaneous injections makes the drug an unlikely candidate for regular use in this group of patients.

Some of the variation in reported results of drug therapy may be due to differences in adrenergic function dependent on whether the degeneration is central, peripheral, preganglionic, postganglionic or due to age-related changes in the adrenoceptors on end-organs. In central autonomic degeneration, 'multisystem atrophy', noradrenaline is still present in peripheral sympathetic nerve endings. In these patients, an indirect-acting amine may be successful, and one patient titrated the amount of Bovril (a tyramine-rich meat extract drink) she required in order to stand up.[9]

Erythropoietin has been used with success (it increases haematocrit and blood viscosity).

Summary

- The adrenergic arm of the autonomic system uses noradrenaline (norepinephrine) as its neurotransmitter.
- Adrenaline (epinephrine), unlike noradrenaline, is a circulating hormone.
- These two catecholamines act on the same adrenoceptors: α_1 and α_2 which are blocked by phenoxybenzamine but not by propranolol, and β_1 and β_2 which are blocked by propranolol but not phenoxybenzamine. Noradrenaline is a 20-fold weaker agonist at β_2-receptors than is adrenaline.
- Distinction between receptor classes is made initially by defining the differing ability of two agonists (or antagonists) to mimic (or block) the effects of catecholamines.
- Often these differences correlate with a difference in receptor type on two different tissues: e.g. stimulation of cardiac contractility by β_1-receptors and bronchodilatation by β_2-receptors.
- The distinction between α_1- and α_2-receptors corresponds to their principal location on blood vessels (causing vasoconstriction) and neurons.
- Catecholamines themselves can be used in therapy when rapid onset and offset are desired. Selective mimetics at each of the four main receptor subtypes are used for individual locations, e.g: α_1 for nasal decongestion, α_2 for systemic hypotension, α_1 for heart failure or shock, β_2 for bronchoconstriction.
- Both α- and β-blockade are used in hypertension; selective β-blockade is used in angina and heart failure.

---

[8] Effective doses may not affect blood volume and may work by sensitising vascular adrenoceptors.

[9] Karet F E et al 1994 Bovril and moclobemide: a novel therapeutic strategy for central autonomic failure. Lancet 344: 1263–1265.

GUIDE TO FURTHER READING

Ahlquist R P 1948 A study of adrenotropic receptors. American Journal of Physiology 153: 586–600

Astiz M E, Rackow E C 1998 Septic shock. Lancet 351: 1501–1505

Bernard G D et al 2001 Efficacy and safety of recombinant human activated protein C for severe sepsis. New England Journal of Medicine 344: 699–709

Brown M J 1995 To β-block or better block? British Medical Journal 311: 701–702

Califf R M, Bengtson J R 1994 Cardiogenic shock. New England Journal of Medicine 330: 1724–1730

Evans T W, Smithies M 1999 ABC of intensive care. Organ dysfunction. British Medical Journal 318: 1606–1609

Ewan P W 1998 Anaphylaxis. British Medical Journal 316: 1442–1445

Insel P A 1996 Adrenergic receptors — evolving concepts and clinical implications. New England Journal of Medicine 334: 580–585.

Lynn W A 1999 Severe sepsis. In: Pusey C (ed) Horizons in medicine. Royal College of Physicians of London, London, p 55–68

Wheeler A P, Bernard G D 1999 Treating patients with severe sepsis. New England Journal of Medicine 340: 207–214

23

Arterial hypertension, angina pectoris, myocardial infarction

SYNOPSIS

Hypertension and coronary heart disease (CHD) are of great importance. Hypertension affects above 20% of the total population of the USA with its major impact on those over age 50. CHD is the cause of death in 30% of males and 22% of females in England and Wales. Management requires attention to detail, both clinical and pharmacological.

The way drugs act in these diseases is outlined and the drugs are described according to class.

- Hypertension and angina pectoris: how drugs act
- Drugs used in both hypertension and angina

  Diuretics
  Vasodilators
     organic nitrates, calcium channel blockers, ACE inhibitors, angiotensin II-receptor antagonists
  Adrenoceptor blocking drugs, α and β
  Peripheral sympathetic nerve terminal
  Autonomic ganglion-blocking drugs
  Central nervous system
  Treatment of angina pectoris

- Acute coronary syndromes and myocardial infarction
- Arterial hypertension
- Sexual function and cardiovascular drugs
- Phaeochromocytoma

Hypertension: how drugs act

Consider the following relationship:

Blood pressure =
$$\text{cardiac output} \times \text{peripheral resistance}$$

Therefore drugs can lower blood pressure by:

- Dilatation of arteriolar *resistance vessels.* Dilatation can be achieved through direct relaxation of vascular smooth muscle cells, by stimulation of nitric oxide (NO) production, or by blocking (suppressing) endogenous vasoconstrictors, noradrenaline (norepinephrine) and angiotensin.
- Dilatation of venous *capacitance vessels;* reduced venous return to the heart (preload) leads to reduced cardiac output, especially in the upright position
- Reduction of *cardiac contractility* and *heart rate.*
- Depletion of *body sodium.* This reduces plasma volume (transiently), and reduces arteriolar response to noradrenaline (norepinephrine)

Modern antihypertensive drugs lower blood pressure with minimal interference with homeostatic control, i.e. change in posture, exercise.

Angina pectoris: how drugs act

Angina can be viewed as a problem of supply and demand. Drugs used in angina pectoris are those that either increase supply of oxygen and nutrients, or reduce the demand for these — or both.

Supply can be increased by: cardiac work and myocardial oxygen need by:

- dilating coronary arteries
- slowing the heart (coronary flow, uniquely, occurs in diastole, which lengthens as heart rate falls).

Demand can be reduced by:

- reducing afterload, (i.e. peripheral resistance), so reducing the work of the heart in perfusing the tissues
- reducing preload, (i.e. venous filling pressure); according to Starling's Law of the heart, workload and therefore oxygen demand varies with stretch of cardiac muscle fibres
- slowing the heart.

Drugs used in hypertension and angina

Two groups of drugs, β-adrenergic blockers and calcium channel blockers, are used in both hypertension and angina. Several drugs for hypertension are used also in the treatment of heart failure.

Diuretics (see also Ch. 26)

Diuretics, particularly the thiazides, are useful antihypertensives. They cause an initial loss of sodium with a parallel contraction of the blood and extracellular fluid volume. The effect may reach 10% of total body sodium but it is not maintained. After several months of treatment, the main blood pressure lowering effect appears to reflect a reduced responsiveness of resistance vessels to endogenous vasoconstrictors, principally noradrenaline. While this hyposensitivity may be a consequence of the sodium depletion, thiazides are generally more effective antihypertensive agents than loop diuretics, despite causing less salt loss, and evidence suggests an independent action of thiazides on an unidentified ion-channel on vascular smooth muscle cell membranes. Maximum effect on blood pressure is delayed for several weeks and other drugs are best added after this time. Adverse metabolic effects of thiazides on serum potassium, blood lipids, glucose tolerance, and uric acid metabolism led to suggestions that they should be replaced by newer agents not having these effects. It is, however, now recognised that unnecessarily high doses of thiazides have been used in the past and that with low doses, e.g. bendrofluazide (bendroflumethiazide) 1.25–2.5 mg/d or less (or hydrochlorothiazide 12.5–25 mg), thiazides are both effective and well-tolerated. Moreover, they are not only by far the cheapest antihypertensive agents available worldwide but have proved to be the most effective in several outcome trials in preventing the major complications of hypertension, myocardial infarction and stroke. The characteristic reduction in renal calcium excretion induced by thiazides may, in long-term therapy, also reduce the occurrence of hip fractures in older patients and benefit women with postmenopausal osteoporosis.

Vasodilators

ORGANIC NITRATES

Organic nitrates (and nitrite) were introduced into medicine in the 19th century.[1] Denitration in the smooth muscle cell releases nitric oxide (NO), which is the main physiological vasodilator, normally produced by endothelial cells. *Nitrodilators* (a generic term for drugs that release or mimic the action of NO) activate the soluble guanylate cyclase in vascular smooth muscle cells and cause an increase in intracellular cyclic GMP (guanosine monophosphate) con-

---

[1] Murrell, W 1879 Nitroglycerin as a remedy for angina pectoris. Lancet 1: 80–81. Nitroglycerin was actually first synthesised by Sobrero in 1847 who noted when he applied it to his tongue it caused a severe headache.

centrations. This is the second messenger that alters calcium fluxes in the cell, decreases stored calcium, and induces relaxation. The result is a generalised dilatation of venules (capacitance vessels) and to a lesser extent of arterioles (resistance vessels), causing a fall of blood pressure that is postural at first; the larger coronary arteries especially dilate. Whereas some vasodilators can 'steal' blood away from atheromatous arteries, with their fixed stenoses, to other, healthier arteries, nitrates probably have the reverse effect as a result of their supplementing the endogenous NO. Atheroma is associated with impaired endothelial function, resulting in reduced release of NO and, possibly, its accelerated destruction by the oxidised LDL in atheroma (see Ch. 25).

The venous dilatation causes a reduction in venous return, a fall in left ventricular filling pressure with reduced stroke volume, but cardiac output (per min) is sustained by the reflex tachycardia induced by the fall in blood pressure.

Pharmacokinetics. The nitrates are generally well absorbed across skin, and the mucosal surface of the mouth or gut wall. Nitrates absorbed from the gut, however, are subject to extensive first-pass metabolism in the liver, as is shown by the substantially larger doses required by that route over sublingual application (this also explains why swallowing a sublingual tablet of glyceryl trinitrate terminates its effect). They are first denitrated and then conjugated with glucuronic acid. The $t\frac{1}{2}$ periods vary (see below) but for glyceryl trinitrate (GTN) it is 1–4 minutes.

Tolerance to the characteristic vasodilator headache comes and goes quickly (hours).[2] Ensuring that a continuous steady-state plasma concentration is avoided prevents tolerance. This is easy with occasional use of glyceryl trinitrate, but with nitrates having longer $t\frac{1}{2}$ (see below) and sustained release formulations it is necessary to plan the dosing to allow low plasma concentration for 4–8 h, e.g. over-

night; alternatively transdermal patches may be removed for a few hours if tolerance is suspected.

Uses. Nitrates are chiefly used to relieve angina pectoris and sometimes left ventricular failure. An excessive fall in blood pressure will reduce coronary flow as well as cause fainting due to reduced cerebral blood flow, and so it is important to avoid accidental overdosing. Patients with angina should be instructed on the signs of overdose — palpitations, dizziness, blurred vision, headache and flushing following by pallor — and what to do about it (below).

The discovery that coronary artery occlusion by thrombosis is itself 'stuttering' — developing gradually over hours — and associated with vaso-spasm in other parts of the coronary tree has made the use of isosorbide dinitrate (Isoket) by continuous i.v. infusion adjusted to the degree of pain, a logical, and effective, form of analgesia for unstable angina.

Transient relief of pain due to spasm of other smooth muscle (colic), can sometimes be obtained, so that relief of chest pain by nitrates does not prove the diagnosis of angina pectoris.

Nitrates are contraindicated in angina due to anaemia.

Adverse effects. Collapse due to fall in blood pressure resulting from overdose is the commonest side effect. The patient should remain supine, and the legs should be raised above the head to restore venous return to the heart.

Nitrate headache, which may be severe, is probably due to the stretching of pain-sensitive tissues around the meningeal arteries resulting from the increased pulsation that accompanies the local vasodilatation. If headache is severe the dose should be halved. Methaemoglobinaemia occurs with heavy dosage.

Interactions. An important footnote to the use of nitrates (and NO-dilators generally) has been the marked potentiation of their vasodilator effects observed in patients taking the phosphodiesterase (PDE) inhibitor sildenafil (Viagra). This agent targets an isoform of PDE (PDE-5) expressed in the blood vessel wall. Other methylaxanthine PDE inhibitors, such as theophylline, do not cause a similar interaction because they are rather weak inhibitors of PDE-5, even at the doses effective in asthma. A

---

[2] Explosives factory workers exposed to a nitrate-contaminated environment lost it over a weekend and some chose to maintain their intake by using nitrate impregnated headbands (transdermal absorption) rather than have to accept the headaches and reacquire tolerance so frequently.

number of pericoital deaths reported in patients taking sildenafil have been attributed to the substantial fall in blood pressure that occurs when used with a nitrate. This is an ironic twist for an agent in first-line use in erectile dysfunction that was originally developed as a drug to treat angina.[3]

GLYCERYL TRINITRATE (see also above)

Glyceryl trinitrate (1879) (trinitrin, nitroglycerin, GTN) ($t\frac{1}{2}$ 3 min) is an oily, nonflammable liquid that explodes on concussion with a force greater than that of gunpowder. Physicians meet it mixed with inert substances and made into a tablet, in which form it is both innocuous and fairly stable. But tablets more than 8 weeks old or exposed to heat or air will have lost potency by evaporation and should be discarded. Patients should also be warned to expect the tablet to cause a burning sensation under the tongue if it is still contains active GTN. An alternative is to use a nitroglycerin spray (see below); formulated as a pressurised liquid GTN has a shelf life of at least 3 years.

GTN is the drug of choice in the treatment of an attack of angina pectoris. The tablets should be chewed and dissolved under the tongue, or placed in the buccal sulcus, where absorption is rapid and reliable. Time spent ensuring that patients understand the way to take the tablets and that the feeling of fullness in the head is harmless, is time well spent. The action begins in 2 min and lasts up to 30 min. The dose in the standard tablet is 300 micrograms, and 500 or 600 microgram strengths are also available; patients may use up to 6 mg daily in total but those who require more than 2–3 tablets per week should take a long-acting nitrate preparation. GTN is taken at the onset of pain and as a prophylactic immediately before any exertion likely to precipitate the pain. Sustained-release buccal tablets are available (Suscard), 1–5 mg. Absorption from the gastrointestinal tract is good, but there is such extensive hepatic first-pass metabolism that

the sublingual or buccal route is preferred; an oral metered aerosol that is sprayed under the tongue (nitrolingual spray) is an alternative.

For prophylaxis, GTN can be given as an oral (buccal, or to swallow, Sustac) sustained-release formulation or via the skin as a patch (or ointment); these formulations can be useful for victims of nocturnal angina.[4]

Venepuncture: the ointment can assist difficult venepuncture and a transdermal patch adjacent to an i.v. infusion site can prevent extravasation and phlebitis and prolong infusion survival.

Isosorbide dinitrate (Cedocard) ($t\frac{1}{2}$ 20 min) is used for prophylaxis of angina pectoris and for congestive heart failure (tabs sublingual, and to swallow). An i.v. formulation 500 micrograms/ml (Isoket) is available for use in *left ventricular failure* and *unstable angina*.

Isosorbide mononitrate (Elantan) ($t\frac{1}{2}$ 4 h) is used for prophylaxis of angina (tabs to swallow). Hepatic first-pass metabolism is much less than for the dinitrate so that systemic bioavailability is more reliable.

Pentaerythritol tetranitrate (Peritrate) ($t\frac{1}{2}$ 8 h) is less efficacious than its metabolite pentaerythritol trinitrate ($t\frac{1}{2}$ 11 h).

CALCIUM CHANNEL BLOCKERS

Calcium is involved in the initiation of smooth muscle and cardiac cell contraction and in the propagation of the cardiac impulse. Actions on cardiac pacemaker cells and conducting tissue are described in Chapter 24.

Vascular smooth muscle cells. Contraction of these cells requires an influx of calcium across the cell membrane. This occurs through ion channels

---

[3] It has been argued that deaths on sildenafil largely reflect the fact that it is used by patients at high cardiovascular risk. But recent postmarketing data shows that death is 50 times more likely after sildenafil taken for erectile failure than alprostadil, the previous first-line agent. Mitka M 2000 Journal of the American Medical Association 283: 590.

[4] Useful, but not always safe. Defibrillator paddles and nitrate patches make an explosive combination, and it is not always in the patient's interest to have the patch as unobtrusive as possible (Canadian Medical Association Journal 1993 148: 790).

that are largely specific for calcium and are called 'slow calcium channels' to distinguish them from 'fast' channels that allow the rapid influx and efflux of sodium.

Activation of calcium channels by an action potential allows calcium to enter the cells. There follows a sequence of events which results in activation of the contractile proteins, myosin and actin, with shortening of the myofibril and contraction of smooth muscle. During relaxation calcium is released from the myofibril and, as it cannot be stored in the cell, it passes out again through the channel. Calcium channel (also called calcium entry) blockers inhibit the passage of calcium through the voltage-dependent L- (for 'long-opening') class membrane channels in cardiac muscle and conducting tissue, and vascular smooth muscle, reduce available intracellular calcium and cause the muscle to relax.[5]

There are three structurally distinct classes of calcium channel blocker:

- Dihydropyridines (the most numerous)
- Phenylalkylamines (principally verapamil)
- Benzothiazepine (diltiazem).

The differences between their clinical effects can be explained in part by their binding to different parts of the L-type calcium channel. All members of the group are vasodilators, and some have negative cardiac inotropic action and negative chronotropic effect via pacemaker cells and depress conducting tissue. The attributes of individual drugs are described below.

The therapeutic benefit of the calcium blockers in hypertension and angina is due mainly to their action as vasodilators. Their action on the heart gives non-dihydropyridines an additional role as Class 4 antiarrhythmics.

Pharmacokinetics. Calcium channel blockers in general are well absorbed from the gastrointestinal tract and their systemic bioavailability depends on the extent of first-pass metabolism in the gut wall and liver, which varies between the drugs. All undergo metabolism to less active products, predominantly by cytochrome P-450 CYP3A, which is the source of interactions with other drugs by enzyme induction and inhibition. As their action is terminated by metabolism, dose adjustments for patients with impaired renal function are therefore either minor or unnecessary.

Indications for use

- *Hypertension:* amlodipine, isradipine, nicardipine, nifedipine, verapamil
- *Angina:* amlodipine, diltiazem, nicardipine, nifedipine, verapamil
- *Cardiac arrhythmia:* verapamil
- *Raynaud's disease:* nifedipine
- *Prevention* of ischaemic neurological damage following subarachnoid haemorrhage: nimodipine.

Adverse effects. Headache, flushing, dizziness, palpitations and hypotension may occur during the first few hours after dosing, as the plasma concentration is increasing, particularly if the initial dose is too high or increased too rapidly. Ankle oedema may also develop. This is probably due to a rise in intracapillary pressure as a result of the selective dilatation by calcium blockers of the precapillary arterioles. Thus the oedema is not a sign of sodium retention. It is not relieved by a diuretic but disappears after lying flat, e.g. overnight. In theory the oedema should also be attenuated by combining the calcium blocker with another vasodilator which is more effective (than calcium blockers) at relaxing the postcapillary venules, e.g. a nitrate or an ACE inhibitor. Bradycardia and arrhythmia may occur. Gastrointestinal effects include constipation, nausea and vomiting; palpitation and lethargy may be felt.

There has been some concern that the shorter-acting calcium channel blockers may adversely affect the risk of myocardial infarction and cardiac death. The evidence is based on case-control studies which cannot escape the possibility that sicker patients, i.e. with worse hypertension or angina, received calcium channel blockade. The safety and efficacy of the class has been strengthened by the recent findings of two prospective comparisons with other antihypertensives.[6]

---

[5] Several calcium-selective channels have been described in different tisues, e.g. the N (present in neuronal tissue) and T (transient, found in brain, neuronal and cardiovascular tissue); the drugs discussed here selectively target the L channel for its cardiovascular importance.

Interactions are quite numerous. The drugs in this group in general are extensively metabolised, and there is risk of decreased effect with enzyme inducers, e.g. rifampicin, and increased effect with enzyme inhibitors, e.g. cimetidine. Conversely, calcium channel blockers decrease the plasma clearance of several other drugs by mechanisms that include delaying their metabolic breakdown. The consequence, for example, is that diltiazem and verapamil cause increased exposure to carbamazepine, quinidine, statins, ciclosporin, metoprolol, theophylline and (HIV) protease inhibitors. Verapamil increases plasma concentration of digoxin, possibly by interfering with its biliary excretion. Beta-adrenoceptor blockers may exacerbate atrioventricular block and cardiac failure. Grapefruit juice raises the plasma concentration of dihydropyridines (except amlodipine) and verapamil.

Individual calcium blockers

Nifedipine ($t\frac{1}{2}$ 2 h) is the prototype dihydropyridine. It selectively dilates arteries with little effect on veins; its negative myocardial inotropic and chronotropic effects are much less than those of verapamil. There are sustained-release formulations of nifedipine that permit once daily dosing with minimal peaks and troughs in plasma concentration so that adverse effects due to rapid fluctuation of concentrations are also lessened. Various methods have been used to prolong, and smooth, drug delivery, and bioequivalence between these formulations cannot be assumed; prescribers should specify the brand to be dispensed. The adverse effects of calcium blockers with a short duration of action may include the hazards of activating the sympathetic system each time a dose is taken. The dose range for nifedipine is 30–90 mg daily. In addition to the adverse effects listed above, gum hypertrophy may occur. Nifedipine can be taken 'sublingually', by biting a capsule and squeezing the contents under the tongue. In point of fact, absorption is still largely from the stomach after this

manoeuvre; it should not be used in a hypertensive emergency because the blood pressure reduction is unpredictable and sometimes large enough to cause cerebral ischaemia (see p. 492).

Amlodipine has a $t\frac{1}{2}$ (40 h) sufficient to permit the same benefits as the longest-acting formulations of nifedipine without requiring a special formulation. Its slow association with L-channels and long duration of action render it unsuitable for emergency reduction of blood pressure where frequent dose adjustment is needed. On the other hand an occasional missed dose is of little consequence. Amlodipine differs from all other dihydropyridines listed in this chapter in being safe to use in patients with cardiac failure (the PRAISE[7] Study).

Verapamil ($t\frac{1}{2}$ 4 h) is an arterial vasodilator with some venodilator effect; it also has marked negative myocardial inotropic and chronotropic actions. It is given thrice daily as a conventional tablet or daily as a sustained-release formulation. Because of its negative effects on myocardial conducting and contracting cells it should not be given to patients with bradycardia, second or third degree heart block, or patients with Wolff–Parkinson–White syndrome to relieve atrial flutter or fibrillation. Amiodarone and digoxin increase the AV block. Verapamil increases plasma quinidine concentration and this interaction may cause dangerous hypotension.

Diltiazem ($t\frac{1}{2}$ 5 h) is given thrice daily, or once or twice daily if a slow-release formulation is prescribed. It causes less myocardial depression and prolongation of AV conduction than does verapamil but should not be used where there is bradycardia, second or third degree heart block or sick sinus syndrome.

Isradipine ($t\frac{1}{2}$ 8 h) is given once or twice daily (it is similar to nifedipine).

Nicardipine ($t\frac{1}{2}$ 4 h) is given × 3/d.

---

[6] Both the NORDIL and INSIGHT trials (Lancet 2000 356: 359–365, 366–372) confirmed that a calcium channel blocker (diltiazem and nifedipine respectively) had the same efficacy as older therapies (diuretics and/or β-blockers) in hypertension with no evidence of increased sudden death.

[7] PRAISE = Prospective Randomised Amlodipine Survival Evaluation (see Packer M et al 1996 The effect of amlodipine on morbidity and mortality in severe chronic heart failure. New England Journal of Medicine 335: 1107–1114).

Nimodipine has a moderate cerebral vasodilating action. Cerebral ischaemia after subarachnoid haemorrhage may be partly due to vasospasm; clinical trial evidence indicates that nimodipine given after subarachnoid haemorrhage reduces cerebral infarction (incidence and extent).[8] Although the benefit is small, the absence of any more effective alternatives has led to the routine administration of nimodipine (60 mg every 4 hours) to all patients for the first few days following subarachnoid haemorrhage. No benefit has been found in similar trials following other forms of stroke.

Other members include *felodipine, isradipine, lacidipine, lercanidipine, nisoldipine.*

ANGIOTENSIN CONVERTING ENZYME (ACE) INHIBITORS AND ANGIOTENSIN (AT) II RECEPTOR ANTAGONISTS

Renin is an enzyme produced by the kidney in response to a number of factors including adrenergic activity (β_1-receptor) and sodium depletion. Renin converts a circulating glycoprotein (angiotensinogen) into the biologically inert angiotensin I, which is then changed by angiotensin converting enzyme (ACE or kininase II) into the highly potent vasoconstrictor angiotensin II. ACE is located on the luminal surface of capillary endothelial cells, particularly in the lungs; and there are also renin-angiotensin systems in many organs, e.g. brain, heart, the relevance of which is uncertain.

Angiotensin II acts on two G-protein coupled receptors, of which the angiotensin 'AT_1' subtype accounts for all the classic actions of angiotensin. As well as vasoconstriction these include stimulation of aldosterone (the sodium-retaining hormone) production by the adrenal cortex. It is evident that angiotensin II can have an important effect on blood pressure. In addition, it stimulates cardiac and vascular smooth muscle cell growth, contributing probably to the progressive amplification in hypertension once the process is initiated. The AT_2 receptor subtype is coupled to inhibition of muscle growth or proliferation, but appears of minor importance in the adult cardiovascular system. The

recognition that the AT_1-receptor subtype is the important target for drugs antagonising angiotensin II has led, a little confusingly, to two alternative nomenclatures for these drugs: either AT_1-receptor blockers, or angiotensin II receptor antagonists (AIIRA).

Bradykinin (an endogenous vasodilator occurring in blood vessel walls) is also a substrate for ACE. Potentiation of bradykinin contributes to the blood pressure lowering action of ACE inhibitors in patients with low-renin causes of hypertension. Either bradykinin or one of the neurokinin substrates of ACE (such as substance P) may stimulate cough (below). The AT_1 blockers differ from the ACE inhibitors in having no effect on bradykinin and do not cause cough. Those that achieve complete blockade of the receptor are slightly more effective than ACE inhibitors at preventing angiotensin II vasoconstriction. ACE inhibitors are more effective at suppressing aldosterone production in patients with normal or low plasma renin.

Uses

Hypertension. The antihypertensive effect of ACE inhibitors and AT_1 receptor blockers results primarily from vasodilatation (reduction of peripheral resistance) with little change in cardiac output or rate; renal blood flow may increase (desirable). A fall in aldosterone production may also contribute to the blood pressure lowering action of ACE inhibitors. Both classes slow progression of glomerulopathy. Whether the long-term benefit of these drugs in hypertension exceeds that to be expected from blood pressure reduction alone remains controversial.

ACE inhibitors and AT_1-receptor blockers are most useful in hypertension when the raised blood pressure results from excess renin production (e.g. renovascular hypertension), or where concurrent use of another drug (diuretic or calcium blocker) renders the blood pressure renin-dependent. The fall in blood pressure can be rapid, especially with short-acting ACE inhibitors, and low initial doses of these should be used in patients at risk: those with impaired renal function, or suspected cerebrovascular disease. These patients may be advised to omit any concurrent diuretic treatment for a few days before the first dose. The antihypertensive effect increases progressively over weeks with continued adminis-

---

[8] Packard J D et al 1989 British Medical Journal 289: 636.

tration (as with other antihypertensives) and the dose may be increased at intervals of 2 weeks.

Cardiac failure (see p. 517). ACE inhibitors have a useful vasodilator and diuretic-sparing (but not diuretic-substitute) action in all grades of heart failure. Their reduction of mortality in this condition, due possibly to their being the only vasodilator which does not reflexly activate the sympathetic system, has made the ACE inhibitors more critical to the treatment of heart failure than of hypertension, where they are not usually an essential part of management. The AT_1 blockers have not yet been introduced for the treatment of cardiac failure. This may only be a matter of time, but the establishment of new drugs for cardiac failure encounters the problem of demonstrating efficacy against a background of existing ACE inhibitor therapy, where a placebo control is no longer ethically acceptable.

Diabetic nephropathy. In patients with type I (insulin dependent) diabetes, hypertension often accompanies the diagnosis of frank nephropathy and aggressive blood pressure control is essential to slow the otherwise inexorable decline in renal function that follows. ACE inhibitors appear to have a specific renoprotective effect, possibly because of the role of angiotensin II in driving the underlying glomerular hyperfiltration in these patients.[9] These drugs are now considered first-line treatment for hypertensive type I diabetics, although most patients will need a second or third agent to reach the new BP targets for these patients (see below). There is also evidence that ACE inhibitors have a proteinuria-sparing effect in type I diabetics with 'normal' BP, but here it is less clear whether this effect extends beyond just a BP-lowering effect.[10] For hypertensive type 2 diabetics with nephropathy, there are better data to support use of AT_1-receptor blockers than ACE inhibitors for a renoprotective effect independent of the blood pressure lowering effect.

Myocardial infarction (MI). Following a myocardial infarction, the left ventricle may fail acutely from the loss of functional tissue or in the long-term from a process of 'remodelling' due to thinning and enlargement of the scarred ventricular wall. Angiotensin II plays a key role in both of these processes and an ACE inhibitor given after an MI markedly reduces the incidence of heart failure. The effect is seen even in patients without overt signs of failure, but who have low left ventricular ejection fractions during the convalescent phase (3–10 days) following their MI. Patients such as this receiving captopril in the SAVE trial,[11] had a 37% reduction in progressive heart failure over the 60-month follow-up period compared to placebo. The benefits of ACE inhibition after MI are additional to those conferred by thrombolysis, aspirin and β-blockers.

Cautions. Certain constraints apply to the use of ACE.

- *Heart failure:* severe hypotension may result in patients taking diuretics, or who are hypovolaemic, hyponatraemic, elderly, have renal impairment or with systolic blood pressure < 100 mmHg. A test dose of captopril 6.25 mg by mouth may be given because its effect lasts only 4–6 h. If tolerated, the preferred long-acting ACE inhibitor may then be initiated in low dose.
- *Renal artery stenosis* (whether unilateral, bilateral renal or suspected from the presence of generalised atherosclerosis): an ACE inhibitor may cause renal failure and is *contraindicated.*
- *Aortic stenosis/left ventricular outflow tract obstruction:* an ACE inhibitor may cause severe, sudden hypotension and, depending on severity, is relatively or absolutely *contraindicated.*
- *Pregnancy* represents a *contraindication* (see below).
- *Angioedema* may result (see below).

Adverse effects

ACE inhibitors cause persistent dry cough in 10–15% of patients. Urticaria and angioedema (< 1

[9] For a review, see: Cooper M E 1998 Pathogenesis, prevention and treatment of diabetic nephropathy. Lancet 352: 213–219.

[10] The EUCLID study group 1997 The EUCLID study. Randomised, placebo-controlled trial of lisinopril in normotensive patients with insulin-dependent diabetes and normoalbuminuria or microalbuminuria. Lancet 349: 1787–1792.

[11] Swedberg K P et al 1992 New England Journal of Medicine 327: 669–677.

in 100 patients) are much rarer, occurring usually in the first weeks of treatment. The angioedema varies from mild swelling of the tongue to life-threatening tracheal obstruction, when s.c. adrenaline (epinephrine) should be given. The basis of the reaction is probably pharmacological rather than allergic, due to reduced breakdown of bradykinin.

Impaired renal function may result from reduced glomerular filling pressure, systemic hypotension or glomerulonephritis, and plasma creatinine should be checked before and during treatment. Hyponatraemia may develop, especially where a diuretic is also given; clinically significant hyperkalaemia (see effect on aldosterone above) is confined to patients with impaired renal function. ACE inhibitors are fetotoxic in the second trimester, causing reduced renal perfusion, hypotension, oligohydramnios and fetal death. Neutropenia and other blood dyscrasias occur. Other reported reactions include rashes, taste disturbance (dysguesia), musculoskeletal pain, proteinuria, liver injury and pancreatitis.

AT$_1$ receptor blockers are contraindicated in pregnancy, but avoid most other complications — particularly the cough and angioedema. They are the only antihypertensive drugs for which there is no 'typical' side effect.

Interactions. Hyperkalaemia can result from use with potassium-sparing diuretics. Renal clearance of lithium is reduced and toxic concentrations of plasma lithium may follow. Severe hypotension can occur with diuretics (above), and with chlorpromazine, and possibly other phenothiazines.

Individual drugs

Captopril (Capoten) has a t$\frac{1}{2}$ of 2 h and is partly metabolised and partly excreted unchanged; adverse effects are more common if renal function is impaired; it is given twice or thrice daily. Captopril is the shortest-acting of the ACE inhibitors, one of the few where the oral drug is itself active, not requiring de-esterification after absorption.

Enalapril (Innovace) is a prodrug (t$\frac{1}{2}$ 35 h) that is converted to the active enalaprilat (t$\frac{1}{2}$ 10 h). Effective 24-h control of blood pressure may require twice daily administration.

Other members include *cilazapril, fosinopril, imidapril, lisinopril, moexipril, perindopril, quinapril, ramipril,* and *trandolapril.* Of these, lisinopril has a marginally longer t$\frac{1}{2}$ than enalapril, probably justifying its popularity as a once-daily ACE inhibitor. Some of the others are longer-acting, with quinapril and ramipril having also a higher degree of binding to ACE in vascular tissue. The clinical significance of these differences is disputed. In the Heart Outcomes Prevention Evaluation (HOPE) Study of 9297 patients, ramipril reduced, by 20–30%, the rates of death, myocardial infarction, and stroke in a broad range of high-risk patients who were not known to have a low ejection fraction or heart failure.[12] The authors considered that the results could not be explained entirely by blood pressure reduction.

Losartan was the first AT$_1$ receptor antagonist licensed in the UK. It is a competitive blocker with a noncompetitive active metabolite. The drug has a short t$\frac{1}{2}$ (2 h) but the metabolite is much longer lived (t$\frac{1}{2}$ 10 h) permitting once daily dosing. Other AT$_1$ receptor antagonists in clinical use include *candesartan, eprosartan, irbesartan, telmisartan* and *valsartan.* Some of these appear more effective than losartan, which is generally used in combination with hydrochlorothiazide. In a landmark study this combination was 25% more effective than atenolol plus hydrochlorothiazide in preventing stroke.[13]

This class of drug is very well tolerated; in clinical trials their side effect profiles are indistinguishable or even better than placebo. Unlike the ACE inhibitors they do not produce cough, and are a valuable alternative for the 10–15% of patients who discontinue their ACE inhibitor for this reason. AT$_1$ receptor antagonists are used to treat hypertension but any role in cardiac failure or after myocardial infarction (as have ACE inhibitors) remains to be established.

The cautions listed for the use of ACE inhibitors (above) apply also to AT$_1$ receptor blockers.

[12] Yusuf S, Sleight P, Pogue J et al 2000 Effects of an angiotensin-converting-enzyme inhibitor, ramipril, on cardiovascular events in high-risk patients. The Heart Outcomes Prevention Evaluation Study Investigators. New England Journal of Medicine 342: 145–53.
[13] Dahlof B et al 2002 Cardiovascular morbidity and mortality in the Losartan Intervention for Endpoint reduction in hypertension study (LIFE): a randomised trial against atenolol. Lancet 359: 995–1010.

Other vasodilators

Several older drugs are powerfully vasodilating, but precluded from routine use in hypertension by their adverse effects. Minoxidil and nitroprusside still have special indications.

Minoxidil is a vasodilator selective for *arterioles* rather than for veins, similar to diazoxide and hydralazine. Like the former, it acts through its sulphate metabolite as an ATP-dependent potassium channel opener. It is highly effective in severe hypertension, but causes increased cardiac output, tachycardia, fluid retention and hypertrichosis. The hair growth is generalised and although a cosmetic problem in women, it has been exploited as a topical solution for the treatment of baldness in men.

Sodium nitroprusside is a highly effective anti-hypertensive agent when given i.v. Its effect is almost immediate and lasts for 1–5 min. Therefore it must be given by a precisely controllable infusion. It dilates both *arterioles* and *veins*, which would cause collapse if the patient stands up, e.g. for toilet purposes. There is a compensatory sympathetic discharge with tachycardia and tachyphylaxis to the drug. The action of nitroprusside is terminated by metabolism within erythrocytes. Specifically, electron transfer from haemoglobin iron to nitroprusside yields *methaemoglobin* and an unstable nitroprusside radical. This breaks down, liberating *cyanide* radicals capable of inhibiting cytochrome oxidase (and thus cellular respiration). Fortunately most of the cyanide remains bound within erythrocytes but a small fraction does diffuse out into the plasma and is converted to thiocyanate. Hence, monitoring plasma *thiocyanate* concentrations during prolonged (days) nitroprusside infusion is a useful marker of impending systemic cyanide toxicity. Poisoning may be obvious as a progressive metabolic acidosis or manifest as delirium or psychotic symptoms. Toxic subjects are also reputed to emit the characteristic bitter almond smell of hydrogen cyanide. Clearly nitroprusside infusion should not be undertaken without meticulous regard for the manufacturer's recommendations and precautions; outside specialist units it may be safer overall to choose another more familiar drug.

Sodium nitroprusside is used in hypertensive emergencies, refractory heart failure and for controlled hypotension in surgery. An infusion[14] may begin at 0.3–1.0 micrograms/kg/min and control of blood pressure is likely to be established at 0.5–6.0 micrograms/kg/min; close monitoring of blood pressure is mandatory usually with direct arterial monitoring of blood pressure; rate changes of infusion may be made every 5–10 min.

Diazoxide is chemically a thiazide but has no appreciable diuretic effect; indeed, like other potent arterial vasodilators it causes salt and water retention. It reduces peripheral arteriolar resistance through activation of the ATP-dependent potassium channel (c.f. nicorandil and minoxidil), with little effect on veins. The $t_{\frac{1}{2}}$ is 36 h.

The principal use of diazoxide has been in the emergency treatment of severe hypertension. The maximum effect after an i.v. bolus occurs within 5 min and lasts for at least 4 h. The dangers from excessive hypotension are now recognised to outweigh the benefit, and emergency use of diazoxide is almost obsolete.

Because it stimulates the same potassium channel in the pancreatic islet cells as is blocked by sulphonylureas, diazoxide causes hyperglycaemia. This effect renders diazoxide unsuitable for chronic use in hypertension, but a useful drug to treat insulinoma. Long-term oral administration causes the same problem of hair growth seen with minoxidil (see below and 'alopecia').

Hydralazine now has little use long-term for hypertension, but it may have a role as a vasodilator (plus nitrates) in heart failure. It reduces peripheral resistance by directly relaxing *arterioles*, with negligible effect on veins. In common with all potent arterial vasodilators, its hypotensive action is accompanied by a compensatory baroreceptor-mediated sympathetic discharge, causing tachycardia and increased cardiac output. There is also renin release with secondary salt and water retention,

---

[14] Light causes sodium nitroprusside in solution to decompose; hence solutions should be made fresh and immediately protected by an opaque cover, e.g. metal foil. The fresh solution has a faint brown colour; if the colour is strong it should be discarded.

which antagonises the hypotensive effect (so-called 'tolerance' on long-term use). Therefore, hydralazine, when used, is combined with a β-blocker and diuretic. The t½ is 1 h.

In most hypertensive emergencies (except for dissecting aneurysm) hydralazine 5–20 mg i.v. may be given over 20 min, when the maximum effect will be seen in 10–80 min; it can be repeated according to need and the patient transferred to oral therapy within 1–2 days.

Prolonged use of hydralazine at doses above 50 mg/day may cause a systemic lupus-like syndrome, more commonly in white than in black races, and in those with the slow acetylator phenotype.

Three other vasodilators find a role outside hypertension.

Nicorandil is an effective vasodilator through two actions. It acts as a *nitrate* by activating cyclic GMP (see above) but also opens the ATP-dependent *potassium channel* to allow potassium efflux and hyperpolarisation of the membrane which reduces calcium ion entry and induces muscular relaxation. It is indicated for use in *angina,* where it has similar efficacy to β-blockade, nitrates or calcium channel blockade. It is administered orally and is an alternative to nitrates when tolerance to these is a problem, or to the other classes when these are contraindicated by asthma or cardiac failure. Adverse effects to nicorandil are similar to those of nitrates, with headache reported in 35% of patients. It is the only antianginal drug for which at least one trial has demonstrated a beneficial influence upon outcome.[15]

Papaverine is an alkaloid present in opium, but is structurally unrelated to morphine. It inhibits phosphodiesterase and its principal action is to relax smooth muscle throughout the body, especially in the vascular system. It is occasionally injected into an area where local vasodilatation is desired, especially into and around arteries and veins to relieve spasm during vascular surgery and when setting up i.v. infusions. It is also used to treat male erectile dysfunction (see p. 546).

Alprostadil is a stable form of prostaglandin E_1. It is effective in psychogenic and neuropathic penile erectile dysfunction by direct intracorporeal injection (see p. 545) and is used i.v. to maintain patency of the ductus arteriosus in the newborn with congenital heart disease.

Vasodilators in heart failure (see p. 517)

Vasodilators in peripheral vascular disease

The aim has been to produce peripheral arteriolar vasodilatation without a concurrent significant drop in blood pressure, so that an increased blood flow in the limbs will result. Drugs are naturally more useful in patients in whom the decreased flow of blood is due to *spasm* of the vessels (Raynaud's phenomenon) than where it is due to *organic obstructive* changes that may make dilatation in response to drugs impossible (arteriosclerosis, intermittent claudication, Buerger's disease).

Vasodilators such as *naftidrofuryl* (Praxilene) and *oxpentifylline (pentoxifylline)* (Trental) increase blood flow to skin rather than muscle; they have also been successfully used in the treatment of *venous leg ulcers* (varicose and traumatic).

Intermittent claudication. Patients should 'stop smoking and keep walking' — i.e. take frequent exercise within their capacity. Other risk factors should be treated vigorously, especially hyperlipidaemia, and patients should also receive aspirin 75–150 mg daily as an antiplatelet agent. Most patients with intermittent claudication succumb to ischaemic or cerebrovascular disease, and therefore a major objective of treatment should be prevention of such outcomes. *Naftidrofuryl* or *oxpentifylline (pentoxifylline)* may be tried but should be withdrawn if there is no benefit in a few weeks. Naftidrofuryl has several actions. It is classed as a metabolic enhancer since it activates the enzyme succinate dehydrogenase, increasing the supply of ATP and reducing lactate levels in muscle. It also blocks $5HT_2$-receptors and inhibits serotonin-

---

[15] The Impact Of Nicorandil in Angina (IONA) study was a double-blind, randomized, placebo-controlled trial conducted in the United Kingdom in which high-risk patients with stable angina were assigned placebo or nicorandil 10–20 mg. Over a mean follow-up of 1.6 years, significantly more placebo-treated patients suffered an acute coronary syndrome or coronary death (15.5% vs 13.1%, $P = 0.01$).

induced vasoconstriction and platelet aggregation. Oxpentifylline is thought to improve oxygen supply to ischaemic tissue by improving erythrocyte deformability and reducing blood viscosity, in part by reducing plasma fibrinogen. Neither of these drugs is a direct vasodilator, as is the third drug used for intermittent claudication, *inositol nicotinate*. The evidence in favour of any benefit is stronger for the first two, for which meta-analyses provide some evidence of efficacy (increase in walking distance). Most vasodilators act selectively on healthy blood vessels, causing a 'steal' of blood from atheromatous vessels.

Night cramps occur in the disease and *quinine* has a somewhat controversial reputation in their prevention. Nevertheless, meta-analysis of six double-blind trials of nocturnal cramps (not necessarily associated with peripheral vascular disease) shows that the number, but not severity or duration of episodes, is reduced by a night-time dose.[16] The benefit may not be seen for 4 weeks (see ticlopidine).

Raynaud's phenomenon may be helped by nifedipine, reserpine (an α-adrenoceptor blocker, in low doses) and also by topical glyceryl trinitrate; indeed any vasodilator is worth trying in resistant cases; enalapril (ACE inhibitor) seems to lack efficacy. In severe cases, especially patients with ulceration, intermittent infusions over several hours of the endogenous vasodilator, prostacyclin (epoprostenol), achieves long-lasting improvements in symptoms.

β-adrenoceptor blockers exacerbate peripheral vascular disease and Raynaud's phenomenon by reducing perfusion of a circulation that is already compromised. Switching to a β_1-selective blocker is unhelpful, since the adverse effect is due to reduced cardiac output rather than unopposed α-receptor induced vasoconstriction.

Adrenoceptor blocking drugs

Adrenoceptor blocking drugs occupy the adreno-

---

[16] Man-Son-Hing M, Wells G 1995 Meta-analysis of efficacy of quinine for treatment of nocturnal cramps in elderly people. British Medical Journal 310: 13–17.

ceptor in competition with adrenaline (epinephrine) and noradrenaline (norepinephrine) (and other sympathomimetic amines) whether released in the body or injected; circulating adrenaline and noradrenaline are antagonised more readily than are the effects of adrenergic nerve stimulation.

There are two principal classes of adrenoceptor, α and β: for details of receptor effects see Table 22.1.

α-ADRENOCEPTOR BLOCKING DRUGS

There are two main subtypes of α-adrenoceptor, defined by their relative affinity for the drugs which occupy them:

- Classic α_1-adrenoceptors, on the effector organ (postsynaptic), mediate vasoconstriction
- α_2-adrenoceptors are present both on some effector tissues (postsynaptic), and on the nerve ending (presynaptic). The presynaptic receptors (or *autoreceptors*) mediate a reduction of release of chemotransmitter (noradrenaline), i.e. they provide a negative feedback control of transmitter release. They are also present in the CNS.

The first generation of α-adrenoceptor blockers were nonselective, blocking both α_1- and α_2-receptors. When subjects taking such a drug rise from supine to erect posture or take exercise, the sympathetic system is physiologically activated (via baroreceptors). The normal vasoconstrictive (α_1) effect (to maintain blood pressure) is blocked by the drug and the failure of this response causes the sympathetic system to be further activated and to release more and more transmitter. This increase in transmitter would normally be reduced by negative feedback via the α_2-autoreceptors; but these are blocked too.

The β-adrenoceptors however are not blocked and the excess transmitter released at adrenergic endings is free to act on them, causing a tachycardia that may be unpleasant. It is for this reason that nonselective α-adrenoceptor blockers are not used alone in hypertension.

An α_1-adrenoceptor blocker that spares the α_2-receptor so that negative feedback inhibition of noradrenaline release is maintained, is more useful in hypertension (less tachycardia and postural and exercise hypotension); prazosin is such a drug (below).

For use in prostatic hypertrophy, see page 548.

Uses of α-adrenoceptor blocking drugs

- Hypertension
  — essential: doxazosin, labetalol
  — phaeochromocytoma: phenoxybenzamine; phentolamine (for crises)
- Peripheral vascular disease
- Benign prostatic hypertrophy (to relax capsular smooth muscle that may contribute to urinary obstruction)

Adverse effects. The converse of the benefit in the treatment of prostatism is the adverse effect of micturition incontinence in women. Other adverse effects of α-adrenoceptor blockade are postural hypotension, nasal stuffiness, red sclerae and, in the male, failure of ejaculation. Effects peculiar to each drug are mentioned below.

Notes on individual drugs

Prazosin blocks postsynaptic α_1-receptors but not presynaptic α_2-autoreceptors. It has a curious adverse 'first-dose effect'; within 2 h of the first (rarely after another) dose there may be a brisk hypotension sufficient to cause loss of consciousness. Hence the first dose should be small (0.5 mg) and given before going to bed. This side effect together with a rather short duration of action ($t\frac{1}{2}$ 3 h) has meant that newer longer-acting drugs have largely replaced it.

Doxazosin ($t\frac{1}{2}$ 8 h) was the first α-adrenoceptor blocker suitable for once daily prescribing. The first dose effect is also much less marked, although it is still advisable to start patients at a lower dose than is intended for maintenance. It is convenient, for instance, to prescribe 1 mg daily, increasing after 1 week to twice this dose without repeating the blood pressure measurement at this stage. A slow-release formulation, Cardura XL, can be started at the maintenance dose of 4 mg daily.

Other α blockers are *alfuzosin* and *terazosin*.

Indoramin is an older α_1-blocker, which is a less useful antihypertensive, but still used for prostatic symptoms.[17] It is taken twice or thrice daily.

Phentolamine is a nonselective α-adrenoceptor blocker. It is given i.v. for brief effect in adrenergic hypertensive crises, e.g. phaeochromocytoma or the MAOI-sympathomimetic interaction. In addition to α-receptor block it has direct vasodilator and cardiac inotropic actions. The dose for hypertensive crisis is 2–5 mg i.v. repeated as necessary (in minutes to hours). The use of phentolamine as a diagnostic test for phaeochromocytoma is appropriate only when biochemical measurements are impracticable, since it is less reliable.

Phenoxybenzamine is an irreversible nonselective α-adrenoceptor blocking drug whose effects may last 2 days or longer. The daily dose must therefore be increased slowly. It is impossible to reverse the circulatory effects by secreting noradrenaline (nor-epinephrine) or other sympathomimetic drugs because its effects are insurmountable. This makes it the preferred α-blocker for treating phaeochromocytoma (see p. 495).

It is wise to observe the effects of a single test dose closely before starting regular administration.

Indigestion and nausea can occur with oral therapy, which is best given with food.

Thymoxamine (moxisylyte) is a nonselective α-blocker for which Raynaud's phenomenon is the only extant indication.

Labetalol has both α- and β-receptor blocking actions that are due to different isomers (see under β-adrenoceptor block, below). Its parenteral preparation is valuable in the treatment of hypertension emergencies (see p. 491).

Ergot alkaloids. The naturally occurring alkaloids with effective α-adrenoceptor blocking actions are also powerful α-adrenoceptor agonists, i.e. they are

---

[17] It can be the reflex sympathetic activation, as much as hypotension itself, which causes problems. Many cardiologists have had their efforts at controlling angina in elderly patients sabotaged when the patient visits a urologist for his prostatic symptoms, and is treated with one of the newer, more powerful α_1-blockers.

partial agonists; the latter action obscures the vasodilatation that is characteristic of α-adrenoceptor blocking drugs.

Chlorpromazine has many actions of which α-adrenoceptor block is a minor one, but sufficient to cause hypotension, and to be clinically useful in amphetamine overdose.

β-ADRENOCEPTOR BLOCKING DRUGS

Actions

These drugs selectively block the β-adrenoceptor effects of noradrenaline (norepinephrine) and adrenaline (epinephrine). They may be pure antagonists or may have some agonist activity in addition (when they are described as *partial* agonists).

Intrinsic heart rate. Sympathetic activity (through $β_1$-adrenoceptors) accelerates, and parasympathetic activity (through muscarinic M_2-receptors) slows the heart. If the sympathetic and the parasympathetic drives to the heart are simultaneously and adequately blocked by a β-adrenoceptor blocker plus atropine, the heart will beat at its 'intrinsic' rate. The intrinsic rate at rest is usually about 100/min, as opposed to the usual rate of 80/min, i.e. normally there is parasympathetic vagal dominance, which decreases with age.

The *cardiovascular* effects of β-adrenoceptor block depend on the amount of sympathetic tone present. The chief *cardiac* effects result from reduction of sympathetic drive:

- Reduced automaticity (heart rate)
- Reduced myocardial contractility (rate of rise of pressure in the ventricle)
- Reduced renin secretion from the juxtaglomerular apparatus in the renal cortex.

With reduced rate the cardiac output/min is reduced and the overall cardiac oxygen consumption falls. The results are more evident on the response to exercise than at rest. With acute administration of a pure β-adrenoceptor blocker (i.e. one without any instrinsic sympathomimetic activity, ISA), *peripheral vascular resistance* tends to rise. This is probably a reflex response to the reduced cardiac output, but also because the α-adrenoceptor (vaso-

constrictor) effects are no longer partially opposed by $β_2$-adrenoceptor (dilator) effects; *peripheral flow* is reduced. With chronic use peripheral resistance returns to about pretreatment levels or a little below, varying according to presence or absence of ISA. But peripheral blood flow remains reduced. The cold extremities that accompany chronic therapy are probably due chiefly to reduced cardiac output with reduced peripheral blood flow, rather than to the blocking of peripheral ($β_2$) dilator receptors.

Hepatic blood flow may be reduced by as much as 30% which prolongs the $t\frac{1}{2}$ of the lipid-soluble members whose metabolism is dependent on hepatic flow (i.e. whose first-pass metabolism is extensive and actually dependent on the rate of delivery of blood to the liver), including propranolol itself; also lignocaine (lidocaine), which is liable to be used concomitantly for cardiac arrhythmias.

Effects

Within hours of starting treatment with a β-blocker, *blood pressure* starts to fall. The mechanism(s) remain uncertain, and the consistency of antihypertensive response in many different types of hypertension may reflect a contribution from a variety of mechanisms. β-blockers are most effective in patients who respond also to ACE inhibitors; blockade of renin secretion is likely therefore to be the main cause of blood pressure reduction. An additional contributor may be the 2–3-fold increase in natriuretic peptide secretion caused by β-blockade.

Most of the blood pressure effect occurs quickly (hours, days) but there is often a modest further decrease over several weeks.

A substantial advantage of β-blockade in hypertension is that physiological stresses such as *exercise, upright posture* and *high environmental temperature* are not accompanied by hypotension, as they are with agents that interfere with α-adrenoceptor-mediated homeostatic mechanisms. With β-blockade these necessary adaptive α-receptor constrictor mechanisms remain intact.

At first sight the *cardiac effects* might seem likely to be disadvantageous rather than advantageous, and indeed maximum exercise capacity is reduced. But the heart has substantial functional reserves so that use may be made of the desired properties in the diseases listed below, e.g. angina, without inducing heart failure. Indeed, β-blockade is now becoming routine practice in patients with established mild-to-moderate heart failure. But heart failure due to the drug does occur in patients with seriously diminished cardiac reserve.

Effect on plasma potassium concentration, see page 517.

β-Adrenoceptor selectivity

Some β-adrenoceptor blockers have higher affinity for cardiac β_1-receptors than for cardiac and peripheral β_2-receptors (see Table 23.1). The ratio of the amount of drug required to block the two receptor subtypes is a measure of the *selectivity* of the drug. (See the note to Table 22.1, p. 449, regarding use of the terms *β_1 selective* and *cardioselective*.) The question is whether the differences between selective and nonselective β-blockers constitute clinical advantages. In theory β_1-blockers are less likely to cause bronchoconstriction, but in practice few available

β_1-blockers are sufficiently selective to be safely recommended in asthma. Bisoprolol and nebivolol may be exceptions that can be tried at low doses in patients with mild asthma and a strong indication for β-blockade. There are unlikely ever to be satisfactory safety data to support such use. The main practical use of β_1-selective blockade is in diabetics where β_2-receptors mediate both the symptoms of hypoglycaemia and the counter-regulatory metabolic responses that reverse the hypoglycaemia.

Some β-blockers (antagonists) also have agonist action or ISA, i.e. they are *partial agonists*. These agents cause less fall in resting heart rate than do the *pure* antagonists and as a result may be less effective in severe angina pectoris in which reduction of heart rate is particularly important. There is also less fall in cardiac output and possibly fewer patients experience unpleasantly cold extremities. Intermittent claudication, however, may be worsened by β-blockade whether or not there is partial agonist

---

TABLE 23.1   β-adrenoceptor blocking drugs: properties at therapeutic doses

	Drug	Partial agonist effect (intrinsic sympathomimetic effect)	Membrane stabilising effect (quinidine-like effect)
Division I: nonselective ($\beta_1 + \beta_2$) blockade			
Group I	oxprenolol	+	+
Group II	propranolol	–	+
Group III	pindolol	+	–
Group IV	sotalol		
	timolol	–	–
	nadolol		
Division II: β_1-('cardio')[1]-selective blockade[2]			
Group I	acebutolol	+	+
Group III	esmolol	+	+
Group IV	atenolol		
	bisoprolol	–	–
	metoprolol		
	nebivolol		
	betaxolol		
	celiprolol[3]		
Division III: nonselective β-blockade + α_1-blockade			
Group II	carvedilol	–	+
Group IV	labetalol[3]	–	–

[1] See Table 22.1, page 449 regarding use of the term cardioselective. Note: hybrid agents having β-receptor block plus vasodilatation unrelated to adrenoceptor have been developed, e.g. nebivolol releases nitric oxide.
[2] β_1-selective drugs are considered to be up to 300 times (nebivolol) as effective against β_1-receptors than β_2-receptors. What selectivity really means, however, is that 300 times more of the blocker is required to achieve the same blockade of the β_2-receptor as of the β_1-receptor. Therefore, as the dose (concentration at receptors) rises the benefit of selectivity is gradually lost.
[3] Celiprolol and labetalol both have partial β_2-selective agonist activity.

effect. Both classes of drug can precipitate heart failure and indeed no important difference is to be expected since patients with heart failure already have high sympathetic drive (but note that β-blockade can be used to treat cardiac failure, p. 477, 517).

Abrupt withdrawal may be less likely to lead to a rebound effect if there is some partial agonist action, since there may be less up-regulation of receptors, such as occurs with prolonged receptor block.

Some β-blockers have *membrane stabilising* (quinidine-like or local anaesthetic) effect. This property is clinically insignificant except that agents having this effect will anaesthetise the eye (undesirable) if applied topically for glaucoma (timolol is used in the eye and does not have this action), and in overdose.

The *ankle jerk relaxation time* is prolonged by $β_2$-adrenoceptor block, which may be misleading if the reflex is being relied on in diagnosis and management of hypothyroidism.

Pharmacokinetics

The plasma concentration of a β-adrenoceptor blocker may have a complex relationship with its effect, for several reasons. *First-order kinetics* usually apply to elimination of drug from plasma, but the decline in receptor block is *zero-order*. The practical application is important: within 4 h of giving propranolol 20 mg i.v. the plasma concentration falls by 50%, but the receptor block (as measured by exercise-induced tachycardia) falls by only 35%. The relationship between the concentration of the parent drug in plasma and its effect is further obscured if pharmacologically active metabolites are also present. Additionally, for some of the lipid-soluble β-blockers, especially timolol, plasma $t\frac{1}{2}$ may not reflect the duration of β-blockade since the drug remains bound to the tissues near the receptor when the plasma concentration is negligible.

Most β-adrenoceptor blockers can be given orally once daily in either ordinary or sustained-release formulations because the $t\frac{1}{2}$ of pharmacodynamic effect exceeds the elimination $t\frac{1}{2}$ of the parent substance in the blood.

Lipid-soluble agents are extensively metabolised (hydroxylated, conjugated) to water-soluble substances that can be eliminated by the kidney. Plasma concentrations of drugs subject to extensive hepatic first-pass metabolism vary greatly between subjects (up to 20-fold) because the process itself is dependent on two highly variable factors: speed of absorption and hepatic blood flow, with latter being the rate-limiting factor.

Lipid-soluble agents readily cross cell membranes and so have a high apparent volume of distribution. They also readily enter the central nervous system, e.g. propranolol reaches concentrations in the brain 20 times those of the water-soluble atenolol.

Water-soluble agents show more predictable plasma concentrations because they are less subject to liver metabolism, being excreted unchanged by the kidney; thus their half-lives are greatly prolonged in renal failure, e.g. atenolol $t\frac{1}{2}$ is increased from 7 to 24 h. Patients with renal disease are best not given drugs (of any kind) having a long $t\frac{1}{2}$ and an action terminated by renal elimination. Water-soluble agents are less widely distributed and may have a lower incidence of effects attributed to penetration of the central nervous system, e.g. nightmares.

- The most lipid-soluble agents are propranolol, metoprolol, oxprenolol, labetalol
- The least lipid-soluble (water-soluble) agents are atenolol, sotalol, nadolol
- Others are intermediate.

Classification of β-adrenoceptor blocking drugs

- *Pharmacokinetic:* lipid-soluble, water-soluble, see above.
- *Pharmacodynamic* (Table 23.1). The associated properties (partial agonist action and membrane stabilising action) have only minor clinical importance with current drugs at doses ordinarily used and may be insignificant in most cases. But it is desirable that they be known, for they can sometimes matter and they may foreshadow future developments.

β-adrenoceptor blockers[18] not listed in Table 23.1 include:

---

[18] More than 40 are available worldwide.

- *nonselective* carteolol, bufuralol
- *β_1-receptor selective:* betaxolol, esmolol (ultra-short acting: minutes)
- *β- and α-receptor block:* bucindolol.

Uses of β-adrenoceptor blocking drugs

Cardiovascular uses *Angina pectoris* (β-blockade reduces cardiac work and oxygen consumption).

Hypertension (β-blockade reduces renin secretion and cardiac output): there is little interference with homeostatic reflexes.

Cardiac tachyarrhythmias: β-blockade reduces drive to cardiac pacemakers: subsidiary properties (see Table 24.1) may also be relevant.

Myocardial infarction and β-adrenoceptor blockers. There are two modes of use that reduce acute mortality and prevent recurrence: the so-called 'cardioprotective' effect.

- *Early use* within 6 hours (or at most 12 h) of onset (i.v. for 24 h then oral for 3–4 weeks). Benefit has been demonstrated only for atenolol. Cardiac work is reduced, resulting in a reduction in infarct size by up to 25% and protection against cardiac rupture. Surprisingly, tachyarrhythmias are not less frequent — perhaps because the cardiac β_2-receptor is not blocked by atenolol. Maximum benefit is in the first 24–36 h but mortality remains lower for up to one year. *Contraindications* to early use include bradycardia (< 55/min), hypotension (systolic < 90 mmHg) and left ventricular failure. A patient already taking a β-blocker may be given additional doses.
- *Late use* for secondary prevention of another myocardial infarction. The drug is started between 4 days and 4 weeks after the onset of the infarct and is continued for at least 2 years.
- *Choice of drug.* The agent should be a pure antagonist, i.e. without ISA.

Aortic dissection and after subarachnoid haemorrhage: by reducing force and speed of systolic ejection (contractility) and blood pressure.

Obstruction of ventricular outflow where sympathetic activity occurs in the presence of anatomical abnormalities, e.g. Fallot's tetralogy (cyanotic attacks):

hypertrophic subaortic stenosis (angina); some cases of mitral valve disease.

Hepatic portal hypertension and oesophageal variceal bleeding: reduction of portal pressure (see p. 656).

Cardiac failure (See also chapter 25). There is now clear evidence from prospective trials that β-blockade is beneficial in terms of mortality for patients with all grades of moderate heart failure. Data support the use of both nonselective (carvedilol, α-blocker as well) and β_1-selective (metoprolol and bisoprolol) agents. The survival benefit exceeds that provided by ACE inhibitors over placebo. The negative inotropic effects can still be significant, so the starting dose is low (e.g. bisoprolol 1.25 mg p.o. or carvedilol 3.625 mg b.d.) and may be tolerated only with additional anti-failure therapy e.g. diuretic.

Endocrine uses *Hyperthyroidism:* β-blockade reduces unpleasant symptoms of sympathetic overactivity; there may also be an effect on metabolism of thyroxine (peripheral deiodination from T_4 to T_3. A nonselective agent (propranolol) is preferred to counteract both the cardiac (β_1 and β_2) effects, and tremor (β_2).

Phaeochromocytoma: blockade of β-agonist effects of circulating catecholamines *always in combination* with adequate α-adrenoceptor block. Only small doses of a β-blocker are required.

Other uses

- Central nervous system
  Anxiety with somatic symptoms (nonselective β-blockade may be more effective than β_1-selective).
  Migraine prophylaxis.
  Essential tremor, some cases.
  Alcohol and *opioid* acute *withdrawal* symptoms.
- Eyes
  Glaucoma: (carteolol, betaxolol, levobunolol and timolol eye drops) act by altering production and outflow of aqueous humour.

Adverse reactions due to β-adrenoceptor blockade

Bronchoconstriction (β_2-receptor) occurs as expected, especially in patients with asthma (in whom even eye drops can be **fatal**).[19] In elderly chronic bronchitics there may be gradually increasing broncho-constriction over weeks (even with eye drops). Plainly risk is greater with nonselective agents, but β_1-receptor selective members are not β_1-selective and may precipitate asthma.

Cardiac failure may arise if cardiac output is dependent on high sympathetic drive (but β-blockade can be introduced at very low dose to *treat* cardiac failure (above). The degree of heart block may be made dangerously worse.

Incapacity for vigorous exercise due to failure of the cardiovascular system to respond to sympathetic drive.

Hypotension when the drug is given after myo-cardial infarction.

Hypertension may occur whenever blockade of β-receptors allows pre-existing α-effects to be un-opposed, e.g. phaeochromocytoma.

Reduced peripheral blood flow, especially with non-selective members, leading to cold extremities which, rarely, can be severe enough to cause necrosis; inter-mittent claudication may be worsened.

Reduced blood flow to liver and kidneys, reducing metabolism and biliary elimination of drugs, is liable to be important if there is hepatic or renal disease.

Hypoglycaemia, especially with nonselective mem-bers, which block β_2-receptors, and especially in diabetes and after substantial exercise, due to impair-ment of the normal sympathetic-mediated homeo-static mechanism for maintaining the blood glucose, i.e. recovery from iatrogenic hypoglycaemia is delayed. But since α-adrenoceptors are not blocked, hypertension (which may be severe) can occur as the sympathetic system discharges in an 'attempt' to reverse the hypoglycaemia. In addition, the symptoms of hypoglycaemia, in so far as they are mediated by the sympathetic (anxiety, palpitations), will not occur (though cholinergic sweating will) and the patient may miss the warning symptoms of hypoglycaemia and slip into coma. β_1-selective drugs are preferred in diabetes.

Plasma lipoproteins: HDL-cholesterol falls and triglycerides rise during chronic β-blockade with nonselective agents. β_1-selective agents have much less impact overall. Patients with hyperlipidaemia needing a β-blocker should generally receive a β_1-selective one.

Sexual function: interference is unusual and generally not supported in placebo-controlled trials.

Abrupt withdrawal of therapy can be dangerous in angina pectoris and after myocardial infarction and withdrawal should be gradual, e.g. reduce to a low dose and continue this for a few days. The existence and cause of a β-blocker withdrawal phenomenon is debated, but probably occurs due to up-regulation of β_2-receptors. It is particularly inadvisable to initiate an α-blocker at the same time as withdrawing a β-blocker in patients with ischaemic heart disease, since the β-blocker causes reflex activation of the sympathetic system. The β-blocker withdrawal phenomenon appears to be least common with partial agonists and most com-mon with β_1-selective antagonists. Rebound hyper-tension is insignificant.

Adverse reactions not certainly due to β-adrenoceptor blockade

These include loss of general wellbeing, tired legs, fatigue, depression, sleep disturbances including insomnia, dreaming, feelings of weakness, gut upsets, rashes.

Oculomucocutaneous syndrome occurred with chronic use of practolol (now obsolete) and even occasionally after cessation of use.[20] Other members either do not cause it, or so rarely do so that they are under suspicion only and, properly prescribed, the benefits of their use far outweigh such a very low risk. The mechanism of the syndrome is uncertain.

---

[19] A 36-year-old patient with asthma collected from a pharmacy, chlorphenamine for herself and oxprenolol for a friend. She took a tablet of oxprenolol by mistake. Wheezing began in one hour and worsened rapidly; she experienced a convulsion, respiratory arrest and ventricular fibrillation. She was treated with positive-pressure ventilation (for 11 h) and i.v. salbutamol, aminophylline and hydrocortisone. She survived (Williams I P et al 1980 Thorax 35: 160). There is a logical — or rather *pharmac*ological — link between the use of timolol as eye drops and the risk of asthma. For local administration, a drug needs high potency, meaning that half the maximal response is achieved with a physically small (and therefore locally administrable) amount of drug. The principal determinant of potency of a receptor antagonist is its affinity for the receptor, which in turn reflects how long each molecule remains bound to the receptor — technically, the dissociation rate constant. This is why one drop of timolol down the lacrimal duct (of the wrong patient) can kill!

Overdose

Overdose, including self-poisoning, causes brady-cardia, heart block, hypotension and low output cardiac failure that can proceed to cardiogenic shock; death is more likely with agents having membrane stabilising action (see Table 23.1). Bronchoconstriction can be severe, even fatal, in patients subject to any bronchospastic disease; loss of consciousness may occur with lipid-soluble agents that penetrate the central nervous system. Receptor blockade will outlast the persistence of the drug in the plasma.

Rational treatment includes:

- *Atropine* (1–2 mg i.v. as 1 or 2 bolus doses) to eliminate the unopposed vagal activity that contributes to bradycardia. Most patients will also require direct cardiac pacing.

---

[20] Practolol was developed to the highest current scientific standards; it was marketed (1970) as the first cardioselective β-blocker and only after independent review by the UK drug regulatory body. All seemed to go well for about 4 years (though skin rashes were observed) by which time there had accumulated about 200 000 patient years of experience with the drug, and then, wrote the then Research Director of the industrial developer, 'came a bolt from the blue and we learnt that it could produce in a small proportion of patients a most bizarre syndrome, which could embrace the skin, eyes, inner ear, and the peritoneal cavity' and also the lung (oculomucocutaneous syndrome). The cause is likely to be an immunological process to which a small minority of patients are prone, 'with present knowledge we cannot say it will not happen again with another drug'. That the drug caused this peculiar syndrome was recognised by an alert opthalmologist who ran a special clinic for external eye diseases. In 1974 he suddenly became aware that he was seeing patients complaining of dry eyes but with unusual features. Instead of the damage (blood vessel changes with metaplasia and keratinisation of the conjunctive) being on the front of the eye exposed by the open lids, it was initially in the areas behind and protected by the lids. He noted that these patients were all taking practolol. Quite soon the whole syndrome was defined, as above. Some patients became blind and some required surgery for the peritoneal disorder and a few died as a consequence.

The drug was first restricted to brief use by injection in emergency control of disorders of heart rhythm, but is now obsolete even for that.

The developers acknowledged moral (though not legal) liability for the harm done and paid compensation to affected patients. They were not negligent because current science did not provide a possibility of predicting the effect, i.e. 'state of the art defence' applied. The law did not provide for strict liability or no-fault compensation (see p. 10).

- *Glucagon,* which has cardiac inotropic and chronotropic actions independent of the β-adrenoceptor (dose 50–150 micrograms/kg in glucose 5% i.v., repeated if necessary) to be used at the outset in severe cases (an unlicenced indication).
- If there is no response, i.v. injection or infusion of a β-adrenoceptor agonist is used, e.g. isoprenaline (4 micrograms/min, increasing at 1–3-min intervals until the heart rate is 50–70 beats/min).
- In severe poisoning the dose may need to be high and prolonged to surmount the competitive block.[21]
- Other sympathomimetics may be used as judgement counsels, according to the desired receptor agonist actions (β_1, β_2, α) required by the clinical condition, e.g. dobutamine, dopamine, dopexamine, noradrenaline, adrenaline.
- For bronchoconstriction, salbutamol may be used; aminophylline has nonadrenergic cardiac inotropic and bronchodilator actions and should be given i.v. very slowly to avoid precipitating hypotension.

Treatment may be needed for days. With prompt treatment death is unusual.

Interactions

Pharmacokinetic. Agents metabolised in the liver provide higher plasma concentrations when another drug that inhibits hepatic metabolism, e.g. cimetidine, is added. Enzyme inducers enhance the metabolism of this class of β-blockers. β-adrenoceptor blockers themselves reduce hepatic blood flow (fall in cardiac output) and reduce the metabolism of β-blockers and other drugs whose metabolic elimination is dependent on the rate of delivery to the liver, e.g. lignocaine (lidocaine), chlorpromazine.

Pharmacodynamic. The effect on the blood pressure of sympathomimetics having both α- and β-receptor agonist actions is increased by block of β-

---

[21] For example, 115 mg of isoprenaline i.v. were infused over 65 h to treat one case. Lagerfelt J et al 1976 Acta Medica Scandinavica 199: 517.

receptors leaving the α-receptor vasoconstriction unopposed (adrenaline added to local anaesthetics may cause hypertension); the pressor effect of abrupt clonidine withdrawal is enhanced, probably by this action. Other cardiac antiarrhythmic drugs are potentiated, e.g. hypotension, bradycardia, heart block. Combination with verapamil (i.v.) is hazardous in the presence of atrioventricular nodal or left ventricular dysfunction because the latter has stronger negative inotropic and chronotropic effects than do other calcium channel blockers.

Most NSAIDs attenuate the antihypertensive effect of β-blockers (but not perhaps of atenolol), presumably due to inhibition of formation of renal vasodilator prostaglandins, leading to sodium retention.

β-adrenoceptor blockers potentiate the effect of other antihypertensive particularly when an increase in heart rate is part of the homeostatic response (Ca-channel blockers and α-adrenoceptor blockers).

Non-selective β-receptor blockers potentiate hypoglycaemia of insulin and sulphonylureas.

Pregnancy

β-adrenoceptor blocking agents are used in hypertension of pregnancy, including pre-eclampsia. Both lipid- and water-soluble members enter the fetus and may cause neonatal bradycardia and hypoglycaemia. They are not teratogenic in pregnancy.

Notes on some individual β-adrenoceptor blockers

(For general pharmacokinetics, see p. 476)

Propranolol is available in standard (b.d. or t.i.d.) and sustained-release (once daily) formulations. When given i.v. (1 mg/min over 1 min, repeated every 2 min up to 10 mg) for cardiac arrhythmia or thyrotoxicosis it should be preceded by atropine (1–2 mg i.v.) to prevent excessive bradycardia; hypotension may occur.

Atenolol has a $\beta_1:\beta_2$ selectivity of 1:15. It is widely used for angina pectoris and hypertension, in a dose of 25–100 mg orally once a day. The tendency in the past has been to use higher than necessary doses. When introduced, atenolol was considered not to need dose-ranging, unlike propranolol, but this was in part because the initial dose was already at the top of the dose–response curve. Some 90% of absorbed drug is excreted by the kidney and the dose should be reduced when renal function is impaired, e.g. to 50 mg/day when the glomerular filtration rate is 15–35 ml/min. The $t\frac{1}{2}$ is 7 h.

Bisoprolol is more β_1-selective than atenolol (ratio 1:50). Although a relatively lipid-soluble agent, its $t\frac{1}{2}$ is one of the longest (11 h), and there is not the wide range of dose-requirement seen with propranolol. As with atenolol, it is worth starting at a low dose (5 mg), to avoid causing unnecessary tiredness, and especially when trying to obtain the maximum benefit of its selectivity. There is no need to alter doses when renal or hepatic function is reduced.

Nebivolol resembles bisoprolol in terms of lipophilicity and $t\frac{1}{2}$ (10 h) but is more β_1-selective (ratio 1:300). Its unique feature is a direct vasodilator action (due to the d-isomer of the racemate, the l-isomer being the β_1-antagonist). The mechanism appears to be through direct activation of nitric oxide production by vascular endothelium.

Combined β_1- and α-adrenoceptor blocking drug

Labetalol is a racemic mixture, one isomer is a β-adrenoceptor blocker (nonselective), another blocks α-adrenoceptors; its dual effect on blood vessels minimises the vasoconstriction characteristic of nonselective β-blockade so that for practical purposes the outcome is similar to using a β_1-selective β-blocker (see Table 23.1). It is less effective than drugs like atenolol or bisoprolol for the routine treatment of hypertension, but is useful for some specific indications.

The β-blockade is 4–10 times greater than the α-blockade, varying with dose and route of administration. Labetalol is useful as a parenterally administered drug in the emergency reduction of blood pressure. Ordinary β-blockers may lower blood pressure too slowly, in part because reflex stimulation of unblocked α-receptors opposes the fall in blood pressure. In most patients, even those with severe hypertension, a gradual reduction in blood pressure is desirable to avoid the risk of cerebral or renal hypoperfusion, but in the presence of a great vessel dissection or of fits a more rapid effect is required (below).

Postural hypotension (characteristic of α-receptor blockade) is liable to occur at the outset of therapy and if the dose is increased too rapidly. But with chronic therapy when the β-receptor component is largely responsible for the antihypertensive effect, it is not a problem.

Labetalol reduces the hypertensive response to orgasm in women.

The $t\frac{1}{2}$ is 4 h; it is extensively metabolised in the hepatic first-pass. The drug needs to be taken thrice daily in a dose of 100–400 mg t.d.s.

For emergency control of severe hypertension the most convenient regime is to initiate infusion at 1 mg/min, and titrate upwards at half-hourly intervals as required. The infusion is stopped as blood pressure control is achieved, and re-initiated as frequently as required until regular oral therapy has been successfully introduced.

Serotonin (5-HT) receptor + α-adrenoceptor blocking drugs

Ketanserin appears to act principally to block serotonin vasoconstrictor (subtype 5-HT$_2$) receptors but also has significant α-adrenoceptor blocking activity (its affinity ratio for the two receptors is 1:5). The latter explains its hypotensive action and use in Raynaud's disease. It is not available in many countries and offers no advantages over pure α-blockers such as doxazosin.

Serotonin (5-hydroxytryptamine, 5-HT) is synthesised in enterochromaffin cells, largely in the gut, and also extensively taken up into blood platelets from which it is released to have vascular effects. It has complex effects on the cardiovascular system, varying with the vascular bed and its physiological state; it generally constricts arterioles and veins and induces blood platelet aggregation; it stimulates intestinal and bronchial smooth muscle. Carcinoid tumours secrete serotonin and symptoms may be benefited by serotonin antagonists, e.g. cyproheptadine, methysergide and sometimes by octreotide (see Index). It is a neurotransmitter in the brain.

Peripheral sympathetic nerve terminal

ADRENERGIC NEURON BLOCKING DRUGS

Adrenergic neuron blocking drugs are selectively taken up into adrenergic nerve endings by the active, energy-requiring, saturable amine (noradrenaline) pump mechanism (uptake-1). They accumulate in the noradrenaline storage vesicles from which they are released in response to nerve impulses, diminishing the release of noradrenaline and so all sympathetic function. They do not adequately control supine blood pressure and are prone to interactions with other drugs affecting adrenergic function, e.g. tricyclic antidepressants and topical nasal decongestants. They are virtually obsolete in hypertension.

Guanethidine has been used to reduce intraocular pressure in open angle glaucoma and to reduce thyrotoxic eyelid retraction for cosmetic effect. Other members of the group are debrisoquine and bethanidine. Metaiodobenzylguanidine (MIBG) is used diagnostically as a radioiodinated tracer, to locate chromaffin tumours (mainly phaeochromocytoma) which accumulate drugs in this class (p. 495).

DEPLETION OF STORED TRANSMITTER (NORADRENALINE)

Reserpine is an alkaloid from plants of the genus *Rauwolfia*, used in medicine since ancient times in southern Asia, particularly for insanity; more recently, reserpine was extensively used in psychiatry but is now obsolete. Reserpine depletes adrenergic nerves of noradrenaline primarily by blocking amine storage within vesicles present in the nerve ending, so reducing stores of releasable transmitter. Its antihypertensive action is due chiefly to peripheral action, but it enters the CNS and depletes catecholamine stores there too; this explains the sedation, depression and parkinsonian (extrapyramidal) side effects that can accompany its use. The effects on catecholamine storage persist for days to weeks after it is withdrawn.

It has also had an important veterinary use in preventing the death of domestic male turkeys, which are liable to fatal hypertensive dissecting aortic aneurysms. This can cause serious economic loss. The addition of reserpine to their drinking water reduces their blood pressure and preserves their lives without noticeably moderating their natural rage as may β-adrenoceptor blockers.[22]

INHIBITION OF SYNTHESIS OF TRANSMITTER

Metirosine (α-methyl-p-tyrosine) is a competitive inhibitor of the enzyme tyrosine hydroxylase, which converts tyrosine to dopa; as dopa is further converted to noradrenaline and adrenaline they are similarly depleted by metirosine. It is used as an adjuvant (with phenoxybenzamine) to treat phaeochromocytomas that cannot be removed surgically. Catecholamine synthesis is reduced by up to 80% over 3 days. It also readily penetrates the CNS and depletes brain noradrenaline and dopamine causing reserpine-like side effects (see above). Hence, in patients whose life expectancy is threatened more by tumour invasion than by mild or moderate hypertension, the need for the drug should be weighed carefully.

Autonomic ganglion-blocking drugs

Hexamethonium was the first orally active drug to treat hypertension. Like all agents in this group it blocks sympathetic and parasympathetic systems alike. Severe side effects have rendered them of historical interest only in hypertension therapy.[23]

---

[22] Conference on use of tranquillising agent Serpasil in animal and poultry production 1959 College of Agriculture, Rutgers State University, USA. Wild turkeys have a blood pressure of 120/60 mmHg, but domestic turkeys are hypertensive (204/144 mmHg). Digoxin increases the incidence of aneurysm. It seems that it is the rate of rise of pressure in the aorta that is important in this disease (probably in man also) and that reserpine and β-adrenoceptor blockers benefit by attenuating this.

Trimetaphan, a short-acting agent (given by i.v. infusion, initially at 3–4 mg/min), also has direct vasodilator effect; it is used for producing hypotension to provide a blood-free field during surgery, and can be used for emergency control of hypertension; pressure may be adjusted by tilting the body; it provides 'minute-to-minute' control, when the lack of selectivity is important.

Histamine release during infusion is occasionally a problem.

Central nervous system

α2-ADRENOCEPTOR AGONISTS

Clonidine (Catapres) is an imidazoline which is an agonist to α2-adrenoceptors (postsynaptic) in the brain, stimulation of which suppresses sympathetic outflow and reduces blood pressure. At high doses it also activates peripheral α2-adrenoceptors (presynaptic autoreceptors) on the adrenergic nerve ending; these mediate negative feedback suppression of noradrenaline release. In overdose clonidine can stimulate peripheral α1-adrenoceptors (postsynaptic) and thus cause *hypertension* by vasoconstriction. Clonidine was discovered to be hypotensive, not by the pharmacologists who tested it in the laboratory but by a physician who used it on himself as nose drops for a common cold.[24] The t$\frac{1}{2}$ is 6 h.

Clonidine reduces blood pressure with little postural or exercise related drop. Its most serious handicap is that abrupt or even gradual withdrawal causes rebound hypertension. This is characterised by plasma catecholamine concentrations as high as those seen in hypertensive attacks of phaeochromocytoma. The onset may be rapid (a few hours) or delayed for as long as 2 days; it subsides over 2–3 days. The treatment is either to reinstitute clonidine, i.m. if necessary, or to treat as for a phaeochromocytoma. Clonidine should never be used with a β-adrenoceptor blocker which exacerbates withdrawal hypertension (see phaeochromocytoma). Common

---

[23] Page L H 1981 New England Journal of Medicine 304: 1371. The eminent pharmacologist, Sir John Gaddum, also dubbed the characteristic appearance as 'hexamethonium man'.
[24] Page L H 1981 New England Journal of Medicine 304: 1371.

adverse effects include sedation and dry mouth. Tricyclic antidepressants antagonise the anti-hypertensive action and increase the rebound hypertension of abrupt withdrawal. *Low dose clonidine* (Dixarit, 50–100 microgram/d) also has a minor role in migraine prophylaxis, menopausal flushing and choreas.

Rebound hypertension is a less important problem with longer-acting imidazolines, since omission of a single dose will not trigger the rebound. Such drugs include *moxonidine* and *rilmenidine*. These drugs are said to be selective for an imidazoline receptor, rather than α_2-receptor. However, no such receptor has been identified at the molecular level, and genetic knock-out experiments have shown that it is the α_2-receptor which is required for the blood pressure lowering action of imidazoline drugs. It is unsurprising therefore that no drug has truly succeeded in separating the sedative and hypotensive effects of this class.

FALSE TRANSMITTER

Chemotransmitters and receptors in the CNS are similar to those in the periphery, and the drug in this section also has peripheral actions, as is to be expected.

Methyldopa (Aldomet) probably acts primarily in the brain stem vasomotor centres. It is a substrate (in the same manner as L-DOPA) for the enzymes that synthesise noradrenaline. The synthesis of α-methylnoradrenaline results in tonic stimulation of CNS α_2-receptors since α-methylnoradrenaline cannot be metabolised by monoamine oxidase, and selectively stimulates the α_2-adrenoceptor. Stimulation of this receptor in the hindbrain nuclei concerned with blood pressure control results in a fall in blood pressure, i.e. methyldopa acts in the same way as clonidine. α-Methylnoradrenaline is also produced at peripheral adrenergic endings, but to a lesser extent and peripheral action is clinically insignificant.

Methyldopa is reliably absorbed from the gastrointestinal tract and readily enters the CNS. The $t\frac{1}{2}$ is 1.5 h. Adverse effects, largely expected from its mode of action, include: sedation (frequent), nightmares, depression, involuntary movements, nausea, flatulence, constipation, score or black

tongue, positive Coombs test with occasionally haemolytic anaemia, leucopenia, thrombocytopenia, hepatitis.

Gynaecomastia and lactation occur due to interference with dopaminergic suppression of prolactin secretion. Any failure of male sexual function is probably secondary to sedation. Because of its adverse effects methyldopa is no longer a drug of first choice in routine long-term management of hypertension, but remains popular with obstertricians for the hypertension of pregnancy.

Drug treatment of angina, myocardial infarction and hypertension

Angina pectoris[25]

An attack of angina pectoris[26] occurs when myocardial demand for oxygen exceeds supply from the coronary circulation.

The principal forms relevant to choice of drug therapy are angina of exercise (commonest) and its worsening form, *unstable* (preinfarction or crescendo) angina (see below), which occurs at rest. Variant (Prinzmetal) angina (very uncommon) results from spasm of a large coronary artery.

Antiangina drugs act as follows:

- Organic *nitrates* reduce *preload* and *afterload* and dilate the main coronary arteries (rather than the arterioles).
- *β-adrenoceptor* blocking drugs reduce *myocardial contractility* and *slow* the heart rate. They may increase coronary artery spasm in variant angina
- *Calcium-channel* blocking drugs *reduce cardiac contractility*, *dilate* the coronary arteries (where

---

[25] Angina pectoris: *angina*, a strangling; *pectoris*, of the chest.
[26] For a personal account by a physician of his experiences of angina pectoris, coronary bypass surgery, ventricular fibrillation and recovery, see Swyer G I M 1986 British Medical Journal 292: 337. Compelling and essential reading.

there is evidence of spasm) and *reduce afterload* (dilate peripheral arterioles).

These classes of drug complement each other and can be used together. The combined nitrate and potassium-channel activator, *nicorandil,* is an alternative when any of the other drugs is contraindicated.

SUMMARY OF TREATMENT

- Any contributory cause is treated when possible, e.g. anaemia, arrhythmia.
- Life style is changed so as to reduce the number of attacks. Weight reduction can be very helpful; stop smoking.
- For immediate pre-exertional prophylaxis: *glyceryl trinitrate* sublingually or *nifedipine* (bite the capsule and hold the liquid in the mouth or swallow it).
- For an acute attack: *glyceryl trinitrate* (sublingual) or *nifedipine* (bite capsule, as above).

For long-term prophylaxis:

- A β_1-adrenoceptor blocking drug, e.g. bisoprolol, given continuously (not merely when an attack is expected). Dosage is adjusted by response. Some put an arbitrary upper limit to dose, but others recommend that if complete relief is not obtained the dose should be raised to the maximum tolerated, provided the resting heart rate is not reduced below 55/min; or raise the dose to a level at which an increase causes no further inhibition of exercise tachycardia. In severe angina a pure antagonist, i.e. an agent lacking partial agonist activity, is preferred, since the latter may not slow the heart sufficiently. Warn the patient of the risk of abrupt withdrawal.
- A *calcium-channel blocking* drug, e.g. nifedipine or diltiazem, is an alternative to a β-adrenoceptor blocker: use especially if coronary spasm is suspected or if the patient has myocardial insufficiency or any bronchospastic disease. It can also be used with a β-blocker, or
- A *long-acting nitrate,* isosorbide dinitrate or mononitrate: use so as to avoid tolerance (p. 463).
- *Nicorandil,* a long-acting potassium-channel activator: this does not cause tolerance like the nitrates.

- Drug therapy may be adapted to the time of attacks, e.g. nocturnal (transdermal glyceryl trinitrate, or isosorbide mononitrate orally at night).
- Antiplatelet therapy (aspirin or clopidogrel) reduces the incidence of fatal and of nonfatal myocardial infarction in patients with unstable angina, used alone or with low-dose heparin.
- Surgical revascularisation in selected cases.

In treating angina, it is important to remember not only the objective of reducing symptoms but also that of preventing complications, particularly myocardial infarction and sudden death. This requires vigorous treatment of all risk factors (hypertension, hyperlipidaemia, diabetes mellitus) and, of course, cessation of smoking. There is little evidence that the symptomatic treatments, medical or surgical, themselves affect outcome except in patients with stenosis of the main stem of the left coronary artery, who require surgical inter- vention. Although aspirin has not specifically been studied in patients with stable angina, it is now reasonable to extrapolate from the studies of aspirin in other patient groups.

Myocardial infarction (MI)

(See also Ch. 28)

AN OVERVIEW

The *acute coronary syndromes* (ACS) are now classified on the basis of the ECG and plasma troponin measurements into (1) patients with ST elevation myocardial infarction (STEMI), (2) non-ST elevation myocardial infarction (non-STEMI, by ECG and a positive troponin test) and (3) unstable angina (by ECG and negative troponin test). The present account recognises that this is a rapidly evolving field, but therapeutic strategies are likely to evolve according to these forms of ACS.

A general practitioner or paramedic can appro- priately administer the initial treatment before a definite diagnosis is established or the patient reaches hospital, namely:

- morphine or diamorphine (2.5 or 5 mg *intravenously,* because of the certainty of haematoma formation when intramuscular injections are followed by thrombolytic therapy)

- aspirin 150–300 mg orally
- 60% oxygen.

The immediate objectives are relief of pain and initiation of treatment demonstrated to reduce mortality. Subsequent management of proven myocardial infarction is concerned with treatment of complications, *arrhythmias, heart failure* and *thromboemboli,* and then secondary prevention of further myocardial infarctions.

When STEMI is diagnosed, instituting myocardial reperfusion as early as possible provides the greatest benefit. Most commonly, the basis of this is *thrombolysis* (although its benefit will be increasingly compared with angioplasty, with or without stenting). This is initiated following arrival at hospital, preferably directly to the coronary care unit to avoid further delays, and provided there are no contraindications to thrombolysis (see below). Patients with non-STEMI may still benefit, especially those with left bundle branch block. Several trials have shown that patients without ECG changes (or with ST depression), and patients with unstable angina, benefit only slightly if at all from thrombolytic therapy.

The choice of thrombolytic is in most places dictated by (1) a wealth of comparative outcome data from well designed trials and (2) relative costs. For a first infarct, patients should receive *streptokinase* 1 500 000 units infused over 1 h, unless they are in cardiogenic shock. For subsequent infarcts, the presence of antistreptokinase antibodies dictates the use of the recombinant tissue plasminogen activator (rt-PA) *alteplase* (or reteplase). Human rt-TPA was one of the first naturally-occurring human proteins to be manufactured in bulk by recombinant DNA technology. Both alteplase and streptokinase bind plasminogen and convert it to plasmin, which lyses fibrin. Alteplase has a much higher affinity for plasminogen bound to fibrin than in the circulation. This selectivity does not, however, confer any therapeutic advantage as originally anticipated, since severe haemorrhage following thrombolysis is almost always due to lysis of an appropriate clot at previous sites of bleeding or trauma. Indeed, the tendency for some lysis of circulating *fibrinogen* as well as fibrin by streptokinase gives this drug some anticoagulant activity, which is lacking from alteplase, so that administration of alteplase needs to be accompanied and followed by administration of heparin (see p. 579 for further details of thrombolytics).

Principal contraindications to thrombolysis
<ul><li>Haemorrhagic diathesis</li><li>Pregnancy</li><li>Recent symptoms of peptic ulcer, or GI bleeding</li><li>Recent stroke (previous 3 months)</li><li>Recent surgery (previous 10–14 days), especially neurosurgery</li><li>Prolonged cardiopulmonary resuscitation (during current presentation)</li><li>Proliferative diabetic retinopathy</li><li>Severe, uncontrolled hypertension (DBP > 120)</li></ul>

In addition to thrombolysis and aspirin, a third treatment has been shown to reduce mortality in MI, namely β-blockade. In the ISIS-1 study,[27] atenolol 50 mg was given i.v. followed by the same dose orally. The reduction in mortality is due mainly to prevention of cardiac rupture, which appears interestingly to remain the only complication of MI that is not reduced by thrombolysis. The usual contraindications to β-blockade apply, but most patients with a first MI should be able to receive this treatment.

Other antiplatelet agents. The final common pathway to platelet aggregation and thrombus formation involves the expression of the glycoprotein IIb/IIIa receptor at the cell surface. This receptor binds fibrinogen with high affinity and can be blocked using either a specific monoclonal antibody (*abciximab*) or one of a rapidly expanding class of specific antagonists, e.g. *eptifibatide* and *tirofiban.* Another agent, *clopidogrel,* acts by inhibiting ADP-dependent platelet aggregation. It is more effective than aspirin for the prevention of ischaemic stroke or cardiovascular death in patients at high risk (see p. 582).

---

[27] Randomised trial of intravenous atenolol among 16 027 cases of suspected acute myocardial infarction: ISIS-1. First International Study of Infarct Survival Collaborative Group. Lancet 1986 2: 57–66

These drugs appear to be very useful adjuncts for the treatment of unstable angina, and in the prevention of thrombosis following percutaneous revascularisation procedures such as angioplasty and coronary artery stenting. Their role in preventing infarction in patients with acutely compromised myocardium is likely to expand rapidly.

Unstable angina requires admission to hospital, the objectives of therapy being to relieve pain, and avert progression to myocardial infarction and sudden death. Initial management is with aspirin 150–300 mg chewed or dispersed in water followed by heparin, or one of the low molecular weight preparations, e.g. dalteparin or enoxaparin. Nitrate is given preferably as isosorbide dinitrate by i.v. infusion until the patient has been pain-free for 24 h. A β-adrenoceptor blocker, e.g. metoprolol, should added orally or i.v. unless it is contraindicated, when a calcium channel blocker is substituted, e.g. diltiazem or verapamil. Patients perceived to be at high risk may also receive a glycoprotein II b/III a inhibitor, e.g. eptifibatide or tirofiban.

SECONDARY PREVENTION

(See also Ch. 28)

The best predictor of risk of a myocardial infarction is to have had previous a myocardial infarction. After the measures instituted in the first few hours, the principal objective of treatment therefore becomes prevention of future infarcts. Patients should receive advice about exercise and diet before discharge, and most enter a formal rehabilitation programme after leaving hospital. In particular, patients need to reduce saturated fat intake, and there is increasing evidence of the benefit of increased intake of fish and olive oil.

DRUGS FOR SECONDARY PREVENTION

All patients should receive *aspirin* and a *β-blocker* for at least two years, unless contraindicated. The commonest contraindication to β-blockade after MI is heart failure, although this should now be uncommon after a first MI. In such patients, an *ACE inhibitor* should replace β-blockade. All three of these drug groups have been shown to reduce the incidence of reinfarction by 20–25%, although their benefit has not been shown to be additive. In the 'SAVE' study,[28] captopril 50 mg × 3/d or placebo was started 3–16 days after a myocardial infarction in 2231 patients without overt cardiac failure but with a left ventricular ejection fraction of < 40%. The captopril group had a lower incidence of recurrent myocardial infarction (133) and deaths (228) than the placebo group (170 and 275). Similar results have been achieved in several other trials of ACE inhibitors. An exception was the CONSENSUS-II study, which found no benefit from enalapril. (In this study, large and rapid falls in BP caused by i.v. enalaprilat probably precipitated cardiovascular events in some patients.) Whereas most studies have used echo or isotope scanning to assess cardiac function, the AIRE study showed a reduction in deaths (170 vs 222) in the active group, receiving ramipril 5 mg × 2/d, started 3–10 days after a myocardial infarction in 2006 patients with only *clinical* signs of heart failure.[28] Indeed, in addition to these drugs, most patients should receive a statin, regardless of their plasma cholesterol level. Long-term benefit from LDL reduction after MI has been shown for high-dose simvastatin (20–40 mg/d) and pravastatin (40 mg/d). Patients with previous MI constituted one-third of the Heart Protection Study of 20 536 high-risk patients. Those randomly assigned to simvastatin 40 mg daily or placebo had a 12% reduction in all cause mortality, and 24% reduction in strokes and coronary heart disease.[29]

There is no place for routine antiarrhythmic prophylaxis, and long-term anticoagulation is similarly out of place, except when indicated by arrhythmias or poor left ventricular function.

---

[28] SAVE = Survival and Ventricular Enlargement Trial; AIRE = Acute Infarction Ramipril Efficacy study; CONSENSUS = Cooperative New Scandinavian Enalapril Survival Study. References: Rutherford J D et al 1994 Effects of captopril on ischemic events after myocardial infarction. Results of the Survival and Ventricular Enlargement trial. SAVE Investigators. Circulation 90: 1731–1738. AIRE Study Investigators 1993 Effect of ramipril on mortality and morbidity of survivors of acute myocardial infarction with clinical evidence of heart failure. Lancet 342: 821–828. Swedberg K P et al 1992 Effects of the early administration of enalapril on mortality in patients with acute myocardial infarction. New England Journal of Medicine 327: 678–684.

Arterial hypertension

Clinical evaluation of antihypertensive drugs seeks to answer two types of question:

1. Whether long-term reduction of blood pressure benefits the patient by preventing complications and prolonging life; these studies take years, require enormous numbers of patients and are extremely costly.
2. Whether a drug is capable of effective, safe and comfortable control of blood pressure for about one year. There is now sufficient evidence of the benefit of reducing elevated blood pressure that regulatory authorities do not demand trials of the first kind for all new drugs. Shorter studies are therefore deemed sufficient to allow the introduction of a new drug. However, such trials may not reveal the long-term consequences of some metabolic effects, e.g. on blood glucose, which may adversely affect the risk of coronary heart disease. Placebo effects are prominent in these shorter trials and must be carefully controlled in trial design.

AIM OF TREATMENT

The principal long-term aim in most patients is the prevention of stroke and myocardial infarction; reduction in the latter also requires attention to other risk factors such as smoking and plasma cholesterol. The more immediate aim of treatment is to reduce the blood pressure as near to normal as possible without causing symptomatic hypotension or otherwise impairing wellbeing (quality of life).

When this aim is achieved in *severe cases* there is great symptomatic improvement: retinopathy clears and vision improves; headaches are abolished. A variable amount of irreversible damage has often been done by the high blood pressure before treatment is started; then renal failure may progress despite treatment, left ventricular hypertrophy may not fully reverse and arterial damage leads to ischaemic events (stroke and MI).

It is obviously desirable to start treatment before irreversible changes occur and in *mild and moderately severe* cases this usually means advising treatment for symptom-free people whose hypertension was revealed by screening.

THRESHOLD AND TARGETS FOR TREATMENT

The British Hypertension Society guidelines[30] require that antihypertensive drug therapy be initiated:

- when sustained BP exceeds 160/100 mmHg or
- when BP is in the range 140–159/90–99 mmHg and there is evidence of target organ damage, cardiovascular disease or a 10-year CHD risk over 15% or
- for diabetics when BP exceeds 140/90 mmHg.

The optimal target is to lower BP to or below 140/85 mmHg in nondiabetics and 140/80 mmHg in diabetics. The World Health Organization/International Society for Hypertension sets a more rigorous target of 130/85 mmHg.

Effective treatment reduces the risk of all complications: strokes and myocardial infarction, but also heart failure, renal failure, and possibly dementia. It is easier in individual trials to demonstrate the benefits of treatment in preventing stroke, because the curve relating risk of stroke to blood pressure is almost twice as steep as that for myocardial infarction. What this tells us is *not* that the *relative risk* of myocardial infarction due to hypertension is irreversible but that substantial reduction in the *absolute risk* of myocardial infarction needs attention to hypercholesterolaemia as well as hypertension.[31]

---

[29] The authors estimated that 5 years of statin treatment will prevent 100 major vascular events in *every* 1000 patients with previous myocardial infarction, or 70–80 events in patients with other forms of coronary heart disease or diabetes. There was no upper age limit to this benefit, and no lower limit to the level of LDL at which benefit was seen. Heart Protection Study Collaborative Group 2002 MRC/BHF Heart Protection Study of cholesterol lowering with simvastatin in 20 536 high-risk individuals. Lancet 360: 7–22.

[30] The British Hypertension Society Guidelines are available in summary form in the BMJ 1999 319: 630–635 or online at http://www.bhsoc.org
[31] Relative risk refers to the increased likelihood of a patient having a complication compared to a normotensive patient of the same age and gender. Absolute risk refers to the number of patients out of 100, with the same age, gender and blood pressure, predicted to have a complication of the next 10 years.

Treatment will almost always be lifelong for essential hypertension, since discontinuation of therapy leads to prompt restoration of pretreatment blood pressures. If it does not, one should suspect the original diagnosis of hypertension, which should not be made unless blood pressure is elevated on at least three occasions over 3 months.

The *relative* risks of hypertension and the benefits of treating the condition in the elderly are less than in those under 65s, but the *absolute* risks and benefits are greater. Given the large choice of treatments available, doctors cannot cite improved quality of life as an excuse for not treating hypertension in the elderly. Starting doses, however, should often be halved and, pending further evidence, less challenging targets for blood pressure reduction may be acceptable.

It is obvious that adverse effects of therapy are important in that *very large* numbers of patients must be treated so that *a few* may gain; this is a salient feature of the use of drugs to prevent disease.

PRINCIPLES OF ANTIHYPERTENSIVE THERAPY

General measures may be sufficient to control mild cases as follows:

- Obesity: reduce it
- Alcohol: stay within recommended limits (e.g. 14 units/week for women, 21 units/week for men)
- Smoking: stop it
- Diet: of proven value for the short-term reduction in blood pressure is reduction in fat content, and increase in fruit, vegetables and fibre.[32] There is some additional benefit from reducing intake of salt: avoidance of highly salted foods, and omission of added salt from freshly prepared food.
- Relaxation therapy: worth considering for highly motivated borderline patients.

DRUG THERAPY

Blood pressure may be reduced by any one or more

[32] DASH-Sodium Collaborative Research Group 2001 Effects on Blood Pressure of Reduced Dietary Sodium and the Dietary Approaches to Stop Hypertension (DASH) Diet. N Engl J Med 344: 3–10.

of the actions listed at the beginning of this chapter (p. 46). The large number of different drug classes for hypertension reduces, paradoxically, the likelihood of a randomly selected drug being the best for an individual patient. Patients and drugs can broadly be divided into two groups depending on their renin status and drug effect on this (Fig. 23.1). Type 1, or high-renin patients, are the younger Caucasians (aged < 55), and they respond better to a β-blocker or ACE inhibitor. Other patients are type 2, or low-renin, in whom diuretics or calcium blockers are more likely to be effective as single agents.

Since each drug acts on only one or two of the blood pressure control mechanisms, the factors that are uninfluenced by monotherapy are liable to adapt (homeostatic mechanism), to oppose the useful effect and to restore the previous state. There are two principal mechanisms of such adaptation or tolerance:

1. *Increase in blood volume:* this occurs with any drug that reduces peripheral resistance (increases intravascular volume) or cardiac output (reduces glomerular flow) due to activation of the renin-angiotensin system. The result is that cardiac output and blood pressure rise. Adding a diuretic in combination with the other drug can prevent this compensatory effect.

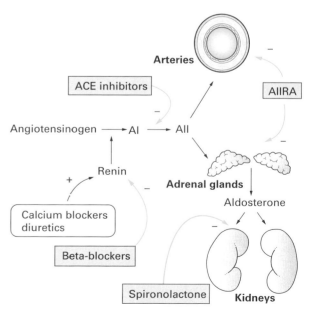

Fig. 23.1 Effects of drugs on the renin-angiotensin system (AIIRA: angiotensin II receptor antagonists)

2. *Baroreceptor reflexes:* a fall in blood pressure evokes reflex activity of the sympathetic system, causing increased peripheral resistance and cardiac activity (rate and contractility). Therefore, whenever high blood pressure is proving difficult to control and whenever a number of antihypertensives are used in combination, the drugs chosen should between them act on all three main determinants of blood pressure, namely:

- *blood volume*
- *peripheral resistance*
- *the heart.*

Such combinations will:

- maximise antihypertensive efficacy by exerting actions at three different points in the cardiovascular system;
- minimise the opposing homeostatic effects by blocking the compensatory changes in blood volume, vascular tone and cardiac function;
- minimise adverse effects by permitting smaller doses of each drug each acting at a different site and having different unwanted effects.

First-dose hypotension is now uncommon and occurs mainly with drugs having an action on veins (α-adrenoceptor blockers, ACE inhibitors) when baroreflex activation is impaired, e.g. old age or with contracted intravascular volume following diuretics.

TREATING HYPERTENSION

A simple stepped regimen in keeping with the 1999 British Hypertension Society guidelines[30] is the AB/CD schema illustrated in Figure 23.2:[33]

1. Depending on the patient's age (see above) use either a β Blocker or thiazide Diuretic as first-line therapy, unless there is a compelling reason to avoid these (e.g. asthma and gout, respectively). If the first drug is effective but not tolerated, switch to the other member of the pair: i.e. ACE inhibitor (or AIIRA) instead of β-blocker, Calcium blocker instead of diuretic.
2. If the blood pressure is not controlled in 4 weeks by the first-line drug then switch to a

drug from the other pair, e.g. a thiazide **D**iuretic should be replaced by a β-**B**locker, and vice versa.

3. If the blood pressure is still not controlled, a second agent should be added, using the opposite pair to the first drug e.g. if the patient is on an **A**CE inhibitor add a **C**alcium channel blocker or thiazide **D**iuretic (**A**+**C** or **A**+**D**), since both vasodilatation or diuresis will stimulate the renin-angiotensin system and turns nonrenin-dependent hypertension into renin-dependent hypertension). The combination **B**+**D** is associated with increased risk of diabetes and should be avoided in at-risk patients (obesity, family history). The combinations **A**+**B** or **C**+**D** usually produce a less than additive effect on blood pressure, but should be tried in patients still uncontrolled on more standard combinations.

4. If blood pressure control is still inadequate on dual therapy **A**+**C**+**D** is the ideal triple regimen.

4a. If additional therapy is required, α-blockade is effective at this stage by blocking the vasoconstrictor component of the baroreflex response to some of the other drugs. A very

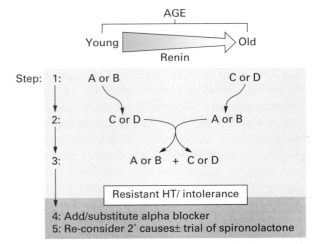

AB/CD Rule for optimisation of antihypertensive treatment

(AB/CD =ACEi, Beta-blocker/Ca⁺⁺-blocker, Diuretic)

Fig. 23.2 Scheme for escalation of anti-hypertensive therapy. A: ACE inhibitor; B: β-adrenoceptor blocker; C: calcium channel blocker; D: diuretic (see text). (From: Dickerson et al. 1999 Lancet 353: 2008–2011.)

---

[33] Dickerson J E C et al 1999 Lancet 353: 2008–2013.

small number of patients may need reversion to an older class of drug such as minoxidil (provided that a loop diuretic and β-blocker can also be given to block the severe fluid retention and tachycardia) or methyldopa.

5. Patients whose blood pressure remains substantially above target on triple therapy are likely to have aldosterone-sensitive hypertension that responds well to *spironolactone*. A particularly effective combination is spironolactone with a second generation AIIRA (e.g. *irbesartan* or *candesartan*).

Treatment and severity

A single drug may adequately treat mild hypertension. The treatment target blood pressures of <140/<85 suggested by the British Hypertension Society[30] will, however, increase the proportion of patients needing two or more drugs. The vast majority of patients with more severe hypertension should be treated by the stepped regimen (above); only rarely are there indications that a more rapid reduction in blood pressure is necessary. This is important so that the efficacy and tolerability of individual drugs can be assessed in each patient.

MONITORING

The blood pressure must be monitored by a doctor or specialist nurse (particularly important in the old) and also sometimes by the patient. 24-hour ambulatory blood pressure monitoring (ABPM) is possible with an increasing number of user-friendly, semi-automatic devices. They are too expensive to be recommended for most patients. 24-h blood pressure predicts outcome better than clinic blood pressure and is therefore useful in influencing the need for extra treatment in difficult or high-risk patients. Home monitoring is a cheaper alternative, providing the sphygmomanometer has been validated. The easy-to-use wrist monitors are unfortunately unreliable in patients receiving drug treatment.

Diuretics and potassium. The potassium-losing (kaliuretic) diuretics used in hypertension deplete body potassium by 10–15%. Potassium chloride supplements are not required routinely, but hypokalaemia will occasionally occur (and should raise suspicion of Conn's syndrome). Uncomplicated patients may not need monitoring if the lowest possible doses are used, e.g. no more than bendrofluazide (bendroflumethazide) 2.5 mg. Vulnerable patients, e.g. the elderly, should be monitored for potassium loss at 3 months and thereafter every 6–12 months. In general a potassium-retaining diuretic (amiloride) in a fixed-dose combination with a thiazide (co-amilozide) is preferred over the use of fixed-dose diuretic/KCl formulations (most supplements, typically 8 mmol of KCl, are in any case inadequate).

Control of potassium balance is particularly important if the patient is also taking digoxin (hypokalemia potentiates the action of digoxin). Because of the risk of hyperkalaemia, amiloride should usually be avoided in patients taking ACE inhibitors unless renal function is normal.

Compliance. Multidrug therapy poses a substantial problem of compliance. Since treatment will be lifelong it is well worthwhile taking the trouble to find the most convenient regimen for each individual. A single daily dose would be ideal and to achieve this sustained-release formulations and fixed-dose combinations are used. Examples include: Tenoretic (atenolol + chlortalidone), Tenif (atenolol + nifedipine) and Zestoretic (lisinopril + hydrochlorothiazide).

TREATMENT OF HYPERTENSION EMERGENCIES

It is important to distinguish three circumstances which may exist separately or together — see the Venn diagram (Figure 23.3)[34] which emphasises the following:

---

[34] J Venn (1834–1923) English logician who 'adopted the diagrammatic method of illustrating propositions by inclusive and exclusive circles' (Dictionary of National Biography). A medical pilgrimage to Cambridge, where Venn worked, should take in Gonville & Caius College (named after its founder, Dr Caius, physician to the Tudor Court and early president of the London College of Physicians in the 16th century); as well as stained glass windows celebrating Venn's circles, the visitor can see a portrait of the most famous medical Caian, William Harvey.

- *Severe hypertension* is not on its own an indication for *urgent* (or large) reductions in blood pressure.
- Blood pressure (BP) can occasionally require *urgent* (emergency) reduction even when the hypertension is not severe, especially where the BP has risen rapidly.
- *Accelerated phase* (malignant) *hypertension* rarely requires urgent reduction, and should instead be regarded as an indication for slow reduction in blood pressure during the first few days.

The indications for *emergency reduction* of blood pressure are rare. They are:

- Hypertensive encephalopathy (including eclampsia)
- Acute left ventricular failure (due to hypertension)
- Dissecting aneurysm.

In these conditions, blood pressure should be reduced over the course of an hour. In patients with a dissecting aneurysm, where the BP may have been completely normal prior to dissection, the target is a BP of 110/70 mmHg. Otherwise even small reductions will usually remove the emergency.

Accelerated phase hypertension was previously called 'malignant' hypertension because the lack of treatment heralded death within a year of diagnosis. It is characterised pathologically by fibrinoid necrosis of the small arteries. An important consequence is the loss of autoregulation of the cerebral and renal circulation, so that any reduction in blood pressure causes a proportional fall in perfusion of these organs. It is therefore vital not to reduce diastolic BP by more than 20 mmHg on the first day of treatment. To ignore this is to risk cerebral infarction.

Treatment. Unless contraindicated, the best treatment for all circles in the Venn diagram is β-*blockade*, e.g. atenolol 25 or 50 mg orally. In emergencies, a vasodilator should be given intravenously, in addition.

A theoretically preferable, but often impractical alternative is i.v. infusion of the vasodilator, nitroprusside (see p. 470). In dissecting aneurysm, vasodilators should not be used unless patients are first β-blocked since any increase in the rate of rise of the pulse stroke is undesirable. *Labetalol* provides a convenient method of treating all patients within the three circles (except asthmatics), using either oral or parenteral therapy as appropriate. It is not the most effective, however, and should be combined with a long-acting formulation of nifedipine, orally, where further blood pressure reduction is required.

Low doses of all drugs should be used if antihypertensive drugs have recently been taken or if renal function is impaired.

Oral maintenance treatment for severe hypertension should be started at once if possible; parenteral therapy is seldom necessary for more than 48 h.

PREGNANCY HYPERTENSION

Effective treatment of pregnancy-induced hypertension improves fetal and perinatal survival. There is a lack of good clinical trial evidence on which to base recommendations of one agent over another. Instead, drug usage reflects longevity of use without obvious harm to the fetus. Hence methyldopa is still the drug of choice for many obstetricians.[35] Calcium-channel blockers (especially nifedipine) are common second-line drugs; parenteral hydralazine is reserved for emergency reduction of blood pressure in late pregnancy, preferably in combination with a β-blocker to avoid unpleasant tachycardia. β-blockers (labetalol and atenolol) are often

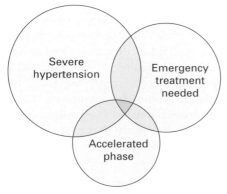

Fig. 23.3 Venn diagram illustrating intersections of three overlapping clinical states defined in the text

[35] Methyldopa: follow-up studies show no intellectual impairment in children up to age 7.5 years (for atenolol, see: Butters L 1990 British Medical Journal 301: 587).

effective and are probably the drugs of choice in the third trimester; there is anecdotal evidence to suggest growth retardation with β-blockade used in first and second trimester. Diuretics reduce the chance of developing pre-eclampsia, but are avoided in pre-eclampsia itself because these patients already have a contracted circulatory volume. ACE-inhibitors (and by implication angiotensin AT_1 receptor antagonists) are absolutely contraindicated during pregnancy, where they cause fetal death, typically mid-trimester. There is no definite evidence that ACE inhibitors — or any of the commonly used antihypertensive drugs — are teratogenic, and women who become pregnant while receiving these should be reassured but should, of course, then discontinue the ACE inhibitor or AT_1 receptor antagonist.

Raised blood pressure and proteinuria (pre-eclampsia) complicates 2–8% of pregnancies and may proceed to fitting (eclampsia), a major cause of mortality in mother and child. Magnesium sulphate halves the risk of progress to eclampsia (typically 4 g i.v. over 5–10 min followed by 1 g/hour by i.v. infusion for 24 hours after the last seizure).[36] Additionally, if a woman has one fit (treat with diazepam), then the magnesium regimen is superior to diazepam or phenytoin in preventing further fits.[37]

Aspirin, in low dose, was reported in early studies to reduce the incidence of pre-eclampsia in at-risk patients, but a more recent meta-analysis has not supported this. Consequently, it is not routinely recommended.

UNWANTED INTERACTIONS WITH ANTIHYPERTENSIVE DRUGS

Specific interactions are described in the accounts of individual drugs. The following are *general examples* for this diverse group of drugs.

Alcohol intake is the commonest contributing factor, or even cause of hypertension, and should always be considered as a cause of erratic or failed

responses to treatment (measurement of the γ-glutamyl transpeptidase and red cell mean corpuscular volume may be useful).

Prostaglandin synthesis. Nonsteroidal anti-inflammatory drugs (NSAIDs), e.g. indomethacin, attenuate the antihypertensive effect of β-adrenoceptor blockers and of diuretics, perhaps by inhibiting the synthesis of vasodilator renal prostaglandins. This effect can also be important when a diuretic is used for *severe left ventricular failure.*

Enzyme inhibition. Ciprofloxacin and cimetidine inhibit hepatic metabolism of lipid-soluble β-adrenoceptor blockers, e.g. metoprolol, labetalol, propranolol, increasing their effect. Methyldopa plus an MAO inhibitor may cause excitement and hallucinations.

Pharmacological antagonism. Sympathomimetics, e.g. amphetamine, phentolamine (present in anorectics and cold and cough remedies) may lead to loss of antihypertensive effect, and indeed to a *hypertensive reaction* when taken by a patient already on a β-adrenoceptor blocker, due to unopposed α-adrenergic stimulation.

Surgical anaesthesia may lead to a brisk fall in blood pressure in patients taking antihypertensives. Antihypertensive therapy should not be routinely altered before surgery, although it obviously can complicate care both during and after the operation. Anaesthetists must be informed.

Sexual function and cardiovascular drugs

All drugs that interfere with sympathetic autonomic activity, including diuretics, can potentially interfere with male sexual function, expressed as a failure of ejaculation or difficulty in sustaining an erection. Nevertheless, placebo-controlled trials have emphasised how common a symptom this is in the untreated male population (approaching sometimes 20–30%). It is also likely that hypertension itself is associated with an increased risk of sexual dysfunction since loss of NO production by the vascular endothelium is an early feature of the pathophysiology of this disease. Laying the blame on antihypertensive medication is probably

---

[36] The Magpie Trial Collaborative Group 2002 Lancet 359: 1877–1890.

[37] The Eclampsia Trial Collaborative Group 1995 Which anticonvulsant for women with eclampsia? Evidence from the Collaborative Eclampsia Trial. Lancet 345: 1455–1463.

incorrect in most instances, especially with drugs from newer drug categories. Calcium channel blockers, ACE inhibitors and angiotensin II (AT_1) receptor antagonists all have reported rates of sexual dysfunction that did not differ from placebos. If symptoms persist with these drugs other causes should be sought. It is important to listen to the patient but also reassure them that the drug is not necessarily to blame; sexual dysfunction as a perceived adverse drug effect is a potent cause of compliance failure. Sildenafil (Viagra) can be safely used in patients receiving any of the commonly used antihypertensive drugs.

As well as the concerns about sexual performance in treated hypertensives there may be concerns about fitness per se to attempt intercourse. The real possibility that it is hazardous is compounded often by their age and concurrent coronary artery disease.

SEXUAL INTERCOURSE AND THE CARDIOVASCULAR SYSTEM

Normal sexual intercourse with orgasm is accompanied by transient but brisk physiological changes, e.g. tachycardia of up to 180 beats/min, with increases of 100 beats/min over less than one min, can occur. Systolic blood pressure may rise by 120 mmHg and diastolic by 50 mmHg. Orgasm may be accompanied by transient pressure of 230/130 mmHg even in normotensive individuals. Electrocardiographic abnormalities may occur in healthy men and women. Respiratory rate may rise to 60/min.

Such changes in the healthy may reasonably be thought to bode ill for the unhealthy (with hypertension, angina pectoris, post myocardial infarction). Sudden deaths do occur during or shortly after sexual intercourse (ventricular fibrillation or subarachnoid haemorrhage), usually in clandestine circumstances such as the bordello or the mistress's boudoir, or when the relationship is between an older man and a younger woman — although this may just reflect reporting bias in the press. In one series, 0.6% of all sudden deaths were (reportedly) attributable to sexual intercourse and in about half of these cardiac disease was present. Clearly it is undesirable that the older patient with coronary heart disease should aspire to the haemodynamic heights attainable in youth.

There are few if any records of sudden cardiovascular death amongst women under these circumstances.

If there is substantial concern about cardiovascular stress (hypertension or arrhythmia) during sexual intercourse in either sex, a dose of labetalol about 2 hours before the event may well be justified (taking account of other therapy already in use). But patients taking a β-blocker long term for angina prophylaxis have shown reductions in peak heart rate during coitus from 122 to 82 beats/min.

Patients suffering from angina pectoris should also use glyceryl trinitrate or isosorbide dinitrate as usual for pre-exertional prophylaxis 10 min before intercourse. They should be aware of the potentially fatal interaction of sildenafil (Viagra) with nitrates (see above, p. 545).

> ### Summary
> - The treatment of both hypertension and angina requires drugs that reduce the work of the heart either directly or by lowering peripheral vascular resistance.
> - β-blockade, which acts mainly through reduced cardiac output, and calcium channel blockade, acting by selective arterial dilatation, may be used in either condition.
> - Other vasodilators are suited preferentially to hypertension (ACE inhibitors, angiotensin AT_1 receptor antagonists and α-adrenoceptor blockers) or to angina (nitrates).
> - The treatment of myocardial infarction requires thrombolysis, aspirin and β-adrenoceptor blockade acutely, with the latter two continued for at least two years as secondary prevention of a further myocardial infarction.
> - Other important steps in secondary prevention include ACE inhibitors and statins in selected patients with cardiac failure and hypercholesterolaemia, respectively.

Pulmonary hypertension

Therapy is determined by the underlying cause. When the condition is secondary to hypoxia accompanying chronic obstructive pulmonary disease, long-term oxygen therapy improves symptoms and prognosis; anticoagulation is essential when the cause is multiple pulmonary emboli.

Primary pulmonary hypertension: verapamil may give symptomatic benefit, also continuous intravenous infusion of prostaglandin. Evidence suggests that endothelin, a powerful endogenous vasoconstrictor, may play a pathogenic role, and bosentan, an endothelin-receptor antagonist may improve exercise tolerance. Heart and lung transplantation is recommended for younger patients.

Phaeochromocytoma

This tumour of chromaffin tissue, usually arising in the adrenal medulla, secretes principally *noradrenaline,* but also variable amounts of *adrenaline.* Symptoms are related to this. Hypertension may be sustained or intermittent. If the tumour secretes only noradrenaline, which stimulates α and β_1 adrenoceptors, rises in blood pressure are accompanied by reflex bradycardia due to vagal activation; this is sufficient to overcome the chronotropic effect of β_1 receptor stimulation. The recognition of bradycardia at the time of catecholamine-induced symptoms (e.g. anxiety, termor or sweating) is useful in alerting the physician to the possibility of this rare syndrome, since physiological sympathetic nervous activation causes is coupled to vagal withdrawal, and causes tachycardia. If the tumour also secretes adrenaline, which stimulates α, β_1 and β_2 adrenoceptors, blood pressure and heart rate change in parallel. This is because stimulation of the vasodilator β_2 receptor in resistance arteries attenuates the rise in diastolic pressure, and vagal activation is insufficient then to oppose the chronotropic effect of combined β_1 and β_2 receptor stimulation in the heart.

Diagnostic tests include measurement of catecholamine metabolites in urine followed by catecholamine concentrations in blood when the urine results are equivocal or high. With modern analytical techniques interference by drugs and diet is less troublesome than formerly.

Antihypertensive drugs may alter catecholamine concentrations (particularly those that induce a reflex increase in sympathetic activity, e.g. vasodilators). False-positive results in tests can then occur and in the past patients have undergone unnecessary operations.[38]

A variety of pharmacological tests is now available, and these are best performed in specialist units to avoid erroneous results, e.g. clonidine suppression test. Provocation tests are dangerous. A phaeochromocytoma may also be stimulated to secrete and cause a hypertensive attack by metoclopramide and by any drug that releases histamine (opioids, curare, trimetaphan). The search for biochemical evidence for a phaeochromocytoma should always precede the radiological hunt for a tumour. The accurate measurement of adrenaline in plasma is itself invaluable in determining whether the tumour is likely to be adrenal or extra-adrenal for only adrenal tumours can synthesise adrenaline. This is because the enzyme which methylates noradrenaline to adrenaline needs to be induced by a concentration of cortisol higher than that which normally circulates. Such a concentration is achieved within the normal adrenal gland by the portocapillary circulation from cortex to medulla. The circulation is progressively disrupted as the tumour grows, so that very large adrenal tumours may cease to secrete adrenaline.

Control of blood pressure preoperatively or when the tumour cannot be removed is achieved by α-adrenoceptor blockade which reverses peripheral vasoconstriction. β-blockade may also be required to control tachycardia in patients with adrenaline-secreting tumours. Since adrenaline secretion, as explained above, tends to fall as tumours enlarge, tachycardia is not usually a major problem. Initiation of α-blocker treatment can unmask tachycardia, since there is no longer baroreceptor induced vagal

---

[38] On the other hand, a positive test must not be ignored. In 1954, a hospital clinical chemistry laboratory was asked to set up a biological assay for catecholamines in the urine. The head of the laboratory tested urine from the lab staff to obtain a reference range for the assay. All were negative except his own which was strongly positive. He felt well and regarded the result as showing insufficient specificity of the test. Two years later a fluorometric assay became available. The urines of the lab staff were tested again with the same result. The head of the laboratory still felt well, but this time he decided to consult a physician colleague. A few days later, before the consultation, he was quietly reading a newspaper at home in the evening when he had a fatal cerebral infarction. Autopsy revealed a phaeochromocytoma. (Robinson R 1980 Tumours that secrete catecholamines. Wiley, Chichester.)

activation to oppose β-receptor stimulation of the heart. A β-receptor blocker should never be given alone, since abolition of the peripheral vasodilator effects of adrenaline leaves the powerful a effects unopposed. The injunction not to use a β-blocker in any patient with a suspected phaeochromocytoma can be circumvented by judicious use of low dose β_1 selective blockade (e.g. bisoprolol 5 mg), which will not prevent adrenaline induced vasodilatation.

For phaeochromocytoma the preferred α blocker is not one of the selective α_1 blockers, as in essential hypertension, but the irreversible α-blocker, *phenoxybenzamine,* whose blockade cannot be overcome by a catecholamine surge. Treatment should be for several weeks, if possible, prior to surgery, to allow the intravascular volume depletion, which is always present in phaeochromocytoma patients, to be reversed.

During surgical removal, *phentolamine* (or sodium nitroprusside) should be at hand to control rises in blood pressure when the tumour is handled. When the adrenal veins have been clamped, volume expansion is often required to maintain blood pressure even after adequate preoperative α-blockade. If a pressor infusion is still needed, isoprenaline is more use than the usual α-agonists, to which the patient will be insensitive due to existing α-receptor blockade.

Metirosine (α-methyltyrosine) has been used with some success to block catecholamine synthesis in malignant phaeochromocytomas.

Metaiodobenzylguanidine (MIBG, an analogue of guanethidine) is actively taken up by adrenergic tissue and is concentrated in phaeochromocytomas. Radioiodinated MIBG (^{123}I-MIBG) allows localisation of tumours and detection of metastases; also selective therapeutic irradiation of functioning metastases or other tumours of chromaffin tissue, e.g. carcinoid.

GUIDE TO FURTHER READING

Blood Pressure Lowering Treatment Trialists Collaboration 2000. Effects of ACE inhibitors, calcium antagonists, and other blood-pressure-lowering drugs: results of prospectively designed overviews of randomised trials. Lancet 355: 1955–1964

Braunstein J B et al 2000 Unstable angina pectoris. New England Journal of Medicine 342: 101–114

British Cardiac Society (and other Societies) 2000 Joint British recommendations on prevention of coronary heart disease in clinical practice: summary. British Medical Journal 320: 705–710

Brown M J 1995 Phaeochromocytoma. In: Weatherall D, Ledingham J, Warrell D (eds) Oxford textbook of medicine. Oxford University Press, Oxford, pp. 2553–2557

Burnier M, Brunner H R 2000 Angiotensin 11 receptor antagonists. Lancet 355: 637–645

Dickerson J E C, Brown M J 1995 Influence of age on general practitioners' definition and treatment of hypertension. British Medical Journal 310: 574

Freemantle N et al 1999 β-blockade after myocardial infarction: systematic review and meta regression analysis. British Medical Journal 318: 1730–1737

Guidelines Subcommittee. 1999 World Health Organization-International Society of Hypertension Guidelines for the Management of Hypertension. Journal of Hypertension 17: 151–183

Maxwell S 1999 Emergency management of acute myocardial infarction. British Journal of Clinical Pharmacology 48: 284–298

Manhapra A, Borzak S 2000 Treatment possibilities for unstable angina. British Medical Journal 321: 1269–1275

Maynard S J et al 2000 Management of acute coronary syndromes. British Medical Journal 321: 220–223

Messerli F H 1995 This day 50 years ago. New England Journal of Medicine 332: 1038–1039 (An account of the hypertension and stroke suffered by US President F D Roosevelt.)

Norwegian Multicentre Study Group 1981 Timolol-induced reduction in mortliaty and reinfarction in patients surviving acute myocardial infarction. New England Journal of Medicine 304: 803 — a classic

O'Brien E et al 2000 Use and interpretation of ambulatory blood pressure monitoring: recommendations of the British Hypertension Society. British Medical Journal 320: 1128–1134

Pahor M et al 2000 Health outcomes associated with calcium antagonists compared with other first-line antihypertensive therapies: meta-analysis of randomised controlled trials. Lancet 356: 1949–1954

Parker J D, Parker J O 1998 Nitrate therapy for stable angina pectoris. New England Journal of Medicine 338: 520–531

Redman C W G, Roberts J M 1995 Management of pre-eclampsia. Lancet 341: 1451–1454

Robson J et al 2000 Estimating cardiovascular risk for primary prevention: outstanding questions for primary care. British Medical Journal 320: 702–704

Safian R D, Textor S C 2001 Renal-artery stenosis. New England Journal of Medicine 334: 431–442

Staessen J A, Wang J-G, Thijs L 2001 Cardiovascular protection and blood pressure reduction: a meta-analysis. Lancet 358: 1305

Stewart P M 1999 Mineralocorticoid hypertension. Lancet 353: 1341–1347

Vaughan O J, Delanty N 2000 Hypertensive emergencies. Lancet 356: 411–417

Ylä-Herttuala S, Martin J F 2000 Cardiovascular gene therapy. Lancet 355: 213–222

24

Cardiac arrhythmia and cardiac failure

SYNOPSIS

The pathophysiology of cardiac arrhythmias is complex and the actions of drugs that are useful in stopping or controlling them may seem equally so. Nevertheless many patients with arrhythmias respond well to therapy with drugs and a working knowledge of their effects and indications pays dividends, for irregularity of the heart-beat is at least inconvenient and at worst fatal. The mechanisms by which the failing heart may be sustained are now better understood; carefully selected and monitored drugs can have a major impact on morbidity and mortality in this condition.

- Drugs for cardiac arrhythmias
- Principal drugs by class
- Specific treatments, including those for cardiac arrest
- Drugs for cardiac failure

Drugs for cardiac arrhythmias

OBJECTIVES OF TREATMENT

In almost no other condition is it as important to remember the dual objectives which are:

- To reduce morbidity and
- To reduce mortality.

Arrhythmias are frequently asymptomatic but may be fatal. Indeed an estimated 70 000 deaths per year are ascribed to ventricular arrhythmias in the United Kingdom. In addition, all antiarrhythmics are also capable of *generating* arrhythmias and should be used only in the presence of clear indications. In addition, antiarrhythmic agents are to a variable degree negatively inotropic (except for digoxin and amiodarone).

A second reason for a careful approach to anti-arrhythmic treatment is the gulf between knowledge of their mechanism of action and their clinical uses. On the side of normal physiology, we can see the spontaneous generation and propagation of the cardiac impulse requiring a combination of specialised conducting tissue and inter-myocyte conduction. The heart also has backstops in case of problems with the variety of pacemakers. By contrast, the available drugs may be considered still to be at an early stage of evolution, and useful antiarrhythmic actions — such as that of adenosine — continue to be discovered by chance.

Doctors and drugs interfere with cardiac electro-physiological actions at their peril. In emergencies, action often needs to be taken by the most junior doctor in the team, and some rote recommendations are then necessary. The diagnosis and elective treatment of chronic, or episodic arrhythmias require greater skill to ensure that the correct balance between risk and benefit is achieved. As will become clear, antiarrhythmic drugs have a hard time proving superior safety or efficacy over other therapeutic (non-drug) options.

SOME PHYSIOLOGY AND PATHOPHYSIOLOGY

There are broadly two types of cardiac tissue.

The first type is ordinary myocardial (atrial and ventricular) muscle, responsible for the pumping action of the heart.

The second type is specialised conducting tissue that initiates the cardiac electrical impulse and determines the order in which the muscle cells contract. The important property of being able to form impulses spontaneously is called *automaticity* and is a feature of certain parts of the conducting tissue, e.g. the sinoatrial (SA) and atrioventricular (AV) nodes. The SA node has the highest frequency of spontaneous discharge, 70 times per minute, and thus controls the contraction rate of the heart, making the cells more distal in the system fire more rapidly than they would do spontaneously, i.e. it is the *pacemaker*. If the SA node fails to function, the next fastest part takes over. This is often the AV node (45 discharges per min) or a site in the His-Purkinje system (25 discharges per min).

Altered rate of automatic discharge or *abnormality of the mechanism* by which an impulse is generated from a centre in the nodes or conducting tissue, is one cause of cardiac arrhythmia, e.g. atrial fibrillation, flutter or tachycardia.

Ionic movements into and out of cardiac cells

Nearly all cells in the body exhibit a difference in electrical voltage between their interior and exterior, the membrane potential. Some cells, including the conducting and contracting cells of the heart, are excitable; an appropriate stimulus alters the properties of the cell membrane, ions flow across it and elicit an action potential. This spreads to adjacent cells, i.e. it is conducted as an electrical impulse and, when it reaches a muscle cell, causes it to contract; this is excitation–contraction coupling.

In the resting state the interior of the cell (conducting and contracting types) is electrically *negative* with respect to the exterior due to the disposition of ions (mainly sodium, potassium and calcium) across its membrane, i.e. it is *polarised*. The ionic changes of the action potential first result in a rapid redistribution of ions such that the potential alters to *positive* within the cell (depolarisation); subsequent and slower flows of ions then restore the resting potential *(repolarisation)*. These ionic movements may be separated into phases which are briefly described here and in Figure 25.1, for they help to explain the actions of antiarrhythmic drugs.[1]

CLASSIFICATION OF ANTI-ARRHYTHMIC DRUGS

This is partially based on the phases of the cardiac cycle depicted in Figure 24.1.

Phase 0 is the rapid depolarisation of the cell membrane that is associated with a fast inflow of sodium ions through channels that are selectively permeable to these ions.

Phase 1 is short initial period of rapid repolarisation brought about mainly by an outflow of potassium ions.

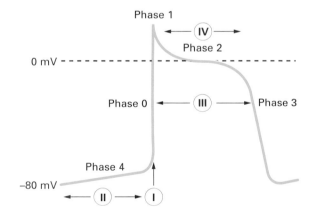

Fig. 24.1 The action potential of a cardiac cell that is capable of spontaneous depolarisation (SA or AV nodal, or His-Purkinje) indicating phases 0–4; the figure illustrates the gradual increase in transmembrane potential (mV) during phase 4; cells that are not capable of spontaneous depolarisation do not exhibit increase in voltage during this phase (see text). The modes of action of antiarrhythmic drugs of classes I, II, III and IV are indicated in relation to these phases

[1] Grace A A, Camm A J 2000 Cardiovascular Research 45: 43–51.

Phase 2 is a period when there is a delay in repolarisation caused mainly by a slow movement of calcium ions from the exterior into the cell through channels that are selectively permeable to these ions ('long-opening' or L-channels).

Phase 3 is a second period of rapid repolarisation during which potassium ions move out of the cell.

Phase 4 begins with the fully repolarised state; for cells that discharge *automatically,* potassium ions then progressively move back into and sodium and calcium ions move out of the cell. The result is that the interior becomes gradually less negative until a (threshold) potential is reached which allows rapid depolarisation (phase 0) to occur, and the cycle is repeated. Automaticity is also influenced by prevailing sympathetic tone. Cells that do not discharge spontaneously rely on the arrival of an action potential from another cell to initiate depolarisation.

In phases 1 and 2 the cell is in an *absolutely refractory* state and is incapable of responding further to any stimulus but during phase 3, the relative refractory period, the cell will depolarise again if a stimulus is sufficiently strong. The orderly transmission of an electrical impulse (action potential) throughout the conducting system may be retarded in an area of disease, e.g. localised ischaemia or previous myocardial infarction. Thus an impulse travelling down a normal Purkinje fibre may spread to an adjacent fibre that has transiently failed to transmit, and pass up it in reverse direction. If this retrograde impulse should in turn re-excite the cells that provided the original impulse, a *re-entrant excitation* becomes established and may cause an arrhythmia, e.g. paroxysmal supraventricular tachycardia.

Most cardiac arrhythmias are probably due either to:

- *impaired conduction* in part of the system leading to the formation of re-entry circuits (> 90% of tachycardias) or
- *altered rate of spontaneous discharge* in conducting tissue. Some ectopic pacemakers appear to depend on adrenergic drive.

CLASSIFICATION OF DRUGS

The Vaughan-Williams[2] classification of anti-arrhythmic drugs is the most commonly used classification. Despite its many peculiarities the classification does provide a useful shorthand for referring to particular groups or actions of drugs.

Class I: sodium channel blockade. These drugs restrict the rapid inflow of sodium during phase 0 and thus slow the maximum rate of depolarisation. Another term for this property is *membrane stabilising activity;* it may contribute to stopping arrhythmias by limiting the responsiveness to excitation of cardiac cells. The class may be subclassified as follows:

A. Drugs that *lengthen* action potential duration and refractoriness (adjunctive class III action), e.g. quinidine, disopyramide, procainamide
B. Drugs that *shorten* action potential duration and refractoriness, e.g. lignocaine (lidocaine) and mexiletine
C. Drugs that have *negligible* effect on action potential duration and refractoriness, e.g. flecainide, propafenone.

One value of the classification is that drugs in class 1B are ineffective for supraventricular arrhythmias, whereas they all have some action in ventricular arrhythmias. The classification is not useful in explaining why the classes differ anatomically in their efficacy.

Class II: catecholamine blockade. Propranolol and other β-adrenoceptor antagonists reduce background sympathetic tone in the heart, reduce automatic discharge (phase 4) and protect against adrenergically stimulated ectopic pacemakers.

Class III: lengthening of refractoriness (without effect on sodium inflow in phase 0). Prolongation of the cardiac action potential and increased cellular refractoriness beyond a critical point may stop a re-entrant circuit being completed and thereby prevent or halt a re-entrant arrhythmia (see above), e.g. amiodarone and sotalol. These drugs act by inhibiting I_{Kr}, the rapidly activating component of the delayed rectifier potassium current (phase 3). The gene, *HERG* (the *human ether-à-go-go-related gene*) encodes a major subunit of the protein responsible for I_{Kr}.

[2] Vaughan Williams E M 1992 Classifying antiarrhythmic actions: by facts or speculation. Journal of Clinical Pharmacology 32: 964–977.

These are the most commonly used antiarrhythmic drugs at this time; new agents in this class include dofetilide and azimilide.

Class IV: calcium channel blockade. These drugs depress the slow inward calcium current (phase 2) and prolong conduction and refractoriness particularly in the SA and AV nodes, which may explain their effectiveness in terminating paroxysmal supraventricular tachycardia, e.g. verapamil.

Although the antiarrhythmics have been entered into this classification according to a characteristic major action, most have other effects as well. For example, quinidine (class I) has major class III effects; propranolol (class II) has minor class I effects, and sotalol (class II) has major class III effects. Amiodarone has class I, II, III and IV effects but is usually classed under III.

Principal drugs by class

(For further data see Table 24.1)

CLASS IA (sodium channel blockade with lengthened refractoriness)

Disopyramide

Disopyramide was the most commonly used drug in this class but is much less so now. It has significant antimuscarinic activity. The drug was thought to be effective in ventricular arrhythmias, especially after myocardial infarction, and in supraventricular arrhythmias, although there are no clinical trials to support this idea.

Pharmacokinetics. Disopyramide is used orally (see Table 24.1) and is well absorbed. It is partly excreted unchanged and partly metabolised. The $t\frac{1}{2}$ is 6 h.

Adverse reactions. The antimuscarinic activity is a significant problem and may lead to dry mouth, blurred vision, glaucoma and micturition hesitancy and retention. Gastrointestinal symptoms, rash and agranulocytosis occur. Effects on the cardiovascular system include hypotension and cardiac failure (negative inotropic effect)

Quinidine

Quinidine is considered the prototype class I drug, although it is now quite rarely used.[3] In addition to its class IA activity, quinidine slightly enhances contractility of the myocardium (positive inotropic effect), and reduces vagus nerve activity on the heart (antimuscarinic effect). At therapeutic doses there is lengthening of ventricular systole which is positively inotropic.

Pharmacokinetics. Absorption of quinidine from the gut is rapid, 75% of the drug is metabolised and the remainder is eliminated unchanged in the urine ($t\frac{1}{2}$ 7 h). Active metabolites may accumulate when renal function is impaired.

Adverse reactions. Quinidine must never be used alone to treat atrial fibrillation or flutter as its antimuscarinic action enhances AV conduction and the heart rate may accelerate. Other cardiac effects include serious ventricular tachyarrhythmias associated with electrocardiographic QT prolongation, i.e. torsades de pointes, the cause of 'quinidine syncope'. Plasma digoxin concentration is raised by quinidine (via displacement from tissue binding and impairment of renal excretion) and the dose of digoxin should be decreased when the drugs are used together. Noncardiac effects, called *cinchonism*, include diarrhoea and other gastrointestinal symptoms, rashes, thrombocytopenia and fever.

CLASS IB (sodium channel blockade with shortened refractoriness)

Lignocaine (lidocaine)

Lignocaine (lidocaine) is used principally for ven-

---

[3] In 1912 K F Wenckebach, a Dutch physician (who described 'Wenckebach block') was visited by a merchant who wished to get rid of an attack of atrial fibrillation (he had recurrent attacks which, although they did not unduly inconvenience him, offended his notions of good order in life's affairs). On receiving a guarded prognosis, the merchant inquired why there were heart specialists if they could not accomplish what he himself had already achieved. In the face of Wenckebach's incredulity he promised to return the next day with a regular pulse, which he did, at the same time revealing that he had done it with quinine (an optical isomer of quinidine). Examination of quinine derivatives led to the introduction of quinidine in 1918 (Wenckebach K F 1923 Journal of the American Medical Association 81: 472).

TABLE 24.1 Drugs for cardiac arrhythmia

	Drug	Usual doses* and interval	Effect on ECG	Usually effective plasma concentration
IA:	Disopyramide	p.o.: 300–800 mg/d in divided doses. i.v.: see specialist literature	Prolongs QRS QT and (±) PR	2–5 mg/l
IB:	Lignocaine (lidocaine)	i.v. loading: 100 mg as a bolus over a few min; i.v. maintenance: 1–4 mg/min	No significant change	1.5–6 mg/l
	Mexiletine	p.o.: initial dose 400 mg, then after 2 h 200–250 mg × 6–8 h. i.v.: see specialist literature	No significant change	0.5–2 mg/l
IC:	Flecainide	p.o.: 100–200 mg × 12 h; and i.v.: see specialist literature	Prolongs PR and QRS	0.2 mg/l
	Propafenone	p.o.: see specialist literature	Prolongs PR and QRS	Active metabolite precludes establishement
II:	Propranolol	p.o.: 10–80 mg × 6 h i.v.: 1 mg over 1 min intervals to 10 mg max. (5 mg in anaesthesia)	Prolongs PR (±). No change in QRS Shortens QT Bradycardia	Not established
	Sotalol	80–160 mg × 2/d	Prolongs QT, PR Sinus bradycardia	Not clinically useful
	Esmolol	i.v.: infusion 50–200 micrograms/kg/min	As for propranolol	0.15–2 mg/l
III:	Amiodarone	p.o.: loading: 200 mg × 8 h for 1 week, then 200 mg × 12 h for 1 week; maintenance 200 mg/d	Prolongs PR, QRS and QT Sinus bradycardia	Not established
IV:	Verapamil	p.o.: 40–120 mg × 8–12 h i.v.: see specialist literature	Prolongs PR	Not clinically useful
Other:	Digoxin	p.o.: initially 1–1.5mg in divided doses over 24 h maintenance: 62.5–500 micrograms/d	Prolongs PR Depresses ST segment Flattens T wave	1–2 micrograms/l
	Adenosine	i.v.: 6 mg initially; if no conversion after 1–2 minutes, give 12 mg and repeat once if necessary. Follow each bolus with saline flush.	Prolongs PR Transient heart block	Not clinically useful

* Doses based on British National Formulary recommendations. Patients with decreased hepatic or renal function may require lower doses (see text).
This table is adapted from that published in the Medical Letter on Drugs and Therapeutics (USA) 1996. We are grateful to the Chairman of the Editorial Board for allowing us to use this material.

tricular arrhythmias, especially those complicating myocardial infarction. Its kinetics render it unsuitable for oral administration and therefore restrict its application to the treatment of acute arrhythmias.

Pharmacokinetics. Lignocaine is used by the i.v, or occasionally the i.m. route; dosing by mouth is unsatisfactory because the $t\frac{1}{2}$ (90 min) is too short to maintain a constant plasma concentration by repeated administration and because the drug undergoes extensive presystemic (first-pass) elimination in the liver.

Adverse reactions are uncommon unless infusion is rapid or there is significant cardiac failure; they include hypotension, dizziness, blurred sight, sleepiness, slurred speech, numbness, sweating, confusion and convulsions.

Mexiletine is similar to lignocaine (lidocaine) but is effective by the oral route ($t\frac{1}{2}$ 10 h). It has been used for ventricular arrhythmias especially those complicating myocardial infarction. The drug is usually poorly tolerated. Adverse reactions are almost universal and dose-related and include nausea, vomiting, hiccough, tremor, drowsiness, confusion, dysarthria, diplopia, ataxia, cardiac arrhythmia and hypotension.

CLASS IC (sodium channel blockade with minimal effect on refractoriness)

Flecainide

Flecainide slows conduction in all cardiac cells including the anomalous pathways responsible for the Wolff–Parkinson–White (WPW) syndrome. Together with encainide and moricizine, it underwent clinical trials to establish if suppression of asymptomatic premature beats with antiarrhythmic drugs would reduce the risk of death from arrhythmia after myocardial infarction.[4] The study was terminated after preliminary analysis of 1727 patients revealed that mortality in the groups treated with flecainide or encainide was 7.7% compared with 3.0% in controls. The most likely explanation for the result was the *induction* of lethal ventricular arrhythmias possibly due to ischaemia by flecainide and encainide, i.e. a *proarrhythmic* effect. In the light of these findings the indications for flecainide are restricted to patients with no evidence of *structural heart disease.* The most common indication, indeed where it is the drug of choice, is *atrioventricular re-entrant tachycardia,* such as AV nodal tachycardia or in the tachycardias associated with the WPW syndrome or similar conditions with anomalous pathways. This should be as a prelude to definitive treatment with radiofrequency ablation. Flecainide may also be useful in patients with paroxysmal atrial fibrillation.

Pharmacokinetics. Its action is terminated by metabolism in the liver and by elimination unchanged in the urine. The $t\frac{1}{2}$ is 14 h in healthy adults but may be over 20 h in patients with cardiac disease, in the elderly and in those with poor renal function.

Adverse reactions. Flecainide is contraindicated in patients with sick sinus syndrome, with cardiac failure, and in those with a history of myocardial infarction who have asymptomatic ventricular ectopic

beats or asymptomatic nonsustained ventricular tachycardia. Minor adverse effects include blurred vision, abdominal discomfort, nausea, dizziness, tremor, abnormal taste sensations and paraesthesiae.

Propafenone

In addition to the defining properties of this class, propafenone also has β-adrenoceptor blocking activity equivalent to a low dose of propranolol. It is occasionally used to suppress nonsustained ventricular arrhythmias in patients whose left ventricular function is normal.

Pharmacokinetics. It is metabolised by the liver and 7% of Caucasian patients are poor metabolisers (it is a substrate for CYP 2D6, see p. 123) who for equivalent doses thus have higher plasma concentrations than the remainder of the population who are extensive metabolisers.

Adverse reactions are similar to those of flecainide and are commoner in poor metabolisers. In addition, conduction block may occur, cardiac failure may worsen and ventricular arrhythmias may be exacerbated, and it should not be used in patients with sustained ventricular tachycardia and poor left ventricular function.

CLASS II (catecholamine blockade)

β-adrenoceptor antagonists (see also Ch. 23)

β-adrenoceptor blockers are effective probably because they counteract the arrhythmogenic effect of catecholamines. The following actions appear to be relevant:

- The rate of automatic firing of the SA node is accelerated by β-adrenoceptor activation and this effect is abolished by β-blockers. Some ectopic pacemakers appear to be dependent on adrenergic drive.
- β-blockers prolong the refractoriness of the AV node which may prevent re-entrant tachycardia at this site.
- Many β-blocking drugs (propranolol, oxprenolol, alprenolol, acebutolol, labetalol) also

---

[4] Cardiac Arrhythmia Suppression Trial (CAST) investigators 1989 New England Journal of Medicine 321: 406.

possess membrane stabilising (class I) properties. *Sotalol* prolongs cardiac refractoriness (class III) but has no class I effects; it is often preferred when a β-blocker is indicated but should be used with care. *Esmolol* (below) is a short-acting β$_1$-selective agent, whose sole use is in the treatment of arrhythmias. Its short duration and β$_1$-selectivity mean that it could be considered in some patients with contraindications to other β-blocking drugs.

- β-adrenoceptor antagonists are effective for a range of supraventricular arrhythmias, in particular those associated with exercise, emotion or hyperthyroidism. Sotalol may be used to suppress ventricular ectopic beats and ventricular tachycardia possibly in conjunction with amiodarone.

Pharmacokinetics. For long-term use, any of the oral preparations of β-blocker is suitable. In emergencies, esmolol may be given i.v. (see Table 24.1). Esmolol has a t$_\frac{1}{2}$ of 9 min, which justifies administration by infusion with rapid alterations in dose, possibly titrated against response.

Adverse reactions. Adverse cardiac effects from overdosage include heart block or even cardiac arrest. Heart failure may be precipitated when a patient is dependent on sympathetic drive to maintain cardiac output (see Ch. 23 for an account of other adverse effects).

Interactions: concomitant i.v. administration of a calcium channel blocker that affects conduction (verapamil, diltiazem) increases the risk of bradycardia and AV block. In patients with depressed myocardial contractility, the combination of oral or i.v. β-blockade and calcium channel blockade (nifedipine, verapamil) may cause hypotension or cardiac failure.

CLASS III (lengthening of refractoriness due to potassium channel blockade)

Amiodarone

Amiodarone is the most powerful antiarrhythmic drug available for the treatment and prevention of both atrial and ventricular arrhythmias. Even short-term use, however, can cause serious toxicity, and its use should always follow a consideration or a trial of alternatives. Amiodarone prolongs the effective refractory period of myocardial cells, the AV node and of anomalous pathways. It also blocks β-adrenoceptors noncompetitively.

Amiodarone is used in chronic ventricular arrhythmias; in atrial fibrillation it both slows the ventricular response and may restore sinus rhythm; it may be used to maintain sinus rhythm after cardioversion for atrial fibrillation or flutter. Amiodarone should no longer be used for the management of re-entrant supraventricular tachycardias associated with the Wolff–Parkinson–White syndrome as radiofrequency ablation is preferable.

Pharmacokinetics. Amiodarone is effective given orally; its enormous apparent distribution volume (70 l/kg) indicates that little remains in the blood. It is stored in fat and many other tissues and the t$_\frac{1}{2}$ of 54 days after multiple dosing signifies slow release from these sites (and slow accumulation to steady state means that a loading dose is necessary, see Table 24.1). The drug is metabolised in the liver and eliminated through the biliary and intestinal tracts.

Adverse reactions. Adverse cardiovascular effects include bradycardia, heart block and induction of ventricular arrhythmia. Other effects are the development of corneal microdeposits which may rarely cause visual haloes and photophobia. These are dose-related, resolve when the drug is discontinued and are not a threat to vision. Amiodarone contains iodine and both hyperthyroidism and hypothyroidism are quite common; thyroid function should be monitored before and during therapy. Photosensitivity reactions are universal. These may be very severe and should be pointed out explicitly to patients when starting this drug. Amiodarone may also cause a bluish discoloration on exposed areas of the skin (occasionally reversible on discontinuing the drug). Less commonly, pulmonary fibrosis and hepatitis occur, sometimes rapidly during short-term use of the drug, and both may be fatal so vigilance should be high. Cirrhosis is reported.

Interaction with digoxin (by displacement from tissue binding sites and interference with its elimination) and with warfarin (by inhibiting its metabolism) increases the effect of both these drugs. β-blockers and calcium channel antagonists augment the depressant effect of amiodarone on SA and AV node function.

CLASS IV (calcium channel blockade)

Calcium is involved in the contraction of cardiac and vascular smooth muscle cells, and in the automaticity of cardiac pacemaker cells. Actions of calcium channel blockers on vascular smooth muscle cells are described with the main account of these drugs in Chapter 23. Although the three classes of calcium channel blocker have similar effects on vascular smooth muscle in the arterial tree, their cardiac actions differ. The phenylalkylamine, verapamil, depresses myocardial contraction more than the others, and both verapamil and the benzothiazepine, diltiazem, slow conduction in the SA and AV nodes.

Calcium and cardiac cells

Cardiac muscle cells are normally depolarised by the fast inward flow of sodium ions, following which there is a slow inward flow of calcium ions through the L-type calcium channels (phase 2, in Fig. 24.1); the consequent rise in free intracellular calcium ions activates the contractile mechanism.

Pacemaker cells in the SA and AV nodes rely heavily on the slow inward flow of calcium ions (phase 4) for their capacity to discharge spontaneously, i.e. for their automaticity.

Calcium channel blockers inhibit the passage of calcium through the membrane channels; the result in myocardial cells is to depress contractility, and in pacemaker cells to suppress their automatic activity. Members of the group therefore may have negative cardiac inotropic and chronotropic actions. These actions can be separated; nifedipine, at therapeutic concentrations, acts almost exclusively on noncardiac ion channels and has no clinically useful antiarrhythmic activity whilst verapamil is a useful antiarrhythmic.

Verapamil

Verapamil (see also p. 466) prolongs conduction and refractoriness in the AV node and depresses the rate of discharge of the SA node. If adenosine is not available, verapamil is a very attractive alternative to it for the termination of narrow complex paroxysmal supraventricular tachycardia. Verapamil should not be given intravenously to patients with broad complex tachyarrhythmias in whom it may be lethal but with due care is very safe in those with narrow complex tachycardia. Adverse effects include nausea, constipation, headache, fatigue, hypotension, bradycardia and heart block.

OTHER ANTIARRHYTHMICS

Digoxin and other cardiac glycosides[5]

Crude digitalis is a preparation of the dried leaf of the foxglove plant *Digitalis purpurea* or *lanata*. Digitalis contains a number of active glycosides (digoxin, lanatosides) whose actions are qualitatively similar, differing principally in rapidity of onset and duration; the pure individual glycosides are used. The following account refers to all the cardiac glycosides but digoxin is the principal one.

Mode of action. Cardiac glycosides affect the heart both directly and indirectly in complex interactions,

---

[5] In 1775 Dr William Withering was making a routine journey from Birmingham (England), his home, to see patients at the Stafford Infirmary. Whilst the carriage horses were being changed half way, he was asked to see an old dropsical woman. He thought she would die and so some weeks later, when he heard of her recovery, was interested enough to enquire into the cause. Recovery was attributed to a herb tea containing some 20 ingredients, amongst which Withering, already the author of a botanical textbook, found it 'not very difficult … to perceive that the active herb could be no other than the foxglove'. He began to investigate its properties, trying it on the poor of Birmingham, whom he used to see without fee each day. The results were inconclusive and his interest flagged until one day he heard that the principal of an Oxford College had been cured by foxglove after 'some of the first physicians of the age had declared that they could do no more for him'. This put a new complexion on the matter and, pursuing his investigation, Withering found that foxglove extract caused diuresis in some oedematous patients. He defined the type of patient who might benefit from it and, equally important, he standardised his foxglove leaf preparations and was able to lay down accurate dosage schedules. His advice, with little amplification, would serve today (Withering W 1785 An account of the foxglove. Robinson, London).

some of which oppose each other. The *direct* effect is to inhibit the membrane-bound sodium-potassium adenosine-triphosphatase (Na^+, K^+-ATPase) enzyme that supplies energy for the system that pumps sodium out of and transports potassium into contracting and conducting cells. By reducing the exchange of extracellular sodium with intracellular calcium, digoxin raises the store of intracellular calcium, which facilitates muscular contraction. The *indirect* effect is to enhance vagal activity by complex peripheral and central mechanisms.

The clinically important consequences are:

- On the contracting cells: increased contractility and excitability
- On SA and AV nodes and conducting tissue: decreased generation and propagation.

Uses. Digoxin is not strictly an *anti*arrhythmic agent but rather it modulates the response to arrhythmias. Its most useful property, in this respect, is to slow conduction through the AV node. The main uses are in:

- Atrial fibrillation, benefiting chiefly by the vagal effect on the AV node, reducing conduction through it and thus slowing the ventricular rate.
- Atrial flutter, benefiting by the vagus nerve action of shortening the refractory period of the atrial muscle so that flutter is converted to fibrillation (in which state the ventricular rate is more readily controlled). Electrical cardioversion is preferred.
- Cardiac failure, benefiting chiefly by the direct action to increase myocardial contractility. Digoxin is still occasionally used in chronic left ventricular or congestive cardiac failure due to ischaemic, hypertensive or valvular heart disease, especially in the short term. This is no longer a major indication following the introduction of other groups of drugs.

Pharmacokinetics. Digoxin is usually administered by mouth. It is eliminated 85% unchanged by the kidney and the remainder is metabolised by the liver. The $t\frac{1}{2}$ is 36 h.

Dose and therapeutic plasma concentration: see Table 24.1. Reduced dose of digoxin is necessary in: renal impairment (see above); the elderly (probably

from decline in renal clearance with age); electrolyte disturbances (hypokalaemia accentuates the potential for adverse effects of digoxin, as does hypomagnesaemia); hypothyroid patients (who are intolerant of digoxin).

Adverse effects. *Abnormal cardiac rhythms* usually take the form of ectopic arrhythmias (ventricular ectopic beats, ventricular tachyarrhythmias, paroxysmal supraventricular tachycardia) and heart block. *Gastrointestinal effects* include anorexia which usually precedes vomiting and is a warning that dosage is excessive. Diarrhoea may also occur. *Visual effects* include disturbances of colour vision, e.g. yellow (xanthopsia) but also red or green vision, photophobia and blurring. *Gynaecomastia* may occur in men and breast enlargement in women with long-term use (cardiac glycosides have structural resemblance to oestrogen). Mental effects include confusion, restlessness, agitation, nightmares and acute psychoses.

Acute digoxin poisoning causes initial nausea and vomiting and *hyperkalaemia* because inhibition of the Na^+, K^+-ATPase pump prevents intracellular accumulation of potassium. The ECG changes (see Table 24.1) of prolonged use of digoxin may be absent. There may be exaggerated sinus arrhythmia, bradycardia and ectopic rhythms with or without heart block.

Treatment of overdose. Overdose with digoxin is now uncommon. For severe digoxin poisoning infusion of the *digoxin-specific binding (Fab) fragment* (Digibind) of the antibody to digoxin, neutralises digoxin in the plasma and is an effective treatment. Because it lacks the Fc segment, this fragment is nonimmunogenic and it is sufficiently small to be eliminated as the digoxin-antibody complex in the urine. It may interfere with the subsequent radioimmunoassay of digoxin in plasma. Phenytoin i.v. may be effective for ventricular arrhythmias, and atropine for bradycardia. Electrical pacing may be needed, but direct current shock may cause ventricular fibrillation.

Interactions. Depletion of body *potassium* from therapy with *diuretics* or with adrenal steroids may lead to cardiac arrhythmias (as may be anticipated from its action on Na^+, K^+-ATPase, above). Verapamil, nifedipine, quinidine and amiodarone raise steady-state plasma digoxin concentrations (see above) and the digoxin dose should be lowered when any of these is added. The likelihood of AV block due to digoxin is increased by verapamil and by β-adrenoceptor blockers.

Adenosine

Adenosine is an endogenous purine nucleotide which slows atrioventricular conduction and dilates coronary and peripheral arteries. It is rapidly metabolised by circulating adenosine deaminase and also enters cells; hence its residence in plasma is brief ($t\frac{1}{2}$ several seconds) and it must be given rapidly i.v. Administered as a bolus injection, adenosine is useful for distinguishing the origin of (ECG) 'broad QRS complex' tachycardias, i.e. whether ventricular, or supraventricular with aberrant conduction. If the latter is the case AV block with adenosine allows the P waves to be seen and the diagnosis to be made; adenosine thus has the same effect as carotid massage (see below). Evidence also indicates that adenosine is effective for terminating paroxysmal supraventricular (re-entrant) tachycardias, including episodes in patients with Wolff–Parkinson–White syndrome. The initial dose in adults is 3 mg over 2 seconds with continuous ECG monitoring, with doubling increments every 1–2 minutes. The average total dose is 125 micrograms/kg. Adenosine is an alternative to verapamil for supraventricular tachycardia and is possibly safer (because adenosine is short-acting and not negatively inotropic), as verapamil is dangerous if used mistakenly in a ventricular tachycardia. Adverse effects from adenosine are not serious because of the brevity of its action but may cause very distressing dyspnoea, facial flushing, chest pain and transient arrhythmias, e.g. bradycardia. Adenosine should not be given to asthmatics or to patients with second or third degree AV block or sick sinus syndrome (unless a pacemaker is in place).

Cardiac effects of the autonomic nervous system

Some drugs used for arrhythmias exert their actions through the *autonomic nervous system* by mimicking or antagonising the effects of the sympathetic or parasympathetic nerves that supply the heart. The neurotransmitters in these two branches of the autonomic system, noradrenaline and acetylcholine, are functionally antagonistic by having opposing actions on cyclic AMP production within the cardiomyocyte. Their receptors are coupled to the two trimeric GTP-binding proteins, Gs and Gi, which stimulate and inhibit adenylyl cyclase, respectively.

The sympathetic division (adrenergic component of the autonomic nervous system), when stimulated, has the following *effects on the heart* (receptor effects):

- Tachycardia due to increased rate of discharge of the SA node
- Increased automaticity in the AV node and His-Purkinje system
- Increase in conductivity in the His-Purkinje system
- Increased force of contraction
- Shortening of the refractory period.

Isoprenaline (isoprotenerol), a β-adrenoceptor agonist, can be used to accelerate the heart when there is extreme bradycardia due to heart block, prior to the insertion of an implanted pacemaker; this is now rarely needed. Adverse effects are those expected of β-adrenoceptor agonists and include tremor, flushing, sweating, palpitation, headache and diarrhoea.

The vagus nerve (cholinergic, parasympathetic), when stimulated, has the following *effects on the heart*:

- Bradycardia due to depression of the SA node
- Slowing of conduction through and increased refractoriness of the AV node
- Shortening of the refractory period of atrial muscle cells
- Decreased myocardial excitability.

These effects are used in the therapy of arrhythmias.

There is also reduced *force of contraction* of atrial and ventricular muscle cells.

The *vagus nerve* may be stimulated *reflexly* by various physical manoeuvres. Vagal stimulation may slow or terminate supraventricular arrhythmias and should if possible be carried out under ECG control.

Carotid sinus massage activates stretch receptors: external pressure is applied gently to one side at a time but never to both sides at once. Some individuals are very sensitive to the procedure and develop severe bradycardia and hypotension.

Other methods include the *Valsalva manoeuvre* (deep inspiration followed by expiration against a closed glottis, which both stimulates stretch receptors in the lung and reduces venous return to the heart); the Muller procedure (deep expiration followed by inspiration against a closed glottis); production of nausea and retching by inviting patients to put their *own fingers* down their throat.

The effects of vagus nerve activity are blocked by *atropine* (antimuscarinic action), an action that is used to accelerate the heart during episodes of sinus bradycardia as may occur after myocardial infarction. The dose is 0.6 mg i.v. and repeated as necessary to a maximum of 3 mg per day. Adverse effects are those of muscarinic blockade, namely dry mouth, blurred vision, urinary retention, confusion and hallucination.

PROARRHYTHMIC DRUG EFFECTS

All antiarrhythmic drugs can also *cause* arrhythmia; they should be used with care and ideally only following advice from a specialist. Such proarrhythmic effects are most commonly seen with drugs that prolong the QT interval or QRS complex of the ECG; hypokalaemia aggravates the danger. Quinidine may cause tachyarrhythmias in an estimated 4–6% of patients. A probable proarrhythmic effect of flecainide resulting in a doubling of mortality was revealed by the Cardiac Arrhythmia Suppression Trial (CAST) (see p. 502).

Digoxin can induce a variety of brady- and tachyarrhythmias (see above).

CHOICE BETWEEN DRUGS AND ELECTROCONVERSION

Direct current (DC) electric shock applied externally is often the best way to convert cardiac arrhythmias to sinus rhythm. Many atrial or ventricular arrhythmias start as a result of transiently operating factors but, once they have begun, the abnormal mechanisms are self-sustaining. When a successful electric shock is given, the heart is depolarised, the ectopic focus is extinguished and the SA node, the part of the heart with the highest automaticity, resumes as the dominant pacemaker.

Electrical conversion has the advantage that it is immediate, unlike drugs, which may take days or longer to act; also, the effective doses and adverse effects of drugs are largely unpredictable, and can be serious.[6]

Uses of electrical conversion: in supraventricular and ventricular tachycardia, ventricular fibrillation and atrial fibrillation and flutter. Drugs can be useful to prevent a relapse, e.g. sotalol, amiodarone.

SPECIFIC TREATMENTS[7]

Sinus bradycardia

Acute sinus bradycardia requires treatment if it is symptomatic e.g. where there is hypotension or escape rhythms; extreme bradycardia may allow a ventricular focus to take over and lead to ventricular tachycardia. The foot of the bed should be raised to assist venous return and atropine should be given i.v. Chronic symptomatic bradycardia is an indication for the insertion of a permanent pacemaker.

Atrial ectopic beats

Reduction in the use of tea, coffee and other methylxanthine-containing drinks, and of tobacco, may suffice for ectopic beats not due to organic

---

[6] To the layman, 'shock' treatment could be interpreted as frights (which stimulate the vagus, as described above), or as the electrical sort. Dr James Le Fanu describes a Belfast doctor who reported a farmer with a solution that covered both possibilities. He had suffered from episodes of palpitations and dizziness for 30 years. When he first got them, he would jump from a barrel and thump his feet hard on the ground at landing. This became less effective with time. His next 'cure' was to remove his clothes, climb a ladder and jump from a considerable height into a cold water tank on the farm. Later, he discovered the best and simplest treatment was to grab hold of his 6-volt electrified cattle fence — although if he was wearing Wellington (rubber) boots he found he had to earth the shock, so besides grabbing the fence with one hand he simultaneously shoved a finger of the other hand into the ground.

[7] See also UK Resuscitation Council guidelines (Fig. 24.2).

heart disease. When action is needed, a small dose of a β-adrenoceptor blocker may be effective.

Paroxysmal supraventricular (AV re-entrant or atrial) tachycardia

For acute attacks, if vagal stimulation (by carotid massage, or swallowing ice-cream) is unsuccessful, *adenosine* has the dual advantage of being effective in most such tachycardias, while having no effect on a ventricular tachycardia. The response to adenosine is therefore of diagnostic value. Intravenous verapamil is an alternative for the acute management of a *narrow complex tachycardia*. If, however, the patient is in circulatory shock as a result of the tachycardia, or drug treatment fails, a DC shock should be delivered, for immediate effect. *Flecainide* or *sotalol* are the drugs of choice for preventing attacks (prophylaxis).

Atrial fibrillation (AF)

The therapeutic options are:

- Treatment vs no treatment
- Conversion vs rate control
- Immediate vs delayed conversion
- Drugs or DC conversion.

The information required is:

- Ventricular rate ('normal' or high)
- Haemodynamic state ('normal' or compromised)
- Atrial size ('normal' or enlarged).

In many patients, AF is an incidental finding on the background of some existing cardiovascular disease, and with a large atrium. With a long history of symptoms, *rate-controlling medication* such as a β-blocker, digoxin or calcium antagonist is indicated. If there appears to be a short history (weeks), and the atrium is not enlarged, or there has been recent onset of heart failure or shock, *cardioversion* should be attempted. *Electrical* (DC) conversion is favoured where treatment is either urgent or likely to be successful in holding the patient in sinus rhythm. *Pharmacological* conversion can often be achieved over hours to days by *amiodarone,* and this drug is also useful in patients who revert rapidly to AF after DC conversion.

When conversion is not urgent, it should be delayed for a month to permit institution of anti-coagulation by warfarin, and this should be continued for 4 weeks thereafter. In patients who have reverted to AF after previous conversions, amiodarone is the drug of choice prior to further attempts at cardioversion. Amiodarone is also used to suppress episodes of paroxysmal supraventricular tachycardia and atrial fibrillation.

Additional treatments in chronic atrial fibrillation. Long-term treatment with warfarin is almost mandatory to reduce embolic complications. The efficacy of aspirin as an antiembolic agent is probably less in this group, but has been shown to be of value in patients where warfarin is considered inappropriate.

Atrial flutter

It is doubtful whether this differs in its origins or sequelae from atrial fibrillation. The ventricular rate is usually faster (typically, half an atrial rate of 300, where 2:1 block is present), which is too fast to leave without treatment. Since, similarly, the patient is unlikely to have been in this rhythm for a prolonged period, there is less likelihood that atrial thrombus has accumulated. Conversion without prior anti-coagulation may occasionally be considered safe but anticoagulation is usually also needed. Patients should not be left in chronic atrial flutter, and DC conversion will usually restore either sinus rhythm or result in atrial fibrillation. The latter is treated as above. Patients who fail to convert, or who revert to atrial flutter should be referred for consideration of radiofrequency ablation that is highly effective and may remove the cause of the atrial flutter > 80% of cases.

Atrial tachycardia with variable AV block

The atrial rate is 120–250/min, and commonly there is AV block. If the patient is taking digoxin, it should be suspected as the possible cause of the arrhythmia, and stopped. If the patient is not taking digoxin, it may be used to control the ventricular rate. These patients should be considered for referral for radiofrequency ablation.

Heart block

The use of permanent pacemakers is beyond the scope of this book. In an emergency, AV conduction may be improved by atropine (antimuscarinic vagal block) (0.6 mg i.v.) or by isoprenaline (β-adrenoceptor agonist) (0.5–10 micrograms/min, i.v.). Temporary pacing wires may be needed prior to referral for pacemaker implantation.

Pre-excitation (Wolff–Parkinson–White) syndrome

This occurs in otherwise healthy individuals, who possess an anomalous (accessory) atrioventricular pathway; they often experience attacks of paroxysmal AV re-entrant tachycardia or atrial fibrillation. Drugs that both suppress the initiating ectopic beats and delay conduction through the accessory pathway are used to prevent attacks e.g. flecainide, sotalol or amiodarone. Verapamil and digoxin may increase conduction through the anomalous pathway and should not be used. Electrical conversion may be needed to restore sinus rhythm when the ventricular rate is very rapid. Radiofrequency ablation of aberrant pathways will almost certainly provide a cure.

Ventricular premature beats

These are common after myocardial infarction. Their particular significance is that the R-wave (ECG) of an ectopic beat, developing during the early or peak phases of the T-wave of a normal beat, may precipitate ventricular tachycardia or fibrillation (the R-on-T phenomenon). About 80% of patients with myocardial infarction who proceed to ventricular fibrillation have preceding ventricular premature beats. Lignocaine (lidocaine) is effective in suppression of ectopic ventricular beats but is not often used as its addition increases overall risk.

Ventricular tachycardia

Ventricular tachycardia demands urgent treatment since it frequently leads to ventricular fibrillation and circulatory arrest. A powerful thump of the fist on the mid-sternum or precordium may very occasionally stop a tachycardia. If there is rapid haemodynamic deterioration, electrical conversion is the treatment of choice. If the patient is in good cardiovascular condition, treatment may begin with lignocaine (lidocaine) i.v. or, should that fail, amiodarone i.v. For *recurrent* ventricular tachycardia, amiodarone or sotalol are preferred. Mexiletine, disopyramide, procainamide, quinidine and propafenone are not usually indicated. These patients should be referred for consideration of the implantation of an implantable cardioverter defibrillator (ICD).

Ventricular fibrillation and cardiac arrest

Ventricular fibrillation is usually caused by myocardial infarction or ischaemia, or serious organic heart disease and is the main cause of cardiac arrest. Guidelines for the management of peri-arrest arrythmias and cardiac arrest are issued by the UK Resuscitation Council and appear in Fig. 24.2 and 24.3. Patients suffering failed *sudden cardiac death* (SCD) should be referred for consideration of the implantation of an ICD.

Long QT syndromes

These are caused by malfunction of ion channels, leading to impaired ventricular repolarisation (expressed as prolongation of the QT interval) and a characteristic ventricular tachycardia, torsade de pointes.[8] The symptoms range from episodes of syncope to cardiac arrest. An enlarging number and variety of *drugs* are responsible for the *acquired* form of the condition (including antiarrhythmic drugs, antibimicrobials, histamine H_1-receptor antagonists, serotonin receptor antagonists), and predisposing factors are female sex, recent heart-rate slowing, and hypokalaemia.[9] *Congenital* forms of the long QT syndrome are due to mutations in the genes encoding for ion channels, some of which may be revealed by exposure to drugs.

Summary

- The treatment of arrhythmias can be directly physical, electrical, pharmacological or

---

[8] Fr. *torsade*, twist + *pointe*, point. 'Twisting of the points', referring to the characteristic sequence of 'up', followed by 'down' QRS complexes. The appearance has been referred to as 'cardiac ballet'.

[9] Viskin S 1999 Lancet 354: 1625–1633.

surgical. Radiofrequency ablation and the use of devices such as permanent pacemakers and ICDs is increasing massively and the use of drugs by themselves declining in relative terms. Drugs are often now used as adjunctive treatments.

- The choice among drugs is influenced partly by theoretical predictions from their action on the cardiac cycle but largely by short and long-term observations of their efficacy and safety.

- All antiarrhythmics can be dangerous, and should not be used unless patients are symptomatic or haemodynamically compromised.

- Adenosine is the treatment of choice for diagnosis and reversal of supraventricular arrhythmias. Verapamil is an alternative for the management of *narrow complex tachycardias.*

- Amiodarone is the most effective drug at reversing atrial fibrillation, and in prevention of ventricular arrhythmias, but has several adverse effects.

- Digoxin retains a unique role as a positively inotropic antiarrhythmic, being most useful in slowing atrioventricular conduction in atrial fibrillation.

Cardiac failure and its treatment

SOME PHYSIOLOGY AND PATHOPHYSIOLOGY

Cardiac output (CO) depends on the rate of contraction of the heart (HR) and the volume of blood that is ejected with each beat, the stroke volume (SV); it is expressed by the relationship:

$$CO = HR \times SV$$

The three factors that regulate the stroke volume are preload, afterload and contractility:

- *Preload* is the load on the heart created by the volume of blood injected into the left ventricle by the left atrium (at the end of ventricular diastole) and that it must eject with each contraction. It

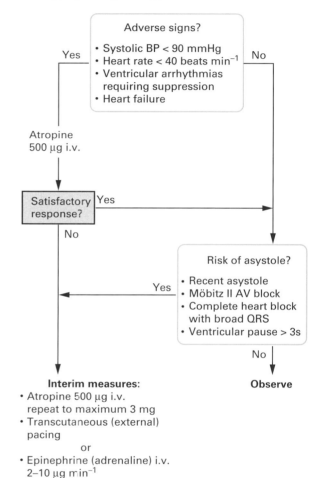

Bradycardia
(includes rates inappropriately slow for haemodynamic state)

If appropriate, give oxygen and establish i.v. access

Adverse signs?

- Systolic BP < 90 mmHg
- Heart rate < 40 beats min^{-1}
- Ventricular arrhythmias requiring suppression
- Heart failure

Atropine 500 µg i.v.

Satisfactory response?

Risk of asystole?

- Recent asystole
- Möbitz II AV block
- Complete heart block with broad QRS
- Ventricular pause > 3s

Observe

Interim measures:
- Atropine 500 µg i.v. repeat to maximum 3 mg
- Transcutaneous (external) pacing
  or
- Epinephrine (adrenaline) i.v. 2–10 µg min^{-1}

Seek expert help
Arrange transvenous pacing

Fig. 24.2 Protocol for the treatment of pericardiac arrest arrhythmias (arrhythmias) in hospitals. With permission, UK Resuscitation Council. The latest versions can be found on www.resus.org.uk

can also be viewed as the amount of stretch to which the left ventricle is subject. As the preload rises so also do the degree of stretch and the length of cardiac muscle fibres. Preload is thus a

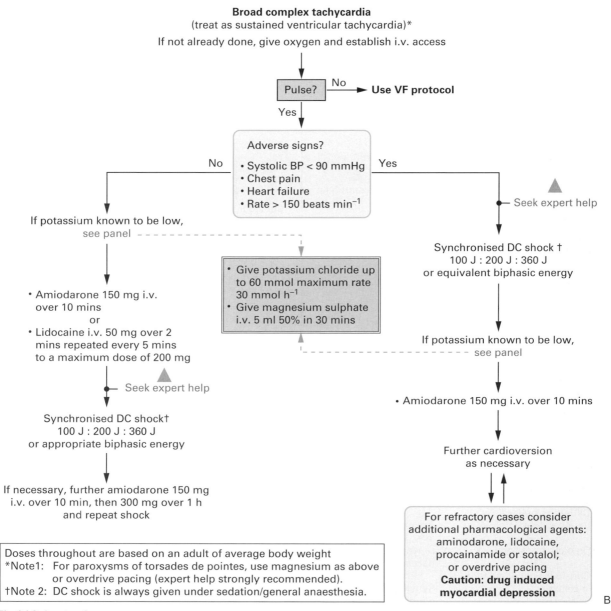

Broad complex tachycardia
(treat as sustained ventricular tachycardia)*

If not already done, give oxygen and establish i.v. access

Pulse? — No → **Use VF protocol**

Yes

Adverse signs?
• Systolic BP < 90 mmHg
• Chest pain
• Heart failure
• Rate > 150 beats min⁻¹

No

If potassium known to be low,
see panel

• Amiodarone 150 mg i.v.
over 10 mins
or
• Lidocaine i.v. 50 mg over 2
mins repeated every 5 mins
to a maximum dose of 200 mg

• Give potassium chloride up
to 60 mmol maximum rate
30 mmol h⁻¹
• Give magnesium sulphate
i.v. 5 ml 50% in 30 mins

Seek expert help

Synchronised DC shock†
100 J : 200 J : 360 J
or appropriate biphasic energy

If necessary, further amiodarone 150 mg
i.v. over 10 min, then 300 mg over 1 h
and repeat shock

Yes

Seek expert help

Synchronised DC shock †
100 J : 200 J : 360 J
or equivalent biphasic energy

If potassium known to be low,
see panel

• Amiodarone 150 mg i.v. over 10 mins

Further cardioversion
as necessary

For refractory cases consider
additional pharmacological agents:
aminodarone, lidocaine,
procainamide or sotalol;
or overdrive pacing
**Caution: drug induced
myocardial depression**

Doses throughout are based on an adult of average body weight
*Note1: For paroxysms of torsades de pointes, use magnesium as above
or overdrive pacing (expert help strongly recommended).
†Note 2: DC shock is always given under sedation/general anaesthesia.

B

Fig. 24.2 (continued)

volume load and can be excessive, e.g. when there is valvular incompetence.
• *Afterload* refers to the load on the contracting ventricle created by the resistance to the blood injected by the ventricle into the arterial system, i.e. the total peripheral resistance. Afterload is thus a *pressure* load and is excessive, e.g. in arterial hypertension.

• *Contractility* refers to the capacity of the myocardium to generate the force necessary to respond to preload and to overcome afterload.

DEFINITION OF CARDIAC FAILURE

Cardiac failure is present when the heart cannot provide all organs with the blood supply appropriate

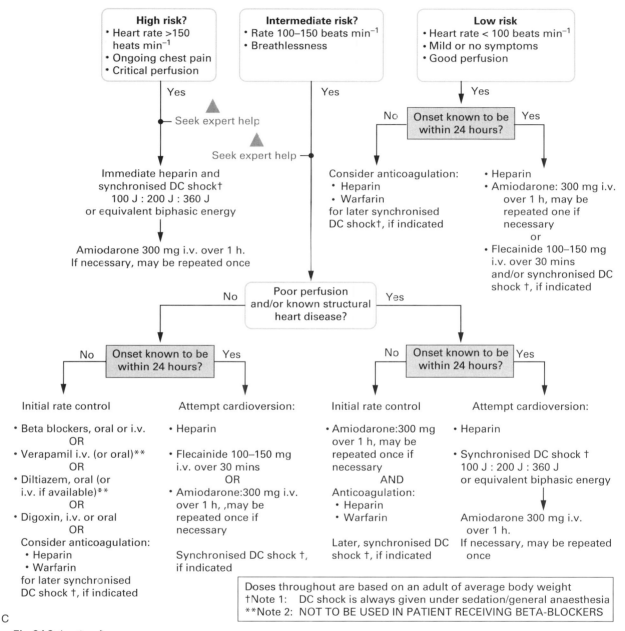

Fig. 24.2 (continued)

to demand. This definition incorporates two elements: firstly, cardiac output may be normal at rest, but secondly, when demand is increased, perfusion of the vital organs (brain and kidneys) is maintained at the expense of other tissues, especially skeletal muscle.

Overall systemic arterial pressure is also maintained until a late stage. These responses follow neuroendocrine activation when the heart begins to fail.

The therapeutic importance of recognising this pathophysiology is that many of the neuroendocrine

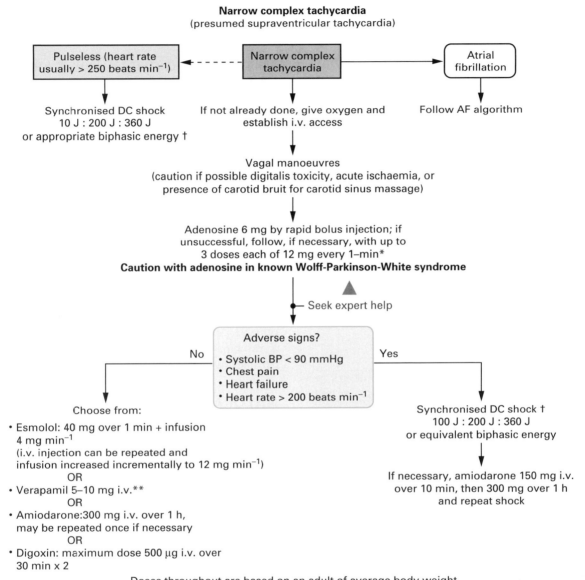

Narrow complex tachycardia
(presumed supraventricular tachycardia)

Pulseless (heart rate usually > 250 beats min⁻¹)

Narrow complex tachycardia

Atrial fibrillation

Synchronised DC shock
10 J : 200 J : 360 J
or appropriate biphasic energy †

If not already done, give oxygen and establish i.v. access

Follow AF algorithm

Vagal manoeuvres
(caution if possible digitalis toxicity, acute ischaemia, or presence of carotid bruit for carotid sinus massage)

Adenosine 6 mg by rapid bolus injection; if unsuccessful, follow, if necessary, with up to 3 doses each of 12 mg every 1–min*
Caution with adenosine in known Wolff-Parkinson-White syndrome

Seek expert help

Adverse signs?
• Systolic BP < 90 mmHg
• Chest pain
• Heart failure
• Heart rate > 200 beats min⁻¹

No

Yes

Choose from:

• Esmolol: 40 mg over 1 min + infusion
  4 mg min⁻¹
  (i.v. injection can be repeated and
  infusion increased incrementally to 12 mg min⁻¹)
          OR
• Verapamil 5–10 mg i.v.**
          OR
• Amiodarone:300 mg i.v. over 1 h,
  may be repeated once if necessary
          OR
• Digoxin: maximum dose 500 μg i.v. over
  30 min x 2

Synchronised DC shock †
100 J : 200 J : 360 J
or equivalent biphasic energy

If necessary, amiodarone 150 mg i.v.
over 10 min, then 300 mg over 1 h
and repeat shock

Doses throughout are based on an adult of average body weight
A starting dose of 6 mg adenosine is currently outside the UK licence for this agent.

*Note 1:	Theophylline and related compounds block the effect of adenosine. Patients on dipyridamole, carbamazepine, or with denervated hearts have a markedly exaggerated effect which may be hazardous.
†Note 2:	DC shock is always given under sedation/general anaesthesia.
**Note 3:	Not to be used in patients receiving beta-blockers.

D

Fig. 24.2 (*continued*)

abnormalities of cardiac failure — particularly, the elevated renin and sympathetic activity — can be caused by drugs used for treatment, as well as by the disease. Renal perfusion is not altered early in heart failure, whereas diuretics and vasodilators *stimulate* renin and noradrenaline production through actions at the juxtaglomerular apparatus in the kidney and on the arterial baroreflex, respectively.

Advanced life support algorithm for the management of cardiac arrest in adults

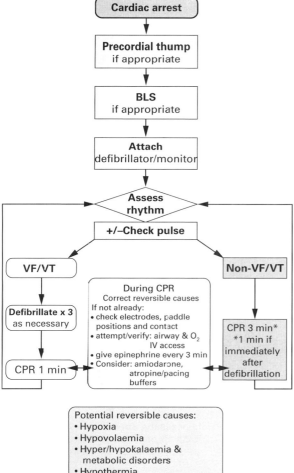

Potential reversible causes:
• Hypoxia
• Hypovolaemia
• Hyper/hypokalaemia & metabolic disorders
• Hypothermia
• Tension pneumothorax
• Tamponade
• Toxic/therapeutic disorders
• Thromboembolic & mechanical obstruction

Fig. 24.3 Advanced cardiac life support. (BLS: basic life support) With permission, UK Resuscitation Council. The latest version can be found on www.resus.org.uk

The earliest endocrine abnormality in almost all types of cardiac disease is increased release of the heart's own hormones, the natriuretic peptides ANP and BNP (A for atrial, B for brain, where it was first discovered), and their concentration in plasma may become a guide to therapy.[10] These peptides normally *suppress* renin and aldosterone production,

but this suppression appears to be overridden in cardiac failure.

THE STARLING CURVE AND CARDIAC FAILURE

The Starling[11] curve originally described the increased contractility of cardiac muscle fibres in response to increased stretch; it can be extrapolated to the whole ventricle to explain the normal relationship between filling pressure and ejection fraction (Fig. 24.4). Most patients with heart failure present in phase 'A' of the relationship, and before the ventricle is grossly dilated (the decompensated phase, 'B'). While diuretic therapy improves the congestive symptoms of cardiac failure which are due to the increased filling pressure *(preload)*, it actually reduces cardiac output in most patients. Depending on whether their predominant symptom is *dyspnoea* (due to pulmonary venous congestion) or *fatigue* (due to reduced cardiac output), patients feel better or worse. It is likely that a principal benefit of using ACE inhibitors in cardiac failure is their diuretic sparing effect.

NATURAL HISTORY OF CHRONIC CARDIAC FAILURE

The severity of cardiac failure can be classified at

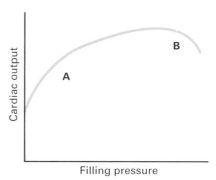

Fig. 24.4 Starling curve of relationship between cardiac filling pressure and cardiac output. In phase A, reduction in blood volume (by diuretics) reduces filling pressure and cardiac output. In phase B, reduction in blood volume reduces filling pressure and increases cardiac output

---

[10] Troughton RW et al 2000 Lancet 355: 1126–1130.

[11] Ernest Henry Starling 1866–1927. Professor of physiology University College, London. He also coined the word 'hormone'.

the bedside according to how much the patient is able to do without becoming dyspnoeic, and this New York Heart Association (NYHA) classification offers also an approximate prognosis, with that of the worst grade (Class 4) being as bad as most cancers.[12] Most patients with cardiac failure die from an arrhythmia, rather than from terminal decompensation, and prognosis is improved most by drugs which do not increase further the heart's exposure to elevated catecholamine concentrations (some vasodilators, but see below).

OBJECTIVES OF TREATMENT

As for cardiac arrhythmias, these are

- To reduce morbidity
- To reduce mortality.

There is some tension between these two objectives in that the action of diuretic and vasodilator drugs, which temporarily improve symptoms, can jeopardise survival. There is a further tension between the needs of treating the features of *forwards* failure, or low output, and *backwards* failure, or the congestive features. The principal symptom of a low cardiac output, fatigue, is difficult to quantify, and patients have tended to have their treatment tailored more to the consequences of venous congestion.

Haemodynamic aims of drug therapy

Acute or chronic failure of the heart may result from disease of the myocardium itself, mainly ischaemic, or an excessive load imposed on it by arterial hypertension, valvular disease or an arteriovenous shunt. The management of cardiac failure requires both the relief of any treatable underlying or aggravating cause, and therapy directed at the failure itself.

The distinction between the capacity of the myocardium to pump blood and the load against which the heart must work is useful in therapy. The failing myocardium is so strongly stimulated to

contract by increased sympathetic drive that therapeutic efforts to induce it to function yet more vigorously are in themselves alone unlikely to be of benefit. Despite numerous attempts over recent years, digoxin remains the only inotropic drug suitable for chronic oral use. By contrast, agents that reduce *preload* or *afterload* are very effective, especially where the left ventricular volume is raised (less predictably so for failure of the right ventricle). The main hazard of their use is a drastic fall in cardiac output in those occasional patients whose output is dependent on a high left ventricular filling pressure, e.g. who are volume depleted by diuretic use or those with severe mitral stenosis.

CLASSIFICATION OF DRUGS

Drugs may be classified as producing:

Reduction of preload

Diuretics increase salt and water loss, reduce blood volume and lower excessive venous filling pressure (see Ch. 26). The congestive features of oedema, in the lungs and periphery, are alleviated; when the heart is grossly enlarged, cardiac output will also increase (see discussion of Starling curve, above).

Nitrates (see also Ch. 23) dilate the smooth muscle in venous capacitance vessels, increase the volume of the venous vascular bed (which normally may comprise 80% of the whole vascular system), reduce ventricular filling pressure, thus decreasing heart wall stretch, and reduce myocardial oxygen requirements. Their arteriolar dilating action is relatively slight. Glyceryl trinitrate may be given sublingually 0.3–1 mg for acute left ventricular failure and repeated as often as necessary or by i.v. infusion, 10–200 micrograms/min. For chronic left ventricular failure isosorbide dinitrate 40–160 mg/d or isosorbide mononitrate 40–80 mg/d may be given by mouth in divided doses. Exercise capacity is improved but tolerance to nitrates may develop with chronic use. Headache, which tends to limit the dose of nitrate used for angina, is less of a problem in cardiac failure perhaps because of pre-existing vasoconstriction.

---

[12] NYHA Class 1 = minimal dyspnoea (except after moderate exercise)
  Class 2 = dyspnoea while walking on the flat
  Class 3 = dyspnoea on getting in/out of bed
  Class 4 = dyspnoea lying in bed.

Reduction of afterload

Hydralazine (see also Ch. 23) relaxes arterial smooth muscle and reduces peripheral vascular resistance. Reflex tachycardia limits its usefulness and lupus erythematosus may be induced when the dose exceeds 100 mg per day.

Reduction of preload and afterload

Angiotensin converting enzyme (ACE) inhibitors (see also Ch. 23) act by:

- reduction of afterload, by preventing the conversion of angiotensin I to the active form, angiotensin II, which is a powerful arterioconstrictor and is present in the plasma in high concentration in cardiac failure
- reduction of preload, because the formation of aldosterone, and thus retention of salt and water (increased blood volume), is prevented by the reduction of angiotensin II.

ACE inhibitors are the only drugs that reduce peripheral resistance (afterload) without causing a reflex activation of the sympathetic system. The CONSENSUS study compared enalapril with placebo in patients with NYHA class IV heart failure; after 6 months 26% of the enalapril group had died, compared with 44% in the control group. The reduction in mortality was found to be among patients with progressive heart failure.[13] There is now evidence from numerous long-term studies showing that ACE inhibition improves survival in and reduces hospital admissions for cardiac failure.[14]

A *test dose* should be given to patients who are in cardiac failure (or who are already taking a diuretic for another reason, e.g. hypertension). Maintenance of blood pressure in such individuals may depend greatly on an activated renin-angiotensin-aldosterone system and a standard dose of an ACE inhibitor can cause a catastrophic fall in blood pressure. Except for *captopril*, most ACE inhibitors (including enalapril) are prodrugs, which are inactive for several hours after dosing. This has favoured the use of captopril

for the initial dose(s) given under medical supervision; captopril also has the shortest $t\frac{1}{2}$ so that hypotension will be reversed the most quickly. Alternatively, some of the many ACE inhibitors now available (see p. 469) have a sufficiently long $t\frac{1}{2}$ to suggest that the initial doses would have a cumulative effect on blood pressure over several days; long-acting ACE inhibitors such as *lisinopril* ($t\frac{1}{2}$ 12 h) and *perindopril* ($t\frac{1}{2}$ 31 h) avoid the risk of sudden falls in blood pressure or renal function (glomerular filtration) after the first dose. These can often be initiated outside hospital in patients who are unlikely to have a high plasma renin (absence of gross oedema or widespread atherosclerotic dicease), although it is prudent to arrange for the first dose to be taken just before going to bed.

Beta-adrenoceptor blockers. The realisation that the course of chronic heart failure can be adversely affected by activation of the renin-angiotensin-aldosterone and sympathetic nervous systems led to exploration of possible benefit from β-adrenoceptors in a condition where, paradoxically, such drugs can have an adverse effect. Clinical trials have, indeed, shown that bisoprolol, carvedilol or metoprolol lower mortality and decrease hospitalisation when *added* to diuretics, digoxin and an ACE inhibitor (see below).

Spironolactone. Plasma aldosterone is elevated in heart failure. Spironolactone acts as a diuretic by competitively blocking the aldosterone-receptor, but in addition it has a powerful effect on outcome in cardiac failure (see below).

Phentolamine or sodium nitroprusside (see Ch. 23) may rarely be used (by i.v. infusion) when *acute* cardiac failure is accompanied by a high blood pressure.

Stimulation of the myocardium

Digoxin improves myocardial contractility (*positive inotropic* effect) most effectively in the dilated, failing heart and in the longer term once an episode of cardiac failure has been brought under control. This effect occurs in patients in sinus rhythm and is separate from its (*negative chronotropic*) action of reducing ventricular rate and thus improving ventricular filling in atrial fibrillation. Over 200

---

[13] The CONSENSUS Trial Study Group 1987 New England Journal of Medicine 316: 1429–1435.
[14] Flather M D et al 2000 Lancet 355: 1575–1587.

years after the first use of digitalis for dropsy, the DIG trial has brought some relief for doctors wishing evidence of long-term benefit.[15] This was a prospective randomised comparison of digoxin with placebo in 7788 patients in NYHA Class II to III heart failure and sinus rhythm, of whom most also received an ACE inhibitor and a diuretic. Overall mortality did not differ between the groups but patients who took digoxin had fewer episodes of hospitalisation for worsening heart failure; unlike all other positive isotropes, digoxin did not increase overall mortality or arrhythmias.

The phosphodiesterase inhibitors, *enoximone* and *milrinone* have positive inotropic effect due to selective myocardial enzyme inhibition and may be used for short-term treatment of severe congestive cardiac failure. Evidence from longer term use indicates that these drugs reduce survival.

Dopamine, dobutamine, dopexamine, xamoterol: see Chapter 22.

DRUG MANAGEMENT OF CARDIAC FAILURE

Chronic cardiac failure

A scheme for the stepwise drug management of chronic cardiac failure is shown in Fig. 24.5. Points to emphasise in this scheme are that *all* patients, even those with mild failure, should receive an *ACE inhibitor* as first-line therapy. Several long-term studies have demonstrated improved survival even in mild cardiac failure. In the SOLVD studies, enalapril was compared with placebo in patients with either clinical features of heart failure, or reduced left ventricular function in the absence of symptoms; treatment reduced serious events (myocardial infarction and unstable angina) by approximately 20% and hospital admissions with progressive heart failure by up to 40%.[16] *Diuretics* are very useful for symptom management but have no impact on survival. For most patients the choice will be a loop diuretic, e.g. frusemide (furosemide) starting at 20–40 mg/d. Because of the potassium-sparing effect of ACE inhibition amiloride is often not required, at least with low doses of a loop diuretic.

There is now overwhelming evidence that *β-blockade* is beneficial in chronic heart failure despite the long-held belief that their negative inotropic effect was a contraindication. Early trials were underpowered but a meta-analysis did suggest a 31% reduction in mortality. Subsequently, the CIBIS-2 and MERIT-HF trials, have independently confirmed that chronic β-blockade has a survival effect of this size in moderate to severe (NHYA III/IV) heart failure.[17] The reduction is additive to ACE inhibition and the survival benefit is largely through a reduction in sudden deaths as opposed to the progressive pump failure benefit seen with ACE inihibitors. The only cautionary note is that patients must be β-blocked very gradually with low starting doses (e.g. bisoprolol 1.25 mg/d or carvedilol 3.125 mg bd) and regular optimisation of other drugs, especially the dose of loop diuretic, to prevent decompensation of their heart failure control.

The use of *spironolactone* has received considerable support from the RALES trial,[18] which implies that ACE inhibition even at high dose does not effectively suppress hyperaldosteronism in

---

[15] The Digitalis Investigation Group 1997 The effect of digoxin on mortality and morbidity in patients with heart failure. New England Journal of Medicine 336: 525–532.
[16] SOLVD = Studies of Left Ventricular Dysfunction. The SOLVD Investigators 1991 Effect of enalapril on survival in patients with reduced left ventricular ejection fractions and congestive heart failure. New England Journal of Medicine 325: 293–302.

[17] Up until 1997, 24 trials of β-blockade in heart failure provided just 3141 patients. MERIT-HF (Lancet 1999 353: 2001) alone contained 3991 patients and CIBIS-2 provided a further 2467 (Lancet 1999 353: 9). Both studies confirmed the one-third reduction in mortality. In MERIT-HF a life was saved for just 27 patient-years of treatment i.e. it was unsually cost effective — more so than ACE inhibitor therapy. The action is probably a class effect of β-blockade given the divergent pharmacology of the drugs used to date.
[18] The RALES trial randomised 1663 patients with stable heart failure to either placebo or spironolactone (New England Journal of Medicine 1999 341: 709). All patients were maintained on their 'optimised' therapy that included ACE inhibitors. After 2 years of follow-up the trial was terminated prematurely due to a 30% reduction of mortality in the spironolactone treated patients; both progressive pump failure and sudden death were significantly reduced. Gynaecomastia or breast discomfort occurred in 10% of treated patients (1% in controls), but significant hyperkalemia occurred in surprisingly few patients. RALES was not adequately powered to decide whether the action of spironolactone is additive to that of a β-blocker.

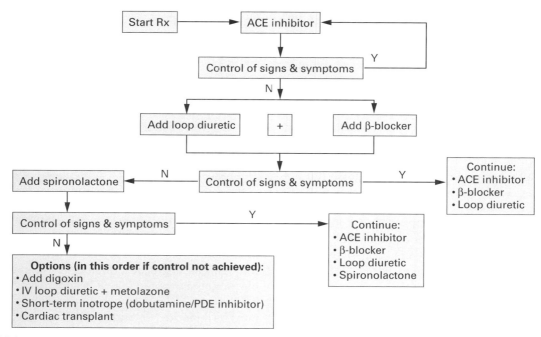

Fig. 24.5 Management of chronic cardiac failure (N = no, Y = yes, Rx = treatment, PDE = phosphodiesterase). Reproduced with permission from Lancet.

heart failure. The benefit is seen at a surprisingly low dose of spironolactone (25 mg/d); it probably reflects both improved potassium and magnesium conservation (both are antiarrythmic) and reversal of fibrosis in the myocardium by aldosterone.

None of the available oral phosphodiesterase inhibitors has become established in routine therapy, because the short-term benefit of the increased contractility has been offset by an increased mortality (presumably due to arrhythmias) on chronic dosing. A similar fate befell flosequinan, a positive inotrope which acted through the phosphatidylinositol system. Their use is restricted to short-term symptom control prior to, for example, transplanation.

Acute left ventricular failure

This is a common medical emergency (despite some possible lessening in frequency with the advent of thrombolysis for myocardial infarction). The approach should be to reassure the intensely anxious patient, who should sit upright with the legs dependent to reduce systemic venous return. A loop diuretic, e.g. *frusemide* (furosemide) 40–80 mg i.v., is the mainstay of therapy and provides benefit both by a rapid and

powerful venodilator effect reducing preload, and by the subsequent diuresis. *Oxygen* should be given, if the patient can tolerate a face mask, and *diamorphine* or *morphine* i.v. which in addition to relieving anxiety and pain, have a valuable venodilator effect.

While there can be a case for short-term use of inotropic drugs (see Ch. 22) for cardiac failure where low output is a predominant feature, it is important to remember that most such drugs substantially increase the risk of arrhythmias when the heart is hypoxic. The pharmacokinetics of digoxin do not lend themselves to emergency use. *Aminophylline* (5mg/kg over 20 min) may be administered i.v., following with great care the precautions regarding dose and monitoring (c.f. acute severe asthma, p. 562). By this stage, the possibility of *assisted ventilation* should be considered: where pulmonary oedema is the main problem, ventilation is likely to be both safer and more effective than inotropic drugs.

CARDIAC TRANSPLANTATION

While this option lies outside the scope of clinical pharmacology, an important element in meeting the objectives of treatment (p. 515) is to recognise when further drug treatment is unlikely to improve symptoms or prognosis. It is the physician who must first consider the possibility of a surgical intervention, which increasingly may involve procedures short of transplantation itself, e.g. bypass grafting or stenting where stenosed vessels contribute to the cardiac failure. On occasion, it can help the patient to be made aware that failure of both the heart and the drugs is not necessarily the end of the road.

Summary

- Cardiac failure is present when the heart cannot provide all organs with the blood supply appropriate to demand.
- Stroke volume is regulated by preload, afterload and contractility.
- In chronic cardiac failure, diuretics and nitrates reduce preload and provide symptomatic relief without affecting outcome.
- ACE inhibitors reduce both preload and afterload and reduce morbidity and mortality by about one-third in all patients.
- β-adrenoceptor blockade, gradually introduced, has an effect equivalent to that of ACE inhibition in patients with moderate or severe heart failure (NYHA III or IV).
- Spironolactone, in low dose, adds further benefit.
- Digoxin improves myocardial contractility most effectively in the dilated, failing heart but also in the longer term, including in patients in sinus rhythm.
- The principal agents for treating acute left ventricular failure are frusemide (furosemide), diamorphine and oxygen.

GUIDE TO FURTHER READING

ABC of heart failure. (A series of 8 articles by various authors, in the British Medical Journal, beginning with 2000 320: 39–42)

Burnier M, Brunner H R 2000 Angiotensin II receptor antagonists. Lancet 355: 637–645

Eisenberg M S, Mengery J 2001 Cardiac resuscitation. New England Journal of Medicine 344: 1304–1313

Grace A A, Camm A J 1998 Quinidine. New England Journal of Medicine 338: 35–45

Hauptman P J, Kelly R A 1999 Digitalis. Circulation 99: 1265–1270

Huikuri H V, Castellanos A, Myerburg R J 2001 Sudden death due to cardiac arrhythmias. New England Journal of Medicine 345: 1473–1482

Hunter J J, Chien K R 1999 Signaling pathways for cardiac hypertrophy and failure. New England Journal of Medicine 341: 1276–1283

Mangrum J M, DiMarco J P 2000 The evaluation and management of bradycardia. New England Journal of Medicine 342: 703–709

Morady F 1999 Radio-frequency ablation as treatment for cardiac arrhythmias. New England Journal of Medicine 340: 534–544

Northridge D 1996 Frusemide or nitrates for acute heart failure? [see comments] Lancet 347: 667–668

Peters N S et al 2002 Atrial fibrillation: strategies to control, combat and cure. Lancet 359: 593–603

Pitt B et al 2000 Effect of losartan compared with captopril on mortality in patients with symptomatic heart failure: randomised trial — the Losartan Heart Failure Survival Study ELITE II. [see comments] Lancet 355: 1582–1587

Podrid P J 1999 Redefining the role of antiarrhythmic drugs. New England Journal of Medicine 340: 1910–1912

Roy D et al 2000 Amiodarone to prevent recurrence of atrial fibrillation. Canadian Trial of Atrial Fibrillation Investigators. New England Journal of Medicine 342: 913–920

Schrier R W, Abraham W T 1999 Hormones and haemodynamics in heart failure. New England Journal of Medicine 341: 577–585

Squire I B, Barnett D B 2000 The rational use of β-adrenoceptor blockers in the treatment of heart failure. The changing face of an old therapy. British Journal of Clinical Pharmacology 49: 1–9

25

Hyperlipidaemias

SYNOPSIS

Correction of blood lipid abnormalities offers scope for a major impact on cardiovascular disease. Drugs play a significant role and have a variety of modes of action. Dietary and lifestyle adjustment are components of overall risk prevention.

- Pathophysiology
- Primary (inherited) and secondary hyperlipidaemias
- Management: risk assessment, secondary and primary prevention, drugs, diet, lifestyle
- Drugs used in treatment: statins; fibric acid derivatives; anion-exchange resins; nicotinic acid and derivatives

SOME PATHOPHYSIOLOGY

The normal function of lipoproteins is to distribute and recycle cholesterol. The pathways of lipid metabolism and transport and their *primary* (inherited) disorders appear in Figure 25.1 and can be summarised thus:

- Cholesterol is absorbed from the intestine and transported to the liver by chylomicron remnants, which are taken up by the low-density lipoprotein (LDL)-receptor-related protein (LRP).
- Cholesterol is then transported to *peripheral tissues* where, for example, it is converted to steroid hormones or used to form cell walls and membranes. Hepatic cholesterol enters the circulation as very-low-density lipoprotein (VLDL) and is metabolised to remnant lipoproteins after lipoprotein lipase removes triglyceride. The remnant lipoproteins are removed by the liver through apolipoprotein E-receptors or LDL-receptors (LDL-R) or further metabolised to LDL and then removed by peripheral tissues or the liver by LDL-R.

- The quantity of cholesterol transported from the liver to peripheral tissues greatly exceeds its catabolism there and mechanisms exist to return cholesterol to the liver. Through this 'reverse transport', cholesterol is carried by high-density lipoprotein (HDL) from peripheral cells to the liver where it is taken up by a process involving hepatic lipase. Cholesterol in the plasma is also recycled to LDL and VLDL by cholesterol-ester transport protein (CETP).

- Cholesterol in the liver is reassembled into lipoproteins, or secreted in bile then recycled by absorption at the terminal ileum or excreted in the faeces.

Lipid disorders

Disorders of lipid metabolism are manifest by elevation of the plasma concentrations of the various lipid and lipoprotein fractions (total and LDL cholesterol, VLDL, triglycerides, chylomicrons) and they result, predominantly, in cardiovascular disease.

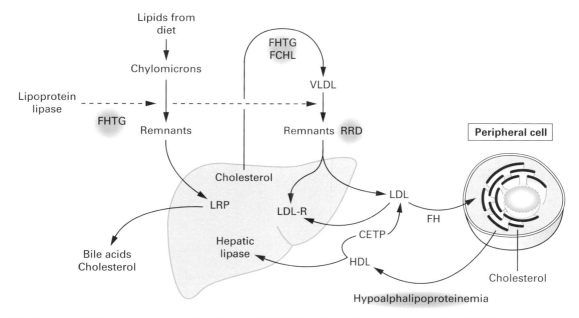

Fig. 25.1 Pathways of lipid transport. Adapted from Knopp R H 1999 New England Journal of Medicine 341: 498–511 (with permission).

This chapter addresses approaches, non-drug as well as drug, to correct abnormal lipid profiles and diminish vascular disease and its consequences.

Deposition of *cholesterol* in the arterial wall is central to the atherosclerotic process. Carriage of VLDL, remnant lipoprotein, and LDL **to** arteries can thus be viewed as potentially **atherogenic.** In the reverse process, HDL carries cholesterol **away** from the arterial wall and can be regarded as **protective** against atherogenesis. Overproduction of VLDL in the liver raises plasma VLDL, remnant lipoprotein and LDL if the capacity to metabolise these lipoproteins is compromised either by a primary (inherited) and/or secondary (environmental) abnormality.

Elevation of *LDL-cholesterol* is associated particularly with risk of coronary heart disease risk, but it is increasingly clear that moderately raised *triglycerides* or *VLDL* or *remnants* in the presence of low HDL-cholesterol may also be atherogenic.

There are five *primary inherited lipoprotein disorders* which disturb lipid matabolism at the points indicated in Figure 25.1. These are:

- *Familial hypertriglyceridemia* (FHTG) (uncommon), including lipoprotein lipase (LPL) deficiency, in which low LPL activity results in decreased removal, and thus increase of serum *triglyceride;* there is increased hepatic secretion and thus raised plasma concentration of *triglyceride-rich VLDL.* Patients are at risk of recurrent acute pancreatitis when plasma triglycerides exceed 10 mmol/l, and especially 20 mmol/l.

- *Familial combined hyperlipidemia* (FCHL) (common and most important) in which there is increased hepatic secretion of apolipoprotein B containing VLDL, and conversion to LDL; in consequence plasma *LDL* and *VLDL* are raised. Patients exhibit macrovascular disease (coronary heart, peripheral and cerebral).

- *Remnant removal disease* (RRD, also called remnant lipaemia, familial dysbetalipoproteinemia) (uncommon) in which there is a defect of apolipoprotein E. This is the major ligand that allows internalisation and subsequent metabolism of remnant particles derived from VLDL and chylomicrons. The consequence is accumulation of VLDL remnants called intermediate density lipoprotein (IDL) with cholesterol and triglycerides usually in the range 6–9 mmol/l. Patients experience severe macrovascular disease (as above).

- *Familial hypoalphalipoproteinemia* (rare) in which the serum concentration of (protective) *HDL is low.* Coronary heart and peripheral vascular disease result.
- *Familial hypercholesterolemia* (FH) (common) is characterised by elevation of *total and LDL-cholesterol* in plasma. In the more severe heterozygous form, this affects about 1:500 of the population (one copy of the LDL-receptor protein is absent or defective). LDL-cholesterol is elevated from childhood. Untreated, half the males will be dead by 60 years, females 10 years later. The principal consequence is coronary heart, but occasionally also peripheral and cerebrovascular disease.

Most commonly, patients present with raised total and LDL-cholesterol of lesser degree which results from overproduction of VLDL in the liver due to a combination of high dietary fat, obesity and individual (inherited) susceptibility; it is thus called *polygenic,* is manifest in adult life, with ather-osclerosis occuring early but not as early as with FH.

Secondary hyperlipidaemias results from: liver and biliary disease, obesity, hypothyroidism, diabetes, diet, alcohol excess, renal disease (nephrotic syndrome) and drugs (including etretinate, HIV protease inhibitors, thiazide diuretics, oral contra-ceptive steroids, glucorticosteroids, β-adrenoceptor antagonists, ciclosporin).

The most severe hyperlipidaemias usually occur in patients with concurrent conditions, e.g. diabetes mellitus with one of the primary hyperlipidaemias.

SITES OF DRUG ACTION

In general, drugs act to reduce the concentration of cholesterol within hepatocytes, causing a compen-satory increase in low-density lipoprotein-receptors (LDL-R) on their surface, and increased uptake of cholesterol-rich LDL particles from the bloodstream (see Fig. 25.1). *Statins* decrease the synthesis of cholesterol and the secretion of VLDL and increase the activity of hepatic LDL-receptors. *Bile-acid-binding resins* deplete the bile acid and thus the cholesterol pool. *Fibrates* decrease the secretion of VLDL and increase the activity of lipoprotein lipase, thereby increasing the removal of tri-glycerides. *Nicotinic acid* decreases the secretion of VLDL and the formation of LDL and increases the formation of HDL.

Management

The management of hyperlipidaemias should be viewed against the background of the following observations.

- Hyperlipidaemias are common; 66% of the adult UK population have a plasma cholesterol concentration in excess of 5.2 mmol/l, the lowest concentration generally associated with cardiovascular risk (in fact, statistical correlation can be shown with cholesterol concentrations well below this value).
- Investigation of hyperlipidaemia must be directed initially at excluding contributory causes, i.e. secondary hyperlipidaemias (see above). None of these should be assumed to be the sole cause, even if present. Long-term decisions on management should be initiated only on the basis at least two fasting blood samples.
- All patients (and their spouses/partners, if appropriate) should receive advice on lifestyle, diet and weight control, which are important components of overall macrovascular risk prevention. Dietary treatment of hypercholesterolaemia has a modest effect at best but diet and weight reduction are more effective for hypertriglyceridaemia. Total fat, especially saturated fat should be reduced (and partially replaced with mono- and polyunsaturated fats); spreads containing plant sterols and stanols, e.g. Benecol, Flora Proactiv, are useful as they can reduce plasma cholesterol by up to 10%. In some individuals, especially those with mixed hyperlipidaemia (elevated cholesterol and triglycerides), successful adherence to dietary advice, and weight loss, produces very significant improvements. Patients with remnant lipaemia (RRD hyperlipidaemia) may respond excellently to diet, weight loss (and possibly the addition of a fibrate).

25 HYPERLIPIDAEMIAS

- Much of the work of lipid clinics is taken up with attending to multiple interacting risk factors such as hypertension, diabetes, thyroid disease and smoking, as well as to the lipid abnormality.

- The decision to use lipid-lowering drugs is made on the basis of the overall absolute CHD risk (see below and footnote 3), e.g. evidence of existing CHD, hypertension, diabetes mellitus, positive family history. The justification is easiest in two cases. Firstly, as *primary* prevention in the relatively small number of patients who are asymptomatic but have significant abnormalities of their lipid profiles; patients with FH and remnant lipaemia are at high risk. The decision to treat is made on the patient's absolute risk as well as the degree of lipid abnormality. Secondly, as *secondary* prevention in patients who have evidence of CHD (previous myocardial infarction, angina pectoris), cerebrovascular or peripheral vascular disease or diabetes mellitus. The Scandinavian '4S' Study[1] of 4444 patients with a total cholesterol 5.8–8.0 mmol/l after a myocardial infarction randomised to receive simvastatin (median dose 27 mg) or placebo found that active treatment reduced total mortality by 30%, deaths from coronary heart disease by 42% and recurrent myocardial infarction risk by 34%. The authors estimated that addition of simvastatin to the treatment regimens of 100 patients with coronary heart disease would, over 6 years, preserve the lives of 4 out of 9 patients who would otherwise die and would prevent a nonfatal myocardial infarction in 7 of an expected 21 cases.

- *Consensus minimum targets* for primary and secondary prevention of CHD with statins are a total plasma cholesterol of < 5 mmol/l (or a reduction of 20–25% if the result is lower) or a LDL-cholesterol of < 3 mmol/l (or a reduction of 30% if that is lower).[2] These may be revised in the light of the Heart Protection Study (see p. 486).

- There is evidence that statins protect against stroke. The benefit is seen in patients with plasma cholesterol > 5.0 mmol/l (or LDL cholesterol > 3.0 mmol/l) who have a history of *ischaemic stroke* or *transient ischaemic attacks*, or CHD or diabetes mellitus.

More controversial is the extent to which primary prevention (treatment of clinically unaffected patients with moderate elevation of cholesterol levels) should include drugs, and whether secondary prevention should ever start with drugs rather than diet. Dietary treatment can lower cholesterol levels in committed subjects, and is obviously less costly than drug treatment. Unfortunately numerous studies have shown that over any substantial period of time (e.g. one year) diet has no clinically significant influence on plasma cholesterol; and the wait for diet to have an effect often results in patients being lost from hospital follow-up after their initial myocardial infarction. Evidence comes from the WOSCOPS study[3] in which pravastatin 40 mg/day and placebo were compared in 6590 men age 50–70 with LDL cholesterol 4–6 mmol/l; pravastatin reduced coronary heart disease (fatal and nonfatal events) by 31%. The authors estimated that treatment of 1000 such subjects each year would prevent 20 myocardial infarctions. Concerns that primary prevention could have a net adverse outcome (that cholesterol reduction increased the risk of cancer or violent deaths) have been laid to rest by a number of outcome trials.

The decision to offer a patient *primary* prophylaxis is influenced by the absolute risk for the individual, the potential risks from the statin therapy and costs to the health provider. As statins so far have an excellent safety record, costs will escalate with a decision to treat lower and lower levels of absolute risk. Current UK recommendations suggest treating patients with a CHD risk of at least 30% over 10 years, and an aspiration to treat those with a 15%

---

[1] Scandinavian Simvastatin Survival Study Group 1994 Randomised trial of cholesterol lowering in 4444 patients with coronary heart disease: the Scandinavian Simvastatin Survival Study (4S). Lancet 344: 1383–1389.

[2] Wood D et al 1998 Joint British recommendations on prevention of coronary heart disease in clinical practice. Heart 80(Suppl): S1–29. (British Cardiac Society, British Hyperlipidaemia Association, British Hypertension Society, British Diabetic Association).

[3] WOSCOPS = West of Scotland Coronary Prevention Study. Shepherd J et al 1995 Prevention of coronary heart disease with pravastatin in men with hypercholesterolemia. New England Journal of Medicine 333: 1301–1307.

10-year risk if resources allow. The large number of additional patients involved by treating at the lower level raises issues of funding and resources (but not the cost-effectiveness of the treatment, which is clear).

The absolute CHD risk is computed using risk equations based on the Framingham cohort;[4] in reality this means consulting a simple colour-coded chart armed with data about the patient including age, sex, smoking status, pretreatment blood pressure and plasma total and LDL cholesterol, and presence or absence of diabetes.[4]

Management may proceed as follows:

1. *Any medical disorder* that may be causing hyperlipidaemia, e.g. diabetes, hypothyroidism, should be treated first.
2. *Dietary adjustment.* The following applies to all patients:

   - Those who are overweight should reduce their total caloric intake, ideally until they have returned to the weight that is appropriate for their height (i.e. body mass index) but realistically with an initial aim of reducing body weight by 10% (see Appetite control p. 696); this automatically assumes reduced intake of alcohol and total (especially animal) fat. Elevated triglyceride concentrations may respond particularly well to alcohol withdrawal.
   - Those who fail to achieve adequate weight reduction or who are already at their ideal weight should reduce their total fat intake; poly- and monounsaturated fats or oils may be taken partially to substitute for the reduction in animal fats. Reduction in dietary cholesterol is a much less important element of the diet, but excess egg yolks should be avoided. Benecol or Flora Proactiv should be added.

3. *Specific types* of hyperlipidaemia are treated thus:

   - Familial hypertriglyceridaemia responds best to dietary modification and weight reduction

(above) together with a fibrate; nicotinic acid may be added.

- Familial combined hyperlipidaemia should be treated with dietary modification and weight reduction (above) together with a statin; nicotinic acid and/or a fibrate may be added in resistant cases.
- Remnant removal disease (remnant lipaemia) responds to dietary modification and weight reduction (above) and a fibrate; nicotinic acid and/or a statin may be added where there is failure to respond.
- Familial or polygenic hypercholesterolaemia is treated by dietary modification and a statin; an anion-exchange resin and/or a fibrate and/or nicotinic acid may be added.
- Familial hypoalphalipoproteinaemia may respond to exercise, weight loss, and nicotinic acid; a fibrate and/or a statin may be added for a small HDL-raising effect but primarily to lower triglycerides and LDL.

Drugs used in treatment

STATINS

These agents block the rate-limiting enzyme for endogenous cholesterol synthesis, hydroxy-methyl-glutaryl coenzyme A *(HMG CoA)* reductase. This results in increased synthesis of LDL-receptors (up-regulation) in the liver and increased clearance of LDL from the circulation; plasma total cholesterol and LDL-cholesterol fall to attain a maximum effect 1 month after commencing therapy. All statins cause a dose-dependent reduction in total and LDL-cholesterol although there are differences in their therapeutic efficacy: for example, at their starting doses LDL-cholesterol falls by average of 17% with *fluvastatin* (20 mg/d), 28% with *simvastatin* (10 mg/d) and 38% with *atorvastatin* (10 mg/d). At higher doses, e.g. atorvastatin 80 mg/d or possibly simvastatin 80 mg/d, a 50% reduction in LDL-cholesterol is possible. The effects of *pravastatin* are similar. There is no tolerance to continued administration of a statin, and because of a circadian rhythm to LDL-receptor synthesis, statins are a little more effective if given in the evening rather than in

---

[4] The cardiac risk program (actually an Excel spreadsheet) and risk assessment charts can be downloaded from the BHS website at http://www.hyp.ac.uk/bhsinfo. They may also be found in the British National Formulary.

the morning. Their efficacy in both primary and secondary prophylaxis of hypercholesterolaemia is probably a class effect, although long-term outcome studies may in time differentiate between the drugs. On current information, with no clear advantages or disadvantages between the different statins, the choice of agent to achieve the suggested total or LDL-cholesterol levels[3] is heavily influenced by their relative cost, and the dose likely to achieve the target. (See also the Heart Protection Study, p. 486.)

Statins are well absorbed after administration orally, and are metabolised in the liver. They are well tolerated, the commonest adverse effect being transient, and usually minor abnormality of liver function tests in some 1% of patients. Asymptomatic elevation of muscle enzymes (creatine phosphokinase, CPK) and myositis (with a generalised muscle discomfort) occur more rarely,[5] but is more frequent when statins are combined with other anti-hyperlidaemic drugs such as fibrates and nicotinic acid; patients should be counseled about myositis when these drugs are co-administered. Myositis is also more likely with co-administered anti-HIV protease inhibitors, and with drugs that interfere with metabolism of some statins, e.g. ciclosporin.

FIBRIC ACID DERIVATIVES (FIBRATES)

The class includes *bezafibrate, ciprofibrate, fenofibrate* and *gemfibrozil*; the original fibrate, clofibrate, is obsolete. The drugs partly resemble short-chain fatty acids and increase the oxidation of these acids in both liver and muscle. In the liver, secretion of triglyceride-rich lipoproteins falls, and in muscle the activity of lipoprotein lipase and fatty acid uptake from plasma are both increased. Fibrates act through a nuclear transcription factor (PPARα) which up-regulates expression of LDL-cholesterol and apolipoprotein A-1 genes, and down-regulates expression of the apolipoprotein C-11 gene. The result is that plasma triglyceride declines by 20–30% and cholesterol by 10–15%; associated with this is a rise in the 'protective' HDL-cholesterol. The latter effect may have contributed to the reduction in nonfatal myocardial infarction with gemfibrozil in both the Helsinki Heart Study[6] and more recent VA-HIT trials.[7] They are the drugs of choice for *mixed hyperlipidaemia* (elevated cholesterol plus triglycerides) but may be used in hyper-

cholesterolaemia, alone or with anion exchange resins or (with care) with statins. There is evidence of varying efficacy among the drugs both in cholesterol-lowering and in additional beneficial effects, such as reduction in blood fibrinogen and urate concentration; the clinical significance of these differences is not yet known.

Fibric acid derivatives are well absorbed from the gastrointestinal tract, extensively bound to plasma proteins and excreted mainly by the kidney as unchanged drug or metabolites. They are contraindicated where hepatic or renal function is severely impaired (but gemfibrozil has been used in uraemic and nephrotic patients without aggravating deterioration in kidney function). Rarely, fibric acid derivatives may induce a myositis-like syndrome; the risk is greater in patients with poor renal function, and in those who are also receiving a statin. Fibrates enhance the effect of co-administered oral anticoagulants.

Anion-exchange resins (bile acid sequestrants)

Colestyramine is an oral anion-exchange resin,[8] which binds bile acids in the intestine. Bile acids are formed from cholesterol in the liver, pass into the gut in the bile and are largely reabsorbed at the terminal ileum. The total bile acid pool is only 3–5 g but, because such *enterohepatic recycling* takes place 5–10 times a day, on average 20–30 g of bile acid are delivered into the intestine every 24 hours. Bile acids bound to colestyramine are lost in the faeces and the depletion of the bile acid pool stimulates conversion of cholesterol to bile acid: the result is a

---

[5] In 30 641 patients in 5 major statin trials, myositis (serum creatinine kinase × 10 normal) occurred in 30 (control 29) and rhabdomyolysis in 2 (control 2). Farmer J A 2001 Lancet 358: 1383–1385.

[6] Frick M H et al 1987 New England Journal of Medicine 317: 1237–1245.

[7] Rubins H B et al 1999 New England Journal of Medicine 341: 410–418.

[8] The resins consist of aggregations of large molecules carrying a fixed positive charge which therefore bind negatively charged ions (anions).

fall in intracellular cholesterol in hepatocytes, and an increase (up-regulation) in both LDL-receptors and cholesterol synthesis. The former has the predominant influence on plasma LDL-cholesterol, which falls by 20–25%. In many patients there is some compensatory increase in hepatic triglyceride output. Anion exchange resins therefore may be used first line for *hypercholesterolaemia* but not when there is significant hypertriglyceridaemia, which may be aggravated in such patients. The powder is taken mixed with water or orange juice and shaken in a closed container.

About half the patients who take colestyramine experience constipation and some complain of anorexia, abdominal fullness and occasionally of diarrhoea; these effects are dose-related but may limit or prevent its use. Because the drug binds anions, drugs such as warfarin, digoxin, thiazide diuretics, phenobarbitone and thyroid hormones should be taken 1 h before or 4 h after colestyramine to avoid impairment of their absorption.

Colestipol is similar to colestyramine.

Nicotinic acid and derivatives

Nicotinic acid acts as an antilipolytic agent in adipose tissue, reducing the supply of free fatty acids and hence the availability of substrate for hepatic triglyceride synthesis and the secretion of VLDL. Nicotinic acid lowers plasma triglyceride and cholesterol concentrations, and raises HDL-cholesterol. Flushing of the skin (preventable by low-dose aspirin) and gastrointestinal upset commonly occur; the unpleasantness may be diminished by gradually building up the oral dose over 6 weeks and in time tolerance develops. Rarely there is major disturbance of liver function.

Acipimox is better tolerated than nicotinic acid, has a longer duration of action but is less effective. Unlike nicotinic acid, it does not reduce circulating

levels of Lp(a), the modest reduction of which (achieved by nicotinic acid) may contribute to overall protection against the complications of atheroma.

OTHER DRUGS

Alpha-tocopherol acetate (vitamin E) has no effect on lipid levels but is a powerful antioxidant. Considerable evidence points to oxidation of LDL as an essential step in the development of atheroma, and therefore interest has centred on the role of either endogenous or therapeutic vitamin E in prevention of atheroma. Reduced concentrations of vitamin E in both blood and fat (vitamin E is a fat soluble vitamin) are found in inhabitants of countries with a high prevalence of ischaemic heart disease, and (within these countries) in patients who develop ischaemic heart disease. A high dose reduced by half the risk of myocardial infarction in 2000 patients with angina and positive coronary angiogram.[9] However most other studies have failed to confirm this finding and there is no indication at present for routine prescribing of α-tocopherol in the treatment or prevention of atherosclerosis.

> **Summary**
>
> - The commonest and most important hyperlipidaemia is hypercholesterolaemia, which is one of the major risk factors for coronary heart disease.
> - Most treatment works by reducing the intracellular concentration of cholesterol in hepatocytes, leading to compensatory increase in low density lipoprotein (LDL) receptors on their surface, and increased uptake of cholesterol-rich LDL particles from the bloodstream.
> - The most effective drugs are the statins, which inhibit the rate-limiting step in cholesterol synthesis.
> - Additional agents may be required for mixed or severe hyperlipidaemia.
> - In outcome trials with these drugs, reductions in blood cholesterol by 25–35% is associated with a 35–45% reduction in risk of coronary heart disease.
> - The main indications for their use are in patients with even slight elevations of cholesterol (> 5mmol/l) after a myocardial infarction or any other macrovascular event, in patients with familial hypercholesterolaemia, and in patients with a significant absolute CHD risk, especially where there is a family history of premature CHD.

---

[9] Stephens N G et al 1996 Randomised controlled trial of vitamin E in patients with coronary disease: Cambridge heart antioxidant study. Lancet 347: 781–786.

SECTION 5

Omega-3 marine triglycerides (Maxepa) contain the triglyceride precursors of two polyunsaturated fatty acids (eicosapentaenoic acid and docosahexaenoic acid) derived from oily fish. They have no place in treating hypercholesterolaemia. Some patients with moderate to severe hypertriglyceridaemia may respond to oral use, although LDL-cholesterol may rise. There is an associated 90 calorie per day energy load.

Orlistat, a weight-reducing agent, lowers the glycaemia of diabetes mellitus to a degree that accords with the weight loss, and improves hyperlipidaemia to an extent greater than would be expected (see p. 696). Since it is a lipase inhibitor there is a risk of steatorrhoea and malabsorption of fat-soluble vitamins A, D and E.

GUIDE TO FURTHER READING

Caro J et al 1997 The West of Scotland coronary prevention study: economic benefit analysis of primary prevention with pravastatin. British Medical Journal 315: 1577–1582.

Hooper L et al 2001 Dietary fat intake and prevention of cardiovascular disease: systematic review. British Medical Journal 322: 757–763

Jönsson B 2001 Economics of drug treatment: for which patients is it cost-effective to lower cholesterol? Lancet 358: 1251

Knopp R H 1999 Drug treatment of lipid disorders. New England Journal of Medicine 341: 498–511

Mansell P, Reckless J P D 1991 Garlic. British Medical Journal 303: 379

Oliver M F 2000 Cholesterol and strokes. British Medical Journal 320: 459–460

Primatesta P, Poulter N 2000 Lipid concentrations and the use of lipid lowering drugs: evidence from a national cross sectional study. British Medical Journal 321: 1322–3125

Sacks F M, Pfeffer M A, Moye L A et al 1996 The effect of pravastatin on coronary events after myocardial infarction in patients with average cholesterol levels. New England Journal of Medicine 335: 1001–1009

White H D et al 2000 Pravastatin therapy and the risk of stroke. New England Journal of Medicine 343: 317–326

26

Kidney and genitourinary tract

The kidneys comprise only 0.5% of body weight, yet they receive 25% of the cardiac output. Drugs that affect renal function have important roles in cardiac failure and hypertension. Disease of the kidney must be taken into account when prescribing drugs that are eliminated by it.

- Diuretic drugs: their sites and modes of action, classification, adverse effects and uses in cardiac, hepatic, renal and other conditions
- Carbonic anhydrase inhibitors
- Cation-exchange resins and their uses
- Alteration of urine pH

Drugs and the kidney
- Adverse effects
- Drug-induced renal disease: by direct and indirect biochemical effects and by immunological effects
- Prescribing for renal disease: adjusting the dose according to the characteristics of the drug and to the degree of renal impairment
- Nephrolithiasis and its management
- Pharmacological aspects of micturition
- Benign prostatic hyperplasia
- Erectile dysfunction

Diuretic drugs

(See also Ch. 23)

Definition. A diuretic is any substance which increases urine and solute excretion. This wide definition, however, includes substances not commonly thought of as diuretics, e.g. water. To be therapeutically useful a diuretic should increase the output of *sodium* as well as of water, since diuretics are normally required to remove oedema fluid, composed of water and solutes, of which sodium is the most important. Diuretics are among the most commonly-used drugs, perhaps because the evolutionary advantages of sodium retention have left an aging population without salt-losing mechanisms of matching efficiency.

Each day the body produces 180 l of glomerular filtrate which is modified in its passage down the renal tubules to appear as 1.5 l of urine. Thus a 1% reduction in reabsorption of tubular fluid will more than double urine output. Clearly, drugs that act on the tubule have considerable scope to alter body fluid and electrolyte balance. Most clinically useful diuretics are organic anions, which are transported directly from the blood into tubular fluid. The following brief account of tubular function with particular reference to *sodium transport* will help to explain where and how diuretic drugs act; it should be read with reference to Figure 26.1.

SITES AND MODES OF ACTION

Proximal convoluted tubule

Some 65% of the filtered sodium is actively transported from the lumen of the proximal tubule by the sodium pump (Na^+, K^+-ATPase). Chloride is absorbed passively, accompanying the sodium; bicarbonate is also absorbed, through the action of carbonic anhydrase. These solute shifts give rise to the iso-osmotic reabsorption of water, with the result that > 70% of the glomerular filtrate is returned to the blood from this section of the nephron. The epithelium of the proximal tubule is described as 'leaky' because of its free permeability to water and a number of solutes. *Osmotic diuretics* such as *mannitol* are solutes which are not reabsorbed in the proximal tubule (**site 1.** Fig. 26.1) and therefore retain water in the tubular fluid. Their effect is to increase water rather than sodium loss, and this is reflected in their special use acutely to reduce intracranial or intraocular pressure and not states associated with sodium overload.

Loop of Henle

The tubular fluid now passes into the loop of Henle where 25% of the filtered sodium is reabsorbed. There are two populations of nephron: those with *short loops* that are confined to the cortex, and the *juxtamedullary nephrons* whose long loops penetrate into the inner parts of the medulla and are principally concerned with water conservation;[1] the following discussion refers to the latter. The physiological changes are best understood by considering first the *ascending* limb. In the thick segment (**site 2,** Fig. 26.1), sodium and chloride ions are transported from the tubular fluid into the interstitial fluid by the three-ion co-transporter system (i.e. $Na^+/K^+/2Cl^-$) driven by the sodium pump. Since the tubule epithelium is 'tight' here i.e. impermeable to water, the tubular fluid becomes dilute, the interstitium becomes hypertonic and fluid in the *descending* limb, which is permeable to water, becomes more concentrated as it approaches the tip of the loop, because the hypertonic interstitial fluid sucks water out of this limb of the tubule. The 'hairpin' structure of the loop thus confers on it the property of a *countercurrent multiplier,* i.e. by active transport of

ions a small change in osmolality laterally across the tubular epithelium is converted into a steep vertical osmotic gradient. The high osmotic pressure in the medullary interstitium is sustained by the descending and ascending *vasa recta,* long blood vessels of capillary thickness which lie close to the loops of Henle and act as *countercurrent exchangers,* for the incoming blood receives sodium from the outgoing blood.[2] *Frusemide (furosemide), bumetanide, piretanide, torasemide* and *ethacrynic acid* act principally at site 2 by inhibiting the three-ion transporter system, thus preventing sodium ion reabsorption and lowering the osmotic gradient between cortex and medulla; this results in the formation of large volumes of dilute urine. These drugs are called the *loop* diuretics.

As the ascending limb of the loop re-enters the renal cortex, sodium continues to be removed from the tubular fluid by the sodium pump, accompanied electrostatically by chloride. Both ions pass into the interstitial tissue (site 3) from which they are rapidly removed because cortical blood flow is high and there are no vasa recta present; consequently the urine becomes more dilute. *Thiazides* act principally at this *cortical diluting segment* of the ascending limb, preventing sodium reabsorption. They inhibit the NaCl co-transporter (called NCCT).

Distal convoluted tubule and collecting duct

In the distal tubule (site 4), sodium ions are exchanged for potassium and hydrogen ions. The sodium ions are transported across the epithelial Na channel (called ENaC), which is stimulated by aldosterone. The aldosterone (mineralocorticoid)

---

[1] Beavers occupying a watery habitat have nephrons with short loops, while those of the desert rat have long loops.
[2] The most easily comprehended countercurrent exchange mechanism (in this case for heat) is that in wading birds in cold climates whereby the veins carrying cold blood from the feet pass closely alongside the arteries carrying warm blood from the body and heat exchange takes place. The result is that the feet receive blood below body temperature (which does not matter) and the blood from the feet which is often very cold, is warmed before it enters the body so that the internal temperature is more easily maintained. The principle is the same for maintaining renal medullary hypertonicity.

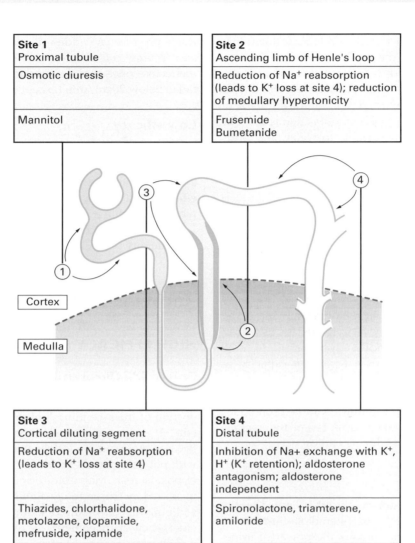

Fig. 26.1 Sites of action of diuretic drugs

receptor is inhibited by the competitive receptor antagonist *spironolactone,* whilst the sodium channel is inhibited by *amiloride* and *triamterene*. All three of these diuretics are potassium sparing because potassium is normally transported into the tubular lumen down the electrochemical gradient created by sodium reabsorption. All other diuretics, acting proximal to site 4, are potassium losing, because an increased sodium load is presented to ENaC, and sodium/potassium exchange is therefore increased. The potassium sparing diuretics are normally considered weak diuretics because site 4 is normally responsible for 'only' 5% of sodium reabsorption, and they usually cause less sodium loss than thiazides or loop diuretics. Patients with genetic abnormalities of ENaC develop severe salt wasting or hypertension, depending on whether the mutation causes loss or gain, respectively, of channel activity. Although ENaC clearly does not have the capacity to compensate for large sodium losses, e.g. during loop diuretic usage, it is the main site of physiological control (via aldosterone) over sodium losses. The reason why amiloride and triamterene are weak diuretics is partly that they compete with sodium for binding to ENaC, and are effective therefore only when sodium intake is low.

The collecting duct then travels back down into the medulla to reach the papilla; in doing so it passes through a gradient of increasing osmotic pressure which tends to draw water out of tubular fluid. This final concentration of urine is under the influence of *antidiuretic hormone* (ADH) whose action is to make the collecting duct permeable to water, and in its absence water remains in the collecting duct; *ethanol* causes diuresis by inhibiting the release of ADH from the posterior pituitary gland.

Diuresis may also be achieved by extrarenal mechanisms, by raising the cardiac output and increasing renal blood flow, e.g. with dobutamine and dopamine.

CLASSIFICATION

The maximum efficacy in removing salt and water that any drug can achieve is related to its site of action, and it is clinically appropriate to rank diuretics according to their *natriuretic* capacity, as set out below. The percentages quoted in this rank order refer to the highest fractional excretion of filtered sodium under carefully controlled conditions and should not be taken to represent the average fractional sodium loss during clinical use.

High efficacy

Frusemide (furosemide) and the other *(loop)* diuretics can cause up to 25% of filtered sodium to be excreted. Their action impairs the powerful urine-concentrating mechanism of the loop of Henle and confers higher efficacy compared to drugs that act in the relatively hypotonic cortex (see below). Progressive increase in dose is matched by increasing diuresis, i.e. they have a *high* 'ceiling' of effect. Indeed, they are so efficacious that overtreatment can readily dehydrate the patient. Loop diuretics remain effective at glomerular filtration rates below 10 ml/min (normal 120 ml/min).

Moderate efficacy

The *thiazide* family, including bendrofluazide (bendroflumethiazide) and the related chlorthalidone, clopamide, indapamide, mefruside, metolazone and xipamide, cause 5–10% of filtered sodium load to be excreted. Increasing the dose beyond a small

range produces no added diuresis, i.e. they have a *low* 'ceiling' of effect. Such drugs tend to be ineffective once the glomerular filtration rate has fallen below 20 ml/min (except metolazone).

Low efficacy

Potassium sparing triamterene, amiloride and spironolactone, cause 5% of the filtered sodium to be excreted. They are usefully combined with more efficacious diuretics to prevent the potassium loss, which other diuretics cause.

Osmotic diuretics, e.g. mannitol, also fall into this category.

Individual diuretics

HIGH EFFICACY (LOOP) DIURETICS

Frusemide (furosemide)

Frusemide (furosemide, Lasix) acts on the thick portion of the ascending limb of the loop of Henle (site 2) to produce the effects described above. Because more sodium is delivered to site 4, exchange with potassium leads to urinary potassium loss and hypokalaemia. Magnesium and calcium loss are increased by frusemide to about the same extent as sodium; the effect on calcium is utilised in the emergency management of hypercalcaemia (see p. 740).

Pharmacokinetics. Frusemide is well absorbed from the gastrointestinal tract and is highly bound to plasma proteins. The $t\frac{1}{2}$ is 2 h, but this rises to over 10 h in renal failure.

Uses. Frusemide is very successful for the relief of oedema. Progressively increasing the dose of frusemide increases urine production. Taken orally it acts within an hour and diuresis lasts up to 6 hours. Enormous urine volumes can result and overtreatment may lead to hypovolaemia and circulatory collapse. Given i.v. it acts within 30 minutes and can relieve acute pulmonary oedema, partly by a vasodilator action which precedes the diuresis. An important feature of frusemide is its efficacy when the glomerular filtration rate is 10 ml/min or less.

The dose is 20–120 mg by mouth per day; i.m. or i.v. 20–40 mg is given initially. For use in renal failure, special high dose tablets (500 mg) are available, and a solution of 250 mg in 25 ml which should be infused i.v. at a rate not greater than 4 mg/min.

Adverse effects are uncommon, apart from excess of therapeutic effect (electrolyte disturbance and hypotension due to low plasma volume) and those mentioned in the general account for diuretics (below). They include nausea, pancreatitis and, rarely, deafness which is usually transient and associated with rapid i.v. injection in renal failure. NSAIDs, notably indomethacin, reduce frusemide-induced diuresis probably by inhibiting the formation of vasodilator prostaglandins in the kidney.

Bumetanide, piretanide and *ethacrynic acid* are similar to frusemide. *Torasemide* is also similar, but has also been demonstrated to be an effective anti-hypertensive agent at lower (non-natriuretic) doses (2.5–5 mg/d) than those used for oedema (5–40 mg). *Ethacrynic acid* is less widely used as it is more prone to cause adverse effects, especially nausea and deafness.

MODERATE EFFICACY DIURETICS

(See also Hypertension, Ch. 23)

Thiazides

Thiazides depress sodium reabsorption at site 3 which is just proximal to the region of sodium–potassium exchange. These drugs thus raise potassium excretion to an important extent. Thiazides lower blood pressure, initially due to reduction in intravascular volume but chronically by a reduction in peripheral vascular resistance. The latter is accompanied by diminished responsiveness of vascular smooth muscle to noradrenaline (norepinephrine); they may also have a direct action on vascular smooth muscle membranes, acting on an as yet unidentified ion channel.

Uses. Thiazides are used for mild cardiac failure, and mild hypertension, or for more severe degrees of hypertension, in combination with other drugs.

Pharmacokinetics. Thiazides are generally well absorbed when taken by mouth and most begin to act within an hour. There are numerous derivatives and differences amongst them lie principally in their duration of action. The relatively water soluble, e.g. cyclopenthiazide, chlorothiazide, hydrochlorothiazide, are most rapidly eliminated, their peak effect occurring within 4–6 h and passing off by 10–12 h. They are excreted unchanged in the urine and active secretion by the proximal renal tubule contributes to their high renal clearance and $t\frac{1}{2}$ of <4 h. The relatively lipid-soluble members of the group, e.g. polythiazide, hydroflumethiazide, distribute more widely into body tissues and act for over 24 h, which can be objectionable if the drug is used for diuresis, though useful for hypertension. With the exception of metolazone, thiazides are not effective when renal function is moderately impaired, because they are not filtered in sufficient concentration to inhibit the NCCT.

Adverse effects in general are discussed below. Rashes (sometimes photosensitive), thrombocytopenia and agranulocytosis occur. Treatment with thiazide-type drugs causes an increase in total serum cholesterol, but on long-term usage even of high doses this is less than 5%. The questions about the appropriateness of use of these drugs for mild hypertension, of which ischaemic heart disease is a common complication, have been laid to rest by their proven success rates in randomised outcome comparisons.

Bendrofluazide (bendroflumethiazide) is a satisfactory member for routine use.
- For a diuretic effect the oral dose is 5–10 mg which usually lasts less than 12 h so that it should be given in the morning. It may be given daily for the first few days then, say, 3 days a week.
- As an antihypertensive 1.25–2.5 mg is given daily; in the absence of a diuresis clinically important potassium depletion is uncommon,

but plasma potassium concentration should be checked in potentially vulnerable groups such as the elderly (see Ch. 24).

Hydrochlorothiazide is a satisfactory alternative. Other members of the group include: benzthiazide, chlorothiazide, cyclopenthiazide, hydroflumethiazide, polythiazide.

Diuretics related to the thiazides. Several compounds, although strictly not thiazides, share structural similarities with them and probably act at the same site on the nephron; they therefore exhibit moderate therapeutic efficacy. Overall, these substances have a longer duration of action, are used for oedema and hypertension and their profile of adverse effects is similar to that of the thiazides. They are listed below.

Chlortalidone acts for 48–72 h after a single oral dose.

Indapamide is structurally related to chlortalidone but lowers blood pressure at subdiuretic doses, perhaps by altering calcium flux in vascular smooth muscle. It has less apparent effect on potassium, glucose or uric acid excretion (see below).

Metolazone is effective when renal function is impaired. It potentiates the diuresis produced by frusemide and the combination can be effective in resistant oedema, provided the patient's fluid and electrolyte loss are carefully monitored.

Xipamide is structurally related to chlortalidone and to frusemide. It induces a diuresis for about 12 h that is brisker than with thiazides, which may trouble the elderly.

LOW EFFICACY DIURETICS

Spironolactone (Aldactone) is structurally similar to aldosterone and competitively inhibits its action in the distal tubule (exchange of potassium for sodium); excessive secretion of aldosterone contributes to fluid retention in hepatic cirrhosis, nephrotic syndrome and congestive cardiac failure (see specific use in chapter 24), in which conditions as well as in primary hypersecretion (Conn's syndrome) spironolactone is most useful. Spironolactone is also useful in the treatment of resistant hypertension, where increased aldosterone sensitivity is increasingly recognised as a contributory factor.

Spironolactone is extensively metabolised and the $t_{1/2}$ is 8 h. The most significant product, canrenone, is available as a drug in its own right, potassium canrenoate. The prolonged diuretic effect of spironolactone is explained by 17 h $t_{1/2}$ of canrenone. Spironolactone is relatively ineffective when used alone but may usefully be combined with a drug that reduces sodium reabsorption proximally in the tubule, e.g. a loop diuretic. Spironolactone (and amiloride and triamterene, see below) also reduces the potassium loss that occurs with loop diuretics, but use in combination with another potassium-sparing diuretic leads to hyperkalaemia. Dangerous potassium retention may also develop if spironolactone is given to patients with impaired renal function. It is given orally in one or more doses totalling 100–200 mg. Maximum diuresis is delayed for up to 4 days. If after 5 days response is inadequate, dose may be increased to 300–400 mg/d. 0.5–1 mg/kg are required in treating hypertension.

The oestrogenic side effects of spironolactone are the major limitation to its long-term use. They are dose-dependent, but in the RALES trial[3] (see Chapter 24) even 25 mg/d caused breast tenderness or enlargement in 10% of men. Women may also report breast discomfort or menstrual irregularities including amenorrhoea. Minor gastrointestinal upset also occurs. These effects are reversible on stopping the drug. Possible human metabolites are carcinogenic in rodents; it seems unlikely after many years of clinical experience that the drug is carcinogenic in humans. In the UK, spironolactone is no longer licenced for use in essential hypertension, but retains its licence for other indications.

Amiloride exerts an inhibitory action on sodium channels under the influence of aldosterone in the distal tubule. Its action is therefore complementary to that of the thiazides and, used with them, it augments sodium loss and but limits potassium loss. One such combination, co-amilozide, (Moduretic) (amiloride 2.5–5 mg plus hydrochlorothiazide 25–50 mg), is used for hypertension or oedema. The maximum effect of amiloride occurs about 6 h after an oral dose with a duration of action > 24 h ($t_{1/2}$ 21 h). The oral dose is 5–20 mg daily.

---

[3] New England Journal of Medicine 1999 341: 709.

Triamterene (Dytac) is a potassium-sparing diuretic which has an action and use similar to that of amiloride. The diuretic effect extends over 10 h. Gastrointestinal upsets occur. Reversible, nonoliguric renal failure may occur when triamterene is used with indomethacin (and presumably other NSAIDs).

INDICATIONS FOR DIURETICS

- *Oedema states* associated with sodium overload, e.g. cardiac, renal or hepatic disease, and also without sodium overload, e.g. acute pulmonary oedema following myocardial infarction. Note that oedema may also be localised, e.g. angioedema over the face and neck or around the ankles following some calcium channel blockers, or due to low plasma albumin, or immobility in the elderly; in none of these circumstances are diuretics indicated.
- *Hypertension,* by reducing intravascular volume and probably by other mechanisms too, e.g. reduction of sensitivity to noradrenergic vasoconstriction.
- *Hypercalcaemia.* Frusemide reduces calcium reabsorption in the ascending limb of the loop of Henle and this action may be utilised in the emergency reduction of elevated plasma calcium in addition to rehydration and other measures (see p. 740).
- *Idiopathic hypercalciuria,* a common cause of renal stone disease, may be reduced by thiazide diuretics
- The *syndrome of inappropriate secretion of antidiuretic hormone secretion* (SIADH) may be treated with frusemide if there is a dangerous degree of volume overload. (see also p. 713).
- *Nephrogenic diabetes insipidus,* paradoxically, may respond to diuretics which, by contracting vascular volume, increase salt and water reabsorption in the proximal tubule, and thus reduce urine volume.

THERAPY

Congestive cardiac failure

The main account appears in Chapter 24 where the emphasis is now on early use of ACE-inhibitors and other therapies which are specifically diuretic-sparing. Nevertheless, because diuretics by mouth are easily given repeatedly, lack of supervision can result in insidious *overtreatment.* Relief at disappearance of the congestive features can mask exacerbation of the low output symptoms of heart failure, such as *tiredness* and *postural dizziness* due to reduced blood volume. A rising *blood urea* is usually evidence of reduced glomerular blood flow consequent on a fall in cardiac output, but does not distinguish whether the cause of the reduced output is overdiuresis or worsening of the heart failure itself. The simplest guide to the success or failure of diuretic regimens is to monitor *body weight,* which the patient can do equipped with just bathroom scales. Fluid intake and output charts are more demanding of nursing time, and often less accurate.

Acute pulmonary oedema: left ventricular failure

(See p. 518)

Renal oedema

The chief therapeutic aims are to reduce dietary sodium intake and to prevent excessive sodium retention using diuretic drugs. Reduction of sodium reabsorption in the renal tubule by diuretics is most effective where glomerular filtration has not been seriously reduced by disease. *Frusemide* and *bumetanide* are effective even when the filtration rate is very low; frusemide may usefully be combined with *metolazone* but the resulting profound diuresis requires careful monitoring. Secondary hyperaldosteronism complicates the nephrotic syndrome because albumin loss causes plasma colloid pressure to fall, and the resulting diversion of intravascular volume to the interstitium activates the renin-angiotensin-aldosterone system; then *spironolactone* may be added usefully to potentiate a loop diuretic and to conserve potassium, loss of which can be severe.

Hepatic ascites (see also p. 656)

Ascites and oedema are due to portal venous hypertension together with decreased plasma colloid osmotic pressure causing hyperalodosteronism as with nephrotic oedema (above). Furthermore, diversion of renal blood flow from the cortex to the medulla favours sodium retention. In addition to dietary sodium restriction, a *loop diuretic* plus *spironolactone* are used to produce a gradual diuresis; too vigorous depletion of sodium with added potassium loss and hypochloraemic alkalosis may cause hepatic coma. Abdominal paracentesis can be very effective if combined with human albumin infusion to prevent further aggravating hypoproteinaemia.

ADVERSE EFFECTS CHARACTERISTIC OF DIURETICS

Potassium depletion. Diuretics, which act at sites 1, 2 and 3 (Fig. 26.1), cause more sodium to reach the sodium–potassium exchange site in the distal tubule (site 4) and so increase potassium excretion. This subject warrants discussion since hypokalaemia may cause cardiac arrhythmia in patients at risk (for instance patients receiving digoxin). The safe lower limit for serum potassium concentration in such patients is normally quoted as 3.5 mmol/l. Whether or not diuretic therapy causes significant lowering of serum potassium depends both on the drug and on the circumstances in which it is used.

- *The loop diuretics* cause a smaller fall in serum potassium than do the thiazides, for equivalent diuretic effect, but have a greater capacity for diuresis, i.e. higher efficacy especially in large dose, and so are associated with greater decline in potassium. If diuresis is brisk and continuous, clinically important potassium depletion is likely to occur.
- *Low dietary intake* of potassium predisposes to hypokalaemia; the risk is particularly notable in the elderly, many of whom ingest less than 50 mmol per day (the dietary normal is 80 mmol).
- Hypokalaemia may be aggravated by other drugs, e.g. β_2-adrenoceptor agonists, theophylline, corticosteroids, amphotericin.
- Hypokalaemia during diuretic therapy is also more likely in *hyperaldosteronism*, whether primary or more commonly secondary to severe liver disease, congestive cardiac failure or nephrotic syndrome.
- Potassium loss occurs with *diarrhoea*, vomiting or small bowel fistula, and may be aggravated by diuretic therapy.
- When a thiazide diuretic is used for *hypertension,*

there is probably no case for routine prescription of a potassium supplement if no predisposing factors are present (see Ch. 24).

Potassium depletion can be minimised or corrected by:

- Maintaining a good dietary potassium intake (fruits, fruit juices, vegetables)
- Combining a potassium-depleting with a potassium-sparing drug
- Intermittent use of potassium-losing drugs, i.e. drug holidays
- Potassium supplements: KCl is preferred because chloride is the principal anion excreted along with sodium when high efficacy diuretics are used. Potassium-sparing diuretics generally defend serum potassium more effectively than potassium supplements. Formulations of the latter include: potassium chloride sustained-release tabs (Slow-K tabs) containing 8 mmol each of potassium and chloride; potassium chloride effervescent tabs (Sando-K tabs) containing 12 mmol of potassium and 8 mmol of chloride. All forms of potassium are irritant to the gastrointestinal tract and in the oesophagus may even cause ulceration. The elderly, in particular, should be warned never to take such tablets dry but always with a large cupful of liquid and sitting upright or standing.

Hyperkalaemia may occur especially if a potassium-sparing diuretic is given to a patient with impaired renal function. Angiotensin-coverting enzyme (ACE) inhibitors and angiotensin II receptor antagonists can also cause modest elevation of plasma potassium. They may cause dangerous hyperkalaemia if combined with KCl supplements or other potassium-sparing drugs, in the presence of impaired renal function. With suitable monitoring, however, the combination can be used safely, as well illustrated by the RALES trial (see p. 517, and footnote 3). Ciclosporin, tacrolimus, indometacin and possibly other NSAIDs may cause hyperkalaemia with the potassium-sparing diuretics.

Hypovolaemia can result from overtreatment. Acute loss of excessive fluid leads to postural hypotension and dizziness. A more insidious state of chronic hypovolaemia can develop especially in the elderly. After initial benefit, the patient becomes sleepy and lethargic. Blood urea concentration rises and sodium concentration may be low. Renal failure may result.

Urinary retention. Sudden vigorous diuresis can cause acute retention of urine in the presence of bladder neck obstruction, e.g. due to prostatic enlargement.

Hyponatraemia may result if sodium loss occurs in patients who drink a large quantity of water when taking a diuretic. Other mechanisms are probably involved, including enhancement of antidiuretic hormone release. Such patients have reduced total body sodium and extracellular fluid and are oedema-free. Discontinuing the diuretic and restricting water intake are effective. The condition should be distinguished from hyponatraemia with oedema which develops in some patients with congestive cardiac failure, cirrhosis or nephrotic syndrome. Here salt and water intake should be restricted because extracellular fluid volume is expanded.

The combination of a potassium-sparing diuretic and ACE inhibitor can also cause severe hyponatraemia, more commonly indeed than life-threatening hyperkalaemia.

Urate retention with hyperuricaemia and, sometimes, clinical gout occurs with the high and moderate efficacy diuretics, but the effect is unimportant or negligible with the low efficacy diuretics. Two mechanisms appear to be responsible. First, diuretics cause volume depletion, reduction in glomerular filtration and increased aborption of almost all solutes in the proximal tubule including urate. Second, diuretics and uric acid are organic acids and compete for the transport mechanism which carries such substances from the blood into the tubular fluid. Diuretic-induced hyperuricaemia can be prevented by allopurinol or probenecid (which also antagonises diuretic efficacy by reducing their transport into the urine).

Magnesium deficiency. Loop and thiazide diuretics cause significant urinary loss of magnesium; potassium-sparing diuretics probably also cause magnesium retention. Magnesium deficiency brought about by diuretics seems rarely to be severe enough to induce the classic picture of neuromuscular irritability and tetany but cardiac arrhythmias, mainly of ventricular origin, do occur and respond to repletion of magnesium (8 mmol of Mg^{++} is given as 4 ml of 50% magnesium sulphate infused i.v. over 10–15 min followed by up to 72 mmol infused over the next 24 h).

Carbohydrate intolerance is caused by those diuretics which produce prolonged hypokalaemia, i.e. the loop and thiazide type. It appears that intracellular potassium is necessary for the formation of insulin, and glucose intolerance is probably due to insulin deficiency. Insulin requirements thus increase in established diabetics and the disease may become mainifest in latent diabetics. The effect is generally reversible over several months.

Treatment of hyperkalaemia

Depends on the severity and the following measures are appropriate:

- Any potassium-sparing diuretic should be discontinued.
- A cation-exchange resin, e.g. polystyrene sulphonate resin (Resonium A, Calcium Resonium, see later) can be used orally (more effective than rectally) to remove body potassium via the gut.
- Potassium may be moved rapidly from plasma into cells by giving:
  (1) Sodium bicarbonate, 50 ml of 8.4% solution through a central line, and repeated in a few minutes if characteristic ECG changes persist.
  (2) Glucose, 50 ml of 50% solution, plus 10 units of soluble insulin by i.v. infusion.
  (3) Nebulised β_2-agonist, salbutamol 5–10 mg, is effective in stimulating the pumping of potassium into skeletal muscle.
- In the presence of ECG changes, calcium gluconate, 10 ml of the 10% solution, should be given i.v. and repeated if necessary in a few minutes; it has no effect on the serum potassium but opposes the myocardial effect of an elevated serum potassium. Calcium may potentiate digoxin and should be used cautiously, if at all, in a patient taking this drug. Sodium bicarbonate and calcium salt must not be mixed in a syringe or reservoir becuse calcium precipitates.
- Dialysis may be needed in refractory cases and is highly effective.

Calcium homeostasis. Renal calcium loss is *increased* by the loop diuretics; in the short term this is not a serious disadvantage and indeed frusemide may be used in the management of hypercalcaemia after rehydration has been achieved. In the long term hypocalcaemia may be harmful especially in elderly patients who tend in any case to be in negative calcium balance. Thiazides, by contrast, *decrease* renal excertion of calcium and this property may influence the choice of diuretic in a potentially calcium deficient or osteoporotic individual, for thiazide use is associated with reduced risk of hip fracture in the elderly. The hypocalciuric effect of the thiazides has also been used effectively in patients with idiopathic hypercalciuria, the commonest metabolic cause of renal stones.

INTERACTIONS

Loop diuretics (especially as i.v. boluses) potentiate ototoxicity of aminoglycosides and nephrotoxicity of some cephalosporins. NSAIDs tend to cause sodium retention which counteracts the effect of diuretics; the mechanism may involve inhibition of renal prostaglandin formation. Diuretic treatment of a patient taking lithium can precipitate toxicity from this drug (the increased sodium loss is accompanied by reduced lithium excretion). Reference is made above to drug treatments which, when combined with diuretics, may lead to hyperkalaemia, hypokalaemia, hyponatraemia, or glucose intolerance.

ABUSE OF DIURETICS

Psychological abnormality sometimes takes the form of abuse of diuretics and/or purgatives. The subject usually desires to slim to become more attractive, or may have anorexia nervosa. There can be severe depletion of sodium and potassium, with renal tubular damage due to chronic hypokalaemia.

OSMOTIC DIURETICS

Osmotic diuretics are small molecular weight substances that are filtered by the glomerulus but not reabsorbed by the renal tubule, and thus increase the osmolarity of the tubular fluid. Consequently they prevent the reabsorption of *water* (and also, by more complex mechanisms, of sodium) principally in the proximal convoluted tubule and probably also the loop of Henle. The result is that urine volume increases according to the load of osmotic diuretic.

Mannitol, a polyhydric alcohol (mol. wt. 452), is most commonly used; it is given i.v. In addition to its effect on the kidney, mannitol encourages the movement of water from inside cells to the extracellular fluid, which is thus transiently expanded before diuresis occurs. These properties define its uses, which are for rapid reduction of intracraninal or intraocular pressure, and to maintain urine flow to prevent renal tubular necrosis. Because it increases circulatory volume, mannitol is contraindicated in congestive cardiac failure and pulmonary oedema.

METHYLXANTHINES

The general properties of the methylxanthines (theophylline, caffeine) are discussed elsewhere (see p. 194). Their mild diuretic action probably depends in part on smooth muscle relaxation in the afferent arteriolar bed increasing renal blood flow, and in part on a direct inhibitory effect on salt reabsorption in the proximal tubule. Their uses in medicine depend on other properties.

Carbonic anhydrase inhibitors

The enzyme *carbonic anhydrase* facilitates the reaction between carbon dioxide and water to form carbonic acid, which then breaks down to *hydrogen* (H^+) and *bicarbonate* (HCO_3^-) ions. This process is fundamental to the production of either acid or alkaline secretions and high concentrations of carbonic anhydrase are present in the gastric mucosa, pancreas, eye and kidney. Because the number of H^+ available to exchange with Na^+ in the proximal tubule is reduced, sodium loss and diuresis occur. But HCO_3^- reabsorption from the tubule is also reduced, and its loss in the urine leads within days to *metabolic acidosis*, which attenuates the diuretic response to carbonic anhydrase inhibition. Consequently, inhibitors of carbonic anhydrase are obsolete as diuretics, but still have specific uses. *Acetazolamide* is the most widely used carbonic anhydrase inhibitor.

Reduction of intraocular pressure. This action is due not to diuresis (thiazides actually raise intraocular pressure slightly). The formation of aqueous humour is an active process requiring a supply of bicarbonate ions, which depends on carbonic anhydrase. Inhibition of carbonic anhydrase reduces the formation of aqueous humour and lowers intraocular pressure. This is a local action and is not affected by the development of acid–base changes elsewhere in the body, i.e. tolerance does not develop. In patients with acute *glaucoma,* acetazolamide can be taken either orally, or intravenously. Acetazolamide is not recommended for long-term use because of the risk of hypokalaemia and acidosis, but *brinzolamide* or *dorzolamide* are effective as eye drops, well tolerated, and thus suitable for chronic use in glaucoma.

High-altitude (mountain) sickness. This condition may affect unacclimatised people at altitudes over 3000 metres especially after rapid ascent; symptoms range from nausea, lassitude and headache to pulmonary and cerebral oedema. The initiating cause is *hypoxia:* at high altitude, the normal hyperventilatory response to falling oxygen tension is inhibited because *alkalosis* is also induced. Acetazolamide induces metabolic *acidosis,* increases respiratory drive, notably at night when apnoetic attacks may occur, and thus helps to maintain arterial oxygen tension; 125–250 mg b.d. may be given orally on the day before the ascent and continued for 2 days after reaching the intended altitude, and 250 mg b.d. is used to treat established high-altitude sickness. (Note that this is an unlicenced indication in the UK). Dexamethasone may be used as an alternative or in addition, 2 mg 6-hourly for prevention, and 4 mg 6-hourly for treatment.

The drug has two other uses. In *periodic paralysis,* where sudden falls in plasma K^+ occur due to its exchange with Na^+ in cells, the rise in plasma H^+ caused by acetazolamide provides an alternative cation to K^+ for exchange with Na^+. Acetazolamide

may be used occasionally as a second-line drug for *tonic-clonic* and *partial epileptic seizures.*

Adverse effects. High doses of acetazolamide may cause drowsiness and fever, rashes and paraesthesiae may occur, and blood disorders have been reported. Renal calculi may develop, because the urine calcium is in less soluble form owing to low citrate content of the urine, a consequence of metabolic acidosis.

Dichlorphenamide is similar, but a more potent inhibitor of carbonic anhydrase.

Cation-exchange resins

Cation-exchange resins are used to treat *hyperkalaemia* by accelerating potassium loss through the gut, especially in the context of poor urine output or prior to dialysis (the most effective means of treating hyperkalaemia). The resins consists of aggregations of big insoluble molecules carrying fixed negative charges, which loosely bind positively charged ions (cations); these readily exchange with cations in the fluid environment to an extent that depends on their affinity for the resin and their concentration. Resins loaded with sodium or calcium exchange these cations preferentially with potassium cations in the intestine (about 1 mmol of potassium per gram of resin); the freed cations (calcium or sodium) are absorbed and the resin plus bound potassium is passed in the faeces. The resin does not merely prevent absorption of ingested potassium, but it also takes up the potassium normally secreted into the intestine and ordinarily reabsorbed.

In hyperkalaemia, oral administration or retention enemas of a polystyrene sulphonate resin may be used. A *sodium* phase resin (Resonium A) should obviously not be used in patients with renal or cardiac failure as sodium overload may result. A *calcium* phase resin (Calcium Resonium) may cause hypercalcaemia and should be avoided in predisposed patients, e.g. those with multiple myeloma, metastatic carcinoma, hyperparathyroidism and sarcoidosis. Enemas should be retained for as long as possible, although patients rarely manage for as long as necessary (at least 9 h) to exchange potassium at all available sites on the resin.

Alteration of urine pH

Alteration of urine pH by drugs is sometimes desirable. The most common reason is in the treatment of poisoning (a fuller account is given on p. 155). A summary of the main indications appears below.

Alkalinisation of urine

- increases the elimination of salicylate, phenobarbitone and chlorophenoxy herbicides, e.g. 2,4-D, MCPA
- reduces irritation of an inflamed urinary tract
- discourages the growth of certain organisms, e.g. *Escherichia coli.*

The urine can be made alkaline by sodium bicarbonate i.v., or by potassium citrate by mouth. Sodium overload may exacerbate cardiac failure, and sodium or potassium excess are dangerous when renal function is impaired.

Acidification of urine

- is used as a test for renal tubular acidosis
- increases elimination of amphetamine, methylene dioxymethamphetamine (MDMA or 'Ecstasy'), dexfenfluramine, quinine and phencyclidine, although it is very rarely needed.

Oral NH_4Cl, taken with food to avoid vomiting, acidifies the urine. It should not be given to patients with impaired renal or hepatic function. Other means include arginine HCl, ascorbic acid and $CaCl_2$ by mouth.

Drugs and the kidney

ADVERSE EFFECTS

The kidneys comprise only 0.5% of body weight, yet they receive 25% of the cardiac output. Thus, it is hardly surprising that drugs can damage the kidney and that disease of the kidney affects responses to drugs.

DRUG-INDUCED RENAL DISEASE

Drugs and other chemicals damage the kidney by:

1. **Direct biochemical effect** Substances that cause direct toxicity include:
   - Heavy metals, e.g. mercury, gold, iron, lead
   - Antimicrobials, e.g. aminoglycosides, amphotericin, cephalosporins
   - Iodinated radiological contrast media, e.g. agents for visualising the biliary tract
   - Analgesics, e.g. NSAID combinations and paracetamol (actually its metabolite, NABQI, in overdose, see p. 287)
   - Solvents, e.g. carbon tetrachloride, ethylene glycol.

2. **Indirect biochemical effect**
   - Cytotoxic drugs and uricosurics may cause urate to be precipitated in the tubule.
   - Calciferol may cause renal calcification by causing hypercalcaemia.
   - Diuretic and laxative abuse can cause tubule damage secondary to potassium and sodium depletion.
   - Anticoagulants may cause haemmorrhage into the kidney.

3. **Immunological effect** A wide range of drugs produces a wide range of injuries.
   - Drugs include: phenytoin, gold, penicillins, hydralazine, isoniazid, rifampicin, penicillamine, probenecid, sulphonamides.
   - Injuries include: arteritis, glomerulitis, interstitial nephritis, systemic lupus erythematosus.

A drug may cause damage by more than one of the above mechanisms, e.g. gold. The sites and pathological types of injury are as follows:

Glomerular damage. The large surface area of the glomerular capillaries renders them susceptible to damage from circulating immune complexes; glomerulonephritis, proteinuria and nephrotic syndrome may result, e.g. following treatment with penicillamine when the patient has made an immune response to the drug. The degree of renal impairment is best reflected in the *creatinine clearance* which measures the glomerular filtration rate because creatinine is eliminated entirely by this process.

Tubule damage. By concentrating 180 l of glomerular filtrate into 1.5 l of urine each day, renal tubule cells are exposed to much greater amounts of solutes and environmental toxins than are other cells in the body. The proximal tubule, through which most water is reabsorbed, experiences the greatest concentration and so suffers most drug-induced injury. Specialised transport processes concentrate acids, e.g. salicylate (aspirin), cephalosporins, and bases, e.g. aminoglycosides, in renal tubular cells. Heavy metals and radiographic contrast media also cause damage at this site. Proximal tubular toxicity is manifested by leakage of *glucose, phosphate, bicarbonate* and *aminoacids* into the urine.

The counter current multiplier and exchange systems of urine concentration (see p. 530) cause some drugs to accumulate in the renal medulla. Analgesic nephropathy is often first evident at this site partly because of high tissue concentration and partly, it is believed, because of ischaemia through inhibition of locally produced vasodilator prostaglandins by NSAIDs. The distal tubule is the site of lithium-induced nephrotoxicity; damage to the medulla and distal nephron is manifested by failure to concentrate the urine after fluid deprivation and by failure to *acidify* urine after ingestion of ammonium chloride.

Tubule obstruction. Given certain physicochemical conditions, crystals can deposit within the tubular lumen. *Methotrexate,* for example, is relatively insoluble at low pH and can precipitate in the distal nephron when the urine is acid. Similarly the uric acid produced by the metabolism of nucleic acids released during rapid tumour cell lysis can cause a fatal *urate nephropathy*. This was a particular problem with the introduction of chemotherapy for leukaemias until the introduction of allopurinol; it is now routinely given before the start of chemotherapy to block xanthine oxidase so that the much more soluble uric acid precursor, hypoxanthine, is excreted instead. Crystal-nephropathy is also a problem with the widely used antiretroviral agent *indinavir.*

Other drug-induced lesions of the kidney include:

- Vasculitis, caused by allopurinol, isoniazid, sulphonamides
- Allergic interstitial nephritis, caused by penicillins (especially), thiazides, allopurinol, phenytoin, sulphonamides
- Drug-induced lupus erythematosus, caused by hydralazine, procainamide, sulfasalazine.

Drugs may thus induce any of the common clinical syndromes of renal injury, namely:

Acute renal failure, e.g. aminoglycosides, cisplatin

Nephrotic syndrome, e.g. penicillamine, gold, captopril (only at higher doses than now recommended)

Chronic renal failure, e.g. NSAIDs

Functional impairment, i.e. reduced ability to dilute and concentrate urine (lithium), potassium loss in urine (loop diuretics), acid–base imbalance (acetazolamide).

PRESCRIBING IN RENAL DISEASE

Drugs may:

- exacerbate renal disease (above)
- be potentiated by accumulation due to failure of renal excretion
- be ineffective, e.g. thiazide diuretics in moderate or severe renal failure; uricosurics.

Problems of safety arise especially in patients with impaired renal function who must be treated with drugs that are potentially toxic and that are wholly or largely eliminated by the kidney.

A knowledge of, or at least access to, sources of pharmacokinetic data is essential for safe therapy for such patients.[4] The profound influence of impaired renal function on the elimination of some drugs is illustrated in Table 26.1.

The $t\frac{1}{2}$ of other drugs, whose activity is terminated by metabolism, is unaltered by renal impairment. Many such drugs, however, produce *pharmacologically active metabolites* which tend to be more water-soluble than the parent drug, are dependent on the kidney for their elimination, and

---

[4] e.g. manufacturers' data, formularies and specialist journals.

accumulate in renal failure, e.g. acebutolol, diazepam, warfarin, pethidine.

The majority of drugs fall into an intermediate class and are partly metabolised and partly eliminated unchanged by the kidney.

Administering the correct dose to a patient with renal disease must therefore take into account both the extent to which the drug normally relies on renal elimination, and the degree of renal impairment; the most convenient and useful guide to the latter is the *creatinine clearance*. These issues are now discussed.

DOSE ADJUSTMENT FOR PATIENTS WITH RENAL IMPAIRMENT

Adjustment of the *initial dose* (or where necessary the *priming* or *loading dose*, see p. 117) is generally unnecessary, for the volume into which the drug has to distribute should be the same in the uraemic as in the healthy subject.

Adjustment of the *maintenance dose* involves either reducing each dose given or lengthening the time between doses.

Special caution is needed when the patient is *hypoproteinaemic* and the drug is usually extensively plasma protein bound, or in advanced renal disease when accumulated metabolic products may compete for protein binding sites; particular care is required in the early stages of dosing until response to the drug can be gauged.

General rules

1. Drugs that are *completely* or *largely* excreted by the kidney or drugs that produce *active, renally-*
eliminated metabolites: give a normal or, if there is special cause for caution (above), a slightly reduced initial dose, and lower the maintenance dose or lengthen the dose interval in proportion to the reduction in creatinine clearance.

2. Drugs that are completely or *largely* metabolised to *inactive* products: give normal doses. When the special note of caution (above) applies, a modest reduction of initial dose and the maintenance dose rate are justified while drug effects are assessed.

3. Drugs that are *partly* eliminated by the kidney and *partly* metabolised: give a normal initial dose and modify the maintenance dose or dose interval in the light of what is known about the patient's renal function and the drug, its dependence on renal elimination and its inherent toxicity.

Recall that the *time* to reach steady-state blood concentration (p. 102) is dependent only on drug $t\frac{1}{2}$ and a drug reaches 97% of its ultimate steady-state concentration in $5 \times t\frac{1}{2}$. Thus if $t\frac{1}{2}$ is prolonged by renal impairment, so also will be the time to reach steady state.

Schemes for modifying drug dosage for patients with renal disease do not altogether remove their increased risk of adverse effects; such patients should be observed particularly carefully throughout a course of drug therapy. Ideally, dosing should be monitored by drug plasma concentration measurements of relevant drugs, where the service is available.

Nephrolithiasis

Calcareous stones result from hypercalciuria, hyperoxaluria and hypocitraturia. Hypercalciuria and hyperoxaluria render urine supersaturated in respect of calcium salts; citrate makes calcium oxalate more soluble and inhibits its precipitation from solution.

Noncalcareous stones occur most commonly in the presence of urea-splitting organisms which create conditions in which magnesium ammonium phosphate (struvite) stones form. Urate stones form when urine is unusually acid (pH < 5.5).

TABLE 26.1 Drug $t\frac{1}{2}$ (h) with normal and with severely impaired renal function

	Normal	Severe renal impairment*
captopril	2	25
amoxicillin	2	14
gentamicin	2.5	> 50
atenolol	6	100
digoxin	36	90

* Glomerular filtration rate < 5 ml/min (normal is 120 ml/min). These are examples of drugs that are excreted almost unchanged; the prolongation of their $t\frac{1}{2}$ indicates that special care must be exercised if they are used in patients with impaired renal function.

Management. Recurrent stone-formers should maintain a urine output exceeding 2.5 l/d. Some benefit from restricting dietary calcium or reducing the intake of oxalate-rich foods (rhubarb, spinach, tea, chocolate, peanuts).

- Thiazide diuretics reduce the excretion of calcium and oxalate in the urine and reduce the rate of stone formation.
- Sodium cellulose phosphate (Calcisorb) binds calcium in the gut, reduces urinary calcium excretion and may benefit calcium stone-formers.
- Allopurinol is effective in those who have high excretion of uric acid in the urine.
- Potassium citrate, which alkalinises the urine, should be given to prevent formation of pure uric acid stones.

Pharmacological aspects of micturition

SOME PHYSIOLOGY

The *detrusor,* whose smooth muscle fibres comprise the body of the bladder, is innervated mainly by parasympathetic nerves which are excitatory and cause the muscle to contract. The *internal sphincter, a* concentration of smooth muscle at the bladder neck, is well developed only in the male and its principal function is to prevent retrograde flow of semen during ejaculation. It is rich in α_1-adrenoceptors, activation of which causes contraction. There is an abundant supply of oestrogen receptors in the distal two-thirds of the female urethral epithelium which degenerates after the menopause causing loss of urinary control.

When the detrusor relaxes and the sphincters close, urine is stored; this is achieved by central inhibition of parasympathetic tone accompanied by a reflex increase in α-adrenergic activity. Voiding requires contraction of the detrusor, accompanied by relaxation of the sphincters. These acts are co-ordinated by a micturition centre probably in the pons.

FUNCTIONAL ABNORMALITIES

The main abnormalities that require treatment are:

- *Unstable bladder* or detrusor instability, characterised by uninhibited, unstable contractions of the detrusor which may be of unknown aetiology or secondary to an upper motor neuron lesion or bladder neck obstruction.
- *Decreased bladder activity* or hypotonicity due to a lower motor neuron lesion or overdistension of the bladder or to both.
- *Urethral sphincter dysfunction* which is due to various causes including weakness of the muscles and ligaments around the bladder neck, descent of the urethrovesical junction and periurethral fibrosis; the result is stress incontinence.
- *Atrophic change* affects the distal urethra in females.

Drugs that may be used to alleviate abnormal micturition

Antimuscarinic drugs such as *oxybutynin* and *flavoxate* are used to treat urinary frequency; they increase bladder capacity by diminishing unstable detrusor contractions. Both drugs may cause dry mouth and blurred vision and may precipitate glaucoma. Oxybutynin has a high level of unwanted effects which limits its use; the dosage needs to be carefully assessed, particularly in the elderly. Flavoxate has less marked side effects but is also less effective. Propiverine, tolterodine and trospium are also antimuscarinic drugs which have been introduced for urinary frequency, urgency and incontinence. Propantheline was formerly widely used in urinary incontinence but had a low response rate and a high incidence of adverse effects; it is now used mainly for adult enuresis. The need for continuing antimuscarinic drug therapy should be reviewed after 6 months.

Tricyclic antidepressants. Imipramine, amitriptyline and nortriptyline are effective, especially for nocturnal but also for daytime incontinence. Their parasympathetic blocking (antimuscarinic) action is probably in part responsible but imipramine may also benefit by altering the patient's sleep profile.

Oestrogens either applied locally to the vagina or taken by mouth may benefit urinary incontinence due to atrophy of the urethral epithelium in menopausal women.

Parasympathomimetic drugs, e.g. bethanechol, carbachol and distigmine, may be used to stimulate the detrusor when the bladder is hypotonic, e.g. due to an upper motor neuron lesion. Distigmine, which is an anticholinesterase, is preferred but, as its effect is not sustained, intermittent catheterisation is also needed when the hypotonia is chronic.

BENIGN PROSTATIC HYPERPLASIA (BPH)

One of the commonest problems in men older than 50, BPH was for a long time helped only by surgical interventions, which themselves were an outstanding example of the different (usually absent) rules that apply in the assessment of surgical compared to pharmacological treatments. Many are the men who would have opted for continuing micturition frequency in preference to the impotence, incontinence or pulmonary emboli that awaited them after transurethral resection; few are the drugs which would survive such complications, whatever the benefits. Now there is a limited choice between medical and surgical approaches, although these have never been formally compared, and the drugs are not a substitute for surgery if urinary retention has occurred. The prostate gland is a mixture of capsular and stromal tissue, rich in α_1-adrenoceptors, and glandular tissue under the influence of androgens. Both these, the α-receptors and androgens, are targets for drug therapy. Because the bladder itself has few α-receptors, it is possible to use selective α_1-blockade without affecting bladder contraction.

Alpha-adrenoceptor antagonists. Prazosin, afluzosin, indoramin, terazosin and doxazosin are all α-adrenoceptor blockers, with selectivity for the α_1-subtype. They cause significant increases (compared to placebo) in objective measures such as maximal urine flow rate, and drugs also improve semi-objective symptoms scores. In normotensive men, they cause generally negligible falls in blood pressure; in hypertensive patients, the fall in pressure can be regarded as an added bonus (provided concurrent treatment is adjusted accordingly). These drugs can cause dizziness and asthenia even in the absence of marked changes in blood pressure. Nasal stuffiness can be a problem — especially in patients who resort to α agonists (e.g. pseudoephedrine) for rhinitis. These adverse events are avoided by using *tamsulosin.* This is selective for the α_{1c}-subclass of adrenoceptors, and therefore does not block the vascular α_1-receptor responsible for the undesired effects of other α blockers. It is taken as a single 400 microgram dose each day.

Finasteride. An alternative drug for such prostatic symptoms is the type II 5α-reductase inhibitor, finasteride, which inhibits conversion of testosterone to its more potent metabolite, dihydrotestosterone. Finasteride does not affect serum testosterone, or most nonprostatic responses to testosterone. It reduces prostatic volume by about 20% and increases urinary flow rates by a similar degree. These changes translate into only modest clinical benefits. Finasteride has a $t\frac{1}{2}$ of 6 h, and is taken as a single 5 mg tablet orally each day. The improvement in urine flow appears over 6 months (as the prostate shrinks in size) and in 5–10% of patients may be at the cost of some loss of libido. The serum concentration of prostate-specific antigen is approximately halved. While this may reflect a real reduction in risk of prostatic cancer, in patients receiving finasteride it is safer to regard as abnormal, values of the antigen in the upper half of the usual range. Lower doses of finasteride have been used successfully to halt the development of baldness.[5] Other antiandrogens, such as the gonadorelin agonists, are used in the treatment of prostatic cancer, but the need for parenteral administration makes them less suitable for BPH.

---

[5] Paradoxically, it has also been used as a treatment for hirsutism in women. Tartagni M et al 2000 Fertility and Sterility 73: 718–723.

ERECTILE DYSFUNCTION

Erectile dysfunction (ED), the inability to achieve or maintain a penile erection sufficient to permit satisfactory sexual intercourse, is estimated to affect over 100 million men worldwide, with a prevalence of 39% in those of 40 years.[6] Its numerous causes include cardiovascular disease, diabetes mellitus and other endocrine disorders, alcohol and substance abuse, and psychological factors (14%). While the evidence is not conclusive, drug therapy is thought to underlie 25% of cases, notably from *antidepressants (SSRI* and *tricyclic), phenothiazines, cyproterone acetate, fibrates, levodopa, histamine H_2-receptor* blockers, phenytoin, carbamazepine, allopurinol, indomethacin, and possibly *β-adrenoceptor blockers* and *thiazide diuretics.*

Sexual arousal releases neurotransmitters from the endothelial cells of the penis which relax the smooth muscle of the arteries, arterioles and trabeculae of its erectile tissue, greatly increase blood flow to it and facilitate rapid filling of the sinusoids and expansion of the corpora cavernosa. The venous plexus that drains the penis thus becomes compressed between the engorged sinusoids and the surrounding and firm tunica albuginea, causing the almost total cessation of venous outflow. The penis becomes erect, with an intracavernous pressure of 100 mmHg. The principal neurotransmitter is nitric oxide, which acts by raising intracellular concentrations of cyclic guanosine monophosphate (cGMP) to relax vascular smooth muscle. The *isoenzyme phosphodiesterase type 5* (PDE5) is selectively active in penile smooth muscle and terminates the action of cGMP by converting it to the inactive non-cyclic GMP.

Sildenafil (Viagra) is a highly selective inhibitor of PDE5 ($\times 70$ more so than isoenzymes 1, 2, 3 and 4 of PDE), which prolongs the action of cGMP, and thus the vasodilator and erectile response to normal sexual stimulation. Its emergence as an agent for erectile dysfunction is an example of serendipity in drug development. Sildenafil was originally being developed for another indication but when the clinical trials ended the volunteers declined to return surplus tablets for they had discovered that the drug conferred unexpected benefits on their sexual lives. Its development for erectile dysfunction followed.

Sildenafil is well absorbed orally, reaches a peak in the blood after 30–120 min and has a $t\frac{1}{2}$ of 4 h. The drug should be taken 1 hour before intercourse in an initial dose of 50 mg (25 mg in the elderly); thereafter 25–100 mg may be taken according to response, with a maximum of one 100 mg dose per 24 h. Food may delay the onset and offset of effect. Sildenafil is effective in 80% of patients with ED.

Adverse effects are short-lived, dose-related, and comprise headache, flushing, nasal congestion and dyspepsia. High doses can inhibit PDE6 which is needed for phototransduction in the retina, and some patients report transient colour vision disturbance. (The more recently developed PDE5 inhibitors, cialis and vardenafil, appear less likely to cause visual upset.) Priapism[7] has been reported.

Sildenafil is *contraindicated* in patients who are taking organic nitrates, for their metabolism is blocked and severe and acute hypotension result. Patients with recent stroke or myocardial infarction or whose blood pressure is known to be < 90/50 mmHg should not use it. Sildenafil is a substrate for the P450 isoenzyme CYP3A4 (and to a lesser extent CYP2C9) which gives scope for interaction with inhibitors or inducers of this system. The metabolic inhibitors erythromycin, saquinavir and ritonavir (protease inhibitors used for AIDS), and cimetidine, for example, produce substantial rises in the plasma concentration of sildenafil.

Alprostadil is a stable form of prostaglandin E1, a powerful vasodilator (see also p. 281), and is effective for psychogenic and neuropathic ED. Alprostadil increases arterial inflow and reduces venous outflow by contracting the corporal smooth muscle that occludes draining venules. The site of injection is along the dorsolateral aspect of the proximal third of the penis, alternating sides and sites for each injection. The duration and grade of erection are dose-related. The patient package insert from the manufacturer provides some helpful

---

[6] Feldman H A et al 1994 Journal of Urology 151: 54–61.

[7] In Greek mythology, Priapus was a god of fertility. He was also a patron of seafarers and shepherds.

drawings. The dose is arrived at by titration (5–20 micrograms) initially in the doctor's surgery, aiming for an erection lasting not more than one hour. It may also be introduced through the urethra (0.125–1 mg). Painful erection is the commonest adverse effect.

Papaverine, an alkaloid (originally extracted from opium but devoid of narcotic properties), is also a nonspecific phosphodiesterase inhibitor. It is effective (up to 80%) for psychogenic and neurogenic ED by self-injection into the corpora cavernosa of the penis shortly before intercourse (efficacy may be increased by also administering the α-adrenoceptor blocker, phentolamine).[8] (Papaveretum, whose actions are principally those of its morphine content, has occasionally been supplied in error, to the surprise, distress and hazard of the subject.) A physician who prescribes papaverine for this purpose must be ready to treat the occasional case of priapism (defined as erection lasting more than 4 h) by aspirating the corpora cavernosa and injecting an α-adrenoceptor agonist, e.g. metaraminol.

Apomorphine, a dopamine antagonist, is given by subcutaneous injection. Nausea can occur.

Summary

- The actions of drugs on the kidney are of an importance disproportionate to the low prevalence of kidney disorders.
- The kidney is the main site of loss, or potential loss, of all body substances. It is among the functions of drugs to help reduce losses of desirable substances and increase losses of undesired substances.
- The kidney is also at increased risk of toxicity from foreign substances because of the high concentrations these can achieve in the renal medulla.
- Diuretics are among the most commonly used drugs, perhaps because the evolutionary advantages of sodium retention have left an aging population without salt-losing mechanisms of matching efficiency.

Summary (continued)

- Loop diuretics, acting on the ascending loop of Henle, are the most effective, and are used mainly to treat the oedema states. Potassium is lost as well as sodium
- Thiazides, acting on the cortical diluting segment of the tubule, have lower natriuretic efficacy, but slightly greater antihypertensive efficacy than loop diuretics. Potassium loss is rarely a significant problem with thiazides, and thiazides reduce loss of calcium. Potassium retention with even hyperkalaemia can occur with potassium-sparing diuretics, which block sodium transport in the last part of the distal tubule, either directly (e.g. amiloride) or by blocking aldosterone receptors (spironolactone).
- Drugs have little ability to alter the filtering function of the kidney, when this is reduced by nephron loss.
- Prostatic enlargement is the main disease of the lower urinary tract where drugs can be used to postpone, or avoid, surgery. The symptoms of benign prostatic hyperplasia are partially relieved either by α$_1$-adrenoceptor blockade or by inhibiting synthesis of dihydrotestosterone in the prostate.
- Drugs are effective for the relief of erectile dysfunction, notably sildenafil, a highly-specific phosphodiesterase inhibitor.

GUIDE TO FURTHER READING

Bihl G, Meyers A 2001 Recurrent renal stone disease — advances in pathogenesis and clinical management. Lancet 358: 651–656

Brater D C 1998 Diuretic therapy. New England Journal of Medicine 339: 387–395

Dumont L, Mardirosoff C, Tramèr MR 2000 Efficacy and harm of pharmacological prevention of acute mountain sickness: quantitative review. British Medical Journal 321: 267–272

Hackett P H, Roach R C 2001 High-altitude sickness. New England Journal of Medicine 345: 107–114

Kirby R 1999 Benign prostatic hyperplasia. British Medical Journal 318: 343–344

Klahr S, Miller S B 1998 Acute oliguria. New England Journal of Medicine 338: 671–675

Lepon H, Williford W O, Barry M J et al 1996 The efficacy of terazosin, finasteride, or both in benign prostatic hyperplasia. New England Journal of Medicine 335: 533–539

Levin E R, Gardiner D G 1998 Natriuretic peptides. New England Journal of Medicine 339: 321–328

---

[8] Brindley G S 1986 Pilot experiments on the actions of drugs injected into the human corpus cavernosum penis. British Journal of Pharmacology 87: 495 — an account of self-experimentation with 17 drugs.

Lue T F 2000 Erectile dysfunction. New England
    Journal of Medicine 342: 1802–1813

Morgentaler A 1999 Male impotence. Lancet 354:
    1713–1718

Orth S R, Ritz E 1998 The nephrotic syndrome. New
    England Journal of Medicine 338: 1202–1211

Pak C Y C 1998 Kidney stones. Lancet 351: 1797–1801

Ralph D, McNicholas T 2000 UK management
    guidelines for erectile dysfunction. British Medical
    Journal 321: 499–503

27

Respiratory system

SYNOPSIS

- Cough: modes of action and uses of antitussives
- Respiratory stimulants: their place in therapy
- Pulmonary surfactant
- Oxygen therapy: its uses and dangers
- Histamine, antihistamines and allergies
- Bronchial asthma: types, modes of prevention, agents used for treatment and their use in asthma of varying degrees of severity
- Infections, see Ch. 13

Cough

There are two sorts of cough: the useful and the useless. Cough is useful when it effectively expels secretions or foreign material from the respiratory tract, i.e. when it is *productive;* it is useless when it is unproductive and persistent. Useful cough should be allowed to serve its purpose and suppressed only when it is exhausting the patient or is dangerous, e.g. after eye surgery. Useless persistent cough should be stopped. Asthma, rhinosinusitis, oesophageal reflux or a combination of the last two is the commonest underlying reason for persistent cough. Recently, eosinophilic bronchitis has been recognised as a possibly significant cause; it

responds well to inhaled or oral corticosteroid. Clearly the overall approach to persistent cough must involve attention to underlying factors.

Clinical assessment of the frequency and intensity of cough of disease by recordings made via a microphone allows objective assessment of antitussives, despite the huge spontaneous fluctuations in both. Such recording has shown patients' own reports of their cough to be too unreliable to provide valid drug comparisons. Placebo effects in cough are considerable.

SITES OF ACTION FOR TREATMENT

Peripheral sites

On the *afferent* side of the cough reflex: by reducing input of stimuli from throat, larynx, trachea, a warm moist atmosphere has a demulcent[1] effect on the pharynx.

On the *efferent* side of the cough reflex: measures to render secretions more easily removable (mucolytics, postural drainage) will reduce the amount of coughing needed, by increasing its efficiency.

The best *antitussive* of all is removal of the cause of the cough itself, e.g. treatment of underlying conditions such as asthma, postnasal drip or gastro-oesophageal reflux. In patients with hypertension or cardiac failure, a common cause of a dry cough is treatment with an ACE inhibitor.

---

[1] Latin: *demulcere,* to caress soothingly.

Central nervous system

Agents may act on:

- the medullary paths of the cough reflex (opioids)
- the cerebral cortex
- the subcortical paths (opioids and sedatives in general).

Cough is also under substantial voluntary control and can be inducible by psychogenic factors (such as anxiety not to cough when it is socially disadvantageous to do so, e.g. during the quiet parts of a musical concert) and reduced by a placebo. Considerations such as these are relevant to practical therapeutics.

COUGH SUPPRESSION

Antitussives that act peripherally

Smokers should stop smoking.

When the cough arises above the larynx, syrups and lozenges that glutinously and soothingly coat the pharynx (demulcents) may be used, e.g. simple linctus (mainly sugar-based syrup). Small children are prone to swallow lozenges and so a confection on a stick may be preferred.

Linctuses are demulcent preparations that can be used alone and as vehicles of other specific antitussive agents. That their exact constitution is not critical was known and taught to medical students in 1896.

> Many of you know that this (simple) linctus used to be very much thicker than it is now, and very likely the thicker linctus was more efficacious. The reason why it was made thinner was this. It was discovered that a large number of children came to the surgery complaining of cough, and they were given the linctus, but instead of their using it as a medicine, they took it to an old woman out in Smithfield, who gave them each a penny, took their linctus, and made jam tarts with it.[2]

When cough arises below the larynx water aerosol inhalations and a warm environment often give relief — the archetypal 'steam' inhalation. Compound benzoin tincture[3] is often used to give the inhalation a therapeutic smell (aromatic inhalation). This manoeuvre may have more than a placebo effect by promoting secretion of a dilute mucus that gives a protective coating to the inflamed mucous membrane. Menthol and eucalyptus are alternatives.

Local anaesthetics can also be used topically in the airways to block the mucosal cough receptors (modified stretch receptors and C fibre endings) directly. Nebulised lignocaine, for example, reduces coughing during fibreoptic bronchoscopy and is also effective in the intractable cough that may accompany bronchial carcinoma.

Antitussives that act centrally

The most consistent means of suppressing cough irrespective of its cause is blockade of the *medullary cough centre* itself. *Opioids,* such as methadone and codeine, are very effective although part of this antitussive effect could reflect their sedatory effect on higher nervous centres; nevertheless antitussive potency of an opiate is generally poorly correlated with its potency at causing respiratory depression. There are also *nonopioid* targets too, since *dextromethorphan* (the d-isomer of the codeine analogue levorphanol) and *pholcodine* have an antitussive effect that is not blocked by naloxone. These opiates also have no significant analgesic or respiratory-depressant effects at the doses required for their antitussive action confirming that opiate receptors are not involved.

Opioids are usually formulated as *linctuses* for antitussive use. Deciding on which agent to use depends largely on whether sedation and analgesia may be useful actions of the linctus. Hence methadone or diamorphine linctus may be preferred in patients with advanced bronchial carcinoma. In contrast, pholcodine, being nonsedating and nonaddictive, is widely incorporated into over-the-counter linctuses.

Sedation generally reduces the sensitivity of the cough reflex. Hence older sedating antihistamines, e.g. diphenhydramine, can suppress cough by non-H_1-receptor actions; often the doses needed cause

---

[2] Brunton L 1897 Lectures on the action of medicines. Macmillan, London.

[3] Friar's Balsam.

substantial drowsiness so that combination with other drugs, such as pholcodine and dextromethorphan, is common in over-the-counter cough remedies.

MUCOLYTICS AND EXPECTORANTS

Normally about 100 ml of fluid is produced from the respiratory tract each day and most of it is swallowed. Respiratory mucus consists largely of water and its slimy character is due to glycoproteins cross-linked together by disulphide bonds. In pathological states much more mucus may be produced; an exudate of plasma proteins which bond with glycoproteins and form larger polymers results in the mucus becoming more viscous. Patients with chest diseases such as cystic fibrosis and bronchiectasis have difficulty in clearing their chest of viscous sputum by cough because the bronchial cilia are rendered ineffective. Drugs that liquefy mucus can provide benefit.

Mucolytics

Carbocisteine and *mecysteine* have free sulphydryl groups that open disulphide bonds in mucus and reduce its viscosity. They are given by orally or by inhalation (or instillation) and may be useful chiefly where particularly viscous secretion is a problem (cystic fibrosis, care of tracheostomies). Mucolytics may cause gastrointestinal irritation and allergic reaction.

Water inhalation as an aerosol (breathing over a hot basin), though cheap, is not to be despised, and is good expectorant therapy in bronchiectasis. Simply *hydrating* a dehydrated patient can have a beneficial effect in lowering sputum viscosity.

Dornase alfa is phosphorylated glycosylated recombinant human deoxyribonuclease. It is given daily by inhalation of a nebulised solution containing 2500 units (2.5 mg). It is of modest value only in patients with cystic fibrosis, whose genetic defect in chloride transport causes particularly viscous sputum. The blocked airways, as well as the sputum itself, are a trap for pathogens and the lysis of invading neutrophils leads to substantial levels of free and very viscous DNA within the CF airways.

Choice of Drug Therapy for Cough

As always, it is necessary to have a clear idea of the underlying problem before starting to any therapy. For example, the approach to cough due to invasion of a bronchus by a neoplasm differs from that due to postnasal drip from chronic sinusitis or to that due to chronic bronchitis. The following are general recommendations:

- **Simple suppression of useless cough**
Codeine, pholcodine, dextromethorphan and methadone linctuses can be used in large, infrequent doses. In children, cough is nearly always useful and sedation at night is more effective to give rest than is codeine. A sedative antihistamine is convenient (e.g. promethazine), although sputum thickening may be a disadvantage. In pertussis infection (whooping cough), codeine and atropine methonitrate may be tried.
- **To increase bronchial secretion slightly and to liquefy what is there**
Water aerosol with or without menthol and benzoin inhalation, or menthol and eucalyptus inhalation may provide comfort harmlessly.

    Carbocysteine or another mucolytic orally may occasionally be useful.

    Preparations containing any drug having antimuscarinic action are undesirable because it thickens bronchial secretion. Oxygen inhalation dries secretions, so rendering them even more viscous; oxygen must be bubbled through water and patients having oxygen may need measures to liquefy sputum.
- **Cough originating in the pharyngeal region**
Glutinous sweets or lozenges (demulcents), incorporating a cough suppressant or not, as appropriate, are used.

Expectorants

These are said to encourage productive cough by increasing the volume of bronchial secretion; however there is little clinical evidence to support this, and they may be of no more value than placebo. The group includes squill, guaiphenesin, ipecacuanha, creosotes and volatile oils.

Cough mixtures

Every formulary is replete with combinations of antitussives, expectorants, mucolytics, bronchodilators and sedatives. Although choice is not critical, a knowledge of the active ingredients is important, for some contain sedative antimuscarinic antihistamines or phenypropanolamines (which may antagonise antihypertensives). Use of glycerol or syrup as a demulcent cough preparation, or of simple linctus (citric acid) is probably defensible. The rationale for compound linctus (dextromethorphan, pseudoephedrine, triprolidine) is dubious.

Respiratory stimulants

The drugs used *(analeptics)* are central nervous system stimulants and the therapeutic dose is close to that which causes convulsions. Their use must therefore be carefully monitored.

Doxapram increases the rate and depth of respiration by stimulating the medullary respiratory centres both directly and reflexly through the carotid body. A continuous i.v. infusion of 1.5–4.0 mg/min is given according to the patient's response. Coughing and laryngospasm that develop after its use may represent a return of normal protective responses. Adverse effects include restlessness, twitching, itching, vomiting, flushing and cardiac arrhythmias, and in addition it causes patients to experience a feeling of perineal warmth; in high doses it raises blood pressure.

Aminophylline (a complex of theophylline and EDTA) in addition to its other actions (see also p. 558) is a respiratory stimulant and may be infused slowly i.v. (500 mg in 6 h).

USES

Respiratory stimulants have a much reduced role in the management acute ventilatory failure, with the ready availability of mechanical methods for assisting respiration. Situations where they may still be encountered are:

- Acute exacerbations of chronic lung disease with *hypercapnia*, drowsiness and inability to cough or to tolerate low (24%) concentrations of inspired oxygen (air is 21% O_2). A respiratory stimulant can arouse the patient enough to allow effective physiotherapy and, by stimulating respiration, can improve ventilation–perfusion matching. As a short-term measure, this may be used in conjunction with assisted ventilation without tracheal intubation (BIPAP[4]), and thereby 'buy time' for chemotherapy to control infection and

avoid full tracheal intubation and mechanical ventilation
- *Apnoea* in premature infants; aminophylline and caffeine may benefit some cases.

Avoid respiratory stimulants in patients with *epilepsy* (risk of convulsions). Other relative contraindications include ischaemic heart disease, acute severe asthma ('status asthmaticus'), severe hypertension and thyrotoxicosis.

Irritant vapours, to be inhaled, have an analeptic effect in fainting, especially if it is psychogenic, e.g. aromatic solution of ammonia (Sal Volatile). No doubt they sometimes 'recall the exorbitant and deserting spirits to their proper stations'.[5]

Pulmonary surfactant

The endogenous surfactant system produces stable low surface tension in the alveoli, preventing their collapse. Failure of production of natural surfactant occurs in respiratory distress syndrome (RDS), including that in the neonate. Synthetic phospholipids are now available for intratracheal instillation to act as surfactants: colfosceril palmitate, poractant alfa, and beractant. These need to be stored chilled, and the manufacturer's instructions followed carefully since on reaching body temperature their physicochemical properties rapidly change. Their function is to coat the surface of the alveoli and maintain their patency, and their administration to premature neonates with RDS is a key part in reducing mortality and long-term complications in this condition.

Oxygen therapy

Oxygen used in therapy should be prescribed with the same care as any drug; there should be a well

---

[4] *Bi*-level *P*ositive *A*irways *P*ressure: air (if necessary enriched with oxygen 24% or 28%) is administered through a close fitting face-mask, at a positive pressure of 14–18 cm of water to support inspiration, then at a pressure of 4 cm of water during expiration to help maintain patency of small airways and increase gas exchange in alveoli.

[5] Thomas Sydenham, 1624–89. He was referred to as the 'English Hippocrates' due to his classic description of diseases.

defined purpose and its effects should be monitored objectively.

The absolute indication to supplement inspired air is inadequate tissue oxygenation. As clinical signs may be imprecise, arterial blood gases should be measured whenever suspicion arises. Tissue hypoxia can be assumed when the PaO_2 falls below 6.7 kPa (50 mmHg) in a previously normal *acutely ill* patient, e.g. with myocardial infarction, acute pulmonary disorder, drug overdose, musculoskeletal or head trauma. *Chronically hypoxic* patients may maintain adequate tissue oxygenation with a PaO_2 below 6.7 kPa by compensatory adaptations including an increased red cell mass and altered haemoglobin-oxygen binding characteristics. Oxygen therapy is used as follows:

- *High* concentration oxygen therapy is reserved for a state of low PaO_2 in association with a normal or low $PaCO_2$ *(type I respiratory failure)*, as in: pulmonary embolism, pneumonia, pulmonary oedema, myocardial infarction, and young patients with acute severe asthma. Concentrations of O_2 up to 100% may be used for short periods, since there is little risk of inducing hypoventilation and CO_2 retention.
- *Low* concentration oxygen therapy is reserved for a state of low PaO_2 in association with a raised $PaCO_2$ *(type II failure)*, typically seen during exacerbations of chronic obstructive pulmonary disease. The stimulus to respiration is elevation of the $PaCO_2$ but this control is blunted in chronically hypercapnic patients whose respiratory drive comes from *hypoxia.* Elevating the PaO_2 in such patients by giving them high concentrations of oxygen removes their stimulus to ventilate, exaggerates CO_2 retention and may cause fatal respiratory acidosis. The objective of therapy in such patients is to provide just enough oxygen to alleviate hypoxia without exaggerating the hypercapnia and respiratory acidosis; normally the inspired oxygen concentration should not exceed 28% and in some 24% may be sufficient.
- *Continuous* long-term domiciliary oxygen therapy (LTOT) is given to patients with *severe persistent hypoxaemia and cor pulmonale* due to chronic obstructive pulmonary disease (see later). Patients are provided with an oxygen

concentrator. Clinical trial evidence indicates that taking oxygen for more than 15 h per day improves survival.

Histamine, antihistamines and allergies

Histamine is a naturally-occuring amine that has long fascinated pharmacologists and physicians. It is found in most body tissue in an inactive bound form, predominantly within tissue mast cells, and pharmacologically active free histamine is released in response to stimuli such as physical trauma or IgE-mediated activation. Various chemicals can also cause release of histamine. The more powerful of these (proteolytic enzymes and snake venoms) have no place in therapeutics, but a number of useful drugs, such as d-tubocurarine and morphine, and even some antihistamines, cause histamine release. This *anaphylactoid* (i.e. IgE-independent) effect is usually clinically mild with a transient reduction in blood pressure or a local skin reaction; but significant bronchospasm may occur in asthmatics.

The physiological functions of histamine are suggested by its distribution in the body.

- In body epithelia (the gut, the respiratory tract and in the skin) it is released in response to invasion by foreign substances.
- In glands (gastric, intestinal, lachrymal, salivary) it mediates part of the normal secretory process.
- In most cells near blood vessels it plays a role in regulating the microcirculation.

Histamine acts as a local hormone *(autacoid)* similarly to serotonin or prostaglandins, i.e. it acts within the immediate vicinity of its site of release. In the context of gastric secretion, for example, stimulation of receptors on the histamine-containing cell causes release of histamine which in turn acts on receptors on parietal cells which then secrete hydrogen ions (see Gastric secretion, Ch. 31).

Actions. The actions of histamine which are clinically important are those on:

Smooth muscle. In general, histamine causes smooth muscle to contract (excepting arterioles, but including the larger arteries). Stimulation of the pregnant human uterus is insignificant. A brisk attack of bronchospasm may be induced in subjects who have any allergy, particularly asthma.

Blood vessels. Arterioles are dilated, with a consequent fall in blood pressure. This action, versus contraction of larger arteries, is partly due to nitric oxide release from the vascular endothelium of the arterioles in response to histamine receptor activation. Capillary permeability also increases especially at postcapillary venules, causing oedema. These effects on arterioles and capillaries represent the *flush* and the *wheal* components of the triple response described by Thomas Lewis.[6] The third part, the *flare*, is arteriolar dilatation due to an axon reflex releasing neuropeptides from C-fibre endings.

Skin. Histamine release in the skin can cause itch.

Gastric secretion. Histamine increases the acid and pepsin content of gastric juices. As may be anticipated from the above actions, anaphylactic shock, which is due in large part of histamine release, is characterised by circulatory collapse and bronchoconstriction. The most rapidly effective antidote is adrenaline (epinephrine) (see below), and an antihistamine (H_1-receptor) may be given as well.

Metabolism. Histamine is formed from the amino acid histidine and is inactivated largely by deamination and by methylation. In common with other local hormones, this process is extremely rapid.

HISTAMINE H_1- AND H_2-RECEPTOR ANTAGONISTS

The effects of histamine can be opposed in three ways:

- By using a drug with opposite effects, e.g. histamine constricts bronchi, causes vasodilatation and increases capillary permeability. Adrenaline (epinephrine), by activating α and β_2 adrenoceptors, produces opposite effects — referred to as *physiological antagonism.*
- By *blocking* histamine binding to its site of action (receptors), e.g. using competitive H_1- and H_2-receptor antagonists.

---

[6] Lewis T et al 1924 Heart 11: 209.

- By *preventing the release* of histamine from storage cells; glucocorticoids and sodium cromoglicate can suppress IgE-induced release from mast cells. β_2-agonists have a similar effect.

Drugs that competitively block H_1-histamine receptors were the first to be introduced and are conventionally called the *'antihistamines'*. They effectively inhibit the components of the triple response and partially prevent the hypotensive effect of histamine, but they have no effect on histamine-induced gastric secretion. Indeed, the standard method of testing a patient's capacity to secrete gastric acid used to be to inject histamine after first giving a large dose of a conventional (H_1-receptor) antihistamine to block the other (undesired) effects of the injection. The search for drugs that could selectively block histamine-induced gastric secretion (see Ch. 31) led to the discovery of the H_2-receptor. A third receptor (H_3-receptor) has now been cloned but its clinical importance is uncertain. In summary:

- H_1-receptor: mediates the oedema and vascular effects of histamine (see above)
- H_2-receptor: mediates the effect on gastric secretion.

Thus, *histamine antagonists* are classified as:

- Histamine H_1-receptor antagonists (see account below)
- Histamine H_2-receptor antagonists: cimetidine, famotidine, nizatidine, ranitidine (see Ch. 31).

HISTAMINE H_1-RECEPTOR ANTAGONISTS

The term antihistamine is unsatisfactory because the older first-generation antagonists (see below) show considerable blocking activity against muscarinic receptors, and often serotonin and α-adrenergic receptors as well. These features are a disadvantage when H_1-antihistamines are used specifically to antagonise the effects of histamine, e.g. for allergies. Hence the appearance of second-generation H_1-antagonists that are more selective for H_1-receptors and largely free of antimuscarinic and sedative effects (see below) has been an important advance. They can be discussed together.

Actions. H_1-receptor antihistamines oppose, to varying degrees, the effects of liberated histamine.

They strongly inhibit all components of the triple response (pure H_1-receptor effect), but only partially block the hypotensive effect of high-dose histamine (a mixed H_1- and H_2-receptor effect). They are of negligible use in asthma, in which nonhistamine mediators, such as the cysteinyl-leukotrienes, are the predominant constrictors. The H_1-antihistamines are generally competitive, surmountable inhibitors of the action of histamine. H_1-antihistamines are more effective if used before histamine has been liberated. Reversal of effects of histamine after it has been released is more readily achieved by physiological antagonism with adrenaline (epinephrine), which should be used first in life-threatening allergic reactions.

The older first-generation H_1-antihistamines cause drowsiness and patients should be warned of this, e.g. about driving or operating machinery, and about additive effects with alcohol. Paradoxically, CNS stimulation may occur with absence epilepsy (petit mal) made worse on therapeutic dosing, and seizures following overdosing with these antihistamines. The newer second-generation H_1-antihistamines penetrate the blood–brain barrier poorly and are largely devoid of these effects. Antimuscarinic effects of first-generation H_1-antihistamines are sometimes put to therapeutic advantage in parkinsonism and motion sickness.

Pharmacokinetics. H_1-antihistamines taken orally are readily absorbed. They are mainly metabolised in the liver. Excretion in the breast milk may also be sufficient to cause sedation in infants. They are generally administered orally and can also be given i.m. or i.v.

Uses. The H_1-antihistamines are used for symptomatic relief of allergies such as hay fever and urticaria (see below). They are of broadly similar therapeutic efficacy.

INDIVIDUAL H₁-RECEPTOR ANTIHISTAMINES

Nonsedative second-generation

These newer drugs are relatively selective for H_1-receptors, enter the brain less readily than do the earlier antihistamines and lack antimuscarinic side effects. Differences lie principally in their duration of action.

Cetirizine ($t\frac{1}{2}$ 7 h), *loratadine* ($t\frac{1}{2}$ 15 h) and *terfenadine* ($t\frac{1}{2}$ 20 h) are effective taken once daily and are suitable for general use. *Acrivastine* ($t\frac{1}{2}$ 2 h) is so short acting that it is best reserved for intermittent therapy, e.g. when breakthrough symptoms occur in a patient using topical therapy for hay fever. Other non-sedating antihistamines are desloratadine, fexofenadine, levocetirizine and mizolastine.

Adverse effects. Terfenadine can prolong the QTc interval on the surface ECG. This is especially likely to occur when the recommended dose is exceeded or the drug is administered with substances that block hepatic metabolism. Since this is dependent solely on the 3A4 isoform of cytochrome P450, offending drugs include erythromycin, ketoconazole and even grapefruit juice. Fexofenadine is the active metabolite of terfenadine and appears safe in this respect.

Sedative first-generation agents

Chlorphenamine ($t\frac{1}{2}$ 20 h) is effective when urticaria is prominent, and its sedative effect is then useful.

Diphenhydramine ($t\frac{1}{2}$ 32 h) is strongly sedative and has antimuscarinic effects; it is also used in parkinsonism and motion sickness.

Promethazine ($t\frac{1}{2}$ 12 h) is so strongly sedative that it is used as an hypnotic in adults and children.

Alimemazine, azatadine, brompheniramine, clemastine, cyproheptadine, diphenylpyraline, doxylamine, hydroxyzine and *triprolidine* are similar.

Adverse effects. Apart from sedation, these include: dizziness, fatigue, insomnia, nervousness, tremors, and antimuscarinic effects, e.g. dry mouth, blurred vision and gastrointestinal disturbance. Dermatitis and agranulocytosis can occur. Severe poisoning due to overdose results in coma and sometimes in convulsions.

DRUG MANAGEMENT OF SOME ALLERGIC STATES

Histamine is released in many allergic states, but it is not the sole cause of symptoms, other chemical mediators, e.g., leukotrienes and prostaglandins, also being involved. Hence the usefulness of H_1-receptor antihistamines in allergic states is variable, depending on the extent to which histamine, rather than other mediators, is the cause of the clinical manifestations.

Hay fever. If symptoms are limited to rhinitis, a *glucocorticoid* (beclomethasone, betamethasone, budesonide, flunisolide or triamcinolone), *ipratropium* or *sodium cromoglicate* applied topically as a spray or insufflation is often all that is required. Ocular symptoms alone respond well to sodium cromoglicate drops. When both nasal and ocular symptoms occur, or there is itching of the palate and ears as well, a systemic nonsedative H_1-antihistamine is indicated. Sympathomimetic vasoconstrictors, e.g. *ephedrine,* are immediately effective if applied topically, but rebound swelling of the nasal mucous membrane occurs when medication is stopped. Rarely, a systemic glucocorticoid, e.g. *prednisolone,* is justified for a severely affected patient to provide relief for a short period, e.g. during academic examinations.[7]

Hyposensitisation, by subcutaneous injection of graded and increasing amounts of *grass and tree pollen extracts,* is an option for seasonal allergic hay fever due to pollens (which has not responded to anti-allergy drugs), and of *bee and wasp allergen extracts* for people who exhibit allergy to these venoms (exposure to which can be life threatening). If it is undertaken facilities for immediate cardiopulmonary resuscitation must be available due to the risk of anaphylaxis.

Urticaria, see page 143.

Anaphylactic shock, see page 143.

Bronchial asthma

Asthma affects 10–15% of the UK population; this incidence is increasing.

SOME PATHOPHYSIOLOGY

The bronchi become hyperreactive as a result of a persistent *inflammatory* process in response to a number of stimuli that include biological agents, e.g. allergens, viruses and environmental chemicals, e.g. ozone and glutaraldehyde. Inflammatory mediators are liberated from mast cells, eosinophils, neutrophils, monocytes and macrophages. Some mediators such as histamine are preformed and their release causes an immediate bronchial reaction. Others are formed after activation of cells and produce more sustained bronchoconstriction; these include metabolites of arachidonic acid from both the cyclo-oxygenase, e.g. prostaglandin D_2 and lipoxygenase, e.g. cysteinyl-leukotrienes C4 and D4, pathways. In addition platelet activating factor (PAF) is being increasingly recognised as an important mediator (see p. 280).

The relative importance of many of the mediators is not precisely defined but they interact to produce mucosal oedema, mucus secretion and damage to the ciliated epithelium. Breaching of the protective epithelial barrier allows hyperreactivity to be maintained by bronchoconstrictor substances or by local axon reflexes through exposed nerve fibres. Wheezing and breathlessness result. The bronchial changes also obstruct access of inhaled drug to the periphery, which is why they can fail to give full relief.

Asthma, like many of the common chronic disorders (hypertension, diabetes mellitus), is a polygenic disorder and already genetic loci linked to either increased production of IgE or bronchial hyperreactivity have been reported in some families with an increased incidence of asthma.

Early in an attack there is hyperventilation so that PaO_2 is maintained and $PaCO_2$ is lowered but with increasing airways obstruction the PaO_2 declines and $PaCO_2$ rises, signifying a serious asthmatic episode.

TYPES OF ASTHMA

Asthma associated with specific allergic reactions

This *extrinsic* type is the commonest and occurs in patients who develop allergy to inhaled antigenic substances. They are also frequently *atopic* showing positive responses to skin prick testing with the same antigens. The hypersensitivity reaction in the lung (and skin) is of the immediate type (type 1) involving IgE-mediated mast cell activation. Allergen

---

[7] A man with severe hay fever who received at least one depot injection of corticosteroid each year for eleven years developed avascular necrosis of both femoral heads, an uncommon but serious complication of exposure to corticosteroid. Nasser S M S, Ewan P W 2001 British Medical Journal 322: 1589.

avoidance is particularly relevant to managing this type of asthma.

Asthma not associated with known allergy

Some patients exhibit wheeze and breathlessness in the absence of an obvious allergen or atopy. They are considered to have *intrinsic* asthma and because of a lack of an identifiable allergen, allergen avoidance has no place in their management.

Exercise-induced asthma

Some patients develop wheeze that regularly follows within a few minutes of exercise. A similar response occurs following the inhalation of cold air since the common mechanism appears to be airway drying. Inhalation of a β_2-adrenoceptor agonist, sodium cromoglicate (see below) or one of the newer leukotriene receptor antagonists (see below) prior to either challenge prevents broncho-constriction.

Asthma associated with chronic obstructive pulmonary disease

A number of patients who have persistent airflow obstruction exhibit considerable variation in airways resistance and hence in their benefit from bronchodilators drugs for asthma. It is important to recognise the coexistence of asthma with chronic obstructive pulmonary disease in some patients, and to assess their responses to bronchodilators or glucocorticoids over a period of time (as formal tests of respiratory function may not reliably predict clinical response in this setting).

APPROACHES TO TREATMENT

With the foregoing discussion in mind, the following approaches to treatment are logical:

- Prevention of exposure to allergen(s)
- Reduction of the bronchial inflammation and hyperreactivity
- Dilatation of narrowed bronchi.

These objectives may be achieved as follows:

Prevention of exposure to allergen(s)

This approach is appropriate for extrinsic asthmatics. Identifying an allergen may be aided by the patient's history (wheezing in response to contact with grasses, pollens, animals), by intradermal skin prick injection of selected allergen or by demonstrating specific IgE antibodies in the patient's serum (RAST testing). Avoiding an allergen may be feasible when it is related to some a specific situation, e.g. occupation, but is less feasible if it is widespread, as with house-dust mite.

Reduction of the bronchial inflammation and hyperreactivity

As persistent inflammation is central to bronchial hyperreactivity, the use of *anti-inflammatory* drugs is logical.

Glucocorticoids (see p. 665) bring about a gradual reduction in bronchial hyperreactivity. They are the mainstay of asthma treatment. The exact mechanisms are still disputed but probably include: inhibition of the influx of inflammatory cells into the lung after allergen exposure; inhibition of the release of mediators from macrophages and eosinophils and reduction of the microvascular leakage which these mediators cause. Glucocorticoids used in asthma include *prednisolone* (orally), and *beclomethasone*, *fluticasone* and *budesonide* (by inhalation) (see Ch. 34).

Sodium cromoglicate[8] (cromolyn, Intal) impairs the immediate response to allergen and was formerly thought to act by inhibiting the release of mediators from mast cells. Evidence now suggests that the late allergic response and bronchial hyperreactivity are also inhibited, and points to effects of cromoglicate on other inflammatory cells and also on local axon reflexes. Cromoglicate is poorly absorbed from the gastrointestinal tract but is well absorbed from the lung, and it is given by inhalation (as powder, aerosol or nebuliser); it is eliminated unchanged in the urine and bile.

---

[8] Cromoglicate was introduced in 1968 as the culmination of work carried out by the asthmatic research director of the company (REC Altounyan) on himself. We can admire Dr Altounyan without recommending this as the best way of screening new chemical entities.

Since it does not antagonise the broncho-constrictor effect of the mediators after they have been released, cromoglicate is not effective at terminating an existing attack, i.e. it *prevents bronchoconstriction* rather than induces bronchodilation. Special formulations are used for *allergic rhinitis* and *allergic conjunctivitis*.

Sodium cromoglicate is effective in extrinsic (allergic) asthma including asthma in children, and in exercise-induced asthma but its use has declined since the efficacy and safety of low dose inhaled corticosteroid have become apparent.

It is remarkably nontoxic. Apart from cough and bronchospasm induced by the powder it may rarely cause allergic reactions. Application to the eye may produce a local stinging sensation and the oral form may cause nausea.

Nedocromil sodium (Tilade) is structurally unrelated to cromoglicate but has a similar profile of actions and can be used by metered aerosol in place of cromoglicate.

Other drugs. Ketotifen is a histamine H_1-receptor blocker which may also have some antiasthma effects but its benefit has not been conclusively demonstrated. In common with other antihistamines it causes drowsiness.

Dilatation of narrowed bronchi

This is most effectively achieved by physiological antagonism of bronchial muscle contraction, namely by stimulation of adrenergic bronchodilator mechanisms. Pharmacological antagonism of specific bronchoconstrictors is less effective either because individual mediators are not on their own responsible for a large part of the bronchoconstriction (acetylcholine, adenosine, leukotrienes) or because the mediator is not even secreted during asthma attacks (histamine).

β_2-adrenoceptor agonists. The predominant adrenoceptors in bronchi are of the β_2 type and their stimulation causes bronchial muscle to relax. β_2-adrenoceptor activation also stabilises mast cells. Agonists in widespread use include: *salbutamol, terbutaline, fenoterol, eformoterol* and *salmeterol,* and are discussed in Chapter 22. Salmeterol is longer-acting because its lipophilic side chain anchors the drug in the membrane adjacent to the receptor, slowing tissue washout.

Less selective adrenoceptor agonists such as adrenaline (epinephrine), ephedrine, isoetharine, isoprenaline and orciprenaline are less safe, being more likely to cause cardiac arrhythmias. α-adrenoceptor activity contributes to bronchoconstriction but α-adrenoceptor antagonists have not proved effective in practice.

Theophylline, a methylxanthine, relaxes bronchial muscle, although its precise mode of action is still debated. Inhibition of phosphodiesterase (PDE), especially its type 4 isoform now seems the most likely explanation for its bronchodilator and more recently reported anti-inflammatory effects. Blockade of adenosine receptors is probably unimportant. Other actions of theophylline include chronotropic and inotropic effects on the heart and a direct effect on the rate of urine production (diuresis).

Absorption of theophylline from the gastro-intestinal tract is usually rapid and complete. Some 90% is metabolised by the liver and there is evidence that the process is saturable at therapeutic doses. The $t\frac{1}{2}$ is 8 h, with substantial variation, and it is prolonged in patients with severe cardio-pulmonary disease and cirrhosis. Obesity and prematurity are associated with reduced rates of elimination, whereas tobacco smoking enhances theophylline clearance by inducing hepatic P450 enzymes. Because of these pharmacokinetic factors and low therapeutic index, monitoring of the plasma theophylline concentration is necessary to optimise its therapeutic effect and minimise the risk of adverse reactions; the optimum concentration range is 10–20 mg/l (55–110 mmol/l).

Theophylline is relatively insoluble and it is formulated either as a salt with choline (choline theophyllinate) or complexed with EDTA (aminophylline). Aminophylline is sufficiently soluble to permit i.v. use of theophylline in status asthmaticus. There are numerous sustained-release oral forms for use in chronic asthma. These are not bio-equivalent and patients should not switch between them once they are stabilised on a particular preparation. It has also been used in the past for the emergency treatment of left ventricular failure (see p. 518). At high therapeutic doses some patients experience nausea and diarrhoea, and plasma concentrations above the recommended range risk cardiac arrhythmia and seizures. The latter are prone to occur with rapid intravenous injection, which exposes the heart and brain to high concentrations before distribution is complete. It follows that i.v. injection must be slow (a loading dose of 5 mg/kg over 20 min followed by an infusion of 0.9 mg/kg/h adjusted according to subsequent plasma theophylline concentrations). The loading dose should be avoided in any patient who is already taking a xanthine preparation (always enquire about this before injecting). Enzyme inhibition by erythromycin, ciprofloxacin, allopurinol or oral contraceptives increases the plasma concentration of theophylline; enzyme inducers such as carbamazepine, phenytoin and rifampicin reduce the concentration.

Overdose with theophylline has assumed greater importance with the advent of sustained-release preparations which prolong toxic effects, with peak plasma concentrations being reached 12–24 h after ingestion. Vomiting may be severe but the chief dangers are cardiac arrhythmia, hypotension, hypokalaemia and seizures. Activated charcoal should be given every 2–4 h until the plasma concentration is below 20 mg/l. Potassium replacement is important to prevent arrhythmias. Diazepam is used to control convulsions.

Antimuscarinic bronchodilators. Release of acetylcholine from vagal nerve endings in the airways activates muscarinic (M_3) receptors on bronchial smooth muscle causing bronchoconstriction. Blockade of these receptors with atropine causes bronchodilation, although the preferred antimuscarinics in clinical practise are inhaled *ipratropium* or *oxitropium*. These synthetic compounds, unlike atropine, are permanently charged molecules, which prevents significant absorption after inhalation and thus minimises antimuscarinic effects outside of the lung. They are mostly used in older patients with chronic obstructive pulmonary disease, but are useful in acute severe asthma when combined with β_2-adrenoceptor agonists. Vagally-mediated bronchoconstriction appears to be important in acute asthma, but relatively unimportant for most chronic stable asthmatics.

Leukotriene receptor antagonists e.g. *montelukast* and *zafirlukast*, competitively prevent the bronchoconstrictor effects of cysteinyl-leukotrienes (C4, D4 and E4) by blocking their common cysLT1 receptor. They have similar efficacy to low-dose inhaled glucocorticoid. The paucity of comparisons with established medications consigns them to a second or third line role in treatment. They could be substituted at step 2 or later stages of the current 5-step regimen for asthma (see Fig. 27.1). There are no studies to justify their use as steroid sparing (far less, replacement) therapy. When used occasionally in this way in patients unwilling or unable to use metered-dose inhalers, serial monitoring of spirometry is essential. Montelukast is given once per day and zafirlukast twice per day. Leukotriene receptor antagonists are generally well tolerated, although Churg-Strauss syndrome has been reported rarely with their use. This probably represents unmasking of the disease as glucocorticoids are withdrawn following addition of the leukotriene receptor antagonist. Alerting features to this development are vasculitic rash, eosinophilia, worsening respiratory symptoms, cardiac complications and peripheral neuropathy.

DRUG THERAPY BY INHALATION

The inhaled route has been developed to advantage because the undesirable effects of systemic exposure to drugs, especially glucocorticoids, are substantially reduced. The pharmacokinetic advantages of using the inhaled versus oral route are apparent from the considerable dose reductions possible: 100 micrograms of salbutamol from an aerosol inhaler, for example, will given similar bronchodilatation as 2000 micrograms given orally.

Before a drug can be inhaled, it must first be converted into particulate form and the optimum particle size to reach and be deposited in the small bronchi is around 2 μm. Such particles are delivered to the lung as an *aerosol,* i.e. dispersed in a gas, which can be produced in a number of different ways:

Pressurised aerosol. Drug is dissolved in a low boiling point liquid in a canister under pressure. Opening the valve releases a metered dose of liquid that is ejected into the atmosphere, carrier liquid evaporates instantly leaving an aerosol of the drug that is inhaled. Until recently the vehicle has been a CFC (chlorofluorocarbon), but due to the concerns over depletion of atmospheric ozone these are being replaced by hydrofluoroalkanes (HFAs) which are ozone-friendly.

To ensure optimal drug delivery, it is necessary to coordinate activation of the inhaler with inspiration and a final hold of breath. Many patients, especially the young and the elderly, find this very difficult and 'spacer' devices are often used between the inhaler and lips; these act as an aerosol reservoir and also reduce impaction of aerosol in the oropharynx. Topical deposition can cause local side effects in the mouth, particularly candida with inhaled glucocorticoids; a spacer abolishes this problem.

Nebulisers convert a solution or suspension of drug into an aerosol. *Jet* nebulisers require a driving gas, usually air from a compressor unit for home use, or oxygen in hospital; the solution in the nebulising chamber is broken into droplets by the jet and the larger droplets are filtered off leaving the smaller ones to be inhaled. *Ultrasonic* nebulisers convert a solution into particles of uniform size by vibrations created by a piezo electric crystal.[9] With either method the aerosol is delivered to the patient by a mouthpiece or facemask, so no coordination is called for, and the dose can be altered by changing the strength of the solution. Much larger doses can be administered by nebuliser than by pressurised aerosol.

Dry powder inhalers. The drug is formulated as a micronised powder and placed in a device, e.g. a spinhaler or diskhaler, from which it is inhaled. Patients can often use these when they fail with metered dose aerosols. Inhalation of powder occasionally causes transient bronchoconstriction.

DRUG TREATMENT

This varies with the severity and type of asthma. It is a general rule that the effectiveness of changes in drug and dose should be monitored by serial measurements of the simple respiratory function tests such as peak expiratory flow rate (PEFR) or forced expiratory volume (FEV_1). Neither the patients' feelings nor physical examination are alone sufficient to determine whether there is still room for improvement. When an asthmatic attack is severe, arterial blood gases must also be measured.

Constant and intermittent asthma

The 1997 British Thoracic Society guidelines recommend a five-step approach[10] (summarised in Fig. 27.1) to the drug management of chronic asthma. The scheme starts with a patient requiring occasional β_2-adrenoceptor agonist and follows an escalating scheme of add-on anti-inflammatory treatment. Points to emphasise are: (1) short-acting β_2-adrenoceptor agonists are used throughout as rescue therapy for acute symptoms; (2) patients must be reviewed regularly as they can move up or down the scheme. Particular attention should be paid to inhaler technique, as this is an important cause of treatment failure. Patients who cannot manage inhaled therapy, even with the addition of a spacer device or use of a dry-powder device, can be given oral therapy, although this will be accompanied by more systemic side effects.

An inhaled β_2-adrenoceptor agonist should be used initially. *Salbutamol* or *terbutaline* (1–2 puffs up to q.d.s.) are typical short-acting β_2-adrenoceptor agonists whose bronchodilator effect is prompt in onset (within a few minutes) and lasts 4–6 h. *Salmeterol* and *eformoterol* have a much longer duration of effect (12–24 h) making them useful for nocturnal symptoms; they should not be used as 'rescue' bronchodilator (salmeterol in particular because its bronchodilators action takes 15–30 mins to emerge) nor as a replacement for inhaled glucocorticoid (see step 3). β_2-adrenoceptor agonists all cause dose-dependent tremor especially if given orally rather than inhaled.

Anti-inflammatory agents can commence either with *sodium cromoglicate* or low-dose inhaled *gluco-*

---

[9] Converts electricity into mechanical vibration.
[10] British Thoracic Society 1997 guidelines on the management of asthma. Thorax 52: Supp. 2. Available online at www.brit-thoracic.org.co.uk/guide/guidelines.html.

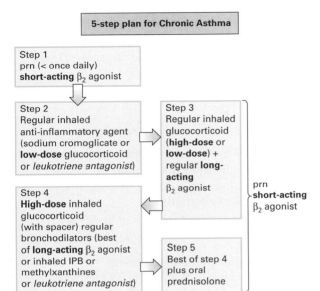

5-step plan for Chronic Asthma

Step 1
prn (< once daily)
short-acting β_2 agonist

Step 2
Regular inhaled
anti-inflammatory agent
(sodium cromoglicate or
low-dose glucocorticoid
or *leukotriene antagonist*)

Step 3
Regular inhaled
glucocorticoid
(**high-dose** or
low-dose) +
regular **long-
acting**
β_2 agonist

Step 4
High-dose inhaled
glucocorticoid
(with spacer) regular
bronchodilators (best
of **long-acting** β_2 agonist
or inhaled IPB or
methylxanthines
or *leukotriene antagonist*)

Step 5
Best of step 4
plus oral
prednisolone

prn
short-acting
β_2 agonist

At all steps the goal is to:
• Minimise symptoms and exacerbations
• Minimise need for additional 'rescue' (short-acting β_2 agonist)
• Achieve PEFR >80% predicted with <20% diurnal variation

Fig. 27.1 Five-step treatment of asthma (British Thoracic Society 1997, with permission)

corticoid (step 2). The inhaled glucocorticoids in current use (*beclomethasone, budesonide* and *fluticasone*) are characterised by low oral bioavailability because of high first-pass metabolism in the liver (almost 100% for fluticasone). This property is important, for it minimises the systemic effects of inhaled glucocorticoid, 80–90% of which is actually swallowed. Precisely for this reason, prednisolone or hydrocortisone would have less advantage if inhaled (over oral administration) since they are absorbed from the gut with relatively little presystemic metabolism. The other important difference between these glucocorticoids and orally administered drugs of the class is their higher potency and lipid solubility. Potency (the physical mass of drug in relation to its effect, see p. 94) is generally unimportant in comparisons of oral drugs, but is essential for locally administered drugs.

Inhaled glucocorticoids are generally safe at low doses. Topical effects (oral candida and hoarseness) are easily eliminated by using a spacer device and rinsing the mouth. High doses (> 1500 microgram day) are reported to carry a slightly increased risk of cataract and glaucoma; this may reflect local aerosol deposition rather than a true systemic effect. Bone turnover is also increased in adults, suggesting a long-term risk of accelerated osteoporosis, and bone growth may be reduced in children (although evidence indicates that normal adult height can be attained[11]). Therefore, it is important that patients are maintained on the *minimum* dose of inhaled glucocorticoid necessary for symptom control.

Oral *prednisolone* is very effective for severe exacerbations and short courses (e.g. 30 mg daily for 5–7 days) are frequently given. Provided symptoms and peak flows respond promptly, more prolonged courses or prolonged reduction of dose is unnecessary. When oral glucocorticoids are used long term (step 5), doses should be adjusted much more slowly. Corticosteroid adverse effects may also be minimised by administering a single morning dose to coincide with the normal peak cortisol concentration (and thus the least suppression of feedback to the hypothalamic-adrenal axis). This is possible because of the long duration of their biological effect (18–36 h) compared with plasma $t\frac{1}{2}$ (3 h for prednisolone). Morning dosing with *inhaled* glucocorticoid may also have a prednisolone-sparing effect. Some patients may get further prednisolone-sparing by addition of nebulised high-dose budesonide, 1–2 mg b.d. or fluticasone 500 micrograms b.d.

Chest infections

Antimicrobials are over prescribed for exacerbations of asthma. Respiratory tract infections do cause increased airflow obstruction and hyperresponsiveness, but viral rather than bacterial pathogens are the commonest culprits. Antimicrobials should be prescribed only if there is high suspicion of a bacterial respiratory tract infection, e.g. purulent sputum. Note that macrolide antibiotics, such as erythromycin and clarithromycin, interfere with theophylline metabolism.

[11] Agertoft L, Pedersen S 2000 New England Journal of Medicine 343: 1064–1069.

ACUTE SEVERE ASTHMA ('STATUS ASTHMATICUS')

This is a life-threatening emergency requiring rapid aggressive treatment. The airways may become refractory to β_2-adrenoceptor agonists after 36–48 h, partly for pharmacological reasons (receptor desensitisation) and partly due to the prolonged respiratory acidosis. The mucous plugs, which are the hallmark of the condition, may also prevent inhaled drugs from reaching the distal airways.

The following lists, with some explanation, the recommendations of the British Thoracic Society[10] for managing acute severe asthma:

Immediate treatment

- *Oxygen* by mask *(humidified,* to help liquefy mucus). CO_2 narcosis is rare in asthma and 60% can be used if the diagnosis is not in doubt. In older patients, or when there is any concern about chronic CO_2 retention, start with O_2 28% and to check that the $PaCO_2$ has not risen before delivering O_2 35%.
- *Salbutamol* by nebuliser in a dose of 2.5–5 mg over about 3 min, repeated in 15 min. *Terbutaline* 5–10 mg is an alternative.
- *Prednisolone* 30–60 mg p.o. or *hydrocortisone* 200 mg i.v.
- *Avoid sedation* of any kind.
- Chest x-ray to exclude pneumothorax.

If life-threatening features are present (absent breath sounds, cyanosis, bradycardia, exhausted appearance or PEFR < 30% predicted):

- *Ipratropium* 0.5 mg should be added to the nebulised β_2-agonist.
- Give i.v. either *salbutamol* 250 microgram over 10 minutes (as nebulised salbutamol may not be reaching the distal airways) or *aminophylline* 5 mg/kg. Aminophylline should not be given to patients already taking oral theophyllines.
- Alert the intensive care unit.

Subsequent management. If the patient is improving, continue:
- 40–60% oxygen
- Prednisolone 30–60 mg daily or hydrocortisone 200 mg 6-hourly
- Nebulised salbutamol or terbutaline 4-hourly.

If the patient is **not** improving after 15–30 minutes:

- Continue oxygen and glucocorticoid
- Give nebulised β_2-adrenoceptor agonist more frequently, up to every 15–30 minutes
- Add ipratropium 0.5 mg to nebuliser and repeat 6-hourly until patient is improving.

If the patient is still not improving give:

- i.v. infusion of β_2-adrenoceptor agonist or aminophylline (0.9 microgram/kg/min)
- i.v. infusion of a β_2-adrenoceptor agonist (as above) as an **alternative**
- Contact the intensive care unit to discuss intubation and mechanical ventilation.

Monitoring response to treatment

- By peak expiratory flow rate (PEFR) every 15–30 minutes
- Oxygen saturation: maintain > 92%
- Repeat blood gas measurements if initial PaO_2 < 8 kPa (60 mm Hg) and/or initial $PaCO_2$ normal or raised (the tachypnoea is expected to reduce $PaCO_2$ in most patients)

Treatment in intensive care unit. Transfer (accompanied by doctor with facilities for intubation) is required if:
- any of the above deteriorates, despite maximal treatment
- the patient becomes exhausted, drowsy, or confused
- coma or respiratory arrest occurs.

Treatment at discharge from hospital. Patients should:
- continue high-dose inhaled glucocorticoid and complete course of oral prednisolone
- be instructed to monitor their own PEFR and not to reduce dose if the PEFR falls, or there is a recurrence of early morning dipping in the reading (patients should not generally be discharged until there is < 25% diurnal variation in PEFR readings).

Warnings

Asthma may be *precipitated* by *β-adrenoceptor blockade* and the use of β-adrenoceptor antagonists is contraindicated altogether in asthmatics; fatal asthma has been precipitated by β-blocker eye-drops, even allegedly β$_1$-selective agents.

Overuse of β$_2$-adrenergic agonists is dangerous. In the mid-1960s, there was an epidemic of sudden deaths in young asthmatics outside hospital. It was associated with the introduction of a high-dose, metered aerosol of isoprenaline (β$_1$- and β$_2$-agonist); it did not occur in countries where the high concentration was not marketed.[12] The epidemic declined in Britain when the profession was warned, and the aerosols were restricted to prescription only. Though the relationship between the use of β$_2$-receptor agonists and death is presumed to be causal, the actual mechanism of death is uncertain; overdose causing cardiac arrhythmia is not the sole factor. The subsequent development of selective β$_2$-receptor agonists was a contribution to safety but a review in New Zealand during the 1980s found that the use of fenoterol (β$_2$-selective) by metered dose inhalation was associated with increased risk of death in severe asthma,[13] and later analysis concluded that it was the most likely cause.[14]

CHRONIC OBSTRUCTIVE PULMONARY DISEASE (COPD)

Whereas asthma is characterised by *reversible* airways obstruction and bronchial hyperreactivity, COPD is characterised by *incompletely reversible* airways obstruction and *mucus hypersecretion*; it is predominantly a disease of the smaller airways. Nevertheless, distinguishing the two can be difficult in some patients and one view is that asthma predisposes smokers to COPD (Dutch hypothesis). In practice, even though — indeed precisely because — most of the airway obstruction is fixed in COPD, it is important to maximise the reversible component. This can be assessed by measuring FEV$_1$ before and after a course of oral prednisolone, e.g. at least 30 mg/day for 2 weeks; reversibility is arbitrarily defined as > 15% rise (and > 200 ml) in FEV$_1$. An important caveat is that patients' symptoms sometimes improve despite little or no demonstrable reversibility, because FEV$_1$ measures large airways function, and in COPD mainly the small airways are affected.

Drugs used to treat COPD are exactly as for asthma, except that antimuscarinics, such as *ipratopium,* are often more effective bronchodilators than β$_2$-agonists in COPD. Patients *with* reversibility should also receive inhaled glucocorticoids. A trial in patients *without* reversibility found that inhaled glucocorticoid had no effect on the decline in their lung function.[15] Mucolytic drugs reduce acute episodes of COPD and days of illness; they are best reserved for patients with recurrent, prolonged or severe exacerbations of the disease.

Quitting smoking remains the only action of proven benefit in preserving lung function in COPD.

Domiciliary oxygen improves survival in hypoxic patients. It is indicated when:

- PaO$_2$ is < 7.3 kPa (56 mmHg) when stabilised on medical treatment
- PaO$_2$ is 7.3–8.0 kPa and
- they suffer an episode of right-sided cardiac failure (cor pulmonale)
- FEV$_1$ is < 1.5 l and FVC > 2 l.

[12] Stolley P D 1972 American Review of Respiratory Diseases 105: 8: 33.

[13] Crane J et al 1989 Lancet 1: 917.

[14] Pearce N et al 1995 Lancet 345: 41–44.

[15] Pauwels R A et al 1999 New England Journal of Medicine 340: 1948.

Summary

- Asthma is characterised by hypersensitivity to the endogenous bronchoconstrictors, acetylcholine and histamine, and by reversible obstruction of the airways.
- Drugs that block the actions of acetylcholine and histamine are weak or ineffective in the treatment of asthma.
- Most antiasthma treatment is therefore aimed either at reducing release of inflammatory cytokines (glucocorticoids and sodium cromoglicate) or at direct bronchodilatation by stimulation of the bronchial β$_2$-adrenoceptors.
- Aggressive use of glucocorticoids, especially by the inhaled route, is the keystone of the modern stepped approach to asthma management.
- Antihistamines conventionally refer to antagonists of the H$_1$-receptor, and have wide applications in the treatment of allergic disorders, and in anaphylaxis.

- The principal adverse effect of older first-generation antihistamines, sedation, is avoided by use of newer second-generation drugs which do not enter the CNS.
- Respiratory distress of the newborn is usually a treatable condition, using synthetic lung surfactant administration, and can often be avoided by prophylactic treatment of the mother with glucocorticoid.
- Smoking cessation and long-term treatment with oxygen are the only interventions that are known to improve survival in chronic obstructive pulmonary disease.

GUIDE TO FURTHER READING

Barnes P J 2000 Chronic obstructive pulmonary disease. New England Journal of Medicine 343: 269–280

Bateman N T, Leach R M 1998 Acute oxygen therapy. British Medical Journal 317: 798–801

Busse W W, Lemanske R F 2001 Asthma. New England Journal of Medicine 344: 350–362

Drazen J M, Elliot I, O'Byrne P 1999 Treatment of asthma with drugs modifying the leukotriene pathway. New England Journal of Medicine 340: 197–206

Holgate S T 2000 Allergic disorders. British Medical Journal 320: 231–234

Hsia F H 1998 Respiratory function of haemoglobin. New England Journal of Medicine 338: 239–247

Irwin R S, Madison J M 2000 The diagnosis and management of cough. New England Journal of Medicine 343: 1715–1721

Kay A B 2001 Allergy and allergic diseases. New England Journal of Medicine 344: 30–37 (part I) 109–113 (part 2)

Poole P J, Black P N 2001 Oral mucolytic drugs for exacerbations of chronic obstructive pulmonary disease. British Medical Journal 322: 1271–1274

Rees P J, Dudley F 1998 Oxygen therapy in chronic lung disease. British Medical Journal 317: 871–874

Rees P J, Dudley F 1998 Provision of oxygen at home. British Medical Journal 317: 935–938

Ware L B, Matthay M A 2000 The acute respiratory distress syndrome. New England Journal of Medicine 342: 1334–1349

Weiner J M, Abramson M J, Puy R M 1998 Intranasal corticosteroids versus oral H_1-receptor antagonists in allergic rhinitis: systematic review of randomised controlled trials. British Medical Journal 317: 1624–1629

BLOOD AND NEOPLASTIC DISEASE

28

Drugs and haemostasis

SYNOPSIS

Occlusive vascular disease is a major cause of morbidity and mortality. There is now better understanding of the mechanisms by which the haemostatic system ensures blood remains fluid within vessels, yet forms a solid plug when a vessel is breached, and of the ways in which haemostasis may be altered by drugs to prevent or reverse (lyse) pathological thrombosis.

- Coagulation system: the mode of action of drugs that promote coagulation and that prevent it (anticoagulants) and their uses
- Fibrinolytic system: the mode of action of drugs that promote fibrinolysis (fibrinolytics) and their uses to lyse arterial and venous thrombi (thrombolysis)
- Platelets: the ways that drugs that inhibit platelet activity are used to treat arterial disease

The haemostatic system is complex but can be separated into the following major components:

- Formation of fibrin (coagulation), which stabilises the platelet plug
- Dissolution of fibrin (fibrinolysis)
- Platelets, which form the haemostatic plug
- Blood vessels.

Drugs that interfere with the haemostatic system (anticoagulants, thrombolytics, antiplatelet agents) are valuable in the management of pathological thrombus formation within blood vessels, or of pathological bleeding. They are classified according to which component of the system they affect.

Coagulation system

The blood coagulation system is shown in simplified form in Figure 28.1. It consists of glycoprotein components that circulate in (necessarily *inactive*) pro-enzyme or pro-cofactor (factors V and VIII) form. The activated enzymes are serine proteases.

Physiological coagulation (the 'extrinsic' pathway) begins when tissue factor (TF, tissue thromboplastin), exposed by vascular injury, activates and complexes with factor VII to activate factors IX and X which complex with VIIIa and Va respectively on membrane surfaces (which provide phospholipid, PL). The Xa/Va complex converts prothrombin to thrombin which converts fibrinogen to fibrin and also activates factors XI, VIII, V and XIII, both accelerating coagulation and cross-linking fibrin (–F–F–F–).

The 'intrinsic' pathway refers to coagulation in vitro. It is initiated when factor XII with the cofactor high molecular weight kininogen (HMWK) comes into contact with a foreign surface, e.g. glass, kaolin. Thus it has no physiological role (and patients lacking factor XII do not have a bleeding disorder).

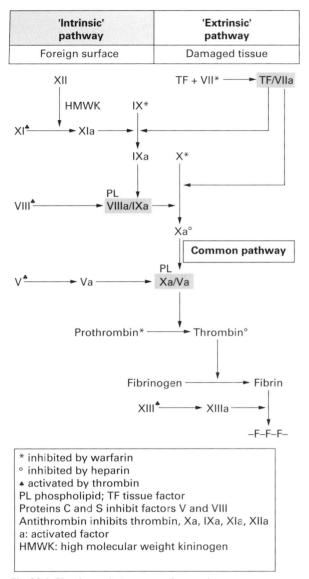

'Intrinsic' pathway	'Extrinsic' pathway
Foreign surface	Damaged tissue

* inhibited by warfarin
° inhibited by heparin
♠ activated by thrombin
PL phospholipid; TF tissue factor
Proteins C and S inhibit factors V and VIII
Antithrombin inhibits thrombin, Xa, IXa, XIa, XIIa
a: activated factor
HMWK: high molecular weight kininogen

Fig. 28.1 Blood coagulation system (see text)

The classical separation of the *intrinsic* and *extrinsic* pathways is a simplification but remains a useful in-vitro phenomenon for monitoring coagulation. Both in vivo and in vitro the systems are dependent on the presence of Ca^{++} ions and key in-vivo steps involve the formation of macromolecular complexes on membrane surfaces, usually those of platelets. Cascade reactions culminate in the generation of fibrin and its polymerisation by factor XIII to form a fibrin clot.

The prothrombin time (PT), which is usually expressed as the International Normalised Ratio (INR) for control of oral anticoagulant therapy, primarily evaluates the *extrinsic* system.

The activated partial thromboplastin time (APTT), also known as the kaolin–cephalin clotting time (KCCT), primarily evaluates the *intrinsic* system. In-vitro coagulation of plasma is initiated by the addition of negatively charged particles such as kaolin with phospholipid, and calcium and exogenous thromboplastin.

Each of these tests is also affected by the *final common pathway*, the endpoint of which is tested by the thrombin time. This tests the formation of a fibrin clot by the addition of exogenous thrombin and calcium. It is sensitive to the level of endogenous fibrinogen and to the presence of inhibitors of thrombin (heparin, FDPs).

VITAMIN K: A CRITICAL CO-FACTOR

Vitamin K (Koagulation vitamin) is essential to normal haemostatic and antithrombotic mechanisms. This vitamin occurs naturally in two forms. Vitamin K_1 (phylloquinone) is widely distributed in plants and K_2 includes vitamin synthesised in the alimentary tract by bacteria, e.g. *Escherichia coli* (menaquinones). Bile is required for the absorption of the natural vitamins K, which are fat-soluble. Leafy green vegetables are a good source of vitamin K_1. The storage pool of vitamin K is modest and can be exhausted in one week, though gut flora will maintain suboptimal production of vitamin K dependent proteins. A synthetic analogue, *menadione*, (K_3) (below) of the natural vitamins also has biological activity in vivo; it is water-soluble.

Vitamin K is necessary for the final stage of the synthesis of six coagulation-related proteins in the liver by γ-carboxylation of glutamic acid residues on the molecule. The γ-carboxyglutamic acid residues permit calcium to bind to the molecule which in turn mediates binding to negatively charged phospholipid surfaces. The vitamin K-dependent proteins are coagulation factors II (prothrombin), VII, IX and X, and the anticoagulant (regulatory) proteins, proteins C and S. During γ-carboxylation of the proteins by the vitamin K dependent carboxylase, the reduced form of vitamin K is converted to an epoxide, an oxidation product, which is subsequently reduced again enzymatically to the active vitamin K, i.e. there exists an interconversion cycle (the vitamin K cycle) between *vitamin K epoxide* and *reduced and active vitamin K* (KH$_2$). When the vitamin is deficient or where its action is inhibited by drugs, coagulation proteins which cannot bind Ca^{++} result; their physiologically critical binding to membrane surfaces fails to occur, and this impairs the coagulation mechanism. This non- or-descarboxylated protein is called 'protein induced in vitamin K absence' or PIVKA.

Deficiency may arise from:

- bile failing to enter the intestine, e.g. obstructive jaundice or biliary fistula
- certain malabsorption syndromes, e.g. coeliac disease, or after extensive small intestinal resection
- reduced alimentary tract flora, e.g. in newborn infants and rarely after broad-spectrum antimicrobials.

The following preparations of vitamin K are available:

Phytomenadione (phytonadione, Konakion), the naturally occurring fat-soluble vitamin K$_1$, acts within about 12 h and should correct the INR within 24–48 h. The i.v. formulation is used in emergency and must be administered slowly as an anaphylactoid reaction with facial flushing, sweating, fever, chest tightness, cyanosis and peripheral vascular collapse may occur. Patients with chronic liver disease and those using histamine H$_2$-receptor antagonists seem to be especially likely to react. Otherwise phytomenadione may be given i.m., s.c. or orally. The preferred route depends on the urgency of correcting the haemorrhagic tendency. The i.m. route should be avoided if the INR is significantly prolonged as local intramuscular haemorrhage may be induced; s.c. absorption is variable and despite the risk of allergic reaction, the intravenous route ensures rapid delivery.

Menadiol sodium phosphate (vitamin K$_3$, Synkavit), the synthetic analogue of vitamin K, being water-soluble, is preferred in malabsorption or in states in which bile flow is deficient. The main disadvantage is that it takes 24 h to act, but its effect lasts for several days. The dose is 5–40 mg daily, orally.

Menadiol sodium phosphate in moderate doses causes haemolytic anaemia and for this reason it should not be given to neonates, especially those that are deficient in glucose-6-phosphate dehydrogenase; their immature livers are unable to cope with the heavy bilirubin load and there is danger of kernicterus.

Fat-soluble analogues of vitamin K which are available in some countries include acetomenaphthone and menaphthone.

Indications for vitamin K or its analogues

- Haemorrhage or threatened bleeding due to the coumarin or indandione anticoagulants. Phytomenadione is preferred for its more rapid action; dosage regimens vary according to the degree of urgency and the original indication for anticoagulation, as described on page 576.
- Haemorrhagic disease of the newborn which develops during the first week of life, usually between days 2–7 (and also late haemorrhagic disease which presents at 6–7 months). Prophylaxis is recommended[1] during the period of vulnerability with vitamin K (phytomenadione, as Konakion) 1 mg by single i.m. injection at birth. Alternatively, vitamin K may be given by mouth as two doses of a colloidal (mixed micelle) preparation of phytomenadione in the first week. Breast-fed babies should receive a further 2 mg at one month of age. Formula-fed babies do not need this last supplement as the formula contains vitamin K. Fears that i.m. vitamin K might cause childhood cancer have been allayed.
- Hypoprothrombinaemia due to intestinal malabsorption syndromes. Menadiol sodium phosphate should be used as it is water-soluble.

DRUGS THAT PREVENT COAGULATION: ANTICOAGULANTS

There are two types of anticoagulant:

Indirect-acting: coumarin[2] and indandione drugs take about 72 h to become fully effective, act for several days, are given orally and can be antagonised (see below) by vitamin K.

---

[1] British National Formulary.

Direct-acting: heparin, hirudin, bivalirudin and argatroban are rapidly effective, act for only a few hours and must be given parenterally.

Indirect-acting anticoagulants

Coumarins include *warfarin* and *acenocoumarol* (nicoumalone). The vitamin K antagonists were discovered as a result of investigation of a haemorrhagic disease of cattle that plagued farmers in the Great Plains of the USA during the 1920s. The disorder which was due to hypoprothrombinaemia was caused by ingestion of spoiled sweet clover hay contaminated by specific toxins. The compound 3, 3'-methylene-bis-4-hydroxycoumarin was purified from bacterial contaminants in the spoiled hay and was found to produce a syndrome similar to vitamin K deficiency.[3] Bishydroxycoumarin (dicoumarol) was introduced into clinical practice as an anticoagulant in the 1940s and other structurally related vitamin K antagonists followed; all share a common ring structure with vitamin K. Warfarin is the most widely used.

Warfarin

Mode of action. During the γ-carboxylation of the coagulant factors II (prothrombin), VII, IX and X (and also the anticoagulant regulatory proteins C and S) in the liver, active vitamin K (KH_2) is oxidised to an epoxide and must be reduced by the enzymes vitamin K epoxide reductase and vitamin K reductase to become active again (the vitamin K cycle). Coumarins are structurally similar to vitamin K and competitively inhibit vitamin K epoxide reductase and vitamin K reductase, so limiting availability of the active reduced form of the vitamin to form coagulant (and anticoagulant) proteins. The overall result is a shift in haemostatic balance in favour of anticoagulation because of the accumulation of clotting proteins with absent or decreased γ-

carboxylation sites (PIVKAs). This shift does not take place until functional vitamin K-dependent proteins made before the drug was administered are cleared from the circulation. The process occurs at different rates for individual coagulation factors (VII $t\frac{1}{2}$ 6 h, IX and X $t\frac{1}{2}$ 24 h, prothrombin $t\frac{1}{2}$ 72 h). Moreover, the anticoagulant proteins C and S have a shorter $t\frac{1}{2}$ than the procoagulant proteins and their more rapid decline in concentration creates a *transient hypercoagulable state*. This can be serious in those who have inherited protein S and C deficiency who may develop skin necrosis and justifies initiating anticoagulation with heparin until the effect of warfarin is well established. Thus the anticoagulant effect of warfarin is delayed and indeed the drug must be administered for 4–5 days before the effect is properly therapeutic. Furthermore, the INR does not reliably reflect anticoagulant protection during this initial phase, because the vitamin K-dependent factors diminish at different rates.

The great advantage of warfarin over heparin is that it can be given orally. Its chief disadvantage is the time lag before it exerts its effect, which is due to its indirect mode of action. A similar time lag is found when the warfarin dose is altered or discontinued as the $t\frac{1}{2}$ of the nonfunctioning proteins is approximately that of functioning proteins.

Pharmacokinetics. Warfarin is readily absorbed from the gastrointestinal tract and like all the oral anticoagulants, is more than 90% bound to plasma proteins. Its action is terminated by metabolism in the liver. Warfarin ($t\frac{1}{2}$ 36 h) is a racemic mixture of approximately equal amounts of two isomers S ($t\frac{1}{2}$ 35 h) and R ($t\frac{1}{2}$ 50 h) warfarin, i.e. it is in effect two drugs. S warfarin is four times more potent than R warfarin. Drugs which interact with warfarin affect these isomers differently.

Uses. Warfarin is the oral anticoagulant of choice, for it is reliably effective and has the lowest incidence of adverse effects. Monitoring of therapy is by the prothrombin time. Usually the test is carried out with a standardised thromboplastin and the result is expressed as the International Normalised Ratio (INR), which is the ratio of the prothrombin time in the patient to that in a normal (non-anticoagulated) person—taking account of the sensitivity of the

---

[2] Coumarins are present in many plants and are important in the perfume industry; the smell of new mown hay and grass is due to coumarins.

[3] Campbell H A, Link K P 1941 Studies on the haemorrhagic sweet clover disease IV: the isolation and crystallisation of the haemorrhagic agent. Journal of Biological Chemistry 138: 21.

thromboplastin used. Oral anticoagulation is commonly undertaken in patients who are already receiving heparin. The INR reliably reflects the degree of prothrombin activity provided that the activated partial thromboplastin time (APTT, a measure of the anticoagulant effect of heparin, see below) is within the therapeutic range (1.5–2.5 times control). Warfarin therapy with an INR in the therapeutic range does not prolong the APTT.

Dose. There is much inter-individual variation in dose requirements. It is usual to initiate therapy with 10 mg daily for 2 days, with the maintenance dose then adjusted according to the INR using an established protocol.[4]

The level of anticoagulation should be adjusted to match the perceived risk of thrombosis, by the following guidelines:[5]

- **INR 2.0–2.5** Prophylaxis of deep vein thrombosis including surgery on high-risk patients (2.0–3.0 for hip surgery and fractured femur operations).
- **INR 2.0–3.0** Treatment of deep vein thrombosis; pulmonary embolism; systemic embolism; prevention of venous thromboembolism in myocardial infarction; mitral stenosis with embolism; transient ischaemic attacks; atrial fibrillation.
- **INR 3.0–4.5** Recurrent deep vein thrombosis and pulmonary embolism; arterial disease including myocardial infarction; mechanical prosthetic heart valves.

Adverse effects. Bleeding is the commonest complication of warfarin therapy. The incidence of major haemorrhage is about 5% per year[6] and an identifiable risk factor is often present, e.g. thrombocytopenia, liver disease or vitamin K deficiency, an endogenous disturbance of coagulation, cancer or recent surgery. Naturally, poor anticoagulant control or drug interaction with warfarin increase the risk. Haemorrhage is most likely to occur in the alimentary and renal tracts, and in the brain in those with cerebrovascular disease.

Cutaneous reactions, apart from purpura and ecchymoses in those who are excessively anticoagulated, include hypersensitivity, rash and alopecia. Skin necrosis due to a mixture of haemorrhage and thrombosis occurs rarely where induction of warfarin therapy is over-abrupt and/or the patient has a genetically determined or acquired deficiency of the anticoagulant protein C or its cofactor protein S; it can be very serious.

Warfarin used in early pregnancy may injure the fetus (other than by bleeding). It causes skeletal disorders (5%) (bossed forehead, sunken nose, foci of calcification in the epiphyses) and absence of the spleen. Women on long-term warfarin should be advised not to become pregnant while taking the drug. Heparin should be substituted prior to conception and continued through the first trimester, after which warfarin should replace heparin, as continued exposure to heparin may cause osteoporosis. Warfarin should be discontinued near term as it exacerbates neonatal hypoprothrombinaemia and its control is too imprecise to be safe in labour; heparin may be substituted at this stage for it can be discontinued just before labour and its anticoagulant effect wears off in about 6 h.

CNS abnormalities (microcephaly, cranial nerve palsies) are reported with warfarin used at any stage of pregnancy and are presumed to be due to intracranial haemorrhage.

Management of bleeding or over-anticoagulation is guided by the clinical state and the INR:[7]

- *Haemorrhage threatening life or major organs.* In addition to blood replacement, rapid reversal of anticoagulation is achieved with prothrombin complex concentrate (containing factors II, IX and X, and given i.v. as 50 units per kg of factor IX) or fresh frozen plasma. If full reversal of anticoagulation is judged necessary, phytomenadione 5 mg is then given by slow i.v. injection. This renders the patient refractory to oral anticoagulant (but not to heparin) for about 2 weeks. The thrombotic risk so created must be assessed for each patient and may be judged

---

[4] Fennerty A et al 1988 British Medical Journal 297: 1285–1288.
[5] British Society for Haematology 1990 Guidelines on oral anticoagulants, 2nd edn. Journal of Clinical Pathology 43: 177–183 (Reproduced with permission).

[6] A study of 261 patients who received warfarin for 221 patient-years reported major haemorrhage in 5.3% after 1 year and 10.6% after 2 years. Gitter M J et al 1995 Mayo Clinic Proceedings 70: 725–733.

unacceptable in some, e.g. those with prosthetic heart valves. For less severe haemorrhage, warfarin should be withheld and phytomenadione 0.5–2 mg may be given by slow i.v. injection if rapid correction of the INR is necessary.

- *INR > 7 but without bleeding.* Correct by withholding warfarin, and giving phytomenadione 0.5 mg by slow i.v. injection if judged appropriate.
- *INR 4.5–7.0.* Manage by withholding warfarin for 1–2 days and then reviewing the INR.
- *INR 2.0–4.5 (the therapeutic range).* Bleeding, e.g. from the nose, alimentary or renal tract, should be fully investigated as a local cause frequently exists.

Withdrawal of oral anticoagulant. The balance of evidence is that abrupt, as opposed to gradual withdrawal of therapy does not of itself add to the risk of thromboembolism, for renewed synthesis of functional vitamin K dependent clotting factors takes several days.

Interactions. Oral anticoagulant control must be precise both for safety and efficacy. If a drug that alters the action of warfarin must be used, the INR should be monitored frequently and the dose of warfarin adjusted during the period of institution of the new drug until a new stable therapeutic dose of warfarin is identified; careful monitoring is also needed on withdrawal of the interacting drug.

The following list, although not comprehensive, identifies medicines that should be avoided and those which may safely be used with warfarin.

- *Analgesics.* Avoid if possible, all NSAIDs including aspirin (but see p. 576, myocardial infarction)because of their irritant effect on gastric mucosa and action on platelets. Paracetamol is acceptable but doses over 1.5 g/d may raise the INR. Dextropropoxyphene inhibits warfarin metabolism and compounds that contain it, e.g. co-proxamol, should be avoided. Codeine, dihydrocodeine and combinations with paracetamol, e.g. co-dydramol, are preferred.

- *Antimicrobials.* Aztreonam, cefamandole, chloramphenicol, ciprofloxacin, co-trimoxazole, erythromycin, fluconazole, itraconazole, ketoconazole, metronidazole, miconazole, ofloxacin and sulphonamides (including co-trimoxazole) increase anticoagulant effect by mechanisms that include interference with warfarin or vitamin K metabolism. Rifampicin and griseofulvin accelerate warfarin metabolism (enzyme induction) and reduce its effect. Intensive broad-spectrum antimicrobials, e.g. eradication regimens for *Helicobacter pylori* (see p. 630), may increase sensitivity to warfarin by reducing the intestinal flora that produce vitamin K.
- *Anticonvulsants.* Carbamazepine, phenobarbital and primidone accelerate warfarin metabolism (enzyme induction); the effect of phenytoin is variable. Clonazepam and sodium valproate are safe.
- *Cardiac antiarrhythmics.* Amiodarone, propafenone and possibly quinidine potentiate the effect of warfarin and dose adjustment is required, but atropine, disopyramide and lignocaine do not interfere.
- *Antidepressants.* Serotonin reuptake inhibitors may enhance the effect of warfarin but tricyclics may be used.
- *Gastrointestinal drugs.* Avoid cimetidine and omeprazole which inhibit the clearance of R warfarin, and sucralfate which may impair its absorption. Ranitidine may be used but INR should be checked if the dose is high. Most antacids are safe.
- *Lipid-lowering drugs.* Fibrates, and some statins, enhance anticoagulant effect. Colestyramine is best avoided for it may impair the absorption of both warfarin and vitamin K.
- *Sex hormones and hormone antagonists.* Oestrogens increase the synthesis of some vitamin K dependent clotting factors and progestogen-only contraceptives are preferred. The hormone antagonists danazol, flutamide and tamoxifen enhance the effect of warfarin.
- *Sedatives and anxiolytics.* Benzodiazepines may be used.

Other vitamin K antagonists. *Acenocoumarol* (nicoumalone) is similar to warfarin but seldom

---

[7] Based on recommendations of the British Society for Haematology.

used; it is eliminated in the urine mainly in unchanged form (t½ 24 h). *Indandione* anticoagulants are practically obsolete because of allergic adverse reactions unrelated to coagulation; phenindione (t½ 5 h) is still available but also seldom used.

Direct-acting anticoagulants: heparin

Heparin was discovered by a medical student, J. McLean, working at Johns Hopkins Medical School in 1916. Seeking to devote one year to physiological research he was set to study 'the thromboplastic (clotting) substance in the body'. He found that extracts of brain, heart and liver accelerated clotting but that activity deteriorated during storage. To his surprise, the extract of liver which he had kept longest not only failed to accelerate but actually retarded clotting. His personal account proceeds:

> After more tests and the preparation of other batches of heparophosphatide, I went one morning to the door of Dr. Howell's office, and standing there (he was seated at his desk), I said 'Dr. Howell, I have discovered antithrombin'. He was most skeptical. So I had the Deiner, John Schweinhant, bleed a cat. Into a small beaker full of its blood, I stirred all of a proven batch of heparophosphatides, and I placed this on Dr. Howell's laboratory table and asked him to call me when it clotted. It never did clot. [It was heparin.][8]

Heparin is a sulphated mucopolysaccharide which occurs in the secretory granules of mast cells and is prepared commercially from a variety of animal tissues (generally porcine intestinal mucosa or bovine lung) to give preparations that vary in molecular weight from 3000 to 30 000 (average 15 000). It is the strongest organic acid in the body and in solution carries an electronegative charge. The low molecular weight (LMW) heparins (mean MW 4000–6500) are prepared from standard heparin by a variety of chemical techniques and commercial preparations (dalteparin, enoxaprin, tinzaparin) contain different fractions and display different pharmacokinetics.

Mode of action. Heparin depends for its anticoagulant action on the presence in plasma of a single chain glycoprotein, *antithrombin* (formerly antithrombin III), a naturally-occurring inhibitor of activated coagulation factors of the intrinsic and common pathways including thrombin, factor Xa and factor IXa (Fig. 28.1). Antithrombin is homologous to members of the α_1-antitrypsin family of serine protease inhibitors (serpins). On intravenous administration heparin binds to antithrombin and this leads to rapid inhibition of the proteases of the coagulation pathway. In the presence of heparin antithrombin becomes vastly more active (approximately 1000-fold) and inhibition is essentially instantaneous. Heparin binding to antithrombin induces a conformational change in antithrombin that locks the heparin in place and is followed by rapid reaction with a target protease. This reaction in turn reduces the affinity of antithrombin for heparin, allowing the heparin to dissociate from the antithrombin/protease complex and to catalyse further antithrombin/protease interactions.

The importance of inhibition of factor Xa is that this factor is a critical step in both the intrinsic and extrinsic coagulation systems and heparin is effective in small quantities. This provides the rationale for giving low dose subcutaneous heparin to prevent thrombus formation. At a molecular level the capacity of heparin to inhibit factor Xa has been found to depend on a specific pentasaccharide sequence which can be isolated in fragments of average MW 5000 (LMW heparins). LMW heparins inhibit factor Xa at a dose similar to standard heparin but have much less antithrombin activity. These fragments are too short to inhibit thrombin which is the principal action of conventional heparin (average MW 15 000). Fibrin formed in the circulation binds to thrombin and protects it from inactivation by the heparin-antithrombin complex, which may provide a further explanation for the higher doses of heparin needed to stop extension of a thrombus than to prevent its formation. Heparin also inhibits thrombin through other inhibitors and, at higher concentrations, accelerates plasminogen activation and inhibits platelet aggregation.

Apart from its anticoagulant properties, heparin inhibits the proliferation of vascular smooth muscle cells and is involved in angiogenesis. Heparin also

---

[8] McLean gives a fascinating account of his struggles to pay his way through medical school, as well as his discovery of heparin in: McLean J 1959 Circulation XIX: 75.

inhibits certain aspects of the inflammatory response; this is evident in the rapid resolution of inflammation that accompanies deep vein thrombosis when heparin is given.

Pharmacokinetics. Heparin is poorly absorbed from the gastrointestinal tract and is given i.v. or s.c.; once in the blood its effect is immediate. Heparin binds to several plasma proteins and to sites on endothelial cells; it is also taken up by cells of the reticuloendothelial system and some is cleared by the kidney. Due to these factors, elimination of heparin from the plasma appears to involve a combination of zero-order and first-order processes, the effect of which is that the plasma biological effect $t\frac{1}{2}$ alters disproportionately with dose, being 60 min after 75 units per kg and 150 min after 400 units per kg.

LMW heparins are less protein bound and have a predictable dose–response profile when administered s.c. or i.v. They also have a longer $t\frac{1}{2}$ than standard heparin preparations.

Monitoring heparin therapy. Control of standard heparin therapy is by the activated partial thromboplastin time (APTT), the optimum therapeutic range being 1.5–2.5 times the control (which is preferably the patient's own pretreatment APTT). An alternative method is to measure the plasma concentration of heparin using an anti-Xa assay aiming for a therapeutic concentration of 0.1–1.0 U/ml. Therapeutic doses of LMW heparin do not prolong the APTT and, having predictable pharmacokinetics, they can be administered using a body-weight adjusted algorithm without laboratory monitoring. If necessary an anti-Xa assay can be used to measure the heparin level.

Dose *Treatment of established thrombosis.* The traditional intravenous regimen of standard unfractionated heparin is a bolus i.v. injection of 5000 units (or 10 000 units in severe pulmonary embolism) followed by a constant rate i.v. infusion of 1000–2000 units per hour. Alternatively 15 000 units may be given s.c. every 12 h but control is less even. The APTT should be measured 6 h after starting therapy and the administration rate adjusted to keep it in the optimum therapeutic ratio of 1.5–2.5; this usually requires daily measurements of APTT preferably

between 0900 h and 1200 h (noon) as the anticoagulant effect of heparin exhibits circadian changes.

The convenience (and cost-effectiveness) of LMW heparin therapy has resulted in widespread changes in practice. Patients with acute venous thromboembolism can be treated safely and effectively with LMW heparin as outpatients. Large-scale studies have demonstrated that outpatient treatment of acute deep vein thrombosis (DVT) with unmonitored body-weight adjusted LMW heparin is as safe and effective as inpatient treatment with adjusted dose intravenous standard heparin.[9,10,11] Further trials have confirmed the safety and efficacy of LMW heparin therapy in acute pulmonary embolism[12] and that 80% of unselected patients with acute thromboembolism can be safely treated as outpatients.[13]

Prevention of thrombosis. Postoperatively or after myocardial infarction 5000 units of unfractionated heparin should be given s.c. every 8 or 12 h without monitoring (this dose does not prolong the APPT), or in pregnancy 5000–10 000 units s.c. every 12 h with monitoring (except for pregnant women with prosthetic heart valves for whom specialist monitoring is needed).

LMW heparins have become the preferred drugs for perioperative prophylaxis because of their convenience. They are as effective and safe as unfractionated heparin at preventing venous thrombosis (see above). Once-daily s.c. administration suffices, as their duration of action is longer than that of conventional heparin and no laboratory monitoring is required. LMW heparins are at least as effective as standard heparin for unstable angina, in combination with aspirin.

Adverse effects *Bleeding* is the principal acute complication of heparin therapy. It is uncommon,

[9] Levine M et al 1996 New England Journal of Medicine 334: 677–681.
[10] Koopman M M W et al 1996 New England Journal of Medicine 334: 682–687.
[11] The Columbus Investigators 1997 New England Journal of Medicine 337: 657–662.
[12] Simonneau G et al 1997 New England Journal of Medicine 337: 663–669.
[13] Lindmarker P, Holmstrom M 1996 Journal of Internal Medicine 240: 395–401.

but patients with impaired hepatic or renal function, with carcinoma, and those over 60 years appear to be most at risk. An APPT ratio > 3 is associated with an 8-fold increased chance of bleeding.

Heparin-induced thrombocytopenia (HIT), characterised by arterial thromboemboli and haemorrhage, occurs in about 2–3% of patients who receive standard heparin for a week or more (less in patients on LMW heparins). It is due to an autoantibody directed against heparin in association with platelet factor 4, causing platelet activation, and occurs most commonly with heparin derived from bovine lung. HIT should be suspected in any patient in whom the platelet count falls by 50% or more after starting heparin, and usually occurs 5 or more days after starting therapy (or sooner if the patient has previously been exposed to heparin). Up to 30% of patients may require amputation or may die.

In patients with HIT and evidence of thrombosis, danaparoid sodium, hirudin or argatroban (see p. 577) should be substituted. Warfarin should not be started until adequate anticoagulation has been achieved with one of these agents and the platelet count has returned to normal as skin necrosis or worsening thromboembolism may result. LMW heparins are unsuitable as the antibody may be cross-reactive.

Osteoporosis may occur, it is dose-related and may be expected with 15 000–30 000 units/day for about 6 months. It is most frequently seen in pregnancy. The relative risk with LMW heparin is not yet established.

Hypersensitivity reactions and skin necrosis (similar to that seen with warfarin) occur but are rare. Transient alopecia has been ascribed to heparin but in fact may be due to the severity of the thromboembolic disease for which the drug was given.

Heparin antagonism. Heparin effects wear off so rapidly that an antagonist is seldom required except after extracorporeal perfusion for heart surgery. *Protamine,* a protein obtained from fish sperm, reverses the anticoagulant action of heparin, when antagonism is needed. It is as strongly basic as heparin is acidic, which explains its immediate action. Protamine sulphate, 1 mg by slow i.v. injection, neutralises about 100 units of heparin derived from mucosa (mucous) or 80 units of heparin from lung;

but if the heparin was given more than 15 min previously, the dose must be scaled down. Protamine itself has some anticoagulant effect and overdosage must be avoided. The maximum dose must not exceed 50 mg. Its effectiveness in patients treated with LMW heparins is unknown.

Heparinoids. Danaparinoid sodium is a mixture of several types of non-heparin glycosaminoglycans extracted from pig intestinal mucosa (84% heparan sulphate). It is an effective anticoagulant for the treatment of deep vein thrombosis (DVT) prophylaxis in high-risk patients and treatment of patients with heparin-associated thrombocytopenia.

USES OF ANTICOAGULANTS

Venous disease

Established venous thromboembolism. An anticoagulant is used to prevent extension of an existing thrombus while its size is reduced by natural thrombolytic activity. Effective anticoagulation prevents formation of fresh thrombus, which is more likely to detach and embolise, particularly if it is in large proximal veins; it also helps to recanalise veins and to clear vein valves of thrombus and should thus prevent long-term consequences such as swelling of the leg and stasis ulceration. The site and extent of thrombosis should be established by venous ultrasound. The majority of patients with proximal vein thrombosis or calf vein thrombosis can be treated with outpatient low molecular weight heparin, weight-adjusted and administered once or twice daily according to manufacturer's recommendations. It should be continued for a total of 4–7 days and until the signs of thrombosis (heat, swelling of the limb) have settled. Warfarin should be started at the same time as the heparin. Patients with a symptomatic pulmonary embolism should be treated in hospital with LMW heparin or high-dose intravenous unfractionated heparin (above).

In patients with an uncomplicated DVT following a precipitating event (e.g. orthopaedic surgery), warfarin may be necessary for only 6 weeks if the patient has returned to normal mobility and the precipitating factor(s) have been eliminated. The patient should wear a well-fitting compression stocking to increase flow in deep veins, should exercise the leg and should be encouraged to mobilise as soon as the discomfort has settled. The risk of recurrence reduces with passage of time after the initial event. In cases of DVT uncomplicated by pulmonary embolus, 3 months of anticoagulant therapy appears adequate. Where there is evidence of pulmonary embolus it is common practice to continue therapy for 6 to 12 months.

Thrombolytic therapy with streptokinase or urokinase i.v. may be used for life-threatening thrombosis, e.g. major pulmonary embolism with compromised haemodynamics (see p. 580).

Anticoagulant therapy may be life-saving in thromboembolic pulmonary hypertension.

Prevention of venous thrombosis. Oral anti-coagulant reduces the risk of thromboembolism in conditions in which there is special hazard, e.g. after surgery. Partly because of the danger of bleeding and partly because of the effort of maintaining control, oral anticoagulants have not been widely adopted. Numerous trials, however, have shown the protective effect of low doses of unfractionated heparin (5000 units every 8–12 h s.c.) and more recently LMW heparin (dose adjusted for body-weight and/or risk) against deep leg vein thrombosis. The significant fact is that it takes a lot less heparin to prevent thrombosis than it does to treat established thrombosis, because heparin acts in low concentration at an early stage in the cascade of coagulation factors which leads to fibrin formation (see above).

Low-dose unfractionated heparin or LMW heparin can be used to prevent venous thromboembolism in other high-risk patients, e.g. those confined to bed and immobilised with strokes, cardiac failure or malignant disease. Spontaneous bleeding has not been a problem with this form of anticoagulant treatment.

Low MW dextrans (see later).

Cardiovascular disease

Acute myocardial infarction. Anticoagulation with heparin is used to reduce the risk of venous thromboembolism, and the risk and size of emboli from mural thrombi following acute myocardial infarction.

Long-term anticoagulation with warfarin to prevent arterial thromboembolism should be considered for any patient who has a large left atrium or a low cardiac output or paroxysmal or established atrial fibrillation (with or without cardiac valvular disease). Where warfarin is considered unsuitable, aspirin may be substituted, for it prevents stroke in patients with atrial fibrillation, though less effectively. The combination of warfarin and aspirin, once regarded as contraindicated, may yet be most effective in patients at high risk of embolism. Heparin is given for 2 h to patients after undergoing angioplasty.

Heparin, aspirin or both are used to prevent myocardial infarction in the acute phase of unstable angina.

Peripheral arterial occlusion. Heparin may prevent extension of a thrombus and hasten its recanalisation; it is commonly used in the acute phase following thrombosis or embolism. There is no case for treating ischaemic peripheral vascular disease with an oral anticoagulant (for prevention, see Antiplatelet drugs).

Long-term anticoagulant prophylaxis

The decision to use warfarin long-term must take into account nondrug factors. The patient should be told of the risks of haemorrhage, including those introduced by taking other drugs, and of the signs of bleeding into the alimentary or urinary tracts. All patients should carry a card stating that they are receiving an oral anticoagulant. Such therapy should be withheld from a patient who is considered to be unlikely or unable to comply with the requirements of regular medication and blood testing. The incidence of haemorrhagic complications is directly related to the level of anticoagulation; safety and good results can be obtained only by close attention to detail. The INR should be monitored at a maximum interval of 8 weeks in patients on a stable maintenance dose and more frequently in patients with an unstable INR.

Surgery in patients receiving anticoagulant therapy

For *elective surgery* warfarin may be withdrawn about 5 days before the operation and resumed about 3 days later if conditions seem appropriate; heparin may be used in the intervening period. In patients with mechanical prosthetic valves, heparin is substituted at full dosage 4 days before surgery, and restarted 12–24 h after the operation. Warfarin is restarted when the patient resumes oral intake. *Emergency surgery:* proceed as for bleeding (p. 571). For *dental extractions:* omission of warfarin for 1–2 days to adjust the INR to the lower limit of the therapeutic range is adequate (INR should be tested just prior to the procedure). The usual dose of warfarin can be resumed the day after extraction.

Aspirin, taken prophylactically for thromboembolic disorders (see below), is commonly discontinued 2 weeks before elective procedures and restarted when oral intake permits.

Contraindications to anticoagulant therapy

Contraindications relate mostly to conditions in which there is a tendency to bleed, and are relative rather than absolute, the dangers being balanced against the possible benefits. They include:

- *Behavioural:* inability or unwillingness to cooperate, dependency on alcohol
- *Neurological:* stroke within 3 weeks, or surgery to the brain or eye
- *Alimentary:* active peptic ulcer, active inflammatory bowel disease, oesophageal varices, uncompensated hepatic cirrhosis
- *Cardiovascular:* severe uncontrolled hypertension
- *Renal:* if function is severely impaired
- *Pregnancy:* in early pregnancy the fetal warfarin syndrome is a hazard and bleeding may cause fetal death in late pregnancy
- *Haematological:* pre-existing bleeding disorder.

Emerging anticoagulant drugs

Recent strategies have sought to develop substances that act at different sites in the coagulation cascade and agents that inhibit thrombin, or prevent thrombin generation, or block initiation of the coagulation process or enhance endogenous anticoagulation have reached the clinical arena.

Novel delivery systems, using synthetic amino acids (e.g. SNAC) to facilitate absorption, allow the oral administration of unfractionated or LMW heparins sufficient to prolong the APTT. These are being evaluated.

Direct inhibitors of thrombin inactivate fibrin-bound thrombin which may promote thrombus extension (as opposed to heparin which acts indirectly through antithrombin) as follows:

Hirudin, a polypeptide originally isolated from the salivary glands of the medicinal leech *Hirudo medicalis,* is now produced by recombinant technology. It is a potent and specific inhibitor of thrombin with which it forms an almost irreversible complex. It is cleared predominantly by the kidneys and has a $t\frac{1}{2}$ of 40 minutes after i.v. administration. No antidote is available for a bleeding patient. It has been used successfully in patients with heparin-induced thrombocytopenia (HIT), thromboprophylaxis in elective hip arthroplasty, unstable angina and myocardial infarction.

Bivalirudin is a semisynthetic bivalent thrombin inhibitor which contains an analogue of the C-terminal of hirudin; this binds to thrombin but having a lower affinity, produces only transient inhibition and hence may be safer. It has been used in patients undergoing coronary angioplasty.

Argatroban, a carboxylic acid derivative, binds noncovalently to the active site of thrombin and is an effective alternative to heparin in patients with HIT.

Other highly selective agents in clinical development include blockers of:

factor IXa, an essential factor for amplification of the coagulation cascade (by active-site-blocked factor IXa or monoclonal antibodies against the factor),

the factor VIIa/tissue factor pathway, the initiating step of coagulation [with recombinant tissue factor pathway inhibitor (TFPI) the analogue of the natural inhibitor], and

factor X or factor Xa and inhibition of factor VIIa within the factor VIIa/tissue factor complex (by NAPc2, a recombinant nematode anticoagulant peptide).

Fibrinolytic (thrombolytic) system

The preservation of an intact vascular system requires not only that blood be capable of coagulating but also that there should be a mechanism for removing the products of coagulation when they have served their purpose of stopping a vascular leak. This is the function of the fibrinolytic system, the essential features of which are shown in Figure 28.2.

The system depends on the formation of the fibrinolytic enzyme *plasmin* from its precursor protein, *plasminogen,* in the blood. During the coagulation process, plasminogen binds to specific sites on fibrin. Simultaneously the natural activators of plasminogen, i.e. *tissue plasminogen activator* (tPA) and *urokinase,* are released from endothelial and other tissue cells and act on plasminogen to form plasmin. The result is that plasmin formation only takes place locally on the fibrin surface but not generally within the circulation where widespread defibrination would occur and the whole coagulation mechanism would be compromised. Since fibrin is the framework of the thrombus, its dissolution clears the clot away.

Fibrinolytics (thrombolytics) can remove established thrombi and emboli. Inhibitors of the fibrinolytic system *(antifibrinolytics)* can be of value in certain haemorrhagic states notably those characterised by excessive fibrinolysis.

DRUGS THAT PROMOTE FIBRINOLYSIS

An important application of fibrinolytic drugs has been to dissolve thrombi in acutely occluded coronary arteries, thereby to restore blood supply to ischaemic myocardium, to limit necrosis and to improve prognosis. The approach is to give a plasminogen activator intravenously by infusion or by bolus injection in order to increase the formation of the fibrinolytic enzyme plasmin. Those currently available include:

Streptokinase is a protein derived from β-haemolytic streptococci: it forms a complex with plasminogen (bound loosely to fibrin) where it converts plasminogen to plasmin. Too rapid administration causes abrupt fall in blood pressure. The $t_{\frac{1}{2}}$ is 20 min.

Anistreplase (anisoylated plasminogen streptokinase activator complex, APSAC), is the plasminogen-streptokinase complex (above) in which the enzyme centre that converts plasminogen to plasmin is protected from deactivation, so prolonging its action.

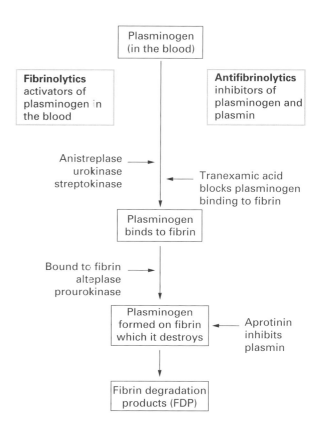

Fig. 28.2 Blood fibrinolytic system

The $t_{\frac{1}{2}}$ is 70 min. It is not available in some countries.

Urokinase made from human fetal kidney cells in tissue culture, is a direct activator of plasminogen. The $t_{\frac{1}{2}}$ is 15 min.

Streptokinase, anistreplase and urokinase are not well absorbed by fibrin thrombi and are called *non-fibrin-selective.* They convert plasminogen to plasmin in the circulation, which depletes plasma fibrinogen and induces a general hypocoagulant state. This does not reduce their local thrombolytic potential but increases the risk of bleeding.

Recombinant prourokinase, as the name suggests, is produced by recombinant DNA technology; on binding to fibrin it converts to urokinase. The $t_{\frac{1}{2}}$ is 7 min.

Alteplase (rt-PA) ($t_{\frac{1}{2}}$ 5 min) is tissue type plasminogen activator produced by recombinant

DNA technology. *Reteplase* (t$\frac{1}{2}$ 15 min) is another recombinant human protein.

Recombinant prourokinase and alteplase are termed *fibrin-selective*, for they bind strongly to fibrin, and are capable of dissolving aging or lysis-resistant thrombi better than nonfibrin-selective agents. These drugs are less likely to produce a coagulation disturbance in the plasma, i.e. they are selective for thrombi.

USES OF THROMBOLYTIC DRUGS

Coronary artery thrombolysis

(See also Ch. 23)

Timing of administration. The earlier thrombolysis is given the better the outcome. Treatment commencing within the first 3 h of onset is a realistic aim but thrombolysis up to 12 h is still worthwhile. Benefit is most striking in patients with anterior myocardial infarction treated within 4 h of onset.

Anistreplase can be given i.v. over 4–5 min (and so more easily out of hospital); its effect persists for 6–9 h. Other agents are normally infused i.v. over 1–3 h with most of the dose being given early in that period. Retelpase is given as a double bolus 30 min apart.

Reduction in mortality (see also Myocardial infarction, p. 485). There is now compelling evidence that streptokinase, anistreplase, alteplase and retelpase reduce mortality with an acceptable frequency of adverse effects.[14] Comparisons between these drugs show no apparent survival advantage of one over the others in respect of survival.[15,16] Both streptokinase and t-PA decrease mortality by about 25% when used alone but by 40–50% when either agent is used with aspirin[17] which reduces the incidence of re-infarction. Those under 75 years appeared to gain most from thrombus dispersal but 'physiological' age is more important than chronological age.

Stroke may complicate myocardial infarction and is considered usually to be embolic, for its incidence correlates with the extent of myocardial infarction. Evidence[18] indicates that the combination of thrombolysis plus aspirin lowers the overall risk of stroke, possibly by limiting the size of the infarct,

or by reducing thromboembolic episodes, or by both.

Thrombolysis may also be valuable in persistent unstable angina and especially where arteriography demonstrates substantial thrombus in coronary arteries.

Adverse effects. *Bleeding* is the most important complication and usually occurs at a vascular lesion, e.g. the site of injection, for fibrinolytic therapy does not distinguish between an undesired thrombus and a useful haemostatic plug. If the contraindications are followed, the incidence of bleeding severe enough to require transfusion is < 1%. Nausea and vomiting may occur.

Multiple microemboli from disintegration of pre-existing thrombus anywhere in the vascular system may endanger life; these commonly originate in an enlarged left atrium, or a ventricular or aortic aneurysm.

Cardiac arrhythmias result from reperfusion of ischaemic tissue. These vary in type and are often transient, a factor which may influence the decision whether or not to treat.

Allergy. Streptokinase and anistreplase are antigenic and anaphylactic reactions with rash, urticaria and hypotension may occur for most people have circulating antibodies to streptococci. Antibodies persist after exposure to these drugs and their re-use should be avoided between 5 days and 12 months as the recommended dose may not overcome immune resistance to plasminogen activation.

Contraindications to thrombolytic drug use (see Myocardial infarction, p. 485).

Noncoronary thrombolysis

Pulmonary embolism. Thrombolysis is superior to heparin at relieving obstructed veins demonstrated radiologically. While a reduction in mortality is thus implied, the numbers of cases reported in clinical trials of thrombolytics have been insufficient to

---

[14] Carins J A et al 1992 Chest 102 (Suppl): 482S–507S.

[15] The International Study Group 1990 Lancet 336: 71–75.

[16] ISIS-3 Collaborative Group 1992 Lancet 339: 753–770.

[17] Carins J A et al 1998 Chest 114: 634S–657S

[18] ISIS-2 Collaborative Group 1988 Lancet 2: 349–360.

provide conclusive statistical proof. There is, nevertheless, a strong impression that thrombolysis is beneficial where pulmonary embolism is accompanied by signs of haemodynamic decompensation (raised jugular venous pressure, pulse rate > 100 beats/min, systolic pressure < 100 mmHg, arterial oxygen desaturation). Alteplase 100 mg may be infused over 2 h, followed by an i.v. infusion of heparin.

Deep vein thrombosis. Thrombolysis may be justified where the affected vessels are proximal and the risk of pulmonary embolism is high. Complete lysis may be achieved in 50% of cases treated within 7 days of onset.

Arterial occlusion Systemic or local thrombolysis may be considered for arterial occlusions distal to the popliteal artery (thrombectomy being the usual therapeutic approach for occlusion of < 24 h duration proximal to this site). Intravenous streptokinase will lyse 80% of occlusions if infusion begins within 12 h, and 60% if it is delayed for up to 3 days.

Ischaemic stroke. There is little evidence of benefit and most trials have shown increased short-term mortality in patients treated with thrombolysis.

Thrombolysis may also be considered for ocular thrombosis (urokinase) and for thrombosed arteriovenous shunts (streptokinase).

DRUGS THAT PREVENT FIBRINOLYSIS

Antifibrinolytics are useful in a number of bleeding disorders.

Tranexamic acid competitively inhibits the binding of plasminogen and t-PA to fibrin and effectively blocks conversion of plasminogen to plasmin (which causes dissolution of fibrin); fibrinolysis is thus retarded. After an i.v. bolus injection it is excreted largely unchanged in the urine; the $t\frac{1}{2}$ is 1.5 h. It may also be administered orally or topically.

The principal indication for tranexamic acid is to prevent the hyperplasminaemic bleeding state that results from damage to certain tissues rich in plasminogen activator, e.g. after prostatic surgery, tonsillectomy, uterine cervical conisation, and

menorrhagia, whether primary or induced by an intrauterine contraceptive device. Tranexamic acid may also reduce bleeding after ocular trauma and in haemophiliacs after dental extraction where it is normally used in combination with desmopressin. The drug benefits some patients with hereditary angioedema presumably by preventing the plasmin-induced uncontrolled activation of the complement system which characterises that condition. Tranexamic acid may be of value in thrombocytopenia (idiopathic or following cytotoxic chemotherapy) to reduce the risk of haemorrhage by inhibiting natural fibrinolytic destabilisation of small platelet plugs; the requirement for platelet transfusion is thereby reduced. It may also be used for overdose with thrombolytic agents.

Adverse effects are rare but include nausea, diarrhoea and sometimes orthostatic hypotension. It is contraindicated in patients with haematuria as it will prevent clot lysis in the urinary tract and result in 'clot colic'.

Aprotinin is a naturally-occurring inhibitor of plasmin and other proteolytic enzymes which has been used to limit bleeding following open heart surgery with extracorporeal circulation, and for the treatment of life-threatening haemorrhage due to hyperplasminaemia complicating surgery of malignant tumours or thrombolytic therapy or in Jehovah's witnesses.[19] It must be administered intravenously or topically.

Platelets

Platelets support haemostasis in three ways: first by sticking to exposed collagen to form a physical barrier at the site of vessel injury; second by accelerating the activation of coagulation proteins and finally by release of storage granule contents promotes vasoconstriction and wound healing.

SOME PHYSIOLOGY

Circulating 'resting' platelets do not stick to healthy endothelium or each other but if a vessel wall is

---

[19] A religious sect that is opposed to blood transfusion on a scriptural basis.

breached they react at the site by four steps: attachment, spreading, secretion and aggregation.

1. Exposure of constituents of the subendothelial matrix most notably collagen initiates platelet attachment which is stabilised by von Willebrand factor.

2. Shape change of the attached platelets, spreading along the fibrils permits multiple tight contacts with the matrix and there is simultaneous release of *thromboxane-A₂* (TXA₂) and *adenosine diphosphate* (ADP) which recruit additional platelets.

3. Agonists in the microenvironment also trigger secretion of the contents of intracellular storage granules which activate circulating platelets and vasoconstriction (including proteins, enzymes, enzyme inhibitors, vasoactive and other peptides and agents that participate in the coagulation process) and translocation of negatively charged phospholipids to the outer surface of the plasma membrane providing a binding site for coagulation proteins (an activity known as 'platelet factor 3').

4. These platelets interact with each other and aggregate through binding of fibrinogen or fibrin to the surface through *glycoprotein (GP) IIb/IIIa* (integrin $\alpha_{IIb}\beta_3$) to form an effective plug to seal the injured vessel which is stabilised by cross linked fibrin

The system that enables platelets to distinguish between healthy and damaged endothelium is shown in simplified form in Figure 28.3. It is a continuation of, and should be studied in conjunction with, the general diagram for eicosanoids on page 281.

Platelet mechanisms

The mechanism which transforms a freely circulating resting platelet (surrounded by fibrinogen and buffeted in the circulation) into an adherent platelet has been a frequent target for drug development. Platelet aggregation does not occur as long as the resting conformation of GP IIb/IIIa is maintained and several external and internal factors dampen activation signals.

1. Cyclic AMP plays a key role. High concentrations of intraplatelet cyclic AMP inhibit platelet adhesion, aggregation and the release of active substances (see above), and low concentrations of cyclic AMP have the opposite effect.

2. The quantity of cyclic AMP within platelets is under enzymatic control, for it is formed by the action of adenylate cyclase and degraded by phosphodiesterase.

3. Platelet adenylate cyclase formation in turn is stimulated by prostacyclin (from the endothelium, also called PGI₂) and inhibited by thromboxane-A₂ (from within platelets, also called TXA₂). Hence the action of thromboxane-A₂ lowers cyclic AMP concentration and promotes platelet adhesion; prostacyclin raises cyclic AMP concentration and prevents platelet adhesion.

4. Prostacyclin and thromboxane-A₂ are derived from arachidonic acid which is a constituent of cell walls, both platelet and endothelial. Cyclo-oxygenase (COX, PGH synthase), an enzyme present in cells at both sites, converts arachidonic acid to cyclic endoperoxides which are further metabolised by prostacyclin synthase to prostacyclin in the endothelium and by thromboxane synthase to thromboxane-A₂ in platelets. Thus prostacyclin is principally

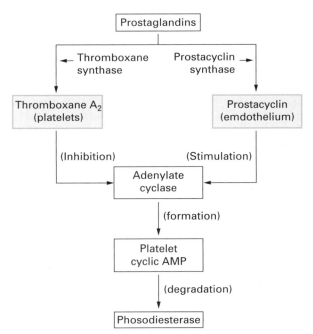

Fig. 28.3 Prostacyclin, thromboxane and the formation of platelet cyclic AMP

formed in the endothelium whereas thromboxane-A_2 is formed mainly in platelets.

5. These differences in the prostaglandins synthesised in endothelium and platelets are important. Intact vascular endothelium does not activate platelets because of the high concentration of prostacyclin in the intima. Subintimal tissues contain little prostacyclin and platelets, under the influence of thromboxane-A_2, immediately adhere and aggregate at any breach in the intima. Atheromatous plaques do not generate prostacyclin—which explains platelet adhesion and thrombosis at these sites.

6. Endothelial cells also produce nitric oxide which raises cyclic GMP levels in platelets to inhibit activation and have on their surface ecto-ADPase (CD39) that metabolises secreted ADP before it can cause platelet activation.

Inhibitors or activators of platelet aggregation act directly or indirectly by altering the rate of formation or degradation of platelet cyclic AMP. Local concentrations of these substances determine whether the platelet adhesion/aggregation process will occur.

DRUGS THAT INHIBIT PLATELET ACTIVITY (ANTIPLATELET DRUGS)

(See also Myocardial infarction Ch. 23)

Aspirin (acetylsalicylic acid) acetylates and thus inactivates COX, the enzyme responsible for the first step in the formation of prostaglandins, the conversion of arachidonic acid to prostaglandin H_2. It follows from the diagram on page 281 (Fig. 15.1) that aspirin can prevent formation of both thromboxane-A_2 (TXA$_2$) and prostacyclin (PGI$_2$). Acylation of COX is irreversible and, as the platelet is unable to synthesise new enzyme, COX activity is irreversibly lost for its lifetime (8–10 d). Therapeutic interest in the antithrombotic effect of aspirin has centred on separating its actions on thromboxane-A_2 and prostacyclin formation, and this can be achieved by using a *low dose*. Thus 75–100 mg/d by mouth is sufficient to abolish synthesis of thromboxane-A_2 without significant impairment of prostacyclin formation, i.e. amounts substantially below the 2.4 g/d used to control pain and inflammation. Low-dose aspirin is yet not without risk:

some 13% of episodes of peptic ulcer bleeds in people over 60 years can be attributed to prophylactic asprin (use in the community about 8%).[20]

Dipyridamole reversibly inhibits platelet phosphodiesterase (see Fig. 28.3) and in consequence cyclic AMP concentration is increased and platelet (thrombotic) reactivity reduced; evidence also suggests that its antithrombotic effect may derive from release of prostaglandin precursors by vascular endothelium. Dipyridamole is extensively bound to plasma proteins and has a $t_{1/2}$ of 12 h.

Ticlopidine is a thienopyridine derivative that inhibits ADP-dependent platelet aggregation. It is converted to its active form by metabolism by the liver and the $t_{1/2}$ of the parent drug is 40 h. Ticlopidine is more effective than aspirin in reducing stroke in patients with transient ischaemic attacks (TIA) but aspirin is safer and less expensive. It is also effective in reducing the risk of the combined outcome of stroke, myocardial infarction (MI) or vascular death in patients with thrombo-embolic stroke, decreasing vascular death and MI in patients with unstable angina, reducing acute occlusion of coronary bypass grafts and improving walking distance and decreasing vascular complications in patients with peripheral vascular disease. It may be used to prevent stroke in patients who are intolerant of aspirin. Neutropenia is the most serious adverse effect (risk 2.4%) and is greatest in the first 12 weeks of therapy; leucocyte counts should be checked every 2 weeks during this period. Diarrhoea and other gastrointestinal symptoms may be induced in a third of patients.

Clopidogrel is also a thienopyridine derivative which is also more effective than aspirin for the prevention of ischaemic stroke, MI or vascular death in patients at high risk but it is not associated with neutropenia. It is more expensive than aspirin though safer than ticlodipine.

Epoprostenol (prostacyclin) may be given to prevent platelet loss during renal dialysis, with or without heparin; it is infused i.v. and s.c ($t_{1/2}$ 3 min). It is a potent vasodilator.

---

[20] Weil J et al 1995 Prophylactic aspirin and risk of peptic ulcer bleeding. British Medical Journal 310: 827–830.

Glycoprotein (GP) IIb-IIIa antagonists. The platelet glycoprotein IIb-IIIa complex is the predominant platelet integrin,[21] a molecule restricted to mega-karyocytes and platelets which mediates platelet aggregation via the binding of adhesive proteins such as fibrinogen and von Willebrand factor (vWF). Where there is hereditary absence of the GP IIb-IIIa complex (Glanzmann's thrombasthenia) platelets are incapable of aggregation by all physiological agonists. GP IIb-IIIa antagonists have been developed as antiplatelet agents and administered intravenously, they inhibit the *final common pathway* of platelet aggregation: binding of fibrinogen or vWF to the GP IIb-IIIa complex. They are more complete inhibitors than either aspirin or clopidogrel which inhibit only the cyclo-oxygenase or ADP pathway respectively. GP IIb-IIIa antagonists also have an anticoagulant effect through inhibition of prothrombin binding to the complex and inhibition of procoagulant platelet-derived microparticle formation. Platelet aggregation is inhibited in a dose-dependent manner.

Abciximab is a human-murine chimeric monoclonal antibody Fab fragment that binds to the GP IIb-IIIa complex with high affinity and slow dissociation rate. After i.v. administration it is cleared rapidly from plasma (t$\frac{1}{2}$ 20 min). Abciximab (0.25 mg/kg bolus then 0.125 microgram/kg/min infusion for 12 h) produces immediate and profound inhibition of platelet activity that lasts for 12–36 h after termination of the infusion. This reduces the risk of death, MI or need for urgent coronary artery bypass grafting after percutaneous coronary angioplasty and benefit is maintained up to 3 years. The dose causes and maintains blockade of > 80% receptors, causing > 80% reduction in aggregation. Patients also receive aspirin and heparin and if a coronary stent has been inserted, either clopidogrel or ticlodipine. Abciximab is also effective in refractory unstable angina prior to percutaneous coronary intervention. It has a potential role in combination with low dose thrombolysis in acute myocardial infarction and as a single agent in stroke.

Eptifibatide is a cyclic heptapeptide based upon the Lys-Gly-Asp sequence. *Tirofiban* and *lamifiban* are nonpeptide mimetics. All three are competitive inhibitors of the GPIIb-IIIa complex with lower affinities and higher dissociation rates than abciximab and short plasma t$\frac{1}{2}$ (2–2.5 h). Platelet aggregation returns to normal 30 min to 4 h after discontinuation. Eptifibatide and tirofiban are effective in acute coronary syndromes. Lamifiban is undergoing clinical development.

Adverse effects. Haemorrhage occurs but is less of a problem with low doses of heparin; it remains a particular risk in patients treated after failed fibrinolytic therapy for acute myocardial infarction. Platelet transfusion after cessation of abciximab is necessary for refractory or life threatening bleeding. After transfusion, the antibody redistributes to the transfused platelets, reduces the mean level of receptor blockade and improves platelet function. Thrombocytopenia may occur from 1 hour to days after commencing treatment in up to 1% of patients. This necessitates platelet counts at 2–4 hours and then daily; if severe, therapy must be stopped and, if necessary, platelets transfused. EDTA-induced pseudothrombocytopenia has been reported and a low platelet count should prompt examination of a blood film for agglutination before therapy is stopped.

Other drugs

Dazoxiben, an inhibitor of thromboxane-A$_2$ but not of prostacyclin synthesis, is being evaluated in cardiovascular disease.

Dextrans, particularly of MW 70 000 (dextran 70), alter platelet function and prolong the bleeding time. Dextrans differ from the other antiplatelet drugs which tend to be used for arterial thrombosis; dextran 70 reduces the incidence of postoperative venous thromboembolism if it is given during or just after surgery. The dose should not exceed 10% of the estimated blood volume. They are rarely used.

USES OF ANTIPLATELET DRUGS

Antiplatelet therapy protects 'at risk' patients against stroke, myocardial infarction or death. A meta-analysis of 145 clinical trials of prolonged

---

[21] Integrins are cell surface adhesion receptors consisting of non-covalently associated alpha- and beta- subunits, now redesignated integrin $\alpha_{IIb}\beta_3$.

antiplatelet therapy versus control and 29 trials between antiplatelet regimens found that the chance of nonfatal myocardial infarction and nonfatal stroke were reduced by one-third, and that there was a one-sixth reduction in the risk of death from any vascular cause.[22] Expressed in another way, in the first month after an acute myocardial infarction (a vulnerable period) aspirin prevents death, stroke or a further heart attack in about 4 patients for every 100 treated. Aspirin is by far the most commonly used antiplatelet agent. The optimum dose is not certain but one not exceeding aspirin 325 mg is acceptable, and 75–100 mg/d may be as effective and preferred where there is gastric intolerance. Aspirin alone (mainly) or aspirin plus dipyridamole greatly reduced the risk of occlusion where vascular grafts or arterial patency was studied systematically.[23]

Many patients who take aspirin for vascular disease may also require an NSAID for, e.g. joint disease, and it may be argued that the NSAID renders aspirin unnecessary as both act by inhibition of prostaglandin G/H synthase. As inhibition by aspirin is *irreversible* and that by NSAIDs may not be, continued use of aspirin in such circumstances seems prudent, especially if NSAID use is intermittent.

Haemostatics

Etamsylate (Dicynene) is given systemically to reduce capillary bleeding, e.g. in menorrhagia.

Adrenaline (epinephrine) may be useful for epistaxis, stopping haemorrhage by local vaso-constriction when applied by packing the nostril with ribbon gauze soaked in adrenaline solution.

Fibrin glue consists of fibrinogen and thrombin contained in two syringes, the tips of which form a common port. The two components are thus delivered in equal volumes to a bleeding point where fibrinogen is converted to fibrin at a rate determined by the concentration of thrombin. Fibrin glue can be used to secure surgical haemostasis, e.g. on a large raw surface, and to prevent external oozing of blood in patients with haemophilia (see also below).

Summary

- Myocardial infarction. Aspirin should be given indefinitely to patients who have survived myocardial infarction. There is as yet no case for using aspirin to prevent myocardial infarction in those without important risk factors for the disease.
- Transient ischaemic attacks (TIAs) or minor ischaemic stroke. There is grave risk of progression to completed stroke and patients should receive aspirin indefinitely. Before starting treatment it is important to exclude intracerebral haemorrhage (by computed tomography) and other conditions that mimic TIAs, e.g. cardiac arrhythmia, migraine, focal epilepsy and hypoglycaemia.
- Unstable angina. The chance of myocardial infarction is high and aspirin should be used with other drugs, i.e. a β-adrenoceptor antagonist, a nitrate, a calcium channel blocker and possibly heparin i.v. as is judged appropriate.
- Arterial grafts, peripheral vascular disease. Aspirin (possibly combined with dipyridamole for grafts) should be given to prevent occlusion. These drugs may also be used to protect against thrombotic occlusion following percutaneous transluminal coronary angioplasty.
- Inhibitors of ADP-dependent platelet aggregation, e.g. ticlopidine, clopidorgrel, and glycoprotein IIb-IIIa antagomists, e.g. abciximab, can be expected to form part of regimens for cardiovascular disease, as evidence accumulates.

Sclerosing agents. Chemicals may be used to cause inflammation and thrombosis in veins so as to induce permanent obliteration, e.g. ethanolamine oleate injection, sodium tetradecyl sulphate (given i.v. for varicose veins) and oily phenol injection (given submucously for haemorrhoids). Local reactions, tissue necrosis and embolus can occur.

Haemophilia

Management of the haemophilia A and haemophilia B (genetic deficiencies of factor VIII or IX) is a matter for those with special expertise but the following points are of general interest.

- Haemorrhage can sometimes be stopped by pressure; edges of superficial wounds should be strapped, not stitched.
- Minor bleeding can be stopped with plasma factor levels of 25–30% but severe bleeding requires a level of at least 50% and surgical

---

[22] Antiplatelet Trialists' Collaboration 1994 British Medical Journal 308: 81.
[23] Antiplatelet Trialists' Collaboration 1994 British Medical Journal 308: 159.

procedures or life-threatening haemorrhage require targets of 75–100%.

- In haemophilia A antihaemophilic globulin (factor VIII) concentrate ($t\frac{1}{2}$ 8–12 h) should be used for bleeding that is more than minor. Administration of each unit of factor VIII per kg body weight raises the plasma level by 2%. Repeat dosing 2–3 times daily is necessary to maintain levels.
- Factor VIII is available as ultrapure recombinant product, ultrapure plasma-derived product, high purity plasma-derived product and intermediate purity plasma-derived product.
- Factor IX ($t\frac{1}{2}$ 18–24 h) should be used for bleeding that is more than minor in haemophilia B (Christmas disease). Administration of each unit of factor IX per kg body weight raises the plasma level by 1%. Maintenance doses are required every 18–24 h.
- Factor IX is available as ultrapure recombinant product, high purity plasma derived product and low purity plasma-derived product.
- Duration of therapy is determined by speed of recovery of the affected joint or resolution of a haematoma. After surgery at least 10–14 days of replacement therapy is required to ensure adequate wound healing and scar formation.
- Recombinant factor VIII or IX concentrates are recommended for all previously untreated patients, those who have been previously treated but remain hepatitis C virus or HIV seronegative, and for mild to moderate severity disease when desmopressin is not sufficient.
- Primary prophylaxis with factor VIII three times weekly or factor IX concentrate twice weekly at doses to keep the factor level above 1–2% beginning in toddlers (through an indwelling venous cannula) results in a significant reduction in spontaneous bleeds and arthropathy.
- Tranexamic acid helps stabilise thrombi in both diseases.
- For patients with high titre factor VIII inhibitors, standard factor IX complex products are first-line therapy but activated factor IX complex concentrates may be necessary for continued, more frequent or more severe bleeding. Porcine factor VIII or recombinant human factor VIIa may be necessary for major bleeds or elective surgery.

The cloning of the factor VIII gene and development of retroviral-vector delivery systems have raised the possibility that the defect in haemophilia A may be corrected by gene therapy. In a sense this is already a reality; patients with haemophilia A who underwent liver transplantation for progressive hepatic disease were found to be producing haemostatic concentrations of factor VIII.

Von Willebrand's disease

Patients with type 2B or severe type 3 von Willebrand's disease, those with severe haemorrhage or patients who require major surgery, need replacement therapy with intermediate purity plasma-derived factor VIII concentrate known to have high molecular weight von Willebrand factor (vWF) multimers.[24] The larger multimers are required for normal biological function. In type 2A and 2B von Willebrand's disease large multimers are absent in plasma, in type 3 von Willebrand's disease all multimers are absent. This is preferred to cryoprecipitate which is rich in vWF but has not undergone any viral inactivation process.

Desmopressin (DDAVP) (see p. 712) 0.3–0.4 micrograms/kg body weight i.v. (also available in a concentrated intranasal form) increases factor VIII and von Willebrand factor levels by 3–5 times baseline in mild to moderate haemophilia A; its use may render transfusion unnecessary after minor procedures such as dental extraction. It is also effective in mild to moderate type 1 von Willebrand's disease for which DDAVP offers nontransfusional treatment. Tachyphylaxis occurs with repeated dosage but stores are repleted after an interval of 2–4 days. Patients with severe deficiency of either factor and patients with any form of haemophilia B do not respond to DDAVP. Adverse effects include flushing, headache, tachycardia, mild hypertension and hyponatraemia.

Homocysteine and vascular disease

High plasma concentrations of homocysteine are associated with increased risk of thrombotic vascular

---

[24] von Willebrands factor is a glycoprotein molecule of 2050 residues which is assembled into multimers (polymers).

events. The association is now known to be causal, strong and directly related. Severe hyperhomocysteinaemia accompanies inherited deficiency of enzymes that metabolise homocysteine, e.g. classical homocystinuria, but lesser degrees have other causes, including nutritional B vitamin deficiency. The normal plasma homocysteine it taken to be 5–15 micromol/l and higher values are associated with thrombotic risk. The high plasma homocysteine of patients with classical homocystinuria responds to treatment with folic acid, vitamin B_{12} and vitamin B_6 (pyridoxine). Clinical trials now in progress will establish whether multivitamin therapy will become a treatment option for patients with mild or moderate hyperhomocysteinaemia, and thrombotic vascular disease.

GUIDE TO FURTHER READING

Atrah H I 1994 Fibrin glue. British Medical Journal 308: 933–934

Antithrombotic Trialists' Collaboration 2002 Collaborative meta-analysis of randomised trials of antiplatelet therapy for prevention of death, myocardial infarction and stroke in high risk patients. British Medical Journal 324: 71–86

Dahlbäck B 2000 Blood coagulation Lancet 355: 1627–1632

Goldhaber S Z 1998 Pulmonary embolism. New England Journal of Medicine 339: 93–104

George J N 2000 Platelets. Lancet 353: 1531–1539

Greaves M 1999 Antiphospholipid antibodies and thrombosis. Lancet 353: 1348–1353

Greer I A 1999 Thrombosis in pregnancy; maternal and fetal issues. Lancet 353: 1258–1265

Hankey G J, Eikelboom J W 1999 Homocysteine and vascular disease. Lancet 354: 407–413

Hardman S M C, Cowie M R 1999 Anticoagulation in heart disease. British Medical Journal 318: 238–244

Lensing A W A et al 1999 Deep-vein thrombosis. Lancet 353: 479–485

Levi M, ten Cate H 1999 Disseminated intravascular coagulation. New England Journal of Medicine 341: 586–592

Mannucci P M 1998 Hemostatic drugs. New England Journal of Medicine 339: 245–253

Mannucci P M, Tuddenham E G D 2001 The haemophilias—from royal genes to gene therapy. New England Journal of Medicine 344: 1773–1779

Scurr J H et al 2001 Frequency and prevention of symptomless deep-vein thrombosis in long-haul flights: a randomised trial. Lancet 357: 1485–1489

Seligsohn U, Lubetski A 2001 Genetic susceptibility to venous thrombosis. New England Journal of Medicine 344: 1222–1231

Shearer M J 1995 Vitamin K. Lancet 345: 229–234

Topol E J, Byzova T V, Plow E F 1999 Platelet GP11b-111a blockers. Lancet 353: 227–231

Vandenbroucke J P et al 2001 Oral contraceptives and the risk of venous thrombosis. New England Journal of Medicine 344: 1527–1535

Weitz J I 1997 Low-molecular-weight heparins. New England Journal of Medicine 337: 688–698

29

Cellular disorders and anaemias

SYNOPSIS

Rational use of haematinic drugs is essential to the correction of anaemia in its various forms. The emergence of haemopoietic growth factors as drugs that stimulate erythroid or myeloid cell lines has opened the way to successful management of other forms of haematological disease.

- Iron: therapy, acute overdose
- Vitamin B$_{12}$ (cobalamins)
- Folic acid
- Haemopoietic growth factors
- Sickle cell anaemia
- Polycythaemia rubra vera
- Aplastic anaemia

Leukaemias and lymphomas: see Chapter 30

Iron

Iron, which was the metal symbolising strength in magical systems, used to be given to people suffering from weakness, and no doubt many were benefited, some psychologically (placebo reactors) and others because the weakness was due to iron deficiency anaemia. The rational use of iron could not begin until both the presence of iron in the 'colouring matter' of the blood and the 'defective nature of the colouring matter' in anaemia were recognised. In fact iron is essential not only to oxygen transport by red cells but as a catalyst for oxidative metabolism in all cells.

Some facts and figures

- Total body iron is 3–5 g (40–50 mg/kg) (male > female).
- Haemoglobin contains about two-thirds of total body iron.
- Stores comprise about one-third (*ferritin*, a water-soluble protein-iron complex, and *haemosiderin*, an insoluble aggregate) in liver, marrow, spleen and muscle.
- 5–10% is present in tissues throughout the body in myoglobin, a variety of heme enzymes (e.g. cytochromes) and non-haem enzymes (e.g. metalloflavoproteins)
- Average Western diet contains 10–15 mg iron/day.
- Normal human absorbs 5–10% dietary iron, i.e. 0.5–1.0 mg/d, which is adequate for an adult male or postmenopausal female but the menstruating or pregnant woman requires 1–3 mg/d.
- Iron deficient or pregnant woman absorbs about 30% of dietary iron.
- Iron is lost from the body mainly in desquamated skin and gut cells and the daily loss in men is under 1 mg/day, in normal menstruating females 1.5 mg/day and in pregnancy averages 2 mg/day.
- Menstrual loss is about 30 mg/period; menstruating women may therefore be in negative iron balance.

IRON KINETICS

Iron absorption takes place predominantly in the duodenum where the acid environment enhances solubility, but also throughout the gut, allowing sustained-release preparations to be used. Most iron in food is present as ferric hydroxide, ferric-protein complexes or haem-protein complexes. Ferrous (Fe^{++}) iron is more readily absorbed than ferric (Fe^{+++}). Thus the simultaneous ingestion of a reducing agent, such as ascorbic acid, increases the amount of the ferrous form; ascorbic acid 50 mg increases iron absorption from a meal by 2–3 times. Food reduces iron absorption due to inhibition by phytates, tannates and phosphates.

Iron balance is determined by the difference between iron absorption and iron loss. Humans lack a mechanism to excrete excess iron and physiological control of iron balance is achieved by *regulation of absorption*. There is a reciprocal relationship between stores and absorption so that, as stores decline absorption increases and vice versa.

The mucosal cells of the proximal small bowel regulate iron absorption. Dietary and administered iron is actively transported into the gut mucosal cell, probably involving a protein DMT1 though the precise details have not been established. Two other proteins, hephaestin and ferroportin 1, appear to be involved in intracellular transport and release into the plasma respectively. *Regulation of absorption* may involve one or more of: (1) control of mucosal uptake; (2) retention of iron in storage form in the mucosal cell and (3) transfer from the mucosal cell to the plasma. Increased erythropoietic activity also stimulates increased absorption. Iron that is not needed by the body may be bound to a protein (apoferritin) as *ferritin* and lost into the gut lumen when the mucosal cell is shed (2–3 days). Iron is eliminated at a near constant rate in the faeces of healthy people.

Iron that is required by the body forms a labile pool within the cell; if this pool is excessive it may stimulate production of more apoferritin in the mucosal cells to bind and lose more iron as ferritin when the cell is shed. Labile pool iron in the Fe^{+++} form enters the plasma bound to a transport globulin, *transferrin*, which delivers it to the sites of physiological need, principally erythrocyte precursors where it is used to form haem. The major pathway of internal iron exchange is a unidirectional flow from plasma *transferrin* to the *erythron* (defined as all red cell elements at any stage of maturity), to the *macrophage* and back to plasma *transferrin*. Over 80% of the iron passing through the transferrin compartment each day is flowing to and from the erythron. Immature red cells acquire iron from transferrin through a specific transferrin receptor located on the cell membrane. Within cells the iron regulatory proteins IRP-1 and IRP-2 control iron availability by translational control of the synthesis of transferrin receptor (increasing uptake) and of ferritin (increasing storage).

There is a small amount of ferritin in the blood in balance with the iron stores. Iron is stored as ferritin (which sequesters iron in a nontoxic but readily mobilised form) and its aggregate, *haemosiderin*, in the cells of the liver, bone marrow and spleen. A measure of the state of iron stores is provided by the amount of ferritin in the serum (normally 20–300 mmol/l) and by the relationship of serum iron concentration (normally 10–30 mmol/l; reduced in iron deficiency) to the binding capacity of transferrin (normally 45–70 mmol/l; increased in iron deficiency). Ferritin is an acute-phase reactant and may be an inaccurate measure of iron stores in inflammatory states, e.g. rheumatoid arthritis. Recently developed techniques to measure the plasma level of soluble transferrin receptor (which is increased in iron deficiency but not by infection or inflammation) may help differentiate the anaemia of iron deficiency from that of chronic disease.

Prolonged heavy excess of iron intake overwhelms the mechanism described and results in haemosiderosis, as there is no physiological mechanism to increase iron excretion in the face of increased absorption. Iron-deficient subjects absorb up to 20 times as much administered iron as those with normal stores. Abnormalities of the small intestine may interfere with either the absorption of iron, as in coeliac disease and other malabsorption syndromes, or possibly with the conversion of iron into a soluble and reduced form, e.g. following loss of acid secretion after a partial gastrectomy.

The formation of insoluble iron salts (such as phosphate and phytate) in the alkaline environment of most of the small intestine explains why much of the iron taken by mouth is not absorbed, even in severe iron deficiency.

Interactions. Iron chelates in the gut with tetracyclines, penicillamine, methyldopa, levodopa, carbidopa, ciprofloxacin, norfloxacin and ofloxacin; it also forms stable complexes with thyroxine, captopril and biphosphonates. These interactions can be clinically important. Ingestion should be separated by 3 hours.

Ascorbic acid increases absorption (see above) but its use (200 mg/day) is not clinically important in routine therapy; desferrioxamine binds iron and reduces absorption (see Poisoning, below); tea (tannins) and bran reduce absorption.

IRON THERAPY

Iron therapy is indicated only for the prevention or cure of iron deficiency. In general terms, making 25 mg of iron per day available to the bone marrow will allow an iron deficiency anaemia to respond with a rise of 1% of haemoglobin (0.15 g Hb/100 ml) per day; a reticulocyte response occurs between 4 and 12 days. An increase in the haemoglobin of at least 2 g/dl after 3 weeks of therapy is a reasonable criterion of an adequate response. Oral preparations are the treatment of choice for almost all patients due to their effectiveness, safety and low cost. Parenteral preparations should be restricted to the few patients unable to absorb or tolerate oral preparations. Red cell transfusion is necessary only in patients with severe symptomatic anaemia or where chronic blood loss exceeds the possible rate of oral or parenteral replacement.

Oral iron therapy. The goal of iron therapy is to repair the haemoglobin deficit and replenish storage iron. When oral therapy is used it is reasonable to assume that about 30% of the iron will be absorbed and to give 180 mg of elemental iron daily for 1–3 months according to the degree of anaemia. Iron stores are less easily replenished by oral therapy than by injection, and oral therapy (at lower dose) should be continued for 3–6 months after the haemoglobin concentration has returned to normal or until the serum ferritin exceeds 50 microgram/l (or as long as blood loss continues).

Contraindications. It is illogical to give iron in the anaemia of chronic infection where utilisation of iron stores is impaired; but such patients may also have true iron deficiency. This may be difficult to diagnose without direct visualisation of stores in a bone marrow aspirate. Iron should not be given in haemolytic anaemias unless there is also haemoglobinuria, for the iron from the lysed cells remains in the body. Moreover the increased erythropoiesis associated with chronic haemolytic states stimulates increased iron absorption and adding to the iron load may cause haemosiderosis.

Iron therapy is needed in:
- Iron deficiency due to dietary lack or to chronic blood loss.
- Pregnancy. The extra iron required by mother and fetus totals 1000 mg, chiefly in the latter half of pregnancy. The fetus takes iron from the mother even if she is iron deficient. Dietary iron is seldom adequate and iron and folic acid (50–100 mg elemental iron plus folic acid 200–500 micrograms/day) should be given to pregnant women from the fourth month. Opinions differ on whether all women should receive prophylaxis or only those who can be identified as needing it. There are numerous formulations. Parents should be particularly warned *not to let children get at the tablets.*
- Abnormalities of the gastrointestinal tract in which the proportion of dietary iron absorbed may be reduced, i.e. in malabsorption syndromes such as coeliac disease.
- Premature babies, since they are born with low iron stores, and in babies weaned late. There is very little iron in human milk and even less in cow's milk.
- Early treatment of severe pernicious anaemia with hydroxocobalamin, as the iron stores occasionally become exhausted by the surge in red cell formation.

Oral iron preparations. There is an enormous variety of official and proprietary iron preparations. For each milligram of elemental iron taken by mouth, ferrous sulphate is as effective as more expensive preparations. It is particularly important to avoid initial overdosage with iron as the resulting symptoms may cause the patient to abandon therapy. A small dose may be given at first and increased after a few days. The objective is to give 100–200 mg of elemental iron per day in an adult (3 mg/kg in a child). Iron given on a full stomach causes less gastrointestinal upset but less is absorbed than if given between meals; however, use with food is commonly preferred to improve compliance. Commonly used preparations, given in divided doses, include:

Ferrous Sulphate Tabs, 200–600 mg/d (providing 67–195 mg/d of elemental iron)

Ferrous Gluconate Tabs, 300–1200 mg daily (providing 35–140 mg/d of elemental iron)

Ferrous Furmarate Tabs, 200–600 mg daily (providing 130–195 mg/d of elemental iron)

Ferrous succinate and *ferrous glycine sulphate* are alternatives.

Choice of oral iron preparation. Oral iron is used both for therapy and for prophylaxis (pregnancy) of anaemia in people who are often feeling little if any ill-health. Because of this, the occurrence of gastrointestinal upset is particularly important as it may cause the patient to give up taking iron. The evidence as to which preparation provides best iron absorption with least adverse effects is conflicting. Gastrointestinal upset is minimal if the daily dose does not exceed 180 mg elemental iron and if iron is given with food.

A suggested course. Start a patient on ferrous sulphate taken on a full stomach once, then twice, then thrice a day. If gut intolerance occurs, stop the iron and reintroduce it with one week for each step. If this seems to cause gastrointestinal upset, try ferrous gluconate, succinate or fumarate. If simple preparations (above) are unsuccessful, and this is unlikely, then the pharmaceutically sophisticated and expensive *sustained-release* preparations may be tried. They release iron slowly and only after passing the pylorus, from resins, chelates (sodium iron edetate) or plastic matrices, e.g. Slow-Fe, Ferrograd, Feospan, so that iron is released in the lower rather than the upper small intestine. Patients who cannot tolerate standard forms even when taken with food may get as much iron with fewer unpleasant symptoms if they use a sustained-release formulation.

Liquid formulations are available for adults who prefer them and for small children, e.g. Ferrous

Sulphate Oral Solution, Paediatric: 5 ml contains 12 mg of elemental iron: but they stain the teeth. Polysaccharide-iron complex (Niferex): 5 ml contains 100 mg of elemental iron. There are numerous other iron preparations which can give satisfactory results.

Sustained-release and *chelated* forms of iron (see above) have the advantage that poisoning is less serious if a mother's supply is consumed by young children, a real hazard.

Iron therapy blackens the faeces but does not generally interfere with modern tests for occult blood (commonly needed in investigation of anaemia), though it may give a false positive with some older occult blood tests, e.g. guaiac test.

Failure of oral iron therapy is most commonly due to poor patient compliance, persistent bleeding and, as with all drug therapy, wrong diagnosis.

Adverse effects. Most patients tolerate oral iron therapy but 10–20% have symptoms that may be attributed to iron, generally gastrointestinal upset. These effects of oral iron include nausea, abdominal pain, and either constipation or diarrhoea. Upper GI effects appear to be dose-related and are best managed by ingestion of the tablet with or after food and/or reduction in the amount of iron content in each dose. This will prolong the necessary period of treatment. Diarrhoea or constipation can usually be treated symptomatically without a change in regimen.

Parenteral iron therapy

This may be required if:

- Iron cannot be absorbed from the intestine
- The patient cannot be relied on to take it or experiences intolerable gut symptoms.

Speed of haemopoietic response is not quicker than that with full doses of oral iron reliably taken and normally absorbed, for both provide as much iron as an active marrow can use, but a course of injected iron is stored and utilised over months. The ionised salts of iron given orally are unsuitable as parenteral preparations as they are powerful protein precipitants and un-ionised iron complexes are used.

Intramuscular iron. Iron sorbitol inj. (50 mg of iron/ml) is an iron-sorbitol-citric-acid complex of MW < 5000 that is rapidly absorbed into the blood from the site of i.m. injection. Iron sorbitol is bound to plasma globulin, transferrin, and is stored in the marrow and liver. It is not substantially taken up in the reticuloendothelial system. Excess unbound iron is excreted in the urine (about 30% of the dose) which may turn black transiently at the time of peak iron excretion or only on standing for some hours.

Intravenous iron. Iron dextran inj. (ferric hydroxide complexed with dextrans; 50 mg/ml) and **iron sucrose inj.** (ferric hydroxide complexed with sucrose; 20 mg/ml) are administered by slow i.v. injection or infusion (not recommended for children).

Oral iron therapy should not be given 24 h before i.m. injections begin and for 5 days after the last i.v. injection; not only is continuation unnecessary, but it may promote adverse reactions by saturating the plasma protein (transferrin) binding capacity so that the injected iron gives a higher unbound plasma iron concentration than is safe.

Doses. The approximate total requirement is ascertained from manufacturers' dosage schedules which relate body weight to the haemoglobin deficit. Iron sorbitol is normally given daily or on alternate days where tolerance is low. It is given by deep i.m. injection, which can be painful. It stains the skin (for up to 2 years) but this can be minimised by inserting the needle through the skin and then moving the skin and subcutaneous tissue laterally before entering the muscle so that the needle track becomes angulated when the needle is withdrawn (the Z-technique).

Adverse effects. General reactions include headache, dizziness, nausea, vomiting, disorientation, pressure sensations in the chest, myalgia, hypotension, a metallic taste, urticaria and hypersensitivity. Intravenous iron may rarely cause anaphylactoid reactions and facilities for cardiopulmonary resuscitation should be available.

Folic acid deficiency may be unmasked by effective iron therapy. Where there is a deficiency of both iron and folic acid, the lack of the latter may not be obvious because haematopoiesis is impaired by insufficiency of iron. If iron is supplied increased erythropoiesis reveals the folic acid deficiency. This is most likely to happen in pregnancy due to high fetal requirements for both haematinics and so folic acid is commonly given to all pregnant patients with anaemia (see below); it also occurs in malabsorption syndromes where both may be malabsorbed.

Acute overdose: poisoning

High doses of iron salts by mouth can cause severe gastrointestinal irritation and even necrosis of the mucous membrane. Autopsy shows severe damage to brain and liver. Iron poisoning is particularly dangerous in children. Sustained-release forms are safer in homes where heedless parents live with small children. Ferrous sulphate is the most toxic.

Typically acute oral iron poisoning has the following phases:

1. 0.5–1 h after ingestion there is abdominal pain, grey/black vomit, diarrhoea, leucocytosis and hyperglycaemia. Severe cases are indicated by acidosis and cardiovascular collapse which may proceed to coma and death.
2. There follows a period of improvement lasting 6–12 h, which may be sustained or which may deteriorate to the next stage.
3. Jaundice, hypoglycaemia, bleeding, encephalopathy, metabolic acidosis and convulsions are followed by cardiovascular collapse, coma and sometimes death 48–60 h after ingestion.
4. 1–2 months later, upper gastrointestinal obstruction may result from scarring and stricture.

Treatment of acute iron poisoning is urgent and immediate efforts must be made to chelate iron in the blood and in the stomach and intestine. Raw egg and milk help to bind iron until a chelating agent is available.

The first step should be to give *desferrioxamine* 1–2 g i.m.; the dose is the same in adults and children. Only after this should gastric aspiration or emesis be performed. If lavage is used, the water should contain desferrioxamine 2 g/l. After emptying the stomach, desferrioxamine 10 g in 50–100 ml water should be left in the stomach to chelate any remaining iron in the intestinal lumen; it is not absorbed.

Subsequently, desferrioxamine should be administered by i.v. infusion not exceeding 15 mg/kg/h (maximum 80 mg/kg/24 h) or further i.m. injections (2 g in sterile water 10 ml) should be given 12-hourly. Poisoning is severe if the plasma iron concentration exceeds the total iron binding capacity (upper limit 75 mmol/l) or the plasma becomes pink due to the large formation of ferrioxamine (see below). If severe poisoning is suspected i.v. rather than i.m. administration of desferrioxamine is indicated without waiting for the result of the plasma concentration.

Desferrioxamine (deferoxamine) (Desferal) (t½ 6 h) is an iron-chelating agent (see Chelating agents, p. 154). During a systematic investigation of actinomycete metabolites, iron-containing substances (sideramines) were discovered. One of these substances was ferrioxamine. The iron in this can be removed chemically, leaving desferrioxamine.

When desferrioxamine comes into contact with ferric iron, its straight-chain molecule twines around it and forms a nontoxic complex of great stability (ferrioxamine), which is excreted in the urine giving it a red/orange colour, and in the bile. It is not absorbed from the gut and must be injected for systemic effect. In acute poisoning, as opposed to chronic overload, desferrioxamine 5 g chelates the iron contained in about 10 tablets of ferrous sulphate or gluconate. It has a negligible affinity for other metals in the presence of iron excess.

Desferrioxamine has been shown to be effective in the therapy of acute iron poisoning and in the treatment and perhaps in the diagnosis of diseases associated with chronic iron accumulation. A topical formulation is available for ocular siderosis.

Serious adverse effects are uncommon but include rashes and anaphylactic reactions; with chronic use cataract, retinal damage and deafness can occur. Hypotension occurs if desferrioxamine is infused too rapidly and there is danger of (potentially fatal) adult respiratory distress syndrome if infusion proceeds beyond 24 h.[1]

Chronic iron overload

Humans are uniquely unable to excrete excess iron so that, if there is uncontrolled iron intake, it progressively accumulates. Grossly excessive parenteral iron therapy or a hundred or more blood transfusions (as in treatment of thalassaemia[2]) can lead to haemosiderosis. Oral iron therapy over many years has also been reported to cause haemosiderosis.

Treatment of chronic iron overload, e.g. haemochromatosis, patients who are transfusion-dependent due to chronic haemolytic anaemias, thalassaemia and refractory anaemias with transfusional iron overload (siderosis). The goal of therapy is the reduction and maintenance of body iron stores at normal or near-normal levels to avoid the tissue damage associated with iron overload.

Iron may be removed by repeated venesection in haemochromatosis where there is no anaemia. A single venesection of 450 ml of blood, in the absence of anaemia, removes 200–250 mg of iron and can be repeated weekly in individuals with haemochromatosis until the ferritin reaches the normal range. After complete removal of the iron load, maintenance therapy in the form of venesection every 3–4 months is required. A small number of patients with haemosiderosis and cardiac failure may require chelator therapy.

Patients with transfusion siderosis require a long-term programme of *chelation therapy*. In patients who are transfusion-dependent from infancy (thalassaemia major, congenital refractory anaemia) chelation therapy is commenced after 10–20 transfusions at about 3 years of age. In older patients with acquired transfusion-dependent anaemias chelation is commenced after 20 transfusions or when the serum ferritin is 2–3 times the upper limit of normal.

Chelation can be effectively carried out only by slow parenteral administration of desferrioxamine s.c. or i.v. through an indwelling catheter with a small portable syringe pump e.g. over 9–12 h

---

[1] Tenenbein M et al 1992 Lancet 339: 699.

[2] A 26-year-old subject with beta-thalassaemia major had been transfused 404 units of blood over his lifetime. His iron stores were so high (estimated at above 100 g) that he triggered a metal detector at an airport security checkpoint (Jim R T S 1979 Lancet 2: 1028).

nocturnally on 5 nights per week. Simultaneous oral administration of ascorbic acid is to be avoided; it increases the availability of free iron for chelation but carries the risk of mobilising iron from relatively safe reticuloendothelial storage sites to a potentially toxic pool in parenchymal cells. This regimen can put a transfusion-dependent patient into the desired negative iron balance. Compliance is often a problem and is typically difficult during teenage years in those with lifelong transfusion-dependence. The expense of chelation therapy over a long period is currently enormous and raises serious ethical problems in economically poor countries where most patients with thalassaemia and haemoglobinopathies live.

A safe, effective, inexpensive, orally-absorbed iron chelating agent would improve compliance and the quality of life of affected patients. Deferiprone, which is the best of many agents examined, is less effective than desferrioxamine, carries a risk of agranulocytosis and may itself cause tissue fibrosis. It remains under clinical trial but may be too toxic for general use.

Vitamin B$_{12}$

PERNICIOUS ANAEMIA

In 1925, it was demonstrated that two factors were required to cure pernicious anaemia: one in the food (extrinsic factor) and one in gastric juice (intrinsic factor).

- *Extrinsic factor,* cyanocobalamin (vitamin B$_{12}$), was isolated in 1948.
- *Intrinsic factor* (a glycoprotein secreted by the parietal cells of the fundus and cardia) acts solely as a vehicle for carrying the important extrinsic factor into the body via receptors in the ileum.

COBALAMINS

Cobalamins comprise a family of compounds which share a complex structure. Vitamin B$_{12}$ is known as *cyano*cobalamin because when originally isolated, an in-vitro artefact had placed a cyan group in the cobalt β position. Vitamin B$_{12}$ is an active cellular coenzyme essential for demethy-

lation of tetrahydrofolate and thus for DNA synthesis. Animals cannot synthesise cobalamin and so are directly or indirectly dependent upon microorganisms for it. Cobalamin is produced in nature only by cobalamin-producing microorganisms, and herbivores obtain their supply from plants contaminated with bacteria and faeces. Carnivores obtain their supply by ingesting the muscular and parenchymal tissues of these animals. Animal protein is the major dietary source of cobalamin in man. Although bacteria in the human colon synthesise cobalamin, it is formed too distally for absorption by the ileal transport system. Rabbits in the wild would suffer from B$_{12}$ deficiency if they did not eat their own faeces.

In the presence of intrinsic factor about 70% of ingested cobalamin is absorbed, in its absence < 2% is absorbed. Some cyanocobalamin may be absorbed by passive diffusion, i.e. independently of intrinsic factor, though less reliably and only with large doses.

Dietary deficiency is virtually confined to people too impoverished to buy meat, and to Vegans, a sect of particularly uncompromising vegetarians.

Deficiency of vitamin B$_{12}$ in the body leads to:
- Megaloblastic anaemia
- Degeneration of the brain, spinal cord (subacute combined degeneration) and peripheral nerves; symptoms may be psychiatric and physical
- Abnormalities of epithelial tissue, particularly of the alimentary tract, e.g. sore tongue and malabsorption.

ABSORPTION AND TRANSPORT

The daily requirement of cobalamin is about 3.0 micrograms. Absorption takes place mainly in the terminal ileum, and it is carried in plasma bound to proteins. Some 90% of recently absorbed or administered cobalamin is carried on transcobalamin II an important transport protein which is rapidly cleared from the circulation (t$\frac{1}{2}$ 6–9 minutes). Hereditary deficiency of transcobalamin II causes severe cobalamin deficiency. About 80% of all circulating cobalamin is bound to transcobalamin I (t$\frac{1}{2}$ 9–12 days) which is possibly a plasma storage form (hereditary deficiency of which is of no consequence). Cobalamin in its reduced form cob(I)alamin functions as a coenzyme for methionine synthase in a reaction that generates tetrahydrofolate, and is critical for DNA and RNA synthessis.

Cobalamin is not significantly metabolised and passes into the bile (there is enterohepatic circulation which can be interrupted by intestinal disease and hastens the onset of clinical deficiency), and is excreted via the kidney. Body stores amount to about 5 mg (mainly in the liver) and are sufficient for 2–4 years if absorption ceases.

INDICATIONS FOR VITAMIN B$_{12}$

Indications for administration are the prevention and cure of conditions due to its deficiency. Hydroxocobalamin is preferred for clinical use.

Pernicious (Addisonian) anaemia. The atrophic gastric mucosa is unable to produce intrinsic factor (and acid) due to an autoimmune reaction to gastric parietal cells and intrinsic factor itself, there is failure to absorb vitamin B$_{12}$ in the terminal ileum so that deficiency results. Despite its name (given when no treatment was known and it was believed to be a neoplastic disorder due to the appearance of the megaloblastic bone marrow), the prognosis of a patient with uncomplicated pernicious anaemia, properly treated with hydroxocobalamin, is little different from that of the rest of the population. The neurological complications, particuarly spasticity, develop only after prolonged severe deficiency but may be permanent; they are rarely seen today. Total removal of the stomach or atrophy of the mucous membrane in a postgastrectomy remnant may, after several years, lead to a similar anaemia.

Malabsorption syndromes. In stagnant loop syndrome (bacterial overgrowth which competes for the available cobalamin and can be remedied by a broad-spectrum antimicrobial), ileal resection, Crohn's disease and chronic tropical sprue affecting the terminal ileum, vitamin B$_{12}$ deficiency is common although megaloblastic anaemia occurs only relatively late. The fish tape worm *Diphyllobothrum latum* which can infest humans who eat raw or partially cooked freshwater fish roe can grow up to 10 meters in the gut and competes for ingested cobalamin.

Tobacco amblyopia has been attributed to cyanide intoxication from strong tobacco which interferes with the coenzyme function of vitamin B$_{12}$; hydroxocobalamin (not cyanocobalamin) may be given.

DIAGNOSIS OF B$_{12}$ DEFICIENCY

The serum concentration of vitamin B$_{12}$ is low (normal 170–925 nanogram/l). In severe deficiency there is pancytopenia, the blood film shows anisopoikilocytosis with oval macrocytes and hypersegmented neutrophils; the marrow is megaloblastic. In many patients with pernicious anaemia antibodies to intrinsic factor can be identified in the serum.

Absorption of radioactive vitamin B$_{12}$ (Schilling test) helps to distinguish between gastric and intestinal causes.

First: the patient is given a small dose of radioactive vitamin B$_{12}$ orally, with a simultaneous large dose of nonradioactive vitamin B$_{12}$ intramuscularly. The large injected dose saturates binding sites so that any of the oral radioactive dose that is absorbed cannot bind and will be eliminated in the urine where it can easily be measured (normally > 10% of the administered dose appears in urine collected for 24 h, if renal function is normal). In pernicious anaemia and in malabsorption, gut absorption and therefore subsequent appearance of radioactivity in the plasma (measured 8–12 h later) and urine are negligible.

Second: the test is repeated with intrinsic factor added to the oral dose. The radioactive vitamin B$_{12}$ is now absorbed in pernicious anaemia (but not in intestinal malabsorption) and is detected in plasma and urine. Both stages of the test are needed to maximise reliability of diagnosis of pernicious anaemia.

CONTRAINDICATIONS TO VITAMIN B$_{12}$

Inconclusively diagnosed anaemia is an important contraindication. Therapy of pernicious anaemia must be both adequate and lifelong, so that accurate diagnosis is essential. Even a single dose of vitamin B$_{12}$ interferes with the haematological picture for weeks (megaloblastic haematopoiesis reverts to normal within 12 hours), although the Schilling test remains diagnostic.

PREPARATIONS AND USE

Hydroxocobalamin is bound to plasma protein to a greater extent than is cyanocobalamin, with the result that there is less free to be excreted in the urine after an injection and rather lower doses at longer intervals are adequate. Thus hydroxoco-balamin is preferred to cyanocobalamin, though the latter can give satisfactory results as the doses administered are much greater than are required physiologically. *Cyanocobalamin* remains available.

The initial dose in cobalamin deficiency anaemias, including uncomplicated pernicious anaemia, is hydroxocobalamin 1 mg i.m. every 2–3 days for 5 doses to induce remission and to replenish stores. Maintenance may be 1 mg every 3 months; higher doses will not find binding sites and will be eliminated in the urine. Higher doses are justified during renal or peritoneal dialysis where hydroxy-cobalamin clearance is increased, and resultant raised plasma methylmalonic acid and homo-cysteine represent an independent risk factor for vascular events in these patients (see later).

Routine low dose supplements of hydroxyco-balamin, folate and pyridoxine fail to control hyperhomocysteinaemia in 75% of dialysis patients but supraphysiological doses are effective: hyd-roxycobalamin 1 mg/d, folic acid 15 mg/d and pyridoxine 100 mg/d.

After initiation of therapy, patients feel better in 2 days, reticulocytes peak at 5–7 days and the haemoglobin, red cell count and haematocrit rise by the end of the first week. These indices normalise within 2 months irrespective of the starting level. Failure to respond implies a wrong or incomplete diagnosis (coexistent deficiency of another hae-matinic). The initial stimulation of haemoglobin synthesis often depletes the iron and folate stores and supplements of these may be needed. *Hypokalaemia* may occur at the height of the erythrocyte response in severe cases. It is attributed to uptake of potassium by the rapidly increasing erythron (erythrocyte mass). Oral potassium should be given prior to initiating therapy in a patient with low or borderline potassiuim levels. Once alternative or additional causes of the anaemia have been excluded, inadequate response should be treated by increased frequency of injec-tions as well as increased amount (because of urinary loss with high plasma concentrations). The reversal of neurological damage is slow (and rarely marked) and the degree of functional recovery is inversely related to the extent and duration of symptoms.

Haemoglobin estimations are necessary at least every 6 months to check adequacy of therapy and for early detection of iron deficiency anaemia due to achlorhydria (common in patients with pernicious anaemia > 60 years) or carcinoma of the stomach, which occurs in about 5% of patients with pernicious anaemia.

When injections are refused or are impracticable (rare allergy, bleeding disorder), administration as snuff or aerosol has been effective, but these routes are less reliable. Large daily oral doses (1000 micro-grams) are probably preferable; depleted stores must be replaced by parenteral cobalamin before switching to the oral preparation; the patient must be compliant; monitoring of the blood must be more frequent and adequate serum vitamin B_{12} levels must be demonstrated.

Adverse effects virtually do not occur, but use of vitamin B_{12} as a 'tonic' is an abuse of a powerful remedy for it may obscure the diagnosis of pernicious anaemia, which is a matter of great importance in a disease requiring lifelong therapy and prone to serious neurological complications. The latter danger is of particular significance when a megaloblastic anaemia due to pernicious anaemia is incorrectly diagnosed as due to folate deficiency; here folic acid, if used alone (see below) may accelerate pro-gression of subacute combined degeneration of the nervous system.

Folic acid (pteroylglutamic acid)

Folic acid[3] was so named because it was discovered as a bacterial growth factor present in spinach leaves. It is one of the B group of vitamins and was soon shown to be the same substance as that

---

[3] Latin: *folium,* a leaf.

present in yeast and liver which cured a nutritional macrocytic anaemia in Indian women.

FUNCTIONS

Folic acid is itself inactive; it is converted into the biologically active coenzyme, tetrahydrofolic acid, which is important in the biosynthesis of amino acids and DNA and therefore in cell division. The formyl derivative of tetrahydrofolic acid is *folinic acid* and this is used to bypass the block when the body fails to effect the conversion of folic acid (see Folic acid antagonists, p. 606). Ascorbic acid protects the active tetrahydrofolic acid from oxidation; the anaemia of scurvy, although usually normoblastic, may be megaloblastic due to deficiency of tetrahydrofolic acid.

Deficiency of folic acid leads to a megaloblastic anaemia because it is necessary for the production of purines and pyrimidines, which are essential precursors of deoxyribonucleic acid (DNA). The megaloblastic marrow of cobalamin deficiency is due to interference with folic acid utilisation and the morphological changes of cobalamin deficiency can be reversed by folic acid. It is vital to realise that folic acid does not provide adequate treatment for pernicious anaemia. Nor does vitamin B_{12} provide adequate treatment for the megaloblastic anaemia of folic acid deficiency, although a partial response may occur because vitamin B_{12} plays a role in folate metabolism.

OCCURRENCE AND REQUIREMENTS

Folic acid is widely distributed, especially in green vegetables, yeast and liver. Daily requirement of folic acid in an adult is some 50–100 micrograms and a diet containing 400 micrograms of polyglutamates will provide this. In childhood the requirement is 50 micrograms per day about $5 \times$ more on a weight-for-weight basis. Body stores last about 4 months.

INDICATIONS

Folic acid is used to prevent or cure deficiency of folate which are due either to a decreased supply or to an increased requirement.

Dietary deficiency. Folate deficiency is extremely common in the setting of general malnutrition in developing countries and is a particular problem in childhood. In Western countries folate deficiency occurs in alcoholics, some slimming diets, the elderly, the infirm and psychiatric patients.

Pregnancy. Folic acid requirement is increased to 300–400 microgram a day. This cannot be met from the diet by one-third of women in Western societies and the problem is greater in less economically developed countries where nutritional deficiency may be aggravated by high red cell turnover due to haemoglobinopathies and endemic malaria. For this reason folic acid is added to iron for prophylaxis of anaemia in pregnancy. The dose needed is about 300 micrograms of folic acid a day, which is insufficient to alter the blood picture of pernicious anaemia and so there is no risk of masking that disease (pernicious anaemia is also very rare in women of reproductive age and is probably incompatible with a successful pregnancy). A large number of preparations of iron with folic acid is available (see also Iron therapy, p. 591). They are suitable only for prevention. Larger doses may be used in therapy of anaemia during pregnancy (see below); it will remit spontaneously some weeks after delivery. Vigorous iron therapy in pregnancy may unmask a folate deficiency. During lactation requirements remain increased.

Prevention of fetal neural tube defect (spina bifida). Folic acid supplementation taken before conception and during the early weeks of pregnancy has been shown in an 8-year trial to prevent the condition in pregnancies subsequent to an affected birth.[4] Women hoping to conceive and who have had an affected child are advised to take folic acid 5 mg/day. To prevent a first occurrence 400 micrograms/day should be taken both before conception, or as soon as possible after diagnosis.[5] In both cases folate supplement should be taken for the first 12 weeks of pregnancy.

---

[4] MRC Vitamin Study research group 1991 Lancet 338: 131.
[5] A supplement of folic acid 5 mg/day is proposed for fuller risk reduction. Wald N J, Law M R, Morris J K et al 2001 Quantifying the effect of folic acid. Lancet 358: 2069–2073.

Premature infants. Supplementation is needed because these infants miss the build-up of folate stores that normally occurs in the last few weeks of pregnancy.

Malabsorption syndromes. Particularly in gluten-sensitive enteropathy and tropical sprue, poor absorption of folic acid from the small intestine often leads to a megaloblastic anaemia.

Drugs. Antiepilepsy drugs, particularly phenytoin, primidone and phenobarbital, occasionally cause a macrocytic anaemia that responds to folic acid. This may be due to enzyme induction by the anti-epileptics increasing the need for folic acid to perform hydroxylation reactions (see Epilepsy) but other factors such as reduced absorption may be involved. Administration of folic acid causes a recurrence of seizures in some patients. Some anti-malarials, e.g. pyrimethamine, may interfere with conversion of folates to the active tetrahydrofolic acid, causing macrocytic anaemia. Methotrexate, another folate antagonist, may cause a megalo-blastic anaemia especially when used long-term for leukaemia, rheumatoid arthritis or psoriasis.

Miscellaneous causes of excess utilisation or loss. In chronic haemolytic states, where erythropoiesis is accelerated, and in myelofibrosis, where haemo-poiesis is inefficient, folate requirement is increased. Extensive shedding of skin cells in exfoliative dermatitis, inflammatory states, e.g. rheumatoid arthritis, and malignant disease (lymphoma), can similarly lead to folate deficiency. Folate loss during chronic haemodialysis may be sufficient to require replacement.

CONTRAINDICATIONS

Imprecisely diagnosed megaloblastic anaemia is the principal contraindication. Tumour cell prolifer-ation in some cancers may be folate dependent and folic acid should be used in malignant disease only where there is confirmed folate deficiency anaemia.

PREPARATIONS AND DOSAGE

Synthetic folic acid is taken orally; for therapy 5 mg daily is usually given for 4 months, or indefinitely if the cause of deficiency cannot be removed; 15 mg/day may be needed in malabsorption states though usually 5 mg is adequate. There is no advantage in giving folinic acid instead of folic acid, except in the treatment of the toxic effects of folic acid antagonists such as methotrexate (folinic acid 'rescue', see p. 608).

- For prophylaxis, with iron, in pregnancy, see page 589
- For prophylaxis in haemolytic diseases and in renal dialysis: 5 mg per day or per week depending on need.

Adverse reactions are rare: allergy occurs, and status epilepticus may be precipitated.

Haemopoietic growth factors

Cloning of growth factor genes and recombinant DNA technology allow the large-scale production of cytokines for clinical use. Growth factors are now available to stimulate both erythroid and myeloid cell lines. These factors are potentially useful when-ever there is cytopenia, whether due to disease or to cytotoxic chemotherapy.

ERYTHROPOIETIN

Erythropoietin is a glycoprotein hormone encoded by a gene on the long arm of chromosome 7 (7q) and 90% is produced in the kidney (the remainder in the liver and other sites) in response to hypoxia. The anaemia of chronic renal failure is largely due to failure of the diseased kidneys to make enough erythropoietin. The principal action of the hormone is to stimulate the proliferation, survival and differ-entiation of erythrocyte precursors. The manu-facture of erythropoietin for clinical use became possible when the human gene was successfully inserted into cultured hamster ovary cells.

Epoetin (recombinant derived human erythro-poietin) must be given s.c. (which may be more effective) or i.v.; the $t\frac{1}{2}$ is 4 h and appears not to be affected by dialysis. Maximum reticulocyte response occurs in 4 days. Self-administration at home three times a week is practicable; the dose is adjusted by response. Iron reserves must be adequate for optimum erythropoiesis, i.e. serum ferritin should exceed 100 micrograms/l. Epoetin is available as two preparations, *epoetin alpha* and *epoetin beta,* which are interchangeable.

Epoetin is effective in the anaemia of chronic renal failure to an extent that it significantly enhances the patients' quality of life. Patients become independent of blood transfusion, with great benefit to blood transfusion services as well as to themselves.

Recombinant erythropoietin has also been used in anaemia of rheumatoid arthritis, prematurity, following cancer chemotherapy, myelodysplasia and zidovudine-treated AIDS, and to improve the quality of presurgical autologous blood collection. Athletes in track events and cycling seeking advantage through increased haemoglobin concentrations have misused it.

Adverse effects. A dose-dependent increase in arterial blood pressure follows the rise in red cell mass and encephalopathy may occur in some previously hypertensive patients. Arteriovenous shunts of dialysis patients, especially those that are compromised, may thrombose as a result of increased blood viscosity.

Iron deficiency may occur, as increased haematopoiesis outstrips available iron stores, and this can be a cause of inadequate response to the hormone; parenteral iron therapy may be needed. Transient influenza-like symptoms may accompany the first i.v. injections.

COLONY-STIMULATING FACTORS

A number of cytokines (see p. 280) stimulate the growth, differentiation and functional activity of myeloid progenitor cells. As the name implies the function of these polypeptides was defined by in-vitro colony assays of bone marrow progenitors. They have effects on all myeloid cells including the multipotential stem cells (but probably not the more immature pluripotential cells), intermediate progenitors and circulating mature cells. Those in clinical use are described below.

Granulocyte colony-stimulating factors: G-CSF, an 18 kDa protein encoded by a gene on the long arm of chromosome 17 (17q), stimulates the proliferation of granulocyte progenitors and activates neutrophil function.

Filgrastim is recombinant human granulocyte colony-stimulating factor. A single dose will cause the neutrophil count to rise 4–5-fold within hours and the increased count persists up to 72 h. The drug is rapidly cleared after i.v. injection ($t\frac{1}{2}$ 2 h) and administration by i.v. infusion or s.c. is necessary to prolong plasma concentration. High concentrations are found in plasma, bone marrow and kidneys. It is degraded to its component amino acids.

G-CSF is widely used to mobilise bone marrow stem cells into the peripheral blood to support both autologous and allogeneic peripheral blood progenitor transplantation. The use of peripheral blood progenitors as opposed to bone marrow progenitors is associated with earlier neutrophil and platelet recovery, fewer red cell transfusions and earlier discharge from hospital.

Another major use of G-CSF is for patients with neutropenia as a result of cytotoxic chemotherapy, to shorten the duration of neutropenia and reduce morbidity due to infection. It is also used for the same purpose after autologous and allogeneic bone marrow transplantation, in aplastic anaemia, AIDS, and congenital, cyclical and idiopathic neutropenia. In combination with epoetin, G-CSF can be effective in the management of some patients with myelodysplastic syndromes. G-CSF not only improves the neutrophil count, but dramatically improves the proportion of patients with a raised haemoglobin in response to epoetin possibly by reduction of erythroid apoptosis (the cause of ineffective erythropoiesis).

Adverse effect. Medullary bone pain occurs with high i.v. doses. Musculoskeletal pain, dysuria, splenomegaly, allergic reactions and abnormality of liver enzymes also occur.

Lenograstim is similar.

Granulocyte-monocyte colony-stimulating factor: GM-CSF, a glycoprotein of 14–35 kDa encoded by a gene on the long arm of chromosome 5 (5q), has a broader spectrum of activity than G-CSF, stimulating both monocyte and granulocyte production with functional effects on the mature cells of both cell lines.

Molgramostim (recombinant human granulocyte-monocyte colony-stimulating factor) has a $t\frac{1}{2}$ of 3 h and administration by i.v. infusion or s.c. is needed to maintain plasma concentration. Molgramostim has also been used to mobilise peripheral blood progenitors and to reduce cytotoxic-induced neutropenia, and in bone marrow transplantation and aplastic anaemia. It is now less widely used than G-CSF. Molgramostim has also been used for neutropenia caused by ganciclovir and for AIDS-related cytomegalovirus retinitis. It appears to be synergistic with amphotericin in the treatment of invasive pulmonary aspergillosis possibly by activation of macrophages to enhance killing of phagocytosed fungi.

Adverse effects. Molgramostim causes medullary bone pain, skin rashes, lethargy and myalgia in 10–20% of patients. It may also cause fever, the interpretation of which presents a clinical dilemma in neutropenic patients who are subject to sepsis. Pleural and pericardial effusions occur after high doses.

Thrombopoietin (TPO), a 36 kDa protein encoded by a gene on the long arm of chromosome 3 (3q) stimulates the growth and differentiation of megakaryocyte progenitors, mature megakaryocytes and primes platlets to respond to stimuli. Recombinant human TPO has been examined in a small number of clinical trials and found to produce a dose-dependent increase in bone marrow megakaryocytes and the peripheral blood platelet count. If it proves nontoxic (concerns include the potential for platelet activation leading to thrombosis, and the risk of myelofibrosis), it may have a role in the treatment of chemotherapy-induced thrombocytopenia.

Hydroxyurea (hydroxycarbamide) in sickle cell anaemia

In sickle cell disease, haemoglobin S (HbS) when deoxygenated forms polymers which result in the red cells changing from flexible biconcave discs to unyielding sickle shapes that obstruct blood flow. This gives rise to the clinical features of haemolysis with shortened red cell survival, anaemia and painful bone crises. Haemoglobin F (HbF) interferes with the polymerisation process and is protective against the disease.

Hydroxyurea (hydroxycarbamide) is the first widely available and affordable agent that provides real benefit. It acts by perturbing the maturation of erythrocytes and promoting HbF production. The mode of action may be more complex; reduction in leukocyte counts may reduce vaso-occlusive events; reduced red cell and endothelial adhesiveness may be a direct effect. Beneficial effects have been seen in adults, children and infants. Long-term hydroxyurea (hydroxycarbamide) (at close to myelotoxic doses) raises HbF to 15–20% and reduces the frequency of hospitalisation, pain, acute chest syndrome and blood transfusion. Neurological complications e.g. stroke, may not be reduced. Some 10–20% of patients will fail to respond due to the condition of the bone marrow, or genetic effects (see also p. 607, 613).

Adverse effects. The long-term risk of leukaemogenesis cannot yet be assessed. There appears to be no adverse effects on growth or development.

Polycythaemia rubra vera

The clinical course of polycythaemia rubra vera (PRV) is marked by a high risk of thrombotic complications and a variable incidence of transformation to myelofibrosis or acute myeloblastic leukaemia. The object of treatment is to minimise the risk of thrombosis and to prevent transformation. The following are used.

Phlebotomy. The object is to reduce the haematocrit to less than 0.45 by venesection (300–500 ml) every 2 days. Thereafter the attempt is made to maintain normal status by occasional venesection. Iron deficiency may occur and need treatment although this may result in a need for more frequent venesection.

Additional myelosuppressive therapy is required in most patients. This is indicated if frequent venesection is required to maintain a normal haematocrit or if the platelet count continues high (added risk of thrombosis).

Radiophosphorus (^{32}P, sodium radiophosphate) is given i.v. Phosphorus is concentrated in bone and in cells that are dividing rapidly, so that the erythrocyte precursors in the bone marrow receive most of the β-irradiation. The effects are similar to those of whole-body irradiation, and in PRV, ^{32}P is a treatment option for those > 65 years (accumulation in the gonads precludes its use in younger patients). The maximum effect on the blood count is delayed 1–2 months after a single dose that usually provides control for 1–2 years. It reduces vascular events and delays progression to myelofibrosis. Excessive depression of the bone marrow including leuco-cytes and platelets is the main adverse effect, but is seldom serious. Acute myeloid leukaemia occurs more frequently in patients treated with ^{32}P espe-cially when used in combination with hydroxyurea.

Alkylating agents. Busulfan is a radio-mimetic cytotoxic agent that is effective in PRV, reducing vascular events and delaying myelofibrosis. Its mutagenic potential should restrict its use to older patients. Chlorambucil and combination chemo-therapy should be avoided because of excessive leukaemogenic risk.

Hydroxyurea (hydroxycarbamide). This anti-metabolite is thought to carry a lower risk of leukaemogenesis than either of the above agents but anxieties remain. It effectively reduces the incidence of thrombosis and is regarded as more acceptable therapy for younger patients.

Anagrelide is an oral agent which inhibits platelet aggregation but at lower doses it lowers platelet counts in man due to a marked effect on mega-karyocyte maturation. It is nonmutagenic and effectively controls thrombocytosis in PRV and essential thrombocythaemia (ET). Adverse effects are cardiovascular: headache, forceful heartbeats, fluid retention and arrhythmias.

Interferon alfa is another probably non-leuk-aemogenic alternative for younger patients.

Other features. Pruritus is troublesome and difficult to relieve; it may be helped by H$_1$- and H$_2$-histamine receptor blockers alone or together. Hyperuricaemia, due to cell destruction, is pre-vented by allopurinol; and iron and folate deficiency by replacement doses (due to the rapid response of the myeloproliferative erythron). Aspirin remains controversial. Low-dose aspirin (for antiplatelet action) may be used if the platelet count remains high or thrombosis occurs despite the above treat-ment but is best avoided in patients with a history of haemorrhage.

Aplastic anaemia

Marrow failure (aplastic anaemia) may be primary, of which 75% are idiopathic acquired, and 25% secondary to a variety of agents, including chemicals (e.g. benzene), drugs and infections. Treatment is chosen according to the severity of the cytopenia, the age of the patient, the availability of a suitable bone marrow donor and, less commonly, the cause (if known). Good supportive treatment is important. The major therapeutic choice is between allogeneic bone marrow transplantation and immuno-suppression, e.g. with antilymphocytic globulin and ciclosporin; and perhaps haemopoietic growth factors (see above). Survival rates after allogeneic transplantation are in the region of 75–80% for data collected from transplant centres by the Inter-national Bone Marrow Transplant Registry, though chronic graft-versus-host disease causes continued morbidity.

Immunosuppression is used in patients who are not candidates for bone marrow transplantation due to age or to the lack of a donor (up to 70%). Horse antithymocyte globulin (ATG) or rabbit anti-lymphocyte globulin (ALG) induce haematological responses (transfusion-independence and freedom from infection) in 40–50%. The addition of ciclosporin to ATG or ALG improves response rates to 70–80% and survival rates in responders to 90%. Adverse effects of ATG and ALG include anaphylaxis, exacerbation of cytopenias and serum sickness. Ciclosporin is nephrotoxic. In refractory patients G-CSF and erythropoetin can improve blood counts, as can androgens in some patients.

GUIDE TO FURTHER READING

Andrews N C 1999 Disorders of iron metabolism. New England Journal of Medicine 341: 1986–1995

Botto L D, Moore C A, Khoury M J et al 1999 Neural tube defects. New England Journal of Medicine 341: 1509–1519

Castle W B 1966 Treatment of pernicious anaemia: historical aspects. Clinical Pharmacology and Therapeutics 7: 347

Ferner R E et al 1989 Drugs in donated blood. Lancet 2: 93–94

Oliveri N F 1999 The β-thalassemias. New England Journal of Medicine 341: 99–109

Roy C N, Enns C A 2000 Iron homeostasis: new tales from the crypt. Blood 96: 4020–4027

Spivak J L 2000 The blood in systemic disorders. Lancet 355: 1707–1712

Steinberg M H 1999 Management of sickle cell disease. New England Journal of Medicine 340: 1021–1030

Stock W, Hoffman R 2000 White blood cells: non-malignant disorders. Lancet 355: 1351–1357

Tefferi A 2000 Myelofibrosis with myeloid metaplasia. New England Journal of Medicine 342: 1255–1265

Toh B-H, van Driel I R, Gleeson P A 1997 Pernicious anaemia. New England Journal of Medicine 337: 1441–1448

Weatherall D J, Provan A B 2000 Red cells I: inherited anaemias. Lancet 355: 1169–1175

Weatherall D J, Provan A B 2000 Red cells II: acquired anaemias and polycythaemica. Lancet 355: 1260–1268

Young N S, Maciejewski J 1997 The pathophysiology of acquired aplastic anaemia. New England Journal of Medicine 336: 1365–1372

30

Neoplastic disease and immunosuppression

SYNOPSIS

Neoplastic disease
In most cases, the cause of cancer is multifactorial. About 75% of cancers are due to environmental factors, some of which are within the control of the individual, e.g. tobacco smoking, exposure to sunlight. Growing understanding of cancer genetics and inherited disease suggests that fewer than 10% of cancers are familial. The different systemic modalities used to treat cancer patients are discussed. Immunosuppressive drugs are described here as they share many characteristics with cytotoxics.

- Cancer treatments and outcomes
- Rationale for cytotoxic chemotherapy[1]
- Classes of cytotoxic chemotherapy drugs
- Chemotherapy in clinical practice
- Endocrine therapy
- Immunotherapy and biological therapies
- Emerging anticancer treatments
- Immunosuppression and immunosuppressive drugs

---

[1] Although not in strict accord with the definition of Chapter 11, the word 'chemotherapy' is in general use in this connection and it would be pedantic to avoid it. It arose because some malignant cells can be cultured and the disease transmitted by inoculation, as with bacteria. The more precise term 'cytotoxic chemotherapy' is adopted here.

Neoplastic disease

Cancer treatments and outcomes

Cancers share some common characteristics:

- Growth that is not subject to normal restrictions for that tissue and fails to respond to apoptotic signals (see later) or in which a high proportion of cells are dividing, i.e. there is a high 'growth fraction'
- Local invasiveness
- Tendency to spread to other parts of the body (metastasise)
- Less differentiated cell morphology
- Tendency to retain some characteristics of the tissue of origin.

Cancer treatment employs six established principal modalities:

1. surgery
2. radiotherapy
3. chemotherapy
4. endocrine therapy
5. immunotherapy
6. biological therapy.

Details of the exploitation of all of these techniques, whether alone, sequentially or concurrently is beyond the scope of a book on clinical pharmacology. This account will essentially be confined to the use of drugs (see Table 30.1). It is important however, to understand the *context* in which *systemic therapy* is offered to patients.

SYSTEMIC CANCER CHEMOTHERAPY

Cancers originating from different organs of the body differ in their behaviour and in their response to treatments. Primary surgery and/or radiotherapy to a *localised* cancer offer the best chance of cure for patients. Drug treatments in the past were mainly restricted to patients with disseminated, metastatic ('advanced') disease, where a systemic effect is required. Cytotoxic chemotherapy for advanced disease offers *cure* for only certain types of cancer, e.g. testicular cancers, Wilms tumour. Most often, chemotherapy may prolong life, although patients ultimately die of their disease.

Palliation may be achieved by treatment in terms of both increased survival and improved quality of life as a consequence of symptom control at least in the short term. There remain a number of types of cancer which are unresponsive to currently available drugs. Patients with chemoresistant cancers who are fit enough and willing may be offered experimental treatments within a clinical trial.

Many cancer patients are not cured by their primary treatment, the disease often returning months or years later even though at the time of completing their initial treatment there was no visible evidence of cancer (complete remission). *Adjuvant* therapy attempts to eradicate microscopic cancer by treating patients usually after their primary surgery. This strategy has improved overall survival for patients with, for example, breast and colorectal cancer.

Most treatments currently available are associated with unwanted effects of varying degrees of severity. The risk of causing harm must be weighed against the potential to do good in each individual case. Chemotherapy depends on developing drugs that kill malignant cells or modify their growth and leave those of the host unharmed or, and more usually, harmed but capable of recovery. When there is realistic expectation of cure or extensive life prolongation of good quality life, then it is appropriate to risk severe drug toxicity, e.g. treatment of testicular cancer patients with potentially life-threatening platinum-based combination chemotherapy regimens offers a greater than 85% chance of cure, even for those with extensive, metastatic disease.

Where expectation is confined to palliation in terms of modest life prolongation of less certain quality, then the benefits and costs of treatment must be considered carefully. Preferably, palliative treatments should involve low risk of serious side effects, e.g. 5-fluorouracil-based chemotherapy for advanced colorectal cancer is well tolerated by most patients while improving survival by around 6–9 months.

Clearly, patients must have the potential benefits and harm of treatment carefully explained to them by skilled clinicians and nurses. They may themselves have strong views about aspects of quality and quantity of the life which should be taken into consideration.

TABLE 30.1   Benefits achieved with cytotoxic chemotherapy for common cancers

Curable: chemosensitive cancers	Improved survival: some degree of chemosensitivity	Equivocal survival benefit: chemoresistant cancers
Teratoma	Colorectal cancer	Pancreatic cancer
Seminoma	Small cell lung cancer	Gastric cancer
High-grade non-Hodgkin's lymphoma	Ovarian cancer	Oesophageal cancer
	Breast cancer	Non-small cell lung cancer
Hodgkin's lymphoma	Cervical cancer	Sarcoma
Wilm's tumour	Endometrial cancer	Bladder cancer
	Low-grade lymphoma	Melanoma
	Myeloma	Renal cancer
		Primary brain cancers
		Nasopharyngeal carcinoma
		Hepatoma
		Astrocytoma

Rationale for cytotoxic chemotherapy

Cytotoxic chemotherapy began with sulphur mustards (oily vesicant liquids) which had been developed and used as chemical weapons in World War I (1914–18). Amongst their actions depression of haemopoiesis and of lymphoid tissues were observed. Preparations for World War II (1939–45) included research to increase the potency and toxicity ('efficacy') of these odious substances. Substitution of a nitrogen atom for the sulphur atom, i.e. making nitrogen mustards, had the desired result. The disappearance of lymphocytes and granulocytes from the blood of rabbits was a useful marker of toxicity and gave rise to the idea of possible efficacy in lymphoid cancers.

> The problem was fundamental and simple: could one destroy a tumour with this group of cytotoxic agents before destroying the host?[2]

Nitrogen mustards, as anticancer alkylating agents, were first tested on experimental lymphoma in mice and the results were sufficiently encouraging to warrant a therapeutic trial in man. 'The response of the first patient was as dramatic as that of the first mouse', following 10 days treatment. But severe bone marrow damage occurred and, disappointingly, as the bone marrow recovered so did the tumour; in addition, with further courses, the tumour rapidly became resistant.

> Twenty years later (1963) we can appreciate how accurately this first patient reflected the future trials and tribulations of therapy with alkylating agents.[2]

Other classes of cytotoxic agents, e.g. antimetabolites, were subsequently identified and used to treat cancer patients. Their efficacy evidently was limited by their relative nonselectivity for proliferating cells: the narrow therapeutic index of cytotoxic agents means that escalation of drug doses is constrained by damage to normal cells and maximum doses which can be safely administered to patients are often suboptimal to achieve total

cancer cell killing. Even so, cytotoxic chemotherapy agents remain the mainstay of systemic anticancer treatment, since an understanding of their pharmacology has enabled clinicians to exploit the benefits of these drugs by various means (see below).

Classes of cytotoxic chemotherapy drugs

Cytotoxic chemotherapy drugs exert their effect by inhibiting cell proliferation. All proliferating cells, whether normal and malignant, cycle through a series of phases of: synthesis of DNA (S phase) mitosis (M phase) and rest (G_1 phase). Noncycling cells are quiescent in G_0 phase (Fig. 30.1). Cytotoxic drugs interfere with cell division at various points of the cell cycle, e.g. synthesis of nucleotides from purines and pyrimidines, of DNA and RNA, and interference with mitosis. They are potentially mutagenic. Such drugs ultimately induce cell death by the process of **apoptosis**.[3,4] This is a process by which single cells are removed from the midst of living tissue by fragmentation into membrane-bound particles and phagocytosed by other cells, without disturbing its architecture or function, or eliciting an inflammatory response. The instructions for the response are built into the cell's genetic material, i.e. 'programmed cell death'.[5]

In general cytotoxics are most effective against *actively cycling cells* and least effective against resting or quiescent cells. The latter are particularly problematic in that, although inactive, they retain the capacity to proliferate and may start cycling again after a completed course of chemotherapy, often leading to rapid regrowth of the cancer at a later date.

Cytotoxic drugs can be classified as either:

- *Cell cycle nonspecific:* these kill cells whether resting or actively cycling (as in a low growth

---

[2] Gilman A 1963 American Journal of Surgery 105: 574.

[3] Greek: *apo,* off; *ptosis,* a falling
[4] Bellamy C O et al 1995 Cell death in health and disease: the biology and regulation of apoptosis. Seminars in Cancer Biology 6 (1): 3–16.
[5] *Dysregulated* apoptosis is also involved in the *pathogenesis* of many forms of neoplastic disease, notably many lymphomas; understanding its mechanisms and the defective processes offers scope for novel approaches to the treatment of cancer.

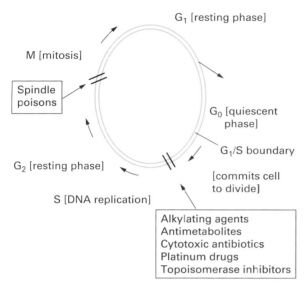

Most cytotoxic chemotherapy drugs inhibit the processes of DNA replication or mitosis

Fig. 30.1 The cell cycle

fraction cancer such as solid tumours, e.g. alkylating agents, doxorubicin and allied anthracyclines)

- *Cell cycle (phase) specific:* these kill only cells that are actively cycling (often because their site of action is confined to one phase of the cell cycle, e.g. antimetabolite drugs).

A list of drugs currently in clinical use appears in Table 30.2.

Table 30.3 provides detail of toxicity of individual agents. The following is an overview of the mode of action and toxicity and use of the principal groups of cytotoxic drugs.

ALKYLATING AGENTS

Alkylating agents (nitrogen mustards and ethyeneimines) act by transferring alkyl groups to DNA in the N–7 position of guanine during cell division. There follows either DNA strand breakage or crosslinking of the two strands so that normal synthesis is prevented.

Examples include: busulfan, carmustine, chlorambucil, cyclophosphamide, ifosfamide, lomustine, melphalan, mustine (mechlorethamine), thiotepa, treosulfan.

Systemic adverse effects of alkylating agents include nausea and vomiting, and bone marrow depression (delayed with carmustine and lomustine), cystitis[6] (cyclophosphamide, ifosfamide) and pulmonary fibrosis (especially busulfan). Male infertility and premature menopause may occur. Myelodysplasia and secondary neoplasia are particularly associated with alkylator therapy (due to sublethal damage to normal cells) especially when accompanied by radiotherapy. These agents are used widely in the treatment of both haematological and nonhaematological cancers, with varying degrees of success.

PLATINUM DRUGS

This family of drugs (including cisplatin, carboplatin, oxaliplatin) crosslink DNA similarly to alkylating agents. The parent drug, *cisplatin,* is associated with a variety of adverse effects, including severe emetogenicity, nephrotoxicity and ototoxicity. Renal damage can be ameliorated by carefully hydrating patients and emetogenicity is now effectively controlled with $5\text{-}HT_3$-receptor (serotonin) antagonists. Although second- (carboplatin) and third- (oxaliplatin) generation platinum agents are now available with improved toxicity profiles, cisplatin remains a highly effective treatment for, in particular, germ cell tumours, when many patients may be cured.

ANTIMETABOLITES

Antimetabolites are synthetic analogues of normal metabolites and act by competition, i.e. they 'deceive' or 'defraud' bodily processes.

Methotrexate, for example, a *folic acid antagonist,* competitively inhibits dihydrofolate reductase, preventing the synthesis of tetrahydrofolic acid (the coenzyme that is important in synthesis of amino and nucleic acids). This drug also provides a cogent illustration of the need to exploit every possible

---

[6] A metabolite, acrolein, of cyclophosphamide and ifosfamide causes haemorrhagic cystitis. A high urine volume plus use of mesna (sodium 2-mercaptoethanesulphonate) which provides free thiol groups that bind acrolein, are used to prevent this serious complication.

TABLE 30.2   Drugs commonly used as standard treatments for different types of cancer

Cancer type	Drugs of choice
Bladder (urinary)	*Local:* instillation of doxorubicin or BCG (Bacille Calmette-Guérin)
	Systemic: MVAC: methotrexate + vinblastine + doxorubicin + cisplatin
Brain	
anaplastic astrocytoma	Procarbazine + lomustine + vincristine
glioblastoma	Carmustine or lomustine
Breast	CMF: cyclophosphamide + methotrexate + 5-fluorouracil
	AC: doxorubicin (Adriamycin) + cyclophosphamide
	Docetaxel;
	Paclitaxel ± trastuzumab (Herceptin)
	Tamoxifen
Cervical	Cisplatin + cyclophosphamide; Bleomycin + ifosfamide + cisplatin
Choriocarcinoma	Methotrexate ± folinic acid
	Dactinomycin
Colorectal	5-fluorouracil ± folinic acid
	Irinotecan ± 5-fluorouracil/folinic acid
	Oxaliplatin + 5-fluorouracil ± folinic acid
Endometrial	Doxorubicin + cisplatin + cyclophosphamide
Ewing's sarcoma∞	CAV: Cyclophosphamide (or ifosfamide) + doxorubicin (Adriamycin) + vincristine
Gastric	ECF: epirubicin + cisplatin + 5-fluorouracil
Head and neck, squamous cell	Cisplatin + 5-fluorouracil; Methotrexate
Islet cell (pancreas)	Streptozotocin + 5-fluorouracil
Kaposi's sarcoma	Etoposide or interferon alfa or vinblastine
	ABV: doxorubicin (Adriamycin) + bleomycin + vincristine or vinblastine
Leukaemias	
Acute lymphocytic leukaemia (ALL)	*Induction:* vincristine + prednisolone + asparaginase ± doxorubicin
	CNS prophylaxis: intrathecal methotrexate with cranial irradiation ± systemic high-dose methotrexate with folinic acid rescue ± intrathecal cytarabine ± intrathecal hydrocortisone
	Maintenance: methotrexate + mercaptopurine; bone marrow transplant
Acute myelogenous leukaemia (AML)	*Induction:* cytarabine + either daunorubicin or idarubicin *Postinduction:* high-dose cytarabine ± other drugs such as etoposide; bone marrow transplant
Chronic lymphocytic leukaemia (CLL)	Chlorambucil ± prednisolone; Fludarabine
Chronic myelogenous leukaemia (CML)	
Chronic phase	Hydroxyurea (hydroxycarbamide); imatinib; bone marrow transplant; interferon alfa
Accelerated	imatinib; Bone marrow transplant
Hairy cell leukaemia	Pentostatin or cladribine or interferon alfa
Lung, small cell (oat cell)	CAV: cyclophosphamide + doxorubicin (Adriamycin) + vincristine
	EP: etoposide + cisplatin
Lung (non-small cell)	MIC: mitomycin + ifosfamide + cisplatin
	MVP: mitomycin + vinblastine + cisplatin
	Cisplatin + gemcitabine; vinorelbine
Lymphomas	
Hodgkin's disease	MOPP: mustine (chlormethine) + vincristine + procarbazine + prednisolone;
	ABVD: doxorubicin (Adriamycin) + bleomycin + vinblastine + dacarbazine
Non-Hodgkin's lymphoma	
Diffuse large-cell lymphoma	CHOP: cyclophosphamide + doxorubicin* + vincristine (Oncovin) + prednisolone
Follicular lymphoma	Cyclophosphamide or chlorambucil + prednisolone; Rituximab
Metastatic melanoma	Dacarbazine
Mycosis fungoides	PUVA (psoralen + ultraviolet A)
	Mustine (topical);
	Interferon alfa; electron beam radiotherapy; methotrexate
Myeloma	Melphalan (or cyclophosphamide) + prednisolone;
	Vincristine + adriamycin + dexamethasone; high dose melphalan + autograft
Oesophageal	Cisplatin + 5-fluorouracil
Osteogenic sarcoma∞	Doxorubicin + cisplatin + etoposide + ifosfamide
Ovary	Carboplatin ± paclitaxel
	Topotecan; liposomal doxorubicin (caelyx)
Pancreas	Gemcitabine
Prostate	Leuprorelin (or goserelin) ± flutamide

TABLE 30.2 *(continued)*	
Renal	Interferon alfa
	Interleukin-2
Sarcomas, adult soft tissue	Doxorubicin + dacarbazine ± cyclophosphamide ± ifosfamide
Testicular	BEP: bleomycin + etoposide + cisplatin
Wilm's tumour	Dactinomycin + vincristine ± doxorubicin ± cyclophosphamide

Reproduced by courtesy of the Medical Letter on Drugs and Therapeutics, New York (abbreviated; numerous alternative regimens omitted).
∞ Drugs have major activity only when combined with surgical resection, radiotherapy or both.
* The original name, **h**ydroxy**d**oxyrubicin, gave rise to this acronym.

means of enhancing selectivity. Where it is desired to maximise the effect of methotrexate a potentially fatal dose is given and is followed 24 h later by a dose of tetrahydrofolic (folinic) acid as calcium folinate (Ca Leucovorin), to bypass and terminate its action. This is called *folinic acid 'rescue'*, since if it is not given the patient will die. The therapeutic justification for this manoeuvre is that high concentrations of methotrexate are obtained and that the bone marrow cells recover better than the tumour cells and some degree of useful selectivity is achieved.

Purine antagonists (azathioprine, mercaptopurine, tioguanine) and *pyrimidine antagonists* (cytarabine, fludarabine, 5-fluorouracil) similarly deprive cells of essential metabolites.

Antimetabolites cause gastrointestinal toxicity including stomatitis and diarrhoea as well as bone marrow depression; renal impairment potentiates the toxicity of methotrexate. Active excretion of methotrexate by the renal tubule is blocked by salicylate, which also displaces it from plasma protein, increasing the risk of toxicity. Hepatic dysfunction potentiates the toxicity of 5-fluorouracil, since it is primarily metabolised by the liver.

5-Fluorouracil has been the mainstay of treatment of gastrointestinal tract tumours for the last 50 years. Combined with cyclophosphamide and methotrexate, the so-called CMF regimen is a gold standard treatment for many women with either early or advanced breast cancer.

CYTOTOXIC ANTIBIOTICS

These antibiotics interfere with DNA and or RNA synthesis.

Examples include: bleomycin, dactinomycin, daunorubicin, doxorubicin, epirubicin (and the related

mitozantrone), idarubicin, plicamycin (mithramycin), mitomycin and streptozotocin (most often used to treat islet-cell pancreatic tumours).

Cytotoxic antibiotics depress the bone marrow, cause gastrointestinal upsets and stomatitis, alopecia, cardiomyopathy (daunorubicin and doxorubicin) and pulmonary fibrosis and skin rashes (bleomycin). Some of these effects are dose-dependent, for example, doxorubicin-induced cardiomyopathy. Others may be potentiated by concomitant use of radiotherapy.

TOPOISOMERASE INHIBITORS

Doxorubicin is a nonspecific inhibitor of topoisomerase I and II. Topotecan and irinotecan selectively inhibit topoisomerase I, an enzyme required for DNA replication. These agents have clinical efficacy in relapsed ovarian and colorectal cancer, respectively. Dose limiting toxicity is bone marrow depression and, in the case of irinotecan, delayed diarrhoea. Administration of irinotecan may be complicated by an acute cholinergic reaction, reversible by administering atropine s.c.

SPINDLE POISONS

The plant *alkaloids* (vincristine, vinblastine, vindesine and vinorelbine) and *taxoids* (paclitaxel, docetaxel) inhibit microtubule assembly and cause cell cycle arrest in mitosis. They particularly cause bone marrow depression, peripheral neuropathy (vincristine) and alopecia. Etoposide blocks the cell cycle before mitosis.

MISCELLANEOUS AGENTS

Asparaginase starves tumour cells dependent upon a supply of the amino acid, asparagine (except those able to synthesise it for themselves); its use is almost confined to acute lymphoblastic leukaemia. Other cytotoxic agents in clinical use include *procarbazine, dacarbazine, hydroxyurea (hydroxycarbamide)*.

Chemotherapy in clinical practice

DRUG USE AND TUMOUR CELL KINETICS

Evidence from leukaemia in laboratory animals shows that:

- survival time is inversely related to the initial number of leukaemia cells, or to the number remaining after treatment
- a single leukaemia cell is capable of multiplying and eventually killing the host.

Cytotoxic drugs act against all cells which are multiplying. Bone marrow, mucosal surfaces (gut), hair follicles, reticuloendothelial system, germ cells, are all dividing more rapidly than many cancers and so are also damaged by cytotoxic drugs, as is shown by the occurrence of adverse effects experienced by patients receiving chemotherapy. In contrast to haematological cancers, most solid tumours in man divide slowly and recovery from cytotoxic agents is slow, while normal marrow and gut recover rapidly. This rapid recovery of normal tissues is exploited in devising intermittent courses of chemotherapy.

In cancer, the normal feedback mechanisms which mediate cell growth are defective and cell proliferation continues unchecked. Cancer cells continue to multiply, at first exponentially. Cancers with high growth fractions (e.g. acute leukaemias, high-grade lymphomas) may visibly enlarge at an alarming rate, but may also be highly sensitive to cytotoxic chemotherapy. In later stages, the growth rate of many cancers slows and the volume-doubling time becomes prolonged due to several factors, most of which conspire to render the advanced cancer less susceptible to drugs:

- Increased cell cycle (division) time
- Decrease in the number of cells actively dividing, with more in the resting state (decrease in growth fraction)
- Increased cell death within the tumour as it ages
- Overcrowding of cells leading to necrotic, avascular areas which cannot easily be penetrated by drugs.

Whilst selectivity of drugs for cancer cells is generally low compared with selectivity of antimicrobial drugs, in some tumours it can be substantial, as in lymphoma, in which the tumour cell kill with some drugs is 10 000 times greater than that of marrow cells. Cell destruction by cytotoxic drugs follows first-order kinetics, i.e. a given dose of drug kills a constant *fraction* of cells (not a constant *number*) regardless of the number of cells present. Thus treatment reducing a cell population from 1 000 000 to 10 000 (a two log cell kill) will reduce a cell population of 100 to 1. Furthermore, cell chemosensitivity within a cancer is not homogeneous due to random mutations as the tumour grows and cells remaining after initial doses are likely to become resistant to treatment. Therefore, combining several drugs may be more effective than administration of a single agent, with repeated administration to the limit of patient tolerance.

The selection of drugs in combination chemotherapy is influenced by:

- Choosing drugs which act at different biochemical sites in the cell
- Using drugs that attack cells at different phases of the growth cycle (see Fig. 30.1)
- The desirability of attaining synchronisation of cell cycling to achieve maximum cell kill. For example, cells are killed or are arrested in mitosis by vincristine, which is then withdrawn. Cells then enter a new reproductive cycle more or less synchronously and when the majority are judged to be in a phase sensitive to a particular phase-specific drug, e.g. methotrexate or cytarabine, it is given.
- Lack of evidence of cross-resistance (see below)
- Non-overlapping adverse effect profiles
- Empirical evidence of efficacy against a particular tumour type.

Considerations of pharmacokinetics in relation to cell kinetics are of great importance, as drug treatment alters the activity of both malignant and normal cells.

DRUG RESISTANCE

Resistance to a chemotherapy agent may be present at the outset (primary resistance), or may develop with repeated drug exposure (acquired resistance). Increasing dosage is limited by toxicity, e.g. to bone marrow, which does not become tolerant. Therefore *combination chemotherapy* is more commonly used in an attempt to overcome the problems of resistance rendering a tumour unresponsive.

Multiple drug resistance (MDR) of a cancer is not uncommon. MDR is most frequently due to increased expression of an ATP-dependent membrane efflux pump called *P-glycoprotein* (Pgp) which is a member of a class of membrane proteins called the ATP-binding cassette superfamily. Pgp is a protective mechanism possessed by many normal cells against environmental toxins and has broad specificity for hydrophobic compounds. Long-lived cells such as the haemopoietic stem cell, cells on excretory surfaces such as biliary hepatocytes, proximal renal tubule and intestinal cells and the cells of the blood–brain barrier all have high expression of Pgp and the protein is clearly an important protective mechanism for both individual cells and organisms. Pgp can be blocked by a number of agents including immunosuppressants (ciclosporin) and calcium channel blockers (verapamil and nifedipine). The MDR phenomenon illustrates how tumour cells adapt and enhance normal cell mechanisms to deal with the effects of chemotherapy and how repeated cycles of chemotherapy select out a population of cells which have developed adaptive survival mechanisms e.g. in myeloma where MDR proteins are rare at diagnosis but common at progression.

Cytotoxic drugs vary in their capacity to stimulate P-glycoprotein and some, e.g. cisplatin, do not induce this type of resistance.

In those tumours where cures can be achieved by chemotherapy (acute lymphoblastic leukaemia in childhood, Hodgkin's lymphoma, choriocarcinoma) it is essential that optimal doses of chemotherapy be administered and dose intensity maintained in order to avoid the emergence of chemoresistance.

IMPROVING EFFICACY OF CHEMOTHERAPY

In order to attain maximum selectivity for killing cancer cells while limiting damage to the host, various methods have been adopted with a view to widening the narrow therapeutic index of cytotoxic agents:

- Regional (as opposed to systemic) administration of drugs: intrathecal, intra-arterial liver perfusion.
- Regional delivery of drug by altered formulation e.g. Caelyx is a formulation comprising high concentrations of doxorubicin encased in liposomes.
- High-dose chemotherapy which is bone marrow ablative can be administered if stem cells are harvested prior to drug exposure and then returned to the patient on completion of treatment.
- Circadian rhythms exist in cell metabolism and proliferation and those of leukaemic cells differ from normal leucocytes. Evidence is increasing that the time of day at which therapy is administered does influence the outcome; for example, maintenance chemotherapy of some leukaemias is more effective if given in the evening (chronomodulation).
- In large solid tumours, the proportion of cells multiplying is often small. These may be better removed by surgery (debulked) even if this is incomplete, and what remains treated by cytotoxic drugs.

ADVERSE EFFECTS OF CHEMOTHERAPY

Principal adverse effects (see Table 30.3) are manifest as, or follow damage to, the following:

- Nausea and vomiting
- Bone marrow and lymphoreticular system: pancytopenia and immunosuppression (depression of both antibody and cell-mediated immunity), leading to opportunistic microbial infection
- Gut epithelium and other mucosal surfaces: diarrhoea, mouth ulcers

- Hair: alopecia due to effect on hair bulb (recovers 2–6 months after ceasing treatment); prevention by scalp hypothermia helps with certain drugs, e.g. vindesine
- Delayed wound healing
- Local toxicity if extravasation occurs
- Specific organ damage
- Germ cells and reproduction: sterility, teratogenesis, mutagenicity
- Second malignancies.

The first six occur immediately or in the short term and are liable to be troublesome with any vigorously pursued regimen.

Nausea and vomiting. This is common, can be extremely severe and prolonged and cause patients to refuse treatment. Effective management is of the utmost importance. Vomiting may be immediate, commonly beginning in 1–5 hours, or may be delayed, lasting several days, depending on the agent. Since emetogenicity is largely predictable, preventive action can be taken. The most effective drugs are competitive antagonists at serotonin (5-HT$_3$) receptors (ondansetron) and at the dopamine D$_2$-receptor (metoclopramide). They may be used in combination with a benzodiazepine (anxiety is a major factor in promoting emesis when the patient knows that it will occur, as with cisplatin), or dexamethasone, which benefits by an unknown mechanism. Other effective agents include prochlorperazine, domperidone and nabilone.

Combinations, e.g. benzodiazepine plus dexamethasone, plus a 5-HT$_3$ (ondansetron) or dopamine D$_2$-receptor blocker (metoclopramide) are often more effective than a single drug.

Routes of administration are chosen as commonsense counsels, e.g. prophylaxis may be intravenous or oral, but when vomiting occurs injections and suppositories are available.

Bone marrow suppression is the single most important dose-limiting factor with cytotoxic agents. Repeated blood monitoring is essential and transfusion of any/all formed elements of the blood may be needed, e.g. platelet transfusion for thrombocytopenic bleeding or where the platelet count falls below $10 \times 10^9/1$. Cell growth factors, e.g. the natural granulocyte colony stimulating factor (filgrastim), are effective in neutropenia.

Septicaemia is often an opportunistic infection by Gram-negative bacteria from the patient's own flora, e.g. from the gut, which has been injured by the drugs. Vigorous antimicrobial prophylaxis and therapy, often in combination, are used. Infections with virus (herpes zoster), fungus (candida) and protozoa (pneumocystis) are also prominent. Fever in a patient under this treatment requires collection of samples for microbiological studies and urgent treatment.

Immune responses. Vigorous and prolonged chemotherapy can impair the immune responsiveness of patients for as long as 3 years after ceasing therapy. Purine analogues (e.g. fludarabine), high dose chemoradiotherapy and allogeneic bone marrow transplant produce profound immunosuppression with significant risk of opportunistic infection (e.g. herpes zoster, *Pneumocystis carinii* pneumonia) and third party graft-versus-host disease following unirradiated blood transfusion. Use of living vaccines is contraindicated.

Gonadal cells and reproduction. Sterility may occur. The mutagenic effects of anticancer drugs mean that reproduction should be avoided during and for several months after therapy (but both men and women have reproduced normally whilst undergoing chemotherapy). When treatment may cause permanent sterility, men are offered the facility for prior storage of sperm. Cryopreservation of ovarian tissue is now also feasible. Most cytotoxic drugs are teratogenic and should not be used during pregnancy. Contraceptive advice should be given before cancer chemotherapy begins.

Urate nephropathy. Rapid destruction of malignant cells releases purines and pyrimidines, which are converted to uric acid and may crystallise in and block the renal tubule (urate nephropathy). In practice this occurs only when there is a large cell mass and the tumour is very sensitive to drugs, e.g. acute leukaemias and high-grade lymphomas. High fluid intake, alkalinisation of the urine and use of allopurinol (p. 296) during the early stages of chemotherapy avert this outcome.

TABLE 30.3 Adverse effects of some cytotoxic drugs, hormones and biological agents (reproduced and adapted by courtesy of the Medical Letter on Drugs and Therapeutics, New York)

Drug	Dose-limiting effects are in bold type	
Cytotoxic agents	**Acute toxicity**	**Delayed toxicity**
Asparaginase	Nausea and vomiting; fever, chills; headache; hypersensitivity; anaphylaxis; abdominal pain; hyperglycaemia leading to coma	CNS depression or hyperexcitability; acute haemorrhagic pancreatitis; coagulation defects; thrombosis; renal damage; hepatic damage
Bleomycin	Nausea and vomiting; fever; anaphylaxis and other allergic reactions; phlebitis at injection site	**Pneumonitis and pulmonary fibrosis;** rash and hyperpigmentation; stomatitis; alopecia; Raynaud's phenomenon; cavitating granulomas; haemorrhagic cystitis
Busulfan	Nausea and vomiting; rarely diarrhoea	Bone marrow depression; pulmonary infiltrates and fibrosis; alopecia; gynaecomastia; ovarian failure; hyperpigmentation; azoospermia; leukaemia; chromosome aberrations; cataracts; hepatitis; seizures and veno-occlusive disease with high doses
Carboplatin	Nausea and vomiting	**Bone marrow depression;** peripheral neuropathy (uncommon); hearing loss; transient cortical blindness; haemolytic anaemia
Carmustine	Nausea and vomiting; local phlebitis	**Delayed leukopenia and thrombocytopenia** (may be prolonged); pulmonary fibrosis (may be irreversible); delayed renal damage; reversible liver damage; leukaemia; myocardial ischaemia
Chlorambucil	Nausea and vomiting; seizures	**Bone marrow depression;** pulmonary infiltrates and fibrosis; leukaemia; hepatic toxicity; sterility
Cisplatin	Nausea and vomiting; diarrhoea; anaphylactic reactions	**Renal damage;** ototoxicity; bone marrow depression; haemolysis; hypomagnesaemia; peripheral neuropathy; hypocalcaemia; hypokalamia; Raynaud's disease; sterility; teratogenesis; hypophosphataemia; hyperuricaemia
Cyclophosphamide	Nausea and vomiting; Type I (anaphylactoid) hypersensitivity; facial burning with i.v. administration; visual blurring	**Bone marrow depression;** alopecia; haemorrhagic cystitis; sterility (may be temporary); pulmonary infiltrates and fibrosis; hyponatremia; leukaemia; bladder cancer, inappropriate antidiuretic hormone secretion; cardiac toxicity
Cytarabine	Nausea and vomiting; diarrhoea; anaphylaxis; sudden respiratory distress with high doses	**Bone marrow depression;** conjunctivitis; megaloblastosis; oral ulceration; hepatic damage; fever; pulmonary oedema and central and peripheral neurotoxicity with high doses; rhabdomyolysis; pancreatitis when used with asparaginase; rash
Dacarbazine	Nausea and vomiting; diarrhoea; anaphylaxis, pain on administration	**Bone marrow depression;** alopecia; flu-like syndrome; renal impairment; hepatic necrosis; facial flushing; paraesthesiae; photosensitivity; urticarial rash
Dactinomycin	Nausea and vomiting; hepatic toxicity with ascites; diarrhoea; severe local tissue damage and necrosis on extravasation; anaphylactic reaction	**Stomatitis; oral ulceration; bone marrow depression;** alopecia folliculitis; dermatitis in previously irradiated areas
Daunorubicin	Nausea and vomiting; diarrhoea; red urine (not haematuria); severe local tissue damage and necrosis on extravasation; transient ECG changes; anaphylactoid reaction	**Bone marrow depression; cardiotoxicity** (may be delayed for years); alopecia; stomatitis; anorexia; diarrhoea; fever and chills; dermatitis in previously irradiated areas; skin and nail pigmentation; photosensitivity
Docetaxel	Nausea and vomiting; hypersensitivity reactions	**Bone marrow depression;** fluid retention; peripheral neuropathy; alopecia; arthralgias; myalgias; cardiac toxicity; mild GI disturbances; mucositis

TABLE 30.3 *(continued)*

Drug	Dose-limiting effects are in bold type	
Cytotoxic agents	**Acute toxicity**	**Delayed toxicity**
Doxorubicin	Nausea and vomiting; red urine (not haematuria); severe local tissue damage and necrosis on extravasation; diarrhoea; fever; transient ECG changes; ventricular arrhythmia; anaphylactoid reaction	**Bone marrow depression; cardiotoxicity** (may be delayed for years); alopecia; stomatitis; anorexia; conjunctivitis; acral (extremities) pigmentation; dermatitis in previously irradiated areas; hyperuricaemia
Etoposide	Nausea and vomiting; diarrhoea; fever; hypotension; anaphylactoid reactions; phlebitis at infusion site	**Bone marrow depression;** rashes; alopecia; peripheral neuropathy; mucositis and hepatic damage with high doses; leukaemia
Fludarabine	Nausea and vomiting	**Bone marrow depression;** CNS effects; visual disturbances; renal damage with higher doses; pulmonary infiltrates; tumour lysis syndrome (profound immunosuppression)
5-Fluorouracil	Nausea and vomiting; diarrhoea; hypersensitivity reaction	**Oral and GI ulcers; bone marrow depression;** diarrhoea; neurological defects, usually cerebellar; cardiac arrhythmias; angina pectoris; alopecia; hyperpigmentation; palmar-plantar erythrodysaesthesia; conjunctivitis; heart failure; seizures
Gemcitabine	Mild nausea and vomiting; allergic reactions	**Bone marrow depression, mainly affecting platelets;** rash; fluid retention; oedema
Hydroxyurea (hydroxycarbamide)	Nausea and vomiting; allergic reactions to tartrazine dye (e.g. in medicinal formulations)	**Bone marrow depression;** stomatitis; dysuria; alopecia; rare neurological disturbances; pulmonary infiltrates
Idarubicin	Nausea and vomiting; tissue damage on extravasation	**Bone marrow depression;** alopecia; stomatitis; myocardial toxicity; diarrhoea
Ifosfamide	Nausea and vomiting; confusion; coma; nephrotoxicity; metabolic acidosis and renal Fanconi's syndrome; cardiac toxicity with high doses	**Bone marrow depression; haemorrhagic cystitis** (prevented by concurrent mesna); alopecia; inappropriate ADH secretion; neurotoxicity (somnolence, hallucinations, blurring of vision, coma)
Irinotecan	Nausea and vomiting; cholinergic syndrome; hypersensitivity reactions; anaphylaxis; diarrhoea	**Bone marrow depression; diarrhoea;** colitis; ileus; alopecia; renal impairment; teratogenic
Lomustine	Nausea and vomiting	**Delayed (4–6 weeks) leukopenia and thrombocytopenia (may be prolonged);** transient elevation of transaminase activity; neurological reactions; pulmonary fibrosis; renal damage; leukaemia
Melphalan	Mild nausea; hypersensitivity reactions	**Bone marrow depression (especially platelets);** pulmonary infiltrates and fibrosis; amenorrhoea; sterility; leukaemia
Methotrexate	Nausea and vomiting; diarrhoea; fever; anaphylaxis; hepatic necrosis	**Oral and gastrointestinal ulceration,** perforation may occur; **bone marrow depression;** hepatic toxicity including cirrhosis; renal toxicity; **pulmonary infiltrates and fibrosis;** osteoporosis; conjunctivitis; alopecia; depigmentation; menstrual dysfunction; encephalopathy; infertility; lymphoma; teratogenesis
Mitomycin	Nausea and vomiting; tissue necrosis; fever	**Bone marrow depression (cumulative);** stomatitis; alopecia; acute pulmonary toxicity; pulmonary fibrosis; hepatotoxicity; renal toxicity; amenorrhoea; haemolytic-uraemic syndrome; bladder calcification (with intravesical administration)

TABLE 30.3 *(continued)*

Drug	Dose-limiting effects are in bold type	
Cytotoxic agents	**Acute toxicity**	**Delayed toxicity**
Mitoxantrone	Blue-green pigment in urine; blue-green sclerae; nausea and vomiting; stomatitis; fever; phlebitis	**Bone marrow depression;** cardiotoxicity; alopecia; white hair; skin lesions; hepatic damage; renal failure; extravasation necrosis
Mustine (chlormethine)	Nausea and vomiting; local reaction and phlebitis	**Bone marrow depression;** alopecia; diarrhoea; oral ulcers; leukaemia; amenorrhoea; sterility; hyperuricaemia; teratogenic
Oxaliplatin	Nausea and vomiting; pharyngolaryngeal dysaesthesia; allergic reaction	**Bone marrow depression;** diarrhoea; mucositis; liver function abnormalities; **sensory peripheral neuropathy;** cold dysaesthesia; renal impairment; fever; alopecia
Paclitaxel	Anaphylaxis, dyspnoea, hypotension, angioedema, urticaria (probably due to vehicle)	**Bone marrow depression;** peripheral neuropathy; alopecia; arthralgias; myalgias; cardiac toxicity; mild GI disturbances; mucositis
Procarbazine	Nausea and vomiting; CNS depression; disulfiram-like effect with alcohol; adverse reactions typical of a MAO inhibitor	**Bone marrow depression;** stomatitis; peripheral neuropathy; pneumonitis; leukaemia
Streptozotocin	Nausea and vomiting; local pain	**Renal damage;** hypoglycaemia; hyperglycaemia; liver damage; diarrhoea; bone marrow depression (uncommon); fever; eosinophilia; nephrogenic diabetes insipidus
Topotecan	Nausea and vomiting	**Bone marrow depression;** alopecia; rash; dyspnoea; headache; paraesthesia; transient raised liver enzymes
Vinblastine	Nausea and vomiting; local reaction and phlebitis with extravasation	**Bone marrow depression;** alopecia; stomatitis; loss of deep tendon reflexes; jaw pain; muscle pain; paralytic ileus
Vincristine	Tissue damage with extravasation	**Peripheral neuropathy;** alopecia; mild bone marrow depression; constipation; paralytic ileus; jaw pain; inappropriate ADH secretion; optic atrophy
Vinorelbine	Nausea and vomiting	**Bone marrow depression;** alopecia
Hormones Aminoglutethimide	Drowsiness; nausea; dizziness; rash	Hypothyroidism (rare); bone marrow depression; fever; hypotension; masculinisation
Flutamide	Nausea; diarrhoea	Gynaecomastia; hepatotoxicity
Goserelin	Transient increase in bone pain and urethral obstruction in patients with metastatic prostatic cancer; hot flushes	Impotence; testicular atrophy; gynaecomastia
Leuprolelin (LHRH analogue)	Transient increase in bone pain and ureteral obstruction in patients with metastatic prostatic cancer; hot flushes	Impotence; testicular atrophy; gynaecomastia; peripheral oedema
Medroxyprogesterone acetate	Nausea; urticaria; headache; fatigue	Menstrual changes; gynaecomastia; hot flushes; weight gain; hirsutism; insomnia; fatigue; depression; oedema; weight gain thrombophlebitis and thromboembolism; sterile abscess
Tamoxifen	Hot flushes; nausea and vomiting; transiently increased bone or tumour pain; hypercalcaemia; hyperglycaemia	Vaginal bleeding and discharge; rash; thrombocytopenia; peripheral oedema; depression; dizziness; headache; decreased visual acuity; corneal changes; retinopathy; purpuric vasculitis; thromboembolism; endometrial cancer

TABLE 30.3 *(continued)*

Drug	Dose-limiting effects are in bold type	
Biological agents	**Acute toxicity**	**Delayed toxicity**
BCG (Bacilli Calmette-Guérin)	Bladder irritation; nausea and vomiting; fever; sepsis	Granulomatous pyelonephritis; hepatitis; urethral obstruction; epididymitis; renal abscess
Trastuzumab (Herceptin)	Fever; chills; nausea and vomiting; pain; hypersensitivity and pulmonary reactions	**Bone marrow depression; cardiomyopathy; ventricular dysfunction; congestive cardiac failure;** diarrhoea
Interferon alfa	Fever; chills; myalgias; fatigue; headache; arthralgias; hypotension	Bone marrow depression; anorexia; neutropenia; anaemia; confusion; depression; renal toxicity; hepatic toxicity; facial and peripheral oedema; cardiac arrhythmias
Interleukin-2	Fever; fluid retention; **hypotension; respiratory distress;** rash, anaemia, thrombocytopenia; nausea and vomiting; diarrhoea, capillary leak syndrome, nephrotoxicity; myocardial toxicity, hepatotoxicity; erythema nodosum; neutrophil chemotactic defects	Neuropsychiatric disorders; hypothyroidism; nephrotic syndrome; possibly acute leucoencephalopathy; brachial plexopathy; bowel perforation
Isotretinoin	Fatigue; headache; nausea and vomiting; pruritis	Teratogenic; cheilitis; xerostomia; rash; conjunctivitis and eye irritation; anorexia; hypertriglyceridaemia; pseudotumour cerebri
Octreotide	Nausea and vomiting; diarrhoea	Steatorrhoea; gallstones
Rituximab	Fever; chills; rigors; hypotension; bronchospasm	**Bone marrow depression;** angioedema; precipitation of angina or arrhythmia with pre-existing heart disease

Carcinogenicity (second malignancies). Many cytotoxic drugs are carcinogenic, and a patient may be cured of the primary disease only to succumb to a second, treatment-induced cancer 5–20 years later. Whether this is due to a mutagenic effect, to immunosuppression, or both, remains undecided. Alkylating agents are particularly incriminated and also some antimetabolites (mercaptopurine) and cytotoxic antibiotics (doxorubicin). The risk can be as high as 10–20 times that of unexposed people and the cancers include leukaemia, lymphoma and squamous carcinoma.

In Hodgkin's lymphoma life is greatly prolonged by chemotherapy, but in ovarian cancer it is not; these aspects are plainly relevant to acceptance of risk of second tumours.

HAZARDS TO STAFF HANDLING CYTOTOXIC AGENTS

The urine of some nurses and of pharmacists who prepare infusions and injections of anticancer drugs was found to contain drugs even to the extent of being sometimes mutagenic to bacteria. When they stopped handling the drugs the contamination ceased. It can be assumed that absorption of even small amounts of these drugs is harmful (mutagenesis, carcinogenesis), especially when it occurs repeatedly over long periods.

Contamination occurs from spilt drugs and carelessly handled syringes (there should be a swab on the tip of the needle when expelling air); even opening an ampoule can create an aerosol. Used ampoules, syringes and absorbent swabs constitute a hazard, as may body wastes of treated patients.

Precautions appropriate to different drugs range from simply avoiding spillage, through gloves, surgical masks, goggles and aprons, to the use of laminar flow cabinets. Special training of nominated drug handlers is essential. Pregnant staff should not handle these drugs.

INTERACTIONS OF CYTOTOXICS WITH OTHER DRUGS

Many examples of *therapeutic* interactions (drug combinations) are shown in Table 30.2. Non-therapeutic interactions can be serious. A combination of cytotoxics causing dangerous degree of immunosuppression represents an adverse pharmacodynamic interaction. There is also a general case for alertness with drugs that inhibit the metabolism or renal excretion of other drugs. Cimetidine, an inhibitor of several P450-mediated oxidation reactions, delays the breakdown and increases the toxicity of 5-fluorouracil, and similarly, the xanthine oxidase inhibitor allopurinol increases toxicity of mercaptopurine and cyclophosphamide. The renal tubular excretion of methotrexate is reduced by competition with NSAIDs, leading to methotrexate toxicity.

Endocrine therapy

HORMONAL INFLUENCE ON CANCER

The possibility of interfering with cancer other than by surgery, e.g. by endocrine manipulation, was first tested in 1895 when a Scottish surgeon faced with a woman aged 33 years with advanced breast cancer.

> put it to her husband and herself as to whether she should have performed the operation of removal of the [fallopian] tubes and ovaries. Its nature was fully explained to them both, and also that it was a purely experimental one … She readily consented … as she knew and felt her case was hopeless. [Eight months after operation] all vestiges of her previous cancerous disease had disappeared. [The surgeon concluded, after treating two further cases, that there may be ovarian influences in breast cancer and added that] whether [this is] accepted or not, I am sure I shall be acquitted of having acted thoughtlessly or recklessly.[7]

The treatment had indeed been based on reason. The author, 20 years previously, had agreed to take charge of a Scottish landowner 'whose mind was affected'. His duties 'were at times exciting, but never onerous', and, having the time and the interest to observe the weaning of lambs on a local farm, he observed a similarity 'up to a point' between the proliferation of epithelial cells of the milk ducts in lactation and in cancer; he learned that some farmers practised oophorectomy to prolong lactation in cows; and he had the idea that cancer of the breast might be due to an abnormal ovarian stimulus and that removal of the ovaries might have a therapeutic effect on cancer of the genital tract.

In 1941[8] it was shown that prostatic cancer with metastases was made worse by androgen and made better by oestrogen (stilboestrol). Activity of this cancer is particularly readily observable since the plasma prostate-specific antigen (PSA) concentration provides a reliable marker. Indeed the availability of some means of reliably measuring effect is crucial to the use of drugs in cancer.

HORMONAL AGENTS

The growth of some cancers is hormone-dependent and may be inhibited by surgical removal of gonads, adrenals and/or pituitary. The same effect is increasingly achievable, at less cost to the patient, by administering hormones, or hormone antagonists, of oestrogens, androgens or progestogens and inhibitors of hormone synthesis.

Breast cancer cells may have receptors for oestrogen, progesterone and androgen and hormonal manipulation benefits some 30% of patients with metastatic disease; when a patient's tumour is oestrogen-receptor positive the response is about 60%, and when negative it is only 10%. After treatment of the primary cancer, endocrine therapy with *tamoxifen*, 20 mg/d, is the adjuvant therapy of choice for postmenopausal women who have disease in the lymph nodes; both the interval before the development of metastases and overall survival are increased. Adjuvant therapy with cytotoxic drugs and/or tamoxifen is recommended for node-negative patients with large tumours or other adverse prognostic factors.

Cytotoxic chemotherapy is more useful in younger women, with tamoxifen, increasingly, as adjuvant therapy. The optimum duration of dosing with tamoxifen is not yet established, but is likely to be for 5 years or more.

For those who do not respond to tamoxifen, second-line therapy includes progestogens, e.g. *megestrol* or *medroxyprogesterone*. Should fluid reten-

---

[7] Beatson G T 1896 Lancet 2: 104, 162.
[8] Huggins C et al 1941 Cancer Research 1: 293.

tion prove a problem with these, *formestane* may be substituted in postmenopausal women (it inhibits aromatase, an enzyme involved in the convertion of androgens to oestrogens). *Aminoglutethimide* and *trilostane,* which similarly inhibit the conversion of androgens to oestrogens (and have largely replaced adrenalectomy for breast cancer), are also used for postmenopausal women; concurrent glucocorticoid replacement therapy is, however, essential.

Prostatic cancer is androgen-dependent and metastatic disease can be helped by orchidectomy, or by a gonadorelin analogue, e.g. *buserelin, goserelin, leuprorelin* or *triptorelin.* These cause a transient stimulation of luteinising hormone and thus testosterone release, before inhibition occurs; some patients may experience exacerbation of tumour effects, e.g. bone pain, spinal cord compression. Where this can be anticipated, prior orchidectomy or antiandrogen treatment, e.g. with *cyproterone* or *flutamide,* is protective.

Benign prostatic hypertrophy is also androgen-dependent and drug therapy includes use of *finasteride,* an inhibitor of the enzyme (5α-reductase) which activates testosterone (see p. 544).

Adrenocortical steroids are used for their action on specific cancers and also to treat some of the complications of cancer, e.g. hypercalcaemia, raised intracranial pressure. Their principal use is in cancer of the lymphoid tissues and blood. In leukaemias they may also reduce the incidence of complications such as haemolytic anaemia and thrombocytopenia. A glucocorticoid is preferred, e.g. prednisolone, as high doses are used and mineralocorticoid actions are not needed and cause fluid retention.

In general, endocrine therapy carries less serious consequences for normal tissues than do cytotoxic agents.

Immunotherapy

Immunotherapy derives from an observation in the 19th century that cancer sometimes regressed after acute bacterial infections, i.e. in response to nonspecific immunostimulant effect. But, in general, it appears that the immune response to cancer appears to be attenuated. Attempts have been made to stimulate the host's own immune system aspiring more effectively to kill cancer cells.

Exploration of immunotherapy has involved:

- Nonspecific stimulation of active immunity with vaccines, e.g. BCG (Bacille Calmette-Guérin[9]) instilled into the urinary bladder for bladder cancer. More modern approaches involve the injection of tumour cells or tumour cell extracts combined with an immune stimulant such as BCG.
- Passive immunotherapy strategies with monoclonal antibodies raised against specific tumour-associated antigens. Targeted antibodies have the advantage of high cancer specificity and low host toxicity. Examples include *rituximab,* an anti-CD20 monoclonal antibody licensed for the treatment of low-grade, follicular lymphomas and *trastuzumab* (Herceptin), which specifically binds to the her2/neu (erbB2) receptor, which is overexpressed by some breast cancers. In combination with conventional cytotoxic chemotherapy, trastuzumab significantly improves the survival of advanced breast cancer patients when compared to cytotoxic chemotherapy alone.

Biological therapy

Naturally-occurring substances which regulate cell function are increasingly used to treat cancer. They include:

Cytokines, produced in response to a variety of stimuli, such as antigens, e.g. virus, cancer. These substances regulate cell growth and activity, and immune responses, and can be synthesised by recombinant DNA technology. They include:

- *Interleukins* which stimulate proliferation of T-lymphocytes and activate natural killer cells. Interleukin-2 is used in metastatic renal cell carcinoma.

---

[9] An attenuated strain of *Mycobacterium bovis* used to prepare the BCG vaccine for immunisation against tuberculosis.

- *Interferons*. Interferon alfa is used for chronic granulocytic leukaemia, hairy cell leukaemia, renal-cell carcinoma and Kaposi's sarcoma. It may also be an effective aduvant therapy for patients at high risk of melanoma recurrence.

Haemopoietic growth factors or cell colony-stimulating factors are used to assist recovery of leukopenic patients, e.g. *filgrastim* (recombinant human granulocyte colony stimulating factor, G-CSF) and *molgramostim* (recombinant human granulocyte macrophage-colony stimulating factor, GM-CSF) (see p. 598).

Emerging anticancer treatments

Our understanding of the biological processes which govern carcinogenesis is growing rapidly and provides the basis for identifying novel cellular targets for anticancer drug development. New approaches that are designed to exploit biological derangements unique to the cancer cell are being tested in clinical trials. Examples include:

- Matrix metalloproteinase inhibitors that are designed to inhibit invasion of cancer cells and prevent formation of metastases.
- Inhibitors of angiogenesis. Tumours require nutrition and produce angiogenic signals that lead to new vessel formation; the strategy is to prevent new blood vessel formation essential for tumour growth.
- Signal transduction inhibitors. An example is farnesyl transferase, an enzyme crucial for the activation of the oncogene, *ras*, which is frequently overexpressed in cancers. Inhibitors of this enzyme appear effectively to inhibit cancer cell growth.
- Designer molecular therapy. A tyrosine kinase inhibitor, imatinib, is specifically designed to block the dysregulated tyrosine kinase hyperactivity produced by the Philadelphia chromosome that is specific for chronic granulocytic leukaemia; clinical trials support its efficacy in this disease.

- Agents that promote apoptosis are being developed for clinical use.

Chemoprevention of cancer

Since many cancers are currently incurable, it would seem preferable to prevent cancer occurring if possible. Individuals changing aspects of their own lifestyles may significantly influence their risk of developing particular cancers. Chemical interventions to reduce cancer risk may be considered for the population as a whole, or for groups at high risk of a specific cancer. Some vitamins and derivatives and dietary micronutrients may inhibit the development of cancers, e.g. beta-carotene, isotretinoin, folic acid, ascorbic acid, alphatocopherol. Large-scale trials of these substances and derivatives are in progress. Isotretinoin appears to prevent second primary squamous cell tumours of the head and neck. The antioestrogen, tamoxifen, when used as an adjuvant therapy in women undergoing surgery for primary breast cancer, was shown to reduce the risk of cancer occurring in the contralateral breast. This oral agent with few unwanted effects is now being tested in women at high risk of developing breast cancer as a chemopreventive strategy. See also aspirin (p. 283).

CANCER 'CURES': UNPROVEN REMEDIES

So long as conventional medicine cannot cure all patients with cancer some will be willing to try anything that they think might help.[10]

This is perfectly understandable and many patients use unproven methods, including medicines (see complementary medicine). Innumerable methods are and have been offered for cancer. A prominent remedy was *laetrile*, a preparation of apricot seeds (pits, pips), which contains amygdalin (a β-glucoside) which incorporates cyanide. It was claimed to relieve pain, prolong survival and even to induce complete remission of cancer. Benefit was reputed to result from release of cyanide in the body which was claimed to kill cancer cells but not normal cells. Although it was claimed that laetrile had no toxic effects, an 11-month-old girl died after swallowing tablets (1–5) being used by her father. The toxicity was due to metabolic formation of hydrocyanic acid in the intestine. There is no serious evidence that laetrile is effective.

As has so often been the case in the past, and no doubt will continue to be in the future, the calm evaluation of such claims is obstructed by a mixture of emotionalism and exploitation.

Interestingly, despite criticism of overpermissive laxity of the drug regulatory authority (FDA) in the USA, the public is unwilling to accept the opinion of the FDA when it advises against the use of drugs such as laetrile. It is important that these interventions be tested for efficacy and toxicity in the same way as conventional drugs are subject to rigorous clinical trials.

There is a long and generally dishonourable history of the promotion of cancer 'cures', but as each new one appears the medical profession must yet again be willing to look dispassionately at the possibility that this time there really may be something in it, whilst avoiding the tragic raising of hopes that will not be realised — a sad and difficult task.

Immunosuppression

Suppression of immune responses mediated via mononuclear cells (lymphocytes, plasma cells) is used in therapy of:

- Autoimmune and collagen and connective tissue disease (see below)
- Organ transplantation; to prevent immune rejection.

Cytotoxic cancer chemotherapeutic agents are immunosuppressive because they interfere with mononuclear cell multiplication and function. But they are generally too toxic for the above purposes and the following are principally used for intended immunosuppression:

---

[10] Editorial. British Medical Journal 1977 1: 3.

- Adrenocortical steroids
- Azathioprine (see below)
- Ciclosporin, tacrolimus (see below)
- Some alkylating agents: cyclophosphamide and chlorambucil (see Table 30.2)
- Antilymphocyte immunoglobulin (see below).

With the exception of *ciclosporin* and *tacrolimus*, all the above cause nonspecific immunosuppression so that the general defences of the body against infection are impaired.

Adrenal steroids destroy lymphocytes, reduce inflammation and impair phagocytosis (see Ch. 34).

Cytotoxic agents destroy immunologically competent cells. *Azathioprine*, a prodrug for the purine antagonist mercaptopurine, is used in autoimmune disease because it provides enhanced immunosuppressive activity. Cyclophosphamide is a second choice. Bone marrow is depressed as is to be expected.

Ciclosporin

Ciclosporin is polypeptide obtained from a soil fungus. It acts selectively and reversibly by preventing the transcription of interleukin-2 and other lymphokine genes, thus inhibiting the production of lymphokines by T-lymphocytes (that mediate specific recognition of alien molecules). Ciclosporin spares nonspecific function, e.g. of granulocytes, that are responsible for phagocytosis and metabolism of foreign substances. It does not depress haemopoiesis.

Pharmacokinetics. Ciclosporin is about 40% absorbed from the gastrointestinal tract and is extensively metabolised in the liver mainly by the cytochrome P450 3A system; the $t\frac{1}{2}$ is 27 h.

Uses. Ciclosporin is used to prevent and treat rejection of organ transplants (kidney, liver, heart–lung) and bone marrow transplants. It may be given orally or i.v. In the context of transplantation. administration continues indefinitely and must be carefully monitored, including measurement of plasma concentration and renal function. It is generally stopped after 6 months in patients who have received a bone marrow transplant unless there is ongoing chronic graft-versus-host disease.

Ciclosporin may also be used for severe, resistant psoriasis in hospitalised patients.

Adverse reactions. Ciclosporin constricts the pre-glomerular afferent arteriole and reduces glomerular filtration; acute or chronic renal impairment may develop if the trough plasma concentration consistently exceeds 250 mg/l. In the main, renal changes resolve if the drug is withdrawn. Hypertension develops in about 50% of patients, more commonly when a corticosteroid is co-administered but possibly due in part to mineralocorticosteroid action of ciclosporin. The blood pressure can be controlled by standard antihypertensive therapy without need to discontinue ciclosporin. Other adverse effects include gastrointestinal reactions, hepatotoxicity, hyperkalaemia, hypertichosis, gingival hypertrophy and convulsions. The clinical syndrome of thrombotic thrombocytopenic purpura may rarely follow cyclosporin therapy.

Interactions. Careful attention to co-administered drugs is essential as many may interact. The plasma concentration of ciclosporin, and risk of toxicity, is increased by drugs that include ketoconazole, erythromycin, chloroquine, cimetidine, oral contraceptives, anabolic steroids and calcium channel antagonists. Grapefruit juice also elevates plasma ciclosporin concentrations; flavonoids in the juice inhibit the cytochrome that metabolises ciclosporin. Drugs that reduce the plasma concentration of ciclosporin, risking loss of effect, include enzyme-inducing antiepileptics (e.g. phenytoin, carbamazepine, phenobarbital) and rifampicin. Inherently nephrotoxic drugs add to the risk of renal damage with ciclosporin, e.g. aminoglycoside antibiotics, amphotericin, NSAIDs (diclofenac). Potassium-sparing diuretics add to the risk of hyperkalaemia.

Tacrolimus is a macrolide immunosuppressant agent that is isolated from a bacterium. It acts like ciclosporin and is used to protect and treat liver and kidney grafts when conventional immunosuppressants fail. Such rescue treatment may be graft- or life-saving. Tacrolimus may cause nephrotoxicity, neurotoxicity, disturbance of glucose metabolism, hyperkalaemia and hypertrophic cardiomyopathy.

Antilymphocyte immunoglobin is used in organ graft rejection, a process in which lymphocytes are involved; it is made by preparing antisera to human lymphocytes in animals (horses or rabbits); allergic reactions are common. It largely spares the patient's response to infection. It is also used in the treatment of severe aplastic anaemia and frequently produces a good partial response either as a single agent or in combination with ciclosporin. It is the treatment of choice for patients with severe aplastic anaemia for whom no bone marrow donor can be found or who are too old or unfit for bone marrow transplant.

Mycophenolate selectively blocks the proliferation of T and B lymphocytes and acts like azathioprine; it is being evaluated in combination immunosuppressive regimens for organ transplantation.

USES

Diseases in which immunosuppression may be useful include: tissue transplantation, inflammatory bowel disease, rheumatoid arthritis, chronic active hepatitis, systemic lupus erythematosus, glomerulonephritis, nephrotic syndrome, some haemolytic anaemias and thrombocytopenias, uveitis, myasthenia gravis, polyarteritis, polymyositis, systemic sclerosis, Behçet's syndrome.

HAZARDS OF LIFE ON IMMUNOSUPPRESSIVE DRUGS

Impaired immune responses render the subject more liable to *bacterial* and *viral* infections. Treat all infection early and vigorously (using bactericidal drugs where practicable); use human gamma globulin to protect if there is exposure to virus infections, e.g. measles, varicella. For example, patients who have not had chickenpox and are receiving therapeutic (as opposed to replacement) doses of corticosteroid are at risk of severe chickenpox; they should receive varicella-zoster immunoglobulin if there has been contact with the disease within the previous 3 months.

Carcinogenicity is also a hazard, generally after 4–7 years of therapy. The cancers most likely to occur are those thought to have viral origin (leukaemia, lymphoma, skin). Where cytotoxics are used there is the additional hazard of mutagenicity, which may induce cancer.

Hazards also include those of long-term corticosteroid therapy, and of cytotoxics in general (bone marrow depression, infertility and teratogenesis).

Whilst the hazards may be acceptable to the patient who has grave life-endangering disease, they give more cause for concern when immunosuppressive regimens are proposed in younger patients with less serious disease, e.g. rheumatoid arthritis, ulcerative colitis.

ACTIVE IMMUNISATION DURING IMMUNOSUPPRESSIVE THERAPY

Response to nonliving antigens (tetanus, typhoid, poliomyelitis) is diminished and giving one or two extra doses may be wise. *Living vaccines* are *contraindicated* in patients who are immunosuppressed by drug therapy or indeed by disease (AIDS, leukaemia, reticulosis) as there is a risk of serious generalised infection.

IMMUNOSTIMULATION

See Immunotherapy, page 617.

GUIDE TO FURTHER READING

Bataille R, Harousseau J-L 1997 Multiple myeloma. New England Journal of Medicine 336: 1657–1664

Clemons M, Goss P 2001 Estrogen and the risk of breast cancer. New England Journal of Medicine 344: 276–285

Corrie P G 1999 Chemotherapy in practice. Medicine 27: 24-29

Crown J, O'Leary M 2000 The taxanes: an update. Lancet 355: 1176–1178

Emery J, Lucassen A, Murphy M 2001 Common hereditary cancers and implications for primary care. Lancet 358: 56–63

Greenwald P 2002 Cancer chemoprevention. British Medical Journal 324: 714–718

Heaney M L, Golde D W 1999 Myelodysplsia. New England Journal of Medicine 340: 1649–1660

Jänne P A, Mayer R J 2000 Chemoprevention of colorectal cancer. New England Journal of Medicine 342: 1960–1968

Lowenberg B, Downing J R, Burnett A 1999 Acute myeloid luekaemia. New England Journal of Medicine 341: 1051–1062

Mullan F 1985 Seasons of survival: reflections of a (32-year-old) physician with cancer. New England Journal of Medicine 313: 270–273

Pui C-H, Evans W E 1998 Acute lymphoblastic leukaemia. New England Journal of Medicine 399: 605–615

Renehan A G, Booth C, Potten C S 2001 What is apoptosis, and why is it important? British Medical Journal 322: 1536–1538

Savage D G, Antman K H 2002 Imatinib mesylate — a new oral targeted therapy. New England Journal of Medicine 346: 683–693

Shapiro C L, Recht A 2001 Side effects of adjuvant treatment of breast cancer. New England Journal of Medicine 344: 1997–2008

Stewart A K, Schuh A C 2000 White cells: impct of unerstanding the molecular basis of haematological malignant disorders on clinical practice. Lancet 355: 1447–1453

Tamm I, Dörken B, Hartman G 2001 Antisense therapy in oncology: new hope for an old idea? Lancet 358: 489–497

GASTRO-INTESTINAL SYSTEM

31

Oesophagus, stomach and duodenum

SYNOPSIS

Approximately one-third of the population in Western societies experiences regular dyspepsia, although more than half self-medicate with over-the-counter antacid preparations and do not seek medical advice. Up to 50% of those who do will have demonstrable pathology, most commonly gastro-oesophageal reflux or peptic ulceration. The remainder, in whom no abnormality is found, are diagnosed as having nonulcer dyspepsia. The pathophysiology and treatment differ for each of these three conditions.

Drugs for peptic ulcer

- Neutralisation of secreted acid
- Reduction of acid secretion
- Enhancing mucosal resistance
- Eradication of *Helicobacter pylori*
- NSAIDs and the stomach

Gastro-oesophageal reflux and vomiting

- Antiemesis and prokinetic drugs
- Treatment of various forms of vomiting

Peptic ulcer

Peptic ulcer occurs when there is an imbalance between the damaging effects of gastric acid and pepsin, and the defence mechanisms, which protect the gastric and duodenal mucosa from these substances (Fig. 31.1). The exact mechanisms are still poorly understood. A major cause of peptic ulcer is use of nonsteroidal anti-inflammatory drugs (NSAIDs), particularly in the elderly.

Treatment of peptic ulceration has traditionally centred around measures to neutralise gastric acid, to inhibit its secretion, or to enhance mucosal defences. More recently, recognition of the central role of *Helicobacter pylori* has revolutionised treatment. Smoking is a major environmental factor and patients who smoke should be advised to stop.

ACID SECRETION BY THE STOMACH

Gastric acid is secreted by the parietal cells in gastric mucosa. The basolateral membranes of these cells contain receptors for the three main stimulants of acid secretion, namely *gastrin* (from antral G cells), *histamine* (from enterochromaffin-like cells) and *acetylcholine* (from vagal efferents). The action

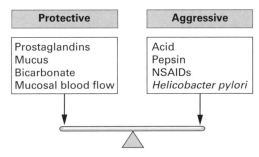

Fig. 31.1 Factors involved in maintaining acid balance

of all these is to stimulate the gastric acid (proton) pump, which is the *final common pathway* for acid secretion. The pump is an H^+/K^+ ATPase, and when stimulated it translocates from cytoplasmic vesicles to the secretory canaliculus of the parietal cell and uses energy, derived from hydrolysis of ATP, to transport H^+ out of parietal cells in exchange for K^+. Hydrogen ions combine with chloride ions to form HCl, which is secreted into the gastric lumen.

On average, patients with duodenal ulcer produce about twice as much HCl as normal subjects, but there is much overlap, and about half the patients with duodenal ulcer have acid outputs in the normal range. Patients with gastric ulcer produce normal or reduced amounts of acid.

INHIBITION AND NEUTRALISATION OF GASTRIC ACID

Healing of gastric and duodenal ulcers by antisecretory drugs and antacids is dependent upon:

- the degree of gastric acid suppression and
- the duration of treatment.

Proton pump inhibitors, which are the most potent antisecretory drugs, heal the majority of peptic ulcers within 4 weeks whereas the less powerful H_2-receptor antagonists require up to twice as long to achieve the same healing rate. Antacids modify intragastric pH only transiently, yet relatively small daily doses (around 120 mmol) will heal ulcers if they are taken for long enough. By the end of three months 85% of peptic ulcers will have healed, regardless of the treatment, but the stronger agents provide much more rapid symptom relief. In addition, numerous studies have shown a high rate of placebo response in ulcer healing.

Antacids

Antacids are basic substances that reduce gastric acidity by neutralising HCl. The hydroxide is the most common base but trisilicate, carbonate and bicarbonate are also used. Therapeutic efficacy and adverse effects depend also on the metallic ion with which the base is combined, and this is usually aluminium, magnesium or sodium. Calcium and bismuth have largely been abandoned for this purpose because of systemic toxicity. Preparations containing calcium may cause rebound acid hypersecretion and, with prolonged use hypercalcaemia and alkalosis. This may rarely be associated with renal failure (the 'milk–alkali syndrome'). Some bismuth preparations may be absorbed, causing encephalopathy and arthropathy; this is not a problem with bismuth chelate (see below).

Antacids protect the gastric mucosa against acid (by neutralisation) and pepsin (which is inactive above pH 5, and which in addition is inactivated by aluminium and magnesium). Continuous elevation of pH by intermittent administration is limited by gastric emptying. If the gastric contents are liquid, half will have left in about 30 minutes, whatever their volume.

Antacids are generally used to relieve dyspeptic symptoms and they are taken intermittently when symptoms occur. Side effects and inconvenience limit their use as ulcer healing agents.

INDIVIDUAL ANTACIDS

Magnesium oxide and **hydroxide** react quickly with gastric HCl, but cause diarrhoea, as do all magnesium salts (which are also used as purgatives). Magnesium carbonate is rather less effective.

Magnesium trisilicate reacts slowly, to form magnesium chloride, which reacts with intestinal secretions to form the carbonate: chloride is liberated and reabsorbed. Systemic acid–base balance is thus not significantly altered.

Aluminium hydroxide reacts with HCl to form aluminium chloride; this in turn reacts with intestinal secretions to produce insoluble salts, especially phosphate. The chloride is released and reabsorbed so systemic acid–base balance is not altered. It tends to constipate. Sufficient aluminium may be absorbed from the intestine to create a risk of encephalopathy in patients with chronic renal failure. Hypophosphataemia and hypophosphaturia may result from impaired absorption due to phosphate binding.

Sodium bicarbonate reacts with acid and relieves pain within minutes. It is absorbed and causes alkalosis which in short-term use may not cause symptoms. Sodium bicarbonate can release enough CO_2 in the stomach to cause discomfort and belching, which may or may not have a psychotherapeutic effect, according to the circumstances. Excess sodium intake may be undesirable in patients with cardiac or renal disease (see below).

Alginic acid may be combined with an antacid to encourage adherence of the mixture to the mucosa, e.g. for reflux oesophagitis.

Dimeticone is sometimes included in antacid mixtures as an antifoaming agent to reduce flatulence. It is a silicone polymer that lowers surface tension and allows the small bubbles of froth to coalesce into large bubbles that can more easily be passed up from the stomach or down from the colon. It helps distended mountaineers to belch usefully at high altitudes.

Adverse effects of antacid mixtures

Those that apply to individual antacids are described above but the following general points are also relevant.

Some antacid mixtures contain *sodium,* which may not be readily apparent from the name of the preparation. Thus they may be dangerous for patients with cardiac or renal disease. For example, a 10 ml dose of magnesium carbonate mixture or of magnesium trisilicate mixture contains about 6 mmol of sodium (normal daily dietary intake is approx. 120 mmol of sodium).

Aluminium- and *magnesium*-containing antacids may interfere with the absorption of other drugs by binding with them or by altering gastrointestinal pH or transit time. Reduced biological availability of iron, digoxin, warfarin and some NSAIDs has been ascribed to this type of interaction. It is probably advisable not to co-administer antacids with drugs that are intended for systemic effect by the oral route.

Choice and use of antacids

No single antacid is satisfactory for all circumstances and mixtures are often used. They may contain sodium bicarbonate for quickest effect, supplemented by magnesium hydroxide or carbonate. Sometimes magnesium trisilicate or aluminium hydroxide is added, but these are often used alone, though they are relatively slow-acting.

Disturbed bowel habit can be corrected by altering the proportions of magnesium salts, which cause diarrhoea, and aluminium salts, which constipate.

Tablets are more convenient for the patient at work but they act more slowly unless they are chewed; a liquid may be more acceptable for frequent use. Patients will find their own optimal pattern of use.

H$_2$ receptor antagonists

These drugs bind selectively and competitively to the histamine H$_2$ receptor on the basolateral membrane of the parietal cell. As well as inhibiting gastric acid release from histamine they inhibit acetylcholine- and gastrin-mediated acid secretion. This inhibitory effect can be overcome, particularly when gastrin levels are high, as occurs postprandially. In addition, tolerance may develop, probably as a result of down-regulation of receptors. Peptic ulcer healing with H$_2$ receptor antagonists correlates best with suppression of *nocturnal* acid secretion and these drugs are often given in a single evening dose. The usual ulcer-healing course is 8 weeks.

Cimetidine

Cimetidine was the first H$_2$ receptor antagonist to be used in clinical practice. It is rapidly absorbed from the gastrointestinal tract and its plasma $t\frac{1}{2}$ is 2 h.

Adverse effects and interactions are few in short-term use. Minor complaints include headache, dizziness, constipation, diarrhoea, tiredness and muscular pain. Bradycardia and cardiac conduction defects may also occur. Cimetidine is a weak antiandrogen, and may cause gynaecomastia and sexual dysfunction in males. In the elderly particularly, it may cause CNS disturbances including lethargy, confusion and hallucinations. Cimetidine inhibits cytochromes P450, in particular CYP 1A2 and CYP 3A4 and there is potential for increased effect from any drug with a low therapeutic index that is inactivated by these isoenzymes, e.g. warfarin, phenytoin, lidocaine, propranolol, 5-fluorouracil and theophylline.

Ranitidine, famotidine, nizatidine

The modes of action, uses and therapeutic efficacy of these histamine H_2 receptor antagonists are essentially those of cimetidine. Differences from cimetidine lie chiefly in dose and profile of unwanted effects. Ranitidine ($t\frac{1}{2}$ 2 h) is 50%, famotidine ($t\frac{1}{2}$ 3 h) is 25% and nizatidine ($t\frac{1}{2}$ 1 h) is 10% metabolised, in each case the remainder being excreted unchanged by the kidney.

The drugs are well tolerated but headache, dizziness, reversible confusion, constipation and diarrhoea may occur. In addition, urticaria, sweating and somnolence are reported with nizatidine. The drugs do not inhibit hepatic microsomal enzymes and do not block androgen receptors.

H_2 receptor antagonists are available as over-the-counter preparations in the UK, albeit of lower strength than those available on prescription. The potential danger is that patients with serious pathology such as gastric carcinoma will self-medicate, allowing their disease to progress. Pharmacists are trained to advise patients to consult their doctor if they have recurrent symptoms or other worrying manifestations such as weight loss.

Proton pump inhibitors (PPIs)

This class of drugs inactivates the H^+/K^+ ATPase (proton pump) in parietal cells, which is the final common pathway for acid production. *Omeprazole* was the first preparation to be used in clinical practice and *esomeprazole, lansoprazole, pantoprazole* and *rabeprazole* were subsequently introduced. All are similar in efficacy and mode of action.

Omeprazole

Omeprazole is a prodrug, in common with all PPIs. It enters the parietal cell from the blood by nonionic diffusion but becomes ionised in the acid milieu around the secretory canaliculus, where it is trapped and concentrated. In this form it is a highly chemically reactive species which binds to sulphydryl groups on Na^+/K^+ ATPase. This irreversibly inactivates the enzyme causing profound inhibition of acid secretion: a single 20 mg dose reduces gastric acid output by 90% over 24 h. Omeprazole is degraded at low pH and must be given in enteric-coated granules. Systemic availability increases with dose and also with time, due to decreased inactivation of the prodrug as gastric acidity is reduced.

Adverse effects include nausea, headache, diarrhoea, constipation and rash but are uncommon. Omeprazole inhibits the 2C family of the cytochrome P450 system, decreasing the metabolism of warfarin, diazepam, carbamazepine and phenytoin, and enhancing the action of these drugs (but inhibition is less than with cimetidine).

Concern has arisen that long-term use of powerful antisecretory drugs may increase the risk of gastric neoplasia. Differing mechanisms have been proposed. When acid secretion is suppressed, gastrin is released as a normal homeostatic response. Gastrin stimulates growth of the gastric epithelium, including the enterochromaffin cells which could transform into carcinoid tumours; some rats developed these tumours after prolonged exposure to high doses of omeprazole. Furthermore, prolonged hypochlorhydria favours colonisation of the stomach by bacteria, which have the potential to convert ingested nitrates into carcinogenic nitrosamines. Surveillance studies to date have not provided evidence that this is a real hazard, and it is certainly unlikely with short-term use, e.g. up to 8 weeks.

Other theoretical concerns relate to reduced absorption of vitamin B_{12} and increased susceptibility to gastrointestinal infections as a result of prolonged hypochlorhydria. There is as yet no real evidence for these being a clinical problem.

Proton pump inhibitors are widely used and possible adverse effects from very long term exposure, e.g. resistant symptoms from gastro-oesophageal reflux disease, are not yet known.

Antimuscarinic drugs, e.g. pirenzepine, formerly widely used to suppress acid secretion, are now obsolete.

Enhancing mucosal resistance

Drugs can increase mucosal resistance by:

- protecting the base of a peptic ulcer (bismuth chelate, sucralfate)
- 'cytoprotection' (misoprostol).

Bismuth chelate

Tripotassium dicitratobismuthate, bismuth subcitrate, (De-Nol) This substance was originally thought to act mainly by chelating with protein in the ulcer base to form a coating, which protects the ulcer from the adverse influences of acid, pepsin and bile. Subsequently, bismuth chelate was found to possess an additional valuable action, namely activity against *Helicobacter pylori,* especially when combined with an antimicrobial (see below).

Bismuth chelate is used for benign gastric and duodenal ulcer and has a therapeutic efficacy approximately equivalent to histamine H_2 receptor antagonists. Ulcers remain healed for longer after bismuth chelate than after the histamine H_2 receptor antagonists, and this may relate to the ability of the former but not the latter to eradicate *Helicobacter pylori.*

Adverse effects. Bismuth chelate, particularly as a liquid formulation, darkens the tongue, teeth and stool; the effect is less likely with the tablet, which is thus more acceptable. There is little systemic absorption of bismuth from the chelated preparation, but bismuth is excreted by the kidney and it is prudent to avoid giving the drug to patients with impaired renal function. Urinary elimination continues for months after bismuth is discontinued.

Sucralfate

This is a complex salt of sucrose sulphate and aluminium hydroxide. In the acid environment of the stomach, the aluminium moiety is released so that the compound develops a strong negative charge and binds to positively charged protein molecules that transude from damaged mucosa. The result is a viscous paste that adheres selectively and protectively to the ulcer base. It also binds to and inactivates pepsin and bile acids. Sucralfate has negligible acid neutralising capacity, which explains why it is ineffective in gastro-oesophageal reflux disease (see below). Its therapeutic efficacy in healing gastric and duodenal ulcers is approximately equal to that of the histamine H_2 receptor antagonists.

Adverse effects. Sucralfate may cause constipation but is otherwise well tolerated. The concentration of aluminium in the plasma may be elevated but this appears to be a problem only with long-term use by uraemic patients, especially those undergoing dialysis. As the drug is effective only in acid conditions, an antacid should not be taken 30 min before or after a dose of sucralfate. Sucralfate interferes with absorption of co-administered ciprofloxacin, theophylline, digoxin, phenytoin and amitriptyline, possibly by binding due to its strong negative charge.

Misoprostol

Endogenous prostaglandins contribute importantly to the integrity of the gastrointestinal mucosa by a number of related mechanisms (see Chapter 15). Misoprostol is a synthetic analogue of prostaglandin E_1 which protects against the formation of gastric and duodenal ulcers in patients who are taking NSAIDs, presumably by these 'cytoprotective' mechanisms (see below). The drug also heals chronic gastric and duodenal ulcers unrelated to NSAIDs, but here the mechanism appears related to its antisecretory properties rather than to a cyto-protective action.

Adverse effects. Diarrhoea and abdominal pain, transient and dose-related, are the commonest. Women may experience gynaecological disturbances such as vaginal spotting and dysmenorrhoea; the drug is *contraindicated* in pregnancy or for women planning to become pregnant, for the products of conception may be aborted. Indeed, women have resorted to using misoprostol (illicitly) as an abortifacient in parts of the world where provision of contraceptive services is poor.[1]

Liquorice derivatives (carbenoxolone) and degly-cyrrhizinised liquorice, formerly used for peptic ulcer, are now obsolete.

HELICOBACTER PYLORI ERADICATION

Colonisation of the stomach with *Helicobacter pylori* is seen in virtually all patients with duodenal ulcer and 70–80% of those with gastric ulcers;[2] this close association is not seen in ulcers complicating NSAID therapy. In patients with duodenal ulcer there is an associated antral gastritis whereas with gastric ulcer, gastritis is more diffuse throughout the stomach. It is not known how *Helicobacter pylori* predisposes to peptic ulceration, but chronic infection with the organism, which establishes itself within and below the mucus layer, is associated with hypergastrinaemia and hyperacidity. The hypergastrinaemia may result from reduced antral production of somatostatin, which inhibits gastrin formation. Production of ammonia by urease by *Helicobacter pylori* may also play a role. With more extensive gastritis there is a reduction in parietal cell mass and decreased acid secretion. Although all patients colonised with *Helicobacter pylori* develop gastritis, only about 20% have ulcers or other lesions, and host factors are likely to be important.

Other possible effects of long-term infection with *Helicobacter pylori* include gastric carcinoma and lymphoma, particularly of the MALT (Mucosa Associated Lymphoid Tissue) type. Eradication of the organism may lead to resolution of the latter tumour.

Helicobacter pylori can be detected histologically from antral biopsies obtained at gastroscopy, or biochemically. In the CLO test an endoscopic biopsy specimen is incubated in a medium containing urea and an indicator which chages colour if ammonia is produced. Proton pump inhibitors and bismuth compounds suppress but do not eradicate *Helicobacter pylori*, and results may be falsely negative if any of these tests is carried out within a month of taking these drugs.

---

[1] Gonzales C H et al 1998 Lancet 351: 1624–1627.
[2] First reported by B Marshall and R Warren (Lancet 1983 I: 1273 and 1273–1274). The association was initially greeted with widespread disbelief and sometimes hostility. Warren reports: "I was just doing my day-to-day pathology. I like looking for funny things and this day, I saw a funny thing and started wondering." In a gastric biopsy he saw "numerous bacteria in close contact with the surface epithelium … They appeared to be actively growing and not a contaminant." The story of *Helicobacter pylori* had begun. (Lancet 2001 345: 694.)

TREATMENT OF *HELICOBACTER PYLORI* INFECTION

Successful eradication of *Helicobacter pylori* infection usually results in long-term remission of the ulcer because reinfection rates are low, particularly in areas of low endemicity. The organism is sensitive to *metronidazole, amoxicillin, clarithromycin, tetracycline* and *bismuth salts*, but eradication is difficult because of its location below the mucus layer. Numerous regimens have been proposed but none can offer more than 80–90% efficacy (see also Table 11.1). Therapy with one or two drugs is ineffective and current regimens comprise three or four drugs. The efficacy of antimicrobials can be increased considerably by mucosal protection with a proton pump inhibitor, ranitidine or bismuth citrate (in the latter case, in addition to its antimicrobial action). It is important that treatment be as short, simple and palatable as possible to encourage compliance, because failure to complete the course encourages antimicrobial resistance. Regimens containing bismuth compounds as the only mucosal protectant are less popular because they involve dosing four times daily and are unpalatable to some. Effective regimens include:

- Proton pump inhibitor or ranitidine bismuth citrate[3] (as Ranitidine Bismutrex) b.d. + clarithromycin 500 mg b.d. + amoxycillin 1g b.d. for 7 days.
- Proton pump inhibitor or ranitidine bismuth citrate b.d. + clarithromycin 500 mg b.d. + metronidazole 400 mg b.d. for 7 days.

Metronidazole resistance is a particular problem, with a prevalence of up to 80% in some countries, particularly sub-Saharan Africa. It probably reflects extensive use of this antimicrobial for pelvic and other infections, and is more common in women. Resistance to clarithromycin is less common but it may reach 10–15% of some communities.

It is not usually necessary to check for successful eradication unless the patient continues to have symptoms. Under these circumstances the urea breath test[4] is a useful noninvasive technique.

---

[3] A complex of ranitidine with bismuth and citrate from which ranitidine and bismuth are released.

Antimicrobial regimens used in eradication are not without risk for cases of antibiotic-associated (pseudomembraneous) colitis have resulted.

A cautionary note. *Helicobacter pylori* infection is acquired in early childhood, probably by the faecal–oral route. The prevailing wisdom that 'the only good *Helicobacter pylori* is a dead *Helicobacter pylori*' is now tempered by the possibility that the organism (or at least certain subtypes) may perform a useful function. This view is based on evidence that gastro-oesophageal reflux symptoms may sometimes be worsened, and response to proton pump inhibitors diminished, after eradication of *Helicobacter pylori.* More worrying is the increased incidence of carcinoma at the gastro-oesophageal junction which correlates epidemiologically with reduced prevalence of *Helicobacter pylori* infection.

In summary, *Helicobacter pylori* eradication therapy is:

- *indicated* for gastric and duodenal ulcer not associated with NSAID use, and gastric lymphoma (especially MALT lymphoma),
- *not indicated* for reflux oesophagitis, and
- *equivocal* in value for nonulcer dyspepsia, after incidental detection, and for prophylaxis of gastric cancer.

NSAIDs and the stomach

Some 500 million prescriptions for NSAIDs are written each year in the UK, and 10–15% of patients develop dyspepsia whilst taking these drugs. Gastric erosions develop in up to 80%, but these are usually self-limiting. Gastric or duodenal ulcers occur in 1–5%. The incidence increases sharply with age in those over 60, and the risk of ulcers and their complications is doubled in patients over 75 and those with cardiac failure or a history of peptic ulceration or bleeding. Ibuprofen may be less prone to cause these problems than other NSAIDs.

---

[4] The urea breath test measures radiolabelled CO_2 in expired air after ingestion of labelled urea, exploiting the fact that the organism produces urease and can convert urea to ammonia.

MECHANISM OF GASTRIC MUCOSAL TOXICITY

Aspirin and the other NSAIDs exert their anti-inflammatory effect through inhibition of the enzyme cyclo-oxygenase (COX) (see Chapter 15). This enzyme is present in two isoforms. COX-1 is involved in the formation of prostaglandins, which *protect* the gastric mucosa, while COX-2 is induced in response to inflammatory stimuli and is involved in the formation of *cell-damaging cytokines.* Most NSAIDs inhibit both isoforms so the beneficial anti-inflammatory effect is offset by the potential for gastric mucosal injury by depletion of prostaglandins. The latter leads to deleterious effects including reduction of mucosal blood flow and a reduced capacity to secrete protective mucus and bicarbonate ion. Aspirin is particularly potent in this respect, perhaps due to the fact that it inhibits COX irreversibly, unlike the other NSAIDs where inhibition is reversible and concentration dependent. Gastrointestinal bleeding can complicate use of low-dose aspirin.

NSAIDs are weak organic acids and the acid milieu of the stomach facilitates their nonionic diffusion into gastric mucosal cells. Here the neutral intracellular pH causes the drugs to become ionised and they accumulate in the mucosa because they cannot diffuse out in this form. Nabumetone differs from other NSAIDs in that it is nonacidic, and therefore is not so avidly concentrated in gastric mucosa, which may partially explain why this drug has less tendency to produce peptic ulceration.

TREATMENT OF NSAID-INDUCED PEPTIC ULCERS

Withdrawal of NSAIDs and acid suppression with standard doses of antisecretory drugs will allow prompt resolution of these ulcers, which should not recur unless the drugs are resumed. Many patients are prescribed NSAIDs inappropriately when their symptoms could be controlled by paracetamol or by local treatment. Topical NSAID creams applied over an affected joint may be helpful, but peptic ulcers can complicate therapy with NSAIDs administered as rectal suppositories. Prodrugs such as sulindac, which are metabolised to form anti-inflammatory derivatives, can also produce ulcers.

PREVENTION OF NSAID-INDUCED PEPTIC ULCERS

This is particularly relevant for the elderly and other high-risk patients (see above). The synthetic prostaglandin misoprostol in a dose of 800 micrograms daily in 2–4 divided doses reduces the incidence of gastric and duodenal ulceration and their complications by about 40% when co-administered with NSAIDs. Abdominal pain and diarrhoea limit its use; halving the dose reduces the incidence of adverse effects, but at the expense of a reduced protective effect. The proton pump inhibitors, in healing doses, are similar in efficacy to the higher dose of misoprostol. H$_2$ receptor antagonists offer some protection against duodenal ulcers but none against gastric ulcers.

Evidence for the benefit of *Helicobacter pylori* eradication is controversial.

Selective inhibition of COX-2 has the objective of preserving anti-inflammatory activity whilst avoiding gastric mucosal toxicity. *Rofecoxib, celecoxib* and *meloxicam* vary in their selectivity for COX-2. The incidence of peptic ulcers and their complications with rofecoxib is similar to that seen when proton pump inhibitors are co-administered with nonselective NSAIDs. The adverse effect profile of these drugs remains fully to be evaluated.

Gastro-oesophageal reflux disease (GORD)

Transient gastro-oesophageal reflux occurs in almost everybody and it is only when episodes become frequent, with prolonged exposure of the oesophageal mucosa to acid and pepsin, that problems develop. Factors contributing to pathological reflux include:

- Incompetence of the gastro-oesophageal sphincter
- Delayed oesophageal clearance of acid
- Delayed gastric emptying.

The commonest symptom is *heartburn,* and as many as 15% of people in Western populations experience this regularly. Approximately 50% will have oesophagitis, the severity of which does not correlate with symptoms. The other main complications are acute or chronic bleeding, oesophageal stricture and Barrett's metaplasia, which carries an increased risk of oesophageal carcinoma. There is no evidence that *Helicobacter pylori* is involved in pathogenesis of GORD.

MANAGEMENT OF GORD

Patients should be advised to lose weight, if it is appropriate, and smokers to quit, as nicotine relaxes the gastro-oesophageal sphincter. Raising the head of the bed by 15–20 cm helps to diminish nocturnal reflux. Patients should be advised to avoid heavy meals and situations predisposing to reflux (such as lying down or prolonged bending within 3 hours of a meal). Drugs that encourage reflux should be avoided if possible, e.g. those with antimuscarinic activity (tricyclic antidepressants), smooth muscle relaxants (nitrates and calcium channel blockers) or theophylline compounds.

Antacids are helpful in controlling mild reflux symptoms when taken regularly after meals with additional doses as needed. Preparations in which an antacid is combined with alginate are particularly useful: the alginate produces a viscous floating gel, which blocks reflux and protectively coats the oesophagus.

Acid suppression. *H$_2$-receptor antagonists* in conventional peptic ulcer healing doses are useful in the short-term management of mild oesophagitis but are less effective in the longer term and on maintenance treatment only one-third of patients will be in remission. *Proton pump inhibitors* are currently the most effective drugs. Conventional ulcer healing doses rapidly relieve reflux symptoms and heal oesophagitis in the majority of patients. Sometimes higher doses are needed, particularly for maintenance therapy. Over three-quarters of patients will still be in remission after 12 months' treatment with a proton pump inhibitor.

Pro-kinetic drugs. The antidopaminergic compounds *metoclopramide* and *domperidone* can alleviate GORD symptoms by increasing the tone of the gastro-oesophageal sphincter and stimulating gastric emptying (actions that are additional to their central action as antiemetics, see below).

Approaches to treatment. The 'step-up' approach involves starting with lifestyle modification (above) and an antacid, progressing as necessary to a H_2 receptor antagonist and prokinetic drug, and a proton pump inhibitor only in those who fail to respond to less powerful measures. The converse ('step down') approach advocates rapid control of symptoms with a proton pump inhibitor followed by substitution with less potent treatments, which are titrated against symptoms. Evidence suggests that this latter approach may be more cost-effective.

Other oesophageal conditions

Diffuse oesophageal spasm may be helped by isosorbide dinitrate 5 mg sublingually or 10 mg by mouth, or by nifedipine 10 mg sublingually or swallowed.

Achalasia, in which there is failure of relaxation of the lower oesophageal sphincter, may be relieved by balloon dilatation or by injection of botulinum toxin at the gastro-oesophageal junction.

NONULCER DYSPEPSIA

Many patients with nonulcer dyspepsia have abnormalities of gastric emptying and increased pain perception in the gastrointestinal tract, suggesting that the condition is part of the spectrum of irritable bowel syndrome (see Chapter 32). Patients with predominant *epigastric pain* or *reflux* symptoms may improve with simple antacids taken as needed. More severe symptoms may require antisecretory drugs, particularly a proton pump inhibitor, although the response rate is lower (40–50%) than in patients with documented pathology. Where the main symptom is *bloating*, a prokinetic agent (metoclopramide or domperidone, see below) is preferred.

Flatulent patients may benefit from *carminatives,* substances which are held to assist expulsion of gas from the stomach and intestines. Examples are: dimethicone, peppermint, dill, anise and other herbs which are commonly included in liqueurs and (in nonalcoholic solutions) for babies. The problem is not new. The Roman Emperor Claudius (AD 10–54) planned an edict to legitimise the breaking of wind at table, either silently or noisily, after hearing about a man who was so modest that he endangered his health by an attempt to restrain himself [Suetonius (trans) R Graves].

Bitters are substances taken before meals to improve appetite. They have not been scientifically investigated. They include gentian, nux vomica and quinine. Preparations can be found in formularies and at wine merchants (Dubonnet, Campari).

The incidence of *Helicobacter pylori* colonisation in patients with nonulcer dyspepsia is not significantly different from that in the general population and eradication of the organism provides, at best, only one-quarter of patients with prolonged symptomatic improvement (a proportion that is similar to the placebo response for this condition).

Vomiting

If the cause of vomiting cannot be promptly removed, it can be prevented, or at least suppressed by drugs.

The pharmacology of vomiting was little studied until the world war of 1939–45, when motion sickness attained military importance as a possible handicap for sea landings made in the face of resistance. The British military authorities and the Medical Research Council therefore organised an investigation. Whenever there was a prospect of sufficiently rough weather, about 70 soldiers were sent to sea in small ships, again and again, after being dosed with a drug or a dummy tablet and having had their mouths inspected to detect noncompliance. The ships returned to land when up to 40% of the soldiers vomited. 'On the whole the men enjoyed their trips;' some of them, however, being soldiers, thought the tablets were given in order to make them vomit and some 'believed firmly in the efficacy of the dummy tablets'. It was concluded that, of the remedies tested, hyoscine (0.6 mg or 1.2 mg) was the most effective.[5]

---

[5] Holling H E et al 1944 Lancet 1: 127.

SOME PHYSIOLOGY

Useful vomiting occurs as a protective mechanism for eliminating irritant or harmful substances from the upper gastrointestinal tract. The act of emesis is controlled by the vomiting centre in the medulla. Close to it lie other visceral centres, including those for respiration, salivation and vascular control, which give rise to the prodromal sensations of vomiting. These centres are not anatomically discrete but comprise interconnected networks within the nucleus of the tractus solitarius). The *vomiting centre* does not initiate, but rather it coordinates the act of emesis on receiving stimuli from various sources, namely,

- The chemoreceptor trigger zone (CTZ), a nearby area that is extremely sensitive to the action of drugs and other chemicals
- The vestibular system
- The periphery, e.g. distension or irritation of the gut, myocardial infarction, biliary or renal stone
- Cortical centres.

The vomiting centre and the nucleus of the tractus solitarius contain many *muscarinic cholinergic* and *histamine H_1* receptors, and the CTZ is rich in *dopamine D_2* receptors; drugs that block these receptors are effective antiemetics. The precise role and location of $5-HT_3$ receptors (see ondansetron, below) in relation to emesis remains to be defined but both central and peripheral mechanisms may be involved.

ANTIEMESIS DRUGS

These may be classified as shown in Table 31.1.

Antiemetics that act on the vomiting centre have *antimuscarinic* (their principal mode) and antihistaminic action (hyoscine, promethazine); they alleviate vomiting from any cause. In contrast, drugs that act on the CTZ (haloperidol, ondansetron) are effective only for vomiting mediated by stimulation of the chemoreceptors (by morphine, digoxin, cytotoxics, uraemia). The most efficacious drugs act at more than one site (Table 31.1).

Antimuscarinic drugs (including those classed primarily as histamine H_1 receptor antagonists) are described in Chapters 21 and 29. Drugs with antimuscarinic activity probably act both centrally

TABLE 31.1 Classification of antiemesis drugs	
Drug	**Site of action/comment**
Dopamine D_2 receptor antagonists	
domperidone	CTZ and gut
metoclopramide	CTZ and gut
haloperidol	CTZ
phenothiazines, e.g. chlorpromazine, prochlorperazine, thiethylperazine	Vomiting centre and CTZ
$5-HT_3$ receptor antagonists	
ondansetron	CTZ and gut
granisetron	
tropisetron	
Antimuscarinics	
hyoscine and some drugs also classed as histamine H_1 receptor antagonists, e.g. cyclizine, dimenhydrinate, promethazine	Vomiting centre and gut
Other agents	
corticosteroids (dexamethasone, methylprednisolone)	Gut (vomiting due to cytotoxics)
cannabinoids (nabilone)	
benzodiazepines (lorazepam)	

and in the gastrointestinal tract. Phenothiazines and butyrophenones owe their antiemetic efficacy to blockade of *dopamine D_2* receptors but they readily penetrate the brain and may produce unwanted extrapyramidal effects by blocking D_2 receptors in the basal ganglia; many also have antimuscarinic effects.

Metoclopramide

Metoclopramide acts *centrally* by blocking dopamine D_2 receptors in the CTZ, and *peripherally* by enhancing the action of acetylcholine at muscarinic nerve endings in the gut. It raises the tone of the lower oesophageal sphincter, relaxes the pyloric antrum and duodenal cap and increases peristalsis and emptying of the upper gut. The peripheral actions are utilised to empty the stomach before emergency anaesthesia and in labour. If an opioid has been given, metoclopramide may fail to overcome the opioid-induced inhibition of gastric emptying and thus the risk of vomiting and inhaling gastric contents remains. The direct effects on the gut are antagonised by antimuscarinic drugs. The action of metoclopramide is terminated by metabolism in the liver ($t_{1/2}$ 4 h).

Uses. Metoclopramide is used for nausea and vomiting associated with gastrointestinal disorders, and with cytotoxic drugs and radiotherapy. It is also an effective antiemetic in migraine and is used as a prokinetic agent (see above).

Adverse reactions are characteristic of dopamine receptor antagonists and include extrapyramidal dystonia (torticollis, facial spasms, trismus, oculogyric crises) which occurs more commonly in children and young adults, and in those who are concurrently receiving other dopamine receptor antagonists, e.g. phenothiazine drugs. The antimuscarinic drug, benzatropine, given i.v., rapidly abolishes the reaction. Long-term use of metoclopramide may cause tardive dyskinesia in the elderly. Metoclopramide stimulates prolactin release and may cause gynaecomastia and lactation. Restlessness and diarrhoea may also occur.

Domperidone is a selective dopamine D_2 receptor antagonist; unlike metoclopramide it does not possess an acetylcholine-like effect. The $t\frac{1}{2}$ is 7 h. Dopamine does not readily penetrate the blood–brain barrier; this does not limit its therapeutic efficacy, for the CTZ is functionally outwith the barrier, but there is less risk of adverse effects in the central nervous system. Domperidone is used for nausea or vomiting associated with gastrointestinal disorders and with cytotoxic and other drug treatment. It can also be helpful in management of bloating in patients with nonulcer dyspepsia (see above). It may cause gynaecomastia and galactorrhoea.

Ondansetron is a selective 5-HT$_3$ receptor antagonist. Drugs with this activity appear to be highly effective against nausea and vomiting induced by cytotoxic agents and radiotherapy. Evidence suggests that such anticancer treatment releases serotonin (5-HT) from enterochromaffin cells in the gut mucosa (where resides > 80% of the serotonin in the body) which activates specific receptors in the gut and central nervous system to cause emesis.[6] The action of ondansetron is thus partly central and partly peripheral. Ondansetron may be given by i.v.

[6] Cubeddu L X et al 1990 New England Journal of Medicine 322: 810.

injection or infusion immediately prior to cancer chemotherapy (notably with cisplatin), followed by oral administration for up to 5 days ($t\frac{1}{2}$ 5 h). The drug appears to be well tolerated but constipation, headache and a feeling of flushing in the head and epigastrium may occur. *Granisetron* and *tropisetron* are similar.

Nabilone is a synthetic cannabinoid and has properties similar to tetrahydrocannabinol (the active constituent of marijuana) which has an antiemetic action. It is used to relieve nausea or vomiting caused by cytotoxic drugs. Adverse effects include: somnolence, dry mouth, decreased appetite, dizziness, euphoria, dysphoria, postural hypotension, confusion and psychosis. These may be reduced if prochlorperazine is given concomitantly.

Treatment for various forms of sickness

MOTION SICKNESS

Motion sickness is more easily prevented than cured. It is due chiefly to overstimulation of the vestibular apparatus (and does not occur if the labyrinth is destroyed). Other factors also contribute. Visually, a moving horizon can be most disturbing, as can the sensations induced by the gravitational inertia of a full stomach when the body is in vertical movement. That the environment, whether close and smelly or open and vivifying, is important, is a matter of common experience amongst all who have been on a rough sea. Psychological factors, including observation of the fate of one's companions, are also important. Tolerance to the motion occurs, generally over a period of days.

Drugs that are used for motion sickness include the antimuscarinic agents *cinnarizine*, *cyclizine*, *dimenhydrinate*, *hyoscine* and *promethazine*.

For prophylaxis an antiemetic is best taken 1 h before exposure to the motion. About 70% protection may be expected by the right dose given at the right time. Once motion sickness has started, oral administration of drugs may fail, and the i.m., s.c.

or rectal routes are required. Alternatively, hyoscine may be administered as a dermal patch, so avoiding the enteral route. Prevention of symptoms may therefore be possible only at the expense of troublesome unwanted effects: sleepiness, dry mouth, blurred vision.

DRUG-INDUCED VOMITING

If reducing the dose or withdrawing the offending drug are not options then an attempt, often unsatisfactory, may be made to oppose it by another drug. In general, *chlorpromazine* or another phenothiazine or *metoclopramide* is best. Opioid-induced vomiting responds to one of the drugs used for motion sickness (see above); cyclizine and morphine are combined as Cyclimorph.

VOMITING DUE TO CYTOTOXIC DRUGS

Prevention and alleviation of this distressing and often very severe symptom of some forms of cancer treatment may allow an optimal chemotherapeutic regimen to be used, and avoid admitting the patient to hospital. Cisplatin is notably emetic. *Ondansetron* (see above) is highly effective and *dexamethasone* is also efficacious although its mode of action is unclear. *Lorazepam,* despite dose-limiting sedation and dysphoria, is a useful adjunct and provides amnesia which may limit the development of anticipatory vomiting. For severe vomiting due to cytotoxics, ondansetron plus dexamethasone with or without lorazepam (all given i.v.) is the most effective combination and is well tolerated. Metoclopramide may be substituted for ondansetron where a less emetic regimen is used, especially in older patients who are less susceptible to its extrapyramidal reactions.

VOMITING AFTER GENERAL ANAESTHESIA

Postoperative vomiting is related to the duration of anaesthesia and has many causes. *Metoclopramide,* a 5-HT_3 receptor antagonist, e.g. *ondansetron* or a butyrophenone, e.g. *haloperidol* or droperidol, may be used. The condition affects some 30% of patients

and routine prophylaxis seems warranted only where the risk is high, e.g. those with a history of postoperative vomiting or of motion sickness, or where vomiting carries special hazard, e.g. eye surgery.

VOMITING IN PREGNANCY

This reaches a peak at 10–11 weeks and usually resolves by 13–14 weeks of gestation. Nausea alone does not require treatment. Much can be achieved by reassurance that the problem is transient and a discussion of diet, e.g. taking food before getting up in the morning. Rarely, a decision is taken to use a drug, and then a histamine H_1 receptor antagonist or a phenothiazine, e.g. promethazine (see above) is preferred. Although pyridoxine deficiency has not been shown to complicate simple pregnancy vomiting, it may occur in hyperemesis gravidarum which requires i.v. fluids and multivitamin supplement.

VERTIGO

A great range of drugs has been recommended to treat vertigo and labyrinthine disorders but antimuscarinics and phenothiazines are generally preferred. Cyclizine or prochlorperazine may be used to relieve an acute attack. *Betahistine* (a histamine analogue) is used in the hope of improving the blood circulation to the inner ear in Menière's syndrome; also cinnarizine.

GUIDE TO FURTHER READING

Agreus L, Talley N 1997 Challenges in managing dyspepsia in general practice. British Medical Journal 315: 1284–1288

Blaser M J 1998 Helicobacter pylori and gastric diseases. British Medical Journal 316: 1507–1510

Cohen S, Parkman H P 1995 Treatment of achalasia — from whalebone to botulinum toxin. New England Journal of Medicine 332: 815–816

Costa S H, Vessey M P 1993 Misoprostol and illegal abortion in Rio de Janeiro, Brazil. Lancet 341: 1258–1261

Danesh J, Pounder R E 2000 Eradication of *Helicobacter pylori* and non-ulcer dyspepsia. Lancet 355: 766–767

De Boer W A, Tytgat G N J 2000 Treatment of *Helicobacter pylori infection.* British Medical Journal 320: 31–34

Fisher R S, Parkman H P 1998 Management of nonulcer dyspepsia. New England Journal of Medicine 339: 1376–1381

Fox J G, Wang T C 2001 *Helicobacter pylori* — not a good bug after all. New England Journal of Medicine 345: 829–832

Galmiche J P et al 1998 Treatment of gastro-oesophageal reflux disease in adults. British Medical Journal 316: 1720–1723

Grunberg S M, Hesketh P J 1994 Control of chemotherapy-induced emesis. New England Journal of Medicine 329: 1790

Mittal R K, Balaban D H 1997 The esophagogastric junction. New England Journal of Medicine 336: 924–932

32

Intestines

SYNOPSIS

Problems of constipation, diarrhoea and irritable bowel syndrome are common. Infective diarrhoeal diseases are a significant cause of morbidity and mortality worldwide, especially in infants and children. The management of these conditions is reviewed.

- Constipation: mode of action and use of drugs
- Diarrhoea (drug treatment importance of fluid and electrolyte replacement)
- Inflammatory bowel disease
- Irritable bowel syndrome

Constipation

The terms purgative, cathartic, laxative, aperient and evacuant are synonymous. They are medicines that promote defaecation largely by reducing the viscosity of the contents of the lower colon and are classified as follows:

- Stool bulking agents
- Osmotic laxatives
- Faecal softeners
- Stimulant laxatives.

STOOL BULKING AGENTS

Dietary fibre comprises the cell walls and supporting structures of vegetables and fruits. Most of the fibre in our diet is in the form of nonstarch poly-saccharides (NSP),[1] which are not digestible by human enzymes. Fibre may be soluble (pectins, guar, ispaghula) or insoluble (cellulose, hemicelluloses, lignin). Insoluble fibre has less effect than soluble fibre on the viscosity of gut contents but is a stronger laxative because it resists digestion in the small bowel and so enters the colon intact. In addition it has a vast capacity for retaining water; thus one gram of carrot fibre can hold 23 grams of water.[2] It has been proposed that as humans have refined the carbohydrates in their diet over the centuries, so they have deprived themselves of fibre, the ensuing *under-filling* of the colon being an important cause of constipation, haemorrhoids and diverticular disease. Stool bulking agents, which add fibre to the diet, are the treatment of choice for simple constipation. They act by increasing the volume and lowering the viscosity of intestinal contents to produce a soft bulky stool, which encourages normal reflex bowel activity. The mode of action of stool bulking agents is thus more physiological than other types of laxative. They

---

[1] The term 'unavailable complex carbohydrate' (UCC) is also used and refers to NSP plus undigested ('resistant') starch.
[2] McConnell A A et al 1974 J Sci Food Agric 25: 1427.

should be taken with liberal quantities of fluid (at least 2 litres daily).

Individual preparations

Bran is the residue left when flour is made from cereals; it contains between 25% and 50% of fibre. The fibre content of a normal diet can be increased by eating wholemeal bread and bran cereals but over-zealous supplementation may cause troublesome wind (from bacterial fermentation in the colon).

Viscous (soluble) fibres, e.g. ispaghula, are effective and more palatable than bran. *Ispaghula husk* contains mucilage and hemicelluloses which swell rapidly in water. *Methylcellulose* takes up water to swell to a colloid about 25 times its original volume and *sterculia,*[3] similarly, swells when mixed with water.

OSMOTIC LAXATIVES

These are but little absorbed and increase the bulk and reduce viscosity of intestinal contents to promote a fluid stool.

Some inorganic salts retain water in the intestinal lumen or, if given as hypertonic solution, withdraw it from the body. When constipation is mild, *magnesium hydroxide* will suffice but *magnesium sulphate* (Epsom[4] salts) is used when a more powerful effect is needed. Both magnesium salts act in 2–4 h. The small amount of magnesium absorbed when the sulphate is frequently used can be enough to cause magnesium poisoning in patients with renal impairment, the central nervous effects of which somewhat resemble those of uraemia. Magnesium sulphate 50% (hypertonic) is available as a single dose retention enema to reduce cerebrospinal fluid pressure in neurosurgery.

Lactulose is a synthetic disaccharide. Taken orally, it is unaffected by small intestinal disaccharidases, is not absorbed and thus acts as an osmotic laxative. Tolerance may develop. Lactulose is also used in

the treatment of hepatic encephalopathy (see Chapter 33).

Osmotic laxatives are frequently used to clear the colon for diagnostic procedures or surgery. Enemas containing phosphate or citrate effectively evacuate the distal colon and can be useful for treating obstinate constipation in elderly or debilitated patients. Oral preparations containing magnesium sulphate and citric acid (Citramag) or polyethylene glycol (Klean Prep) are used in preparation for colonoscopy; they are made up with water to create an isotonic solution and some patients find the large volumes difficult to tolerate. Isotonic mannitol was used for the same purpose in the early days of colonoscopy, but has since been abandoned; hydrogen liberated by the action of colonic bacteria was the cause of several intestinal explosions triggered by the use of diathermy. The stimulant laxative sodium picosulphate (Picolax) is a frequently used alternative to the osmotic preparations. Care should be used with all these preparations in the elderly; they can induce dehydration, hypovolaemia and electrolyte disturbances.

FAECAL SOFTENERS (EMOLLIENTS)

The softening properties of these agents are useful in the management of anal fissure (see below) and haemorrhoids.

Docusate sodium (dioctyl sodium sulphosuccinate) softens faeces by lowering the surface tension of fluids in the bowel. This allows more water to remain in the faeces. It appears also to have bowel stimulant properties but these are relatively weak. Docusate sodium acts in 1–2 days. Poloxamers, e.g. poloxalkol (poloxamer 188), act similarly and are used in combination with other agents.

Liquid paraffin is a chemically inert mineral oil and is not digested. It promotes the passage of softer faeces. It is often presented in emulsions with magnesium hydroxide. Large doses may leak out of the anus causing both physical and social discomfort. Paraffin taken orally over long periods, especially at night, may be aspirated and cause chronic lipoid pneumonia. An unusual case resulted from attempts by a patient, an amateur singer, to lubricate his larynx with liquid paraffin. Because of

---

[3] Named after Sterculinus, a god of ancient Rome, who presided over manuring of agricultural land.
[4] Epsom, a town near London, known for its now defunct mineral spring water, and for horse racing.

these disadvantages its use is declining and it should never be used long term as a laxative.

STIMULANT LAXATIVES

These drugs increase intestinal motility by various mechanisms; they may cause abdominal cramps, should used only with caution in pregnancy, and never where intestinal obstruction is suspected.

Bisacodyl stimulates sensory endings in the colon by direct action from the lumen. It is effective orally in 6–10 h and, as a suppository, acts in 1 h. In geriatric patients, bisacodyl suppositories reduce the need for regular enemas. There are no important unwanted effects.

Sodium picosulphate is similar and is also used to evacuate the bowel for investigative procedures and surgery.

Glycerol has a mild stimulant effect on the rectum when administered as a suppository.

The anthraquinone group of laxatives includes senna, danthron, cascara, rhubarb[5] and aloes. In the small intestine soluble anthraquinone derivates are liberated and absorbed. These are excreted into the colon and act there, along with those that have escaped absorption, probably after being chemically changed by bacterial action.

Patients taking some anthraquinones may notice their urine coloured brown (if acid) or red (if alkaline). Prolonged use can cause melanosis of the colon.

Anthraquinone preparations made from crude plant extracts are to be avoided as their lack of standardisation leads to erratic results.

Senna, available as a biologically standardised preparation, is widely used to relieve constipation and to empty the bowel for investigative procedures and surgery. It acts in 8–12 h.

Danthron is available as a standardised preparation in combination with the faecal softeners poloxamer 188 (co-danthramer) and docusate sodium (as co-danthrusate). It acts in 6–12 h. Evidence from rodent studies indicates a possible carcinogenic risk and long-term exposure to danthron should be avoided.

Drastic purgatives (castor oil, cascara, jalap,[6] colocynth, phenolphthalein and podophyllum) are obsolete.

Suppositories and enemas

Suppositories (bisacodyl, glycerin) may be used to obtain a bowel action in about 1 hour. Enemas produce defaecation by softening faeces and distending the bowel. They are used in preparation for surgery, radiological examination and endoscopy.[7] Preparations with sodium phosphate, which is poorly absorbed and so retains water in the gut, are generally used. Arachis oil is included in enemas to soften impacted faeces.

Misuse of laxatives

Dependence (abuse) may arise following laxative use during an illness or in pregnancy, or the individual may have the mistaken notion that a daily bowel motion is essential for health, or that

---

[5] In the late 18th century Britain made approaches to trade with China which were met with indifference; it seems that the mandarins held the belief that the British feared death from constipation if deprived of rhubarb *(Rheum palmatum)*, one of China's exports.

[6] In the 19th century 'young men proceeding to Africa' were advised to take pills named Livingstone's Rousers, consisting of rhubarb, jalap, calomel and quinine. British Medical Journal 1964 2: 1583.

[7] Enemas may arouse complex psychosocial/sexual impulses ranging from frequent use for imagined self-cleansing (colonic lavage) to the extraordinary case of the 'Illinois enema bandit' (USA, 1966–75), a man who broke into women students' accommodation and forcibly administered enemas. His exploits were immortalised in song by Frank Zappa (© 1978 Zappa Family Trust. Reprinted by permission):
'The Illinois Enema Bandit
I heard he's on the loose
I heard he's on the loose
Lord, the pitiful screams
Of all them college-educated women…
Boy, he'd just be tyin' 'em up
(They'd be all bound down!)
Just be pumpin' every one of 'em up with all the bag fulla
The Illinois Enema Bandit Juice…'

the bowels are only incompletely opened by nature, and so indulge in regular purgation. This effectively prevents the easy return of normal habits because the more powerful stimulant purges empty the whole colon, whereas normal defaecation empties only the descending colon. Cessation of use after a few weeks is thus inevitably followed by a few days' constipation whilst sufficient material collects to restore the normal state; the delay may convince the patient of the continued need for purgatives. Laxative dependence, which may be solely emotional at first, may be followed by *physical dependence,* so that the bowels will not open without a purgative. Prolonged abuse can damage gut nerves and lead to an atonic colon.

It is easier to prevent laxative dependence than to cure it; patients feel they understand their own bowels far better than anyone else possibly could, an opinion they seldom extend to other organs, except perhaps the liver. In Britain, there is a belief that nurses have an intuitive understanding of the bowels that is denied to doctors.

Excessive use of stimulant purgatives[8] may, especially in the old, lead to severe water and electrolyte depletion, even to hypokalaemic paralysis, malabsorption and protein-losing enteropathy. Purgatives are dangerous if given to patients with undiagnosed abdominal pain, inflammatory bowel disease or obstruction. Nor should they be used to empty the rectum of hardened faeces, for they will fail and cause pain. Initial treatment should be with enemas, but digital removal, generally ordered by a senior and performed by a junior doctor, may occasionally be required. A bulking agent or a faecal softener will help to prevent recurrence.

Diarrhoea

Diarrhoea ranges from a mild and socially inconvenient illness to a major cause of death and malnutrition among children in less developed countries; acute diarrhoea from gastroenteritis causes 4–5 million deaths throughout the world annually. Drugs have a place in its management but the first priority of therapy is to preserve fluid and electrolyte balance.

SOME PHYSIOLOGY

In the normal adult, 7–8 litres of of water and electrolytes are secreted daily into the gastrointestinal tract. This, together with dietary fluid, is absorbed by epithelial cells in the small and large bowel. Water follows the osmotic gradients which result from shifts of electrolytes across the intestinal epithelium, and sodium and chloride transport mechanisms are central to the causation and management of diarrhoea, especially that caused by bacteria and viruses. The energy for the process is provided by the activity of Na^+/K^+ ATPase.

Absorption of sodium into the epithelium is effected by:

- *Sodium-glucose-coupled entry.* Glucose stimulates the absorption of sodium and the resulting water flow also sweeps additional sodium and chloride along with it *(solvent drag).* This important mechanism remains active in diarrhoea of various aetiologies and improvement of sodium and water absorption by glucose (and amino acids) is the basis of oral rehydration regimens (see below). Absorption of sodium and water in the colon is stimulated by short-chain fatty acids (see below, cereal-based ORT).
- *Sodium-ion-coupled entry.* Na^+ and Cl^- enter the epithelial cell, either as a pair or, as seems more likely, there is a double exchange: Na^+ (extracellular) with H^+ (intracellular) and Cl^- (extracellular) with $2OH^-$ or $2HCO_3^-$ (intracellular). Oral rehydration solutions (see below) contain sodium, chloride and bicarbonate.

Secretion is the opposite process to that of absorption. In response to various stimuli, crypt cells actively transport chloride into the gut lumen and sodium and water follow. This stimulus-secretion coupling is modulated by cyclic AMP and GMP, calcium, prostaglandins and leukotrienes.

---

[8] The Roman Emperor Nero (AD 37–68) murdered his severely constipated aunt by ordering the doctors to give her 'a laxative of fatal strength'. He 'seized her property before she was quite dead and tore up the will so that nothing could escape him'. (Suetonius (trans) R Graves).

Diarrhoea results from an imbalance between secretion and reabsorption of fluid and electrolytes; it has numerous causes, including infections with enteric organisms (which may stimulate secretion or damage absorption), inflammatory bowel disease and nutrient malabsorption due to disease. It also commonly occurs as a manifestation of disordered gut motility in the absence of demonstrable disease (see below). Rarely it is due to secretory tumours of the alimentary tract, e.g. carcinoid tumour or vipoma (a tumour which secretes VIP, vasoactive intestinal peptide).

Motility patterns in the bowel. An important factor in diarrhoea may be loss of the normal segmenting contractions that delay passage of contents, so that an occasional peristaltic wave has a greater propulsive effect. Segmental contractions of the smooth muscle in the bowel mix the intestinal contents. Patients with diarrhoea commonly have less spontaneous segmenting activity in the sigmoid colon than do people with normal bowel habit, and patients with constipation have more. Antimotility drugs (see below) reduce diarrhoea by increasing segmentation and inhibiting peristalsis.

FLUID AND ELECTROLYTE TREATMENT

Oral rehydration therapy (ORT) with glucose-electrolyte solution is sufficient to treat the vast majority of episodes of watery diarrhoea from acute gastroenteritis. As a simple, effective, cheap and readily administered therapy for a potentially lethal condition, ORT must rank as a major advance in therapy. It is effective because glucose-coupled sodium transport continues during diarrhoea and so enhances replacement of water and electrolyte losses in the stool.

Oral rehydration salts (ORS) The WHO/UNICEF recommended formulation is:

Sodium chloride	3.5 g/l
Potassium chloride	1.5 g/l
Sodium citrate	2.9 g/l
Anhydrous glucose	20.0 g/l

This provides sodium 90 mmol/l, potassium 20 mmol/l, chloride 80 mmol/l, citrate 10 mmol/l, glucose 111 mmol/l (total osmolarity 311 mmol/l).[9]

Several other formulations exist, some with less sodium (see national formularies).[10]

Rehydration therapy with commercial soft drinks alone will fail because their sodium content is too low (usually less than 4 mmol/l). The glucose may be replaced by another substrate such as glycine or rice powder. Indeed *cereal-based* ORS, relying on starch (to produce glucose) from many sources (rice, wheat, corn, potato) have the advantage of controlling diarrhoea much more effectively than the glucose-based preparations. This may be because undigested starch is fermented in the colon to short-chain fatty acids, which stimulate colonic sodium and water absorption. Thus almost every household in the world can find the essential components of an effective oral rehydration mixture: cereals and salt.

Most cases can be adequately treated by assiduous attention to oral intake, but fluid and electrolyte depletion is especially dangerous in children and intravenous fluid replacement in hospital may be needed. Antimotility drugs are inappropriate for severe diarrhoea in young children; any marginal effect they may have is liable to be counterbalanced by hazardous adverse effects (see below).

ANTIDIARRHOEAL DRUGS

There are two types of drug which are often used in combination.

Antimotility drugs

These act on bowel muscle to delay the passage of gut contents so allowing time for more water to be absorbed.

Codeine ($t\frac{1}{2}$ 3 h) activates opioid receptors on the smooth muscle of the bowel to reduce peristalsis and increase segmentation contractions. Tolerance may develop with prolonged use, as may dependence (rarely). It should be avoided in patients with

---

[9] Solutions with lower sodium content and thus reduced total osmolarity (250 mmol/l) are associated with less need for unscheduled intravenous fluid infusion, lower stool volume and less vomiting, and may now be preferred. Hahn S et al 2001 British Medical Journal 323: 81–85.
[10] The higher sodium content of the WHO/UNICEF formulation is based on sodium concentrations in diarrhoeal stools, but low-sodium, high-glucose formulations may be preferred for infants, whose faecal losses of sodium are less.

diverticular disease as it increases intraluminal pressure.

Diphenoxylate (t½ 3 h) is structurally related to pethidine and affects the bowel like codeine. The drug is offered mixed with a trivial dose of atropine (to discourage abuse) as co-phenotrope (Lomotil). The drug can cause nausea, vomiting, abdominal pain and CNS depression. Following overdose with Lomotil respiratory depression may be serious, and can occur up to 16 h after ingestion because gastric emptying is delayed.

Loperamide (t½ 10 h) is structurally similar to diphenoxylate. Its precise mode of action remains obscure but it impairs propulsion of gut contents by effects on intestinal circular and longitudinal muscle that are at least partly due to an action on opioid receptors. Loperamide may cause nausea, vomiting and abdominal cramps. Its potential for abuse appears to be low.

The actions of codeine, diphenoxylate and loperamide are antagonised by naloxone.

Warning. Antimotility drugs should not be used for acute diarrhoea in children, especially babies, or in patients with active inflammatory bowel disease, for there is danger of causing paralytic ileus and, in babies, respiratory depression.

Drugs that directly increase the viscosity of gut contents

Kaolin and chalk are adsorbent powders. Their therapeutic efficacy is marginal as is shown by the fact that they are often combined with an opioid. *Bulk-forming agents* such as ispaghula, methylcellulose and sterculia (see above) are useful for diarrhoea in diverticular disease, and for reducing the fluidity of faeces in patients with ileostomy and colostomy.

TRAVELLERS' DIARRHOEA

So familiar is diarrhoea to travellers that it has acquired regional popular names: the Aztec 2-step, Montezuma's Revenge, Delhi Belly, Rangoon Runs, Tokyo Trots, Gyppy Tummy, Hong-Kong Dog, Estomac Anglais and Casablanca Crud, all indicate some of the areas deemed dangerous by visitors. The Mexican name 'turista' indicates the principal sufferers.

Most cases are infective, and up to half of the diarrhoea that afflicts visitors to tropical and sub-tropical countries is associated with enterotoxigenic strains of *Escherichia coli;* other bacteria including *Shigella* and *Salmonella* spp, viruses including the Norwalk family, and parasites (particularly *Giardia lamblia*) have also been implicated. Recognition that transmission is almost invariably by ingestion of contaminated food and water points to the most effective way of reducing the risk.

Acute watery diarrhoea *in adults* can usually be controlled by oral rehydration solutions and one of the antimotility drugs, although in mild cases the abdominal bloating produced by the latter may be less acceptable than the loose stools. While diarrhoea usually lasts only 2–3 days, this may still be socially inconvenient, and if symptomatic remedies fail, an aminoquinolone, e.g. ciprofloxacin 500 mg b.d. will be effective. The use of antimicrobials for travellers' diarrhoea continues to evoke controversy (see below) but most sufferers will appreciate the relief that even one or two tablets can bring.

Prophylactic antimicrobial therapy has been shown to reduce the incidence of attacks of diarrhoea but its routine use carries the risk of hindering the diagnosis of serious infection. A wider issue is the possible development and spread of antibiotic-resistant organisms. Thus any benefits to the individual must be weighed against the risk to *the community* in the future. In most instances prophylactic antimicrobials should not be used but ciprofloxacin (500 mg once daily) may be justified for individuals who must remain well while travelling for short periods to high-risk areas.

SPECIFIC INFECTIVE DIARRHOEAS

Chemotherapy is available for certain specific organisms, e.g. amoebiasis, giardiasis, typhoid fever (see Index).

DRUG-INDUCED DIARRHOEA

Antimicrobials are the commonest drugs that cause diarrhoea, probably due to alteration of bowel flora. It may range from a mild inconvenience to life-threatening *antibiotic-associated* (*pseudomembranous colitis*), due to colonisation of the bowel with *Clostridium difficile*. The condition particularly affects elderly patients in hospital. Clindamycin and third generation cephalosporins are especially prone to cause this complication, whereas it is uncommon with the quinolone and aminoglycoside groups. Treatment is with vancomycin or metronidazole.

Magnesium-containing antacids may also produce diarrhoea, as may NSAIDs and lithium.

SECRETORY DIARRHOEAS

Octreotide, a synthetic peptide which shares amino acid homology with somatostatin (see p. 710), inhibits the release of peptides that mediate certain alimentary secretions, and may be used to relieve diarrhoea due to carcinoid tumours and vipomas.

Inflammatory bowel disease

The pathogenesis of inflammatory bowel disease is still poorly understood. Immune mechanisms are probably involved, and potential antigens include intestinal bacteria and intestinal epithelium. Abnormalities in inflammatory mediators have also been described; it has been suggested that an imbalance between proinflammatory and anti-inflammatory cytokines may determine susceptibility, although the abnormalities observed could simply be secondary to the disease process.

The main drugs used in the treatment of ulcerative colitis and Crohn's disease are the *aminosalicylates* and *corticosteroids*. Their mode of action is obscure. Other immunosuppressives also have a role and recent studies into the mechanisms of inflammation are leading to the introduction of novel therapies to inhibit the inflammatory process.

In acute exacerbations of inflammatory bowel disease a gastrointestinal infection should always be excluded by stool microscopy and culture, and testing for *Clostridium difficile* toxin. Measures to correct anaemia, fluid and electrolyte abnormalities and to improve the general nutritional state are also important. Antidiarrhoeals should be used with extreme caution in active colitis and are contra-indicated if the disease is severe. They can lead to toxic dilatation of the colon, with perforation.

ULCERATIVE COLITIS

Aminosalicylates

Aminosalicylates maintain remission in patients with ulcerative colitis (relapses are reduced by a factor of 3), and may also be used for treatment of an acute attack (corticosteroids may also be needed).

Sulfasalazine (salicylazosulfapyridine, Salazopyrin) consists of two compounds, sulpha-pyridine and 5-aminosalicylic acid, joined by an azo-bond. Sulfasalazine is poorly absorbed from the small intestine and colonic bacteria split the azo-bond to release the component parts. The therapeutically active moiety is 5-aminosalicylic acid (5-ASA). Sulphapyridine is well absorbed, is acetylated in the liver and excreted in the urine; it has no therapeutic action in colitis but contributes to a mechanism for delivering 5-ASA to the colon.

Sulfasalazine is also used as a disease-modifying agent in rheumatoid arthritis (see p. 292), the condition for which it was originally introduced in the 1930s. It is available as a tablet, retention enema or suppository.

Adverse effects are due largely to the sulph-onamide moiety and include headache, malaise, anorexia, nausea and vomiting; these are dose-related and commoner in slow acetylators (of the sulphonamide). Allergic reactions include rash, fever and lymphadenitis; rarely leucopenia and agranulo-cytosis occur. Males may become infertile due to oligospermia and reduced sperm motility; this reverses if salazopyrin is replaced with mesalazine.

Mesalazine. Patients intolerant of salazopyrin usually tolerate mesalazine, which is 5-ASA. Mesalazine is absorbed rapidly and completely in the upper jejunum, and is presented in various formulations which delay its release. *Asacol* tablets are coated in a resin, which dissolves only at a pH of 7 or higher, favouring its release in the ileum and colon. In contrast *Pentasa* has a slow-release but pH independent coating so that 5-ASA is liberated throughout the gastrointestinal tract. 5-ASA that enters the blood is rapidly cleared by acetylation in the liver and renal excretion. In addition to oral formulations, mesalazine is available as an enema.

The profile of adverse effects includes nausea, abdominal pain, watery diarrhoea (which can lead to diagnostic confusion in patients with inflammatory bowel disease) and interstitial nephritis. Renal function should be monitored regularly in patients taking 5-ASA, particularly preparations extensively released in the small intestine.

Two other 5-ASA preparations effectively delay release of the active moiety until the preparation reaches the colon: **Olsalazine** is two molecules of 5-ASA acid linked by an azo-bond, while **balsalazide** comprises one molecule of 5-ASA acid linked by an azo-bond to an inert carrier. 5-ASA is liberated after cleavage of the azo-bonds by colonic bacteria.

Corticosteroids

Enemas and suppositories. When ulcerative colitis is restricted to the *left hemicolon,* exacerbations that do not respond to an aminosalicylate alone can often be controlled by steroid enemas. Properly administered, these will reach the splenic flexure, and for this to occur the patient should be instructed to lie down for at least 30 minutes after insertion of the enema. The foam-based preparations appear to coat the colonic mucosa more efficiently than the aqueous formulations.

In patients with disease limited to the distal few centimetres of the rectum, steroid enemas may be ineffective because they will be delivered proximal to the inflamed segment. In this situation steroid suppositories are often helpful. Patients with distal colitis are prone to faecal loading above the inflamed segment and this can lead to overflow diarrhoea and worsening of inflammation. Faecal loading can be detected on straight abdominal x-ray and is treated with laxatives; this is safe provided the inflammatory process is restricted to the distal colon. On no account should antidiarrhoeals be used as these will exacerbate the problem. Adequate quantities of dietary fibre and fluid should be encouraged, and stool bulking agents can also be helpful in protecting against faecal loading.

Systemic corticosteroid. *Moderately severe attacks* of ulcerative colitis should be treated with *systemic* corticosteroid, and oral preparations usually suffice. It is important to give enough drug to bring the inflammatory process under control (starting dose prednisolone 60 mg/d). A response should start within 10–14 d and if it does not the patient should be admitted to hospital for more intensive treatment including intravenous corticosteroid. Once remission has been attained the dose can be tailed down over a period of 6–8 weeks. It is important not to do this too quickly; the rapidly tailing regimes used for treating asthma are not appropriate for inflammatory bowel disease.

Severe attacks of ulcerative colitis should be treated in hospital with intravenous corticosteroid. The main danger is toxic dilatation of the colon and perforation, which can occur insidiously. Regular measurements of abdominal girth and straight x-ray of the abdomen are useful in monitoring response, which should be seen within 72 h. If there is no improvement a trial of ciclosporin (see below) may induce response. Treatment otherwise is by emergency colectomy.

Ciclosporin may induce remission in some patients with severe ulcerative colitis unresponsive to corticosteroid. The drug is given in a dose of 2–4 mg/kg i.v. until remission is attained. Renal function should be monitored closely as ciclosporin is nephrotoxic (see p. 620). For maintenance therapy *azathioprine* (see below) is often substituted. Ciclosporin use only delays surgery for many patients; after 1 year 50% will have relapsed and undergone colectomy.

Smoking aggravates Crohn's disease but (perversely) improves ulcerative colitis. Nicotine patches may provide benefit in ulcerative colitis but the effect is not sufficiently great to justify their routine use in management.

Maintenance of remission

Corticosteroids can be reduced slowly (see above) and maintenance therapy with an aminosalicylate started. If the disease is corticosteroid dependent, azathioprine or another immunosuppressive agent may be used (see below). Surgery is indicated if medical therapy fails to control the disease or is associated with unacceptable adverse effects.

CROHN'S DISEASE

Treatment depends on the site of disease. Management of *colonic* Crohn's disease is very similar to that of ulcerative colitis, with aminosalicylate and corticosteroid. These drugs are of less value in maintaining remission in Crohn's disease than in ulcerative colitis, although they do help to reduce recurrence of disease at sites of surgical anastamoses. Topical enema preparations are less useful because of the patchy distribution of inflammation and rectal sparing.

In contrast to ulcerative colitis, about 50% of patients with Crohn's colitis will respond to *metronidazole* given for up to 3 months, although adverse effects including alcohol intolerance, and peripheral neuropathy from such prolonged therapy often limit its use. The drug is also helpful in controlling perianal and small bowel disease and it decreases the incidence of anastamotic recurrence after surgery. Other antimicrobials, particularly *ciprofloxacin* may also be effective.

Crohn's disease of the *small bowel* classically affects the ileocaecal region, although any part of the gastrointestinal tract may be involved, from the mouth downwards. Patients with small bowel involvement are frequently malnourished and specialist dietetic input is essential; enteral or parenteral nutrition may be required. Osteoporosis is common, particularly if corticosteroid consumption has been high.

Sulfasalazine, olsalazine and balsalazide are ineffective in small bowel Crohn's disease because these drugs are designed to liberate 5-ASA in the colon. Mesalazine preparations release 5-ASA higher in the gut and control mild to moderate exacerbations of ileocaecal disease in approximately 50% of patients, although high doses are needed (Asacol 2.4 g in divided doses, Pentasa 2 g b.d.).

In *more severe disease* corticosteroids are needed to induce remission (prednisolone 60 mg/day until remission induced, tailing the dose by 5 mg/week). Approximately 75% of patients respond. Budesonide, a potent topically active corticosteroid, is an alternative which can be administered either orally or as an enema. The oral preparation is presented as a delayed release formulation which delivers drug to the terminal ileum and ascending colon. Extensive first pass metabolism in the liver limits its systemic availability and potential for adverse effects. Budesonide is also useful as maintenance therapy of the 30% of patients with Crohn's disease who are steroid dependent.

Maintenance of remission may require addition of azathioprine or another immunosuppressive drug (see below). Tobacco smoking definitely contributes to relapse and should be strongly discouraged.

Crohn's disease may be complicated by intestinal strictures, fistulae and intra-abdominal abscesses. Surgery is often necessary but strictures may be amenable to endoscopic balloon dilatation and abscesses can be drained under radiographic control.

Dietary therapy

There is evidence that liquid diets based on amino-acids (elemental diets) or oligopeptides for 4–6 weeks are as effective as corticosteroids in controlling Crohn's disease although relapse is common when the treatment stops. Elemental preparations are not particularly palatable and they often have to be administered through a nasogastric tube, which is not popular with patients. They are worth trying in steroid resistant cases, and are particularly favoured by paediatricians who prefer to avoid adrenal steroid because of its adverse effects on growth.

Antibodies to tumour necrosis factor (TNF)

TNFα causes activation of immune cells and release of inflammatory mediators. The inhibitors of TNF, infliximab and etanercept (see p. 293), have been found to benefit Crohn's disease. A single dose of anti-TNFα will induce remission in approximately one-third of patients with Crohn's disease resistant to conventional therapies, with improvement in a further third. A further dose after 8 weeks appears to produce longer lasting remissions. This treatment is also useful in treating Crohn's fistulae. Adverse reactions include headache, nausea and malaise; repeat infusions after prolonged intervals (1–2 years) may lead to hypersensitivity reactions. Its efficacy and potential for adverse effects in the long term (including development of malignancy) remain to be established. There is no good evidence that anti-TNFα antibodies are effective for ulcerative colitis.

Immunosuppressive drugs

Azathioprine is effective as a steroid sparing agent in maintenance therapy of Crohn's disease. Use of this drug in a dose of up to 2 mg/kg may allow corticosteroid to be withdrawn altogether. It is also used for the same purpose in ulcerative colitis although evidence for its efficacy in this disorder is less persuasive. As the onset of action of azathioprine is delayed for about 8 weeks, it is not effective for inducing remission, and reduction in steroid dose in the first few weeks of azathioprine treatment may lead to relapse. Azathioprine can cause bone marrow suppression and the blood count should be monitored weekly for the first two months of therapy and every 2 months thereafter for as long as the drug is taken.

Intolerance of azathioprine is shown by malaise, abdominal discomfort and sometimes fever. Pancreatitis occurs in up to 5%. These effects are usually due to the imidazole side chain of the molecule, and *mercaptopurine* (which is azathioprine without the side chain) may be better tolerated. The dose is 1–1.5 mg/kg.

Ciclosporin. There is no good evidence that ciclosporin is effective in Crohn's disease.

Methotrexate can be helpful in controlling relapses of Crohn's disease unresponsive to corticosteroid or azathioprine. It has also been used with benefit in ulcerative colitis. Its short- and long-term use are limited by a wide profile of adverse effects including bone marrow suppression and pulmonary and hepatic fibrosis (see p. 291).

Other conditions

MICROSCOPIC COLITIS

This condition presents with diarrhoea: the colonic mucosa is macroscopically normal but histologically shows either lymphocytic infiltration of the mucosa (lymphocytic colitis) or subendothelial fibrosis (collagenous colitis). Treatment with aminosalicylate induces remission in about 50% and corticosteroid may also be needed.

BILE SALT MALABSORPTION

Failure of the terminal ileum to reabsorb bile salts may result from Crohn's disease, or ileal resection,

and it occurs in many patients with microscopic colitis. Bile salts in the colon cause *diarrhoea* which is relieved by colestyramine. The dose required is titrated against symptoms, starting with 8 g bd. Colestyramine can also bind to many drugs and reduce their bioavailability (see p. 131).

IRRITABLE BOWEL SYNDROME (IBS)

This condition affects 20% of the population and is the commonest reason for referral to a gastroenterologist. It is manifested by a variety of gastrointestinal symptoms including disordered bowel habit (constipation, diarrhoea or both), abdominal pain and bloating. Upper gastrointestinal symptoms manifest as nonulcer dyspepsia (see Chapter 31). All these symptoms occur in the absence of demonstrable pathology in the gastrointestinal tract, although patients with IBS often have abnormalities of gut motility. Another feature of the condition is visceral hypersensitivity; patients with IBS have lower thresholds for pain from colonic distension induced by inflating balloons placed in the bowel. A proportion of patients develop their IBS symptoms after an episode of gastroenteritis and in many emotional stress is an important precipitating factor. Associated psychopathology, with anxiety and sometimes depression, are common.

The mainstay of treatment, after investigation when appropriate, is to reassure the patient of the entirely benign nature of the disorder and the good prognosis. Those with predominant *constipation* should be encouraged to increase the fluid and fibre content of their diet. Unprocessed bran can lead to troublesome bloating and wind and a bulking agent such as ispaghula husk is often better tolerated.

Diarrhoea can be treated with an antimotility drug such as loperamide, the dose being adjusted to symptoms. Codeine phosphate is effective although it may cause sedation.

Antispasmodics (see below) are given for *abdominal pain,* although there is little objective evidence for their efficacy from controlled clinical trials. The generation of evidence is complicated by the variable nature of IBS symptoms, the patients who suffer from them, and the high rate of placebo response in this condition. There are two main classes of antispasmodic, the antimuscarinic drugs and drugs which are direct smooth muscle relaxants.

Antimuscarinic drugs

These drugs block cholinergic transmission at parasympathetic postganglionic nerve endings and cause smooth muscle to relax. The synthetic antimuscarinics *dicyclomine* and *propantheline* are probably the most useful in IBS, but therapeutic efficacy is often limited by other anticholinergic effects. The drugs are contraindicated in patients with glaucoma and prostatism, and should be avoided in patients with gastro-oesophageal reflux.

Other smooth muscle relaxants

Mebeverine is a reserpine derivative which has a direct effect on colonic muscle activity, especially, it appears, on colonic hypermotility. As it does not possess antimuscarinic activity, it does not exhibit the troublesome unwanted effects of that group of drugs.

Alverine and peppermint oil also have direct smooth muscle relaxing activity.

A trial of low dose *amitryptiline* (10–25 mg at night) is worthwhile in patients who do not respond to antispasmodics, and associated depression will be helped by conventional doses of this or other antidepressants. Relaxation therapy, hypnotherapy and cognitive behaviour therapy have a place in selected cases.

DIVERTICULAR DISEASE

Diverticular disease affects 5–10% of Western people over the age of 45; the incidence rises to 80% in those over 80. Colonic dysmotility with increased intracolonic pressure, and diets high in refined carbohydrate and low in fibre are important pathogenic factors. Some patients experience abdominal pain from dysmotility whilst others remain asymptomatic. Infection of diverticula occurs in a minority, giving potential for rupture or abscess formation.

Symptomatic diverticular disease often responds to an increase in dietary fibre, and addition of a stool bulking agent. Antispasmodic drugs are helpful in controlling the pain of colon spasm but antimotility drugs encourage stasis of bowel contents, increase intracolonic pressure, and should be avoided. *Diverticulitis* requires treatment with broad spectrum antimicrobials for 7–10 days (e.g.

ciprofloxacin and metronidazole, or ampicillin, gentamycin and metronidazole).

PROTECTION AGAINST COLON CARCINOMA

Certain drugs may develop a protective role against colonic cancer. The reasoning is based on the observation that expression of the cyclo-oxygenase isoenzyme COX-2 is increased in colon cancer tumours, and also in familial adenomatous polyposis, a premalignant condition. Evidence suggests that aspirin and other NSAIDs may exert a protective effect through inhibiting this enzyme; the protective dose of aspirin is probably higher than that used in cardiovascular disease and, clearly, any benefits must be weighed against risks from complications, notably gastrointestinal bleeding. Selective COX-2 inhibitors may possess advantage in this situation.

ANAL FISSURE

Anal fissures are often intensely painful due to sphincter spasm. Anaesthetic ointments and stool softening agents have been widely used, with surgery (lateral internal sphinterotomy) for severely affected cases, but this procedure can cause incontinence from loss of sphincter control. An alternative is topical application of nitrate which heals two-thirds of fissures. Preparations should be diluted to 0.2% as such use may be complicated by headache; tolerance can develop. Intrasphincteric injection of botulinum toxin has also been shown to be effective.

GUIDE TO FURTHER READING

Almroth S, Latham M C 1995 Rational home management of diarrhoea. Lancet 345: 709–711

Eastwood M 1995 The dilemma of laxative abuse. Lancet 346: 1115

Farrell R J, Reppercorn M A 2002 Ulcerative colitis. Lancet 359: 331–340

Ferzoco L B et al 1998 Acute diverticulitis. New England Journal of Medicine 338: 1521–1526

Goyal R K, Hirano I 1996 The enteric nervous system. New England Journal of Medicine 334: 1106–1115

Horwitz B J, Fisher R S 2001 The irritable bowel syndrome. New England Journal of Medicine 344: 1846–1850

Janne P A, Mayer R J 2000 Chemoprevention of colorectal cancer. New England Journal of Medicine 342: 1960–1968

Madoff R D 1998 Pharmacologic therapy for anal fissure. New England Journal of Medicine 338: 257

Midgley R, Kerr D 1999 Colorectal cancer. Lancet 353: 391–399

Podolsky D K 2002 Inflammatory bowel disease. New England Journal of Medicine 347: 417–430

Rabbani G H 2000 The search for a better oral rehydration solution for cholera. New England Journal of Medicine 342: 345–347

Schiller L R 2000 Pathogenesis and treatment of microscopic-colitis syndrome. Lancet 355: 1198–1199

Talky N J, Spiller R 2002 Irritable bowel syndrome: a little understood organic bowel disease? Lancet 360: 555–564

Wright N, Scott B 1997 Dietary treatment of active Crohn's disease. British Medical Journal 314: 454–455

33

Liver, biliary tract, pancreas

SYNOPSIS

The liver is the most important organ in which drugs are structurally altered. Some of the resulting metabolites may be biologically inactive, some active and some toxic (see Chapter 7). The liver is exposed to drugs in higher concentrations than are most organs because most are administered orally and are absorbed from the gastrointestinal tract. Thus the whole dose must pass through the liver to reach the systemic circulation. Because of this the liver is a vulnerable target for injury from chemicals and drugs, and disordered hepatic function is an important cause of abnormal drug handling and response.

Drugs and the liver

- Pharmacodynamic and pharmacokinetic changes
- Prescribing in liver disease
- Drug-induced liver injury
- Aspects of therapy

Bile salts and gallstones
Pancreas and drugs

Effects of liver disease

PHARMACODYNAMIC CHANGES IN LIVER DISEASE

Patients with severe liver disease characteristically show abnormal end-organ response to drugs. For example:

- CNS sensitivity to opioids, sedatives and antiepilepsy drugs is increased.
- The effect of oral anticoagulants is increased because synthesis of coagulation factors is impaired.
- Fluid and electrolyte balance are altered. Sodium retention may be more readily induced by NSAIDs or corticosteroids; ascites and oedema become more resistant to diuretics.

PHARMACOKINETIC CHANGES IN LIVER DISEASE

The liver has a large metabolic reserve, and it is only when disease becomes decompensated that important changes in drug handling occur. *Parenchymal* liver disease e.g. chronic viral or alcoholic liver disease, has more impact on hepatic drug-metabolising enzyme activity than primarily *cholestatic* conditions, e.g. primary biliary cirrhosis, although clearance of drugs eliminated mainly by biliary excretion will be impaired in the latter.

Hepatocellular injury (toxic, infectious) leads to decreased activity of drug-metabolising enzymes, which is reflected in diminished plasma clearance of drugs that are metabolised. There is much variation between patients, and often overlap with healthy subjects.

HEPATIC BLOOD FLOW AND METABOLISM

Complex changes in blood flow occur with liver disease. Resistance to hepatic portal blood flow rises in cirrhosis, and portasystemic and intrahepatic shunts reduce drug delivery to hepatocytes. The pattern of change caused by disease relates to the manner in which the healthy liver treats a drug and there are two general classes:

- *Drugs that are rapidly metabolised and highly extracted in a single pass through the liver.* Clearance of such compounds is normally limited by *hepatic blood flow* but in severe liver disease less drug is extracted from the blood as it passes through the liver due to poor liver cell function, and portasystemic shunts allow a proportion of blood to bypass the liver altogether. Therefore the predominant change in the kinetics of drugs that are given orally is *increased systemic availability.* Accordingly the initial and maintenance doses of such drugs should be smaller than usual. When liver function is severely impaired the $t_{\frac{1}{2}}$ of drugs in this class may also be lengthened.
- *Drugs that are slowly metabolised and are poorly extracted in a single pass through the liver.* The rate-limiting factor for elimination of this type of drug is *metabolic capacity,* and the major change caused by liver disease is *prolongation of $t_{\frac{1}{2}}$.* Consequently the interval between doses of such drugs may need to be lengthened, and the time to reach steady-state concentration in the plasma $(5 \times t_{\frac{1}{2}})$ is increased.

PLASMA PROTEIN-BINDING OF DRUG

Binding of drugs to albumin is reduced when plasma concentrations of the latter are low due to defective synthesis. Additionally, endogenous substances produced in liver disease may displace drugs from plasma protein binding sites. These changes provide scope to enhance the biological activity of drugs, but assume importance only for those that are extensively (> 90%) protein bound.

OTHER CONSIDERATIONS

Patients with severe decompensated liver disease usually have associated renal impairment, with obvious consequences for drugs eliminated predominantly by the kidney. Where facilities exist, dosing should be guided by plasma concentration monitoring, e.g. of theophylline, lidocaine and phenytoin.

These changes in drug response (in particular) and in disposition affect prescribing, as is now discussed.

Prescribing for patients with liver disease

If liver disease is stable and well compensated, prescribing of most drugs is safe. Particular care should attend evidence of:

- Impaired hepatic synthetic function (hypoalbuminaemia, impaired blood coagulation)
- Current or recent hepatic encephalopathy
- Fluid retention and/or renal impairment
- Drugs with
  - high hepatic extraction
  - high plasma protein binding
  - low therapeutic ratio
  - CNS depressant effect.

When a drug undergoes significant hepatic metabolism, a reasonable approach is to reduce the dose to 25–50% of normal and monitor the response carefully. The following are comments on specific examples:

CNS depressants. Sedatives, antidepressants and antiepilepsy drugs should be avoided or used with extreme caution in patients with advanced liver disease, and particularly those with current or recent hepatic encephalopathy. Enhanced sensitivity of the CNS to such drugs is well documented and adds to the pharmacokinetic changes. Treatment of alcohol withdrawal in patients with established liver disease using chlormethiazole is hazardous, especially given i.v. The temptation to give initial large doses to control agitation must be avoided because this drug, which normally has a high hepatic extraction, can readily accumulate to toxic concentrations. Chlordiazepoxide is preferred.

Analgesics. Opiates can precipitate hepatic encephalopathy in patients with decompensated liver disease. If required to control postoperative pain, doses should be reduced to 25–50% of normal. Constant intravenous infusions should be avoided if the patient is not to be insidiously overdosed. Codeine can precipitate hepatic encephalopathy by its constipating effect alone. Aspirin and other NSAIDs may exacerbate impaired renal function and fluid retention by inhibiting prostaglandin synthesis and may also precipitate gastrointestinal bleeding.

Cardiovascular drugs. Propranolol (to prevent variceal bleeding) and diuretics (to treat ascites), see below.

Gastrointestinal system. Antacids that contain large quantities of sodium can precipitate fluid retention to cause ascites. Aluminium- and calcium-based preparations cause constipation and may thereby precipitate hepatic encephalopathy, as can antimotility drugs.

Hormone preparations. Use of contraceptives should be monitored carefully in patients with cholestatic liver disease, because jaundice may be exacerbated; continued use of oral contraceptives during an attack of acute hepatitis can have the same effect. Low oestrogen preparations carry less risk of this complication.

Drug-induced liver damage

The spectrum of hepatic abnormalities caused by drugs is broad, and encompasses the whole range of liver lesions from other causes. Adverse hepatic effects of drugs, classified as elsewhere in this book (see Chapter 8) include:

TYPE A (Augmented)

Liver injury or abnormal function occurs as the dose of some drugs is increased, causing:

- *Interference with bilirubin metabolism and excretion.* Jaundice is induced selectively with minimal or no disturbance of other liver function tests; recovery ordinarily occurs on stopping the drug. Examples are:

  - C-17α-substituted steroids impair bilirubin excretion into the hepatic canaliculi; the block is biochemical not mechanical. These include synthetic anabolic steroids and oestrogens used in oral contraceptives; jaundice due to the latter is rare with the low dose formulations now preferred.
  - Rifampicin impairs hepatic uptake and excretion of bilirubin; plasma unconjugated and conjugated bilirubin may be elevated during the first 2–3 weeks of dosing.
  - Fusidic acid interferes with hepatic bilirubin excretion to cause conjugated hyperbilirubinaemia, particularly in patients with sepsis.

- *Centrilobular necrosis* due to production of reactive metabolites, from *paracetamol* in overdose and also *carbon tetrachloride* (used in dry-cleaning) and other nonmedicinal chemicals.
- *Hepatocellular necrosis* with salicylates, particularly in patients with collagen diseases, when > 2 g/d are taken.
- *Fatty change* in liver cells and *hepatic failure* with tetracyclines with high doses; this is avoided if < 2 g/day is given orally and < 1 g/day i.v.

TYPE B (Bizarre)

Many drugs can cause hepatic damage at therapeutic doses, although the incidence with any single agent is very low. Pathogenesis probably involves stimulation of metabolic pathways leading to production of hepatotoxic reactive metabolites. For some reactions immune mechanisms directed against drug metabolite-altered liver cell antigens are also likely to be involved. Patterns include:

- *Acute hepatocellular necrosis.* This reaction varies from a transient disturbance of liver function tests to acute hepatitis. It can be induced by several drugs including general anaesthetics (halothane), antiepileptics (carbamazepine, phenytoin, sodium valproate, phenobarbital), antidepressants (MAO inhibitors), antiinflammatory drugs (indomethacin, ibuprofen), antimicrobials (isoniazid, sulphonamides, nitrofurantoin) and cardiovascular drugs (methyldopa, hydralazine).

- *Cholestatic hepatitis.* The picture is of obstructive jaundice with a variable component of hepatocellular damage. This pattern is particularly associated with the *phenothiazine neuroleptics,* especially chlorpromazine. The jaundice generally occurs within the first month of therapy, its onset may be insidious or acute with abdominal pain, and can be accompanied by features suggesting allergy (see above). Recovery is usual but occasionally a picture resembling primary biliary cirrhosis (see below) may develop. Cholestatic hepatitis can also be caused by antidiabetic drugs (tolbutamide, glibenclamide, carbimazole, erythromycin and gold, chlorpropamide).

TYPE C (Continued use)

- *Benign liver tumours* may develop when synthetic C17-α-substituted gonadal steroids (e.g. anabolic steroids usually in high dose, and oral contraceptives) are used for more than 5 years; there is also increased risk of hepatocellular carcinoma, although the absolute risk of either complication is very low. These liver tumours are highly vascular and may cause recurrent or acute abdominal pain if they rupture and bleed.

- *Chronic active hepatitis* may develop with prolonged use of methyldopa, isoniazid, dantrolene and nitrofurantoin.

- *Hepatic fibrosis or cirrhosis* may be caused by therapeutic use of methotrexate, e.g. for psoriasis; in the latter case the risk is lessened by giving a large dose weekly rather than a smaller dose daily and by monitoring progress by liver biopsy after every 1.5–2 g of methotrexate. Chronic exposure to amiodarone may lead to cirrhosis; this drug can also cause an alcoholic hepatitis-like picture.

DIAGNOSIS AND MANAGEMENT OF DRUG-INDUCED LIVER INJURY

- Always bear in mind the possibility. Take a careful *drug history,* including over-the-counter and alternative complementary medicine remedies.

- In patients with *hepatitis* a viral aetiology should be excluded.

- *Cholestatic lesions,* which may resolve only slowly on drug withdrawal, have to be differentiated from other causes of obstructive jaundice, both intrahepatic and extrahepatic.

- *Underlying liver disease* can cause diagnostic confusion, e.g. the alcoholic patient receiving antituberculosis drugs. It is wise to measure liver function tests before starting treatment with any drug which has documented hepatotoxic potential.

- Liver biopsy is of only limited use in diagnosis, although certain features, e.g. eosinophil infiltration, may provide a pointer to drug-induced liver disease.

- Diagnostic challenge is extremely dangerous for hepatic reactions because it may precipitate fulminant hepatic failure; the procedure is safer for cholestatic reactions.

- Monitoring liver function tests in the early weeks of therapy is useful in detecting an impending reaction to some drugs e.g. isoniazid. Minor abnormalities (serum transaminases less than twice normal) are often self-limiting and progress can be monitored. Elevations greater than three-fold should be an indication for drug withdrawal, even if the patient is asymptomatic.

COMPLICATIONS OF CIRRHOSIS

Variceal bleeding

Varices are dilated anastamoses between the portal and systemic venous systems which form in an attempt to decompress the portal venous system when the pressure within undergoes sustained elevation. Those in the lower oesophagus or gastric body are prone to rupture because they are thin-walled and lie just below the mucosa.

Portal pressure is a function of *resistance* in the portal venous system and the *flow* of blood through it. In cirrhosis, portal venous resistance is increased, and inflow of blood is increased by splanchnic vasodilatation and elevation of cardiac output. Variceal bleeding is increasingly likely as the pressure gradient between the portal and systemic venous systems rises beyond 12 mmHg.

Up to 50% of patients with portal hypertension bleed from oesophageal or gastric varices and half die from complications of their first bleed. Hypovolaemia must be corrected with plasma expanders and blood transfusion. Sepsis is common; the incidence rises from 20% at 48 hours to over 60% at 7 days and antimicrobial prophylaxis should be given with ciprofloxacin (1 g/day). Some 70% will stop bleeding spontaneously but over half rebleed within 10 days.

Acute variceal bleeding

Management involves measures directed at the varices and also to reduce portal pressure by pharmacological methods and blood shunting procedures.

Direct treatment of varices by endoscopy is preferred. *Band ligation,* in which the varices are strangulated by application of small elastic bands has fewer complications than *sclerotherapy,* which involves injecting sclerosant into and around the varices but may lead to oesophagitis, stricture or embolisation of sclerosant. Either technique can control bleeding in about 90% of patients, and rebleeding is reduced if this direct treatment is combined with reduction of portal pressure (see below).

Direct pressure on varices can be applied by inserting an inflatable triple-lumen (Sengstaken) tube which abuts the gastro-oesophageal junction, and controls bleeding in 90%; rebleeding is common when the tube is withdrawn and its use may be accompanied by aspiration, oesophageal ulceration or perforation.

Reduction of portal pressure. *Vasopressin* (antidiuretic hormone, see p. 711), in addition to its action on the renal collecting ducts (through V_2 receptors), constricts smooth muscle (V_1 receptors) in the cardiovascular system (hence its name), and particularly in splanchnic blood vessels, so reducing blood flow in the portal venous system. Unfortunately, coronary vasoconstriction can also occur, and treatment has to be withdrawn from 20% of patients because of myocardial ischaemia. Glyceryl trinitrate (transdermally, sublingually, or intravenously) reduces the cardiac risk and, advantageously, further reduces portal venous resistance and pressure.

Vasopressin is rapidly cleared from the circulation and must be given by continuous i.v. infusion. The synthetic analogue, *terlipressin* (triglycyl-lysine-vasopressin) is now preferred. This prodrug (or hormogen) is converted in vivo to the vasoactive *lysine vasopressin* which has biological activity for 3–4 hours, and is effective by bolus injections 4-hourly, usually for 48–72 hours. It is a useful adjunct to endoscopic therapy and reduces rebleeding.

Somatostatin and its synthetic analogue *octreotide* reduce portal pressure by decreasing splanchnic blood flow. Octreotide has the advantage of a longer duration of action so that it can be given as a bolus injection rather than the constant intravenous infusion needed for administration of somatostatin. Its can be used as an alternative to terlipressin, having similar efficacy and indications for use.

Patients who continue to bleed despite the above measures require surgery (ligation or transection of varices) or placement of a stent between intrahepatic branches of the portal and (systemic) hepatic veins under radiological control. The latter is now the technique of choice for the 10–15% of patients with acute bleeding resistant to conventional treatment, and also for long-term management of patients who are difficult to help by other methods (see below).

Prevention of variceal bleeding

Endoscopic therapy as (above), preferably by band ligation, and repeated at weekly intervals until all varices are obliterated, is currently the treatment of choice; it reduces the incidence of rebleeding by 50–60%.

Pharmacological therapy. Nonselective β-blockers, e.g. propranolol or nadolol, reduce cardiac output (β$_1$ receptor antagonism) and induce splanchnic vasoconstriction (β$_2$ receptor antagonism allowing unopposed α-adrenergic vasoconstriction). Recurrent bleeding is reduced by about 40%. As propranolol is extensively extracted in a single pass through the liver, its systemic availability may be unpredictable in patients with cirrhosis and portal hypertension due to variations in hepatic blood flow and portal/systemic shunts. Ideally, the dose of propranolol (given b.d.) should be adjusted by measuring the portal/systemic venous pressure gradient; if this is not feasible, the resting pulse rate is monitored, aiming at a 25% reduction. Decreased cardiac output can exacerbate impaired renal function and fluid retention. Nadolol, having a longer duration of action, is given only once daily.

ASCITES

About 50% of patients with cirrhosis develop ascites within 10 years of diagnosis and 50% of these will die within 2 years. The process by which ascites forms in cirrhosis is not fully understood but appears to involve the accumulation of vasodilator substances, activation of the renin-angiotensin-aldosterone system (causing renal *retention* of sodium and water), and the production of antidiuretic hormone (causing *hyponatraemia* due to dilution, not deficiency, of plasma sodium).

Management of ascites

The aim is to induce *natriuresis* with consequent loss of water. Fluid restriction is unnecessary unless the plasma sodium falls below 120 mmol/l. The initial management must include a diagnostic tap of the ascitic fluid as spontaneous bacterial peritonitis complicates up to 25% of patients on presentation.

A combination of bed-rest (which lowers plasma renin activity) and dietary sodium restriction are effective in about 10% of patients but *diuretic therapy* is usual. The most useful drug is *spironolactone* but its maximum effect can take up to 2 weeks to develop as it is metabolised to products with long duration of action, e.g. canrenone t$\frac{1}{2}$ 10–35 h. A loop diuretic, e.g. *frusemide (furosemide),* is therefore given in combination, which also helps to counteract hyperkalaemia induced by spironolactone. A dose ratio of spironolactone 100 mg and frusemide 40 mg o.d. works well, and can be increased every 3–4 days to a maximum of spironolactone 400 mg + frusemide 160 mg.

Body weight and urinary sodium excretion should be monitored. Patients who have oedema as well as ascites exhibit rapid weight loss. When ascites only is present weight loss should not exceed 0.5 kg/day, which is the maximum rate that fluid can move from the peritoneal cavity into the circulation. Creating a negative fluid balance runs the risk of hypovolaemia, electrolyte disturbance, renal impairment and eventually hepatic encephalopathy. Patients should lose weight if their urinary sodium excretion exceeds that provided by the diet; those who do not respond despite high urinary sodium outputs are almost certainly receiving additional sodium in their diet or medications, e.g. antacids. Should spironolactone cause painful gynaecomastia, amiloride is a useful substitute (10–40 mg/day) with a more rapid onset of action.

Abdominal paracentesis is useful particularly when ascites is tense; rapid drainage of 5 litres leads to prompt relief of discomfort and improves circulatory dynamics. Provided renal function is not compromised, extensive paracentesis is safe and can be used as an adjunct to diuretic therapy to shorten hospital stay. When more than 5 litres are drained it is customary to infuse colloid or albumin (6–8 g per litre of fluid removed) to prevent hypovolaemia.

HEPATIC ENCEPHALOPATHY

Infection, gastrointestinal bleeding or injudicious use of sedatives and diuretics can precipitate hepatic encephalopathy in cirrhotic patients. The pathophysiology is complex but *ammonia* appears to hold a central role. Derived mainly from the action of colonic urease-containing bacteria, ammonia is normally extracted from the portal blood by the liver, but when there is portal/systemic shunting and impaired hepatic metabolism, it reaches high concentration in the blood and adversely affects the brain. Theraputic measures that limit production of ammonia have therefore been developed.

Lactulose acts as an osmotic laxative to expedite clearance of potentially toxic substances from the gastrointestinal tract. In addition, colonic bacteria metabolise it to lactic and acetic acids which inhibit the growth of ammonia-producing organisms and, by lowering pH, reduce nonionic diffusion of ammonia (a basic substance) from the colon into the bloodstream. The correct dose is that which produces 2–4 soft acidic stools daily (usually 30–60 ml daily). Exceeding this dose can dehydrate the patient. As lactulose is intended for long-term use, there is no rational basis for giving it to patients after paracetamol overdose, as prophylaxis against hepatic encephalopathy.

Reduction of dietary protein reduces ammonia production and has long been used to prevent hepatic encephalopathy. Any potential benefit against encephalopathy must be tempered by the knowledge that most patients with severe liver disease are malnourished. Protein from vegetable sources is often better tolerated than animal-derived protein, at least in part due to its higher fibre content which accelerates transit through the gut.

Neomycin and *metronidazole* both inhibit urease-producing bacteria and are useful, but their long-term use is limited by toxicity.

Immune-mediated liver disease

AUTOIMMUNE ACTIVE CHRONIC HEPATITIS

This chronic inflammatory disease of the liver is characteristically associated with circulating auto-antibodies and high serum immunoglobulin concentrations. Untreated, it progresses to cirrhosis, but the condition responds well to immunosup-

pressives. Some 80% will benefit from *prednisolone* which should be continued in the long term, as most patients relapse if the drug is withdrawn. *Azathioprine* (1 mg/kg daily) is effective as a steroid sparing agent, and usually permits reducing of prednisolone to 5–10 mg/d. Increasing azathioprine to 2 mg/kg allows further reduction in prednisolone dose but haematological toxicity may result and the blood count must be monitored every 2 months.

PRIMARY BILIARY CIRRHOSIS (PBC)

This chronic cholestatic liver disease affects 1 in 4000 people in the United Kingdom. Pruritus is a common early symptom, and can be helped by *colestyramine*. Chronic cholestasis leads to malabsorption of fat-soluble vitamins, particularly vitamin D, and deficiency of which must be corrected to avoid osteomalacea.

The aetiology of PBC is unknown but high titres of antimitochondrial antibody in the majority suggest involvement of immune mechanisms. There is no effective treatment. Adverse effects outweigh benefits from prednisolone, but budesonide is currently under assessment as it is highly extracted by the liver and thus poorly available to the systemic circulation. Ursodeoxycholic acid 10–15 mg/kg/d improves biochemical liver function tests, but appears not to lengthen survival or prevent complications.

Viral hepatitis

HEPATITIS A

Passive immunity can be obtained by i.m. injection of globulin containing antibody to the virus (*normal immunoglobulin*; prepared from pooled plasma from known immune donors) which confers temporary protection for travellers visiting areas where the virus is endemic. Active immunisation with *Hepatitis A vaccine* is now preferable; protective antibody takes about two weeks to develop.

HEPATITIS B

Chronic carriage in the UK occurs in about 5% of those infected but is more common in the immunocompromised and in other high-risk groups including male homosexuals and intravenous drug abusers. In parts of Asia and Africa, chronic carriage occurs in up to 50% of the population. Worldwide there are about 300 million chronic carriers of hepatitis B virus and it is the most important cause of *primary hepatocellular carcinoma.*

Interferon alfa (see p. 263) given for 4–6 months gives long-term clearance of hepatitis B virus from the plasma in 25–40% of patients. The effect is characteristically preceded by elevations in serum transamininases which reflects immune-mediated destruction of virus-infected hepatocytes; if liver function is impaired prior to therapy use of interferon alfa should be monitored carefully because it may precipitate hepatic failure.

Lamivudine, a nucleoside analogue, inhibits replication of hepatitis B virus DNA and reduces hepatic inflammation. The serum of about 17% of patients converts from positive to negative for antibodies to hepatitis B after one year of therapy. Long-term treatment is probably necessary and the drug is well tolerated.

Hepatitis B immunisation

Hepatitis B vaccine (inactivated B virus surface antigen adsorbed on aluminium hydroxide adjuvant) provides active immunity against hepatitis B infection, and in countries of low endemicity it is given to individuals at high risk, including healthcare professionals. Immunity is conferred for at least 5 years and can be supplemented by booster injections.

Hepatitis B immunoglobulin (pooled plasma selected for high titres of antibodies to the virus) provides passive immunity for post-exposure prophylaxis e.g. after accidental needlestick injury.

In countries with high prevalence of hepatitis B the virus is transmitted vertically (from mother to baby). Passive immunoprophylaxis with immune globulin given to the baby at birth, followed by vaccination, is effective at preventing chronic carriage. Mass vaccination should lead to a reduction in the incidence of primary hepatocellular carcinoma, but cannot yet be implemented in third world countries for want of funding.

HEPATITIS D

This virus replicates only in the presence of hepatitis B. Interferon alfa is less effective than in other forms of viral hepatitis, giving sustained responses in about 15% of patients.

HEPATITIS C

Most individuals infected with the hepatitis C virus become long-term carriers. Chronic infection with hepatitis C virus affects an estimated 170 million individuals worldwide. Up to one-third of these will progress to cirrhosis with its attendant complications including hepatocellular carcinoma, over a period of 30–40 years. In the western world hepatitis C infection arises mainly from intravenous drug abuse.

Treatment with *interferon alfa* leads to suppression of circulating hepatitis C viral RNA and improvement in hepatic inflammation in about 40%, but at least half relapse on cessation of treatment. Combination of interferon alfa with *ribavirin* greatly enhances the response, achieving sustained remission in up to 70%; age, duration of infection and viral genotype are among the factors that determine the response. Interferon alfa is cleared rapidly, mainly by the kidney ($t^{1/2}$ 4 h), and must be given by s.c. injection three times per week. Increasing the molecular weight of the drug by conjugation with polyethylene glycol (pegylation) prolongs the $t^{1/2}$ to 40 h, allowing single weekly injections. Pegylation also appears to enhance the efficacy of interferon alfa, possibly by increasing exposure time to the virus.

Treatment should last 6–12 months but should cease after 3 months if any virus RNA persists. Depression, agitation, headache and malaise may limit treatment. Its use is currently restricted to patients with severe necroinflammatory changes on liver biopsy (who are thought to be most at risk of progressing to cirrhosis).

Gallstones

Ursodeoxycholic acid can be used to dissolve cholesterol gallstones; it supplements the bile acid pool and thus improves the solubility of cholesterol in bile. Its use is limited to patients with a functioning gallbladder who have small stones that are not calcified. The dose is 8–12 mg/kg/day p.o., treatment takes up to 2 years and recurrence is common.

Pancreas

DIGESTIVE ENZYMES

In pancreatic *exocrine insufficiency,* the aim of therapy is to prevent weight loss and diarrhoea and, in children, to maintain adequate growth. The problem of getting enough enzyme to the duodenum concurrently with food is not as simple as it might appear. Gastric emptying varies with the composition of meals, e.g. high fat, calories or protein cause delay, and the pancreatic enzymes taken by mouth are destroyed by gastric acid. On the other hand, only one-tenth of the normal pancreatic output is sufficient to prevent steatorrhoea. Acid suppression by proton pump inhibitors improves the efficacy of pancreatic enzyme supplements.

Preparations are of animal origin and variable potency. *Pancreatin,* as Cotazym and Nutrizym, appears to be satisfactory. A reasonable course is to start the patient on the recommended dose of a reliable formulation and to vary this according to the individual's needs, and the size and composition of meals. Enteric-coated formulations (pancreatin granules, tablets) are available. High-potency pancreatic enzymes should not be used in patients with cystic fibrosis as they may cause ileocaecal and large bowel strictures.

ACUTE PANCREATITIS

Many drugs have been tested for specific effect, and none has shown convincing benefit. The main requirements of therapy are:

- To provide adequate *analgesia.* Opioids are generally satisfactory; their potential disadvantage of contracting the sphincter of Oddi (and retarding the flow of pancreatic secretion) appears to be outweighed by their analgesic efficacy; buprenorphine is often preferred.
- To correct *hypovolaemia* due to the exudation of large amounts of fluid around the inflamed pancreas. Plasma may be required, or blood if the haematocrit falls; in addition large volumes of electrolyte solution may be needed to maintain urine flow.

DRUGS AND THE PANCREAS

Adverse effects are most commonly manifest as *acute pancreatitis.* The strongest association is with *alcohol* abuse. High plasma calcium, including that caused by hypervitaminosis D, and parenteral nutrition also increase the risk. Corticosteroids, didanosine, azathoipurine, diuretics (including thiazides and frusemide), sodium valproate, mesalazine and paracetamol (in overdose) have also been causally related.

GUIDE TO FURTHER READING

Dusheiko G 1999 A pill a day, or two, for hepatitis B? Lancet 353: 1032–1033

Jalan R, Hayes P C 1997 Hepatic encephalopathy and ascites. Lancet 350: 1309–1315

Krige J E J, Beckingham I J 2001 Portal hypertension — 1: varices. British Medical Journal 322: 348–351; also Portal hypertension — 2: ascites, encephalopathy, and other conditions. 322: 416–418

Koff R S 1998 Hepatitis A. Lancet 351: 1643–1649

Lauer G M, Walker B D 2001 Hepatitis C virus infection. New England Journal of Medicine 345: 41–52

Lee W M 1997 Hepatitis B virus infection. New England Journal of Medicine 337: 1733–1745

Martin P-Y et al 1998 Nitric oxide as a mediator of haemodynamic abnormalities and sodium and water retention in cirrhosis. New England Journal of Medicine 339: 533–541

Mas A, Rodes J 1997 Fulminant hepatic failure. Lancet 349: 1081–1085

Ryder S D, Beckingham I J 2001 Chronic viral hepatitis. British Medical Journal 322: 219–221

Sharara A I, Rockey D C 2001 Gastroesophageal variceal haemorrhage. New England Journal of Medicine 345: 669–681

Schafer D F, Sorrell M F 1999 Hepatocellular
    carcinoma. Lancet 353: 1253–1257
Steer M L et al 1995 Chronic pancreatitis. New
    England Journal of Medicine 332: 1482–1490
Steinberg W, Tenner S 1994 Acute pancreatitis. New
    England Journal of Medicine 330: 1198–1210

Tilg H, Diehl A M 2000 Cytokines in alcoholic and
    non-alcoholic steatohepatitis. New England
    Journal of Medicine 343: 1467–1476
Trauner M et al 1998 Molecular pathogenesis of
    cholestasis. New England Journal of Medicine 339:
    1217–1227

ENDOCRINE SYSTEM, METABOLIC CONDITIONS

34

Adrenal corticosteroids, antagonists, corticotropin

In 1855, Dr Thomas Addison, assisted in his observations by three colleagues, published his famous monograph 'On the constitutional effects of disease on the suprarenal capsules' (Addison's disease). It was not until the late 1920s that the vital importance of the adrenal cortex was appreciated and the distinction between the hormones secreted by the cortex and medulla.

By 1936, numerous steroids were being crystallised from cortical extracts, but not enough could be obtained to provide supplies for clinical trial.

In 1948 *cortisone* was made from bile acids in quantity sufficient for clinical trial, and the dramatic demonstration of its power to induce remission of rheumatoid arthritis was published the following year. In 1950 it was realised that cortisone was biologically inert and that the active natural hormone is hydrocortisone *(cortisol).* Since then an embarrassingly large number of synthetic steroids has been made and offered to the clinician. They are derived from natural substances (chiefly plant sterols), the constitutions of which approach most nearly to that of the steroids themselves. A principal aim in research is to produce steroids with more selective action than hydrocortisone, which induces a greater variety of effects than desired in any patient who is not suffering from adrenal insufficiency.

About the same time as cortisone was introduced, *corticotropin* became available for clinical use.

Adrenal steroids and their synthetic analogues

Hormones normally produced by the adrenal cortex include hydrocortisone (cortisol) and some androgens and oestrogens, the synthesis and release of which is controlled by the hypothalamic-pituitary system, and aldosterone, whose biosynthesis is largely dependent on the renin-angiotensin system.

Numerous analogues have been made in which the major actions have been separated.

When the adrenal cortex fails (Addison's disease) adrenocortical steroids are available for *replacement therapy*, but their chief use in medicine is for their *anti-inflammatory* and *immunosuppressive effects* *(pharmacotherapy)*. These are obtained only when the drugs are given in doses far above those needed for physiological replacement. Various metabolic effects, which are of the greatest importance to the normal functioning of the body, then become adverse effects. Much successful effort has gone into separating *glucocorticoid* from *mineralocorticoid* effects[1] and some steroids, e.g. dexamethasone, have virtually no mineralocorticoid activity. But it has not yet proved possible to separate the glucocorticoid effects from each other, so that if a steroid is used for its anti-inflammatory action the risks, e.g. of osteoporosis, diabetes, remain.

In the account that follows, the effects of hydrocortisone will be described and then other steroids in so far as they differ. In the context of this chapter 'adrenal steroid' means a substance with hydrocortisone-like activity. Androgens are described in Chapter 37.

MECHANISM OF ACTION

Glucocorticoids diffuse into the cell but access to the receptor may be prevented, for example in kidney, by the enzyme 11-beta hydroxysteroid dehydrogenase, which converts active cortisol into inactive cortisone. When activated, the receptors translocate to the nucleus where they can upregulate gene transcription by dimerising on specific DNA response elements and recruiting co-activator proteins, but can also oppose other transcription factor function, for example NFκB and AP-1, by protein–protein interaction. The anti-inflammatory actions of glucocorticoids are mediated mainly by this latter mechanism, suggesting that one day drugs may be found which have the beneficial

effects of steroids with less of the undesired properties.

Glucocorticoids inhibit pathways that normally lead to production of prostaglandins, leukotrienes and platelet activating factor. These mediators would normally contribute to increased vascular permeability and subsequent changes including oedema, leucocyte migration, fibrin deposition.

ACTIONS OF HYDROCORTISONE

Plainly, there is a distinction between replacement therapy (physiological effects) and the higher doses of pharmacotherapy.

On inorganic metabolism (mineralocorticoid effects): increased retention of sodium by the renal tubule, and increased potassium excretion in the urine.

On organic metabolism (glucocorticoid effects):

- *Carbohydrate metabolism:* gluconeogenesis is increased and peripheral glucose utilisation (transport across cell membranes) may be decreased (insulin antagonism) so that hyperglycaemia and sometimes glycosuria result. Latent diabetes becomes overt.
- *Protein metabolism: anabolism* (conversion of amino acids to protein) is decreased but catabolism continues unabated or even faster, so that there is a negative nitrogen balance with muscle wasting. Osteoporosis (reduction of bone protein matrix) occurs, growth slows in children, the skin atrophies and this, with increased capillary fragility, causes bruising and striae. Healing of peptic ulcers or of wounds is delayed, as is fibrosis.
- *Fat deposition:* this is increased on shoulders, face and abdomen.
- *Inflammatory response* is depressed, regardless of its cause, so that as well as being of great benefit in 'useless' or excessive inflammation, corticosteroids can be a source of danger in infections by limiting useful protective inflammation. Neutrophil and macrophage function are depressed, including the release of chemical mediators and the effects of these on capillaries.

---

[1] The mere introduction of a double bond transforms hydrocortisone to prednisolone, a big biological change: see Table 34.1 for relative potencies 1.0:1.0 to 4:0.8.

- *Allergic responses* are suppressed. The antigen–antibody interaction is unaffected, but its injurious inflammatory consequences do not follow.
- *Antibody production* is reduced by heavy doses.
- *Lymphoid tissue* is reduced (including leukaemic lymphocytes).
- *Renal excretion* of urate is increased.
- *Blood eosinophils* are reduced in number.
- *Euphoria or psychotic states* may occur, perhaps due to CNS electrolyte changes.
- *Anti-vitamin D action,* see calciferol (p. 738).
- *Reduction of hypercalaemia* chiefly where this is due to excessive absorption of calcium from the gut (sarcoidosis, vitamin D intoxication).
- *Urinary calcium excretion* is increased and renal stones may form.
- *Growth reduction* where new cells are being added (growth in children), but not where they are replacing cells as in adult tissues.
- *Suppression of hypothalamic/pituitary/adrenocortical feedback system* (with delayed recovery) occurs with chronic use, so that abrupt withdrawal leaves the patient in a state of adrenocortical insufficiency.

Normal daily secretion of hydrocortisone is 10–30 mg. The exogenous daily dose that completely suppresses the cortex is hydrocortisone 40–80 mg, or prednisolone 10–20 mg, or its equivalent of other agents. Recovery of function is quick after a few days' use; but when used over months recovery takes months. A steroid-suppressed adrenal continues to secrete aldosterone.

INDIVIDUAL ADRENAL STEROIDS

The relative potencies[2] for glucocorticoid and mineralocorticoid (sodium-retaining) effects which are shown in Table 34.1 are central to the choice of agent in relation to clinical indication.

All drugs in Table 34.1 except aldosterone are active when swallowed, being protected from hepatic first-pass metabolism by high binding to

---

[2] *Potency* (the weight of drug in relation to its effect) rather than *efficacy* (strength of response): see page 94. If a large enough dose of a glucocorticoid, e.g. prednisolone, were administered, the Na^+-retention would be almost as great as that caused by a mineralocorticoid. This is why, in practice, different (more selective, and potent) glucocorticoids, not higher doses of prednisolone, need to be used when maximal stimulation of glucocorticoid receptors is desired (e.g. in the treatment of acute transplant rejections).

Compound (tablet strength, mg)		Approximate relative potency		
		Anti-inflammatory (glucocorticoid) effect	Sodium-retaining (mineralocorticoid) effect	Equivalent[1] dosage (for anti-inflammatory effect, mg)[2]
Cortisone	(25)	0.8	1.0	25
Hydrocortisone	(20)	1.0	1.0	20
Prednisolone	(5)	4	0.8	5
Methylprednisolone	(4)	5	minimal	4
Triamcinolone	(4)	5	none	4
Dexamethasone	(0.5)	30	minimal	0.75
Betamethasone	(0.5)	30	negligible	0.75
Fludrocortisone	(0.1)	15	150	irrelevant
Aldosterone	none	none	500[3]	irrelevant

TABLE 34.1 Relative potencies of adrenal steroids

[1] Note that these equivalents are in approximate inverse accord with the tablet strengths.
[2] The doses in the final column are in the lower range of those that may cause suppression of the hypothalamic/pituitary/adrenocortical axis when given daily continuously. Much higher doses, e.g. prednisolone 40 mg, can be given on alternate days or daily for up to 5 days without causing clinically significant suppression.
[3] Injected.

plasma proteins. Some details of preparations and equivalent doses are given in the table. Injectable and topical forms are available (creams, suppositories, eye drops).

The selectivity of hydrocortisone for the glucocorticoid receptor is not due to a different binding affinity of hydrocortisone to the two receptors but to the protection of the mineralocorticoid receptor by locally high concentrations of the enzyme 11β-hydroxysteroid dehydrogenase, which converts cortisol (hydrocortisone) to the inactive cortisone. This enzyme is inhibited by one of the components of liquorice, and can occasionally harbour a genetic defect. Therefore both acquired (in liquorice addicts) and inherited syndromes of 'pseudohyperaldosteronism' can occasionally occur.

Hydrocortisone (cortisol) is the principal naturally occurring steroid; it is taken orally; a soluble salt can be given i.v. for rapid effect in emergency (whether due to deficiency, allergy or inflammatory disease). A suspension (Hydrocortisone Acetate Inj.) can be given intra-articularly.

Parenteral preparation for systemic effect: the soluble Hydrocortisone Sodium Succinate Inj. is used for quick (1–2 h) effect; for continuous effect about 8-hourly administration is appropriate. Prednisolone Acetate Inj. i.m. is an alternative, once or twice a week.

Oral tablet strengths, see Table 34.1.

Prednisolone is predominantly anti-inflammatory (glucorticoid), biologically active, and has little sodium-retaining activity; it is the standard choice for anti-inflammatory pharmacotherapy, orally or i.m.

Prednisone is a prodrug, i.e. it is biologically inert and converted into prednisolone in the liver. Since there is 20% less on conversion there seems to be no point in using it.

Methylprednisolone is similar to prednisone; it is used i.v. for megadose pulse therapy (see below).

Fluorinated corticosteroids: triamcinolone has virtually no sodium retaining (mineralocorticoid) effect but has the disadvantage that muscle wasting

may occasionally be severe and anorexia and mental depression may be more common at high dose.

Dexamethasone and betamethasone are similar, powerful predominantly anti-inflammatory steroids. They are longer-acting than prednisolone and are used for therapeutic adrenocortical suppression.

Fludrocortisone has a very great sodium-retaining effect in relation to its anti-inflammatory action, and only at high doses need the nonelectrolyte effects be considered. It is used to replace aldosterone where the adrenal cortex is destroyed (Addison's disease). Fludrocortisone is also the drug of choice in most patients with *autonomic neuropathy*, in whom volume expansion is easier to achieve than a sustained increase in vasoconstrictor tone. Much higher doses of fludrocortisone (0.5–1.0 mg) are required when the cause of hypotension is a salt-losing syndrome of renal origin, e.g. following an episode of interstitial nephritis.

Aldosterone (t½ 20 min), the principal natural salt-retaining hormone, has been used i.m. in acute adrenal insufficiency. After oral administration, it is rapidly inactivated in the first pass through the liver but has no place in routine therapeutics, as fludrocortisone is as effective and is active orally.

Spironolactone (see p. 534) is a competitive aldosterone antagonist which also blocks the mineralocorticoid effect of other steroids; it is used in the treatment of *primary hyperaldosteronism* and as a diuretic, principally when severe oedema is due to *secondary hyperaldosteronism*, e.g. cirrhosis, congestive cardiac failure.

Beclomethasone and budesonide are used by inhalation for asthma (see p. 561). About 90% of an inhalation dose is swallowed and these steroids are inactivated by hepatic first-pass; the rest, absorbed from the mouth and lungs, gives very low systemic plasma concentration. The risk of suppression of the hypothalamic/pituitary/adrenal axis is thus minimal (but it can happen). This property of extensive hepatic first-pass metabolism with low systemic availability is also an advantage in the topical treatment of inflammatory bowel disease with minimal risk of systemic adverse effects.

PHARMACOKINETICS OF CORTICOSTEROIDS

Absorption of the synthetic steroids given *orally* is rapid. The t$\frac{1}{2}$ in plasma of most is 1–3 h but the maximum biological effect occurs after 2–8 h. Administration is usually 2 or 3 times a day. They are metabolised principally in the liver (some undergoing hepatic first-pass metabolism, see above) and some are excreted unchanged by the kidney. The t$\frac{1}{2}$ is prolonged in hepatic and renal disease and is shortened by enzyme induction to an extent that can be clinically important.

Topical application (skin, lung, joints) allows absorption which can be enough to cause systemic effects.

In the blood, adrenal steroids are carried in the free (biologically active) form (5%) and also bound (95% in the case of hydrocortisone) to *transcortin* (a globulin with high affinity, but low binding capacity) and, when this is saturated, to albumin (80% in the case of hydrocortisone). The concentration of transcortin is increased by oestrogens, e.g. pregnancy, hormonal contraception, other oestrogen therapy; if these substances are taken, the total plasma hydrocortisone will be found to be raised, but the amount of free hydrocortisone may be normal, being controlled by the physiological feedback mechanism. Patients may be wrongly suspected of having Cushing's syndrome if the fact that they are taking oestrogen is unrecognised and only the total is measured (as is usual).

In patients with very low serum albumin, steroid doses should be lower than usual owing to the reduced binding capacity. In addition, low albumin concentration may be caused by liver disease, which also augments the effects of steroids by delaying metabolism (t$\frac{1}{2}$ of prednisolone may be doubled).

DOSAGE SCHEDULES

Various spaced-out schedules have been used in the aspiration of reducing hypothalamic/pituitary/adrenal (HPA) suppression by allowing the plasma steroid concentration to fall between doses to provide time for pituitary recovery, e.g. prednisolone 40 on alternate days. But none has been successful in both completely avoiding suppression and at the same time controlling symptoms. The following are examples:

- Where a *single daily dose* is practicable it should be given in the early morning (to coincide with the natural activation of the HPA axis).
- *Alternate day schedules* are worth using, especially where immunosuppression is the objective (organ transplants) rather than anti-inflammatory effect (rheumatoid arthritis).
- *Short courses* (a few days) may be practicable for some conditions without significant suppression, e.g. acute asthma of moderate severity.
- Another variant is to give *enormous doses* (grams, not mg), orally or i.v., e.g. methylprednisolone 1.0 g i.v. on 3 successive days, at intervals of weeks or months (megadose pulses). The technique is used particularly in collagen diseases.

> **Choice of adrenal steroid: summary**
>
> - **For oral replacement therapy** in adrenocortical insufficiency, *hydrocortisone* should be used to supply glucocorticoid and some mineralocorticoid activity. In Addison's disease a small dose of a hormone with only mineralocorticoid effect *(fludrocortisone)* is normally needed in addition. Prednisolone on its own is not effective replacement therapy.
> - **For anti-inflammatory and antiallergic (immunosuppressive) effect,** *prednisolone*, *triamcinolone* or *dexamethasone*. It is not possible to rank these in firm order of merit. One or other may suit an individual patient best, especially as regards incidence of adverse effects such as muscle wasting. *By inhalation:* beclomethasone or budesonide.
> - **For hypothalamic/pituitary/adrenocortical suppression,** e.g. in adrenal hyperplasia, prednisolone or dexamethasone.

ADVERSE EFFECTS OF SYSTEMIC ADRENAL STEROID PHARMACOTHERAPY

These consist largely of too intense production of the physiological or pharmacological actions listed under actions of hydrocortisone. Some occur only with systemic use and for this reason local therapy, e.g. inhalation, intra-articular injection, is preferred where practicable.

Unwanted effects generally follow prolonged administration and virtually do not occur with 1 or 2 doses though some occur with a few days' use, e.g. spread of infection. The undesired effects recounted below should never be experienced in replacement therapy, but are sometimes unavoidable when the steroid is used as pharmacotherapy. Obviously, the nature of unwanted effects depends on the choice of steroid. Fludrocortisone (mineralocorticoid) in ordinary doses does not cause osteoporosis and prednisolone (glucocorticoid) does not normally cause oedema.

In general, serious unwanted effects are unlikely if the daily dose is below the equivalent of hydrocortisone 50 mg or prednisolone 10 mg.

The principal adverse effects of chronic corticosteroid administration are:

Endocrine. To greater or lesser degree features of *Cushing's syndrome* result in moon face, characteristic deposition of fat on the body, oedema, hypertension, striae, bruising, acne, hirsutism. Major skin damage can result from minor injury of any kind. *Diabetes mellitus* may appear. *Hypothalamic/pituitary/adrenal (HPA) suppression* is dependent on the corticosteroid used, its dose, duration and the time of administration. A single morning dose of less than 20 mg of prednisolone may not be followed by suppression, whereas a dose of 5 mg given late in the evening is likely to suppress the essential early morning activation of the HPA axis (circadian rhythm). Substantial suppression of the HPA axis can occur within a week (but see Withdrawal of steroid therapy, below).

Musculoskeletal. *Proximal myopathy* and *tendon rupture* may occur. *Osteoporosis* develops insidiously leading to fractures of vertebrae, ribs, femora and feet. Pain and restriction of movement may occur months in advance of radiographic changes. A biphosphonate, with or without vitamin D, is useful for prevention and treatment. *Growth* in children is impaired. *A vascular necrosis of bone* (femoral heads) is a serious complication (at higher doses); it appears to be due to restriction of blood flow through bone capillaries.

Immune. *Suppression of the inflammatory response to infection and immunosuppression* causes some patients to present with atypical symptoms and signs and quickly to deteriorate. The incidence of infection is increased with high dose therapy, and any infection can be more severe when it occurs. *Candidiasis* may appear, particularly in the alimentary tract. Previously dormant *tuberculosis* may become active insidiously. Intra-articular injections demand the strictest asepsis. *Live vaccines* become dangerous. Developing *chickenpox* may result in a *severe form of the disease* and patients who have not had chickenpox should receive varicella-zoster immune globulin within 3 days of exposure. Similarly, exposure to *measles* should be avoided.

Gastrointestinal. Patients taking continuous steroid, especially in combination with a nonsteroidal anti-inflammatory drug (NSAID), have an excess incidence of *peptic ulcer* and *haemorrhage* of about 1–2%. It is plainly unreasonable to seek to protect all such patients by routine prophylactic antiulcer therapy, i.e. to treat 98 patients unnecessarily in order to help two. But such therapy (proton pump inhibitor, histamine H_2-receptor blocker, sucralfate) is appropriate when ulcer is particularly likely, e.g. a patient with rheumatoid arthritis taking an NSAID, or for patients with a history of peptic ulcer disease. There is increased incidence of *pancreatitis.*

Central nervous system. *Depression and psychosis* can occur during the first few days of high dose administration, especially in those with a history of mental disorder. Other effects include *euphoria, insomnia,* and *aggravation of schizophrenia* and *epilepsy.* Long-term treatment may result in *raised intracranial pressure with papilloedema,* especially in children.

Ophthalmic effects may include *posterior subcapsular lens cataract* (risk if dose exceeds prednisolone 10 mg/day or equivalent for above a year), *glaucoma* (with prolonged use of eye drops), and *corneal* or *scleral* thinning.

Other effects include menstrual disorders, delayed tissue healing (including myocardial rupture after myocardial infarction), thromboembolism, and paradoxically, hypersensitivity reactions including anaphylaxis.

ADRENAL STEROIDS AND PREGNANCY

Adrenal steroids are teratogenic in animals. Although a relationship between steroid pharmacotherapy and cleft palate and other fetal abnormalities has been suspected in man, there is no doubt that many women taking a steroid throughout have both conceived and borne normal babies. Adrenal insufficiency due to hypothalamic/ pituitary suppression in the newborn occurs only with high doses to the mother. Dosage during pregnancy should be kept as low as practicable and fluorinated steroids are best avoided as they are more teratogenic in animals (dexa- and betamethasone, triamcinolone and various topical steroids, e.g. fluocinolone). Hypoadrenal women who become pregnant may require an increase in hydrocortisone replacement therapy by about 10 mg per day to compensate for the increased binding by plasma proteins that occurs in pregnancy. Labour should be managed as described for major surgery (below).

PRECAUTIONS DURING CHRONIC ADRENAL STEROID THERAPY

The most important precaution during replacement and pharmacotherapy is to see the patient regularly with an awareness of the possibilities of adverse effects including fluid retention (weight gain), hypertension, glycosuria, hypokalaemia (potassium supplement may be necessary) and back pain (osteoporosis); and of the serious hazard of patient noncompliance.

Mild withdrawal symptoms (iatrogenic cortical insufficiency) include conjunctivitis, rhinitis, weight loss, arthralgia and itchy skin nodules.

Patients must always
- carry a card giving details of therapy
- be impressed with the importance of compliance
- know what to do if they develop an intercurrent illness or other severe stress: double their next dose and to tell their doctor. If a patient omits a dose then it should be made up as soon as possible so that the total daily intake is maintained, because every patient should be

taking the minimum dose necessary to control the disease.

Treatment of intercurrent illness

The normal adrenal cortex responds to *severe stress* by secreting more than 300 mg/day of cortisol. Intercurrent illness is stress and treatment is urgent, particularly of *infections;* the dose of corticosteroid should be doubled during the illness and gradually reduced as the patient improves. Effective chemotherapy of bacterial infections is specially important.

Viral infections contracted during steroid therapy can be overwhelming because the immune response of the body may be largely suppressed. This is particularly relevant to immunosuppressed patients exposed to varicella/herpes zoster virus, which may cause fulminant illness; they may need passive protection with varicella/zoster immunoglobulin, VZIG, as soon as practicable. Continuous use of prednisolone 20 mg/day (or the equivalent) is immunosuppressive. But a corticosteroid may sometimes be useful in therapy after the disease has begun (thyroiditis, encephalitis) and there has been time for the immune response to occur. It then acts by suppressing unwanted effects of immune responses and excessive inflammatory reaction.

Vomiting requires parenteral administration.

In the event of *surgery* being added to that of adrenal steroid therapy the patient should receive hydrocortisone 100–200 mg i.m. or i.v. with premedication. If there is any sign suggestive that the patient may collapse, e.g. hypotension, during the operation, i.v. hydrocortisone (100 mg) should be infused at once. Otherwise, if there are no complications, the dose is repeated 6-hourly for 24–72 h and then reduced by half every 24 h until normal dose level is reached.

Minor operations, e.g. dental extraction, may be covered by hydrocortisone 20 mg orally 2–4 h before operation and the same dose afterwards.

In all these situations an i.v. infusion should be available for immediate use in case the above is not enough. These precautions should be used in patients who have received substantial treatment with corticosteroid within the past year, because their hypothalamic/pituitary/adrenal system, though sufficient for ordinary life, may fail to respond adequately to severe stress. If steroid therapy has been very prolonged, these precautions should be taken for as long as 2 years after stopping it. This will mean that some unnecessary treatment is given, but collapse due to acute adrenal insufficiency can be fatal and the ill-effects of short-lived increased dosage of steroid are less grave, being confined to possible increased incidence and severity of infection.

DOSAGE AND ROUTES OF ADMINISTRATION

Dosage depends very much on the purpose for which the steroid is being used and on individual response. There is no single schedule that will suit every case but examples appear below.

Systemic commencing doses

- *For a serious disease* such as systemic lupus, dermatomyositis: prednisolone up to 0.75–2.0 mg/kg/d orally in divided doses.
- *If life-threatening*, prednisolone up to 70 mg, or its equivalent of another steroid. The dose is then increased if necessary until the disease is controlled or adverse effects occur; as much as prednisolone 2–3 mg/kg/d can be needed. Cyclophosphamide or azathioprine (see p. 292) are valuable adjuncts; they may enhance the initial control of the disease and have a sparing effect on the maintenance dose of prednisolone required.
- More usually now, megadose pulses (methylprednisolone 1.0 g i.v. daily for 3 days) are used, followed by oral maintenance with prednisolone and/or a steroid-sparing agent (above).
- *For less dangerous disease,* such as rheumatoid arthritis: prednisolone 7.5–10.0 mg daily, adjusted later according to the response.
- In some special cases, including *replacement* of adrenal insufficiency, dosage is given in the account of the treatment of the disease.
- *For continuous therapy* the minimum amount to produce the desired effect must be used. Sometimes imperfect control must be accepted by the patient because full control, e.g. of rheumatoid arthritis, though obtainable, involves use of doses that must lead to long-term toxicity, e.g. osteoporosis, if

continued for years. The decision to embark on such therapy is a serious matter for the patient.

Topical applications (creams, intranasal, inhalations, enemas) are used in attempts, often successful, to obtain local, whilst avoiding systemic, effects; suspensions of solutions are also injected into joints, soft tissues and subconjunctivally. All these can, with heavy dose, be sufficiently absorbed to suppress the hypothalamus and cause other unwanted effects. Individual preparations are mentioned in the text where appropriate.

The relatively high selectivity of *inhaled beclomethasone* in asthma is due to a combination of route of administration, high potency and rapid conversion to inactive metabolites by the liver of any drug that is absorbed (see asthma, skin); but yet hypothalamic/pituitary suppression and systemic toxicity occasionally occur.

Contraindications to the use of adrenal steroids for suppressing inflammation are all relative, depending on the advantage to be expected. They should be used only for serious reasons if the patient has: diabetes, a history of mental disorder or peptic ulcer, epilepsy, tuberculosis, hypertension or heart failure. The presence of any infection demands that effective chemotherapy be begun before the steroid, but there are exceptions (some viral infections, see above). Topical corticosteroid applied to an inflamed eye (with the very best of intention) can be *disastrous* if the inflammation is due to herpes virus.

Steroids containing fluorine (see above) intensify diabetes more than others and so should be avoided in that disease.

Long-term use of adrenal steroids in children presents essentially the same problems as in adults except that growth is retarded approximately in proportion to the dose. This is unlikely to be important unless therapy exceeds 6 months; there is a spurt of growth after withdrawal. Intermittent dosage schedules (alternate day) may reduce the risk (rarely, corticotropin may be preferred, see p. 675).

Some other problems loom larger in children than in adults. Common childhood viral infections may be more severe, and if a nonimmune child taking an adrenal steroid is exposed to one, it is wise to try to prevent the disease with the appropriate specific immunoglobulin (if available).

Live virus vaccination is unsafe in immunosuppressed subjects, e.g. systemic prednisolone > 2 mg/kg per day for > 1 week in the preceding 3 months, as it may cause the disease, but active immunisation with killed vaccines or toxoids will give normal response unless the dose of steroid is high, when the response may be suppressed.

Raised intracranial pressure may occur more readily in children than in adults.

Fixed-dose combinations of adrenal steroids with other drugs in one tablet should never be used as they abrogate the principles for the use of such formulations (p. 118).

Indications for use of adrenal steroids

- Replacement of hormone deficiency
- Inflammation suppression
- Immunosuppression
- Suppression of excess hormone secretion

USES OF ADRENOCORTICAL STEROIDS

REPLACEMENT THERAPY

Acute adrenocortical insufficiency (Addisonian crisis)

This is an emergency and hydrocortisone sodium succinate 100 mg should be given i.v. immediately it is *suspected*, or the patient may die.

- An i.v. infusion of sodium chloride solution (0.9%) is set up immediately and a second 100 mg of hydrocortisone is added to the first litre, which may be given over 2 h (several litres of fluid may be needed in the first 24 h).
- The patient should then receive hydrocortisone 50–100 mg i.v. or i.m. 6-hourly for 24 h; then 12-hourly, initiating oral use when appropriate; then a total of 40–60 mg a day orally in 2 or 3 doses.

Other treatment to restore electrolyte balance will depend on the circumstances. The cause of the

crisis should be sought and treated; it is often an infection. When the dose of hydrocortisone falls below 40 mg a day, supplementary mineralocorticoid (fludrocortisone) may be needed (see below).

The hyperkalaemia of Addison's disease will respond to the above regimen and must not be treated with insulin because of the risk of severe hypoglycaemia.

Chronic primary adrenocortical insufficiency (Addison's disease)

Hydrocortisone orally is used (15–40 mg total daily) in the lowest dose that maintains wellbeing and body weight, with two-thirds of the total dose in the morning and one-third in the evening to mimic the natural *diurnal rhythm* of secretion.[3] Plainly corticotropin is useless.

Some patients do well on hydrocortisone alone, with or without added salt, but most patients require a small amount of mineralocorticoid as well (fludrocortisone, 50–200 micrograms once a day, orally). If the dose of fludrocortisone should exceed 500 micrograms a day, an unlikely event, then its glucocorticoid effect must be taken into account.

The dosage of the hormones is determined in the individual by following general clinical progress and particularly by observing: weight, blood pressure, appearance of oedema, serum sodium and potassium concentrations and haematocrit. The dose of fludrocortisone can be adjusted against the plasma renin activity (routinely assayed in a number of chemical pathology laboratories by the radioimmunoassay of the amount of angiotensin I produced during a timed incubation of a plasma sample). Renin is secreted (by the juxtoglomerular apparatus of the kidney) in response to incomplete reversal of the sodium depletion in patients

---

[3] But this can be associated with an unphysiologically low plasma concentration of hydrocortisone in the late afternoon (with loss of wellbeing). Such patients may be best managed on 3 equal doses per day. *Air travellers* on long flights across longitude east to west (> 12 h, i.e. longer day): take an extra dose near the end of the flight. For west to east flights (> 8 h, i.e. shorter day): the normal evening dose may be taken sooner and the usual dose taken on the 'new' morning. *Night workers* may adjust their dosage to their work pattern (Drug and Therapeutics Bulletin 1990 28: 71).

receiving inadequate replacement therapy. If any complicating disease arises, such as infection, a need for surgery or other stress, the hydrocortisone dosage should immediately be doubled, see above.

If there is vomiting, the replacement hormone must be given parenterally without delay.

There are no contraindications to replacement therapy. The risk lies in withholding rather than in giving it.

Some patients (particularly those with hypopituitarism), when first treated, cannot tolerate full doses of hydrocortisone because they become euphoric or otherwise mentally upset; 10 mg a day may be all they can take. The dose can usually soon be increased if it is done slowly. If diabetes is present the full dose is used and the diabetes controlled with insulin.

Chronic secondary adrenocortical insufficiency

This occurs in *hypopituitarism*. In theory the best treatment is corticotropin, but the disadvantages of frequent injection are such that hydrocortisone is preferred. Usually less hydrocortisone is needed than in primary insufficiency. Special sodium-retaining hormone is seldom required, for the pituitary has little control over aldosterone production which responds principally to plasma potassium concentration and to the renin-angiotensin system. Thyroxine and sex hormones are given when appropriate. The general conduct of therapy does not differ significantly from that in primary adrenal insufficiency.

Iatrogenic adrenocortical insufficiency: abrupt withdrawal

(See also Withdrawal of corticosteroid pharmacotherapy, below) This occurs in patients who have recently received prolonged pharmacotherapy with a corticosteroid which inhibits hypothalamic production of the corticotropin releasing hormone and so results in *secondary* adrenal failure. It is treated by reinstituting therapy or as for acute insufficiency, as appropriate. To avoid an acute crisis on stopping, steroid therapy must be withdrawn gradually to allow the hypothalamus,

the pituitary and the adrenal to regain normal function. Also, when patients taking corticosteroids have an infection or surgical operation (major stress) they should be treated as for primary insufficiency.

After the use of large doses of hormone to suppress inflammation or allergy, sudden withdrawal may not only lead to an adrenal insufficiency crisis but to relapse of the disease, which has only been suppressed, not cured. Such relapse can be extremely severe, sometimes life-threatening.

PHARMACOTHERAPY

Suppression of adrenocortical function

In *adrenogenital syndrome and adrenal virilism,* an attempt may be made to suppress excess adrenal androgen secretion by inhibiting pituitary corticotropin production by means of prednisolone or dexamethasone. Suppression of androgen production is effective if there is adrenal hyperplasia, but not if an adrenal tumour is present. Hairiness, which women especially dislike in themselves, is often unaffected even though good suppression is achieved, and menstruation recommences.

Use in inflammation and for immunosuppression

Only a brief survey can be given here.

Drugs with primarily *glucocorticoid effects,* e.g. prednisolone, are chosen, so that dosage is not limited by the mineralocorticoid effects that are inevitable with hydrocortisone. But it remains essential to use only the *minimum* dose that will achieve the desired effect. Sometimes therapeutic effect must be partly sacrificed to avoid adverse effects, for it has not yet proved possible to separate the glucocorticoid effects from each other; indeed it is not known if it is possible to eliminate catabolic effects and at the same time retain anti-inflammatory action. In any case, in some conditions, e.g. nephrotic syndrome, the clinician cannot specify exactly what action they want the drug developer to provide.

Further specific uses

The decision to give a corticosteroid commonly depends on knowledge of the likelihood and amount of benefit (bearing in mind that very prolonged high dose inevitably brings serious complications such as osteoporosis), on the severity of the disease and on whether the patient has failed to respond usefully to other treatment. It often requires expertise that can be imparted only by those with wide experience of the disease concerned. The following are examples.

Adrenal steroids are used in all or nearly all cases of:

- *Exfoliative dermatitis* and pemphigus, if severe
- *Collagen diseases,* if severe, e.g. lupus erythematosus (systemic), polyarteritis nodosa, polymyalgia rheumatica and cranial giant cell arteritis (urgent therapy to save sight), dermatomyositis
- *Acute severe asthma*
- *Acute lymphatic leukaemia* (see p. 617)
- *Acquired haemolytic anaemia*
- *Severe allergic reactions* of all kinds, e.g. serum sickness, angio-oedema, trichiniasis. Alone they will not control acute manifestations of anaphylactic shock as they do not act quickly enough
- *Organ transplant rejection*
- *Acute spinal cord injury:* early, brief, and high dose (to reduce the oedema/inflammation)
- *Autoimmune active chronic hepatitis:* a corticosteroid improves wellbeing, liver function and histology; *prednisolone* will benefit some 80% and should be continued in the long term, as most patients relapse if the drug is withdrawn.

Adrenal steroids are used in some cases of:

- *Rheumatic fever*
- *Rheumatoid arthritis*
- *Ankylosing spondylitis*
- *Ulcerative colitis and proctitis*
- *Regional enteritis* (Crohn's disease)
- *Bronchial asthma and hay-fever* (allergic rhinitis): also some bronchitics with marked airways obstruction.
- *Sarcoidosis.* If there is hypercalcaemia or threat to a major organ, e.g. eye, adrenal steroid

administration is urgent. Pulmonary fibrosis may be delayed and central nervous system manifestations may improve.

- *Acute mountain/altitude sickness,* to reduce cerebral oedema.
- Prevention of *adverse reaction to radiocontrast media* in patients who have had a previous severe reaction.
- *Blood diseases due to circulating antibodies,* e.g. thrombocytopenic purpura (there may also be a decrease in capillary fragility with lessening of purpura even though thrombocytes remain few); agranulocytosis.
- *Eye diseases.* Allergic diseases and nongranulomatous inflammation of the uveal tract. But bacterial and virus infections may be made worse and use of steroids to suppress inflammation of infection is generally undesirable, is best left to ophthalmologists and must be accompanied by effective chemotherapy; this is of the greatest importance in herpes virus infection. Corneal integrity should be checked before use (by instilling a drop of fluorescein). Prolonged use of corticosteroid eye drops causes glaucoma in 1 in 20 of the population (a genetic trait). Application is generally as hydrocortisone, prednisolone or fluorometholone drops, or subconjunctival injection.
- *Nephrotic syndrome.* Patients with *minimal change disease* respond well to daily or alternate day therapy. With a total of prednisolone 60 mg/d, 90% of those who will lose their proteinuria will have done so within 4–6 weeks, and the dose is tapered off over 3–4 months. Longer courses only induce adverse effects. Relapses are common (50%) and it is then necessary to find a minimum dose of steroid that will keep the patient well. If a steroid is for any reason undesirable, cyclophosphamide or chlorambucil may be substituted. *Membranous nephropathy* may respond to high dose corticosteroid with or without chlorambucil.
- *A variety of skin diseases,* such as eczema. Severe cases may be treated by occlusive dressings if a systemic effect is not wanted, though absorption can be substantial (see Ch. 16).

- *Acute gout* resistant to other drugs (see p. 297).
- *Hypercalcaemia* of sarcoidosis and of vitamin D intoxication responds to prednisolone 30 mg daily (or its equivalent of other steroid) for 10 days. Hypercalcaemia of myeloma and some other malignancies responds more variably. Hyperparathyroid hypercalcaemia does not respond.
- *Raised intracranial pressure due to cerebral oedema,* e.g. in cerebral tumour or encephalitis (probably an anti-inflammatory effect which reduces vascular permeability and acts in 12–24 h): give dexamethasone 10 mg i.m. or i.v. (or equivalent) initially and then 4 mg 6-hourly by the appropriate route, reducing dose after 2–4 days and withdrawing over 5–7 days; but much higher doses may be used in palliation of inoperable cerebral tumour.
- *Preterm labour:* (to mother) to enhance fetal lung maturation.
- *Aspiration of gastric acid* (Mendelsohn's syndrome).
- *Myasthenia gravis:* see page 439.
- *Cancer,* see Chapter 30.

Use in diagnosis: dexamethasone suppression test. Dexamethasone acts on the hypothalamus (like hydrocortisone), to reduce output of corticotropin releasing hormone (CRH), but it does not interfere with measurement of corticosteroids in blood or urine. Normal suppression of cortisol production after administering dexamethasone indicates that the hypothalamic/pituitary/adrenal axis is intact. Failure of suppression implies pathological hyper-secretion of ACTH by the pituitary or of cortisol by the adrenal. Dexamethasone is used because its action is prolonged (24 h). There are several ways of carrying out the test.

WITHDRAWAL OF PHARMACOTHERAPY

The longer the duration of therapy the slower must be the withdrawal. For use of less than 1 week (e.g. in severe asthma), although there is some hypo-thalamic suppression, withdrawal can be safely accomplished in a few steps. After use for 2 weeks,

if rapid withdrawal is desired, a 50% reduction in dose may be made each day; but if the patient has been treated for a longer period, reduction in dose is accompanied by the dual risk of a flare up of the disease and of iatrogenic hypoadrenalism; then withdrawal should be done very slowly, e.g. 2.5–5 mg prednisolone or equivalent at intervals of 3–7 days.

An alternative scheme is to try halving the dose weekly until 25 mg prednisolone or equivalent is reached, after which it may be reduced by about 1 mg every third to seventh day. Paediatric tablets (1 mg) can be useful during withdrawal.

But these schemes may yet be found too fast (giving rise to the occurrence of fatigue, 'dish-rag' syndrome, or relapse of disease) and the rate may need to be even as slow as prednisolone 1 mg per day (or equivalent) per mouth, particularly as the dose approaches the level of physiological require-ment (equivalent of prednisolone 5–7.5 mg daily).

The long tetracosactride test (see later) or measurements of plasma corticotropin concen-tration may be used to assess recovery of adrenal responsiveness, but a positive result should not be taken to indicate full recovery of the patient's ability to respond to stressful situations; the latter is best shown by an adequate response to insulin-induced hypoglycaemia (which additionally tests the hypothalamic/pituitary capacity to respond).

Corticotropin should not be used to hasten recovery of the atrophied cortex since its effects cause further suppression of the hypothalamic-pituitary axis, on the recovery of which the patient's future depends. Complete recovery of normal hypothalamic/pituitary/adrenal function sufficient to cope with severe intercurrent illnesses or surgery is generally complete in 2 months but may take as long as 2 years.

There have been many *reports of collapse,* even coma, occurring within a few hours of omission of steroid therapy, e.g. due to patients' ignorance of the risk to which their physicians are exposing them or failing to have their tablets with them and other trivial causes; but it is not invariable. Patients must be instructed on the hazards of omitting therapy and, during intercurrent disease, i.m. preparations should be freely used. Anaesthesia and surgery in adrenocortical insufficiency is dis-cussed on page 676.

Inhibition of synthesis of adrenal and other steroid hormones

These agents have use in diagnosis of adrenal disease and in controlling excessive production of corticosteroids, e.g. by corticotropin producing tumours of the pituitary (Cushing's syndrome) or by adrenocortical adenoma or carcinoma where the cause cannot be removed. They must be used with special care since they can precipitate acute adrenal insufficiency. Some members inhibit other steroid synthesis.

Metyrapone inhibits the enzyme, steroid 11β-hydroxylase, that converts 11-deoxy precursors into hydrocortisone, corticosterone and aldosterone. It affects synthesis of aldosterone less than that of glucocorticoids.

Trilostane blocks the synthetic path earlier (3β-hydroxysteroid dehydrogenase) and thus also inhibits aldosterone synthesis.

Formestane is a specific inhibitor of the aromatase which converts androgens to oestrogens. A depot injection of 250 mg i.m. is given twice a month in the treatment of some patients with carcinoma of the breast who relapse on tamoxifen.

Aminoglutethimide blocks even earlier, preventing the conversion of cholesterol to pregnenolone. It therefore blocks synthesis of all steroids, hydrocortisone, aldosterone and sex hormones (including the conversion of androgens to oestrogens); it has a use in breast cancer.

Ketoconazole is an effective antifungal agent by virtue of its capacity to block sterol/steroid synthesis (ergosterol in the case of fungi). In man it inhibits steroid synthesis in gonads and adrenal cortex and it has been used in Cushing's syndrome and prostatic cancer.

COMPETITIVE ANTAGONISM OF ADRENAL STEROIDS

Spironolactone antagonises the sodium-retaining effect of aldosterone and other mineralocorticoids. It is used to treat primary and secondary hyperaldosteronism (p. 538).

Adrenocorticotrophic hormone (ACTH) (corticotropin)

Natural corticotropin is a 39-amino-acid polypeptide secreted by the anterior pituitary gland; it is obtained from animal pituitaries.

The physiological activity resides in the first 24 amino acids (which are common to many species) and most immunological activity resides in the remaining 15 amino acids.

The pituitary output of corticotropin responds rapidly to physiological requirements by the familiar negative-feedback homeostatic mechanism. Since the $t\frac{1}{2}$ of corticotropin is 10 min and the adrenal cortex responds rapidly (within 2 min) it is plain that adjustments of steroid output can be quickly made.

Synthetic corticotropins have the advantage that they are shorter amino acid chains (devoid of amino acids 25–39) and so are less likely to cause serious allergy, though this can happen. In addition they are not contaminated by animal proteins which are potent allergens.

Tetracosactride (tetracosactrin) consists of the biologically active first 24 amino acids of natural corticotropin (from man or animals and so it has similar properties, e.g. $t\frac{1}{2}$ 10 min.

ACTIONS

Corticotropin stimulates the synthesis of corticosteroids (of which the most important is hydrocortisone) and to a lesser extent of androgens, by the cells of the adrenal cortex. It has only a minor (transient) effect on aldosterone production, which can proceed *independently*; in the absence of corticotropin the cells of the inner cortex atrophy.

The release of natural corticotropin by the pituitary gland is controlled by the hypothalamus via *corticotropin releasing hormone* (CRH or corticoliberin), production of which is influenced by environmental stresses as well as by the level of circulating hydrocortisone. High plasma concentration of any steroid with glucocorticoid effect prevents release of corticotropin releasing hormone and so of corticotropin, lack of which in turn results in adrenocortical hypofunction. This is the reason why catastrophe may follow sudden withdrawal of steroid therapy in the chronically treated patient who has an atrophied cortex.

The effects of corticotropin are those of the steroids (hydrocortisone, androgens) liberated by its action on the adrenal cortex. Prolonged heavy dosage causes the clinical picture of Cushing's syndrome.

Uses. Corticotropin is used principally in diagnosis and rarely in treatment. It is inactive if taken orally and has to be injected like other peptide hormones.

Diagnostic use: as a test of the capacity of the adrenal cortex to produce cortisol; with the short test, the plasma cortisol (hydrocortisone) concentration is measured before and after an i.m. injection of tetracosactride (Synacthen); a normal response is a rise of more than 200 nanomol/l in the plasma concentration of hydrocortisone. Longer variants of the test in cases of difficulty involve use of the depot (sustained-release) formulation i.m. For example, 1 mg of the depot is injected daily for 3 days at 9.00 am, with a short tetracosactride test performed on day 3.

Therapeutic use is seldom appropriate because the peptide hormone has to be injected; selective glucocorticoid action (without mineralocorticoid effect) cannot be obtained, and clinical results are irregular. Corticotropin can not be relied on to restore adrenal cortisol output when a steroid is being withdrawn after prolonged therapy, as it does not restore function in the suppressed hypothalamic/pituitary part of the HPA axis.

Preparations

Tetracosactride Injection is a powder dissolved in water immediately before injection i.v., i.m. or s.c.

Tetracosactride Zinc Injection (Synacthen Depot) in which the hormone is adsorbed on to zinc phosphate from which it is slowly released. This is the form used in the long tetracosactride test.

Summary

- Cortisol and aldosterone produced in the adrenal cortex have a major role in physiology and pharmacology.
- Physiological concentrations of cortisol are essential for supporting the circulation and glucose production. Physiological concentrations of aldosterone are essential to prevent excessive sodium loss.
- For systemic pharmacological uses, prednisolone or other synthetic adrenocorticosteriods are used because they are more selective glucocorticoids, i.e. have less sodium-retaining activity.
- For local administration (skin, lung), more potent, fluorinated steroids may be required.
- Glucocorticoids inhibit the transcriptional activation of many of the inflammatory cytokines, giving them a versatile role in the treatment of many types of inflammation.
- Fludrocortisone is a valuable treatment for many sodium-losing states, and for most causes of autonomic neuropathy.

GUIDE TO FURTHER READING

Boscaro M et al 2001 Cushing's syndrome. Lancet 357: 783–791

English J et al 1983 Diurnal variation in prednisolone kinetics. Clinical Pharmacology and Therapeutics 33: 381

Freidy J F 1988 Reactions to contrast media and steroid pretreatment. British Medical Journal 296: 809

Hench P S et al 1949 The effect of a hormone of the adrenal cortex (17-hydroxy-11-dehydrocorticosterone: Compound E) and of pituitary adrenocorticotrophic hormone on rheumatoid arthritis. Proceedings of the Staff Meetings of the Mayo Clinic 24: 181, 277 (acute rheumatism). The classic studies of the first clinical use of an adrenocortical steroid in inflammatory disease. See also page 298 for an account by E C Kendall of the biochemical and pharmaceutical background to the clinical studies. Kendall writes of his collaboration with Hench, 'he can now say "17-hydroxy-11-dehydrocorticosterone" and in turn I can say "the arthritis of lupus erythematosus". In sophisticated circles, however, I prefer to say, "the arthritis of L.E."'.

Hilditch K 2000 My Addison's disease. British Medical Journal 321: 645 (A patient's account of the disease.)

Lamberts S W J, Bruining H A, de Jong F H 1997 Corticosteroid therapy in severe illness. New England Journal of Medicine 337: 1285–1292

Lipworth B J 2000 Therapeutic implications of non-genomic glucocorticoid activity. Lancet 356: 87–88

Lavin M J et al 1986 Use of steroid eye drops in general practice. British Medical Journal 292: 1448

Marx J 1995 How the glucocorticoids suppress immunity. Science 270: 232–233

Mitchell A, O'Keane V 1998 Steroids and depression. British Medical Journal 316: 244–245

Newton R W et al 1978 Adrenocortical suppression in workers manufacturing synthetic glucocorticoids. British Medical Journal 1: 73

35

Diabetes mellitus, insulin, oral antidiabetes agents, obesity

SYNOPSIS

Diabetes mellitus affects 1–2% of many national populations. Its successful management requires close collaboration between the patient and the doctor.

- Diabetes mellitus and insulin
- Insulins in current use (including choice, formulations, adverse effects, hypoglycaemia, insulin resistance)
- Oral antidiabetes drugs
- Treatment of diabetes mellitus
- Diabetic ketoacidosis
- Surgery in diabetic patients
- Obesity and overweight

Diabetes mellitus and insulin

HISTORY

Insulin (as pancreatic islet cell extract) was first administered to a 14-year-old insulin-deficient patient on 11 January 1922 in Toronto, Canada. An adult sufferer from diabetes who developed the disease in 1920 and who, because of insulin, lived until 1968, has told how:

Many doctors, after they have developed a disease, take up the speciality in it … But that was not so with me. I was studying for surgery when diabetes took me up. The great book of Joslin said that by starving you might live four years with luck. [He went to Italy and, whilst his health was declining there, he received a letter from a biochemist friend which said] there was something called 'insulin' appearing with a good name in Canada, what about going there and getting it. I said 'No thank you; I've tried too many quackeries for diabetes; I'll wait and see'. Then I got peripheral neuritis … So when [the friend] cabled me and said, 'I've got insulin — it works — come back quick', I responded, arrived at King's College Hospital, London, and went to the laboratory as soon as it opened … It was all experimental for [neither of us] knew a thing about it … So we decided to have 20 units a nice round figure. I had a nice breakfast. I had bacon and eggs and toast made on the Bunsen. I hadn't eaten bread for months and months … by 3 o'clock in the afternoon my urine was quite sugar free. That hadn't happened for many months. So we gave a cheer for Banting and Best.[1]

But at 4 pm I had a terrible shaky feeling and a terrible sweat and hunger pain. That was my first experience of hypoglycaemia. We remembered that

---

[1] F G Banting and C H Best of Toronto, Canada (see also Journal of Laboratory and Clinical Medicine 1922 7: 251).

Banting and Best had described an overdose of insulin in dogs. So I had some sugar and a biscuit and soon got quite well, thank you.[2]

Diabetes mellitus is classified broadly as:

Type I (formerly, insulin dependent diabetes mellitus, IDDM) which typically occurs in younger people who cannot secrete insulin

Type 2 (formerly, non-insulin dependent diabetes mellitus, NIDDM), which typically occurs in older, often obese people who retain capacity to secrete insulin but who are resistant to its action. These terms and abbreviations are used in this chapter.

Sources of insulin

Insulin is synthesised and stored (bound to zinc) in granules in the β-islet cells of the pancreas. Daily secretion amounts to 30–40 units, which is about 25% of total pancreatic insulin content. The principal factor that evokes insulin secretion is a high blood glucose concentration.

Insulin is a polypeptide with two peptide chains (A chain, 21 amino acids and B chain, 30) linked by two disulphide bridges. The basic structure having metabolic activity is common to all mammalian species but there are minor species differences, which result in the development of antibodies in all patients treated with animal insulins, as well as to unavoidable impurities in the preparations, minimal though these now are.

- **Bovine** insulin differs from human insulin by three amino acids and is more antigenic to man than is
- **Porcine** insulin differs from human by only one amino acid
- **Human** insulin (1980) is made either by enzyme modification of porcine insulin, or by using recombinant DNA to synthesise the proinsulin, precursor molecule for insulin. This is done by artificially introducing the DNA into either *Escherichia coli* or yeast.

The three forms of human insulin have the same amino acid sequence, but are separately designated

as insulin *emp* (Enzyme Modified Porcine), *prb* (Proinsulin Recombinant in Bacteria) and *pyr* (Precursor insulin Yeast Recombinant). Although one of the incentives for introducing human insulin was avoidance of insulin antibody production, the allergies to older insulins were largely caused by impurities in the preparations, and are avoided equally well by using the highly purified, mono-component porcine and bovine insulins. Other preparations have been withdrawn. There is no systematic difference in activity between human and animal insulin, but any change in preparation prescribed to a patient should be monitored with care (see below).

Insulin receptors

Insulin binds to the α subunit of its receptor. The β subunit is a tyrosine kinase which is activated by insulin binding and is autophosphorylated. Tyrosine kinase also phosphorylates other substrates so that a signalling cascade is initiated and biological response ensues. Insulin receptors are present on the surface of the target cells (mostly liver, muscle, fat). Receptors vary in number inversely with the insulin concentration to which they are exposed, i.e. with high insulin concentration the number of receptors declines (*down-regulation*) and responsiveness to insulin also declines (insulin resistance); with low insulin concentration the number of receptors increases (*up-regulation*) and responsiveness to insulin increases. Type 2 diabetes patients have insulin resistance.

Hyperinsulinaemia predates the onset of diabetes and the resistance is thought to be secondary to down-regulation of insulin receptors as well as postreceptor, intracellular events. Obesity is a major factor in the development of insulin resistance. Patients may recover insulin responsiveness as a result of dieting so that the insulin secretion decreases, cellular receptors increase and insulin sensitivity is restored.

Actions of insulin

The effects of stimulation of the insulin receptors include activation of glucokinase and glucose phosphatase. Insulin also increases glucose transport

---

[2] Abbreviated from Lawrence R D 1961 King's College Hospital Gazette 40: 220. Transcript from a recorded after dinner talk to students' Historical Society.

as well as its utilisation, especially by muscle and adipose tissue. Its effects include:

- *Reduction in blood glucose* due to increased glucose uptake in the peripheral tissues (which convert it into glycogen or fat), and reduction of hepatic output of glucose (diminished breakdown of glycogen and diminished gluconeogenesis). When the blood glucose concentration falls below the renal threshold (10 mmol/l or 180 mg/100 ml) glycosuria ceases, as does the osmotic diuresis of water and electrolytes. Polyuria with dehydration and excessive thirst are thus alleviated. As the blood glucose falls, appetite is stimulated.

- *Other metabolic effects.* In addition to enabling glucose to pass across cell membranes, the transit of amino acids and potassium into the cell is enhanced. Insulin regulates carbohydrate utilisation and energy production. It enhances protein synthesis. It inhibits breakdown of fats (lipolysis). An insulin-deficient diabetic (Type 1) becomes dehydrated due to osmotic diuresis, and is ketotic because fats break down faster than the ketoacid metabolites can be metabolised.

Uses

- Diabetes mellitus is the main indication.
- Insulin promotes the passage of potassium simultaneously with glucose into cells, and this effect is utilised to correct hyperkalaemia (see p. 537).
- Insulin-induced hypoglycaemia can also be used as a test of anterior pituitary function (growth hormone and corticotropin are released).

Pharmacokinetics

- Insulin, naturally secreted by the pancreas, enters the portal vein and passes straight to the liver, where half of it is taken up. The rest enters and is distributed in the systemic circulation so that its concentration (in fasting subjects) is only about 15% of that entering the liver.
- When insulin is injected s.c. it enters the systemic circulation and both liver and other peripheral organs receive the same concentration.

This difference may have clinical importance and this is why some continous infusion pumps (see below) deliver insulin intraperitoneally rather than subcutaneously.

In conventional use, insulin is injected (s.c., i.m. or i.v.) as it is digested if swallowed. It is absorbed into the blood[3] and is inactivated in the liver and kidney; about 10% appears in the urine. The $t\frac{1}{2}$ is 5 min.

In addition to needles and syringes, alternative techniques for insulin administration have been developed, some availing themselves of the kinetics of insulin: insulin pens (supplied preloaded or with replaceable cartridges), external infusions and implantable pumps. These latter are convenient for an accurately controlled continuously functioning biofeedback system, but pose difficulties for routine replacement in insulin deficiency. Therefore sustained-release (depot) formulations are used to provide an approach reasonably near to natural function and compatible with the convenience of daily living. An even closer approach is provided by the development of (at present inevitably expensive) miniaturised infusion pumps which can be used by reliable patients.

DIFFERENCES BETWEEN HUMAN AND ANIMAL INSULINS

Human insulin is absorbed from subcutaneous tissue slightly more rapidly than animal insulins and it has a slightly shorter duration of action.

Human insulin is less immunogenic than bovine, but not porcine, insulin. When changing from animal to human insulin, patients taking < 100 units of animal insulin are likely to require 10% less human insulin, and if taking > 100 units animal insulin, 25% less human insulin.

There has been concern that patients taking human insulin may experience more frequent and more severe hypoglycaemic attacks, especially when

---

[3] Peak plasma insulin (s.c.) concentration is attained in 60–90 min. Absorption is slower if there is peripheral vascular disease or smoking, and faster if the patient takes a hot bath or uses an ultraviolet light sunbed (which may induce a hypoglycaemic fit) or exercises. The effects are due to changes in peripheral blood flow.

transferring from animal insulins. Such occurrences are likely to be due to management problems rather than to pharmacological differences.

There is some evidence of a lessened awareness of hypoglycaemia with human insulin, i.e. the counter-regulatory physiological responses to animal and human insulin may differ. It is claimed that with human insulin patients experience less adrenergic symptoms (sweating, tremor, palpitations), which are such a useful warning, although the neurological (neuroglycopenic) symptoms (dizziness, headache, inability to concentrate) are unchanged. It now seems likely that the reduced awareness is a paradoxical response to improved glycaemic control. Thus patients with a normal level of glycosylated haemoglobin (HbA1c) show no reduction in glucose uptake in the brain during episodes of hypoglycaemia that trigger a symptomatic and neuroendocrine response in patients with elevated levels of HbA1c (see Boyle et al 1995, in Guide to Further Reading).

PREPARATIONS OF INSULIN (Fig. 35.1)

There are three major factors:

- Strength (concentration)
- Source (human, porcine, bovine)
- Formulation
  — short-acting solution of insulin for use s.c., i.m. or i.v.
  — intermediate and longer acting (sustained release) preparations in which the insulin has been physically modified by combination with protamine or zinc to give an amorphous or crystalline suspension; this is given s.c. and slowly dissociates to release insulin in its soluble form (given i.m., which is not advised, the time course of release would be different).

Dosage is measured in *international units* now standardised by chemical assay.

Diabetes mellitus may be managed from a choice of four types of insulin (animal or human) preparations, having:

1. *Short duration* of action (and rapid onset): Soluble Insulin (neutral insulin). The most recent addition to this class of insulin, insulin lispro (Humalog), is a modified human insulin in which the reversing of two amino acids has

resulted in a very rapid onset of action (within 15 minutes of injection). Insulin aspart is similar.

2. *Intermediate duration* of action (and slower onset): Isophane Insulin, a suspension with protamine; Insulin Zinc Suspensions, amorphous or a mixture of amorphous and crystalline

3. *Longer duration* of action: Insulin Zinc Suspension, crystalline, or Protamine Zinc Insulin (insulin in suspension with both zinc and protamine).

4. A *mixture* of soluble and isophane insulins, officially called *biphasic* insulins. The short-acting analogue insulins are now also available in mixtures. Other mixtures are available, but infrequently used.

Insulin nomenclature

This is potentially confusing. The problems have arisen because insulin is a naturally occuring molecule (differing slightly among species), which has been formulated in many ways — partly catering for differing patient requirements, and partly reflecting a variety of manufacturing processes used by pharmaceutical companies. Fortunately, there has been considerable rationalisation of the preparations but it may be helpful to explain some remaining ambiguities.

- *Soluble* and *neutral* insulin are the same; the British National Formulary favours the former term, but neutral is the INN (internationally approved) name, dating back to when there were acid and neutral pH formulations of soluble insulin. Human, porcine and beef are available.
- *Isophane* insulin is the only approved name for suspensions of insulin with protamine. Human, porcine and beef are available; the latter is rarely used.
- *Biphasic* insulins are, with one exception, proprietary mixtures of soluble (neutral) insulin and isophane insulin, which provide soluble (neutral) insulin at concentrations between 10% and 50% of the total insulin concentration. Human, porcine and beef are available, but most preparations in this group are of human insulin. These preparations remove the need for patients to mix soluble and isophane insulins, without

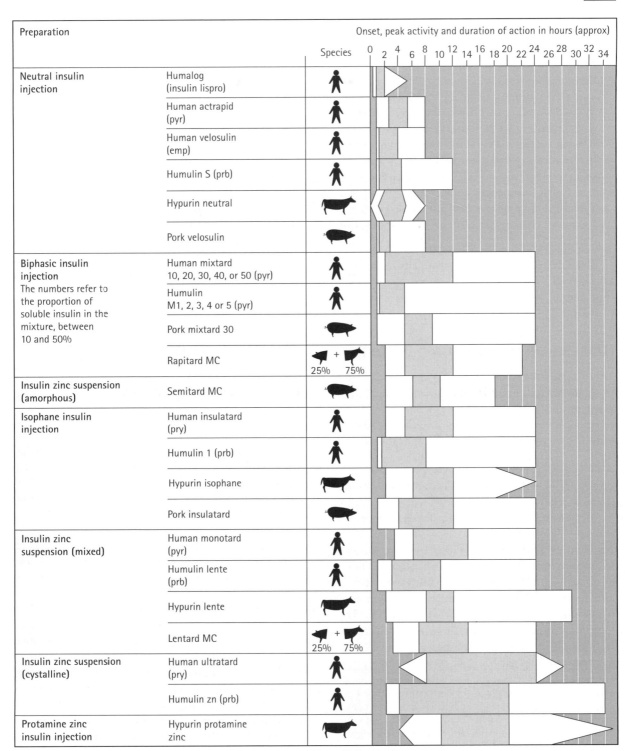

Preparation		Species	Onset, peak activity and duration of action in hours (approx)
Neutral insulin injection	Humalog (insulin lispro)	👤	
	Human actrapid (pyr)	👤	
	Human velosulin (emp)	👤	
	Humulin S (prb)	👤	
	Hypurin neutral	🐄	
	Pork velosulin	🐖	
Biphasic insulin injection The numbers refer to the proportion of soluble insulin in the mixture, between 10 and 50%	Human mixtard 10, 20, 30, 40, or 50 (pyr)	👤	
	Humulin M1, 2, 3, 4 or 5 (pyr)	👤	
	Pork mixtard 30	🐖	
	Rapitard MC	🐖 + 🐄 25% 75%	
Insulin zinc suspension (amorphous)	Semitard MC	🐖	
Isophane insulin injection	Human insulatard (pry)	👤	
	Humulin 1 (prb)	👤	
	Hypurin isophane	🐄	
	Pork insulatard	🐖	
Insulin zinc suspension (mixed)	Human monotard (pyr)	👤	
	Humulin lente (prb)	👤	
	Hypurin lente	🐄	
	Lentard MC	🐖 + 🐄 25% 75%	
Insulin zinc suspension (cystalline)	Human ultratard (pry)	👤	
	Humulin zn (prb)	👤	
Protamine zinc insulin injection	Hypurin protamine zinc	🐄	

(prb) – produced from prc insulin synthesised by bacteria using recombinant DNA technology;
(pyr) – produced from a precursor synthesised by yeast using recombinant DNA technology;
(emp) – produced by enzymatic modification of porcine insulin.

Fig. 35.1 Insulin chart. Reproduced with permission of the Monthly Index of Medical Specialities. This chart is subject to change as companies develop their products.

losing the flexible administration of the right amount of soluble (neutral) insulin to cover the meal following the dose.

• *Mixed insulin zinc suspension* is, confusingly, the approved name for proprietary mixtures of crystalline and amorphous zinc suspension. Mixed insulins are not, therefore, the same as biphasic insulins. While the different proprietary formulations in this group do have differing time courses of action (see Fig. 35.1) depending on their (unstated) proportions of amorphous and crystalline suspension, it is not expected that doctors or patients would vary the formulation prescribed.

The important thing is for the doctor to get to know well a range that will serve most patients. (For insulin regimens and injection techniques, see p. 691.)

NOTES FOR PRESCRIBING INSULIN

There is no need to change a stabilised diabetic from animal to human insulin. Unexplained requirement of above 100 units/d is usually due to non-compliance and less often to antibodies since the withdrawal of the older insulin preparations.

Allergy still occurs to additives (protamine), to the preservative, e.g. phenol, cresol, or to insulin itself. It may take the form of local reactions (inflammatory or fat atrophy) or of insulin resistance.

Antibodies to insulin, provided they are moderate in amount, may be actually advantageous. They act as a carrier or store, binding insulin after injection and releasing it slowly as the free insulin in the plasma declines. In this way they smooth and prolong insulin action. But too high antibody concentrations cause insulin resistance.

---

[4] An adverse effect of easy self-monitoring is that a minority of obsessional patients, told of the desirability of blood glucose concentrations being kept in the normal range to prevent diabetic complications, become obsessed with monitoring, and experience great anxiety when they find what are, in fact, normal fluctuations. They then anxiously change their insulin doses daily and as a result induce frequent hypoglycaemia, e.g. one patient had 33 episodes in 44 days, many with loss of consciousness (Beer S F et al 1989 British Medical Journal 298: 362).

Compatibility. Soluble insulin may be mixed in the syringe with insulin zinc suspensions (amorphous, crystalline) and with isophane and mixed (biphasic) insulin, and used at once: but there are insulins in which protamine is used as a carrier, and spare protamine will bind some of the short-acting neutral insulin, thus blunting its effects.

Intravenous insulin. Only Soluble (neutral, clear) Insulin Inj. should be used.

The standard strength of insulin preparations is 100 units per ml in a large and growing number of countries. Even very low doses can be accurately measured with modern special syringes. Solutions of 40 units and 80 units remain available in many countries, and healthcare providers should be aware of this.

Insulins in current use

CHOICE OF PREPARATION

That insulin preparations should be both precise and of uniform strength all over the world is vital to the health and safety of millions of diabetics. Advances in technology now allow biological standardisation in animal insulin to be replaced by physicochemical methods (high performance liquid chromatography: HPLC).

Soluble insulin inj. (neutral, regular insulin) is an aqueous solution of insulin. It is simple to use, being given s.c. 2–3 times a day, 30 min before meals. There is little risk of serious hypoglycaemic reaction if it is used sensibly. If a meal must be delayed, then the insulin injection should be delayed. The dose can easily be adjusted according to self-performed blood glucose measurements.[4] For these reasons it is often used initially to balance diabetics needing insulin and always for the treatment of diabetic ketoacidosis. The biggest disadvantages of soluble insulin for long-term use are the need for frequent injections, and the occurrence of high blood glucose before breakfast.

Soluble insulin is neutral, adjusted to pH 7.0. Acid formulations of soluble insulin are no longer available.

Intravenous soluble (neutral) insulin is used in diabetic ketoacidosis. It may be given intermittently (i.v. or i.m.) but continous infusion is preferred. If the insulin is infused by drip in physiological saline (40 units/l) as much as 60–80% can be lost due to binding to the fluid container and tubing. It is necessary to take this into account in dosing. Polygeline (Haemaccel) may be added to bind the insulin in competition with the apparatus and so carry it into the body.

Use of a slow-infusion pump with a concentrated solution (insulin 1.0 unit/ml) is recommended. Insulin loss is minimised and control of dose is more accurate than when more dilute solutions are used. (For i.v. doses see diabetic ketoacidosis, below.) Insulin is suitable for adimistration by continuous i.v. infusion because its short $t\frac{1}{2}$ (5 min) means that the plasma concentration rapidly reaches steady state after initiating the infusion or altering its rate ($5 \times t\frac{1}{2}$, see p. 101). Long-acting (sustained-release) preparations must not be given i.v.

Insulin zinc suspensions and isophane insulin (see Fig. 35.1) are sustained-release formulations in which rate of release is controlled by modifying particle size. Neutral pH, soluble insulin can be mixed with them without altering the time course of effect of either and these formulations can be a great convenience.

Duration of action. Patients live by a 24-hour cycle and plainly insulins having a duration of action exceeding 24 hours can cause problems, especially early morning hypoglycaemia.

DOSE AND USAGE

The total daily output of endogenous insulin from pancreatic islet cells is 30–40 units (determined by the needs of completely pancreatectomised patients), and most insulin-deficient diabetics will need 30–50 unit/day (0.5–0.8 units/kg) of insulin (two-thirds in the morning and one-third in the evening).

Initial treatment for a Type 1 (IDDM) patient, who does not present with ketoacidosis, will usually be outside hospital with two injections of intermediate-acting insulin, or a mixed insulin. Other permutations, including soluble insulin before each meal,

and an intermediate-acting insulin at bedtime, can follow later. The following is a guide to initial daily dose requirements:

- 0.3 units/kg (16–20 units daily)
- increasing to 0.5 units/kg.

The dose is adjusted according to the usual monitoring of blood[5] glucose (or urine, if glucose meters are unavailable). Daily (total) dose increments should be 4 units at 3–4-day intervals.

If it is decided to give the patient only one injection per day, then 10–14 units of an intermediate-acting isophane suspension may be given. Dose increments (4 units) may be made on alternate days. Soluble insulin (neutral) may be added, or mixed (biphasic) insulins may be used, according to the patient's response.

When stable, patients usually receive either a biphasic insulin or a mixture of soluble, short-acting human insulin, and a longer-acting suspension of insulin with protamine or zinc.

Excessive dose of insulin leads to overeating and obesity; it also leads to hypoglycaemia (especially nocturnal), that may be followed by rebound morning hyperglycaemia that is mistakenly treated by increased insulin, thus establishing a vicious cycle (Somogyi effect).

Physical activity increases carbohydrate utilisation and insulin sensitivity, so that hypoglycaemia is likely if a well-stabilised patient changes suddenly from an inactive existence to a vigorous life. If this is likely to happen the carbohydrate in the diet may be increased and/or the dose of insulin reduced by up to one-third and then readjusted according to need. This is less marked in patients on oral agents.

See also Selection of therapy and Ketoacidosis (below).

ADVERSE EFFECTS OF INSULIN

Adverse effects of insulin are mainly those of overdose.[6] Because the brain relies on glucose as its

---

[5] The normal (fasting) blood glucose range is 3.9–5.8 mmol/1 (70–105 mg/100 ml).
[6] Suicidal overdose (in diabetics) is well recorded. Surgical excision of the skin and subcutaneous tissue at the injection site of an enormous dose of long-acting insulin has been used effectively.

source of energy, an adequate blood glucose concentration is just as essential as an adequate supply of oxygen, and *hypoglycaemia* may lead to coma, convulsions and even death (in 4% of diabetics under 50 years of age).

It is usually easier to differentiate hypoglycaemia from severe diabetic ketosis than from other causes of coma, which are as likely in a diabetic as in anyone else. It is unsound to advocate blind administration of i.v. glucose to comatose diabetics on the basis that it will revive them if they are hypoglycaemic and do no harm if they are hyperglycaemic. A minority of comatose insulin-dependent diabetics have hyperkalaemia and added glucose can cause a brisk and potentially hazardous rise in serum potassium (mechanism uncertain), in contrast to nondiabetics in whom glucose causes a fall in serum potassium.

Hypoglycaemia may manifest itself as disturbed sleep (nightmares) and morning headache. For details of treatment see below.

Other adverse reactions to insulin are *lipodystrophy* (atrophy or hypertrophy) at the injection sites (rare with purified pork and human insulin), after they have been used repeatedly. These are unsightly, but otherwise harmless. The site should not be used further, for absorption can be erratic, but the patient may be tempted to continue if local anaesthesia has developed, as it sometimes does. Lipoatrophy is probably allergic and lipohypertrophy is due to a local metabolic action of insulin. Local allergy also is manifested as itching or painful red lumps.

Generalised allergic reactions are very rare, but may occur to any insulin (including human) and to any constituent of the formulation. Change of brand of insulin, especially to highly purified preparations (or to one with a different mode of manufacture) may rectify allergic problems. But zinc occurs in all insulins (though very little in soluble insulin) and can be the allergen.

TREATMENT OF A HYPOGLYCAEMIC ATTACK

Prevention depends very largely upon patient education, but it is an unavoidable aspect of intensive glycaemic control. Patients should not miss meals, must know the early symptoms of an attack, and always carry glucose with them.[7] Treatment is

to give sugar, either by mouth if the patient can still swallow or glucose (dextrose) i.v. (20–50 ml of 50% solution, i.e. 10–25 g; this concentration is irritant especially if extravasation occurs and the veins of diabetics are precious, so compress the vein immediately after completion of injection; administration of 50–125 ml of 20% glucose is less thrombotic, if available. The response is usually dramatic. The patient should be given a meal to avoid relapse. But if the patient does not respond within 30 min, it may be because of cerebral oedema, which recovers slowly and may require treatment with i.v. dexamethasone. If the patient has been severely hypoglycaemic or if very large amounts of insulin or sulphonylurea have been taken, then 20% glucose should be given by i.v. infusion. Very severe attacks sometimes damage the central nervous system permanently. (See also use of glucagon, below.)

After recovery from a severe attack and elucidation of the cause, the patient's treatment regimen should be carefully reviewed with appropriate educational input.

Hypoglycaemia due to other causes, e.g. alcohol, is treated similarly.

INSULIN RESISTANCE AND HORMONES THAT INCREASE BLOOD GLUCOSE

Insulin resistance may be due to a decline in number and/or affinity of receptors (see above) or to defects in postreceptor mechanisms.

A diabetic patient requiring more than 200 units/day is rare and regarded as insulin resistant (occasional patients have needed as much as 5000 units/day). Insulin resistance has become much less frequent with the wide availability of purified, mono-component and human insulins. If the requirement is acquired and genuine, it is due to antibodies binding insulin in a biologically inactive complex (though it can dissociate as with protein binding of drugs). De novo insulin resistance occurs in a small number of genetic syndromes, e.g. in combination with the skin condition acanthosis nigricans.

---

[7] In the early stages of insulin treatment, it can be very useful training to allow a patient to experience hypoglycaemia once by delaying a meal.

Where animal insulins are still in use, change to a highly purified pork or human insulin may be successful in reducing resistance. Responsiveness to insulin may sometimes be restored by immunosuppression, e.g. an adrenocortical steroid (prednisolone 20–40 mg/d) over weeks (or a few months), to suppress antibody production. Obviously, if this is successful, insulin dosage will have to be reduced in accordance with the unpredictable reduction in antibodies. Patients need to be carefully monitored to avoid severe hypoglycaemia. Ketoacidosis also reduces the effect of insulin.

Glucagon $(t\frac{1}{2}\ 4\,\text{min})$ is a polypeptide hormone (29 amino acids) from the α-islet cells of the pancreas. It is released in response to hypoglycaemia and is a physiological regulator of insulin effect, acting by causing the release of liver glycogen as glucose. Glucagon has been used to treat insulin-induced hypoglycaemia, but in about 45 min from onset of coma the hepatic glycogen will anyway be exhausted and glucagon will be useless. Its chief advantage is that, as it can be given s.c. or i.m. (1.0 mg), glucagon can be used in a severe hypoglycaemic attack by somebody, e.g. a member of the patient's family, who is unable to give an i.v. injection of glucose. If a comatose patient does not recover sufficiently in 20 min to allow oral therapy, i.v. glucose is essential. Glucagon is ineffective in substantial hepatic insufficiency.

Glucagon has a positive cardiac inotropic effect by stimulating adenylyl cyclase; it appears to have value in acute overdose of β-adrenoceptor blockers (see Index).

Adrenaline (epinephrine) raises the blood sugar by mobilising liver and muscle glycogen; it does not antagonise the peripheral actions of insulin. Glycosuria and diabetic symptoms may occur in patients with phaeochromocytoma.

Adrenal steroids, either endogenous or exogenous, antagonise the actions of insulin, although this effect is only slight with the primarily mineralocorticoid group; the glucocorticoid hormones increase gluconeogenesis and reduce glucose uptake and utilisation by the tissues. Patients with Cushing's syndrome thus develop diabetes very readily and may be resistant to insulin. Patients with Addison's disease, hypothyroidism and hypopituitarism are abnormally sensitive to insulin action.

Oral contraceptives can impair carbohydrate tolerance.

Growth hormone antagonises the actions of insulin in the tissues. Acromegalic patients may develop insulin-resistant diabetes.

Thyroid hormone increases the requirements for insulin.

Oral antidiabetes drugs

Oral antidiabetes drugs are of two kinds: *sulphonamide* derivatives (sulphonylureas) and *guanidine* derivatives (biguanides). They are used by 30% of all diabetics. Unlike insulin they are not essential for life.

Following the observation in 1918 that guanidine had hypoglycaemic effect, guanides were tried in diabetes in 1926, but were abandoned a few years later for fear of hepatic toxicity.

In 1930 it was noted that sulphonamides could cause hypoglycaemia, and in 1942 severe hypoglycaemia was found in patients with typhoid fever during a therapeutic trial of sulphonamide. In the 1950s a similar observation was made during a chemotherapeutic trial in urinary infections. This was followed up and effective drugs soon resulted. The first sulphonylureas were introduced into clinical practice in 1954.

MODE OF ACTION

Sulphonylureas block the ATP-sensitive potassium channels on the β-islet cell plasma membrane. This results in the release of stored insulin in response to glucose. They do not increase insulin formation. Sulphonylureas appear to enhance insulin action on liver, muscle and adipose tissue by increasing insulin receptor number and by enhancing the post-receptor complex enzyme reactions mediated by insulin. The principal result is decreased hepatic glucose output and increased glucose uptake in muscle. They are ineffective in totally insulin-deficient patients and for successful therapy probably require about 30% of normal β-cell function to be present. Their main adverse effects are hypoglycaemia and weight gain.

Secondary failure (after months or years) occurs due to declining β-cell function and to insulin resistance.

Biguanides. These agents have been in use since 1957. *Metformin* is the only biguanide in current use, and is a major agent in the management of Type 2 diabetes. Its cellular mode of action is uncertain but the most important effect is reduction of hepatic glucose production. Other effects include enhancement of peripheral insulin sensitivity increaseing glucose uptake in peripheral tissues; biguanides are ineffective in the absence of insulin. Rare complications are hypoglycaemia and lactic acidosis. Secondary failure is not a problem. Metformin can be used in combination with either insulin or other oral hypoglycaemic agents.

Thiazolidinediones. *Pioglitazone* and *rosiglitazone* reduce peripheral insulin resistance, leading to a reduction of blood glucose concentration. These drugs stimulate the nuclear hormone receptor, peroxisome proliferator-activated receptor (PPARγ), which causes differentation of adipocytes.[8] They should be initiated only by a physician experienced in treating Type 2 diabetes and should always be used in combination with metformin or with a sulphonylurea (if metformin is inappropriate). The drugs can cause 3–4 kg weight gain in the first year of use, with peripheral oedema in 3–4% of patients. Other adverse effects of the class have included abnormal liver function, and relevant tests should be monitored during the first year.

---

[8] The importance of PPARγ in insulin sensitivity was confirmed with the finding, in Cambridge, of two families presenting with severe insulin resistance in whom rare mutations of the PPARγ gene caused loss of PPARγ activity (Barroso I, Gurnell M, Crowley VE, et al 1989 Dominant negative mutations in human PPARγ associated with severe insulin resistance, diabetes mellitus and hypertension. Nature 402: 880–882.)

INDIVIDUAL DRUGS

Absorption from the alimentary tract is good for all the oral agents. It is advisable to take drugs ~30 min before a meal. These three groups of drugs are effective only in the presence of insulin. If a patient fails to respond to one drug, response to another as single treatment is unlikely. Proceeding to a combination of drugs from different classes may then be effective.

Sulphonylureas (see also Table 35.1)

Several sulphonylureas are available. Choice is determined by the duration of action as well as the patient's age and renal function, and unwanted effects. The long-acting sulphonylureas, e.g. glibenclamide, are associated with a greater risk of hypoglycaemia; for this reason they should be avoided in the elderly for whom the shorter-acting alternatives, such as gliclazide or tolbutamide, should be used. As chlorpropamide is both long-acting and has more unwanted effects than the other sulphonylureas (see below) it is no longer recommended. In patients with impaired renal function, gliclazide, glipizide or tolbutamide are preferred since they are not excreted by the kidney. Generally, it is prudent to start at the lowest recommended dose in order to minimise risk of hypoglycaemia.

TABLE 35.1 Principal oral antidiabetes drugs

Drug	Total daily dose (mg)	Dosing schedule (doses/day)	Duration of action (h)
Sulphonylureas			
glibeclamide	2.5–20	1–2	12–24
gliclazide	40–320	1–2	12–24
glipizide	2.5–40	1–2	12–24
glimepiride	1–6	1	16–24
Biguanide			
metformin	500–3000	2–3	8–12
Thiazolidinedione			
rosiglitazone	2–8	1–2	12–24
pioglitazone	15–30	1	16–24
Meglitinide			
repaglinide	0.5–16	3	3–4
nateglinide	60–180	3	2–3
α-glucosidase inhibitor			
acarbose	50–300	3	3–4

Other sulphonylureas include tolbutamide, gliquidone, glibornuride, tolazamide.

Sulphonamides, as expected, potentiate sulphonylureas by direct action and by displacement from plasma proteins.

Gliclazide is a commonly used second generation sulphonylurea. If more than 80 mg is prescribed, the drug should be taken twice daily before meals.

Glimepiride is designed to be used once daily and to provoke less hypoglycaemia than glibenclamide.

Repaglinide is a very short-acting oral hypoglycaemic agent whose action, like the sulphonylureas, is mediated through blockade of ATP-dependent potassium channels. It affects only postprandial insulin profiles, and should in theory reduce risk of hypoglycaemia.

Biguanides (see also Table 35.1)

Metformin ($t\frac{1}{2}$ 5 h) is taken with or after meals. Its chief use is in the obese patient with Type 2 diabetes either alone or in combination with a sulphonylurea. It has a mild anorexic effect which helps to reduce weight in the obese. The action of metformin is terminated by excretion by the kidney and it should not be used in the presence of renal impairment.

Minor adverse gut reactions are common, including nausea, diarrhoea, and a metallic taste in the mouth. These symptoms are usually transient or subside after reduction of dose. Heavy prolonged use can cause vitamin B_{12} deficiency due to malabsorption. With a biguanide, ketonuria may occur in the presence of normal blood sugar. This is not generally severe and responds to reduction of dose. More serious, but rare, is *lactic acidosis,* which occurs in 0.03 cases per 1000 patient years. When this condition does occur, it is usually against the background of a serious underlying medical state such as renal impairment, liver failure or cardiogenic or septic shock. Lactic acidosis is treated with large (i.v.) doses of isotonic sodium bicarbonate.

Thiazolidinediones (see also Table 35.1)

Pioglitazone, is indicated once daily in patients not controlled by metformin alone. It is contraindicated by cardiac or hepatic failure. Weight gain and oedema are the main adverse effects.

Rosiglitazone is similar and is administered once or twice daily.

PRECAUTIONS WITH ORAL AGENTS

Hypoglycaemia is the most common adverse effect with sulphonylureas, but is less common than with insulin therapy. It can be severe, and prolonged (for days), and may be fatal in 10% of cases, especially in the elderly and in patients with heart failure. Erroneous alternate diagnoses such as stroke may be made.

Renal and hepatic disease. A biguanide should not be used in patients with either condition as the risk of lactic acidosis is too great. Sulphonylureas are potentiated in these diseases and a drug with a short $t\frac{1}{2}$ (i.e. not glibenclamide) should be used in low dose.

Age adds to the hazard of oral agents.

Other adverse effects are rare but include skin rashes, gastrointestinal upset, minor derangement of haematological and hepatic indices.

OTHER ORAL AGENTS

Acarbose is an α-glucosidase inhibitor which reduces digestion of complex carbohydrates and slows their absorption from the gut; in high doses it may cause actual malabsorption. Acarbose reduces glycaemia after meals, and may improve overall glycaemic control. The usual dose is 50–300 mg daily. Adverse effects are mainly flatulence and diarrhoea, which lead to a high discontinuation rate. The drug may be combined with a sulphonylurea.

Dietary fibre and diabetes. The addition of gel-forming (soluble) but unabsorbable fibre (guar gum, a hydrocolloidal polysaccharide of galactose and mannose from seeds of the 'cluster bean') to the diet of diabetics reduces carbohydrate absorption and flattens the postprandial blood glucose curve. Reduced need for insulin and oral agents are reported, but adequate amounts (taken with lots of water) are unpleasant (flatulence) and patient compliance is therefore poor.

Treatment of diabetes mellitus

Doctor, nurse and patient are faced with a lifetime of collaboration. Compliance is not a one-sided process, and the patients need all the consideration and support they can get. They should learn about their disease and its management, including home monitoring of blood glucose, and about the need for appropriate diet, exercise and avoidance of smoking.

All Type 1 patients need immediate insulin therapy. Initial therapy in Type 2 patients should be by dietary means alone, for 2–3 months but most patients will need oral antidiabetes drugs in addtion.

The *aims of treatment* are:

- to alleviate symptomatic hyperglycaemia and improve quality of life, while avoiding hypoglycaemia
- to avoid ketosis and infections
- to keep
  - the fasting blood glucose ≤ 6 mmol/l
  - the 1-hour postprandial concentration < 9 mmol/l
  - the glycosylated haemoglobin HbA1c as close to normal as possible
- In addition to optimal glycaemic control other cardiovascular risk factors should be corrected:
  - optimal blood pressure control $< 130/80$ mmHg
  - cholesterol < 5.2 mmol/l
  - triglycerides < 2.0 mmol/l
- by this regimen to avoid or delay long-term microvascular and macrovascular complications, and reduce mortality.

Each patient must be assessed individually; only an outline of the general principles involved can be given here.

Diet. Patients should be allowed to follow their own preferences as far as is practicable. They should receive dietary advice on a high complex carbohydrate diet (~65% of total calories) with low fat ($< 30\%$ of calories) with emphasis on reduction in saturated fat in favour of mono- and poly-unsaturates. Calories should be restricted and patients encouraged to achieve an ideal body weight. Diet should contain ~40 g of fibre/day, with plenty of fresh fruit and vegetables.

The way in which carbohydrate is distributed through the day should correspond with the type of drug treatment, and especially the type of insulin in Type 1 patients.

Type 1 patients are initially underweight, whereas the reverse is true of Type 2. While carbohydrate intake needs to be controlled in both types, overall energy intake is restricted initially only in the obese Type 2 patients. Other general factors which influence the diet, in both Types 1 and 2, are the

- High incidence of ischaemic heart disease in diabetics, requiring restriction of saturated fat intake
- Need to reduce protein intake in patients with established nephropathy.

Weight. Older overweight diabetics (70% of Type 2) have a relative deficiency of insulin but seldom develop ketosis. In these patients, a hypocaloric (weight-reducing) diet is vital, as weight loss dramatically improves glycaemic control and indeed, glycosuria may cease when their weight is reduced. It is also likely that effective dieting helps to prevent macrovascular disease through improved control of blood lipids and blood pressure. Exercise is similarly, beneficial. Biguanide treatment particularly helps weight reduction. Weight loss is associated with an increase in numbers of insulin receptors and so an increase in responsiveness to insulin. The use of anorectic agents is discussed later in the chapter (p. 696).

Young patients with Type 1 diabetes are often underweight and need insulin to restore normal weight. Calorie restriction is not initially required in these patients. The blood of these young diabetics contains negligible insulin and they readily become ketotic.

SELECTION OF THERAPY FOR DIABETES

Patients are treated with:

- Diet alone
- Diet plus oral agent(s)

- Diet plus insulin
- Diet plus oral agent (metformin) plus insulin
- For ketoacidosis: soluble insulin, urgently.

Diabetic patients under 30 years: almost all need insulin; the exception is the rare single-gene disorder of Maturity Onset Diabetes of the Young (MODY) due usually to mutations in the glucokinase gene.

Diabetic patients over 30 years: approximately one-third need insulin, one-third oral agents and one-third diet only.

Type 1 diabetes: human insulin is preferred for new patients (for regimen see below).

Type 2 diabetes: careful trial is the only sure way of deciding who can be maintained on oral therapy rather than on insulin. About 30% of patients will be adequately managed without oral therapy. When diet alone has failed to control Type 2 diabetes, it is necessary to add an oral agent; the choice should fall first on

- metformin for the *obese* patient: the usual regimen is metformin 500 mg once or twice daily after meals, increasing at 2–4-weekly intervals to a maximum of 3 g daily.
- a sulphonylurea for the *nonobese*: an example regimen would be gliclazide 80 mg orally (or 40 mg in the small or aged) before the main meal of the day. The dose is adjusted, according to response, at 2–4-weekly intervals by increments of 40–80 mg, to a maximum of 320 mg. If control is incomplete, metformin may be added.

Insulin treatment in Type 2 diabetes. When oral therapy fails, insulin treatment should be used alone or in combination with metformin. There is little advantage from adding insulin to a sulphonylurea. The advent of thiazolidinediones offers an alternative to combining metformin with insulin, but more experience of these drugs is required before their combination with metformin can be routinely recommended. It is important to stop the thiazolidinedione, if not effective, before progressing to insulin. Definitive evidence that institution of insulin will reduce complications is lacking; however, there is an improvement in quality of life, with few patients requesting to stop insulin once they have

started, and the improved glycaemic control can be assumed also to improve outcome. Initial treatment with a single injection of intermediate-acting insulin (see Fig. 35.1) at night, or twice daily, may control hyperglycaemia. Fluctuations in blood glucose levels may be controlled with twice daily mixed insulin or by multiple injections.

Re-evaluation of the requirement for drugs can be made after the patient has been controlled and stable for 3–6 months, but complete withdrawal of oral agents is unusual.

Monitoring of patients taking oral agents should be as close as those on insulin. The prognosis of poorly controlled type 2 diabetes is serious.

Prevention of complications in Type 2 diabetes: the United Kingdom Prospective Diabetes Study (UKPDS)[9,10] This landmark study in Type 2 diabetes confirmed that good glycaemic control and aggressive blood pressure reduction independently improve outcome. For every 1% reduction in HbA1c there was a 21% reduction in diabetes related deaths, and 37% reduction in microvascular disease. The study disproved concerns about long-term safety of sulphonylureas, but suggested that metformin might be the preferred first-line pharmacological therapy in obese patients. Of highest importance was the finding that effective blood pressure control — regardless of type of antihypertensive drug — was more influential than glycaemic control in preventing macrovascular complications. Reduction of blood pressure in 758 patients to a mean of 144/82 mmHg achieved 32% reduction in deaths related to diabetes and 37% reduction in microvascular end points, compared to 390 patients treated to a blood pressure of 154/87 mmHg.

Type 1 treatment. The range of insulin formulations available allows flexible adjustment of the

[9] UK Prospective Diabetes Study (UKPDS) Group 1998 Effect of intensive blood-glucose control with metformin on complications in overweight patients with type 2 diabetes (UKPDS 34). Lancet 352: 854–865.
[10] UK Prospective Diabetes Study (UKPDS) Group 1998 Tight blood pressure control and risk of macrovascular and microvascular complications in type 2 diabetes. British Medical Journal 317: 703–713.

regimen to the patient's way of life. No single regimen suits all patients but one of the following regimens can suit most patients (see Fig. 35.1):

- Three doses of soluble insulin (before the main meals) plus an intermediate-acting insulin at bedtime
- A biphasic or intermediate-acting insulin (see Fig. 35.1) twice a day before morning and evening meals
- A single morning dose of a biphasic or intermediate-acting insulin before breakfast may suffice for some patients.

Injection technique has pharmacokinetic consequences according to whether the insulin is delivered into the subcutaneous tissue or (inadvertently) into muscle. The introduction of a range of appropriate length needles and pen-shaped injectors has enabled patients to inject perpendicularly to the skin without risk of intramuscular injection. The absorption of insulin is as much as 50% more rapid from shallow i.m. injection. Clearly factors such as heat or exercise which alter skin or muscle blood flow can markedly alter the rate of insulin absorption.

Patients should standardise their technique to ensure injection is s.c. Inadvertent i.m. injection of an overnight dose of an extended duration insulin can lead to inadequate early morning control of blood glucose. Sites of injection should be rotated to minimise the now rare local complications (lipodystrophy). Absorption is faster from arm and abdomen than it is from the thigh and buttock.

Complications of diabetes. A well-controlled diabetic is less liable to ketosis and infections. It is now certain that good control of glycaemia mitigates the serious microvascular complications, retinopathy, nephropathy, neuropathy and cataract. Too tight control of glycaemia can increase the frequency of attacks of hypoglycaemia.

SOME FACTORS AFFECTING CONTROL OF DIABETES

Intercurrent illnesses cause fluctuations in the patient's metabolic needs. If these are severe, e.g. myocardial infarction, it is prudent to substitute

insulin for oral agents. An appropriate starting dose is biphasic (mixtard) insulin 10–15 units twice daily. Infections cause an increase in insulin need (about 20%), which may drop briskly on recovery. In patients with poor glycaemic control, it is preferable to use an insulin infusion and sliding scale, as described below for diabetic ketosis.

Surgery, see later.

Menstruation and oral contraception: insulin needs may rise slightly.

Use of glucocorticoids: insulin needs are increased.

In pregnancy close control of diabetes is of the first importance to avoid fetal loss at all stages, and in the first trimester to reduce fetal malformations. Insulins requirements increase steadily after the third month. Ideally, women of childbearing age should be advised to conceive during a period of stable, euglycaemic control.

During labour soluble insulin should be given by continuous infusion at about 1–2 unit/h with i.v. infusion of 5% glucose 1.0 litre in 8 h). Substantially less, e.g. 25%, insulin is likely to be needed immediately after delivery, when timing and dose of insulin injections should be carefully reconsidered lest hypoglycaemia occurs. Insulin need remains lower during the first 6 weeks of lactation.

Blood glucose estimations are necessary during pregnancy, for glycosuria is not then a reliable guide. The renal threshold for glucose (also of lactose) falls, so that glycosuria and lactosuria may occur in the presence of a normal blood glucose.

Maternal hyperglycaemia leads to fetal hyperglycaemia with consequent fetal islet cell hyperplasia, high birthweight babies, and postnatal hypoglycaemia.

Premature labour: use of β_2-adrenoceptor agonists and of dexamethasone (to prevent respiratory distress syndrome in the prematurely newborn) causes hyperglycaemia and increased insulin (and potassium) need.

Current practice for women on oral hypoglycaemic agents who are planning, or starting, a pregnancy is to change to insulin and continue on it throughout pregnancy. There is no definitive evidence that oral drugs are associated with fetal malformations.

INTERACTIONS WITH NONDIABETES DRUGS

The subject is ill-documented, but whenever a diabetic under treatment takes other drugs it is prudent to be on the watch for disturbance of control.

β-adrenoceptor blocking drugs impair the sympathetic mediated (β_2-receptor) release of glucose from the liver in response to hypoglycaemia and also reduce the adrenergic-mediated symptoms of hypoglycaemia (except sweating). Insulin hypoglycaemia is thus both more prolonged and less noticeable. A diabetic needing β-adrenoceptor blocker should be given a β_1-selective member, e.g. bisoprolol.

Thiazide diuretics at a higher dose than generally now used in hypertension can precipitate diabetes, and it is wise to use low doses especially in established diabetes.

Hepatic enzyme inducers may enhance the metabolism of sulphonylureas that are metabolised in the liver (tolbutamide). Cimetidine, an inhibitor of drug metabolising enzymes, increases metformin plasma concentration and effect.

Monoamine oxidase inhibitors potentiate oral agents and perhaps also insulin. They can also reduce appetite and so upset control.

Interaction may occur with *alcohol* (hypoglycaemia with any antidiabetes drug).

Salicylates and *fibrates* can increase insulin sensitivity.

The action of *sulphonylureas* is intensified by heavy sulphonamide dosage and some sulphonamides increase free tolbutamide concentrations, probably by competing for plasma protein binding sites. These examples suffice to show that the possibility of interactions of practical clinical importance is a real one.

DRUG-INDUCED DIABETES

Diazoxide (see p. 470) is chemically similar to thiazide diuretics, but stimulates the ATP dependent K^+ channel that is blocked by the sulphonylureas. Therefore its chronic use as an antihypertensive agent is precluded by the development of diabetes. Indeed its use in therapeutics should now be confined to the rare indication of treating hypoglycaemia due to islet-cell tumour (insulinoma). Adrenocortical steroids are also diabetogenic.

Diabetic ketoacidosis

The condition is discussed in detail in medical texts and only the more pharmacological aspects will be dealt with here. Nevertheless, it should be emphasised that the patients are always severely dehydrated and that *fluid replacement* is the first priority.

In severe ketoacidosis the patient urgently needs *insulin* to stop ketogenesis. The objective is to supply, as continuously as possible, a moderate amount of insulin.

Soluble insulin, preferably from the same species the patient has been using (never a sustained-release form), should be given by continuous i.v. infusion of a 1 unit/ml solution of insulin in isotonic sodium chloride. It is best to use a pump, which allows independent control of insulin and electrolyte administration more readily than an i.v. drip. If a pump is not available, the insulin should be added in a concentration of 1 unit/ml to 50–100 ml of sodium chloride in a burette. The infusion rate is determined by a sliding scale, as illustrated in Table 35.2. The rate is adjusted hourly using the same scale. If an i.v. drip is used instead of a pump the concentration should be lower (40 units/l). Stringent precautions against septicaemia are necessary in these patients. Continuous infusion i.m. (not s.c.) can also be equally effective, provided the patient is not in shock and provided there is not an important degree of peripheral vascular disease.

Intermittent doses i.v. or i.m. may be used when circumstances demand. If the i.m. route is used, a priming dose of 10 units should be given at the outset and then 6–10 units hourly.

TABLE 35.2 Sliding scale of insulin doses according to blood glucose concentrations in ketoacidosis (see text)

Blood glucose (mmol/l)	Infusion rate (ml/h = units/hour for 50 ml syringe containing 50 units of insulin)
≥ 22.0	10.0 (+ check pump and connections)
19–21.9	8.0
16–18.9	6.0
12–15.9	4.0
8–11.9	2.0 (+ change from saline to glucose infusion if blood glucose < 10mmol/l)
4–7.9	1.0
< 3.9	0.5 (+ increase glucose infusion)

Progress. When the patient can eat and drink s.c. insulin is restarted. The rate of fall of blood glucose/hour is proportional to the rate of infusion of insulin over the range of 1–10 units/h. A reasonable rate of fall during treatment is 4–5.5 mmol/l (75–100 mg/100 ml) per hour.

Intravenous fluid and electrolytes.[11] Patients are often more deficient in water than in saline and although initial replacement is by isotonic (0.9%) sodium chloride solution, occurrence of hypernatraemia is an indication for half isotonic (0.45%) solution. A patient with diabetic ketoacidosis may have a fluid deficit of above 5 litres and may be given:

- 1 litre in the first hour,
- followed by 2 litres in 4 hours,
- then 4 litres in the next 24 hours, watching for signs of fluid overload.

Note that fluid replacement causes a fall in blood glucose by dilution.

Glucose should be given only when its concentration in blood falls below the renal threshold, in practice starting when the blood glucose falls to 10 mmol/l. If glucose is used at concentrations above the renal threshold it merely increases the diabetic osmotic diuresis, causing further dehydration and potassium and magnesium loss (but see Hypoglycaemia, above). When the blood glucose

[11] In this situation glucose solution does not provide water replacement since the normal capacity to metabolise glucose is fully taken up.

level falls to 10 mmol/l, the fluid replacement should be changed from saline to 5% glucose, at the same rate as detailed above.

Potassium. Even if plasma potassium is normal or high, patients have a substantial total body *deficit*, and the plasma concentration will fall briskly with i.v. saline (dilution) and insulin which draws potassium into cells within minutes. Potassium chloride should be added to the second and subsequent litres of fluid according to plasma potassium (provided the patient is passing urine):

- < 3.5 mmol/l add 40 mmol/l of fluid
- 3.5–5.0 mmol/l add 20 mmol/l of fluid
- > 5.0 mmol/l none.

Bicarbonate (isotonic) should be used only if plasma pH is < 7.0 and peripheral circulation is good; insulin corrects acidosis.

Success in treatment of diabetic ketoacidosis and its complications (hypokalaemia, aspiration of stomach contents, infection, shock, thromboembolism, cerebral oedema) depends on close, constant, informed supervision.

Mild diabetic ketosis. If the patient is fully conscious and there has been no nausea or vomiting for at least 12 h, intravenous therapy is unnecessary. It is reasonable to give small doses of insulin s.c. 4–6-hourly and fluids by mouth.

Hyperosmolar diabetic coma occurs chiefly in non-insulin-dependent diabetics who fail to compensate for their continuing, osmotic glucose diuresis. It is characterised by severe dehydration, a very high blood sugar (> 33 mmol/l : 600 mg/100 ml) and lack of ketosis and acidosis. Treatment is with isotonic (0.9%) saline, at half the rate recommended for ketoacidotic coma, and with less potassium than in severe ketoacidosis. Insulin requirements are less than in ketoacidosis, where the acidosis causes resistance to the actions of insulin, and should generally be half those shown in Table 35.2. Patients are more liable to thrombosis and prophylactic heparin is used.

Surgery in diabetes patients

Principles of management:

- Surgery constitutes a major stress
- Insulin needs increase with surgery
- Avoid ketosis
- Avoid hypoglycaemia

High blood glucose concentration matters little over short periods, except in the critically ill. The programme for control should be agreed between anaesthetist and physician whenever diabetic patients must undergo general anaesthesia or modify their diets. There are many different techniques that can give satisfactory results.

TYPE I DIABETES (IDDM)

Elective major surgery

- Admit to hospital the day before surgery
- Arrange operation for morning
- Evening before surgery: give patient's usual insulin
- Day of operation: omit morning s.c. dose; set up i.v. infusion: glucose 5–10% + KCl 20 mmol/l, infuse at 100 ml/h; insulin 20 units may be added to 1 litre of infusate or infused by pump at a basal rate of 2–3 units/h and adjusted according to a sliding scale.
- Modify regimen during and after surgery according to monitoring; insulin doses should be adjusted according to similar scale as in Table 35.2
- Stop i.v. infusion one hour after first postsurgical s.c. insulin
- Insulin requirements may be high, 10–15 units/h, in cases of serious infection, corticosteroid use, obesity, liver disease.

Minor surgery

For example, simple dental extractions (for multiple extractions or when there is infection the patient should be admitted to hospital). A suitable postoperative diet of appropriate calorie and carbo-hydrate content must be arranged. Plan the operation for between 12 noon and 5 pm (17.00 h). Omit the usual dose of long-acting insulin on the morning of the operation and substitute soluble insulin, one-quarter of the usual total daily dose, before a light breakfast 6 h preceding the operation. Arrange a light evening meal after the operation and soluble insulin, 10–20 units s.c., according to the blood glucose. Return to the normal routine the next day.

Emergency surgery

When a surgical emergency is complicated by diabetic ketosis, an attempt should be made to control the ketosis before the operation. Management during the operation will be similar to that for major surgery except that more insulin will be needed.

In other cases small doses of soluble insulin are given 2–4-hourly (where pumps are not available), keeping the blood glucose between 5 and 8 mmol/l.

TYPE 2 DIABETES (NIDDM)

Elective and emergency surgery, and minor surgery if NIDDM is poorly controlled: use the same regimen as for IDDM.

Minor surgery: If NIDDM is well controlled, omit the oral hypoglycaemic agent on the morning of surgery. If the surgery is more than trivial, monitor blood glucose carefully, and use soluble insulin s.c. or by infusion if blood glucose rises. If vomiting is likely, use insulin.

Miscellaneous

Most patients with both Type 1 and Type 2 succumb to either the macrovascular or microvascular complications — especially ischaemic heart disease and diabetic nephropathy, respectively. Indeed diabetes is the major indication for dialysis and transplantation. As discussed in other chapters, the treatment of hypertension and hyperlipidaemia is particularly important in patients with diabetes. Patients with diabetic nephropathy should receive either an ACE inhibitor or angiotensin receptor

Summary

- Diabetes mellitus is important in global terms because of its chronicity, and high incidence and frequency of major complications. It is of two kinds: Type 1 (previously, insulin dependent diabetes mellitus) and Type 2 (previously, non-insulin dependent diabetes).
- Type 1 diabetes is commoner among young, thin patients with diabetes. Insulin may also be required when glycaemic control is not achieved by oral drugs in Type 2 pateints.
- Insulin is given s.c. to stable patients, usually as a biphasic mixture of soluble, short-acting human insulin, and a longer-acting suspension of insulin with protamine or zinc.
- In the treatment of diabetic ketoacidosis, in the perioperative patient, and at other times of changing insulin requirement, insulin is best given by i.v. infusion of the soluble form.
- Diet plays a major role in the treatment of Type 2 diabetes with obesity.
- There is now a clear difference in the choice of first-line drug, if a drug is required, in Type 2 diabetes. A sulphonylurea is used for the nonobese, and metformin (a biguanide) for the obese.
- Aggressive treatment of Type 1, and probably Type 2, successfully reduces microvascular complications. Close attention to associated risk factors, especially hyperlipidaemia and hypertension, is important in reducing risk of macrovascular disease.

12.0% to 17.9% in the USA. Obesity predisposes to several chronic diseases including hypertension, hyperlipidaemia, diabetes mellitus, cardiovascular disease and osteoarthritis, and aspects of these are discussed in the relevant sections of this book.

The body mass index[15] (BMI) correlates highly with the amount of body fat; individuals whose BMI lies between 25 and $30 \, kg/m^2$ are considered overweight and those in whom it exceeds $30 \, kg/m^2$ are defined as obese. Management of the condition involves a variety of approaches from nutritional advice to lifestyle alteration, drugs and, in extreme instances, gastric surgery. An evidence-based algorithm coordinates these.[16] The present account concentrates on pharmacological interventions.

Drugs for obesity act either on the gastrointestinal tract to lower nutrient absorption or centrally to reduce food intake by decreasing appetite or increasing satiety (appetite suppressants).

antagonist, with the evidence for the latter being particularly strong that they are superior to other antihypertensive agents in reducing progression to renal failure.[12] Addition of an ACE inhibitor to other drugs may also improve overall outcome in patients with diabetes.[13] Most impressively, the Heart Protection Study showed that addition of simvastatin 40 mg daily to the treatment of 4000 patients with diabetes reduced all cardiovascular complications by 30%[14] (see p. 486).

Obesity and appetite control

Overweight and obesity are the commonest nutritional disorders in developed countries. Between 1991 and 1998 the incidence of obesity rose from

[12] Three trials compared an angiotensin blocker with other blood pressure lowering drugs, and found a 20% reduction in the proportion of patients in whom proteinuria worsened or serum creatinine doubled during follow-up:
1. Parving H H, Lehnert H, Brochner-Mortensen J, Gomis R, Andersen S. Arner P 2001 The effect of irbesartan on the development of diabetic nephropathy in patients with type 2 diabetes. *New England Journal of Medicine* 345: 870–878.
2. Brenner B M, Cooper M E, de Zeeuw D et al 2001 Effects of losartan on renal and cardiovascular outcomes in patients with type 2 diabetes and nephropathy. *New England Journal of Medicine* 345: 861–869.
3. Lewis E J, Hunsicker L G, Clarke W R et al 2001 Renoprotective effect of the angiotensin-receptor antagonist irbesartan in patients with nephropathy due to type 2 diabetes. *New England Journal of Medicine* 345: 851–860.
[13] The HOPE study included patients with diabetes as one of its high risk group of cardiovascular patients, in whom ramipril reduced further coronary heart disease endpoints by about 30%. Yusuf S, Sleight P, Pogue J et al 2000 Effects of an angiotensin-converting-enzyme inhibitor, ramipril, on cardiovascular events in high-risk patients. The Heart Outcomes Prevention Evaluation Study Investigators *New England Journal of Medicine* 342: 145–153.
[14] Heart Protection Study Collaborative Group 2002 MRC/BHF Heart Protection Study of cholesterol lowering with simvastatin in 20 536 high-risk individuals. Lancet 360: 7–22
[15] The weight in kilograms divided by the square of the height in metres.
[16] http//www.nhlbi.nih.gov/guidelines/obesity/practgde.htm

ORLISTAT

Orlistat is a pentanoic acid ester that binds to and inhibits gastric and pancreatic lipases; the resulting inhibition of their activity prevents the absorption of about 30% of dietary fat compared with a normal 5% loss. Weight loss is due to calorie loss but drug-related adverse effects also contribute by diminishing food intake. The drug is not absorbed from the alimentary tract.

Clinical trials show that patients who adhere to a low-calorie diet and take orlistat lost on average 9–10 kg after one year (compared to 6 kg in those who took placebo); in the following year those who remained on orlistat regained 1.5–3.0 kg (4–6 kg with placebo). Orlistat has found a place in the management of obesity in the UK but, not surprisingly, this is subject to stringent guidance from the National Institute for Clinical Excellence, namely that it be initiated only in individuals:

- aged 18–75 years
- with BMI 28 kg/m^2 or more who also have cardiovascular risk factors or 30 kg/m^2 or more without such comorbidity and
- who have lost at least 2.5 kg body weight by dieting and increasing physical activity in the previous month.

The dose is 120 mg, taken immediately before, during or 1 h after each main meal, up to thrice daily. If a meal is missed, or contains no fat, the dose of orlistat should be omitted.

Treatment should be accompanied by counselling advice and proceed beyond 3 months only in those who have lost > 5% of their initial weight, beyond 6 months in those who have lost > 10%, should not normally exceed 1 year, and never more than 2 years.

Adverse effects include flatulence and liquid, oily stools, leading to faecal urgency, abdominal and rectal pain. Symptoms may be reduced by adhering to a reduced-fat diet. Low plasma concentrations of the fat-soluble vitamins A, D and E have been found. Orlistat is contraindicated where there is chronic intestinal malabsorption or cholestasis.

SIBUTRAMINE

Sibutramine was originally developed as an anti-depressant and it inhibits the reuptake of nor-adrenaline and serotonin at nerve endings, increasing the concentration of these neurotransmitters at postsynaptic receptors in the brain that affect food intake. It is also thought to stimulate energy expenditure.

The drug is rapidly absorbed from the gastro-intestinal tract and extensively metabolised in the liver by cytochrome P450 3A4. These metabolites have a t$\frac{1}{2}$ of 14–16 h and are responsible for its effects.

When taken with dietary advice, sibutramine can be expected to cause a loss of 5–7% of initial body weight but this tends to be regained once the drug is stopped.

Sibutramine should be prescribed only for individuals with BMI 27 kg/m^2 or more who have other cardiovascular risk factors or 30 kg/m^2 or more in their absence. It should be discontinued if weight loss after 3 months is < 5% of initial weight, if weight stabilises at < 5% of initial weight thereafter or if users regain more than 3 kg after previous weight loss. It should not be given for more than 1 year.

The dose is 10–15 mg day by mouth.

Adverse effects include constipation, dry mouth and insomnia which occur in > 10% of users. Less commonly, nausea, tachycardia, palpitations, raised blood pressure, anxiety, sweating and altered taste may occur. Blood pressure should be monitored closely throughout its use (twice weekly in the first 3 months). *Contraindications* include severe hypertension, peripheral occlusive arterial or coronary heart disease, cardiac arrhythmia, prostatic hypertrophy and those with severe hepatic or renal impairment. It should not be used to treat obesity of endocrine origin or those with a history of major eating disorder or psychiatric disease. Concomitant use with tricyclic antidepressants should be avoided (CNS toxicity).

The noradrenergic drugs fenfluramine, dexfenfluramine and phenteramine were formerly prescribed as appetite suppressants but were withdrawn when their use was associated with cardiac valve disease and pulmonary hypertension.

Considerable interest continues to surround the adipocyte-derived hormone leptin (Greek, *leptos*, thin) which acts on the hypothalamus to control appetite and energy expenditure by informing neuroendocrine pathways of the state of energy stores in adipose tissue. Plasma leptin correlates with indices of obesity in humans, with most obese patients being resistant to their elevated levels of leptin, rather than deficient in leptin production. The use of therapeutic doses of leptin is under evaluation; physiological doses are effective in rare patients with inherited leptin deficiency. Further understanding of the leptin pathway may open avenues for new agents to control appetite and obesity.

GUIDE TO FURTHER READING

Atkinson M A, Eisenbarth G S 2001 Type 1 diabetes: new perspectives on disease pathogenesis and treatment. Lancet 358: 221–229

Boyle P J et al 1995 Brain glucose uptake and unawareness of hypoglycemia in patients with insulin-dependent diabetes mellitus. New England Journal of Medicine 333: 1726–1731

Clark C M Jr, Lee D A 1995 Prevention and treatment of the complications of diabetes mellitus. New England Journal of Medicine 332: 1210–1217

Dornhorst A 2001 Insulinotropic meglitinide analogues. Lancet 358: 1709–1716

Diabetes Control and Complications Trial Research Group 1993 The effect of intensive treatment of diabetes on the development and progression of long-term complications in insulin-dependent diabetes mellitus. New England Journal of Medicine 329: 977–986

Fajans S S, Bell G I, Polonski K S 2001 Molecular mechanisms and clinical pathophysiology of maturity-onset diabetes in the young. New England Journal of Medicine 345: 971–980

Garner P 1995 Type I diabetes mellitus and pregnancy. Lancet 346: 157–161

Owens D R, Zinman B, Bolli G B 2001 Insulins today and beyond. Lancet 358: 739–746

Report 1998 Clinical management of overweight and obese patients with particular reference to the use of drugs. Royal College of Physicians of London: London

Stevens A B et al 1989 Motor vehicle driving amongst diabetics taking insulin and non-diabetics. British Medical Journal 299: 591

Stumvoll M et al 1995 Metabolic effects of metformin in non-insulin-dependent diabetes mellitus. New England Journal of Medicine 333: 550–554

Willett W C, Dietz W H, Colditz G A 1999 Guidelines for healthy weight. New England Journal of Medicine 341: 427–434

Williams G 1994 Management of non-insulin-dependent diabetes mellitus. Lancet 343: 95–100

Wright J R 2002 From ugly fish to conqueror of death: J J R Macleod's fish insulin research, 1922–24. Lancet 359: 1238–1242

Yanovski S Z, Yanovski J A 2002 Obesity. New England Journal of Medicine 346: 591–602

36

Thyroid hormones, antithyroid drugs

SYNOPSIS

- Thyroid hormones (thyroxine/levothyroxine T_4, liothyronine T_3)
- Use of thyroid hormone: treatment of hypothyroidism
- Antithyroid drugs and hyperthyroidism: thionamides, drugs that block sympathetic autonomic activity, iodide and radioiodine ^{131}I, preparation of patients for surgery, thyroid storm (crisis), exophthalmos
- Drugs that cause unwanted hypothyroidism
- Calcitonin, see Chapter 38

Thyroid hormones

L-thyroxine (T_4 or tetraiodo-L-thyronine) and liothyronine (T_3 or triiodo-L-thyronine) are the natural hormones of the thyroid gland. T_4 is a less active precursor of T_3, which is the major mediator of physiological effect. In this chapter T_4 for therapeutic use is referred to as levothyroxine (the rINN, see p. 83) rather than levothyroxine (the former usage).

For convenience, the term 'thyroid hormone' is used to comprise T_4 plus T_3. Both forms are available for oral use as therapy.

Calcitonin: see page 741.

PHYSIOLOGY AND PHARMACOKINETICS

Thyroid hormone synthesis requires oxidation of dietary iodine, followed by iodination of tyrosine to mono- and diiodotyrosine; coupling of iodotyrosines leads to formation of the *active molecules,* tetraiodotyrosine, (T_4 or L-thyroxine) and triiodotyrosine (T_3 or L-thyronine).

These active thyroid hormones are stored in the gland within the molecule of thyroglobulin, a major component of the intrafollicular colloid. They are released into the circulation following reuptake of the colloid by the apical cells and proteolysis. The main circulating thyroid hormone is T_4. About 80% of the released T_4 is deiodinated in the peripheral tissues to the biologically active T_3 (30–35%) and biologically inactive *reverse* T_3 (45–50%); thus most circulating T_3 is derived from T_4. Further deiodination, largely in the liver, leads to loss of activity.

In the blood both T_4 and T_3 are extensively (99.9%) bound to plasma proteins (thyroxine-binding globulin, TBG, and thyroxine-binding prealbumin, TBPA). The concentration of TBG is raised by oestrogens (including doses used in oral contraceptives), prolonged use of neuroleptics, and in pregnancy. The concentration of TBG is lowered by adrenocortical and androgen (including anabolic steroid) therapy and by urinary protein loss in nephrotic syndrome. Phenytoin and salicylates compete with thyroid hormone for TBG binding sites. Effects such as these would interfere with the assessment of the clinical significance of measurements of total thyroid hormone concentration but the availability of free thyroid hormone assay (free thyroxine index) largely avoids such complicating factors. Normal values are: free T_4 9–25 pmol/l, free T_3 3–9 pmol/l.

T_4 and T_3 are well absorbed from the gut, except in myxoedema coma when parenteral therapy is required.

T_4 **(levothyroxine):** a single dose reaches its maximum effect in about 10 days (its binding to plasma proteins is strong as well as extensive) and passes off in 2–3 weeks ($t\frac{1}{2}$ 7 d in euthyroid subjects; 14 d in hypothyroid; 3 d in hyperthyroid).

T_3 **(liothyronine)** is about 5 times as biologically potent as T_4; a single dose reaches its maximum effect in about 24 h (its binding to plasma proteins is weak) and passes off in one week ($t\frac{1}{2}$ 2 d in euthyroid subjects).

PHARMACODYNAMICS

Thyroid hormone passes into the cells of target organs, combines with specific nuclear receptors there and induces characteristic metabolic changes:

- *Protein synthesis* during growth
- Increased *metabolic rate* with raised oxygen consumption
- Increased *sensitivity to catecholamines* with proliferation of β-adrenoceptors (particularly important in the cardiovascular system).

Levothyroxine for hypothyroidism

The main indication for levothyroxine is treatment of *deficiency* (cretinism, and adult hypothyroidism) from any cause. The adult requirement of hormone is remarkably constant, and dosage does not usually have to be altered once the optimum is found. Patients should be monitored at annual intervals. Monitoring needs to be more frequent in children, who may need more as they grow. Similarly, pregnant women should be monitored monthly, and require 50–100% increase in their normal dose of levothyroxine.

Early treatment of neonatal hypothyroidism (cretinism) (1:5000 births) is important if permanent mental defect is to be avoided. It must be lifelong.

Hypothyroidism due to panhypopituitarism requires replacement with adrenocortical as well as with thyroid hormones. Use of levothyroxine alone can cause acute adrenal insufficiency.

Small doses of levothyroxine in normal subjects merely depress pituitary thyroid stimulating hormone (TSH) production and consequently reduce the output of thyroid hormone by an equivalent amount.

Levothyroxine has been used in the treatment of nontoxic nodular goiter. In such patients it suppresses TSH secretion, and treatment is given on the assumption that nodular (like normal) thyroid tissue growth is dependent on TSH. The long-term value of levothyroxine in these patients remains unproven, and withdrawal of therapy leads to return of the goitre. Levothyroxine should not be used to treat obesity (see Obesity).

Treatment of hypothyroidism

Levothyroxine Tabs contain pure L-thyroxine sodium and should be used. The initial oral dose in young patients without cardiac disease is 50–100 micrograms daily; but in the old and patients with heart disease or hypertension, this should be achieved gradually (to minimise cardiovascular risk due to a too sudden increase in metabolic demand), starting with 12.5–25 micrograms daily for the first 2–4 weeks, and then increasing by 12.5 micrograms monthly until symptoms are relieved. The usual replacement dose at steady state is 75–125 micrograms in women, and 100–200 micrograms in men, as a single daily dose. This is usually sufficient to reduce plasma TSH to normal concentrations (0.3–3.5 mU/l) which is the *best indicator* of adequate treatment. Patients who appear to need more are probably not taking their tablets consistently. The maximum effect of a dose is not reached for about 10 days and passes off over about 2–3 weeks. Absorption is more complete and less variable if levothyroxine is taken well apart from food.

Tablets containing physiological mixtures of levothyroxine and liothyronine have not been sufficiently studied to recommend in preference to levothyroxine alone.

Hypothyroid patients tend to be *intolerant of drugs* in general owing to delayed metabolism.

Liothyronine Tabs. Liothyronine is the most rapidly effective thyroid hormone, a single dose giving maximum effect within 24 h and passing off over 24–48 h. It is not used in routine treatment of hypothyroidism because its rapid onset of effect can induce heart failure. Its main uses are in myxoedema coma and psychosis, both rare conditions. A specialised use is during the withdrawal of levothyroxine replacement (to permit diagnostic radioiodine scanning) in patients with thyroid carcinoma.

Myxoedema coma follows prolonged total hormone deficiency and constitutes an emergency. Intravenous therapy is mandatory because of impaired absorption of drugs in this condition. Liothyronine 5–20 micrograms is given every 12 hours. Hydrocortisone i.v. is also needed, as prolonged hypothyroidism may be associated with adrenocortical insufficiency.

Subclinical hypothyroidism. This term refers to patients with a normal free T_4 but elevated TSH. The indications for considering treatment in these patients are: symptoms of hypothyrodism, presence of a goitre, detectable thyroid antibodies or hypercholesterolaemia.

Adverse effects of thyroid hormone parallel the increase in metabolic rate. The symptoms and signs are those of hyperthyroidism. Symptoms of myocardial ischaemia, atrial fibrillation or heart failure are liable to be provoked by too vigorous therapy or in patients having serious ischaemic heart disease who may even be unable to tolerate optimal therapy. Should they occur levothyroxine must be discontinued for at least a week and begun again at lower dosage. Only slight overdose is needed to precipitate atrial fibrillation in patients over 60 years.

In pregnancy a hypothyroid patient should be carefully assessed and monitored monthly; a 50–100% increase in dose of levothyroxine may be required; breast feeding is not contraindicated though the baby's thyroid status should be watched.

Antithyroid drugs and hyperthyroidism

Drugs used for the treatment of hyperthyroidism include:

- **Thionamides** which block the synthesis of thyroid hormone
- **Iodine:** *radioiodine* which destroys the cells making thyroid hormone; *iodide*, an excess of which reduces the production of thyroid hormone temporarily by an unknown mechanism (it is also necessary for the formation of hormone, and both excess and deficiency can cause goitre).

THIONAMIDES (THIOUREA DERIVATIVES) CARBIMAZOLE, METHIMAZOLE, PROPYLTHIOURACIL

Mode of action

The major action of thionamides is to *reduce the formation of thyroid hormone* by inhibiting oxidation and organification (incorporation into organic form) of iodine (iodotyrosines), and by inhibiting the coupling of iodotyrosines to form T_4 and T_3. These actions result in intrathyroidal iodine deficiency. Maximum effect is delayed until existing hormone stores are exhausted (weeks, see below). With high dosage the reduction in hormone synthesis leads to hypothyroidism.

Carbimazole and methimazole (the chief metabolite of carbimazole) ($t\frac{1}{2}$ 6 h) and propylthiouracil ($t\frac{1}{2}$ 2 h) are commonly used, but $t\frac{1}{2}$ matters little since the drugs accumulate in the thyroid and act there for 30–40 h; thus a single daily dose suffices.

Propylthiouracil differs from other members of the group in that it also inhibits peripheral conversion of T_4 to T_3, but only at the high doses used in treatment of thyroid storm (p. 705).

Doses

- *Carbimazole*, orally 40 mg total/day (or methimazole 30 mg) until euthyroid (usually

4–6 weeks); then *either* titrate ('titration regimen') by decrements initially of 10 mg every 4–6 weeks to a maintenance dose of 5–10 mg daily; *or* continue ('block-replace regimen') 40 mg once daily, and add levothyroxine 75–125 micrograms/day, with monitoring of free T_4 and TSH.

- *Propylthiouracil*, orally, 600 mg total/day until euthyroid: maintenance 50–100 mg total/day. Much higher doses (up to 2.4 g/day) with frequent administration are used for thyroid storm.

Use

It is probable that no patient is wholly refractory to these drugs. Failure to respond is likely to be due to the patient not taking the tablets or to wrong diagnosis. The drugs are used in hyperthyroidism as

- principal therapy,
- adjuvant to radioiodine to control the disease until the radiation achieves its effect,[1]
- to prepare patients for surgery.

Clinical improvement is noticeable in 2–4 weeks, and the patient should be euthyroid in 4–6 weeks. The best guides to therapy are the patient's symptoms (decreased nervousness and palpitations), increased strength and weight gain, and pulse rate.

Symptoms and signs are, of course, less valuable as guides if the patient is also taking a β-adrenoceptor blocker, and reliance is then put on biochemical tests.

With optimal treatment the gland decreases in size, but overtreatment leading to low hormone concentrations in the blood activates the pituitary feedback system, inducing TSH secretion and goitre.

Adverse reactions

The thionamide drugs are all liable to cause minor and major adverse effects. *Minor* are rash, urticaria, arthralgia, fever, anorexia, nausea, abnormalities of taste and smell. *Major* are agranulocytosis, thrombocytopenia, acute hepatic necrosis, cholestatic hepatitis, lupus-like syndrome, vasculitis.

---

[1] Use of a thionamide during the week before and after radioiodine therapy may impair the response to radiation (Velkeniers B et al 1988 Lancet 1: 1127) (see Mode of action of thionamides, above).

Blood disorders (< 3/10 000 patient years) are most common in the first 2 months of treatment. Routine leucocyte counts have been advocated in order to detect blood dyscrasia before symptoms develop; but agranulocytosis may be so acute that the counts give no warning. Patients must be advised to stop the drug and have a leucocyte count performed if symptoms of a sore throat, fever, bruising or mouth ulcers develop. Any suggestion of anaemia should be investigated. Cross allergy between the drugs occurs sometimes, but must not be assumed for agranulocytosis. Treatment of agranulocytosis consists of drug withdrawal, admission to hospital, and administration of broad-spectrum antibimicrobials plus granulocyte colony stimulating factor (where available).

Pregnancy. If a pregnant woman has hyperthyroidism (2/1000 pregnancies) she should be treated with the smallest possible amount of these drugs because they cross the placenta; with overtreatment fetal goitre occurs. Surgery in the second trimester may be preferred to continued drug therapy.

During *breast feeding*, propylthiouracil is the treatment of choice because little passes into breast milk.

CONTROL OF ANTITHYROID DRUG THERAPY

The aim of drug therapy is to control the hyperthyroidism until a natural remission takes place. The duration of therapy that minimises the relapse rate is controversial, and 12–18 months' total therapy before withdrawal as a routine is commonly advised. Longer (minimum 24 months) treatment is usual for young patients with large, vascular goitres, because of the higher risk of recurrence. Most patients enter remission, but some will relapse — usually during the first three months after withdrawal from treatment. Approximately 30–40% of patients remain euthyroid 10 years later. If hyperthyroidism recurs, there is little chance of a second course of thionamide achieving long-term remission.

The use of levothyroxine concurrently with an antithyroid drug ('block and replace regimen') facilitates of maintenance of a euthyroid state, and reduces the frequency of clinic visits. There is no good evidence that the choice of titration or block-replace regimen influences the relapse rate.

β-adrenergic blockade. There is increased tissue sensitivity to catecholamines in hyperthyroidism with an increase in either the number of β-adrenoceptors or the second messenger response (i.e. intracellular cyclic AMP synthesis) to their stimulation. Therefore some of the unpleasant symptoms are adrenergic.

Quick relief can be obtained with a β-adrenoceptor blocking drug (judge dose by heart rate) though these do not block all the metabolic effects of the hormone, e.g. on the myocardium, and the basal metabolic rate is unchanged. For this reason they should not be used as sole therapy except in mild thyrotoxicosis in preparation for radioiodine treatment, and should be continued in these patients until the radioiodine has taken effect. They do not alter the course of the disease, nor biochemical tests of thyroid function. Any effect on thyroid hormonal action on peripheral tissues is clinically unimportant. It is desirable to choose a drug that is *nonselective* for β_1 and β_2 receptors and *lacks partial agonist effect* (e.g. propranolol 20–80 mg 6–8-hourly, or timolol 5 mg once daily). Usual contraindications to β-blockade (see p. 478) should be observed, especially asthma.

IODINE (IODIDE AND RADIOACTIVE IODINE)

Iodide is well absorbed from the intestine, is distributed like chloride in the body and is rapidly excreted by the kidney. It is selectively taken up and concentrated (about × 25) by the thyroid gland, but more in hyperthyroidism and less in hypothyroidism. A deficiency of iodide reduces the amount of thyroid hormone produced, which stimulates the pituitary to secrete TSH. The result is hyperplasia and increased vascularity of the gland, with eventual goitre formation.

Effects

Iodide effects are complex and related to dose and to thyroid status of the subject.

In hyperthyroid subjects a moderate excess of iodide may enhance hormone production by providing 'fuel' for hormone synthesis. But a substantial excess inhibits hormone release and promotes storage of hormone and involution of the gland, making it firmer and less vascular so that surgery is

easier. The effect is transient and its mechanism uncertain.

In euthyroid subjects with normal glands an excess of iodide from any source can cause goitre (with or without hyperthyroidism), e.g. use of iodide-containing cough medicines, iodine-containing radiocontrast media, amiodarone, seaweed eaters.

A euthyroid subject with an autonomous adenoma (hot nodule) becomes hyperthyroid if given iodide.

Uses

Iodide (large dose) is used for thyroid storm (crisis) and in preparation for thyroidectomy because it rapidly benefits the patient by reducing hormone release and renders surgery easier and safer (above).

Potassium iodide in doses of 60 mg orally 8-hourly (longer intervals allow some escape from the iodide effect) produces some effect in 1–2 days, maximal after 10–14 days, after which the benefit declines as the thyroid adapts. A similar dose is used for 3 days to cover administration of some 131- or 123-Iodine containing isotopes, for instance metaiodobenzylguanidine (MIBG) (see p. 492).

Iodine therapy maximises iodide stores in the thyroid, which delays response to thionamides. Prophylactic iodide (1 part in 100 000 parts) may be added to the salt, water or bread where goitre is endemic.

In economically deprived communities a method of prophylaxis is to inject iodised oil i.m. every 3–5 years; given early enough to women, this prevents endemic cretinism; but occasional hyperthyroidism occurs (see Autonomous adenoma, above).

As an antiseptic for use on the skin, providone-iodine (a complex of iodine with a sustained-release carrier, povidone or polyvinyl-pyrrolidone) is used. It can be applied repeatedly and used as a surgical scrub.

Bronchial secretions. Iodide is concentrated in bronchial and salivary secretions. It acts as an expectorant (see Cough, p. 550).

Organic compounds containing iodine are used as contrast media in *radiology*. It is essential to ask patients specifically whether they are allergic to iodine before they are used. An i.v. test dose ought to be given half an hour before the full i.v. dose if there is history of any allergy. Despite this, severe anaphylaxis, even deaths, occur every year in busy radiology departments, and iodine containing contrast media are being superseded by so-called nonionic preparations.[2]

Adverse reactions

Patients vary enormously in their tolerance of iodine; some are intolerant or allergic to it both orally and when put on the skin.

Symptoms of iodism include: a metallic taste, excessive salivation with painful salivary glands, running eyes and nose, sore mouth and throat, a productive cough, diarrhoea, and various rashes that may mimic chicken-pox. Elimination can be enhanced by inducing a saline diuresis.

Goitre can occur (see above) with prolonged use of iodide-containing expectorant by bronchitics and asthmatics. Such therapy should therefore be intermittent, if it is used at all.

Topical application of iodine-containing antiseptics to neonates has caused hypothyroidism. Iodide intake above that in a normal diet will depress thyroid uptake of administered radioiodine, because the two forms will compete.

In the case of diet, medication and water soluble radio-diagnostic agents, interference with thyroid function will cease 2–4 weeks after stopping the source, but with agents used for cholecystography it may last for 6 months or more (tissue binding).

RADIOIODINE (^{131}I)

^{131}I is treated by the body just like the ordinary nonradioactive isotope, so that when swallowed it is concentrated in the thyroid gland. It emits mainly β radiation (90%), which penetrates only 0.5 mm of tissue and thus allows therapeutic effects on the thyroid without damage to the surrounding structures, particularly the parathyroids. It also emits

some gamma rays, which are more penetrating and can be detected with a radiation counter. ^{131}I has a physical (radioactive) $t_{1/2}$ of 8 days.

^{131}I is the preferred initial treatment for hyperthyroidism caused by Graves' disease in North America. It is contraindicated in children and pregnant or breast-feeding women, and can induce or worsen ophthalmopathy. It is used in combination with surgery in some cases of thyroid carcinoma, especially those in which metastases are sufficiently differentiated to take up iodide selectively.

In hyperthyroidism the beneficial effects of a single dose may be felt in one month, and patients should be reviewed at 6 weeks to monitor for onset of hypothyroidism. The maximal effect of radioiodine may take 3 months. β-adrenoceptor blockade and, in severe cases, an antithyroid drug (but see footnote 1) will be needed to render the patient comfortable whilst waiting; this is more likely when radioiodine is used for treatment of patients with relapsing thyrotoxicosis. Very rarely radiation thyroiditis causes excessive release of hormone and thyroid storm. Repeated doses are sometimes needed.

The *adverse effects* of radioiodine are as for iodism, above. In the event of *inadvertent overdose,* large doses of sodium or potassium iodide should be given to compete with the radioiodine for thyroid uptake and to hasten excretion by increasing iodide turnover (increased fluid intake and a diuretic are adjuvants).

Radioiodine offers the advantages that treatment is simple and carries no immediate mortality. However, it is slow in acting and it is difficult to judge the dose that will render the patient euthyroid.

In the first year after treatment 20% of patients will become hypothyroid. After this 5% of patients become hypothyroid annually, perhaps because the capacity of thyroid cells to divide is permanently abolished so that cell renewal ceases. Patients must therefore be followed up indefinitely after radioiodine treatment, for most are likely to need treatment for hypothyroidism eventually. Because such follow-up over years may fail and because the onset of hypothyroidism may be insidious and not easily recognised, some physicians prefer deliberately to render patients hypothyroid with the first dose and to educate them on the use of replacement therapy which is safe and effective.

---

[2] The newer preparations approximately triple the cost of diagnostic investigations requiring contrast media. With a fatality rate of ~1/50 000 in patients receiving the older agents, hospitals are faced with an interesting cost-benefit equation.

Risks

Medical experience had eliminated the fear that radioiodine causes carcinoma of the thyroid, and led to its use in patients of all ages. However the Chernobyl disaster revived concern about exposure of children and it would be wise again to restrict radioiodine treatment to adults. Pregnant women should not be treated with radioiodine (^{131}I) because it crosses the placenta.

There is a theoretical risk of teratogenic effect and patients should not reproduce for an arbitrary 12 months after treatment.

Larger doses of radioiodine are used for thyroid carcinoma than for hyperthyroidism, and there is an increased incidence of late leukaemia in these patients. The treatment of thyroid carcinoma is highly specialised.

Tests

Radioiodine uptake can be used to test thyroid function, though technetium would be more usual. Scanning may be used for the identification of solitary nodules, and in the differential diagnosis of Graves' disease from the less common thyroiditides (e.g. de Quervain's thyroiditis). In the latter, excessive thyroid hormone release caused by follicular cell damage can cause clinical and biochemical features of hyperthyroidism, but ^{131}I uptake is reduced.

PREPARATION FOR SURGERY

Preparation of hyperthyroid patients for surgery can be satisfactorily achieved by making them euthyroid with one of the above drugs plus a β-adrenoceptor blocker for comfort (see below) and safety,[3] and adding iodide for 7–10 days before operation (not sooner) to reduce the surgically inconvenient vascularity of the gland.

In an emergency, the patient is prepared with a β-adrenoceptor blocker (e.g. propranolol 6-hourly, with dose titration to eliminate tachycardia) for 4 days. This is continued through the operation and for 7–10 days after. Iodide should also be given, as above (see p. 703). The important differences with this second technique are that the gland is smaller and less friable, although the patient's tissues are still

---

Choice of treatment of hyperthyroidism

There are three possible lines of treatment, each with its special advantages and disadvantages:
- Antithyroid drugs
- Radioiodine
- Surgery, after preparation as below.

Antithyroid drugs are generally preferred provided the goitre is small and diffuse. A nodular goitre is generally large enough to be a source of complaint, relapses when drug therapy is withdrawn (nodules are autonomous), and is best treated surgically. These drugs do not decrease thyroid size; it may even increase (see above). They may be used in pregnancy.

Radioiodine is now commonly used for adult patients of all ages; but not in pregnancy. It affects both diffuse and nodular goitre. The goitre becomes smaller. Monitoring indefinitely for subsequent hypothyroidism is essential. Hyperthyroidism due to a single hyperfunctioning adenoma ('hot nodule') is also suitable for this treatment, and higher doses may be used since the function of the rest of the gland is already suppressed by the familiar negative feedback regulatory process.

Surgery is generally a second choice for thyrotoxicosis. It may be indicated if obstruction of neck veins or trachea exists or is thought to be likely in the future, if the thyroid contains a nodule of uncertain nature, or in young patients with relapsing thyrotoxicosis, with preference for surgery.

---

hyperthyroid, and it is essential, in order to avoid a hyperthyroid crisis or storm, that the adrenoceptor blocker be continued as above without the omission of even a single 6-hourly dose of propranolol.

Thyroid storm

Thyroid crisis, or storm, is a life-threatening emergency due to liberation of large amounts of hormone into the circulation. Surgical storm is rare with modern methods of preparing hyperthyroid patients for surgery. Medical thyroid storm may occur in patients who are untreated or incompletely treated. It may be precipitated by infection, trauma, surgical emerg-

---

[3] No patient should be operated on with a resting pulse of 90/min or above, and no dose of β-adrenoceptor blocker, including the important postoperative dose, should be omitted. Toft A D et al 1978 New England Journal or Medicine 298: 643.

encies or operations, radiation thyroiditis, toxaemia of pregnancy or parturition. Treatment is urgently required to save life.

Propranolol should be given immediately (i.v. slowly, 1 mg/min to max of 10 mg, in severe cases, preceded by atropine 1–2 mg i.v. to prevent excessive bradycardia). Large doses of an antithyroid agent, preferably propylthiouracil 300–400 mg 4-hourly down a nasogastric tube or per rectum, are required. After this is initiated, iodide is used to inhibit further hormone release from the gland (600 mg–1.0 g iodide orally in the first 24 h) (see Potassium iodide). Large doses of adrenocorticoid, e.g. dexamethasone 2 mg 6-hourly, are given to inhibit both release of thyroid hormone from the gland and peripheral conversion of T_4 to T_3. Mental disturbance may be treated by chlorpromazine; hyperthermia by cooling and aspirin; heart failure in the ordinary way.

Exophthalmos of hyperthyroidism

The cause may be related to an immunoglobulin that attacks the external ocular muscles and retrobulbar tissue. Antithyroid drugs do not help. TSH secretion is not responsible (it is high in primary thyroid gland failure in which exophthalmos rarely occurs). The patient should be rendered euthyroid. Mild to moderate cases regress spontaneously. Artificial tears (hypromellose) are useful when natural tears and blinking are inadequate to maintain corneal lubrication. In severe cases, high systemic doses of prednisolone, alone or in combination with another immunosuppressive (azathioprine) may help. A course of low-dose orbital radiation achieves rapid regression of ophthalmopathy, and may take the place of prolonged immunosuppressant treatment. In urgent cases orbital decompression by surgery is necessary.

Treatment of subclinical hyperthyroidism

This term is sometimes used of patients with normal serum T_4 and T_3 but undetectable TSH levels. Some of these patients progress to frank hyperthyroidism, with an increased risk of atrial fibrillation and osteoporosis in the elderly. This is most likely in patients with nodular goitres. In the remainder, treatment is unnecessary, but thyroid-function tests should be performed every six months.

Drugs that cause hypothyroidism

In addition to drugs used for their antithyroid effects, the following substances can cause hypothyroidism: lithium (for mania/depression), amiodarone (cardiac antiarrhythmic), PAS (for tuberculosis), phenylbutazone (antirheumatic), iodide (see above), cobalt salts (for anaemia), resorcinol (for leg ulcers). Effects are generally reversible on withdrawal.

Miscellaneous

Treatment of thyroiditis (Hashimoto's thyroiditis, subacute thyroiditis of de Quervain). Where hyperthyroidism is a feature, treatment is by a β-adrenoceptor blocking drug. Antithyroid drugs should not be used. Where there is permanent hypothyroidism, the treatment is thyroid hormone replacement.

Calcitonin: see Chapter 38.

Summary

- Autoimmune disease of the thyroid can cause over- or underproduction of thyroid hormone.
- Hypothyroidism is readily treated by oral administration of levothyroxine 50–200 micrograms daily. This needs to be continued indefinitely.
- The treatment of hyperthyroidism due to Graves' disease is either 12 months treatment with carbimazole or propylthiouracil or a single diagnosis of [131]I. These drugs do not have a place in the 5–10% of patients in whom thyrotoxicosis is due to a toxic adenoma or to subacute thyroiditis.
- The natural history of Graves' disease is of alternating remission and relapse. Progression to hypothyroidism can occur, especially after ^{131}I treatment. Such patients should have long-term follow-up, and are likely to require thyroid hormone replacement therapy.
- Severe forms of thyroid eye disease should be treated with steroids and immunosuppressants or low-dose radiotherapy. Urgent surgical decompression can be required for exophthalmos.

GUIDE TO FURTHER READING

Cooper D S 2001 Subclinical hypothyroidism New England Journal of Medicine 345: 260–265

Dayan C M 2001 Interpretation of thyroid function tests. Lancet 2001: 619–624

Franklyn J A et al 1990 Thyroxine replacement treatment and osteoporosis. British Medical Journal 300: 693–694

Lazarus J H 1997 Hyperthyroidism. Lancet 349: 339–343

Lindsay R S, Toft A D 1997 Hypothyroidism. Lancet 349: 413–417

Mandel S J et al 1990 Increased need for thyroxine during pregnancy in women with primary hypothyroidism. New England Journal of Medicine 323: 91–96

Mazzaferri E L 1993 Management of a solitary thyroid nodule. New England Journal of Medicine 328: 553–559

Pashke R, Ludgate M 1997 The thyrotropin receptor in thyroid diseases. New England Journal of Medicine 337: 1675–1681

Surks M I, Sievert R 1995 Drug therapy: drugs and thyroid function. New England Journal of Medicine 333: 1688–1694

Toft A D 1994 Thyroxine therapy. New England Journal of Medicine 331: 174–180

Toft A D 2001 Subclinical hyperthyroidism. New England Journal of Medicine 345: 512–516

Weetman A P 2000 Medical Progress: Graves' Disease. New England Journal of Medicine 343: 1236–1248

37

Hypothalamic, pituitary and sex hormones

SYNOPSIS

- Hypothalamic and pituitary hormones (anterior and posterior)
- Sex hormones and antagonists
  Androgens
  Antiandrogens
  Anabolic steroids
  Oestrogens
  Antioestrogens
  Progesterone and progestogens
  Antiprogestogens
  Danazol
- Fertility regulation
  Infertility
  Contraception by drugs and hormones
  Development of new contraceptives
- Menstrual disorders
- Myometrium
  Ergot and derivatives
  Oxytocin
  Uterine relaxants
  Prostaglandins
  Hormones, analogues and antagonists

These hormones, analogues (agonists) and antagonists can be used:

- to analyse the functional integrity of endocrine control systems
- as replacement in hormone deficiency states
- to modify malfunction of endocrine systems
- to alter normal function where this is inconvenient, e.g. contraception.

The scope of the specialist endocrinologist continues to increase in amount and in complexity and only an outline is appropriate here.

Hypothalamic and pituitary hormones

Hypothalamus: hormone-releasing hormones, hormone-releasing inhibiting hormones, gonadorelin.

Anterior pituitary: growth hormone, gonadotrophic hormones, corticotropin, thyrotrophin,

Posterior pituitary: vasopressin, oxytocin.

Once the structure of natural hormones, local or systemic (including hormone-releasing hormones), is defined it becomes possible to synthesise not only the hormones themselves[1] but also analogues and antagonists. Thus, increasingly, substances become available differing in selectivity and duration of action, and active by various routes of administration.

---

[1] Hormones can be synthesised directly in the chemical laboratory or by inserting mammalian genes into microbes, e.g. *Escherichia coli* recombinant DNA technology.

Hypothalamus and anterior pituitary

Some agents have restricted commercial availability. The $t\frac{1}{2}$ of the polypeptide and glycoprotein hormones listed below is 5–30 min; they are digested if swallowed.

Corticotrophin releasing hormone (CRH), corticoliberin, is a hypothalamic polypeptide that has diagnostic use. It increases ACTH secretion in Cushing's disease secondary to pituitary ACTH-secreting adenoma. It has no therapeutic use.

Corticotrophin, adrenocorticotrophic hormone (ACTH), see page 675.

Thyrotrophin releasing hormone (TRH) protirelin, is a tripeptide formed in the hypothalamus and controlled by free plasma T_4, T_3 concentration. It has been synthesised and can be used in diagnosis to test the capacity of the pituitary to release thyroid stimulating hormone (TSH), e.g. to determine whether hypothyroidism is due to primary thyroid gland failure or is secondary to pituitary disease or to a hypothalamic lesion. TRH is also a potent prolactin-releasing factor.

Thyroid stimulating hormone (TSH) thyrotrophin, a glycoprotein of the anterior pituitary, controls the synthesis and release of thyroid hormone from the gland, and also the uptake of iodide. There is a negative feedback of thyroid hormones on both the hypothalamic secretion of TRH and pituitary secretion of TSH.

Antithyroid drugs, by reducing thyroid hormone production, cause increased formation of TSH which is the cause of the thyroid enlargement that sometimes occurs during antithyroid drug therapy. GHRH and somatostatin both regulate growth hormone secretion.

Sermorelin is an analogue of the hypothalamic growth hormone releasing hormone (somatorelin); it is used in a diagnostic test for growth hormone secretion from the pituitary.

Somatostatin, growth hormone release inhibiting hormone, occurs in other parts of the brain as well as in the hypothalamus, and also in some peripheral tissues, e.g. pancreas, stomach. In addition to the action implied by its name, it inhibits secretion of thyrotrophin, insulin, gastrin and serotonin.

Octreotide is a synthetic analogue of somatostatin having a longer action ($t\frac{1}{2}$ 1.5 h). **Lanreotide** is much longer acting, and is administered only twice a month. Uses include acromegaly, carcinoid (serotonin secreting) tumours and other rare tumours of the alimentary tract. An unlicensed use of octeotride is the termination of variceal bleeding (see p. 655). Radiolabelled somatostatin is used to localise metastases from neuroendocrine tumours which often bear somatostatin receptors.

Somatropin, growth hormone (Genotropin, Humatrope), is a biosynthetic form (191 amino acids) of growth hormone prepared by recombinant DNA technology, as is somatrem. Naturally occurring human growth hormone obtained from dead people is no longer used because of the risk of transmitting Creutzfeldt-Jacob disease, the lethal prion infection. Growth hormone acts on many organs to produce a peptide (somatomedin) which causes muscle, bone and other tissues to increase growth, i.e. protein synthesis, and the size and number of cells.

It is used in children with growth hormone deficiency, while the bone epiphyses are still open, to prevent dwarfism and provide normal growth. Use simply to avoid low height for social reasons is controversial, and at ~£15 000 ($20 000) p.a. is certainly hard to justify. Growth hormone therapy should be confined to specialist clinics.

The use of growth hormone in growth hormone deficient adults is problematic. Treatment improves exercise performance and increases lean body mass. It may improve overall quality of life. Perceived advantages need to be weighed against the cost of many thousands of pounds per year. There is a need for large, prolonged and detailed clinical studies before growth hormone can be considered for use to improve the quality of life of otherwise healthy elderly people. Possibilities of abuse have also arisen, e.g. creation of 'super' sports people. Less dubious, but not yet a licensed indication, is the potential for accelerated wound healing reported in children with large cutaneous burns.[2]

In *acromegaly,* excess growth hormone causes diabetes, hypertension and arthritis. The former two lead to a 2-fold excess in cardiovascular mortality. Surgery is the treatment of choice. Growth hormone secretion is reduced by octreotide and other somatostatin analogues and to a lesser degree by bromocriptine (see Index).

Gonadorelin: gonadotrophin releasing hormone (GnRH) releases luteinising hormone (LH) and follicle-stimulating hormone (FSH). Its full abbreviation is thus LH-FSH-RH, but it is commonly represented as LH-RH for brevity, or GnRH. It has use in assessment of pituitary function. Intermittent pulsatile administration evokes secretion of gonadotrophins (LH and FSH) and is used to treat infertility. But continuous use evokes tachyphylaxis due to down-regulation of its receptors, i.e. gonadotrophin release and therefore gonadal secretions are reduced. Longer-acting analogues, e.g. buserelin, goserelin, nafarelin, deslorelin and leuprorelin are used to suppress androgen secretion in prostatic carcinoma. Other uses may include endometriosis, precocious puberty and contraception. All these drugs need to be administered by a parenteral route, by i.m. injection or intranasally. Their use should generally be in the hands of a specialist endocrinologist, oncologist or gynaecologist.

Follicle stimulating hormone (FSH) stimulates development of ova and of spermatozoa. It is prepared from the urine of postmenopausal women; menotrophin (Pergonal) also contains a small amount of LH, and urofollitrophin (Metrodin) is FSH alone. They are used in female and male hypopituitary infertility.

Chorionic gonadotrophin (human chorionic gonadotrophin: HCG) is secreted by the placenta and is obtained from the urine of pregnant women. Its predominant action is that of luteinising hormone (LH) (interstitial cell stimulating hormone) which induces progesterone production by the corpus luteum and, in the male, gonadal testosterone production. It is used in hypopituitary anovular and other infertility in both sexes (for LH effect is not confined to women despite its name). It is also used for cryptorchidism in prepubertal boys (6 years of age; if it fails to induce testicular descent, there is time for surgery before puberty to provide maximal possibility of a full functional testis). It may also precipitate puberty in men where this is delayed.

Prolactin is secreted by the lactotroph cells of the anterior pituitary gland. Its control is by tonic hypothalamic inhibition through prolactin inhibitory factor (PIF), probably dopamine, opposed by a prolactin releasing factor (PRF) in both women and men and, despite its name, it influences numerous biological functions (as many as 80), though not all of physiological importance. Prolactin secretion is controlled by an inhibitory dopaminergic path. Hyperprolactinaemia may be caused by drugs (with antidopaminergic actions e.g. metoclopramide), hypothyroidism, or prolactin secreting adenomas. Medical treatment is with bromocriptine 2.5–20 mg daily (in divided doses), cabergoline 500 micrograms to 2 mg weekly, or quinagolide 25–150 micrograms at bedtime.

HYPOPITUITARISM

In hypopituitarism there is a partial or complete deficiency of hormones secreted by the anterior lobe of the pituitary. The posterior lobe hormones (see below) may also be deficient in a few cases, e.g. when a tumour has destroyed the pituitary. Patients suffering from hypopituitarism may present in coma, in which case treatment is as for a severe acute adrenal insufficiency. Maintenance therapy is required, using hydrocortisone, thyroxine, oestradiol and progesterone (in women) and testosterone (in men). For growth hormone see above.

Infertility: see page 721.

Posterior pituitary hormones and analogues

Vasopressin: antidiuretic hormone (ADH)

Vasopressin is a nonapeptide ($t\frac{1}{2}$ 20 min) with two separate G-protein coupled target receptors

---

[2] Gilpin D A et al 1994 Annals of Surgery 220: 19.

responsible for its two roles. The V_1 receptor on vascular smooth muscle cells is coupled to calcium-ion entry. This receptor is not usually stimulated by physiological concentrations of the hormone. The V_2 receptor is coupled to adenylyl cyclase, and regulates opening of the water channel, aquaporin, in cells of the renal collecting duct.

Secretion of the antidiuretic hormone is stimulated by any increase in the osmotic pressure of the blood supplying the hypothalamus and by a variety of drugs, notably *nicotine*. Secretion is inhibited by a fall in blood osmotic pressure and by alcohol.

In large nonphysiological doses (pharmaco-therapy) vasopressin causes *contraction of all smooth muscle,* raising the blood pressure and causing intestinal colic. The smooth-muscle stimulant effect provides an example of tachyphylaxis (frequently repeated doses give progressively less effect). It is not only inefficient when used to raise the blood pressure, but is also dangerous, since it causes constriction of the coronary arteries and sudden death has occurred following its use.

For replacement therapy of *pituitary diabetes insipidus* the longer acting analogue desmopressin is used.

Desmopressin

Desmopressin (des-amino-D-arginine vasopressin) (DDAVP) has two major advantages: the vasocon-strictor effect has been reduced to near insignificance and the duration of action with nasal instillation, spray or s.c. injection, is 8–20 h (t½ 75 min) so that, using it once to twice daily, patients are not incon-venienced by frequent recurrence of polyuria during their waking hours and can also expect to spend the night continuously in bed. The adult dose for intranasal administration is 10–20 micrograms daily. The dose for children is about half that for adults. The bioavailability of intranasal DDAVP is 10%. It is also the only peptide for which an oral formulation is currently available, albeit with a bioavailability of only 1%. The tablets of DDAVP are prescribed ini-tially at 300–600 micrograms daily in three divided doses. The main complication of DDAVP is hypona-traemia which can be prevented by allowing the patient to develop some polyuria for a short period during each week. The requirement for DDAVP may decrease during intercurrent illness.

Nephrogenic diabetes insipidus, as is to be expected, does not respond to antidiuretic hor-mone.

In *bleeding oesophageal varices* in hepatic cirrhosis, use is made of the vasoconstrictor effect of vaso-pressin (as terlipressin, a vasopressin prodrug): see page 654.

In *haemophilia* desmopressin can enhance blood concentration of factor VIII. Felypressin is used as a vaso constriction with local anaesthetics.

DIABETES INSIPIDUS: VASOPRESSIN DEFICIENCY

Diabetes insipidus (DI) can be due to either pituitary or renal causes. The pituitary may be damaged by trauma, tumours, haemorrhage or infarction. Nephrogenic DI has a larger number of causes including drugs (lithium, demeclocycline) and several diseases affecting the renal medulla. The DNA sequencing of the preceptor and aquaporins has also allowed identification of mutations in these which cause congenital DI.

Desmopressin replacement therapy is the first choice. *Thiazide diuretics* (and chlortalidone) also have paradoxical antidiuretic effect in diabetes insipidus. That this is not due to sodium depletion is suggested by the fact that the nondiuretic thiazide, diazoxide (see Index), also has this effect. It is probable that changes in the proximal renal tubule result in increased reabsorption and in delivery of less sodium and water to the distal tubule, but the mechanism remains incompletely elucidated. Some cases of the nephrogenic form, which is not helped by antidiuretic hormone, may be benefited by a thiazide.

Chlorpropamide (but not other sulphonylureas) and *carbamazepine* are effective in *partial* pituitary diabetes insipidus, i.e. some natural hormone pro-duction remains, because they act on the kidney potentiating the effect of vasopressin on the renal tubule. Hypoglycaemia may occur with chlorpropamide.

Evidently all these drugs may cause difficulty due to their other actions that are not desired, and none is drug of first choice for this disease.

SYNDROME OF INAPPROPRIATE ANTIDIURETIC HORMONE SECRETION (SIADH)

A variety of tumours, e.g. oat-cell lung cancer, can make vasopressin, and of course they are not subject to normal homeostatic mechanisms. SIADH also occurs in some CNS and respiratory disorders (infection). Dilutional hyponatraemia follows, i.e. low plasma sodium with an inappropriately low plasma osmolality and high urine osmolality. When the plasma sodium approaches 120 mmol/l treatment should be with fluid restriction (< 500 ml/day). Treatment is primarily of the underlying disorder accompanied by fluid restriction. Chemotherapy to the causative tumour or infection is likely to be the most effective treatment. Demeclocycline, which inhibits the renal action of vasopressin, is useful Infusion of isotonic or hypertonic saline must be reserved for extreme emergencies, associated with stupor, and undertaken with great caution. Rapid correction of hyponatraemia must be avoided because of the risk of central pontine myelinolysis; the rate of correction must not exceed 12 mmol/l per 24 h.

Oxytocin: see page 731.

Sex (gonadal) hormones and antagonists: steroid hormones

Steroid hormone receptors (for gonadal steroids and adrenocortical steroids) are complex proteins inside the target cell. The steroid penetrates, is bound and translocates into the cell nucleus, which is the principal site of action and where RNA/protein synthesis occurs. Compounds that occupy the receptor without causing translocation into the nucleus or the replenishment of receptors act as antagonists, e.g. spironolactone to aldosterone, cyproterone to androgens, clomiphene to oestrogens.

Selectivity. Many synthetic analogues, although classed as, e.g. androgen, anabolic steroid, progestogen, are nonselective and bind to several types of receptor as agonist, partial agonist, antagonist.

The result is that their effects are complex, as will be seen in the following account.

PHARMACOKINETICS

Steroid sex hormones are well absorbed through the skin (factory workers need protective clothing) and the gut. Most are subject to extensive hepatic metabolic inactivation (some so much that oral administration is ineffective or requires very large doses if a useful amount is to pass through the liver and reach the systemic circulation). There is some enterohepatic recirculation, especially of oestrogen, and this may be interrupted by severe diarrhoea to cause loss of efficacy. There are some nonsteroid analogues that are more slowly metabolised. Sustained-release (depot) preparations are used. The hormones are carried in the blood extensively bound to sex-hormone-binding globulin. In general the plasma $t\frac{1}{2}$ relates to the duration of cellular action, which is implied in the recommended dosage schedules.

Androgens

Testosterone is the natural androgen secreted by the interstitial cells of the testis; it is necessary for normal spermatogenesis, for the development of the male secondary sex characteristics, and for the growth, at puberty, of the sexual apparatus. It is converted by hydroxylation to the active dihydrotestosterone.

Protein *anabolism* is increased by androgens, i.e., androgens increase the proportion of protein laid down as tissue, especially muscle (and, combined with training, increase strength). Growth of bone is promoted, but the rate of closure of the epiphyses is also hastened, causing short stature in cases of precocious puberty or of androgen overdose in the course of treating hypogonadal children.

INDICATIONS FOR ANDROGEN THERAPY

The prime indication is *testicular failure* which may be primary or secondary (due to lack of pituitary gonadotrophins). In either case replacement with androgens is often necessary.

Unfortunately, the sterility is not remedied, although loss of libido and of secondary sex characteristics can be greatly improved. Impotence is helped if it is hypogonadal, but not if it has a psychological cause (which is often the case).

For *male contraception* androgens are under trial; they inhibit pituitary gonadotrophin production and have a direct testicular action.

If androgen is given to a boy with delayed puberty, a growth spurt and sexual development will occur. Such treatment is not usually indicated until the age of 16 years since up to that age natural delay in pituitary secretion may be responsible and normal development may yet occur.

In *hepatic cirrhosis* degradation of oestrogens in the liver may be impaired, leading to raised blood concentrations of oestrogen with feminisation; androgens may help such patients. They may also stop the itching of *biliary obstruction*. Androgens may also help in some cases of *anaemia* due to bone marrow failure. Androgens are now little used in *metastatic breast cancer* because of their virilising effects.

PREPARATIONS AND CHOICE OF ANDROGENS

- *Testosterone* given orally is subject to extensive hepatic first-pass metabolism and is therefore most successful as an implant, but this is superseded by testosterone esters, e.g. enanthate, which may be given orally or as depot injections; these esters do not injure the liver (see below). Skin patches are available.
- *Mesterolone* provides oral therapy; its molecular structure is such that its hypothalamic feedback inhibition of pituitary gonadotrophin secretion is less and it does not cause liver injury (see below).
- See also: anabolic steroids, danazol (p. 715).

ADVERSE EFFECTS

Adverse effects are mainly those to be expected of a male sex hormone (including hypothalamic-pituitary suppression of gonadotrophin production); increased libido may lead to undesirable sexual activity, especially in mentally unstable patients, and virilisation is obviously undesired by most women. Androgens have a weak salt and water retaining activity, which is not often clinically important. Liver injury (cholestatic) can occur, particularly with 17 α-alkyl derivatives (ethylestrenol, stanozolol, danazol, oxymetholone); it is reversible; these agents should be avoided in hepatic disease.

Effects on *blood lipids* are complex and variable, and the balance may be to disadvantage.

In patients with malignant disease of bone androgen administration may be followed by hypercalcemia. The less virilising androgens are used to promote anabolism and are discussed below.

Antiandrogens (androgen antagonists)

Plainly oestrogens and progestogens are physiological antagonists to androgens. But compounds which compete selectively for androgen receptors have been made.

Cyproterone

Cyproterone is a derivative of progesterone; its combination of structural similarities and differences results in the following:

- Competition with testosterone for receptors in target peripheral organs (but not causing feminisation as do oestrogens); it reduces spermatogenesis even to the level of azoospermia (reverses over about 4 months after the drug is stopped); abnormal sperm occurs during treatment.
- Competition with testosterone in the central nervous system, reducing sexual drive and thoughts, and causing impotence.
- Some agonist progestogenic activity on hypothalamic receptors, inhibiting gonadotrophin secretion, which also inhibits testicular androgen production.

Uses. Cyproterone is used for reducing male hypersexuality and in prostatic cancer and severe female hirsutism. A formulation of cyproterone plus ethinylestradiol (Dianette) is offered for this latter purpose as well as for severe acne in women; this preparation acts as an oral contraceptive but does not have a UK licence, and should not be used primarily for this purpose. Plainly, long-term use of the drug poses both medical and ethical problems.[3] It is even advised that for management of male hypersexuality formally witnessed written consent be obtained.

Cyproterone causes hepatomas in rats.

Cyproterone is plainly unsuitable for male contraception (see actions above).

Flutamide and bicalutamide are nonsteroidal antiandrogens available for use in conjunction with the gonadorelins (e.g. goserelin) in the treatment of prostatic carcinoma. Finasteride (p. 544), which inhibits conversion of testosterone to dihydro-testosterone, has localised antiandrogen activity in tissues where dihydrotestosterone is the principal androgen: this makes it a useful drug in the treatment of *benign prostatic hypertrophy.*

Spironolactone (p. 534) also has antiandrogen activity and may help hirsutism in women. Androgen secretion may be diminished by continued use of a gonadorelin (LH-RH) analogue (see p. 714).

Ketoconazole (antifungal) interferes with androgen and corticosteroid synthesis and may be used in prostatic carcinoma.

Anabolic steroids

(See also above)

Androgens are effective protein anabolic agents, but their clinical use for this purpose is limited by the amount of virilisation that women will tolerate. Attempts made to separate anabolic from androgenic action have been only partially successful and *all anabolic steroids also have androgenic effects.* They have been used to treat osteoporosis in women but are no longer recommended for this purpose.

The itching of *chronic biliary obstruction* may be relieved by stanozolol 5–15 mg/day. There remains, however, a risk of increasing the degree of jaundice (see p. 653).

They benefit some patients with *aplastic anaemia.*

Hereditary angioedema (lack of inhibition of the complement Cl esterase) may be prevented by androgens (stanozolol and danazol are used).

Anabolic steroids can prevent the calcium and nitrogen loss in the urine that occurs in patients bedridden for a long time and they have therefore been used in the treatment of some severe fractures. The use of anabolic steroids in conditions of general wasting despite nutritional support may be justifiable in extreme debilitating disease, such as severe ulcerative colitis, and after major surgery. In the later stages of malignant disease they may make the patient feel and look less wretched. Their general use as tonics is scandalous, as is their use in sport (see Index).[4]

Anabolic steroids do not usefully counter the unwanted catabolic effects of the adrenocortical hormones.

None of these agents is free from virilising properties in high doses; acne and greasy skin may be the early manifestation of virilisation (see also, Adverse effects of androgens, p. 714; and Drugs and sport).

Oestrogens have only modest anabolic effect.

Administration should generally be intermittent in courses of 3–12 weeks with similar intervals, to reduce the occurrence of unwanted effects, especially liver injury.

There is little to choose between the principal available drugs, nandrolone (Durabolin) (i.m. once a week) and stanozolol (Stromba) (orally), except that the latter is contraindicated in liver disease.

---

[3] Individual problems can be quite trying and revealing. A 26-year-old woman with severe facial hirsutism was prescribed cyproterone from days 5 to 15 of each menstrual cycle. After 4 months, she reported to her doctor that her male Rottweiler would not leave her alone and repeatedly tried to mount her during these 10 days of each month. The patient managed to keep her Rottweiler and lose her hair by having the dog castrated (Cotterill J A 1992 Lancet 340: 986).

[4] While the misuse of anabolic steroids in sport is well known (infamous), a report has drawn attention to the practice among some teenagers of using the drugs to improve their appearance and handsomeness, giving themselves the 'macho' look which they think girls like. (Nilsson S 1995 Androgenic anabolic steroid use among male adolescents in Falkenberg. European Journal of Clinical Pharmacology 48: 9–11).

Oestrogens

Estrone and estradiol are both natural oestrogens. Oestrogens are responsible for the normal development of the female genital tract, of the breast and of the female secondary sex characteristics. The pubertal growth spurt is less marked in females than in males, probably because oestrogens have less protein anabolic action than do androgens, although they are as effective in promoting closure of epiphyses.

Blood oestrogen concentrations must be above a critical level for the maintenance of both proliferative and (together with progesterone) secretory phases of the uterine endometrium. If the oestrogen level falls too low then the endometrium can no longer be maintained and uterine bleeding follows. Thus uterine bleeding may be stopped temporarily by giving large doses of oestrogens, or started by abrupt withdrawal (oestrogen-withdrawal bleeding). Bleeding may occur despite a high blood oestrogen concentration if large doses are given for a long time, due to infarctions in the greatly hypertrophied endometrium. Oestrogens are necessary for the maintenance of normal pregnancy and for the accompanying breast hyperplasia. The vagina is more sensitive to oestrogens than is the endometrium.

PHARMACOKINETICS: see page 713

PREPARATIONS OF OESTROGENS

The dose varies according to whether replacement of physiological deficiencies is being carried out *(replacement therapy)* or whether *pharmacotherapy* is being used.

- *Ethinylestradiol* (t½ 13 h) is a synthetic agent of first choice for pharmacological (mainly contraceptive) uses; it is effective by mouth.
- *Estradiol* and *estriol* are orally active mixed natural oestrogens.
- *Conjugated estrogens* (Premarin) are orally active mixed natural oestrogens containing 50–65% oestrone obtained from the urine of pregnant mares.[5]
- *Estropipate* (piperazine oestrone sulphate) is an orally active synthetic conjugate.

- *Stilboestrol* (diethylstilbestrol) is the first synthetic oestrogen: its use is confined to androgen dependent cancers (breast, prostate).

CHOICE OF OESTROGEN

Ethinyloestradiol, or its methylated derivative mestranol, is a satisfactory first choice for pharmacotherapy. The weaker endogenous oestrogens, oestradiol, oestrone or the conjugated equine oestrogens are preferable for physiological replacement. It remains uncertain whether all oestrogens have exactly similar hormonal and nonhormonal effects, including adverse effects.

Transdermal formulations of estradiol are available. They can be effective and convenient for women who dislike taking oral therapy. Both oestradiol and oestriol can be taken vaginally as a cream, ring, pessary or tablet.

INDICATIONS FOR OESTROGEN THERAPY

Replacement therapy in hypoestrogenaemia. This term refers to decreased oestrogen production due to ovarian disease, or to hypothalamic/pituitary disease (hypogonadotropic hypogonadism). Treatment is by cyclic oestrogen (conjugated oestrogens 0.625/1.25 mg daily or ethinylestradiol 20–30 micrograms daily for 21 days) plus a progestogen, medroxyprogesterone 2.5 to 10 mg daily for the last 10 to 14 days of oestrogen treatment. An alternative treatment is the oral contraceptive (see p. 721).

Unless the cause of the hypo-ovarian state is primary ovarian failure, treatment should be stopped after every third cycle to see if spontaneous menstruation will occur.

Postmenopausal hormone replacement therapy (HRT)

HRT refers to the use of oestrogen treatment in order to reverse or prevent problems due to the loss of ovarian hormone secretion after the menopause,

---

[5] The mares are bred on 480 farms in the prairie provinces of Canada. The 80 000 foals that are produced each year have a less medicinal future than their mothers' urine: they are weaned at 120 days and sold for meat.

whether physiological or induced. The tissues sensitive to oestrogen include brain, bone, skin, cardiovascular and genitourinary. Consequently the two aims of HRT are:

- To reduce the everyday symptoms of oestrogen loss: hot flushes, sleeplessness, lethargy and depression, vaginal dryness
- To prevent the long-term complications associated with oestrogen deficiency: osteoporotic fractures (see Chapter 38) and coronary heart disease

Only the first is a proven indication for HRT. In addition, HRT must avoid causing disorders due to oestrogen excess, especially endometrial and breast cancer.

All types of HRT (oestrogen with or without progestogen) are effective in reducing the hot flushes experienced by more than 50% of postmenopausal women. The benefit is most during the first year of treatment when 80% of women report a reduced likelihood of flushes, and becomes less as the frequency of flushing diminishes, even in the placebo treated groups in trials. The other major value from HRT is the relief of vaginal dryness. Vaginal administration is the most effective route for treatment of dyspareunia and related symptoms.

Because most women do not suffer the long-term complications of oestrogen loss during the 5–10 years that HRT might be taken, it has been much more difficult to evaluate the second objective of HRT, i.e. reduction in coronary heart disease. For many years, the value of HRT seemed to be supported by the epidemiological data, which compared the incidence of fractures or coronary events in women taking, or not taking, HRT. These data suffered from the major flaws that most of the women were receiving 'unopposed' oestrogens (no progestogen), and that it was difficult to rule out the confounding effect of self-selection for HRT. In other words, taking HRT in such studies was simply a marker for women who took more care over their health. Concerns about the undesirable effects of progestogens, and the thrombotic effects of oestrogen, necessitate prospective randomized controlled trials to resolve questions about long-term benefits. The first of these, and a preliminary report from a second, are not favourable.

In the Heart and Estrogen/progestin Replace-ment Study (HERS)[6] daily therapy with conjugated oestrogen and progestin did not reduce the incidence of coronary events during four years of follow-up. The trial was too small to be informative about hip fractures but there was no difference in overall fracture rate between the groups. More recently, the Women's Health initiative primary prevention study in 27 000 (following a preliminary report) women has issued a warning letter that women on HRT are at increased risk of cardiovascular events during the first two years. A trial of unopposed oestrogen in 664 postmenopausal women with previous strokes has also found no benefit, and indeed a 2-fold greater risk of fatal strokes during 3 years of follow-up.[7] These trials do not yet exclude a long-term benefit of HRT as might be expected from the beneficial effects of oestrogen on LDL, HDL and vascular tone; the effects may be outweighed in trials of secondary prevention by the increased risk of clotting. Advice for the present is not to initiate HRT solely on grounds of preventing coronary disease, stroke or fractures. On the other hand, HRT should not be withdrawn from patients who need symptomatic treatment.

Other unproven benefits of long-term treatment are reduced risk of senile dementia and prevention of colon cancer.

Preparations used for HRT. There are three types of regimen:

---

[6] Hulley et al 1998 JAMA 280: 605–613. 2763 women with coronary disease were randomised to placebo or conjugated equine oestrogens plus medroxyprogesterone acetate. After 4 years 172 women in the hormone group and 176 women in the placebo group had a myocardial infarction or CHD death. There were significantly more events in the hormone group in the first year, but fewer in years 4 and 5. There were significantly more thromboembolic events in the hormone group (34) than controls (12). There was no difference in fracture incidence (130 vs 138), but the study was not powered to examine hip fractures, the commonest site of osteoporosis. The number of hip fractures overall (23) means that a substantial benefit of treatment could have been missed.

[7] Viscoli et al 2001 New England Journal of Medicine 345: 1243–1249. Women received estradiol 1 mg or placebo. There were 99 strokes or deaths in the estradiol group vs 93 in controls. Twelve of the strokes in the estradiol group were fatal compared to four in controls.

1. Women without a uterus take continuous oestrogen alone.
2. Other women require oestrogen combined with progestogen to prevent endometrial proliferation.
   a. In the commonest, 'sequential' regimen, women take oestrogen without break, and add a progestogen from approximately the 14th to 28th day of each cycle (different preparations vary in the exact length of progestogen prescribing). The first course is started on the 1st day of mentruation (if present), and 28-day cycles of treatment follow thereafter without interval.
   b. In the 'continuous' regimen, *appropriate only for women who have been amenorrhoeic for more than one year,* fixed dose combinations of oestrogen and progestogen are taken without a break. Continuous combination HRT regimens will eventually induce amenorrhoea in most women, thereby eliminating one of the major deterrents to HRT use, withdrawal bleeding.

Special calendar packs of the various regimens are available. The oral preparations, Prempak C and Femoston, use, respectively, conjugated oestrogen and oestradiol as their oestrogen. Progestogens are used mainly by mouth and include dihydrogesterone, medroxyprogesterone, norgestrel and norethisterone. Individual progestogens can be given orally in combination with an oestrogen given by sub-cutaneous depot injection or by transdermal patch. One patch (Estracombi) provides both hormones but obviously the doses cannot be separately titrated to provide the minimum necessary to prevent both flushing and (if undesired) withdrawal bleeding.

A popular alternative to oestrogen therapy is the drug tibolone (Livial), which is a synthetic steroid with weak oestrogenic, progestogenic and andro-genic properties. It is administered as a daily oral dose of 2.5 mg to suppress vasomotor symptoms and to prevent postmenopausal osteoporosis. The main adverse effect is vaginal bleeding, which needs investigation if persistent. Vasomotor menopausal symptoms may occasionally be helped by low doses of clonidine (Dixarit).

Contraception. HRT in routine use *does not provide contraception* and any potentially fertile woman who needs to use HRT should take appropriate precautions. A woman is considered potentially fertile for 2 years after her last menstrual period if she is under 50 years, and for 1 year if she is over 50 years. A woman who is under 50 years and free of all risk factors for venous and arterial disease can use a low-oestrogen combined oral contraceptive pill to provide both relief of menopausal symptoms and contraception; it is recommended that the oral contraceptive be stopped at 50 years of age since there are more suitable alternatives.

Adverse effects of HRT

The commonest reasons for withdrawal are *irregular* or *withdrawal bleeding* and *breast pain*. Concerns about musculoseletal symptoms and weight gain were not substantiated in the long-term trials.

The more serious complications are venous *thromboembolism* and *cancer of the endometrium or breast*. These risks are small in absolute terms, particularly so for the risks of cancer during the first 5 years of treatment.

For venous thromboembolism, the excess risk is 4/1000 woman years, which may be considered clinically insignificant except in women with pre-disposing factors, e.g. previous personal or family history of thromboembolism, or recent surgery.

Carcinoma of the endometrium is associated only with *unopposed* oestrogens, which increase risk by 2-fold during 5 years rising to 7-fold with longer treatment. Because endometrial cancer is uncom-mon, the absolute risk is about one-tenth that of thromboembolic disease; the risk reduces over 5–10 years after stopping treatment.

Carcinoma of the breast can occur with any type of HRT. Some 45 in every 1000 women aged 50 years will have breast cancer over the next 20 years, rising by only 2, 6 and 12 cases, respectively, for women who take HRT for 5, 10 or 15 years. A family history of breast cancer does not increase the risks from HRT.

The risk of gallstones may be increased up to 2-fold. HRT does not increase risk of ovarian cancer.

Blood lipids: the effect of oestrogens is on balance favourable, but the addition of a progestogen (unless gestodene or desogestrel) reverses the balance.

Contraindications to oestrogen therapy include women who may have an oestrogen-dependent neoplasm, e.g. breast cancer, who may be pregnant, or have a disposition to thromboembolism. Hypertension, liver disease or gallstones, migraine, diabetes, uterine fibroids or endometriosis may all be made worse by oestrogen. These are not necessarily absolute contraindications, and HRT should not for instance be denied to a polysymptomatic woman with mild hypertension. If necessary, it may be permissible to treat both the hypertension and the postmenopausal symptoms with separate drugs.

Pharmacotherapy

Contraception: see p. 721.

Menstrual disorders: see p. 729.

Vaginitis. Senile vaginitis usually responds to daily use of an oestrogen pessary or cream (which can also be used in small girls with vaginitis). Absorption can occur sufficiently to cause systemic effects in both the subject and her male sexual partner.

Inhibition of lactation. Oestrogens are no longer recommended because of associated risk of thromboembolism.

Androgen-dependent carcinoma. Diethylstilbestrol (stilboestrol) is rarely used to treat prostate cancer because of its adverse effects. It is occasionally used in postmenopausal women with breast cancer. Toxicity is common.

To reduce sexual urge in men whose activities are qualitatively or quantitatively unacceptable to the community and/or to themselves is an occasional indication for oestrogens: 1 mg of stilboestrol daily should be enough (see also Antiandrogen (cyproterone) and benperidol).

Epistaxis: as a last resort in recurrent cases, e.g. telangiectasia.

Atrophic rhinitis may benefit, as also may acne.

Antioestrogens

Selective antagonists of the oestrogen receptor are used either to induce gonadotrophin release in anovulatory infertility, or to block stimulation of oestrogen-receptor-positive carcinomas of the breast

Clomifene is structurally related to stilboestrol; it is a weak oestrogen agonist having less activity than natural oestrogens, so that its occupation of receptors results in antagonism, i.e. it is a partial agonist. Clomifene blocks hypothalamic oestrogen receptors so that the negative feedback of natural oestrogens is prevented and the pituitary responds by increased secretion of gonadotrophins, which may induce ovulation. Clomifene is administered during the early follicular phase of the menstrual cycle (50 mg daily on days 2–6) and is successful in inducing ovulation in about 85% of women. *Multiple ovulation with multiple pregnancy* may occur and this is its *principal adverse effect*. There have also been reports of an increased incidence of ovarian carcinoma following multiple exposure, and the number of consecutive cycles for which clomiphene may be used to stimulate ovulation should be limited to 12.

Cyclofenil acts similarly to clomiphene.

Tamoxifen is a nonsteroid competitive oestrogen antagonist on target organs. Although available for anovulatory infertility (20 mg daily on days 2, 3, 4 and 5 of the cycle) its main use now is in the treatment of *oestrogen-dependent breast cancer.* Treatment with tamoxifen delays the growth of metastases and increases survival; if tolerated it should be continued for 5 years.

Tamoxifen is also the hormonal treatment of choice in women with oestrogen-receptor-positive metastatic breast cancer. Approximately 60% of such patients respond to initial hormonal manipulation, whereas less than 10% of oestrogen-receptor-negative tumours respond.

Severe adverse effects are unusual with tamoxifen but patients with bony metastases may experience an exacerbation of pain, sometimes associated with hypercalcaemia; this reaction commonly precedes tumour response. Amenorrhoea commonly develops in premenopausal women. Patients should be told of the small risk of endometrial cancer and encouraged to report relevant symptoms early. They can be reassured that the benefits of treatment far outweigh the risks.

Progesterone and progestogens

Progesterone (t½ 5 min) is produced by the corpus luteum and converts the uterine epithelium from the proliferative to the secretory phase. It is thus necessary for successful implantation of the ovum, and is essential throughout pregnancy in the last two-thirds of which it is secreted in large amounts by the placenta. It acts particularly on tissues that are sensitised by oestrogens. Some synthetic progestogens are less selective, having varying oestrogenic and androgenic activity, and these may inhibit ovulation, though not very reliably.

Progestogens are of two principal kinds:

- *Progesterone and its derivatives:* dydrogesterone, hydroxyprogesterone, medroxyprogesterone (t½ 28 h), etc.
- *Testosterone derivatives:* norethisterone and its prodrug ethynodiol (t½ 10 h), levonorgestrel, desogestrel, gestodene, gestronol, norgestimate.

All can virilise directly or via metabolites (except progesterone and dydrogesterone) and fetal virilisation to the point of sexual ambiguity has occurred with vigorous use during pregnancy (see also Contraception, p. 721).

Megestrol is used only in cancer; it causes tumours in the breasts of beagle dogs.

PHARMACOKINETICS: see p. 714

USES

The clinical uses of progestational agents are ill-defined, apart from contraception, the menopause and postmenopausal hormone replacement therapy (see above).

Other possible uses include

- *menstrual disorders*, e.g. menorrhagia,

endometriosis, dysmenorrhoea and premenstrual syndrome (doubtful efficacy)
- *breast and endometrial cancer.*

PREPARATIONS

Available progestogens (some used only in combined formulations) include:

- *oral:* norethisterone, dydrogesterone, gestodene, desogestrel, levonorgestrel, megestrol, medroxyprogesterone
- *suppositories or pessaries:* progesterone
- *injectable:* progesterone, hydroxyprogesterone, medroxyprogesterone.

Adverse effects of prolonged use include virilisation (see above), raised blood pressure and adverse trend in blood lipids. Gestodene, desogestrel and norgestimate may have less affinity for androgen receptors and therefore less unfavourable effect on blood lipids; however the first two of these may have a higher risk of thrombosis.

Antiprogestogens

Menstruation (in its luteal phase) is dependent on progesterone, and uterine bleeding follows antagonism of progesterone. Pregnancy is dependent on progesterone (for implantation, endometrial stimulation, suppression of uterine contractions and placenta formation), and abortion follows progesterone antagonism in early pregnancy.

Mifepristone is a pure competitive antagonist at progesterone and glucocorticoid receptors. Clinical trials of oral use in hospital outpatients have shown it to be safe and effective in terminating pregnancy. Efficacy is enhanced if its use is followed by administration of a prostaglandin (gemeprost) (vaginally) to produce uterine contractions (the success rate is raised from 85% to above 95%). Adverse effects of the combined treatment include nausea and vomiting, dizziness, asthenia, abdominal pain; uterine bleeding may be heavy. Mifepristone also offers the opportunity for mid-trimester terminations. These are likely to become increasingly frequent as the number of inherited syndromes amenable to antenatal diagnosis at this stage increases.

Guidelines may vary in detail and the following are general regimens.

- For gestation up to a week where the fetus is deemed viable, mifepristone 600 mg by mouth followed 36–48 hours later by gemeprost 1 mg by vagina
- For mid-trimester medical abortion (13–24 weeks), mifepristone 600 mg by mouth followed 36–48 hours later by gemeprost 1 mg every 3 hours by vagina to a maximum of 5 mg.

Other progesterone derivatives

Danazol (Danol) is a derivative of the progestogen, ethisterone. It has partial agonist androgen activity and is described as an 'impeded' androgen; it has little progestogen activity. It is a relatively selective inhibitor of pituitary gonadotrophin secretion (LH, FSH) affecting the surge in the mid-menstrual cycle more than basal secretion. This reduces ovarian function, which leads to atrophic changes in endometrium, both uterine and elsewhere (ectopic), i.e. endometriosis. In males it reduces spermatogenesis. Androgenic unwanted effects occur in women (acne, hirsutism and, rarely, enlargement of the clitoris).

It is chiefly used for: *endometriosis, fibrocystic mastitis, gynaecomastia,* precocious puberty, menorrhagia and hereditary angioedema (p. 715).

Gestrinone is similar.

Fertility regulation

Infertility

The treatment of infertility in either sex is a highly specialised business, requiring a detailed understanding of reproductive physiology and analysis of the cause.

Depending on the cause, the following agents, already described, are used:

For women: to procure ovulation
- Hypothalamic hormone: gonadorelin (p. 711)
- Anterior pituitary hormones: follicle stimulating hormone (p. 711); chorionic gonadotrophin (p. 711)
- Antioestrogens: clomiphene, etc. (p. 719)
- Bromocriptine for hyperprolactinaemia (p. 711).

For men: to enhance spermatogenesis: the same agents as for ovulation are used; androgens are not useful unless there is hypogonadism.

Contraception by drugs and hormones

The requirements of a successful hormonal contraceptive are stringent, for it will be used by millions of healthy people who wish to separate sexual relations from physical reproduction. The following represent the ideal.

- It must be *extremely safe* as well as *highly effective*
- Its action must be quick in onset and quickly and *completely reversible,* even after years of continuous use
- It must not affect *libido.*

The fact that alternative methods are less reliable implies that their use will lead to more unwanted pregnancies with their attendant inconvenience, morbidity and mortality, and this must be taken into account in deciding what risks of hormonal contraception are acceptable.

POSSIBLE MODES AND SITES OF ACTION

1. *Direct inhibition of spermatogenesis:* this presents many problems including the lag in onset of effect due to storage of mature spermatozoa until they are ejaculated or die of old age.
2. *Indirect inhibition of spermatogenesis* by suppression of hypothalamic/pituitary activity, which controls it, e.g. by progestogen-androgen combinations; see gonadorelin.
3. *Immunological techniques* (vaccines), to induce antibodies to pituitary gonadotrophins, sperm,

or other components of the reproductive process in either sex; these are being developed.

4. *Inhibition of ovulation* presents a different and easier biological problem. There is no need to suppress continuous formation of the gametes, as in the male, but only to prevent their release from the ovary approximately 13 times a year. Either the pituitary gonadotrophin may be inhibited or the ovary may be made unresponsive to it.

5. *Prevention of fertilisation:* the female genital tract may be made inhospitable to spermatozoa, e.g. by altering cervical mucus or fallopian tube function.

6. *Antizygotic drugs:* compounds effective in the rat have been developed.

7. *Inhibition of implantation:* implantation does not occur unless the endometrium is in the right state, and this depends on a delicate balance between oestrogen and progesterone. This balance can readily be disturbed.

8. *Use of spermicides in the vagina* (They are used in combination with barrier methods. This is strictly *chemical* rather than hormonal contraception; as also are intrauterine devices that contain copper, which is gametocidal).

Hormonal contraception in women comprises

- Oestrogen and progestogen (combined and phased administration)
- Progestogen alone

COMBINED CONTRACEPTIVES (THE 'PILL'[8])

Combined oestrogen-progestogen oral contraceptives have been extensively used since 1956. The principal mechanism is inhibition of ovulation (4, above) through inhibition of gonadotrophin secretion from the hypothalamus. In addition the endometrium is altered, so that implantation is less likely (7, above) and cervical mucus becomes more viscous and impedes the passage of the spermatozoa (5, above).

Oestrogens alone are not completely reliable. At the necessary dose, they can also cause thromboembolism and endometrial cancer.

Progestogens used alone inhibit ovulation in up to 40% of cycles, render cervical mucus less easily penetrable by sperm and induce a premature secretory change in the endometrium so that implantation does not occur. There is liable to be break-through bleeding and some are a cause of raised blood pressure and an adverse trend in blood lipids and arterial disease.

An appropriate dose of oestrogen + progestogen gives excellent reliability with good menstrual cycle control. The following account applies to these combined preparations.

The combination is conveniently started on the first day of the cycle (first day of menstruation) and continued for 21 days (this is immediately effective, inhibiting the first ovulation). It is followed by a period of 7 days when no pill is taken, and during which bleeding usually occurs. Thereafter, regardless of bleeding, a new 21-day course is begun, and so on, i.e. active tablets are taken daily for 3 weeks out of 4.[9] For easy compliance, some combined pills are packaged so that the woman takes one tablet every day without interruption (21 active then 7 dummy).

In some instances, the course is not started on the first day of menstruation but on the 2nd to the 5th day (to give a full month between the menses at the outset). An alternative method of contraception should then be used until the 7th pill has been taken, since the first ovulation may not have been suppressed in women who have short menstrual cycles.

---

[8] The word 'pill' has gained currency in both professional and popular usage to mean 'oral contraceptive', losing its original precise technical pharmaceutical meaning.

[9] Despite rigid adherence to it, women occasionally conceive on this regimen, i.e. their follicles develop early. Where this has occurred yet the women wishes to continue on hormonal contraception, a safer regimen is 24 days hormone administration with a 4-day interval.

[10] It may also be prudent to tell the patient how the pill works: 'Her medical records showed that over the previous 3 months, she had received 6 months supply of a contraceptive pill. Had she lost some, or had someone else taken the pills? After a shy pause, she confided that she was taking two pills a day — one for her husband and one for her lover.' Lancet 2000 356: 1118.

The pill should be taken about the same time (to within 12 hours) every day to establish a routine.[10] The monthly bleeds that occur 1–2 days after the cessation of active hormone administration are hormone withdrawal bleeds not natural menstruation. They are not an essential feature of oral contraception, but women are accustomed to monthly bleeds and they provide monthly reassurance of the absence of pregnancy.

Numerous field trials have shown that progestogen-oestrogen combinations, if taken precisely as directed, are the most reliable reversible contraceptive known. (The only close competitors are depot progestogens and progestogen-releasing intrauterine devices.)

Important aspects

Subsequent fertility. After stopping the pill, fertility that is normal for the age the woman has now reached is restored, although conception may be delayed for a few months longer in younger and as much as a year in older users than if other methods had been used.

Effect on an existing pregnancy. Although progestogens can masculinise the female fetus, the doses for contraception are so low that risk of harming an undiagnosed pregnancy is extremely low, probably less than 1 in 1000 (the background incidence of birth defects is 1–2%).

Carcinoma of the *breast* and *cervix* may be unaffected or very slightly increased in incidence; *hepatoma* (very rare) is increased. The risk to life seems to be less than that of moderate smoking (10 cigarettes/day). Carcinoma of the *ovary* and the *endometrium* are substantially *reduced*. Total incidence of cancer is unaltered.

Effect on menstruation (it is not true menstruation, see above) is generally to regularise it, and often to diminish blood loss, but amenorrhoea can occur. In some women 'break-through' intermenstrual bleeding occurs, especially at the outset, but this seldom persists for more than a few cycles. *Premenstrual tension* and *dysmenorrhoea* are much reduced.

Libido is greatly subject to psychosocial influences, and removal of fear of pregnancy may permit enthusiasm for the first time. It is likely that direct pharmacological effect (reduction) is rare. There is evidence that the normal increase in female-initiated sexual activity at time of ovulation is suppressed.[11]

Cardiovascular complications. Incidence of *venous thromboembolism* is increased in pill users. It is lowest in the 20–35 microgram pill and rises progressively with the 50 microgram and 100 microgram preparations; it is not known if there is any difference between doses of 20–35 micrograms. The small increase in *hypertension, cerebrovascular event and acute myocardial infarction* is principally confined to *smokers*.

Increased arterial disease also appears to be associated with the type of progestogen in the combined pill. The '3rd generation' pills (see later) appear to carry a higher risk of venous thrombosis,[12] but may have a lower risk of arterial thrombosis because their lower androgen activity leads to slightly higher HDL levels than older pills.[13] The progestogen-only pill does not significantly affect coagulation.

Major surgery (in patients taking oestrogen-progestogen contraceptives and postmenopausal hormone replacement therapy). Because of the added risk of venous thromboembolism (surgery causes a fall in antithrombin) it has been advised that these oral contraceptives should be withdrawn, if practicable, 4 weeks before all lower limb operations or any major elective surgery (and started again at the first menstruation to occur more than 2 weeks after surgery). But increase in clotting factors may persist for many weeks and there is also the risk of pregnancy to be considered (plainly, alternative contraception should be used). An

---

[11] Adams D B et al 1978 New England Journal of Medicine 299: 1145.
[12] Estimated to be 30 thromboembolic episodes per 100 000 women taking the pill compared with 15 per 100 000 with 2nd generation pills (the background rate is 8 per 100 000).
[13] Spitzer W O et al 1996 Third generation oral contraceptives and risk of venous thromboembolic disorders: an international case-control study. British Medical Journal 312: 83–88.

alternative for emergencies is to use low molecular weight heparin (though this may not reverse all the oestrogen effects on coagulation) and other means (mechanical stimulation of venous return) to prevent postoperative thrombosis. A similar problem arises with *prolonged immobilisation* from other causes.

Hepatic function may be impaired as may drug-metabolising capacity ($t\frac{1}{2}$ of antipyrine, a general indicator of the drug-metabolising capacity, may increase by 30%). Gallbladder disease is more common, and highly vascular hepatocellular adenomas occur (rare).

Cervical ectropion (erosion) incidence is double (it is a harmless condition).

Crohn's disease is more frequent.

Decreased glucose tolerance occurs, perhaps due to a peripheral effect reducing the action of insulin.

Plasma lipoproteins may be adversely affected; least where the progestogen is desogestrel or low-dose norethisterone.

Plasma proteins. Oestrogens cause an increase in proteins, particularly the globulins that bind hydrocortisone, thyroxine and iron. As a result, the total plasma concentration of the bound substances is increased, though the concentration of free and active substance remains normal. This can be misleading in diagnostic tests, e.g. of thyroid function. This effect on plasma proteins passes off about 6 weeks after cessation of the oestrogen.

Other adverse effects

Often more prominent at the outset and largely due to oestrogen, these include: nausea and, rarely, vomiting; breast discomfort, fluid retention, headache (including increase in migraine), lethargy, abdominal discomfort, vaginal discharge or dryness. Depression may occur but most depression in pill users is not due to the contraceptive.

The above account gives rise to guidelines for use:

Absolute contraindications include:

- A personal history of thromboembolic venous, arterial or cardiac disease or severe or multiple risk factors for these
- Transient cerebral ischaemic attacks without headache
- Infective hepatitis, until 3 months after liver function tests have become normal, and other liver disease including disturbances of hepatic excretion, e.g. cholestatic jaundice, Dubin-Johnson and Rotor syndromes
- Migraine, if there is a typical aura, focal features, or if it is severe and lasts > 72 hours despite treatment, or is treated with an ergot derivative (use with caution is acceptable if there is no aura, focal features, or if it is controlled with a $5HT_1$ receptor agonist)
- Carcinoma of the breast or of the genital tract, past or present
- Other conditions including: systemic lupus erythematosus, porphyria, following evacuation of a hydatidiform mole (until urine and plasma gonadotrophin concentrations are normal), undiagnosed vaginal bleeding.

Relative contraindications or uses with caution, include:
- Family history of venous thromboembolism, arterial disease or a known prothrombotic condition, e.g. factor V Leiden (pretreatment coagulation investigation is advised).
- Diabetes mellitus which may be precipitated or become more difficult to control (avoid if there are diabetic complications).
- Hypertension (avoid if blood pressure exceeds 160/100)
- Smoking > 40 cigarettes per day (15 cigarettes/day enhances the risks of circulatory disease (× 3), and constitutes an *absolute contraindication* for women over 35 years.
- Age over 35 years (avoid if > 50 years)
- Obesity (avoid if body mass index exceeds 39 kg/m^2)
- Long-term immobility, e.g. due to leg plaster, confinement to bed
- Breast feeding (until weaning or for 6 months after birth).

Duration of use does not enhance risks of itself. The increase in risk with increased duration of use is due to increasing age. The approaching menopause presents an obvious problem. Because cyclic bleeding will continue to occur under the influence of the drugs even after the natural menopause, the only way of deciding whether contraception can be permanently abandoned is by abandoning it (and using another technique) for 3 months annually to see if natural menstruation is resumed; or stop the combined pill for one month and measure LH/FSH concentration in the blood, which indicates the state of pituitary function.

Benefits additional to contraception

Side-effects are commonly assumed always to be unpleasant aspects of drug action, but they can sometimes also be pleasant.

The oestrogen-progestogen pill is associated with *reduced* risk of functional ovarian cysts and cancer, of endometrial cancer and of benign breast disease; there is a reduced risk of uterine fibroids and they bleed less; menses are regular and blood loss is not excessive; menses are accompanied by less premenstrual tension and dysmenorrhoea. When oestrogen is combined with the antiandrogen cyproterone acetate as the progestogenic agent 'Dianette', the combined pill is useful treatment for acne in young women.

Conclusions

- Pregnancy carries risk.
- Serious adverse effects of the combined pill are rare and 'several times a rare event is still a rare event'.[14]
- Precise figures on risk with current low-dose formulations are not available. The major studies, involving, e.g. 23 000 women, used higher dose formulations and cannot be repeatedly replicated (cost, logistics) to keep up with developments.
- Overall mortality amongst users (having low risk factors) is either unaffected or only slightly increased.

---

[14] Guillebaud J 1989 The pill. Oxford University Press. A general reference for all practical aspects of use.

Formulations of oestrogen-progestogen combination

Oestrogen: ethinylestradiol or mestranol

Progestogen
- 2nd generation: norethisterone, levonorgestrel
- 3rd generation: desogestrel, gestodene, norgestimate

Combined oral contraceptives are defined as 2nd or 3rd generation by the progestogen component (1st generation progestogens are obsolete). Those containing a fixed amount of an oestrogen and a progestogen in each active tablet are termed 'monophasic'. Other pills employ variable ratios between oestrogen and progestogen, in 2 (*biphasic*) or 3 (*triphasic*) periods within the menstrual cycle. The dose of progestogen is low at the beginning and higher at the end, the oestrogen remaining either constant or rising slightly in mid-cycle. The objective is to achieve effective contraception with minimal distortion of natural hormonal rhythms. The advantages claimed for these techniques are diminished adverse metabolic changes, e.g. blood lipids, and a particularly reliable monthly bleeding pattern without loss of contraceptive efficacy. Preparations include BiNovum, TriNovum, Logynon.

It is now appreciated that the earlier preparations had much more oestrogen than was necessary for efficacy. It seems probable that 20 micrograms is about the limit below which serious loss of efficacy can be expected. Indeed in patients whose hepatic enzymes are likely to be induced, e.g. those taking antiepileptic or some antirheumatic drugs, it is advisable to use a preparation containing 50 micrograms or more of oestrogen to avoid loss of efficacy due to increased oestrogen metabolism (elimination of breakthrough bleeding is a guide to adequacy of dose).

Choice of oestrogen-progestogen combination

There is a wide choice of formulations:

- *Low oestrogen* (20 micrograms) plus *low progestogen*, e.g. Loestrin 20, Mercilon, Femodette

- *Low oestrogen* plus *high progestogen*, e.g. Ovran 30, Eugynon 30
- *High oestrogen* (50 micrograms) plus *low* or *high progestogen*, e.g. Ovran, Norinyl-1.

In general, users should be prescribed the lowest total hormone dose that suits them (good cycle control and minimal side-effects) and should make a start with the first preparation given above, recognising that compliance is particularly important with the 20 microgram dose.

Common problems

Missed pill. The following refers to the *combined pill* (see later for the progesterone-only pill).

- If an omitted dose is remembered within 12 hours it should be taken at once and the next dose at the usual time, and all should be well.
- If more than 12 hours have elapsed, the above procedure should be followed but an *additional* barrier method of contraception should be used for 7 days (or abstinence). Whereas the protective effect of cervical mucus returns within 48h, this 7-day period is needed to ensure effective suppression of an ovulation that may have been initiated by the missed pill.[15]

  Plainly a regimen in which a pill is taken every day (dummy pills) may confuse the subject who will then need advice.

Intercurrent gut upset. Obviously a patient may vomit the dose; if vomiting occurs more than 3 hours after a pill, behave as for a missed pill (above). The hormones are rapidly absorbed and only severe diarrhoea would interfere significantly with efficacy.[16] But if there is doubt, it would be prudent to use a barrier method during and for 7 days after the episode.

Changing of preparation. If a woman is unhappy on one preparation she may be changed to another containing a different dose of oestrogen and/or progestogen. The new preparation should start the day after she has finished a cycle on the previous preparation. If this is done no extra risk of pregnancy occurs.

Break-through bleeding (bleeding on days of active pill taking) can mean a higher dose of oestrogen or progestogen is required. Note that missed or late pills, drug interaction (see later) or sexually transmitted infection, e.g. due to chlamydia, can also cause breakthrough bleeding.

PROGESTOGEN-ONLY CONTRACEPTION

The oral formulation ('mini-pill') is taken every day; it must be taken at the same time each day (to within 3 hours). Oral progestogen-only contraception is less effective but safer (no effect on blood coagulation) than combined formulations.

Subdermal implantations that release hormone for several years are in use; they can be removed surgically if adverse effects develop or pregnancy is desired. For example, a flexible rod containing etonorgestrel (Implanton) inserted into the lower surface of the upper arm provides contraception for 3 years (2 years for overweight women because they have lower blood concentrations). The rod must be removed when its effective period has elapsed.

Intramuscular progestogen. A 3-month depot injection is equal in efficacy to the combined pill and is an alternative. It works by inhibiting ovulation, and also renders cervical mucus impenetrable to sperm.

Progestogen-only contraception is particularly appropriate to women having an absolute contra-indication for oestrogen, e.g. history of thrombo-embolism, smokers over 35 years (who refuse to give it up), and for diabetics. Hypertension is not an absolute contraindication to the more effective combined pill since only a proportion of women have oestrogen dependent hypertension (and often such women are normotensive until exposed to increased levels of oestrogen). It is used by *lactating women* as it interferes with the milk less than the combined pill.

---

[15] If these 7 days run beyond the beginning of the routine intended pill-free days, the next cycle (packet) should follow without a gap, thus postponing the menses by a month (Family Planning Association).

[16] Orme M et al 1991 Unintended pregnancies and contraceptive use. British Medical Journal 302: 789.

A missed oral dose allows even less latitude than the combined pill. If a dose is more than *3 hours late* it should be taken at once and a barrier method used for 7 days. Act similarly where there has been vomiting, severe diarrhoea, or if an enzyme-inducing drug has been taken.

A significant limitation to the use of the progestogen-only pill is erratic uterine bleeding which many women understandably dislike. There may be no bleeding for months or there may be frequent and irregular bleeding. Ectopic pregnancy may be more frequent due to a fertilised ovum being held up in a functionally depressed fallopian tube. Other adverse effects are generally less than the combined pill (blood coagulation is unaffected), data on breast cancer are conflicting but are largely reassuring. Ovarian cysts occur more frequently in progesterone-only pill users.

The progestogens used (alone) orally include norgestrel, levonorgestrel, ethynodiol, norethisterone, desogestrel (e.g. Noriday, Micronor, Femulen). Medroxyprogesterone (Depo-Provera) ($t\frac{1}{2}$ 28 h) is a sustained-release (aqueous suspension) deep i.m. injection given 3-monthly. When injected between day 1 and day 5 of the menstrual cycle, contraception starts immediately. If given after day 5, a barrier contraceptive is needed for 7 days. Depo-Provera can be started within 5 days of childbirth or abortion; however, starting it so soon after childbirth may cause heavy bleeding and so waiting until 6 weeks postpartum is probably better.

Medroxyprogesterone acetate and its metabolites are excreted in breast milk, so women who breast-feed should wait until 6 weeks post partum before starting Depo-Provera, when the infant's enzyme system should be more mature. *Norethisterone enantate* 200 mg (Noristerat) is shorter acting than Depo-Provera, 8 weeks, and is used to provide contraception after administration of the rubella vaccine, and until a partner's vasectomy has taken effect. It can also be used in the longer-term but only on a 'named patient' basis.

POSTCOITAL ('morning after pill')[17] AND EMERGENCY CONTRACEPTION

Overall risk of pregnancy following a single act of unprotected intercourse on any day in the menstrual cycle is 2–4%. The risk from a single act is highest (20–30%) in the days before and just after ovulation. Pregnancy may be prevented before implantation by disrupting the normal hormonal arrangements; the mode of action is probably by delaying or preventing ovulation or by preventing implantation of the fertilised ovum.

Postcoital contraception may be successful up to *72 hours* after a single act of unprotected intercourse. A common technique is to take one tablet of levonoegestrel 750 micrograms (Levonelle 2) as soon as possible after intercourse and then a second tablet 12 hours (but not more than 16 hours) later.[18] With this regimen, vomiting is rare but if it occurs within 3 hours of either dose, another table should be taken immediately. It is available 'over the counter', i.e. off prescription, in the UK from trained pharmacists.

If pregnancy is present the treatment will not cause abortion, and evidence suggests that it does not harm a fetus. The procedure is not licenced for use more than once in a cycle.

DRUG INTERACTION WITH STEROID CONTRACEPTIVES

Particularly now that the lowest effective doses are in use there is little latitude between success and failure if the absorption, distribution and metabolism are distrubed. Any additional drug-taking must be looked at critically lest it reduces efficacy.

Enzyme induction. The rifamycins, *rifampicin* and *rifabutin*, are potent inducers of hepatic drug-metabolising enyzmes. The classic example of failure with the combined pill is break-through bleeding and pregnancy in young women being treated with rifampicin for tuberculosis, or meningitis including eradication of the carrier state. The enhanced metabolism of the steroids results in contraceptive failure. *Antiepileptics* (phenytoin and carbamazepine but not sodium valproate) create a similar risk. Indeed, all drugs that induce metabolising enzymes (see p. 113) whether prescribed or self-administered (alcohol, tobacco smoking) constitute a risk to

---

[17] A popular term that misleads women (see text below).
[18] Levonorgestrel prevented 95% of expected pregnancies if it was taken within 24 h, 85% if taken within 48 h and 58% if taken within 72 h (Grimes D et al 1998 Lancet 352: 428–433).

contraceptive efficacy and prescribing should be specifically reviewed for the effect. Pregnancies have occurred in women taking a contraceptive who commence an antiepileptic drug and doctors have been sued (for negligence) successfully in a court of law.

Broad spectrum antimicrobials, e.g. ampicillin, doxycillin, can reduce the efficacy of combined oral contraceptives by diminishing the bacterial flora that metabolise ethinylestradiol in the large bowel and make it available for recycling. Additional contraceptive measures should be taken during a *short* course of antimicrobial, and for 7 days thereafter. When the course is *long*, i.e. > 3 weeks the bacteria have time to recover by developing resistance and additional precautions are unnecessary after the first 14 days.

HYPOTHALAMIC/PITUITARY HORMONE APPROACH TO CONTRACEPTION

(See gonadorelin)

OTHER METHODS OF CONTRACEPTION

Copper intrauterine devices are widely used and highly effective (> 99% at one year) for 5 and some for 10 years. They are especially useful in the over-40s in whom oral contraceptives may become progressively contraindicated and for whom one IUD will last into the menopause. The IUD prevents implantation of the fertilised ovum, and has an additional antifertilisation effect enhanced by the toxic effect of copper ions on the gametes.

Norplant consists of six nonbiodegradable flexible silicone capsules, which release levonorgestrel at a rate of around 30 micrograms per day over a period of five years. It is no longer available for new use but some women who have had the system implanted may retain it till the year 2004. The shorter-acting (2–3 years) single rod containing etonogestrel (Implanon) is now preferred.

Vaginal preparations, used to immobilise or kill (spermicide) spermatozoa, are used to add safety to various mechanical contraceptives. They are very unreliable and should be used alone only in an emergency. Substances used include nonoxinols (surfactants that alter the permeability of the sperm liporotein membrane) as pessary, gel or foam.

Oil-based lubricants cause failure of rubber condoms and contraceptive diaphragms; many 'lubricants', e.g. hand or baby creams, wash off readily, but are nevertheless oil-based. Barrier contraceptive devices made of polyurethane, e.g. the female condom (femidom), are not so affected.

RISKS OF CONTRACEPTION IN RELATION TO BENEFIT

The death rate from taking oral contraceptives is less than that from playing cricket or football (in Britain) and much less than those from swimming (750 men, 250 women per annum in Britain). A car driver may expect, on average, to be admitted to hospital once in 20 years due to a road accident. A woman would have to use oral contraceptives for 2000 years for a similar chance due to a thrombotic episode.

Any danger oral contraceptives may have for the individual must also be seen in relation to their benefits, not only to the individual, but to the community, e.g. fewer self-induced and criminal abortions, fewer unwanted children, slowing down

---

Summary

- Many of the pituitary hormones and their hypothalamic releasing factors are used in diagnosis or therapy.
- Vasopression (antidiuretic hormone) is used both for its vasoconstrictor effect (in the treatment of oesophageal varices) and for its antidiuretic action.
- The main therapeutic use of pituitary hormones is of growth hormone (anterior pituitary) and those from the posterior pituitary: oxytocin and vasopressin.
- The main hypothalamus-pituitary target organ axis for therapeutic intervention is that controlling reproductive hormones, especially in women.
- Suppression of oestrogen and/or androgen production is used in the treatment of tumours stimulated by these: breast and prostate.
- Therapy in women is used to suppress ovulation (contraceptives), to stimulate ovulation (fertility treatment) or to mimic ovarian endocrine function (postmenopausal hormone replacement therapy, HRT).

of the speed of increase of world population with less hunger and misery.

MALE CONTRACEPTION (systemic)

Suppression of spermatogenesis may be achieved by interfering with:

- extragonadal endocrine control, i.e. the hypothalamic/pituitary/gonadal axis
- direct action on gonadal spermatogenesis
- vaccines to produce antibodies to sperm.

Approaches include androgen or combinations of androgen with danazol, or progestogen, or oestrogen, also gonadorelin.

In practice, the condom and vasectomy are the only commonly used forms of male contraception

Menstrual disorders

Amenorrhoea, primary or secondary, requires specialist endocrinological diagnosis. Where the cause is failure of hormone production, cyclical replacement therapy is indicated.

Menorrhagia can be associated with both ovulatory and anovulatory ovarian cycles. It is important to distinguish the menstrual consequences of each cycle. Ovulatory ovarian cycles give rise to regular menstrual cycles whereas anovulatory cycles result in irregular menstruation or, extremely, amenorrhoea. This distinction is critical in management. Both ovulatory and anovulatory cycles can give rise to excessive menstrual loss in the absence of any other abnormality; so called dysfunctional uterine bleeding. Endocrine disorders do not cause excessive menstrual loss, with the exception of the endocrine consequences of anovulation. Equally, haemostatic disorders are rare causes of menorrhagia. One consequence of excessive menstrual loss is iron deficiency anaemia. In the western world menorrhagia is the commonest cause of iron deficiency anamea.

Medical treatment of menorrhagia is either nonhormonal or hormonal therapy. As there is no hormonal defect the use of hormonal therapy does not correct an underlying disorder but merely imposes an external control of the cycle. For many women, cycle control is as important an issue as the degree of menorrhagia.

The two main first-line treatments for menorrhagia associated with ovulatory cycles are *nonhormonal* namely, *tranexamic acid* (an antifibrinolytic) and a nonsteroidal anti-inflammatory drug e.g. *mefenamic acid* 500 mg when the blood loss becomes heavy, followed by 250 mg t.d.s. for 3 days. The effectiveness of these treatments has been shown in randomised trials and reported in systematic reviews of treatment. Tranexamic acid reduces menstrual loss by about a half and nonsteroidal anti-inflammatory drugs reduced it by about a third. Both have the advantage of only being taken during menstruation itself and are particularly useful in those women who either do not require contraception or do not wish to use a hormonal therapy. They are also of value in treating excessive menstrual blood loss associated with the use of nonhormonal intrauterine contraceptive devices.

Hormonal therapy should be regarded as a third choice treatment only in women not requiring contraception as a parallel objective. Progestogens are effective only if given for 21 days in each cycle. Combined oral contraceptives are useful for anovulatory bleeding as they impose a cycle. The levonorgestrel releasing intrauterine system (Mirena) is advocated as an alternative to surgery.[19]

THE TIMING OF MENSTRUATION

Sometimes there are pressing reasons to prevent menstruation at the normal time but obviously this cannot be done at the last moment.

---

[19] Two studies have examined the effect of offering this treatment to women on waiting lists for hyserectomy. In the first of these studies 50 women were offered this treatment, and 82% (41/50) were removed from the waiting list as a result (Barrington JW, Bowen-Simpkins P 1997 British Journal of Obstetrics and Gynaecology 104: 614–616). Lahteenmaki P et al (British Medical Journal 1998 316: 1122–1126) randomised women on surgical waiting lists to continue with their current regimen or to use a levonorgestrel releasing intrauterine system; 64% of women using the system cancelled their surgery compared with 14% of women not using the system.

Menstruation can be postponed by giving oral norethisterone 5 mg t.d.s., starting 3 days before the expected onset; bleeding occurs 2–3 days after withdrawal. Users of the combined oral contraceptive pill (having a 7-day break) can simply continue with active pills where they would normally stop for 7 days.

Although there is no evidence that harm follows such manoeuvres, it is obviously imprudent to practise them frequently.

Note. These uses of progestogen should not be undertaken if there is any possibility of pregnancy.

Endometriosis. Medical treatments for endometriosis have focused on the hormonal alteration of the menstrual cycle in an attempt to produce a pseudo-pregnancy, pseudo-menopause, or chronic anovulation. Each of these situations is believed to cause a suboptimal milieu for the growth and maintenance of endometrium and, by extension, of implants of endometriosis. *Danazol* 600 to 800 mg per day causes anovulation by attenuating the midcycle surge of luteinising hormone secretion, inhibiting multiple enzymes in the steroidogenic pathway, and increasing serum free testosterone concentrations.

Medroxyprogesterone causes the decidualisation of endometrial tissue, with eventual atrophy. Adverse effects occur at low (20–30 mg) or high (100 mg/day) dose including abnormal uterine bleeding, nausea, breast tenderness, fluid retention, and depression. These resolve after the discontinuation of the drug. *Gestrinone* 5–10 mg/week is an antiprogestational steroid that causes a decline in the concentrations of oestrogen and progesterone receptors, and a 50% decline in serum oestradiol concentrations. Androgenic side effects, such as a deepening of the voice, hirsutism, and clitoral hypertrophy, are potentially irreversible.

A combination of an oestrogen and a progestogen induces a hormonal pseudo-pregnancy. The oral contraceptive is used either continuously or cyclically (21 active pill followed by 7 days of placebo). Both regimens are effective; the amenorrhea of continuous administration is advantageous for women with dysmenorrhea. *Gonadotropin-releasing hormone (GnRH) agonists* diminish the secretion of follicle-stimulating hormone and luteinising hormone, resulting in hypogonadotropic hypogonadism, endometrial atrophy and amenorrhea. The GnRH agonist can be given

intranasally, subcutaneously, or intramuscularly, with a frequency of administration ranging from twice daily to every three months. The side effects are the menopausal-type symptoms of hypoestrogenism (such as transient vaginal bleeding, hot flushes, vaginal dryness) and can be prevented by concurrent administration of HRT in postmenopausal doses.

Although most treatments for endometriosis are directed at the implant themselves, the symptoms can be also treated directly. Nonsteroidal anti-inflammatory drugs (NSAID) such as diclofenac, ibuprofen, mefenamic acid, are often given to relieve the pain associated with endometriosis. These drugs are frequently the first-line treatment in women with pelvic pain whose cause has not yet been proved to be endometriosis.

Dysmenorrhoea is due to uterine contractions resulting from excess prostaglandins in the uterus during ovulatory cycles. It can be treated by suppressing ovulation (using the combined pill or norethisterone); also by using inhibitors of prostaglandin synthesis, e.g. aspirin, indometacin, naproxen. The analgesic prostaglandin synthase inhibitor (NSAID) may need to be given for several days before menstruation or only at the time of the pain.

Premenstrual tension syndrome may be due to an imbalance of natural oestrogen and progesterone secretion but knowledge of the syndrome remains imprecise. Psychosocial factors can be important. Placebo effects are strong. Drugs are not necessarily the preferred treatment. There is evidence for and against:

- *Restriction of salt and fluid plus a thiazide diuretic* in the second half of the menstrual cycle where symptoms suggest fluid retention
- *Pyridoxine* (vitamin B_6, a coenzyme): try 100 mg/d orally (not more) for 3 months and abandon if there is no benefit. It may help depression and irritability particularly
- Oestrogen-progestogen oral contraceptive combination
- Bromocriptine, especially where there is breast pain
- Prostaglandin synthase inhibition. e.g. mefenamic acid.

Cyclical breast pain or mastalgia, when severe, may respond to continuous use of gamolenic acid (Efamast) (orally); it is an essential unsaturated fatty acid for cell membranes (patients have low concentrations); it may act by reducing cellular uptake of prolaction and ovarian hormones. Danazol and bromocriptine also help.

Myometrium

Oxytocics, i.e. drugs that hasten childbirth, and prostaglandins induce uterine contractions. They are used to induce abortion, to induce or augment labour, and to minimise blood loss from the placental site.

OXYTOCICS

Oxytocin is a peptide hormone of the posterior pituitary gland. It stimulates the contractions of the pregnant uterus, which becomes much more sensitive to it at term. Patients with posterior pituitary disease (diabetes insipidus) can, however, go into labour normally.

Oxytocin is reflexly released from the pituitary following suckling (also by manual stimulation of the nipple) and causes almost immediate contraction of the myoepithelium of the breast; it can be used to enhance milk ejection (nasal spray). The only other clinically important effect is on the blood pressure, which may fall if an overdose is given.

Synthetic oxytocin (Syntocinon) is pure and is not contaminated with vasopressin as is the natural product, which is obsolete.

Oxytocin is used i.v. in the induction of labour and sometimes for uterine inertia, haemorrhage or during abortion. It produces, almost immediately, rhythmic contractions with relaxation between, i.e. it mimics normal uterine activity.

The decision to use oxytocin requires special skill. It has a $t\frac{1}{2}$ of 6 min and is given by i.v. infusion using a pump (see below); it must be closely supervised; the dose is adjusted by results; overdose can cause uterine tetany and even rupture. The utmost care is required.

Oxytocin is structurally close to vasopression and it is no surprise that it also has antidiuretic activity (p. 711). Serious water intoxication can occur with prolonged i.v. infusions, especially where accompanied by large volumes of fluid. The association of oxytocin with neonatal jaundice appears to be due to increased erythrocyte fragility causing haemolysis.

Oxytocin has been supplanted by the ergot alkaloid, *ergometrine*, as prime treatment of postpartum haemorrhage.

Ergometrine is used to contract the uterus. It is an α-adrenoceptor and dopamine receptor agonist and acts almost immediately when injected i.v. The uterus is stimulated at all times, but is much more sensitive in late pregnancy (see also ergotamine, p. 327).

Ergometrine and oxytocin differ in their actions on the uterus. In moderate doses oxytocin produces slow generalised contractions with full relaxation in between; ergometrine produces faster contractions superimposed on a tonic contraction. High doses of both substances produce sustained tonic contraction. It will be seen, therefore, that oxytocin is more suited to induction of labour and ergometrine to the prevention and treatment of postpartum haemorrhage, the incidence of which is reduced by its routine prophylactic use (generally i.m.).

There are advantages in a mixture of oxytocin and ergometrine (Syntometrine).

PROSTAGLANDINS

(For a general account of the prostaglandins see Chapter 15)

Prostaglandins that soften the uterine cervix (by an action on collagen) and have a powerful oxytocic effect include:

Dinoprost (prostaglandin $F_2\alpha$, $PGF_2\alpha$) (Prostin F2 alpha) and **dinoprostone** (prostaglandin E_2; PGE_2) (Prostin E2). They are used to induce labour and to terminate pregnancy, including missed or partial abortion and in the treatment of hydatidiform mole; they are given by intra- or extra-amniotic injection, by vaginal tablet, or intracervical gel, by i.v. infusion or by mouth. Their safe and effective use (including choice of route) requires special skill.

Adverse effects include vomiting, diarrhoea, headache, pyrexia and local tissue reaction.

Gemeprost (prostaglandin E$_1$ analogue) (Cervagem) is used intravaginally to soften the cervix before operative procedures in the first trimester of pregnancy and for abortion, alone and in combination with an antiprogestogen (mifepristone, p. 720).

Carboprost (prostaglandin F$_2\alpha$ analogue) is used for postpartum haemorrhage (resistant to ergometrine and oxytocin) for its oxytocin action. It is highly effective. Adverse effects include hypertension, asthma and pulmonary oedema.

INDUCTION OF ABORTION

Gemeprost, administered vaginally as pressaries is the preferred prostaglandin for the medical induction of late therapeutic abortion. Gemeprost ripens and softens the cervix before surgical abortion, particularly in primigravida. *Misoprostol* by mouth or by vaginal administration or gemeprost may be given to induce medical abortion (an unlicensed indication in the UK). Pretreatment with *mifepristone* (see p. 720) can facilitate the process, by sensitising the uterus to the prostaglandin so that abortion occurs in a shorter time and with a lower dose of prostaglandin.

INDUCTION AND AUGMENTATION OF LABOUR

Oxytocin is administered by slow i.v. infusion as below, usually in conjunction with amniotomy, and *dinoprostone* by vaginal tablets, pressaries and vaginal gels. *Misoprostol* may be used orally or vaginally to induce labour (an unlicenced indication in the UK)

The UK National Institute for Clinical Excellence has recommended that:

- dinoprostone is preferable to oxytocin for induction of labour in women with intact membranes, regardless of parity or cervical favourability;
- dinoprostone or oxytocin are equally effective for the induction of labour in women with ruptured membranes, regardless of parity or cervical favourability;
- intravaginal dinoprostone preparations are preferable to intracervical preparations;
- oxytocin should not be started for 6 hours

following administration of vaginal prostaglandins;
- when used to induce labour, the recommended dose of oxytocin by intravenous infusion[20] is initially 0.001–0.002 units/minute increased at intervals of at least 30 minutes until a maximum of 3–4 contractions occur every 10 minutes (0.012 units/minute is often adequate); the maximum recommended rate is 0.032 units/minute (licensed max. 0.02 units/minute)

PREVENTION AND TREATMENT OF UTERINE HAEMORRHAGE

Bleeding due to incomplete abortion can be controlled with ergometrine and oxytocin (Syntometrine) given intramuscularly. Their combination is more effective in early pregnancy than either drug alone.

For the routine management of the third stage of labour ergometrine 500 micrograms with oxytocin 5 units (Syntometrine 1 ml) is given by intramuscular injection on delivery of the anterior shoulder or, at the latest, immediately after the baby is delivered. In pre-eclampsia, oxytocin may be given alone by intramuscular injection. The same regimens are used for the treatment of postpartum haemorrhage. The same drugs may be given intravenously for excessive uterine bleeding caused by uterine atony. Carboprost is an alternative for haemorrhage unresponsive to ergometrine and oxytocin.

UTERINE RELAXANTS

β_2-adrenoceptor agonists relax the uterus and are given by i.v. infusion by obstetricians *to inhibit premature labour*, e.g. isoxsuprine, terbutaline, ritodrine, salbutamol. Their use is complicated by the expected cardiovascular effects, including tachycardia, hypotension. Less easy to explain, but more devastating on occasion to the patient, is severe left ventricular failure. Possibly the combination of fluid overload (due to the vehicle) and increased oxygen demand by the heart are factors,

---

[20] Oxytocin should be used in standard dilutions of 10 units/500 ml (infusing 3 ml/hour delivers 0.001 unit/minute) or, for higher doses, 30 units/500 ml (infusing 1 ml/hour delivers 0.001 unit/minute).

and the risk is higher in the presence of multiple pregnancy, pre-existing cardiac disease or maternal infection. It is important to administer the β_2-agonist with minimum fluid volume using a syringe pump with 5% dextrose (*not saline*) as diluent, and to monitor the patient closely for signs of fluid overload.

The dose of ritodrine for intravenous administration is: initially 50 micrograms/minute, increased gradually according to response by 50 micrograms/minute every 10 minutes until contractions stop or maternal heart rate reaches 140 beats per minute; continue for 12–48 hours after contractions cease (usual rate 150–350 micrograms/minute).

GUIDE TO FURTHER READING

Bagatell C J, Bremner W J 1996 Androgens in men — uses and abuses. New England Journal of Medicine 334: 707–714, 1415

Barrett-Connor E 1998 Hormone replacement therapy. British Medical Journal 317: 457–461

Christin-Maitre S, Bouchard P, Spitz I M 2000 Medical termination of pregnancy. New England Journal of Medicine 342: 946–956

Collaborative Group on Hormone Factors in Breast Cancer 1996 Breast cancer and hormonal contraceptives: collaborative reanalysis of individual data on 53 297 women with breast cancer and 100 239 women without breast cancer from 54 epidemiological studies. Lancet 347: 1703, 1713

Glasier A 1997 Emergency postcoital contraception. New England Journal of Medicine 337: 1058–1064

Goldberg A B, Greenberg M B, Darney P D 2001 Misoprostol and pregnancy. New England Journal of Medicine 344: 38–47

Greendale G A, Lee N P, Arriola E R 1999 The menopause. Lancet 353: 571–580

Gruber C J et al 2002 Production and actions of estrogens. New England Journal of Medicine 346: 340–352

Huirne J A F, Lambalk C B 2001 Gonadotrophin-releasing-hormone-receptor antagonists. Lancet 358: 1793–1802

Kemmeren J A, Algra A, Grobbee D E 2001 Third generation oral contraceptive and risk of venous thrombosis. British Medical Journal 323: 131–137

Kubba A, Guillebaud J, Anderson R A, MacGregor E A 2000 Contraception. Lancet 356: 1913–1919

Lamberts S W, de Herder W W, van der Lely A J 1998 Pituitary insufficiency. Lancet 352: 127–134

Manson J E, Martin K A 2001 Postmenopausal hormone-replacement therapy. New England Journal of Medicine 345: 34–40

Mendelsohn M E, Karas R H 1999 The protective effects of estrogen on the cardiovascular system. New England Journal of Medicine 340: 1801–1811

Olive D L, Pritts E A 2001 Treatment of endometriosis. New England Journal of Medicine 345: 266–275

Prentice A 1999 Medical management of menorrhagia. British Medical Journal 319: 1343–1345

Vance M L, Mauras N 1999 Growth hormone therapy in adults and children. New England Journal of Medicine 341: 1206–1216

Vessey M P et al 1989 Mortality among oral contraceptive users: 20 year follow-up of women in a cohort study. British Medical Journal 299: 1487–1491

Wyatt K et al 2001 Efficacy of progesterone and progestogens in management of premenstrual syndrome: systematic review. British Medical Journal 323: 776–780

38

Vitamins, calcium, bone

SYNOPSIS

The principally *pharmacological* aspects of vitamins are described here. The *nutritional* aspects, physiological function, sources, daily requirements and deficiency syndromes (primary and secondary) are to be found in any textbook of medicine.

- Vitamin A: retinol
- Vitamin B: complex
- Vitamin C: ascorbic acid
- Vitamin D, calcium, parathyroid hormone, calcitonin, bisphosphonates, bone
- Treatment of calcium and bone disorders
- Vitamin E: tocopherol

Vitamins are substances that are essential for normal metabolism and must be chiefly supplied in the diet.

Humans cannot synthesise vitamins in the body except some vitamin D in the skin and nicotinamide from tryptophan. Lack of a particular vitamin may lead to a specific deficiency syndrome. This may be *primary* (inadequate diet), or *secondary,* due to failure of absorption (intestinal abnormality or chronic diarrhoea), or to increased metabolic need (growth, pregnancy, lactation, hyperthyroidism).

Vitamin deficiencies are commonly multiple, and complex clinical pictures occur. There are numerous single and multivitamin preparations to provide prophylaxis and therapy.

It has often been suggested, but never proved,

that subclinical vitamin deficiencies are a cause of much chronic ill-health and liability to infections. This idea has led to enormous consumption of vitamin preparations, which, for most consumers, probably have no more than placebo value. Fortunately most of the vitamins are comparatively nontoxic, but prolonged administration of *vitamins A and D* can have serious ill-effects.

Vitamins fall into two groups:

- **water-soluble vitamins:** the B group and C
- **fat-soluble vitamins:** A, D, E and K

Vitamin A: retinol

Vitamin A is a generic term embracing substances having the biological actions of retinol and related substances (which are called *retinoids*). The principal functions of retinol are to:

- sustain normal epithelia
- form retinal photochemicals
- enhance immune functions
- protect against infections and probably some cancers.

Deficiency of retinol leads to metaplasia and hyperkeratosis throughout the body. This metaplasia is reminiscent of the early stage of transformation of normal tissue to cancer.

Retinol and derivatives are used in doses above those needed for nutrition, i.e. pharmacotherapy, in dyskeratotic skin diseases (psoriasis, acne) and in leukaemia.

Tretinoin is retinoic acid. It is used in acne by topical application, see page 313, and orally to induce remission in promyelocytic leukaemia.

Isotretinoin is a retinoic acid isomer ($t\frac{1}{2}$ 20 h). It is used orally in acne (see p. 313). It is effective in preventing second primary tumours in patients who have been treated for squamous cell carcinoma of the head and neck.

Acitretin is a retinoic acid derivative ($t\frac{1}{2}$ 48 h). It is used orally for *psoriasis*, see p. 313.

Retinol itself is used in prevention and treatment of deficiency ($t\frac{1}{2}$ 7–14 d).

Adverse effects

Toxic effects occur with prolonged high intake (in children 25 000–500 000 IU daily). A diagnostic sign of *chronic poisoning* is the presence of painful tender swellings on the long bones. Anorexia, skin lesions, hair loss, hepatosplenomegaly, papilloedema, bleeding and general malaise also occur. Vitamin A is very cumulative (it is stored in liver and fat) and effects take weeks to wear off. Most cases of vitamin A poisoning have been due to mothers administering large amounts of fish-liver oils to their children in the belief that it was good for them.

Chronic overdose also causes an increased liability of biological membranes and of the outer layer of the skin to peel. An extreme example of this is the case of the hungry Antarctic explorer who in 1913 ate the liver of his husky sledge dogs. His feet felt sore and

the sight of my feet gave me quite a shock, for the thickened skin of the soles had separated in each case as a complete layer … I did what appeared to be the best thing under the circumstances: smeared the new skin with lanoline … and with bandages bound the skin soles back in place.[1]

Vitamin A and its derivatives are *teratogenic* at above physiological doses, i.e. with pharmacotherapy (for precautions, see use in acne and psoriasis, p. 313). Misguided pregnant health enthusiasts may take enough self-prescribed supplements to hazard a fetus. The Teratology Society advises that supplements should not exceed 8000 IU (2400 micrograms) per day.

Acute overdose: Travellers have been made ill by eating the livers of Arctic carnivores:

Eskimos never eat polar-bear liver, knowing it to be toxic, and husky dogs, with instinctive wisdom, also avoid it. Those who pooh-pooh the Eskimos' fears of the husky dogs' instincts and are tempted to enjoy a man's portion of polar-bear liver — appetites get sharp near the North Pole — will consume anything up to 10 000 000 IU of vitamin A (normal daily requirement is 5000 IU). This is too much of a good thing, and the diner will probably soon find himself drowsy then overcome by headache and vomiting, and finally losing the outer layer of his skin.[2]

Vitamin B complex

A number of widely differing substances are now, for convenience, classed the 'vitamin B complex'. Those used for *pharmacotherapy* include the following:

Thiamine (B_1) is used orally for nutritional purposes, but is given i.v. in serious emergencies, e.g. Wernicke-Korsakoff syndrome, when it can cause anaphylactic shock; the injection should be given over 10 min (or i.m.).

Cobalamins (B_{12}): see Chapter 29.

Folic acid: see Chapter 29.

Pyridoxine (B_6) is a coenzyme (including decarboxylases) for transamination and is concerned with many metabolic processes. Normal adult requirements are about 2 mg/d. As pharmacotherapy,

---

[1] Shearman J C 1978 Vitamin A and Sir Douglas Mawson. British Medical Journal 1: 283.

[2] Editorial 1962 British Medical Journal 1: 855.

pyridoxine is given to treat certain pyridoxine-dependent inborn errors of metabolism, namely homocystinuria, hereditary sideroblastic anaemia and primary hyperoxaluria. Deficiency may be induced by drugs such as isoniazid, hydralazine and penicillamine; pyridoxine 10 mg/day prevents the development of peripheral neuritis without interfering with therapeutic action.

Pyridoxine has also been used for a variety of conditions including premenstrual tension, vomiting in pregnancy and radiation sickness in doses sometimes exceeding 100 mg/day. Concerns that prolonged exposure to high doses may be harmful, e.g. causing sensory neuropathy, have not been resolved.

Niacin (nicotinic acid, nicotinamide) (B_7) is an essential part of codehydrogenases I and II, and so it is present in every living cell. It is used in some hyperlipidaemias, see page 527.

Adverse effects do not occur with standard doses of nicotinamide. *Nicotinic acid*, which is converted into nicotinamide, causes peripheral vasodilatation accompanied by an unpleasant flushing and itching, and the patient may faint.

Vitamin C: ascorbic acid

Deficiency of ascorbic acid leads to *scurvy*,[3] which is characterised by petechial haemorrhages, haematomas, bleeding gums (if teeth are present) and anaemia. It has a memorable place in the history of therapeutic measurement.

Scurvy had been a scourge for thousands of years, particularly amongst sailors on long voyages. In 1753, Dr James Lind performed a simple controlled therapeutic trial on 12 sailors with advanced scurvy. They were all on the same basic diet and were living in the same quarters on board ship at sea. He divided them into pairs and dosed each pair separately on cider, sulphuric acid, sea-water, vinegar, a concoction of garlic, mustard, balsam and myrrh, and two oranges and a lemon. The pair receiving

the oranges and lemon recovered and were back on duty within a week; of the others, only the pair taking cider was slightly improved. The efficacy of oranges and lemons in the prevention and cure of scurvy was repeatedly confirmed. Eventually the British Navy provided a regular daily allowance of lemon juice, unfortunately later replaced by the cheaper lime[4] juice which contained insufficient ascorbic acid to prevent scurvy completely.

Function

Ascorbic acid is required for the synthesis of collagen. It is also a powerful reducing agent (antioxidant) and plays a part in intracellular oxidation-reduction systems, and in mopping up oxidants (free radicals) produced endogenously or in the environment, e.g. cigarette smoke (see Vitamin E).

Indications for ascorbic acid

- The prevention and cure of scurvy
- Urinary acidification (rarely appropriate)
- Methaemoglobinaemia, for its properties as reducing agent (see below)
- Coryza: it is possible that large daily doses (1 g or more/d) of ascorbic acid (daily nutritional requirement 60 mg) may reduce the incidence and severity of coryza (common cold). Reliable trials in this disease are difficult and the results are inconclusive. To justify use of such doses in populations, benefit must be shown to be clinically, as well as statistically, significant; and harm insignificant. This has not been achieved.

Adverse effects

High doses may cause sleep disturbances, headaches and gut upsets. Ascorbic acid is partly eliminated in the urine unchanged and partly metabolised to oxalate. Doses above 4 g/d, which have been taken over long periods in the hope of preventing coryza, increase urinary oxalate concentration sufficiently to from oxalate stones. Intravenous ascorbic acid

---

[3] Only man (and other primates), guinea-pigs, the Indian fruit bat and the red-vented bulbul (a bird) get scurvy; other animals are able to synthesise ascorbic acid for themselves.

[4] Hence the term 'limey' for British sailors; generally used pejoratively, but obsolete except in Australia.

may precipitate a haemolytic attack in subjects with glucose-6-phosphate dehydrogenase deficiency.

METHAEMOGLOBINAEMIA

A reducing substance is needed to convert the methaemoglobin (ferric iron) back to oxyhaemoglobin (ferrous iron) whenever enough has formed seriously to impair the oxygen-carrying capacity of the blood. Ascorbic acid is nontoxic (it acts by direct reduction) but is less effective than *methylene blue* (methylthioninium chloride). Both can be given orally, i.v. or i.m. Excessive doses of methylene blue can cause methaemoglobinaemia (by stimulating NADPH-dependent enzymes).

Methaemoglobinaemia may be induced by *oxidising drugs:* sulphonamides, nitrites, nitrates (may also occur in drinking water), primaquine, -caine local anaesthetics, dapsone, nitrofurantoin, nitroprusside, vitamin K analogues, chlorates, aniline and nitrobenzene. In the rare instance of there being urgency, methylene blue 1 mg/kg slowly i.v. benefits within 30 min. (Ascorbic acid competes directly with the chemical cause but is inadequate in severe cases, which are the only ones that need treatment.)

In the *congenital form,* oral methylene blue with or without ascorbic acid gives benefit in days to weeks.

Methylene blue turns the urine blue and high concentrations can irritate the urinary tract, so that fluid intake should be high when big doses are used.

Sulphaemoglobinaemia cannot be treated by drugs. It can be caused by sulphonamides, nitrites or nitrates.

Vitamin D, calcium, parathyroid hormone, calcitonin, bisphosphonates, bone

The agents are closely interrelated and will be discussed together.

VITAMIN D

Vitamin D comprises a number of structurally related sterol compounds having similar biological properties in that they prevent or cure the vitamin D deficiency diseases, rickets and osteomalacia. The important forms are:

- **D₂** or **ergocalciferol** (calciferol) made by ultraviolet irradiation of ergosterol
- **D₃** or **colecalciferol** made by ultraviolet irradiation of 7-dehydrocholesterol; it is the form that occurs in natural foods and is formed in the skin.

Vitamins D_2 and D_3 are made more active by two hydroxylation reactions: (a) 25-hydroxylation in the *liver,* and (b) 1α-hydroxylation in the *kidney* (under the control of parathormone) to form, 1α-25-dihydroxycholecalciferol; this, the most active natural form of vitamin D, is available as **calcitriol.** In renal disease this final rate-limited renal α-hydroxylation is inadequate, and administration of the less biologically active precursors is therefore liable to lack efficacy.

Subsequently there was introduced a 1α-hydroxylated form (1α-hydroxycholecalciferol) **alfacalcidol** (One-Alpha), that requires only hepatic hydroxylation to become the highly active 1α-25-dihydroxycholecalciferol (calcitriol). Alfacalcidol (and of course calcitriol) is therefore effective in renal failure since the defective renal hydroxylation stage is bypassed. Its extraordinary potency and efficacy is indicated by the usual adult maintenance dose, often only 0.25–1 micrograms/d.

In addition there is a structural variant of vitamins D_2 and D_3 **dihydrotachysterol** (ATIO, Tachyrol), which is also biologically activated by hepatic 25-hydroxylation.

Advantages of alfacalcidol and dihydrotachysterol include a fast onset and short duration of clinical effect (days) which renders them suitable for rapid adjustment of plasma calcium, e.g. in hypoparathyroidism. Such factors are not relevant to the slower adjustment of plasma calcium (weeks) with vitamins D_2 and D_3 in the ordinary management of vitamin D deficiency.

Actions are complex. Vitamin D promotes the active transport (absorption) of calcium and therefore of phosphate from the gut, to control, with parathormone, the mineralisation of bone and to promote the renal tubular reabsorption of calcium and phosphate. The plasma calcium concentration rises. After a dose of D_2 or D_3 there is a lag of about 21 h before the intestinal effect begins and this is probably due to the time needed for its metabolic conversion to the more active forms. But with the biologically active calcitriol the lag is only 2 h.

A large single dose of vitamin D has biological effects for as long as 6 months (because of metabolism and storage). Thus the agent is cumulative and overdose by a mother anxious that her child shall have strong bones can cause serious toxicity.

Indications for vitamin D are the prevention and cure of rickets of all kinds and osteomalacia, and the symptomatic treatment of some cases of hypoparathyroidism; also psoriasis.

Calcitriol is licensed for the management of postmenopausal osteoporosis.

In osteomalacia secondary to steatorrhoea or renal disease there is defective absorption of calcium from the gut and large amounts of vitamin D are often needed to enhance absorption.

Use of vitamin D as pharmacotherapy should in general be accompanied by monitoring of plasma calcium.

Dose and preparations (1.0 microgram = 40 units). Simple vitamin D deficiency can be prevented by taking an oral supplement of only 10 micrograms (400 units) of *ergocalciferol* daily. Vitamin D deficiency is not uncommon in Asians consuming unleavened bread and in the elderly living alone; it can be prevented by taking an oral supplement of ergocalciferol 20 micrograms (800 units) daily. Vitamin D in deficiency caused by intestinal malabsorption or chronic liver disease usually requires vitamin D in pharmacological doses, such as ergocalciferol tablets up to 1 mg (40 000 units) daily. The maximum antirachitic effect of vitamin D is delayed for 1–2 months and the plasma calcium concentration reflects the dosage given days or weeks before. Frequent changes of dose are therefore not required.

The hypocalcaemia of hypoparathyroidism may require ergocalciferol in doses up to 2.5 mg (100 000 units) daily to achieve normocalcaemia but the dose is difficult to titrate and hypercalcaemia from overdose may take weeks to resolve. The synthetic vitamin D derivatives, *alfacalcidol* and *calcitriol*, are therefore preferred as their rapid onset and offset of action makes for easier control of plasma calcium. Supplementary calcium by mouth may also be needed.

Alfacalcidol or calcitriol, *but not* ergocalciferol, should be prescribed if patients with severe renal impairment require vitamin D therapy (see above).

Calcipotriol and *tacalcitol* are vitamin D analogues available as creams or ointments for the treatment of psoriasis (p. 313).

Symptoms of overdose are due mainly to excessive rise in plasma calcium. General effects include: malaise, drowsiness, nausea, abdominal pain, thirst, constipation and loss of appetite. Other long-term effects include ectopic calcification almost anywhere in the body, renal damage and an increased calcium output in the urine; renal calculi may be formed. It is dangerous to exceed 10 000 units daily of vitamin D in an adult for more than about 12 weeks.

Vitamin D toxicity may arise from well-meaning, but needless, administration by parents. The US Food and Drug Administration warns that intake of fortified diet supplements should not exceed 400 units a day.

Patients with *sarcoidosis* are intolerant of vitamin D possibly even to the tiny amount present in a normal diet, and to that synthesised in their skin by sunlight. The intolerance may be due to over-production of calcitriol (see above) by macrophages activated by interferon; the overproduction is reversed by corticosteroid, which is also used in the treatment of severe hypervitaminosis D (see below).

Epileptic patients taking drugs that are enzyme inducers can develop osteomalacia (adults) or rickets (children). This may be due to enzyme induction increasing vitamin D metabolism and causing deficiency, or there may be inhibition of one of the hydroxylations that increase biological activity.

Treatment of calcium and bone disorders

HYPOCALCAEMIA

In acute hypocalcaemia requiring systemic therapy

calcium gluconate inj. is given as a 10% solution, 10–20 ml at the rate of about 2 ml per min and followed by a continuous i.v. infusion containing 40 ml (9 mmol) per day with monitoring of plasma calcium. It must not be given i.m. as it is painful and causes necrosis. *Calcium glubionate* (Calcium Sandoz) can be given by deep i.m. injection in adults.

For chronic use, e.g. hypoparathyroidism, alfacalcidol or calcitriol are needed. Dietary calcium is increased by giving calcium gluconate (an effervescent tablet is available) or lactate. *Aluminium hydroxide* binds phosphate in the gut causing hypophosphataemia, which stimulates renal formation of the most active vitamin D metabolite and usefully enhances calcium absorption.

Adverse effects of intravenous calcium may be very dangerous. An early sign is a tingling feeling in the mouth and of warmth spreading over the body. Serious effects are those on the heart, which mimic and synergise with digitalis (fatal cardiac arrest may occur in digitalised animals) and it would seem advisable to avoid i.v. calcium in any patient on a digitalis glycoside (except in severe symptomatic hypocalcaemia). The effect of calcium on the heart is antagonised by potassium and similarly the toxic effects of a high serum potassium in acute renal failure may be to some extent counteracted with calcium.

HYPERCALCAEMIA

Treatment of severe acute hypercalcaemia causing symptoms is needed whether or not the cause can be removed; generally a plasma concentration of 3.0 mmol/l (12 mg/100 ml) needs urgent treatment if there is also clinical evidence of toxicity (individual tolerance varies greatly).

Temporary measures

After taking account of the patient's cardiac and renal function, the following measures may be employed selectively:

- *Physiological saline solution* is important, firstly to correct sodium and water deficit and secondly to promote sodium-linked calcium diuresis in the proximal renal tubule. Initially, 0.9% saline 500 ml should be given i.v. every 4–6 h for

2–3 days and continued at a rate of 2 l/day until plasma calcium falls below 3.0 mmol/l and the oral intake is adequate. The regimen requires careful attention to fluid and electrolyte balance, including potassium. Furosemide may be added to the regimen once salt depletion has been corrected.

- Bisphosphonates (see later). Pamidronate[5] is infused according to the schedule in Table 38.1; it is active in a wide variety of hypercalcaemic disorders. Fall in serum calcium begins in 1–2 d, reaches a nadir in 5–6 d and lasts 20–30 d. Etidronate may be given i.v. in hypercalcaemia of malignant disease. It acts in 1–2 d and a dose lasts 3–4 weeks; it may also provide benefit for neoplastic metastatic disease in bone. Clodronate (oral or i.v.) or zoledonic acid (i.v.) are alternatives.
- *Calcitonin* (see below). When the hypercalcaemia is at least partly due to mobilisation from bone, calcitonin can be used to inhibit bone resorption, and it may enhance urinary excretion of calcium. The effect develops in a few hours, and responsiveness may be lost over a few days (but may sometimes be restored by an adrenal steroid).
- An *adrenocortical steroid*, e.g. prednisolone 20–40 mg/d orally, is effective in particular situations; it reduces the hypercalcaemia of vitamin D intoxication (which is due to excessive intestinal absorption of calcium) and of sarcoidosis (principally by its disease-modifying effect). Steroid may be effective in the hypercalcaemia of malignancy where the disease itself is responsive, e.g. myeloma of lymphoma. Most patients with hyperparathyroidism do not respond.

TABLE 38.1 Treatment of hypercalcaemia with disodium pamidronate

Calcium (mmol/l)	Pamidronate (mg)
<3.0	15–30
3.0–3.5	30–60
3.5–4.0	60–90
>4.0	90

Infuse slowly, e.g. 30 mg in 250 ml 0.9% saline over 1 hour. Expect response in 3–5 days.

[5] formerly called aminohydroxypropylidenediphosphonate disodium, APD.

- *Phosphate* i.v. is quickly effective but lowers calcium by precipitating calcium phosphate in bone and soft tissues and inhibiting osteoclastic activity; it should be used only when other methods have failed.
- *Trisodium edetate* (therapeutically equivalent to disodium edetate) i.v. chelates calcium and the inert complex is excreted by glomerular filtration. Although it is rapidly effective, it causes pain in the limb receiving the infusion and may cause renal damage.
- *Dialysis* is quick and effective and is likely to be needed in severe cases or with renal failure.

The above measures are temporary only, giving time to tackle the cause.

Long-term use

To bind dietary calcium in the gut *sodium cellulose phosphate* (Calcisorb) is an oral ion exchange substance with a particular affinity for calcium. Bound calcium is eliminated in the faeces. It is used particularly for patients who overabsorb dietary calcium and who develop hypercalciuria and renal stones.

Inorganic phosphate, e.g. sodium acid phosphate (Phosphate Sandoz) taken orally also binds calcium in the gut.

HYPERCALCIURIA

In renal stone formers, in addition to general measures (low calcium diet, high fluid intake), urinary calcium may be diminished by a thiazide diuretic (with or without citrate to bind calcium) and oral phosphate (see above). See also Nephrolithiasis (p. 543).

PARATHYROID HORMONE

Parathyroid hormone acts chiefly on kidney increasing renal tubular resorption and bone resorption of calcium; it increases calcium absorption from the gut, indirectly, by stimulating the renal synthesis of 1α-25-dihydroxycholecalciferol (see Vitamin D). It increases the rate of bone remodelling (mineral and collagen) and osteocyte activity with, at high doses, an overall balance in favour of resorption (osteoclast activity) with a rise in plasma calcium con-

centration (and fall in phosphate); but, at low doses, the balance favours bone formation (osteoblast activity).

CALCITONIN

Calcitonin is a peptide hormone produced by the C cells of the thyroid gland (in mammals). It acts on bone (inhibiting osteoclasis) to reduce the rate of bone turnover, and on the kidney to reduce reabsorption of calcium and phosphorus. It is obtained from natural sources (pork, salmon, eel), or synthesised. The $t\frac{1}{2}$ varies according to source; $t\frac{1}{2}$ human is 10 min. Antibodies develop particularly to pork calcitonin and neutralise its effect; synthetic salmon calcitonin *(salcatonin)* is therefore preferred for prolonged use; loss of effect may also be due to down-regulation of receptors. Calcitonin is used (s.c., i.m. or intranasally) to control hypercalcaemia (rapid effect), Paget's disease of bone (relief of pain, and to relieve compression of nerves, e.g. auditory cranial), metastatic bone cancer pain, and post-menopausal osteoporosis.

Adverse effects include allergy, nausea, flushing and tingling of the face and hands.

BISPHOSPHONATES

Bisphosphonates are synthetic, nonhydrolysable analogues of pyrophosphate in which the central oxygen atom of the -P-O-P- structure is replaced with a carbon atom to give the -P-C-P- group.

Actions. These compounds are effective calcium chelators that rapidly target exposed bone mineral surfaces in vivo, where they can be released by bone-resorbing osteoclasts, resulting in inhibition of osteoclast function and osteoclast apoptosis. The bisphosphonates *(alendronate, clodronate, etidronate, pamidronate, risedronate, tiludronate and zoledronate)* inhibit the activation and function of osteoclasts and possibly directly stimulate formation of bone by the osteoblasts. They also bind strongly to hydroxyapatite crystals and, in high doses, can inhibit the mineralisation of bone. The doses at which effects on mineralisation occur are not related to antiresorptive efficacy. There is wide variation between these compounds in terms of their capacity to inhibit resorption relative to that of inhibiting mineralisation. Etidronate, for instance, must be administered cyclically to prevent demineralisation whereas alendronate, more recently available, does not appear to interfere with mineralisation at antiresorptive doses and can be used continously.

Pharmacokinetics. Bisphosphonates are poorly absorbed after oral ingestion. Absorption is further impaired by food, drinks and drugs containing calcium, magnesium, iron or aluminium salts. A proportion of bisphosphonate that is absorbed is rapidly incorporated into bone; the remaining fraction is excreted unchanged by the kidneys. Once incorporated into the skeleton, bisphosphonates are released only when the bone is resorbed during turnover. They may be given orally or i.v.

Uses. Three bisphosphonates *(alendronate, etidronate, risedronate)* are currently licensed in the UK for the treatment of osteoporosis (zoledronate is also effective), and the others are used in Paget's disease of bone, and hypercalcaemia due to cancer (pamidronate, clodronate, zoledronate). Bisphosphonates may also provide benefit for neoplastic disease that has spread to bone; evidence indicates that clodronate by mouth and pamidronate i.v. are effective in the secondary prevention of bone metastases due to multiple myeloma and breast cancer.

Adverse effects include gastrointestinal disturbances, with oesophageal irritation being a particular problem with alendronate. This should be given at least 30 minutes before food, with the patient remaining erect during this period. Alendronate can be taken weekly (70 mg) instead of daily (10 mg). Disturbances of calcium and mineral metabolism (e.g. vitamin D deficiency, parathyroid hormone dysfunction) should be corrected before starting a bisphosphonate. Increased bone pain (as well as relief), fractures (high dose, prolonged use only) can occur due to demineralisation of bone.

OSTEOPOROSIS

Osteoporosis is an abnormal decrease in amount of bone, but what is there is of normal quality. Low bone mass is reflected in reduced bone mineral density measurements. It occurs most commonly in postmenopausal women and patients taking corticosteroid long-term. Underlying causes such as hyperthyroidism, hyperparathyroidism and hypogonadism (in both sexes) should be excluded before treatment is initiated.

People at risk of osteoporosis, e.g. elderly housebound persons, must maintain an adequate intake of calcium and vitamin D. Calcium dietary supplementation (Ca gluconate, carbonate, hydroxyapatite, citrate, maleate) reduces nett bone loss where intake may be inadequate, i.e. below 800 mg/d, and ergocalciferol 10 micrograms (400 units) by mouth corrects dietary vitamin D deficiency.

Postmenopausal osteoporosis is due to gonadal deficiency; it can be *prevented.* One in 4 women in her 60s and one in 2 in her 70s in the UK experiences an osteoporotic fracture.

- *Oestrogen* arrests the process by reducing bone resorption.
- *Progestogen* arrests the process by increasing bone formation, but therapeutic benefit is less than with oestrogen.

Oestrogen inhibits the age-related loss of bone that occurs in most women after menopause. Observational studies have indicated that the use of oestrogen reduces the risk of vertebral fracture by approximately 50% and the risk of hip fracture by 25–30%. Unopposed oestrogen increases by 10-fold the risk of endometrial cancer, which is diminished by added progestogen. Therefore combinations of oestrogen and progestogen are the mainstay of treatment for postmenopausal osteoporosis; they inhibit the rapid bone loss that occurs immediately after the menopause and should be continued for 5 years.

Longer-term use is more problematic, given the probable increase (though < 2-fold) in the risk of breast cancer associated with extended use. Reasonable candidates are the small proportion of postmenopausal women with documented osteoporosis or osteopenia (decreased bone density) or those at increased risk for osteoporosis (personal or family history of nontraumatic fracture, current smokers, or those with a body-mass index < 22) who do not have a personal or family history of breast cancer or other contraindications and who are willing to try this therapy. With more long-term evidence, *raloxifene* 60 mg daily where affordable will become an attractive option. This selective oestrogen receptor agonist can be used unopposed without apparent increase in risk of breast or endometrial cancer.

Bisphosphonates increase bone mineral density in osteoporosis.

A schema for the prevention of osteoporosis with HRT beyond 5 years, or other options, appears in Figure 38.1

Treatment of osteoporosis. It is usual to start with HRT or a bisphosphonate and, if these are unsuitable, calcitriol, calcitonin or raloxifene may be used. Calcitonin, additionally, is effective for relief of pain for up to 3 months after vertebral fracture where other analgesics fail.

Fracture is the only important outcome of osteoporosis and the evidence to support the efficacy of various interventions appears in Table 38.2.

Corticosteroid-induced osteoporosis. The greatest

TABLE 38.2 Anti-fracture efficacy of interventions in post menopausal osteoporotic women: grades of recommendation

	Spine	Nonvertebral	Hip
Alendronate	A	A	A
Calcitonin	A	B	A
Calcitriol	A	A	ND
Calcium	A	B	B
Calcium plus vitamin D	ND	A	A
Cyclical etidronate	A	B	B
Hip protectors	—	—	A
HRT	A	A	B
Physical exercise	ND	B	B
Raloxifene	A	ND	ND
Risedronate	A	A	A
Tibolone	ND	ND	ND
Vitamin D	ND	B	B

Grade A, meta-analysis of randomised, controlled trials or from at least one randomised, controlled trial, or from at least one well designed, controlled study without randomisation; grade B, from at least one other type of well designed, quasi-experimental study, or from well designed, nonexperimental studies (e.g. comparative studies, correlation studies, case-control studies); grade C, from expert committee reports/opinions and/or clinical experience of authorities. ND, not demonstrated. Data from the Royal College of Physicians and the Bone and Tooth Society.

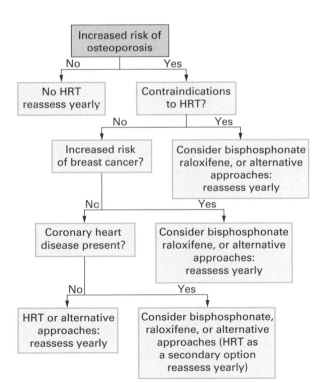

Fig. 38.1 The prevention of osteoporosis. With permission from J Manson, Harvard Medical School and the New England Journal of Medicine

rate of bone loss occurs during the first 6–12 months of corticosteroid use. Patients taking the equivalent of prednisolone 7.5 mg or more each day for 3 months or longer should be considered for prophylactic treatment, and this is mandatory in those over 65 years. Treatment for osteoporosis should be given when a patient taking a corticosteroid sustains a low-trauma fracture. Long-term use of inhaled corticosteroids may reduce bone mineral density and place patients at risk. The treatment options for both the prophylaxis and treatment are: hormone replacement (HRT in women, testosterone in men), a bisphosphonate and calcitriol.

OSTEOMALACIA

Osteomalacia is due to *primary* or *secondary* vitamin D deficiency. In secondary cases, e.g. malabsorption or renal disease, high doses of vitamin D are sometimes needed. Long-term therapy with some *antiepilepsy drugs* may cause osteomalacia see Vitamin D).

PAGET'S DISEASE OF BONE

This disease is characterised by bone resorption and formation (bone turnover) being increased as much as 50 times normal, the results of which are large, vascular, deformed, painful bones which fracture.

Bisphosphonates (etidronate, pamidronate, tiludronate) are effective because of their inhibition of crystal formation, growth and dissolution, such as must occur in bone mineralisation and demineralisation. The response is dose-related and remission after a course may last up to two years. *Calcition* (which inhibits bone resorption) has been largely superseded by the bisphosphonates but is useful to reduce bone blood flow before operation.

Vitamin E: tocopherol

The functions of vitamin E may be to take up (scavenge) the free radicals generated by normal metabolic process and by substances in the environment, e.g. hydrocarbons, and so to prevent them attacking polyunsaturated fats in cell membranes with resultant cellular injury. A deficiency syndrome is now recognised, including peripheral neuropathy with spinocerebellar degeneration; and a haemolytic anaemia in premature infants.

Alpha tocopheryl acetate (Ephynal) pharmacotherapy may benefit the neuromuscular complications of congential cholestasis and abetalipoproteinaemia.

Vitamin K

see page 568.

GUIDE TO FURTHER READING

Bates C J 1995 Vitamin A. Lancet 345: 31–35

Bushinsky D A, Monk R D 1998 Calcium. Lancet 352: 306–311

Cooper C, Eastell R 1993 Bone gain and loss in premenopausal women. British Medical Journal 306: 1357–1358

Delmas P D, Meunier P J 1997 The management of Paget's disease of bone. New England Journal of Medicine 336: 558–566.

Editorial 1962 Arctic offal. British Medical Journal 1: 855

Eastell R 1998 Treatment of postmenopausal osteoporosis. New England Journal of Medicine 338: 736–746.

Fraser D R 1995 Vitamin D. Lancet 345: 104–107

Greenberg E R, Sporn M B 1996 Antioxidant vitamins, cancer and cardiovascular disease. New England Journal of Medicine 334: 1198–1190

Humphrey J H, Rice A L 2000 Vitamin A supplementation in young infants. Lancet 356: 422–424

Manolagas S C et al 1995 Bone marrow, cytokines, and bone remodeling. New England Journal of Medicine 332: 305–311

Manson J E, Martin K A 2001 Postmenopausal Hormone-Replacement Therapy. New England Journal of Medicine 345: 34–40

Meydani M 1995 Vitamin E. Lancet 345: 170–175

Relston S H 1992 Medical management of hypercalcaemia. British Journal of Clinical Pharmacology 34: 11–20

Seeman E 2002 Pathogenesis of bone fragility in women and men. Lancet 359: 1841–1850

Spector T D, Sambrook P N 1993 Steroid osteoporosis. British Medical Journal 307: 519–520

Willett W C, Stampfer M J 2001 What vitamins should I be taking, doctor? New England Journal of Medicine 345: 1819–1824

Index